Multisensory Teaching of Basic Language Skills

Fourth Edition

Multisensory Teaching
of Basic Language Skills
Fourth Edition

edited by

Judith R. Birsh, Ed.D., CALT-QI
Independent Literacy Consultant
New York, New York

and

Suzanne Carreker, Ph.D., CALT-QI
Principal Educational Lead, Lexia Learning Systems
Concord, Massachusetts

with invited contributors

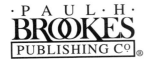

·P·A·U·L·H·
BROOKES
PUBLISHING C⁰ ®

Baltimore • London • Sydney

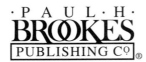

Paul H. Brookes Publishing Co.
Post Office Box 10624
Baltimore, Maryland 21285-0624
USA

www.brookespublishing.com

Typeset by Progressive Publishing Services, York, Pennsylvania.
Manufactured in the United States of America by
Sheridan Books, Inc. Chelsea, Michigan.

Cover photo © iStockphoto.com

The individuals described in this book are composites or real people whose situations are masked
and are based on the authors' experiences. In all instances, names and identifying details have been
changed to protect confidentiality.

A companion activity book, *Multisensory Teaching of Basic Language Skills Activity Book, Fourth Edition*
(ISBN: 9781681253084), by Suzanne Carreker and Judith R. Birsh, is also available from Paul H.
Brookes Publishing Co. (1-800-638-3775; 1-410-337-9580). For more information on the Multisensory
Teaching of Basic Language Skills materials, go to www.brookespublishing.com/birsh.

Library of Congress Cataloging-in-Publication Data

Names: Birsh, Judith R., editor. | Carreker, Suzanne editor.
Title: Multisensory teaching of basic language skills / edited by Judith R. Birsh, Ed.D., Independent
    Literacy Consultant, Certified Academic Language Therapist (CALT), Qualified Instructor (QI),
    New York, New York, and Suzanne Carreker, Ph.D., CALT-QI, Principal Educational Content
    Lead, Lexia Learning Systems, Concord, Massachusetts, with invited contributors.
Description: Fourth Edition. | Baltimore, Maryland : Paul H. Brookes Publishing Company, [2018] |
    "Previous edition copyright (c) 2011"—T.p. verso. | Includes bibliographical references and index.
Identifiers: LCCN 2018005328 (print) | LCCN 2018010368 (ebook) | ISBN 9781681252919 (epub) |
    ISBN 9781681252926 (pdf) | ISBN 9781681252261 (hardcover)
Subjects: LCSH: Dyslexic children—Education—United States. | Dyslexics—Education—United
    States. | Language arts—United States.
Classification: LCC LC4708.85 (ebook) | LCC LC4708.85 .M85 2018 (print) | DDC 371.91/44—dc23
LC record available at https://lccn.loc.gov/2018005328

British Library Cataloguing in Publication data are available from the British Library.

2022   2021   2020   2019   2018

10   9   8   7   6   5   4   3   2   1

Contents

Section III   Beginning Reading/Literacy Skills

About the Online Companion Materials

Purchasers of this book may download, print, and/or photocopy the Reflect, Connect, and Respond questions, Knowledge and Skill Assessment quizzes, and other resources provided in the Online Companion Materials (OCM) for educational use. The questions, quizzes, and Technology Resources lists are included with the print book and are also available at www.brookespublishing.com/birshcarreker/ materials for both print and e-book buyers; additional chapter resources are available online.

Online Companion Materials

Chapter 1

Reflect, Connect, and Respond Questions

Appendix 1.1: Knowledge and Skill Assessment Answer Key

Appendix 1.2: Resources

Chapter 2

Reflect, Connect, and Respond Questions

Appendix 2.1: Knowledge and Skill Assessment Answer Key

A full-color version of Figure 2.1 showing neural activity during reading

Chapter 3

Reflect, Connect, and Respond Questions

Appendix 3.1: Knowledge and Skill Assessment Answer Key

Chapter 4

Reflect, Connect, and Respond Questions

Appendix 4.1: Technology Resources

Appendix 4.2: Knowledge and Skill Assessment Answer Key

Appendix 4.3: Formal Assessment Tools and Resources

Appendix 4.4: Autumn or The Harvest

Chapter 5

Reflect, Connect, and Respond Questions

Appendix 5.1: Technology Resources

Appendix 5.2: Knowledge and Skill Assessment Answer Key

Appendix 5.3: Additional Resources

Appendix 5.4: Activities for Developing Dictionary Skills

Chapter 6

Reflect, Connect, and Respond Questions

Appendix 6.1: Technology Resources

Appendix 6.2: Knowledge and Skill Assessment Answer Key

About the Editors

Judith R. Birsh, Ed.D., Independent Literacy Consultant, Certified Academic Language Therapist (CALT), Qualified Instructor (QI), 333 West 86th Street, New York, New York

Dr. Birsh was the editor of the first three editions of *Multisensory Teaching of Basic Language Skills*. She welcomes Dr. Suzanne Carreker, with her expertise in the field of literacy, as co-editor of the fourth edition. Dr. Birsh's enduring belief that well-prepared, informed teachers are the major influence on effective instruction in the field of reading and dyslexia had its beginning in 1960, when she met her first student who, although 18 years old, read poorly. The quest to find answers to this puzzle led her to a master's degree in remedial reading and a doctorate in reading and language at Teachers College, Columbia University. After training with Aylett R. Cox in Dallas, Texas, she became a Certified Academic Language Therapist and Qualified Instructor, founding and directing the multisensory teaching of basic language skills courses at Teachers College in the Department of Curriculum and Teaching, Program in Learning Disabilities. Since her retirement in 2000, Dr. Birsh has maintained her commitment to teacher preparation as an independent literacy consultant, by giving professional development workshops, consulting with private and public schools, writing articles, and working with students with dyslexia. In 2008, she received the Luke Waites Academic Language Therapy Association Award of Service and the Margaret Byrd Rawson Lifetime Achievement Award from The International Dyslexia Association.

Suzanne Carreker, Ph.D., Certified Academic Language Therapist (CALT), Qualified Instructor (QI), Principal Educational Lead, Lexia Learning Systems, Concord, Massachusetts

Dr. Carreker is developing content for blended-learning reading programs at Lexia Learning Systems. Her passion for teaching reading began with an impromptu opportunity to attend a lecture given by dyslexia pioneer Margaret Byrd Rawson. She taught at Briarwood School in Houston, Texas, and directed teacher preparation programs at Neuhaus Education Center in Houston for 28 years. During her second year of teaching, Dr. Carreker attended a 1-hour workshop presented by the three Neuhaus founders that led to her preparation as a CALT and QI at the center. Dr. Carreker believes that teachers' deep knowledge about reading and skill in teaching reading should not be the result of serendipity. To that end, Dr. Carreker served on the committee for the development of The International Dyslexia Association's (IDA) *Knowledge and Practice Standards for Teachers of Reading* and led the development of the Certification Exam for Effective Teaching of Reading—both guideposts for pre-service and in-service teacher preparation programs. She was the 2009 HBIDA Nancy LaFevers Community Service Award recipient for her contributions to students with dyslexia and related learning differences in the Houston area. In 2018, she received the Margaret Byrd Rawson Lifetime Achievement Award from the IDA.

About the Contributors

Kay A. Allen, M.Ed., Academic Language Therapist, Private Practice; Instructor, Adult Literacy Program, Neuhaus Education Center, 4433 Bissonnet Street, Bellaire, Texas

Ms. Allen served as Executive Director of Neuhaus Education Center from 2000 to 2007 and was Associate Director there from 1985 to 2000. She is a board member of the International Multisensory Structured Language Education Council (IMSLEC) and is coauthor of *Multisensory Reading and Spelling* (Neuhaus Education Center, 1993). She received the Nancy LaFevers Community Service Award from the Houston Branch of The International Dyslexia Association in 2016.

Virginia Wise Berninger, Ph.D., Licensed Psychologist; Professor Emerita, University of Washington, Seattle, Washington

Virginia (Ginger) Berninger taught in urban, suburban, and rural public schools (1967–1977) before her Ph.D. studies specializing in developmental, psycholinguistics, and cognitive psychology; she has been a licensed psychologist since 1983. She completed American Psychological Association–approved predoctoral and postdoctoral training in clinical psychology at Boston's Children's Hospital's Ambulatory Pediatrics and Developmental Evaluation Clinic, specializing in specific learning disabilities, developmental disabilities, and individuals with physical and communication disabilities. She has served on medical school faculties at Harvard University and Tufts University and on the College of Education faculty at the University of Washington (1986–2016; currently Professor Emerita), where she was Director of an APA-approved school psychology program and taught courses on interdisciplinary foundations of education. She was Principal Investigator (PI) of Eunice Kennedy Shriver National Institute of Child Health and Human Development–funded grants from 1989 to 2008 on typical language learners, and later on an interdisciplinary center grant on specific learning disabilities, which conducted research on assessment, instruction, genetics, and brain imaging. She has authored or coauthored numerous peer-reviewed, interdisciplinary publications and participated in many professional development activities in person and online. She currently specializes in consultation and professional development.

Susan H. Blumenthal, Ed.D., Licensed Clinical Psychologist, Private Practice (Retired); Founder, The Learning Difficulties Program, Institute for Contemporary Psychotherapy, New York, New York

Dr. Blumenthal specializes in psychoeducational evaluations and cognitive remediation for adults and adolescents with learning difficulties and academic work output problems. She started an innovative program at the Institute for Contemporary

Psychotherapy to train psychotherapists to work with adult patients on learning disabilities. In addition, she has trained teachers at Teachers College, Columbia University; Hunter College; and Manhattanville College.

Elsa Cárdenas-Hagan, Ed.D., CCC-SLP, CALT, QI, President, Valley Speech Language and Learning Center, Brownsville, Texas

Elsa Cárdenas-Hagan is a bilingual speech-language pathologist, certified academic language therapist, and qualified instructor. She is President of Valley Speech Language and Learning Center and works with the University of Houston–Texas Institute for Evaluation and Statistics. Her research interests include the language and literacy development of Spanish-speaking English learners and interventions for bilingual students. She has authored research articles, book chapters, and interventions for English learners.

Elaine A. Cheesman, Ph.D., Associate Professor Emerita, University of Colorado at Colorado Springs; Dyslexia Therapist, Founding Director, Read to Succeed Adult Reading Clinic, Hartford, Connecticut

Dr. Cheesman specializes in teacher education and instructional technology to support Structured Literacy. Her university courses were among the first to be accredited by The International Dyslexia Association.

Nancy Cushen White, Ed.D., Clinical Professor, Department of Pediatrics, Division of Adolescent & Young Adult Medicine, University of California, San Francisco; private practitioner, Dyslexia Evaluation & Remediation Clinic (DERC); Certified Instructor of Teacher Training Courses, Slingerland Multisensory Structured Language Approach, Slingerland Institute for Literacy; Certified Academic Language Therapist and Qualified Instructor; Licensed Dyslexia Therapist (Texas); Board Certified Educational Therapist

Nancy Cushen White is a Clinical Professor at the University of California at San Francisco (UCSF) and a member of the UCSF Dyslexia Research Center Leadership Team; she also teaches classes in child and adolescent psychiatry. Since 1973, she has used multisensory structured language strategies to teach students of all ages. She worked for 40 years in San Francisco public schools as a classroom teacher, special education teacher, and program consultant in special education curriculum. Currently, Dr. Cushen White works as a Certified Academic Language Therapist, Board-Certified Educational Therapist, certified Slingerland teacher training course instructor, and dyslexia consultant in her private practice at the Dyslexia Evaluation & Remediation Clinic. She has been a Literacy Intervention Consultant and Case Manager for Lexicon Reading Center in Dubai since 2010. A member of the AB 1369 Work Group (California Department of Education) charged with drafting public school dyslexia guidelines required under the new law, Dr. Cushen White was also recipient of the 2007 Margaret Byrd Rawson Lifetime Achievement Award from The International Dyslexia Association (IDA), the 2014 Etoile DuBard Award of Excellence from the International Multisensory Structured Language Education Council (IMSLEC), and the 2016 Lucius Waites Award of Service from the Academic Language Therapy Association (ALTA). She has served as a national IDA board member and as President of its Northern California Branch. She is an IDA representative to the National Joint Committee on Learning Disabilities; editor of the *Examiner,* IDA's monthly online newsletter; board member of IMSLEC and the Alliance for Certification and Accreditation; advisory board member for IDA's Northern California Branch and for Parents Education Network (PEN), and an advisor for PENs student-organized, student-led SAFE Voices branch.

Carolyn DeVito, M.A., Assistant Executive Director, Montclair Community Pre-K, 49 Orange Road, Montclair, New Jersey

Carolyn DeVito is a long-time professional in the field of early childhood education. She has worked with children ages 3–5 for more than 40 years. For the past 20 years, Ms. DeVito has been Master Teacher and Assistant Executive Director at the Montclair Community Pre-K, which is a National Association for the Education of Young Children (NAEYC)-accredited center. It is also one of 21 centers initially identified by the Center for the Study of Social Policy as an exemplary program in the Strengthening Families Initiative. Ms. DeVito is a member of the adjunct faculty at Kean University in Union, New Jersey, teaching courses in the field of early childhood education.

Mary Lupiani Farrell, Ph.D., Professor, Fairleigh Dickinson University, 1000 River Road, T-RH5-02, Teaneck, New Jersey

Mary Lupiani Farrell earned her Ph.D. at Teachers College, Columbia University. She is a professor at Fairleigh Dickinson University (FDU), where she directs the Center for Dyslexia Studies, through which FDU's International Multisensory Structured Language Education Council (IMSLEC) and International Dyslexia Association (IDA)–accredited Orton-Gillingham teacher training program is provided. Dr. Farrell is also University Director of the Regional Center for Students with Learning Disabilities, a comprehensive support program for colleges students with learning disabilities.

Katherine Garnett, Ed.D., Professor, Department of Special Education, Hunter College in New York City

Professor Garnett founded Hunter's learning disabilities graduate program in 1980. A year later, she launched the HC Learning Lab, nationally recognized in 1996 as an "Exemplary LD Program." Professor Garnett also developed the special education training for The Edison Schools and partnered with Uncommon, Achievement First, and Kipp charter systems. She has spearheaded grant programs; authored articles, chapters, and monographs; served on editorial boards; and consulted with a wide variety of public and private schools, K–12.

Monica Gordon-Pershey, Ed.D., CCC-SLP, Associate Professor, School of Health Sciences, Cleveland State University, 2121 Euclid Avenue, IM324, Cleveland, Ohio

Monica Gordon-Pershey is an associate professor in the School of Health Sciences at Cleveland State University in Cleveland, Ohio. She is a certified speech-language pathologist and holds a doctorate in language and literacy instruction. Her teaching and scholarship focus on language development and disorders. She is the author of over 130 articles, book chapters, and presentations.

Nancy E. Hennessy, M.Ed., Educational Consultant, The Consulting Network, 1008 Martins Point Road, Kitty Hawk, North Carolina

Ms. Hennessy is Past President of The International Dyslexia Association (IDA). She is an experienced teacher, diagnostician, and administrator. While working in public schools, she provided leadership in the development of professional learning systems, innovative programming for students with special needs, and a statewide revision of special education code. She has designed and delivered keynote addresses, workshops, and training to educators nationally and internationally. She coauthored the second edition of Module 6 of *LETRS, Digging for Meaning: Teaching Text Comprehension* (with Louisa C. Moats; Sopris West, 2009) and was a national trainer for *Language Essentials for Teachers of Reading and Spelling (LETRS)*. In addition, she has written articles on varied topics. Ms. Hennessy is an honorary member of the Delta Kappa Gamma Society, the recipient of the North Carolina Branch of IDA's *June Lyday Orton Award* 2012 and the IDA's *Margaret Byrd Rawson Lifetime Achievement Award* in 2011.

Marcia K. Henry, Ph.D., Professor Emerita, Special Education, San Jose State University

Dr. Henry received her doctorate in educational psychology from Stanford University. She was a Fulbright Lecturer/Research Scholar at the University of Trondheim, Norway, in 1991. Dr. Henry served as President of The International Dyslexia Association from 1992 to 1996. She now provides professional development for schools and organizations across the country.

Larry E. Hess, Psy.D., Psychologist (independent practice), 145 East 74th Street, Suite 1C, New York, New York

Dr. Hess is a psychologist in independent practice who has more than 20 years of experience in assessing toddlers, children, adolescents, and young adults. He frequently speaks at conferences and seminars about assessment and learning disorders. He is a graduate of the University of Chicago and of the Illinois School of Professional Psychology. He performed his clinical training at The University of Chicago Medical Center, Northwestern Memorial Hospital, and SUNY–Stony Brook's University Counseling Center and Child and Adolescent Program. He is a member of the International Neuropsychological Society, the New York State Association for Neuropsychology, and the National Academy of Neuropsychology.

Judith C. Hochman, M.A., M.Ed., Ed.D., Founder and Chief Academic Officer, The Writing Revolution, 22 Cortlandt Street, 33rd Floor, New York, New York

Dr. Hochman is Founder and Chief Academic Officer of The Writing Revolution and is Founder of The Windward Teacher Training Institute in White Plains, New York. She is Former Head of The Windward School in White Plains, New York, an independent school for students with learning and language disabilities. Dr. Hochman was also Superintendent of Schools for the Greenburgh-Graham Union Free School District in Hastings, New York.

Betsy MacDermott-Duffy, M.S.Ed., Director of Language Arts and Instruction, The Windward School, 40 Red Oak Lane, White Plains, New York

Betsy MacDermott-Duffy is Director of Language Arts and Instruction at The Windward School and former Director of Curriculum Instruction at The Graham School, both located in Westchester County. She has published several articles in professional magazines, including *Perspectives on Language and Literacy,* the official publication of The International Dyslexia Association. She is also the author of the *Teaching Basic Writing Skills Activity Templates,* published by Voyager-Sopris Learning. In addition to serving as a consultant for educational companies, Ms. Duffy presents at conferences throughout the United States on reading, writing, and vocabulary strategies, as well as executive functioning and the Common Core State Standards (CCSS). She is an International Multisensory Structured Language Education Council (IMSLEC) teacher trainer and holds a certification as a Dyslexia Practitioner. Ms. MacDermott-Duffy has a master's degree in learning disabilities, is certified in advanced graduate study of staff development, and earned a master's degree in school administration and supervision.

Eileen S. Marzola, Ed.D., Education Consultant/Learning Disabilities Specialist, Marzola Education Services, New York, New York

Dr. Marzola received her doctorate in special education (with a focus on learning disabilities) from Teachers College, Columbia University. She taught for more than 35 years at every level from kindergarten through graduate school and has conducted numerous staff development trainings for those interested in improving instructional strategies for struggling learners. Dr. Marzola has been a keynote speaker and presented at many national and international conferences; she has published articles in professional journals and chapters in books about learning disabilities. She was honored by the New York State Federation of the Council for Exceptional Children with the New York State Teacher of the Year Award. Dr. Marzola is Past President of the New York Branch of The International Dyslexia Association and also served on its Board of Directors. She also served on the

Board of Directors of Everyone Reading in New York and created and presented a webinar on comprehension for the New Jersey Department of Education.

Graham F. Neuhaus, Ph.D., Faculty, Department of Social Sciences, University of Houston–Downtown, 1 Main Street, Houston, Texas

Dr. Neuhaus is a faculty member of the Psychology Department of the University of Houston–Downtown, where she teaches, mentors students, and conducts research in the area of automaticity and reading fluency.

Lucy Hart Paulson, M.S., Ed.D., Speech-Language Pathologist, Literacy Specialist

Dr. Paulson is a speech-language pathologist and literacy specialist with years of experience working with young children and their families and teachers in public school, Head Start, private, and university settings. She has a unique and broad-based perspective blending areas of language, literacy, and social communication together, resulting in effective and engaging learning opportunities for children and valuable foundations for teachers. She is the lead author of *Language Essentials for Teachers of Reading and Spelling (LETRS) for Early Childhood Educators, Second Edition* (Voyager Sopris Learning, 2018); *Building Early Literacy and Language Skills* (Sopris West, 2001), a resource and activity guide for young children; and *Good Talking Words* (Sopris West, 1998), a social communication skills program for preschool and kindergarten. In addition, Dr. Paulson served on the faculty of the Communicative Sciences and Disorders Department at the University of Montana, sharing responsibilities for teaching, supervising, research, and service.

Eve Robinson, M.S.Ed., Project Director, Central Jersey Family Health Consortium, Grow NJ Kids Regional Technical Assistance Center North, 161 Madison Avenue, Suite 225, Morristown, New Jersey

Eve Robinson is an experienced early childhood professional who has worked in the field for more than 30 years. She led an exemplary early childhood center, the Montclair Community Pre-K (MCPK), for 13 years as it became nationally and internationally known for its educational approach as well as its support of families. The MCPK was one of only 21 early childhood centers in the United States to be recognized as exemplary by the Center for the Study of Social Policy Strengthening Families Initiative. In addition, Ms. Robinson is a professor at Montclair State University and an appointed member of the Montclair Board of Education.

Jean Schedler, Ph.D., Fellow AOGPE, Educational Consultant and Trainer, Priority PD, Post Office Box 8, Elkton, Maryland

Dr. Schedler partners with schools to develop and implement sustainable reading workshops and school-based programs. As an Academy Graduate of Learning

Forward, her work focuses on the intersection of reading curriculum and professional learning. Dr. Schedler is a former International Dyslexia Association (IDA) Branch President. Her experience includes classroom teacher, reading director in a private school for special needs, adjunct professor, and teacher trainer across grade levels. Dr. Schedler works nationally and internationally with schools, training centers, and educational organizations.

Robin Anderson Singer, M.A., Instructor of Education, Hudson County Community College, 70 Sip Avenue, Jersey City, New Jersey

Ms. Singer prepares prospective teachers in early literacy, early childhood, and special education. She was the lead teacher of the Language Enrichment Program at Pascack Hills High School, an Alphabetic Phonics–based program, created by the Neuhaus Education Center, and also taught at The Stephen Gaynor School, early intervention services, and elementary school districts in New Jersey. She received her M.A. in the education of children with learning disabilities at Teachers College, Columbia University, and began doctoral studies in teacher education teacher development at Montclair State University in Fall 2017. She is the recent recipient of the NISOD Excellence Award, which honors exceptional work of community college faculty.

Lydia H. Soifer, Ph.D., Language and Speech Pathologist; Founder and for its 25-year tenure, Director of The Soifer Center for Learning and Child Development

Dr. Soifer is an assistant professor of pediatrics at Albert Einstein College of Medicine, Bronx, New York, and a faculty member of the Early Intervention Training Institute of the Children's Evaluation and Rehabilitation Center of the Montefiore Hospital Medical Center. As a parent educator, teacher trainer, and staff developer in public and private schools, mainstream, and special education schools, Dr. Soifer's focus has been on the dynamic among the factors influencing a child's ability to learn. Her approach is cognitive-linguistic in nature, with an emphasis on the role of both the teacher's trained and conscious use of language and the student's language abilities in effective teaching and learning. Dr. Soifer is a frequent presenter at national and local conferences and regularly offers courses on language, literacy, and learning, as well as training in her program, *Classroom Language Dynamics.*

Gloria Trabucco, M.A., Founding Teacher/Curriculum Director, Montclair Community Pre-K, Montclair, New Jersey

Ms. Trabucco has been an early childhood educator and administrator for 40 years. Opening Montclair Community Pre-K and developing its curriculum was one of the biggest and most rewarding challenges of her career. She is happy that the field of early childhood education and its teachers are beginning to get the recognition they so deserve.

Colleen Uscianowski, M.S., Ph.D candidate, Adjunct Instructor, Teachers College, Columbia University, 525 W 120th Street, New York, New York

Colleen Uscianowski is an experienced special educator and adjunct lecturer at Hunter College and Teachers College, Columbia University. She is a co-founder of Luminous Learning, a company that creates specialized math materials for students with disabilities. She is currently completing her doctoral degree in Cognitive Studies in Education at Teachers College, Columbia University. Her research focus is on early childhood math and remediation for struggling learners.

Barbara A. Wilson, M.Ed., President, Wilson Language Training, 47 Old Webster Road, Oxford, Massachusetts

Barbara A. Wilson is the co-founder and president of Wilson Language Training, which provides materials and professional learning throughout the country. In 1988, Ms. Wilson authored the Wilson Reading System®, now in its fourth edition, based on reading research and her work at Massachusetts General Hospital Reading Disabilities Clinic, where she taught adults with dyslexia. Ms. Wilson developed and oversees graduate courses and clinical practicums, which lead to Wilson® Dyslexia Practitioner and Therapist certifications, which are accredited International Dyslexia Association (IDA) Tier 3 training programs. More than 25,000 teachers hold Wilson certifications in the United States. This certification is also an integral component for several university programs. Ms. Wilson has authored two other multisensory structured language programs: Fundations® for K–3 students and Just Words® for students in Grades 4–12 and adults. Ms. Wilson provides professional expertise for several organizations and efforts dedicated to reading and dyslexia. She was invited to the White House to speak to the President's Domestic Policy Adviser on Education regarding the issue of literacy in America's middle and high schools, and in 2015, she testified in front of the U.S. House of Representatives' Committee on Science, Space, and Technology in support of H.R. 3033, the Research Excellence and Advancements for Dyslexia (READ) Act, which was later signed into law. Ms. Wilson has been awarded honorary doctorate degrees from two Massachusetts institutions: Becker College and Fitchburg State University.

Beverly J. Wolf, M.Ed., Slingerland Consultant

Ms. Wolf is a former classroom teacher; tutor; Slingerland Consultant for the Renton Public Schools; Dean of Faculty for the Slingerland Institute for Literacy; and head of a Hamlin Robinson School for children with dyslexia. She continues to train teachers in the Slingerland® Adaptation of the Orton-Gillingham Approach and in Prerequisites for Beginning Reading. Ms. Wolf is the author of articles and books about dyslexia and creative activities for the classroom and language-related guides for classroom teachers, most recently, with Virginia Wise Berninger: *Dyslexia, Dysgraphia, OWL LD, and Dyscalculia: Lessons from Science and Teaching* (Paul H. Brookes Publishing Co., 2016).

Foreword

This fourth edition of what I fondly call Birsh's bible (now Birsh's and Carreker's) is even more comprehensive and instructive than previous editions. The improvements include new chapters on a broader range of topics, more current references, and useful technology resource lists. Adoption of the term *Structured Literacy* by the editors and chapter authors squares the content with the International Dyslexia Association's preferred label for literacy instruction that works best with all students and that is essential for students who experience reading disabilities.

Structured Literacy teaching builds knowledge of language at all levels and uses methods that are explicit, systematic, cumulative, and diagnostic-prescriptive. Structured Literacy instruction is teacher led and code focused. It assumes that the learner either can benefit from, or is dependent on, an informed teacher who can unveil the complexities and mysteries of English.

The chapters in this volume address each aspect of language within that framework. Beginning with the precursors of reading and writing, a new chapter on pre-kindergarten instruction complements the others on oral language development, teaching phonology, and teaching letter recognition. The chapters on teaching beginning reading, spelling, and writing, which stress the importance of cumulative learning of the orthographic code, are enhanced by the new chapter on executive functioning. The chapter on math disabilities is also a welcome new addition, as language-based learning difficulties affect performance in math and many students need better instruction in quantitative reasoning.

The section on advanced language and literacy instruction widens the scope of topics to those relevant for intermediate grades through adulthood. Chapters include a thorough treatment of vocabulary instruction and additional information on program and classroom management. These additions accompany updated chapters on morphology, comprehension, and written composition that were valuable in previous editions. The final section on special populations addresses the needs of English language learners, high-functioning adults with dyslexia, and older students with word-level reading disabilities. Thus, an educator can find in this one volume much useful guidance on what to teach, how to teach it, and why specific content and methodologies are vital for students with language learning difficulties.

In my view, the detailed information provided about instruction of each essential component of literacy is unique among books of this kind. Often in my own work as a consultant, author, and teacher of teachers, I have consulted this text for advice about how, exactly, to present linguistic concepts to students who depend on our ability to get the concepts across. Want to know how to teach a written syllable type? A multiple meaning word? A complex sentence? An expository text organizational structure? Read about it here; you can rely on the wisdom of individual authors who are masters of their practice.

Given the comprehensiveness and specificity of the book, the reader may wonder how anyone could teach reading in some other way than that which is described here. With what can Structured Literacy be contrasted? Could someone teach reading in an unstructured and unsystematic manner? Could a teacher lead implicit, haphazard lessons on foundational reading skills? Are there classrooms where no explicit teaching of phoneme awareness, sound–spelling correspondences, morphemes, syntax, or text structure occurs?

The answer to those last three questions unfortunately is "yes." The gulf between common classroom practices and those recommended by research remains very wide (see Kilpatrick, 2015, and Seidenberg, 2017, for discussions of this chasm). After hundreds of millions of dollars have been spent by the National Institutes of Health, the National Science Foundation, and the U.S. Department of Education to support reading research, one might assume that teachers would know the science of reading as a matter of course. After all, treating potential and actual reading failure is an urgent and important public health concern. Teaching all students to read, write, and use language well is one of the primary antidotes for a number of avoidable consequences, including underemployment, criminal behavior, and unwanted pregnancy (World Literacy Foundation, 2015).

Many factors conspire to perpetuate the gulf between popular practices and the teaching approaches supported by science. Schools of education are slow to change and have few incentives to do so. Popular textbooks used in reading courses may have little to no information about language and the psychology of reading development as currently understood but continue to be used. Courses may do nothing to prepare student teachers to address the needs of struggling students. The study of language is seldom required for licensure. Course professors may themselves lack current information based on scientific reading research.

And more understandably, the content is complex and takes a while to learn. One or two courses in a licensing program are seldom enough, even when the content is aligned with research. Adults who read have little intuitive insight into how they accomplished this remarkable feat. They must be formally educated to understand not only the content (e.g., Can you identify the speech sounds in *ooze* and *use*?) but also the hidden cognitive mechanisms by which to translate written symbols into spoken language.

Often the debates educators have about how to teach reading and writing diminish the importance of the issues by relegating them to personal "philosophy" as if every opinion about instruction is equivalent to every other. Yet, as many authors of this volume acknowledge, teaching reading well to *all* children is an urgent social and economic matter. Teachers have to get it right and do it with intensity for as long as it takes. The excellent techniques of instruction that imbue the chapters of this book make the difference not only for white, affluent students in pockets of privilege but also the nonwhite and poor—and those in between. Seventeen percent of Americans are poor by international standards, twice as many as in most developed countries (Merelli, 2017). Rather than being relegated to underfunded and mediocre schools, those children would have a leg up on the future if their teachers understood and were implementing the practices described here. That's why my preferred title for this book is *Good Language, Reading, and Writing Instruction for All.*

Louisa C. Moats, Ed.D.
President
Moats Associates Consulting, Inc.

REFERENCES

Kilpatrick, D.A. (2015). *Essentials of assessing, preventing, and overcoming reading difficulties.* Hoboken, NJ: Wiley.

Merelli, A. (2017). *The US has a lot of money, but it does not look like a developed country.* Retrieved from https://qz.com/879092/the-US-doesn't-look-like-a-developed-country/

Seidenberg, M. (2017). *Language at the speed of sight: How we read, why so many can't, and what can be done about it.* New York, NY: Basic Books.

World Literacy Foundation. (2015). *The economic and social cost of illiteracy: A snapshot of illiteracy in a global context.* Retrieved from https://worldliteracyfoundation.org/wp-content/uploads/2015/02/WLF-FINAL-ECONOMIC-REPORT.pdf

Preface

Reading is reading, or is it? Just a short time ago, it would have been hard to imagine the numerous platforms for reading, writing, and listening to the written word that have emerged recently. However, the reader and writer have to communicate through the words in order to receive or deliver the message. Language is still the medium that has to be mastered for whatever form literacy assumes. Accuracy gets you where you want to go, and fluency gets you there faster.

It is with great optimism and dedication that we present the updated fourth edition of this textbook in the hopes that such a vital resource will encourage many pre-service and in-service teachers and their instructors to explore and discover the richness of the study of the disciplines underlying literacy. Armed with knowledge and practice methods, teachers and other allied professionals will be able to deliver reading instruction to a wide spectrum of students, such as those with dyslexia and other struggling readers who need explicit, direct, systematic, intensive, multisensory lessons, as well as students who confidently soar using the breadth and depth of this information as an added benefit. For our purposes, *multisensory*, as detailed in Chapter 2, refers to instructional strategies that help students to link input from eye, ear, voice, and hand simultaneously during the carefully sequenced teaching of all language systems, so as to foster learning.

Since the last edition of this book was published in 2011, the conversation about reading instruction and learning difficulties has changed, along with ways of communicating and obtaining information. At the head of the education reform agenda is the promotion of data-based decision making of response to intervention (RTI) with the possibilities of helping to address reading difficulties early and identifying dyslexia and related learning disorders. No longer is the IQ discrepancy model of identifying reading disability the sine qua non. Differentiated instruction has risen to prominence as a must for all good teachers to apply in their classrooms. We now know, based on data from assessments of reading skills, at least 15%–20% of the school-age population needs explicit, systematic, evidence-based standard treatment protocols. The responsibility often falls on teachers in general education classrooms, where one half of students with disabilities learn. What today's classrooms call for are well-prepared and clinically experienced teachers (Fuchs, Fuchs, & Stecker, 2010).

In support of well-prepared and clinically experienced teachers, The International Dyslexia Association (IDA; 2018) created the *Knowledge and Practice Standards for Teachers of Reading*. The IDA standards outline what the knowledgeable and skilled teacher of reading should know and be able to do to teach all students to read well. Research has demonstrated that all but the most severe reading difficulties can be resolved or, at least, ameliorated through reading instruction delivered by knowledgeable and skilled teachers of reading. The Certification Exam for Educators of Reading Instruction (CEERI), which aligns with the IDA standards, provides proof of teacher knowledge.

The fourth edition aligns well with the IDA standards and prepares individuals interested in completing the CEERI. The goal of this new edition, like the third edition, is to bring to its readers an updated and expanded version that will continue to provide an explanation of Multisensory Structured Literacy (MSL). By presenting new scientific evidence about our understanding of language learning disabilities, its biological and environmental bases, and studies on responsiveness to remediation from the fields of cognitive psychology, education, and neuroscience, the fourth edition provides the foundation for teacher knowledge about the components of informed, language-based reading instruction and effective teaching strategies.

THE NEW EDITION

One of the major purposes of this new edition is to promote high-quality preparation of teachers for their day-to-day work with students so they can use informed and effective instruction. All of the chapters have been updated with the latest research related to their topics and the strategies for instruction within them. They are aimed at personnel who operate at the highest and most intensive levels of need, recognizing that there are students who will succeed only if this kind of instruction, supported by in-depth knowledge of what to teach and how to teach it, is available regardless of whether they are in elementary, middle, or high school. With these needs in mind, we are pleased to announce the introduction of three new chapters to expand the usefulness of the textbook and to meet the demands for a broader approach to teacher preparation and professional development for a wider range of ages. The first is Chapter 4, "Pre-Kindergarten Literacy," by Eve Robinson, Carolyn DeVito, and Gloria Trabucco, a topic that has drawn well-deserved attention because it creates the platform for every aspect of literacy development as students strive to become good readers and writers. The second is Chapter 8, "The Role of Executive Function in Literacy Instruction," by Monica Gordon-Pershey, which addresses the mental processes that allow individuals to regulate their thinking and behaviors so that they can learn while paying attention and making good choices in the classroom. The third new chapter is Chapter 13, "Math Learning Disabilities," by Katherine Garnett and Colleen Uscianowski, which focuses on the underacknowledged disability known as dyscalculia and how to help children, schools, and families with appropriate interventions.

The chapters have been arranged into specific groupings of topics within five sections. Section I, "Introduction to Multisensory Teaching" contains Chapter 1, "Connecting Research and Practice," by Judith R. Birsh, which leads to Chapter 2, "Structured Literacy Instruction," by Mary Lupiani Farrell and Nancy Cushen White. Section II, "Pre-reading/Literacy Skills" opens with Chapter 3, "Oral Language Development and Its Relationship to Literacy," by Lydia H. Soifer, which sets the necessary background for readers to understand the many facets of language processes involved in literacy. The remainder of this section shows the continuing development of early literacy laid out through Chapter 4, "Pre-Kindergarten Literacy," by Eve Robinson, Carolyn DeVito, and Gloria Trabucco; Chapter 5, "Alphabet Knowledge: Letter Recognition, Letter Naming, and Letter Sequencing" by Kay A. Allen and Graham F. Neuhaus; and Chapter 6, "Teaching Phonemic Awareness" by Lucy Hart Paulson.

Section III, "Beginning Reading/Literacy Skills" ties together information from the previous section and builds on it with knowledge and practice information about the basic tenets of literacy. Section III starts off with Chapter 7, "Assessment of Reading Skills: A Review of Select Key Ideas and Best Practices" by Larry E. Hess and Eileen S. Marzola, which helps to guide the direction and content of instruction, and continues on to Chapter 8, "The Role of Executive Function in Literacy Instruction." Then comes Chapter 9, "Teaching Reading: Accurate Decoding" by Suzanne Carreker, followed by Chapter 10, "Teaching Spelling," also by Suzanne Carreker. Integrated into this section is Chapter 11, "Multi-Modal Handwriting Instruction for Pencil and Technology Tools," by Beverly J. Wolf and Virginia Wise Berninger. The importance of fluency, though promoted in all aspects of literacy instruction, claims an important place in Chapter 12, "Fluency in Learning to Read: Conceptions, Misconceptions, Learning Disabilities, and Instructional Moves" by Katherine Garnett. This section concludes with a new chapter addressing a topic long neglected within educational research: Chapter 13, "Math Learning Disabilities," by Katherine Garnett and Colleen Uscianowski.

Section IV, "Advanced Reading/Literacy Skills" concentrates on the delivery of the content of instruction in Chapter 14, "The History and Structure of Written English," by Marcia K. Henry; Chapter 15, "Working With Word Meaning: Vocabulary Instruction" by Nancy Hennessy; Chapter 16, "Strategies to Improve Reading Comprehension in the Multisensory Classroom" by Eileen S. Marzola; Chapter 17, "Composition: Evidence-Based Instruction" by Judith C. Hochman and Betsy MacDermott-Duffy; and finally, Chapter 18, "Designing the Learning Environment and Planning Multisensory Structured Literacy Lessons" by Judith R. Birsh, Jean Schedler, and Robin Singer.

Section V, "Instructional Strategies for Specific Populations and Skill Areas" provides advanced preparation for teachers with previous experience teaching literacy. It begins with Chapter 19, "Language and Literacy Development Among English Language Learners," in which Elsa Cárdenas-Hagan describes ways to teach reading and spelling English to Spanish-speaking students. In Chapter 20, Barbara A. Wilson explores "Instruction for Older Students With a Word-Level Reading Disability"; this chapter is followed by Susan H. Blumenthal's Chapter 21, "Working with High-Functioning Adults With Dyslexia and Other Learning Challenges." We hope you find this order fits your growing understanding of the complexities and joys of teaching literacy to a wide range of students.

In the fourth edition, each chapter includes Reflect, Connect, and Respond questions, threaded throughout the chapter sections, and ends with a brief Knowledge and Skill Assessment. The goal of the questions is for the reader to review and synthesize the information in the chapters to build deep knowledge of the theory of, and research about, essential components of effective reading instruction, along with deep understanding of how these components can be incorporated and taught in comprehensive reading instruction to all students, especially those students who struggle to learn to read.

Online Companion Materials

Online Companion Materials (OCM) is an exciting new resource available to readers of the fourth edition. By OCM, we mean downloadable accompaniments that the contributors have provided to deepen readers' understanding of each chapter's content. The OCM may include further readings addressing this content, examples of instructional strategies and materials, supplemental questions for the chapter, and the like. Each chapter's OCM will also include a list of the Reflect, Connect, and Respond questions provided in the chapter; answers to the Knowledge and Skill Assessment multiple-choice questions, and, for most chapters, a list of Technology

Resources (discussed next). Because of its online format, the OCM can and will be updated periodically by the contributors.

Each chapter concludes with a bulleted list of the specific resources that can be found within the OCM for that chapter. A full, chapter-by-chapter list of these online resources follows the Table of Contents for this book.

The spotlighted feature of the OCM is Dr. Elaine A. Cheesman's Technology Resources, a curated guide to educational technology that is pertinent to the content of each chapter. (The Technology Resources for each chapter are also provided as chapter appendices in the print textbook.) The educational technology in the guide was carefully evaluated by Dr. Cheesman. The introduction to this feature is found in the following section.

Technology Resources

Smartphones, tablets, and other mobile devices make educational technology more affordable for parents and educators, and more accessible for children, starting in the preschool years. In the evolving world of technology, educational programs include computer software, web-based programs, and mobile applications (apps). Because platforms frequently overlap, this text uses the term "software/apps" as an umbrella term for all applications.

Educational technology includes both assistive technology (AT) and instructional technology, although the boundaries between these categories often overlap. AT allows a person to do a task independently that would be difficult or impossible under typical conditions. Assistive technologies should not replace or supplant instruction. However, children still benefit from opportunities to learn to read, write, and calculate independently. For example, too often, well-meaning educators will suggest that a child with imprecise handwriting type or word-process work, rather than help the child improve his or her letter-writing skills. Thus, the child has fewer opportunities to learn and practice the essential literacy skill of correct letter formation. Assistive technologies should be used to help a student do work independently, without having to rely on assistance from others.

Instructional technology helps the user learn new information or develop automaticity and fluency in previously taught skills. Instructional technology can be used in two ways—to augment teacher-led instruction and to provide opportunities for independent student practice (Winters & Cheesman, 2013). For example, electronic dictionaries can be used as AT because they enable someone to access a word's pronunciation independently, but they can also be used as instructional technology because the program/app can help someone learn new word meanings. Using a program or device to broaden academic vocabulary knowledge falls into the category of instructional technology because the technology helps the user learn new information or practice a previously taught skill. The key is for the teacher to understand student needs and align technology accordingly.

For students with learning disabilities, instructional technology can provide much-needed opportunities for additional individual practice at home and school. Well-designed programs/apps have the potential to increase student motivation, prolong focus, and build confidence (Bennett, 2012; McClanahan, Williams, Kennedy, & Tate, 2012). To motivate learners, software/apps need to be engaging and stimulating. But that is not enough. While software/apps are often very appealing at first glance, they may have significant content flaws or designs that are overly distracting, particularly for students with learning disabilities. A great deal of award-winning software/apps have been created by developers who are technologically savvy but have little or no knowledge of research-based content or effective instruction (Gottwald, 2016). O'Malley, Jenkins, and their colleagues (2013) reported that software/apps that introduce concepts systematically and provide immediate, corrective feedback increase student engagement and improve academic outcomes. To improve student achievement, the software/app must allow students to work at their own pace with interactive, structured, and systematic practice. The activities need a clear focus that is aligned with student needs and emphasize one or more of the areas identified by science as essential for proficient speaking, reading, spelling, composition, math, and organizational skills.

To augment teacher-led instruction, mobile devices—including Android, Chrome, Windows, and Apple platforms—can be linked to an overhead projector for whole-class instruction. Many brand-name projectors have apps that allow one to connect via a Bluetooth or Wi-Fi network. If wireless is not an option, one can connect via a hard-wired connection using HDMI (high definition media interface) or VGA (video graphics adapter or video graphic array) cables and adaptors appropriate for a projector and mobile device. Besides projecting specialized apps, tablets can be used in much the same way as a static or interactive white board. With Wi-Fi, mobile devices can project photos, movies, music clips, and other web-based content.

To assist the parent and educator, all software/apps mentioned in this text have been carefully reviewed to meet the standards identified by researchers in the field. The most effective instructional apps meet these criteria (Ishizuka, 2011; Winters & Cheesman, 2013):

1. The content is accurate and validated by research evidence and does not perpetuate theories unsupported by research evidence, such as colored backgrounds or special "dyslexia" fonts.

2. The design has professional sound and images to support learning.

3. The user interface is straightforward and orderly with minimal distracting images or sounds.

4. The user interface is intuitive and is age- and content-appropriate for the intended users.

5. Practice activities develop automaticity.

6. The feedback for success or error correction is immediate and unobtrusive.

7. Users can access oral or written instructions intuitively.

8. Teachers and parents can access written instructions easily.

9. NO in-app purchases (IAP) for other programs /apps are included.

10. NO advertisements are included.

Individual chapters include suggestions for some of the best specific software programs/apps currently available and features of effective programs/apps to help parents and teachers evaluate the quality of any new program/app that comes on the market in years to come.

Glossary

Robin Singer has added new information and organized the Glossary, which appears at the end of the book. The glossary terms are printed in boldface at first occurrence in the chapters.

UPDATED ACTIVITY BOOK

We have updated the *Multisensory Teaching of Basic Language Skills Activity Book, Fourth Edition* (Carreker & Birsh, 2019), to include activities that are tied directly to former and new chapters in this book. With these varied exercises, teachers can reinforce their new knowledge as they get ready to use this language-rich content and practice their new skills with confidence. Together, the textbook and the activity book can help guide teachers by presenting numerous models of evidence-based practices to use in the complicated task of literacy instruction across the grade levels.

HISTORY OF THE BOOK

The idea for the first edition evolved from an annual gathering of teacher educators that began in 1990. The Committee on Teacher Education Initiatives of The International Dyslexia Association, 60 people representing a wide range of MSL programs that prepared teachers to work with students with dyslexia, met yearly to create an accrediting body for organizations that prepare specialists in the education of individuals with dyslexia. Their aim was to set high professional standards for teachers, clinicians, and teacher education programs in the field of specific language disability or dyslexia already existing in college and university setting, hospitals, and other organizations that have MSL preparation as their function and encourage the growth of new ones. By 1995, the group incorporated as the International Multisensory Structured Language Education Council (IMSLEC). It is presently accrediting programs to ensure that individuals who need effective intervention and their families are indeed receiving help from well-prepared professionals who have been held to exemplary standards of teaching.

Today, IMSLEC accredits programs. Graduates of those programs may apply to The Alliance for Accreditation and Certification to take the National Alliance Registration Exam at either the therapy or teaching level. If successful, they will become either Certified Academic Language Therapists (CALT) or Associate Academic Language Teachers (AALT) and members of the Academic Language Therapy Association, whose members provide quality professional services for students with dyslexia and/or related disorders. Another organization that accredits programs and certifies individuals is the Academy of Orton-Gillingham Practitioners and Educators (AOGPE). Graduates of preparation programs that align with the IDA *Knowledge and Practice Standards* (e.g., IMSLEC, AOGPE, Wilson Language Systems) who successfully completed the CEERI are eligible for certification through the Center for Effective Reading Instruction as a certified Structured Literacy Dyslexia Specialist (SLDS) or a certified Structured Literacy Dyslexia Practitioner (SLDP).

During those early collaborative forums of expert teacher trainers and therapists, it became clear that there was a great need for a comprehensive textbook for MSL instruction that would gather together in one place resources based on research in reading and learning disabilities. In particular, the first edition was designed to reflect the group members' long years of professional experience in the classroom and in one-to-one and small-group practice. It brought together research and clinical experience from the second half of the 20th century, a time rich in innovation in teaching written language skills to children and adults with dyslexia, the most prevalent learning disability. We are truly indebted to the struggling readers who forced us to deconstruct the act of reading to shed light on how to teach those who struggle to grasp even the essential connection of letters and sounds at the outset. Still tuned to the same rich background of experience and dedication, the fourth edition builds on those priorities with contributions from classroom and clinical experience and ongoing research.

CLOSING THOUGHTS

The content and principles of MSL embedded in the chapters of this edition form a solid foundation of knowledge in the critical areas of oral language development, phonology and phonemic awareness, letter knowledge, handwriting, phonics, fluency, vocabulary, comprehension, spelling, and writing skills. As with the earlier editions, users can turn to this text time and again at each step of the way toward becoming expert practitioners. Obviously, all of the information cannot be integrated at once. Multiple readings and intensive practical applications in the everyday work of planning and teaching bring deeper understanding of the multilayered content and theory. With the help of one's own students, much of the complexity becomes clear when successful instructional outcomes occur. Like listening to a great symphony or poem several times, each encounter brings fresh insights and new understanding.

REFERENCES

Bennett, K.R. (2012). Less than a class set. *Learning & Leading with Technology, 39*(4), 22–25.

Carreker, S., & Birsh, J.B. (2019). *Multisensory teaching of basic language skills activity book* (4th ed.). Baltimore, MD: Paul H. Brookes Publishing Co.

Fuchs, D., Fuchs, L.S., & Stecker, P. (2010). The "blurring" of special education in a new continuum of general education placements and services. *Exceptional Children, 76*(3), 301–323.

Gottwald, S. (2016). The curiosities of using mobile devices for literacy instruction. *The Examiner.* Retrieved from http://dyslexiaida.org

International Dyslexia Association, The. (2018, March). *Knowledge and practice standards for teachers of reading.* Retrieved from https://dyslexiaida.org/knowledge-and-practices/

Ishizuka, K. (2011). The app squad: SLS's advisors weigh in on kids' book apps. *School Library Journal.* Retrieved from http://www.slj.com

McClanahan, B., Williams, K., Kennedy, E., & Tate, S. (2012). A breakthrough for Josh: How use of an iPad facilitated reading improvement. *TechTrends: Linking Research and Practice to Improve Learning, 56*(3), 20–28.

O'Malley, P., Jenkins, S., Wesley, B., Donehower, C., Rabuck, D., & Lewis, M.E.B. (2013). *Effectiveness of using iPads to build math fluency.* Paper presented at the Council for Exceptional Children Annual Meeting, San Antonio, Texas.

Winters, D.C., & Cheesman, E.A. (2013). Mobile instructional and assistive technology for literacy. *Perspectives in Language and Literacy, 39*(4), 42–46.

Acknowledgments

We would like to thank Astrid Pohl Zuckerman, Acquisitions Editor at Paul H. Brookes Publishing Co., for her steady guidance and wise advice as we worked on the revisions for this fourth edition. No question ever went unanswered, and those asked multiple times were patiently answered. Melissa Solarz, Associate Editor, Tess Hoffman, Developmental Editor, and Stephanie Henderson, Editorial Assistant, also deserve special praise for their exceptional organizational skills and uncompromising pursuit of accuracy and clarity to help readers understand the content and find the information they are seeking. There are many people whom we wish to acknowledge here.

First of all, we would like to acknowledge contributors who joined together for only the first edition of this book as a trial run because they believed in the need for such a resource for future teachers, and the contributors from the second and third editions, whose influence also hovers over this fourth edition, need acknowledgment as well.

We deeply appreciate the dedication and collaboration of all the current contributors, who worked diligently to revise and expand their chapters to reflect new research and new ideas in literacy instruction. We would like to welcome the new authors, who willingly coordinated their topics with the existing chapters, thus adding needed information to the book in a seamless way. We are excited that this fourth edition will highlight and support Structured Literacy and provide valuable information to educators so they can meet the learning needs of all students.

Thanks go to all of the readers whose suggestions and criticisms helped refine the content of this volume. Ideas came from many teacher educators and professional development providers. They gave helpful suggestions on how to improve the organization of the book and make it more useful. We particularly appreciate the encouragement we were given from the many teachers and teacher educators who hold the book as their beacon for instruction in all of the literacy skills.

And, finally, a broad acknowledgment of all the people across the country, too numerous to mention in person, who are devoting themselves to improving the outcome of reading instruction: teachers, teacher educators, principals, administrators, and parents; researchers, including psychologists, neuropsychologists, pediatricians, and speech-language specialists; and lawmakers. The work of all these constituencies is reflected in this volume.

With love and gratitude to my children,
Andrew, Philip, and Joanne Hope, and to their
children, Alexander, Abigail, Mark, Neena, Charlotte,
and Nikolai, for their sustained patience and inspiration

—*JRB*

With love and gratitude to my greatest
teachers, James and Elsa, and my rock, Larry

—*SC*

Introduction to Multisensory Teaching

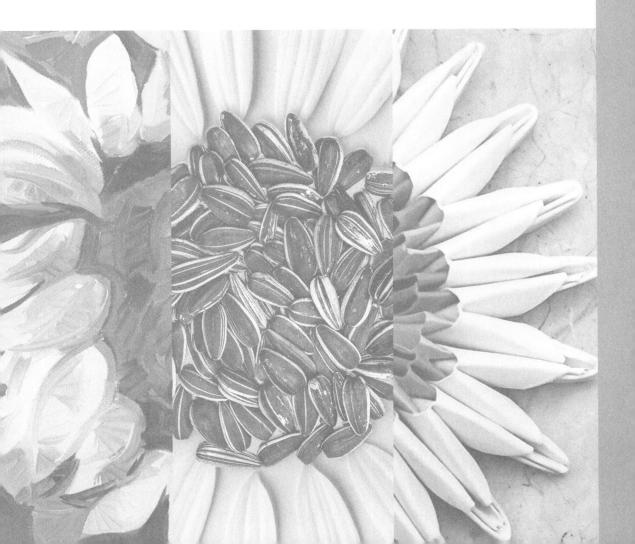

Chapter 1

Connecting Research and Practice

Judith R. Birsh

In the midst of many cultural treasures, reading is by far the finest gem.

—Stanislas Dehaene (2009)

LEARNING OBJECTIVES

1. To describe the importance of aligning the science of reading with best practices for instruction

2. To outline the essential components of reading and elements of effective instruction

3. To explain scientifically based reading research and how it has informed the understanding of dyslexia

4. To summarize the reasons for delivering evidence-based reading instruction to all students

5. To interpret the relationship between teacher preparation and student achievement

Teachers rarely remember how they learned to read, unless they met with difficulty. Some remember they learned by looking at the words and the pictures and putting them together early in first grade. Yet, understanding the complex **linguistic** tasks involved is crucial to their ability to succeed as exemplary teachers of literacy. To many, reading seems a natural act, whereas it is anything but natural. Listening and speaking are hardwired into the brain, but written language has to be acquired through instruction.

This book discusses Structured Literacy instruction, an approach grounded in scientific research for acquiring all literacy skills emphasizing direct, explicit, sequenced, systematic, cumulative, and intensive lessons, while incorporating multisensory instructional strategies. The dissemination of the relevant science of reading is a priority so that committed and motivated teachers receive appropriate information and training in this foundation in how reading works and how children learn (Seidenberg, 2017). New in this edition is a chapter focused on developing pre-kindergarten preparation for literacy; one on the importance of executive function, especially attention and memory, when planning lessons; and another on specific methods, techniques, and activities for the understanding of mathematical thinking and dyscalculia. The underlying premise of all the chapters is to promote the use of student data to drive and differentiate instruction based on specific techniques and activities to develop mastery.

The term **multisensory strategies** means the use of direct instructional strategies involving visual, auditory, and tactile–kinesthetic sensory systems to learn the phonological, morphemic, semantic, and syntactic layers of language along with the articulatory–motor aspects of language. Listening, speaking, reading, and writing are directly involved while the student sees, hears, says, and writes during brief and varied lesson routines (Birsh, 2006).

Mastery of the details within words, sentences, and paragraphs evolves from exposure to expert teachers who have the knowledge and skills to deliver top-notch instruction from elementary school through high school. To be ready for such high-level tasks, teachers need to undergo extensive preparation in the disciplines inherent in literacy: language development, **phonology** and **phonemic awareness,** alphabet knowledge, handwriting, **decoding,** spelling, **fluency, vocabulary, comprehension,** composition, testing and **assessment,** lesson planning, behavior management, history of the English language, use of technology, and the needs of older struggling readers.

The national spotlight on literacy is intense due to several developments. One major concern is the movement toward data analysis and research to improve instruction. For example, following the **No Child Left Behind (NCLB) Act of 2001 (PL 107-110)** legislation and the subsequent Reading First initiative were several changes that affected multiple aspects of education, including literacy. These included 1) **response to intervention (RTI)** (Gersten et al. 2008) as a way of assessing risk of failure, benchmarking progress, and providing **differentiated instruction** to struggling students, including those who struggle with literacy; 2) the creation of the Common Core State Standards Initiative: Preparing America's Students for College and Career (Council of Chief State School Officers [CCSSO] & National Governors Association Center for Best Practices [NGA Center], 2010); and the adoption of The International Dyslexia Association's (IDA; 2018) *Knowledge and Practice Standards for Teachers of Reading.* Using research-based information, each "movement" is an attempt to bring high-level content and best practices to schools to improve the delivery of equable instruction and to uphold high standards for administrators, teachers, parents, and students. Along with these efforts, organizations were formed to change states' licensure for teaching reading and to influence how teachers are prepared in schools of education and through professional development in alternative pathways models of effective instruction, with the help of coaching and mentoring to ensure consistent translation into good practice. Parents organized to improve understanding and ensure better provision of services. Appendix 1.2 lists organizations dedicated to these purposes.

Teachers who have a wide range of experience and a strong foundation of knowledge enhanced by scientifically based reading research from which to make judgments about what to teach, how to teach it, when to teach it, and to whom to teach it, increase the chances of a successful outcome when working with all students but especially with students at risk of failing to learn to read or with those who have already fallen behind (Aaron, Joshi, & Quatroche, 2008; McCardle, Chhabra, & Kapinus, 2008). When an individual struggles with written language, none of the myriad layers of language processing can be taken for granted. Differentiated instruction is language based—intensive, systematic, direct, and comprehensive. Each individual is different and brings unique cognitive and linguistic strengths and weaknesses to the task. Therefore, teachers who work at prevention, intervention, or remediation require a foundation based on scientific evidence and need to be informed about the complex nature of instruction in reading and related skills.

Since the early 1980s, a broad range of individuals have made major contributions to research on the component processes of learning to read, reading disabilities, language disabilities, and models of effective instruction. More research is needed, but teachers must work with what is already known.

THE SCIENCE OF READING

This keen interest in the newly acknowledged science of reading (Kilpatrick, 2015; Seidenberg, 2017) has involved general and special educators, psychologists, linguists, neuroscientists, geneticists, speech-language specialists, parents, and children with and without reading difficulties. Since the previous edition of this book, reading instruction is no longer based on opinion; rather, it is informed by science in an orderly progression of research data that shows what works. This book focuses on scientifically based instruction in reading and related literacy skills. In this chapter, five major concerns from research are explored so that teachers have ways to think about and apply relevant theory and substantiated practices:

1. What is scientifically based reading research, and why is it important?

2. What has scientifically based reading research explained about the components of reading?

3. How has scientifically based reading research advanced understanding of **dyslexia?**

4. How can teachers deliver evidence-based reading instruction with fidelity of implementation so that students learn to read with accuracy, fluency, and comprehension?

5. How does scientifically based reading instruction correspond to the Common Core State Standards and other state standards in furthering reading proficiency and preparing students for college, career, and life?

DEFINITION AND IMPORTANCE
OF SCIENTIFICALLY BASED RESEARCH

Scientifically based research, also referred to as **evidence-based research,** gathers evidence to answer questions and bring new knowledge to a field of study so that effective practices can be determined and implemented. Scientific research is a process.

A scientist develops a theory and uses it to formulate hypotheses. A study is designed to evaluate the hypotheses. The methods used in the study depend on the hypotheses, and these methods result in findings. The scientist then integrates what is found from this particular study into the body of knowledge that has accumulated around the research question. As such, scientific research is a cumulative process that builds on understandings derived from systematic evaluations of questions, models, and theories (Fletcher & Francis, 2004). Lyon and Chhabra (2004) underscored that good evidence is derived from a study that asks clear questions that can be answered empirically, selects and implements valid research methods, and accurately analyzes and interprets data.

Using **randomized controlled trials** is a critical factor in establishing strong evidence for what works (causation) in **experimental research.** This means that individuals in an intervention study are randomly assigned to experimental and control groups. With randomized controlled trials, all variables are held constant (e.g., gender, age, demographics, skill levels) except the one variable that is hypothesized to cause a change. This allows the researcher to show a causal relationship between the intervention and the **outcomes**; in other words, the intervention caused a change, thus establishing what does and does not work. **Quasi-experimental research** attempts to determine cause and effect without strict randomized controlled trials and is valid but less reliable. The **meta-analysis** done by the National Reading Panel (NRP; National Institute of Child Health and Human Development [NICHD], 2000) reviewed both experimental and quasi-experimental studies of instructional practices, procedures, and techniques in real classrooms. The NRP's criteria closely followed accepted practices for evaluating research literature found in other scientific disciplines, such as medicine, and in behavioral and social research (Keller-Allen, 2004). The major recommendations from the meta-analyses were that every child needs to be taught the Big Five—phonemic awareness, **phonics,** fluency, vocabulary, and comprehension—as the basis of literacy instruction beginning in kindergarten.

Peer review and the **convergence of evidence** should also be considered. Peer review stipulates that the results of an intervention study be scrutinized and evaluated by a group of independent researchers with expertise and credentials in that field of study before the results are publicly reported in a journal article, book, or other type of publication. Another avenue of critical review is through presentations and papers that are scrutinized by fellow scientists to bring objectivity, validity, and reliability into the process of educational research (Fletcher & Francis, 2004). Convergence of evidence derives from the identical replication of a study in a similar population by other researchers because the outcomes from a single study are not sufficient to generalize across all populations. Other caveats for educational research are to be clear about the specific intervention, monitor it, and then use valid and reliable outcome measures (Reyna, 2004).

There are two kinds of educational research methodology: qualitative and quantitative. **Qualitative research** involves observing individuals and settings and relies on observation and description of events in the immediate context. **Ethnographic observation** is an example of qualitative research in which researchers observe, listen, and ask questions to collect descriptive data in order to understand the content, context, and dynamics of an instructional setting. Qualitative research can be scientific if it follows the principles of scientific inquiry. It is difficult to say what works or does not work (causation) in qualitative research; however, this kind of research affords a picture of what is happening and a description of the context.

Quantitative research uses large numbers of individuals to generalize findings to similar settings using statistical analyses. Quantitative research must use experimental or quasi-experimental design methods to gather data.

Some debate exists over whether quantitative or qualitative research is better, which obscures the principle. It is not the method of observation (qualitative vs. quantitative) that qualifies a study as providing rigorous evidence; rather, it is the fact that the design follows scientific inquiry. For example, a study must have enough individuals in well-matched groups so that **statistical significance** between groups can be established. Regression-discontinuity (Schochet et al., 2010), which uses a cut-off point instead of random assignment in making comparison groups, and the use of single-case studies (Kratochwill et al., 2010) are now being considered along with randomized controlled trials. This expansion to include both experimental and descriptive research paradigms will be interesting to follow for its effect on the outcomes of interventions in reading.

The U.S. Department of Education, Institute of Education Sciences (2008), is a resource that further explains evidence-based research and provides educational practitioners with tools to distinguish practices supported by rigorous evidence from those that are not. Also, Kilpatrick (2015) and Seidenberg (2017) discussed the progress and the pitfalls in current reading research. Another resource to find out what works in education is the Florida Center for Reading Research web site (http://www.fcrr.org), which provides excellent reviews of programs.

The National Reading Panel

In 1997, the U.S. Congress asked the director of the National Institute of Child Health and Human Development (NICHD), in consultation with the Secretary of Education, to convene a national panel to assess the status of research-based knowledge, including the effectiveness of various approaches for teaching children to read (NICHD, 2000). Thus, unlike previous inquiries, the NRP analyzed experimental and quasi-experimental research literature, using rigorous research standards, to determine how "critical reading skills are most effectively taught and what instructional methods, materials, and approaches are most beneficial for students of varying abilities" (NICHD, 2000, p. 1-1). The NRP intensively reviewed the following topics:

- Phonemic awareness

- Phonics instruction

- Fluency

- Comprehension

- Teacher education and reading instruction

- Computer technology and reading instruction

The findings from the meta-analyses (i.e., longitudinal studies, cognitive and linguistic studies, studies in neurobiology) by the subgroups in this list of topics reviewed by the 14 members of the NRP (NICHD, 2000) revealed consensus among effective educators on what works in reading instruction. As a result of the review of the literature, the panel arrived at strong conclusions (Pressley, 2002) and identified the following five critical components that are essential for teaching young children to read:

1. Phonemic awareness

2. Phonics

3. Vocabulary development

4. Reading fluency, including oral reading skills

5. Reading comprehension strategies

Research by itself cannot improve practice. The importance of converging scientific evidence in reading research and its relationship to practice, however, has begun to gain new prominence in the thinking of not only teacher educators and teachers but also government officials on the federal, state, and local levels charged with educational reform; business people; and parents and caregivers of young children. The 2017 report of the most recent National Assessment of Educational Progress (NAEP) indicated that fourth-grade reading scores have changed little since the 1980s, with about 67% of fourth-grade students performing at or below *basic* level, and only 31% performing at or above *proficient* (National Center for Education Statistics, 2017). Achievement gaps still persist, with no significant changes among racial/ethnic groups, gender, or types of schools (National Center for Education Statistics, 2017). The tests measured knowledge of literary and informational reading comprehension. Teachers must adopt more effective instructional practices and policies to close the reading gap and to solve the problem of pervasive, persistent reading failure.

The ongoing, dynamic process of scientifically based reading research is identifying the causes of reading failure and the practices that help children—including those most at risk—learn to read. Snow (2004) emphasized that knowing which practices work to produce specific results in the critical areas of reading instruction could help many teachers use methods and approaches in their daily work that are consonant with research-based evidence and could thus help significantly more children learn to read proficiently. Layered on top of this important research are the new fields being investigated with a future impact on reading instruction in psychology, linguistics, cognitive science, cognitive neuroscience, and human memory, which Seidenberg said are "being studied in the context of how students acquire, retain, and forget new information and how courses can be structured to promote learning, retention and 'transfer'" (2017, p. 290).

College- and Career-Readiness Standards

The **Common Core State Standards (CCSS)** and other state standards define educational goals for what students should know and be able to do in reading by the end of each grade level so that by high school graduation they will be prepared to succeed in college, career, and adult life. In part, the genesis of these college- and career-readiness standards were studies that documented a steady decrease in the complexity of K–12 textbooks since the 1960s, whereas the complexity of college textbooks has remained the same or has increased (see Williamson, 2008). Because of the gap between students' reading proficiency at the end of high school and the demands of more complex texts, many students face significant challenges related to reading ability in college.

Readiness standards are responsible for the trend of reading increasingly complex texts, beginning in kindergarten and continuing through high school. By the end of high school, students are expected to read grade-appropriate complex text independently and proficiently. Fluent reading, vocabulary, syntactic awareness, general knowledge, and basic comprehension skills and strategies are indispensable as the foundation for reading increasingly complex text. The instruction presented in this book will prepare students for the rigorous reading they will need for college, career, and adult life.

RESEARCH ON THE COMPONENTS OF READING

While researchers were studying learning disabilities such as dyslexia, they learned how reading develops in readers both with and without reading impairments. NICHD-sponsored studies of both struggling and skilled readers led to data on more than 42,000 readers. These findings have straightforward, practical implications for teachers of typically developing readers and those students with dyslexia and other related co-occurring challenges (Lyon, 2004).

There is a broad scientific consensus, based on empirical evidence, on what is needed to become a good reader. Two important sources for this agreement are the National Research Council report (Snow, Burns, & Griffin, 1998) and the NRP report (NICHD, 2000). This consensus on the high-priority skills that children must acquire as they learn to read is based on clear evidence.

The five essential components of reading instruction are sometimes referred to as the building blocks for reading (Partnership for Reading, 2003). Most educators agree that no single reading component is sufficient in itself. Students need to acquire all of the combined essential components in a balanced, comprehensive reading program to become successful readers. The chapters in this book give detailed analyses of the research pertaining to each component and provide the reader with in-depth discussions of approaches for developing and implementing instruction in each of these component areas. Consider the conclusions of the NRP on essential reading skills instruction, along with a few key ideas from the CCSS.

Phonemic Awareness

The Partnership for Reading defined *phonemic awareness* as "the ability to notice, think about and work with the individual sounds in words" (2003, p. 2). The NRP meta-analysis confirmed that phonemic awareness, along with knowing the names and shapes of both lower- and uppercase letters, is a key component "that contributes significantly to the effectiveness of beginning reading and spelling instruction" (NICHD, 2000, p. 2-43). Phonemic awareness plays a vital role in learning to read because it helps children connect spoken language to written language. (See Chapter 6 for a detailed discussion of how to teach phonemic awareness.) It helps expose the underlying sounds in language that consequently relate to the alphabetic symbols on the printed page. Phonemic awareness has a causal relationship with literacy achievement, and understanding it in kindergarten is the single best predictor of later reading and spelling achievement in first and second grade (Catts, Nielsen, Liu, & Bontempo, 2015; de Groot, van den Bos, Minnaert, & van der Meulen, 2015).

In kindergarten, phonemic awareness predicts growth in word-reading ability (Torgesen, Wagner, & Rashotte, 1994). Children at risk because of early speech-language impairments and those with dyslexia perform more poorly on tests of phonemic awareness than typically developing children. When children do not have good word-identification skills, they fall behind in reading, and without appropriate intervention, they have only a 1 in 8 chance of catching up to grade level (Juel, 1988).

Numerous studies of weak readers with highly effective outcomes that provided training intensively in phonemic awareness, phonic decoding, and opportunities to read connected text reported by Kilpatrick stand as a rebuttal to taking a "wait-and-see" approach to early reading difficulties (2015, p. 113). Without the ability to think about and manipulate the individual sounds in words, beginning and especially older struggling readers risk falling behind or never catching up to their peers. Isolating and manipulating sounds in words using oral **segmenting** and **blending** activities helps children learn the **alphabetic principle** as they are learning to read and spell. Learning letter names and shapes is an important adjunct to these skills (see Chapter 5 on alphabet knowledge).

Although phonemic awareness is a means to understanding and using letters and sounds for reading and writing, it is not an end in itself (see NICHD, 2000, p. 2-43). Phonemic awareness stands as one of the major components of a comprehensive program of instruction when taught in small groups and in moderate amounts. Children differ in their need for instruction, but phonemic awareness benefits everyone, especially those with little experience detecting and manipulating speech sounds (see Chapter 5).

Phonics

Systematic and explicit instruction in phonics, the relationship between letters or **letter combinations** in written language (**graphemes**) and the approximately 44 sounds in English spoken language (**phonemes**), has proven effective for improving children's reading (Adams, 1990; NICHD, 2000; Partnership for Reading, 2003). It is best introduced early in kindergarten and first grade, which leads to accurately recognizing familiar words and decoding unfamiliar words. Teaching phonics is beneficial for all children, regardless of socioeconomic status (SES), especially when it is accompanied by memory aids such as **key words** for sounds, pictures, and articulatory gestures (McCardle et al., 2008).

Eden and Moats pointed out the reciprocal relationship between phonemic awareness and reading in that "learning how letters represent sounds (phonology) and seeing words in print (**orthography**) helps novice readers to attend to speech sounds" (2002, p. 1082). Phonics, deemed valuable and essential, should be integrated with other types of reading instruction in a comprehensive program that includes all of the reading components listed previously in this chapter. The NRP found solid support for using systematic phonics rather than an unsystematic approach or no phonics at all because systematic phonics (i.e., a plan or sequence to introducing letter–sound relationships) provided a more significant contribution to children's growth in reading (NICHD, 2000). It has a great impact on children in kindergarten and first grade, with the greatest effects shown with beginning readers who are at risk and have low SES backgrounds (Keller-Allen, 2004). However, **effect sizes** among children from low- and middle-income homes for the outcomes of phonics instruction did not differ, leading Ehri, Nunes, Stahl, and Willows to conclude that "phonics instruction contributes to higher performance in reading" in students from low-SES and middle-SES backgrounds (2001, p. 418). Systematic phonics has its greatest effect in the early grades; that is, in kindergarten and first grade for all beginning readers, children at risk, and children diagnosed with reading disabilities. Phonics instruction at any age, however, facilitates learning to read.

Another important finding of the NRP meta-analysis was that positive results were produced through one-to-one tutoring, in small-group instruction, and in whole-class programs (Ehri et al., 2001). Furthermore, systematic phonics can be taught through **synthetic** phonics, **analytic** phonics, phonics through spelling, analogy phonics, and **embedded phonics.** (It is beyond the scope of this chapter to discuss these approaches in detail; for more information see Ehri, 2004.) Pressley (2002) agreed that phonics instruction calls for more than a one-size-fits-all approach. Many variations are possible as long as the program is both extensive and systematic.

One added benefit of systematic phonics instruction is its impact on beginning readers' comprehension. Subsequent to the NRP report, researchers have found that phonics does indeed have benefits for struggling readers who are older when taught systematically (Connor, Morrison, & Underwood, 2007). In many ways, Chall (1967) said it best when she said students need both phonics and meaning-focused activities in balanced reading programs. (See Chapter 9 for discussion of teaching accurate decoding as part of reading instruction.)

Fluency

Beginning readers need to be fluent in letter naming, knowledge of sounds, and phonemic awareness activities. Fluency, however, was defined by the Partnership for Reading as "the ability to read a text accurately and quickly, recognize words, [and] gain meaning from text" (2003, p. 22). This is a key concept, with well-documented converging evidence supporting the connection between fluency and reading comprehension (Rasinski, 2017; Snow et al., 1998). Without the advantage of fluency, children remain slow and laborious readers. Meaningful improvements in reading fluency are well documented when a range of well-described instructional approaches are used. (See Chapter 12 for a detailed discussion of methods for building fluency.)

Major approaches to teaching fluency include **guided oral reading** procedures that include repeated oral reading, with modeling by the instructor, in which students receive feedback from peers, parents, or teachers. Guided oral reading and encouraging students to read are effective in improving fluency and overall reading achievement (see NICHD, 2000). Gaps in fluency remain in older students, however, in both those with extremely low word-level reading skills and those who have good, compensated word accuracy skills but need remediation to enable them to read faster with sufficient comprehension.

Vocabulary

Knowing word meanings is a major contributor to students' ability to communicate ideas and comprehend text. The NRP analyses confirmed that there is a strong relationship between vocabulary learning and comprehension gains (NICHD, 2000). Although the database of studies on vocabulary instruction and measurement that qualified for the NRP review was small, the panel did find some trends in the data that have implications for instruction:

- Vocabulary should be taught both directly and indirectly.

- Repetition and multiple exposures to vocabulary items are important.

- Learning in rich contexts is valuable for vocabulary learning.

- Vocabulary tasks should be restructured when necessary.

- Vocabulary learning should entail active engagement in learning tasks.

- Computer technology can be used to help teach vocabulary.

- Vocabulary can be acquired through **incidental learning.**

- How vocabulary is assessed and evaluated can have a differential effect on instruction.

- Dependence on a single vocabulary instruction method will not result in optimal learning.

The CCSS promotes the use of **academic vocabulary,** which is different from the vocabulary that is used in everyday conversation. Academic vocabulary is often referred to as the language of the classroom. Words related to the features and structures of informational text, rhetorical devices used in literary text, domain-specific words, grammatical terms, and morphology are examples of academic vocabulary. Such language is an essential part of the oral and written discourse necessary for academic success and should be used liberally throughout the school day. Many of the bolded words in the chapters of this book (collected and defined in the Glossary) are academic vocabulary. See Chapter 15 for research and teaching activities for vocabulary. Each academic content area includes vocabulary specific to that content area; for example, see Chapter 13 on math, which stresses the importance of understanding the many terms used regularly as students learn all levels of math.

Students need a broad daily lexicon to function in and out of school, but to carry them through content courses, they will need academic language to allow them to comprehend what their courses demand by understanding the vocabulary in the material being studied. Chapter 15 describes in detail the most practical and useful ways to teach vocabulary and its impact on comprehension.

Comprehension

Comprehension is making sense of what is read and depends on good **word recognition,** fluency, vocabulary, world knowledge, and verbal reasoning. Good instruction calls for attention to comprehension when children listen to books read aloud and as soon as they begin reading text. Since the 1980s, research on comprehension instruction has supported using specific **cognitive strategies,** either individually or in concert, to help readers understand and remember what they read (NICHD, 2000). Direct instruction of these cognitive strategies in the classroom leads to active involvement of the readers and helps readers across the range of ability. Chapter 16 presents many research-supported strategies as well as other promising methods designed to improve this essential reading skill within a multisensory learning environment.

Metacognition is thinking about thinking. Good readers think about what they are reading in complex ways. The research suggests that students will improve in their ability to comprehend text through modeling and metacognitive instruction by the teacher (Klingner, Morrison, & Eppolito, 2011). Effective strategies include question answering and generation, summarization, graphic and semantic organizers such as story maps, **comprehension monitoring,** and **cooperative learning.** Many opportunities for discussion and writing enhance comprehension. The evidence reviewed by the NRP led the panel to conclude that instruction that provides a "variety of reading comprehension strategies leads to increased learning of the strategies, to specific transfer of learning, to increased memory and understanding of new passages, and in some cases, general improvements in comprehension" (NICHD, 2000, p. 4-52).

The CCSS and other state standards present several important ideas about reading that further develop the solid foundation laid by the NRP. **Close reading, text-dependent questions,** and **evidence** are terms that speak to how the readiness standards have increased rigor to ensure that students are prepared for college and career. Close reading is a deep examination of a text. Text-dependent questions that involve analysis, evaluation, and synthesis require students to look carefully and critically at the text. To answer text-dependent questions, students must find evidence in the text to support a claim. These questions lead students to understand what a text means, how it works, and what the text implies in terms of a deeper meaning, themes, and other ideas. Along with the five essential areas of skills needed to learn to read as outlined in the NRP, the CCSS presented other critical factors needed for proficient reading and academic success. These are described in detail in Textbox 1.1.

TEXTBOX 1.1   Consensus from scientifically based research on learning to read and write

Oral language—Long before children begin to read, they need solid oral language and literacy experiences at home and in preschool that will support them later in acquiring abstract linguistic skills necessary for reading. These include language play, such as saying rhymes; listening to, discussing, and examining books; developing oral vocabulary and verbal reasoning; and learning the purposes of reading, along with gross and fine motor writing activities. Exposure to reading aloud and oral language play fosters development of sounds and symbols and a language about reading. Oral language is the foundation of comprehension and helps the reader use decoding strategies. (See Chapter 3 for more about developing oral language.)

Emergent literacy—Early childhood educators have a great impact on the emergent literacy skills of the children in their classrooms. They promote language development and literacy skills by providing an appropriate learning environment; engaging in language play; conducting read-alouds with emphasis on the sounds in words; developing concepts of print and alphabetic and letter–sound knowledge; providing scaffolded teaching of writing; and using formal and informal assessment. (See Chapter 4 for more about building emergent literacy skills.)

Alphabet knowledge—It is essential that children learn the alphabet and be able to say the names of the letters, recognize letter shapes, and write the letters. They need to know the difference between upper- and lowercase letters. These skills are powerful predictors of reading success. (See Chapter 5 for more about alphabet knowledge.)

Phonemic awareness—Reading development depends on acquiring phonemic awareness and other phonological processes. Phonemic awareness is the ability to understand the sound structure in spoken words. To learn to read, however, children also must be able to pay attention to the sequence of sounds or phonemes in words and to manipulate these sounds. Children learn to do this by engaging in intensive oral play activities of sufficient duration, such as identifying and making rhymes, counting and working with syllables in words, segmenting initial and final phonemes, hearing and blending sounds, analyzing initial and final sounds of words, and segmenting words fully before learning to read and during beginning reading. This training facilitates and predicts later reading and spelling achievement. (See Chapter 6 for more about teaching phonemic awareness.)

Phonics—Along with instruction on letter names, children need well-designed and focused phonics instruction to learn predictable letter-sound correspondences. Fast and accurate decoding of familiar and unfamiliar words and spelling rest on the alphabetic principle: how the written spellings of words systematically represent the phonemes in the spoken words. The efficacy of the code-emphasis approach is supported by decades of research. It requires explicit, systematic, and sequential instruction for at least 25% of students, without which they are likely to fail. (See Chapter 9 for more about decoding and reading instruction.)

Fluency—Fluency and comprehension depend on the accuracy and speed of word recognition; a reader who can read words quickly and accurately without laboring to decode them has developed automaticity. Word accuracy and automaticity are problem areas for most students with reading/learning disabilities. Slow decoders are poor at comprehension due to reduced attentional and memory resources. Adequate oral reading fluency rates with connected texts leads to better comprehension. There are reading fluency goals for first through eighth grade supported by research (Hasbrouck & Tindal, 2006). Overall, fluency needs to be addressed in each of the component sub-skills of reading instruction. (See Chapter 12 for more about developing fluency.)

Morphology—Explicit teaching of morphology and etymology can begin as early as kindergarten and first grade as an important part of literacy instruction. It has been proven to have a significant role in learning word meanings and improving spelling. Exposure to Greek and Latin roots, Anglo-Saxon compounds, and prefixes and suffixes helps students read and spell an unlimited number of words.

Vocabulary development—Vocabulary facilitates phonological awareness and word recognition in students and is important for reading comprehension. The predictive value for vocabulary in later reading comprehension and the relationship between kindergarten and first-grade word knowledge and elementary, middle, and secondary reading performance have been documented. Vocabulary growth benefits from repeated exposure to word meanings and use in context and from studying morphology with direct, explicit instruction across the curriculum. Vocabulary should be taught both directly and indirectly. Wide reading mitigates against reduced exposure to rich vocabulary, which is often the experience of struggling readers. (See Chapter 15 for more about word learning and vocabulary instruction.)

(continued)

TEXTBOX 1.1 *(continued)*

Comprehension—Comprehension depends on accurate, fluent decoding skills and efficient, active comprehension strategies, including monitoring for understanding while reading. Comprehension also depends on activating relevant background knowledge and is related strongly to oral language comprehension and vocabulary growth. Along with providing explicit vocabulary instruction and instruction in how to understand sentence structure, teachers should **model** and use direct teaching of **metacognitive strategies** such as questioning, predicting, making inferences, clarifying misunderstandings, and summarizing. The Common Core State Standards presented other critical factors needed for proficient reading and academic success, such as close reading, a deep examination of a text; text-dependent questions that involve analysis, evaluation, and synthesis by looking carefully and critically at text; and finding evidence in the text to answer text-dependent questions. Written expression reinforces students' comprehension skills. (See Chapter 16 for more about specific strategies for teaching reading comprehension.)

Spelling—English orthography is 87% reliable. When children are familiar with the spelling regularities of English, their reading and spelling are strengthened. Opportunities to apply the predictable and logical rules and spelling patterns that match the reading patterns being learned give children a double immersion in the information. Spelling is an essential and interconnected complement to reading instruction because it enhances reading proficiency by reinforcing sounds and letter patterns (Adams, 1990). Explicit instruction in the sounds of the language and exposure to consistent and frequent letter patterns and spelling rules lead to successful spelling outcomes.

Handwriting—Manuscript and cursive handwriting is a vital component of multisensory instruction of literacy skills and a component skill for developing a functional writing system (Berninger & Wolf, 2009). Formal, multisensory handwriting instruction reinforces students' knowledge of letter shapes and letter formation while connecting them to letter names and sounds in beginning reading. Later, both legibility and fluency aid students in the quality of their compositions, improve spelling, and help in proofreading and notetaking. Motor skills in handwriting can be improved with practice. Including accurate keyboarding is an appropriate use of technology with students. (See Chapter 11 for more about teaching handwriting.)

Written expression—Three areas need to be addressed in written expression: the purpose and structure of sentences, including grammar, word choice, and **sentence expansion**; step-by-step building of paragraphs and compositions with the emphasis on developing ideas for expository text; and revising and editing compositions. Direct, explicit instruction is needed in grammar, punctuation, and capitalization, using multisensory methods differentiated for students' unique abilities and weaknesses. Teaching writing should contain oral language practice activities preliminary to paper-and-pencil tasks. Working on complex ideas for sentence generation has a positive effect on reading comprehension. (See Chapter 17 for more about evidence-based instruction in composition.)

*Executive function in literacy instruction—*There are tools that teachers and parents can use to support learners across all learning contexts to increase the development of language, literacy, and academic skills. By using all learning modalities and joining together visual, auditory, kinesthetic, print-oriented, and interactive activities, students with executive function challenges can build cognitive flexibility. Explicit instruction in academic skills can sharpen their self-regulation and build inhibitory control and working memory. (See Chapter 8 for more about the role of executive function in literacy instruction.)

*Well-prepared teachers able to implement research-based instruction—*Well-prepared, knowledgeable, and accomplished teachers who can screen students for potential problems, analyze their work, monitor progress, set goals and plan efficiently, provide opportunities for constructive feedback, and review and practice while continuing to learn about effective practices are the mainstay of children's success in learning to read and write.

From *Multisensory Teaching of Basic Language Skills, Third Edition* (pp. 9–10).

UNDERSTANDING DYSLEXIA THROUGH READING RESEARCH

Understanding dyslexia is one way to have a sophisticated understanding of the reading process. Following is the definition of *dyslexia* adopted in 2003 by the IDA in collaboration with the NICHD.

> Dyslexia is a specific learning disability that is neurobiological in origin. It is characterized by difficulties with accurate and/or fluent word recognition and by poor spelling and decoding abilities. These difficulties typically result from a deficit in the phonological component of language that is often unexpected in relation to other cognitive abilities and the provision of effective classroom instruction. Secondary consequences may include problems in reading comprehension and reduced reading experience that can impede growth of vocabulary and background knowledge. (Lyon, Shaywitz, & Shaywitz, 2003, p. 2)

Dyslexia is a **specific learning disability** because it is associated with specific cognitive deficits in basic reading skills (Lyon et al., 2003). It affects 80% of those identified with learning disabilities and is one of the most common learning problems in children and adults (Lerner, 1989). Dyslexia is estimated to occur in approximately 5%–17% of the population in the United States (Shaywitz, 1998). Only about one third of fourth- and eighth-grade students score at or above proficient levels of reading on the NAEP assessment (National Center for Education Statistics, 2017). Among these children not showing even partial mastery of grade-level skills in reading, there is a disproportionate representation of students who are from low-SES households and racial minorities and students whose home language is a language other than English. Large numbers of children from every social class, race, and ethnic group, however, have significant difficulties with reading. Children most at risk for reading failure have limited exposure to the English language; have little understanding of phonemic awareness, letter knowledge, **print awareness,** and the purposes of reading; and lack oral language and vocabulary skills. Children from very low-SES households, children with speech and hearing impairments, and children whose parents' or caregivers' reading levels are low are also at risk for reading failure.

As Lyon noted, "Children with **reading disability** differ from one another *and* from other readers along a continuum" (1996, p. 64), with reading disability representing the lower tail of a normal distribution of reading ability (Shaywitz, 2003). An individual with dyslexia typically will have some but not all of the problems that are described next because of individual differences and access to early remediation. The clinical diagnosis of dyslexia with its long-term outcomes is a language-based **learning disability** and is the most widespread form of learning disability. Some common signs of dyslexia are 1) difficulty learning to speak; 2) problems organizing written and spoken language; 3) difficulty learning the letter names and their sounds; 4) inaccurate decoding; 5) slow, laborious reading lacking fluency due to using compensatory systems; 6) conspicuous problems with spelling and writing; 7) difficulty learning a foreign language; 8) having a hard time memorizing number facts; and 9) difficulty with math operations. Dyslexia varies in severity, and the prognosis depends on the severity of the disability, each individual's strengths and weaknesses, and the appropriateness and intensity of intervention. Dyslexia is not caused by a lack of motivation to learn to read, sensory impairment, inadequate instruction, a lack of environmental opportunities, or low intelligence.

Reading involves many regions throughout the brain. The present working definition, based on empirical support, emphasizes that dyslexia is neurobiological in origin because of the involvement of the neural systems in the brain that process the sounds of language and are critical to reading (see Figure 1.1). Dyslexia is manifested by a disruption in these language systems, which leads to **phonological** weaknesses. According to Shaywitz, the phonological weakness occurs "at the lowest level of the language system" (2003, p. 41) and, in turn, impairs decoding. In fact, there are two neural systems for reading: one for word analysis in the parieto-temporal region and the other for automatic, rapid responses localized in the occipito-temporal area that is used by skilled readers for rapid word recognition. Low **phonological processing** skills are the result of left hemisphere posterior processing anomalies typical of children with dyslexia. See Chapter 2 for a more detailed analysis of the reading brain and the neural correlates of typical reading and reading disability using current imagery techniques.

Individuals with dyslexia have difficulty gaining access to and manipulating the sound structure (phonemes) of spoken language. Such a deficit prevents easy and early access to **letter–sound correspondences** and decoding strategies that foster accurate and fluent word decoding and recognition. A vast majority of individuals with dyslexia have a phonological core deficit (Morris et al., 1998; Ramus et al., 2003). Phonological abilities include awareness of the sounds of words in

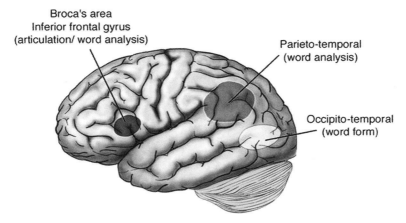

Figure 1.1. The brain system has three important neural pathways: 1) an interior system in the left inferior frontal region (Broca's area) for articulation and slower word analysis; 2) a parieto-temporal region for step-by-step analytic word reading; and 3) an occipital-temporal word-form area for skilled, rapid reading. (From Shaywitz, S. [2003]. *Overcoming dyslexia: A new and complete science-based program for reading problems at any level.* New York, NY: Alfred A. Knopf, p. 78. Copyright © 2003 by Sally E. Shaywitz, M.D. Used by permission of Sally E. Shaywitz, M.D.)

sentences, awareness of **syllables** in words, and awareness of phonemes in words or syllables (see Chapter 6).

Approximately 17%–20% of school-age children are affected to some degree by impairments in phonemic awareness (Lyon, 1999). The result is that individuals with dyslexia have difficulty recognizing both real and **pseudowords** (i.e., nonsense words), which leads to overreliance on context and guessing and prevents building words in memory instead of using the alphabetic principle to **decode** words. Readers with dyslexia may also have difficulties with processes underlying the rapid, precise retrieval of visually presented linguistic information. Measures of letter, digit, and color naming are predictors of later reading fluency (Wolf, Bowers, & Biddle, 2000).

Difficulties with accurate and/or fluent word recognition mean that poor readers lack the ability to read quickly, accurately, and with good understanding (Partnership for Reading, 2003). They fail to grasp the meaning of the text, avoid reading, and fail to develop the necessary vocabulary and **background knowledge** for comprehension.

Poor spelling is a hallmark of dyslexia because of its intimate connection to reading. Educators can identify students with phoneme and word-recognition weaknesses early by administering screening tools for phonemic awareness and other pre-reading skills validated by research and promptly applying appropriate intervention in kindergarten and first grade before failure sets in, thus preventing a pattern of compromised text-reading fluency, deficient vocabulary acquisition, and difficulty with reading comprehension (Eden & Moats, 2002).

Another aspect of the biological origin of dyslexia is that it runs in families. A child with dyslexia will commonly have parents and siblings who also have dyslexia. If a parent has dyslexia, between one quarter and one half of his or her children will likely have dyslexia too (Shaywitz, 2003). According to Olson (2004), genetic influences on reading disability are just as important as shared environmental ones. Both are partly dependent on the quality of instruction available

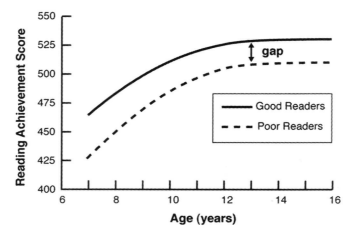

Figure 1.2. Trajectory of reading skills over time in readers with and without dyslexia. The *y* axis indicates Rasch scores (*W* scores) from the Reading subtest of the *Woodcock-Johnson–Revised Tests of Achievement* (Woodcock & Johnson, 1989). Both readers with and without dyslexia improved their reading scores as they get older, but the gap between the two groups remains. Thus, dyslexia is a deficit and not a developmental lag. (Adapted from *Frames of Reference for the Assessment of Learning Disabilities: New View of Measurement Issues* [p. 40] Edited by G. Reid Lyon, Ph.D., © 1994 by Paul H. Brookes Publishing Co., Inc.)

because improper instruction and lack of reading might affect brain processes. A number of genes play a part in individual differences in phonemic awareness, word reading, and related skills. Deficits in phonemic awareness and reading of pseudowords are heritable. Evidence from research on identical and fraternal twins, funded by NICHD and conducted at the Colorado Learning Disabilities Research Center (Olson, 2004), has shown that these genetic constraints can be remediated so that children read normally after engaging in intensive practice with an early emphasis on phonological skills and more time in later grades spent reading for accuracy and fluency to promote continued growth. Olson (2004) suggested that there may be a genetic influence on learning rates for reading and related skills. Children with a family history of dyslexia should be monitored for early signs of oral language problems and attention given to pre-reading language play at home and the opportunity for effective beginning reading instruction at school.

Beginning with data from the Connecticut Longitudinal Study (Shaywitz, 2003), funded by the NICHD, ongoing research has underscored that early identification along with intensive, scientifically based instruction can bring poor readers up to grade level. Unless these readers receive intensive help early on, the gap between good and poor readers stays the same, although both groups progress over time. Children facing reading difficulties at the beginning of school remain poor readers, as depicted in Figure 1.2. As noted by Lyon, a reading disability "reflects a persistent deficit rather than a developmental lag" and "longitudinal studies show that of those children who have a [reading disability] in the third grade, approximately 74% continue to read significantly below grade level in the ninth grade" (1996, p. 64). They are unlikely to catch up without informed teaching. Compounding that dire circumstance is the fact that students who receive help often receive it for a short period of time, inconsistently, and from untrained teachers using methods that lack a scientific base (Shaywitz, 2003).

Dyslexia is recognized in the definition as difficulty in learning to read that is unexpected in relation to other cognitive abilities and the provision of effective classroom instruction. The **Individuals with Disabilities Education Improvement Act (IDEA) of 2004 (PL 108-446)** neither requires nor prohibits discrepancy between IQ score and achievement to determine a specific learning disability such as dyslexia (i.e., use of the **discrepancy model**). In identifying dyslexia, an alternative is the need to compare reading age with chronological age or, in the case of adults, career attainment level. New to the definition is the idea that effective classroom instruction to meet the range of needs children bring to school may be factored in to recognize dyslexia and to tease out reading failure from inadequate instruction, poor preschool preparation, and lack of response to quality instruction. In addition, there are secondary consequences such as weaknesses in vocabulary development and reading comprehension due to less developed accuracy and fluency and a smaller store of background knowledge to support comprehension. Much of this is due to reduced reading experience.

Deficits in attention, problems in short-term verbal memory, and difficulty with word retrieval and mathematics have also been identified in students with dyslexia. These deficits can affect listening and reading comprehension. (For more information about these effects, see Chapter 8 on the role of executive function in literacy and Chapter 16 on strategies to improve reading comprehension.) Students with dyslexia who spell poorly often have difficulty with the motor aspects of writing. Poor pencil grip and messy handwriting persist (Berninger & Wolf, 2009). (See Chapter 11 for more about teaching handwriting.) Expression of ideas clearly in both written and oral form is slow to develop. According to Ramus and colleagues (2003), it is not clear why sensory and motor disorders are often associated with phonological deficits.

Parents and teachers, therefore, should be aware of the manifestations of dyslexia in early childhood, such as difficulty learning to talk and incorrectly pronouncing words. Following directions, retrieving names of things such as letters of the alphabet, **sequencing,** and/or forming letters or numbers also can be areas of poor functioning. Characteristics that may accompany dyslexia include time management and organization problems, lack of social awareness, difficulty with attention (e.g., **attention-deficit/hyperactivity disorder [ADHD]**), poor spatial sense, and difficulty with motor skills.

Many individuals with dyslexia may also have attention disorders. Reading disabilities and attention disorders, however, are distinct. Although they are separate from learning disabilities, attention disorders and organization difficulties frequently co-occur with language-based reading disability. The severity of a reading disability may be compounded by attention disorders (Lyon, 1996). The IDA's web site (http://www.eida.org) is a good resource that explains these symptoms and offers timely and research-based information. See Chapter 8 for hallmarks of how attention disorders affect language skills and Chapter 7 for discussion of the need for a good reading assessment that can determine the existence of an attention disorder affecting progress in school.

Perhaps what puzzles teachers and parents the most is that students who fail to learn how letters represent speech sounds and how sounds are represented by the letters in words often are good thinkers and are talented in other areas. Because dyslexia is domain specific, other cognitive abilities such as reasoning, comprehension, vocabulary, **syntax,** and general IQ score typically are unaffected (Shaywitz & Shaywitz, 2004). In fact, although IQ score and reading in the typical reader influence each other over time, IQ score and reading are not linked in the reader who has dyslexia (Ferrer, Shaywitz, Holahan, Marchione, & Shaywitz, 2010). People with dyslexia may excel in the arts, law, politics, architecture, science, medicine, business, and sports, for example.

REFLECT, CONNECT, and RESPOND
How important is it for students to understand the internal structure of words for their overall reading achievement?

Data from the representative sample of children tested in the Connecticut Longitudinal Study (Shaywitz, Shaywitz, Fletcher, & Escobar, 1990) showed that although boys are identified as having dyslexia four times more often than girls, there are as many girls as boys with dyslexia. Boys are more often referred for special services due to behavior that signals problems, whereas girls in need of help are less likely to be identified (Shaywitz, 2003). There are accurate and reliable screening and identification procedures available that are linked to prevention programs. Early identification and intervention are essential to successful treatment of children who are at risk for reading failure.

There has been a shift in the approach of identifying a specific reading disability. According to Lyon, "Definitions that measure the discrepancy between IQ and achievement do not adequately identify learning disabilities, particularly in the area of beginning reading skills" (1996, p. 64).

There is growing evidence in support of an alternative approach. Fletcher, Coulter, Reschly, and Vaughn stated, "Our most pressing challenge is conveying urgency about preventing disabilities through early screening and effective instruction, and for those who do not respond sufficiently, providing effective special education interventions that change achievement and social/behavioral outcomes" (2004, p. 312). The claim that using RTI as identification criteria can lead to targeting intervention first and assessment second, using formal progress monitoring with data on student response for accountability and planning, and building bridges between general and **special education** (Fletcher et al., 2004) has no evidence yet to support it. However, there are signs that RTI is beginning to be put to the tasks it was designed to carry out, especially in early identification of children at risk (Gillis, 2017).

As mentioned previously, dyslexia persists across the life span and is not a developmental lag. This is most clearly seen in the manifestations of dyslexia among adults (Brozgold, 2002). As in children, it exists across a continuum, with varying indications depending on the individual. Adults with dyslexia show decreased reading efficiency (i.e., slower reading rate and lower accuracy) relative to individuals without dyslexia, despite good intelligence, education, and career achievement. Their **phonetic** decoding is impaired relative to their reading comprehension, which may be better because they rely on context cues and know about the subject that they are reading. When tested, their decoding of pseudowords is impaired. Other language-based difficulties can be observed, such as mispronouncing words and names and word-retrieval difficulty. Written composition is problematic because writing calls on integrating so many language skills. Spelling is likely to be persistently weak. Unless the text is of particular interest, the individual may have ongoing difficulty retaining information that he or she reads. A diagnosis of dyslexia in adults can have significant therapeutic and practical value because it confirms and validates the individual's strengths and weaknesses and leads to interventions and **accommodations,** a plethora of electronic devices to help mitigate these difficulties, and, especially, extended time on tests, which can improve academic skills, vocational functioning, and self-esteem (Brozgold, 2002).

TEACHERS CAN DELIVER EVIDENCE-BASED READING INSTRUCTION TO ALL STUDENTS

Consensus on effective teacher preparation has been widely accepted by scholarly panels, scientific investigators, and noted professional organizations, as indicated previously. What is paramount is being able to teach the elements of language structure well, using research-based instructional practices, to diverse groups of students in need of such instruction.

Effective Instruction Improves Reading and Changes the Brain

Although dyslexia affects individuals over the life span and cannot be cured, reading skills can be increased with the right early intervention and prevention programs. Researchers have drawn attention to the interactions between the neurobiological and environmental factors in students with reading disabilities using **functional magnetic resonance imaging (fMRI).** When children with reading disabilities were given intensive, systematic code-based reading interventions, they demonstrated increased activation in the left occipito-temporal brain region and also made significant gains in reading fluency and comprehension 1 year after the intervention had ended. Shaywitz and colleagues (2004) reported that this outcome provides evidence of the neuroplasticity of the systems for reading and demonstrates that a scientifically based reading intervention brings about significant and durable changes in brain organization so that the brain facilitates the development of those fast-paced neural systems that underlie skilled reading.

Using a scientifically based reading intervention with children who were poor readers who participated in a fMRI study, Shaywitz and colleagues found that the intensive, phonologically based intervention made "significant and durable changes in brain organization so that brain activation patterns resemble those of typical readers" of the neural system for reading (2004, p. 931). The children's reading fluency improved. NICHD-supported research also has found that older individuals with dyslexia can improve with intervention that focuses on remediation of reading and writing skills and other areas of weakness. Sometimes, it is a matter of learning how to learn (see Chapter 21). As children get older, however, Lyon found that "the intensity and duration of reading interventions must increase exponentially" (1999) to achieve the same improvement possible with younger children. In fact, Torgesen and colleagues found that adolescent students will attain grade-level standards only with "instruction sufficiently powerful to accelerate reading development dramatically so that students make more than one year's progress during one year of school" (2007, p. 5).

Effective programs must involve intensive instruction using a systematic, structured language approach. It is crucial that the programs be consistent and of sufficient duration for individuals to make progress in improving reading and related skills (Shaywitz, 2003). (See Chapter 20 for information about instructing older students with word-level reading disabilities.) Although not a substitute for remediation, **modifications** and accommodations, along with robust use of technology to support learning, can pave the way for many poor readers to gain information, expand their world knowledge, and be successful at school or work. They can improve their decoding and comprehension skills at any age but often remain slow readers. Accommodations that build on the strengths of older students and adults with dyslexia can help them to lead successful lives.

Content and Delivery of Reading Instruction Is Critical

It is clear from the consensus of scientifically based reading research that the nature of the educational intervention for individuals with reading disabilities and dyslexia is critical. Characterizing reading and writing as language is central to every aspect of intervention for individuals with language-based learning disabilities. Knowledge of language development and disabilities is essential for those who administer assessments and interpret them, deliver instruction, and design and carry out programs at all levels (Dickman, Hennessy, Moats, Rooney, & Tomey, 2002).

Relationship Between Teacher Preparation and Student Achievement   As teachers learn about underlying concepts and instructional strategies in the components of reading, accompanied by comprehensive instruction and practice, they begin to incorporate these ideas into their everyday work, and student achievement improves (Moats & Foorman, 2003). Evidence shows that student achievement and teacher preparation and domain-specific knowledge are correlated (Darling-Hammond, 2000; Moats & Foorman, 2003; NICHD, 2000).

There is also mounting evidence that teachers are being underprepared in schools of education because these schools are not designating the science of reading, five basic components of reading, and, most important, knowledge of language structure as essential information (Spear-Swerling, Brucker, & Alfano, 2005; Walsh, Glaser, & Wilcox, 2006). Spear-Swerling and colleagues (2005) pointed out that the most experienced and well-trained teachers do not promote student growth unless they use this knowledge and translate it into classroom practice. In a survey, teacher educators were asked how important it was for public school teachers to "teach phonics and phonemic awareness when teaching literacy in the early grades" (Farkas & Duffett, 2010). Only 44% thought it was "absolutely essential" (Farkas & Duffett, 2010).

Too often, content knowledge and depth of training are lacking in the most basic areas of preparation for reading instruction. For example, Cheesman and colleagues (2009) found that the beginning certified teachers they surveyed lacked the ability to differentiate between phonemic awareness and phonics and the ability to segment written words by phonemes. Other studies have found that teachers cannot count speech sounds in words. This raises questions about the quality of preservice teacher education and the availability of quality professional development and mentoring for beginning certified teachers.

A study by Piasta, Connor, Fishman, and Morrison (2009) showed that in addition to teacher knowledge about language and literacy concepts, including elements of explicit decoding instruction, the actual classroom practices that accompanied this specialized knowledge were vital to produce student gains in first-grade word-reading growth. This synergy of both expert teaching practice and the knowledge to call on when responding to student errors is important (Moats, 1999). Through better pre-service and professional development and mentoring, teachers can be sufficiently prepared to deliver effective reading instruction that teaches listening, speaking, reading, and writing using explicit, systematic, cumulative, and multisensory methods based on scientific research to students at risk and students with dyslexia.

Because of well-documented insufficient preparation of classroom teachers and specialists in teaching students who are struggling with reading, the IDA saw the need to adopt and promote standards for "1) content knowledge necessary to teach reading and writing to students with dyslexia or related disorders who are at risk for reading difficulty; 2) practices of effective instruction; and 3) ethical conduct expected of professional educators and clinicians" (2010, p. 3). The IDA *Knowledge and Practice Standards* call for teacher educators to base their courses on the following standards:

- Foundation concepts about oral and written language learning
- Knowledge of dyslexia and other learning disorders
- Interpretation and administration of assessments for planning instruction
- Structured language teaching

   Phonology

   Phonics and word study

   Fluent, automatic reading of text

   Vocabulary

   Text comprehension

   Handwriting, spelling, and written expression

   Ethical standards for the profession

These standards are also appropriate for classroom teachers, who are responsible for recognizing and preventing reading difficulties. The knowledge and practice criteria outlined in detail in this book are aligned with these standards to assist teachers and their instructors in the complex endeavor to become the experts their students deserve. (See also the IDA *Knowledge and Practice Standards for Teachers of Reading, Second Edition* [IDA, 2018].)

> **REFLECT, CONNECT, and RESPOND**
> Will changes in teacher preparation and licensure make a difference in how students are taught to read? Explain your answer.

Elements of Effective Instruction   The importance of critical reading and thinking, highlighted in the CCSS, is predicated on a solid foundation of basic reading skills. Contrary to the belief that comprehension is hard and takes intensive instruction whereas basic reading skills are easily and naturally acquired, Seidenberg (2017) pointed out that science supports the opposite. Writing systems represent only an abstract and partial connection to spoken language; therefore, "[b]asic skills are difficult to acquire" and need exemplary instruction (p. 272). To minimize reading failure, classroom reading approaches must include systematic, explicit instruction in phonemic awareness (orally identifying and manipulating syllables and speech sounds); particular attention to letter–sound knowledge (phonics); spelling integrated with reading; fluency (developing speed and **automaticity** in accurate letter, word, and text reading); vocabulary building; and text comprehension strategies. If such classroom programs prove to be insufficient for students with dyslexia, then these students will need a **Multisensory Structured Literacy (MSL)** program, which incorporates systematic, cumulative, explicit, and sequential approaches taught by teachers trained in language structure at the levels of sounds, syllables, meaningful parts of words, sentence structure, and paragraph and discourse organization (Eden & Moats, 2002). (See Chapter 2 for an introduction to Multisensory Structured Literacy.)

Some commercial programs that fit this description are Alphabetic Phonics, Slingerland, Project Read, LANGUAGE!, the Sonday System, Orton-Gillingham, Wilson Language, the Spalding Method, Lindamood-Bell, Take Flight, Preventing Academic Failure, and Read Write Type. (See the Online Companion Materials for this chapter for more information about MSL programs.) Instruction in these programs is multisensory and engages the learner in visual, auditory, and **kinesthetic** responses and feedback with deliberate and intensive practice in reading and spelling, controlled for what has been taught. Teachers use structured lesson planning and ongoing monitoring of progress to organize instruction and chart the growth in skills. One added benefit to this type of instruction is that it helps students with executive function difficulties deal with them in the classroom while learning the basic skills of reading.

Figure 1.3 shows the content (the structure of the English language) allied with the principles of instruction inherent in all MSL programs. All are in agreement

Content: Structure of the English language	Principles of instruction				
	Simultaneous multisensory VAKT (visual, auditory, kinesthetic, tactile)	Systematic and cumulative	Direct instruction	Diagnostic teaching to automaticity	Synthetic/ analytic instruction
Phonology and phonological awareness	√	√	√	√	√
Sound–symbol association: visual to auditory, auditory to visual, blending, segmenting	√	√	√	√	√
Syllables: types and patterns for division	√	√	√	√	√
Morphology: base words, roots, affixes	√	√	√	√	√
Syntax: grammar, sentence variation, mechanics of language	√	√	√	√	√
Semantics: meaning	√	√	√	√	√

Figure 1.3. Multisensory structured language programs: Content and principles of instruction. (*Key:* VAKT, visual, auditory, kinesthetic, tactile.) (Adapted from *IMSLEC Directory: MSL Training Courses and Graduates* [2010]. Dallas, TX: The International Multisensory Structured Language Education Council, p. 11. Adapted by permission.)

with the IDA (2018) *Knowledge and Practice Standards*. These standards are the metric that will measure effective preparation programs and will lead to certification. After examining what teachers are minimally exposed to in their preparation for their profession, Seidenberg (2017) called for licensure that reflects expertise using similar science-based knowledge and practice standards to those of the IDA. Textbox 1.2 provides a more detailed explanation of the terms used in Figure 1.3.

Personalized Instruction Is Important

The role of technology in MSL instruction is important. Technology will not replace the teacher but will provide the specific practice and additional instructional support that individual students need. It will provide useful data about the type of personalized instruction students require. Personalized learning tells teachers what to teach and indicates the intensity (or acceleration) of instruction. The idea of acceleration is important for older students and for students who are slightly below grade level versus students who are well below grade level.

Intensity of Instruction Matters

From 25 years of prevention and intervention research targeting the five major components of reading, Torgesen (2004) concluded that explicitness and intensity of instruction are the key ingredients in teaching this knowledge and these skills to students who are struggling greatly with reading. He clarified that "explicit instruction is instruction that does not leave anything to chance and does not make assumptions about skills and knowledge that children will acquire on their own" (2004, p. 363).

   In contrast to leaving things to chance or assuming that students are absorbing the necessary concepts to decode new words or comprehend text, explicit instruction calls on teachers to 1) make clear connections between letters and sounds and their consistent, systematic relationships; 2) teach individual word meanings and word-learning strategies; 3) provide modeling for fluent reading and have students engage in repeated oral reading; and 4) learn how to use explicit, carefully sequenced instruction in comprehension strategies. Research has shown that more favorable outcomes are associated with systematic phonics instruction than with an approach emphasizing implicit phonics (Lyon, 1996; NICHD, 2000).

   Furthermore, Torgesen (2004) reinforced the importance of **explicit instruction** for remediation and intervention by including the need for intensity, which is wholly different from general education classroom experiences. Through small-group instruction of one-to-one and one-to-three, with intensity guided by students' rate of progress, students with reading problems have a better chance of closing the grade gap with their peers in reading accuracy and reading comprehension than in large-group configurations (Vaughn & Linan-Thompson, 2003). To make gains, students need to engage in highly structured, sequential activities and be closely monitored in ways that are not possible in the general education classroom. They need to form direct connections between the known and the new, and they need time for explicit practice to build automaticity and fluency. In addition, the curriculum needs a sequential order for instruction and practice.

   Teachers in the general education classroom can also apply these practices with students struggling with reading by incorporating these teaching approaches and rethinking their grouping of students. The instructional practices and curriculum

TEXTBOX 1.2   **Definition of terms**

Content of Structured Language Teaching

Phonology and phonological awareness—Phonology is the study of sounds and how they work within their environment. A phoneme is the smallest unit of sound in a given language that can be recognized as being distinct from other sounds. Phonological awareness is understanding the internal linguistic structure of words. An important aspect of phonological awareness is the ability to segment words into their component phonemes [phonemic awareness].

Sound-symbol association—This is knowing the various sounds in the English language and their correspondence to the letters and combinations of letters that represent those sounds. Sound-symbol association must be taught (and mastered) in two directions: visual to auditory and auditory to visual. In addition, students must master blending sounds and letters into words as well as segmenting whole words into the individual sounds.

Syllable instruction—A syllable is a unit of oral or written language with one vowel sound. Instruction must include teaching the six basic types of syllables in the English language: closed, open, vowel-consonant-*e*, *r*-controlled, vowel pair [or vowel team], and final stable syllable. Syllable division rules must be directly taught in relation to the word structure.

Morphology—Morphology is the study of how morphemes are combined to form words. A morpheme is the smallest unit of meaning in the language. The curriculum must include the study of base words, roots, and affixes.

Syntax—Syntax is the set of principles that dictate the sequence and function of words in a sentence in order to convey meaning. This includes grammar, sentence variation, and the mechanics of language.

Semantics—Semantics is that aspect of language concerned with meaning. The curriculum (from the beginning) must include instruction in comprehending written language.

Principles of Instruction

Simultaneous, multisensory (VAKT)—Teaching is done using all learning pathways in the brain (visual, auditory, kinesthetic, tactile) simultaneously in order to enhance memory and learning.

Systematic and cumulative—Multisensory language instruction requires that the organization of material follow the logical order of the language. The sequence must begin with the easiest and most basic elements and progress methodically to more difficult material. Each step must also be based on those [elements] already learned. Concepts taught must be systematically reviewed to strengthen memory.

Direct instruction—The inferential learning of any concept cannot be taken for granted. Multisensory language instruction requires the direct teaching of all concepts with [continual] student-teacher interaction.

Diagnostic teaching to automaticity—The teacher must be adept at prescriptive or individualized teaching. The teaching plan is based on careful and [continual] assessment of the individual's needs. The content presented must be mastered to the degree of automaticity.

Synthetic and analytic instruction—Multisensory structured language programs include both synthetic and analytic instruction. Synthetic instruction presents the parts of the language and then teaches how the parts work together to form a whole. Analytic instruction presents the whole and teaches how this can be broken down into its component parts.

From McIntyre, C.W., & Pickering, J.S. (1995). Clinical studies of multisensory structured language education for students with dyslexia and related disorders (p. xii). Salem, OR: International Multisensory Structured Language Education Council.

content described in this book fit this model of intervention and remediation. It is encouraging that research evidence has arrived at a consensus on the critical element of instruction and how it should be delivered.

Reading disability has far-reaching consequences, which is why teachers must be prepared to intervene early and intensively until the reader is on target for success. Pre- and in-service teachers must be prepared to work directly with children with reading, writing, and spelling disabilities who also may have co-occurring difficulties, such as difficulties with arithmetic calculation. Without question, general and special education teachers need the tools to identify students with language-based learning disabilities, to intervene with explicit instructional procedures, and to continue to sustain their students with intensive support for as long as they need it.

REFLECT, CONNECT, and RESPOND
Based on what you have read in this chapter, which is the best way for students to attack an unknown word?

CLOSING THOUGHTS: THE IMPACT OF RESEARCH ON PRACTICE

There have been more than 45,000 participants in the NICHD-funded research programs in reading development, reading disorders, and reading instruction. Both children and adults have participated, including more than 22,500 good readers at the 50th percentile and above and about 22,500 struggling readers below the 25th percentile (Lyon, 2004). Researchers have learned from these studies and others how children read, why some children have difficulties, how to prevent difficulties from becoming ingrained, and how to provide intervention when readers continue to struggle.

Reading emerges from substantial and significant oral language experiences from birth onward. (See Chapter 3 for more on oral language development.) The importance of providing oral language and literacy experiences from birth onward, including reading to children, playing with language through rhyming and games, and encouraging writing activities, is well documented. These activities encourage vocabulary development and enhance verbal reasoning and semantic and syntactic abilities. The importance of early assessment and intervention for reading problems is supported by the fact that reading problems identified in Grade 3 and beyond require considerable intervention; children do not simply outgrow reading problems. In fact, 74% of children identified as having a reading disability in Grade 3 still had a reading disability in Grade 9 (Francis, Shaywitz, Stuebing, Shaywitz, & Fletcher, 1996).

The risk factors for dyslexia can be seen in kindergarten and first grade—trouble with letter–sound knowledge, **phonological awareness,** and oral language development. The earliest clue to dyslexia is what Shaywitz described as "a weakness in getting to the sounds of words" (2003, p. 93). Lyon noted that "the best predictor of reading ability from kindergarten and first-grade performance is phoneme **segmentation** ability" (1996, p. 64). It is best to assess all children and intervene first in the classroom, with explicit instruction in phonemic awareness, phonics, and comprehension with an emphasis on fluency in all these competencies.

The instruction should be guided by a carefully constructed, sequenced curriculum that is designed to be explicit about language structure and leaves nothing to chance. The texts chosen for practice need to be controlled and later **decodable texts** so that children are taught to mastery. Developing phonemic awareness is necessary but not the sole component of learning to read. From the beginning, reading instruction must include attention to phonics principles for accurate and rapid decoding and active use of comprehension strategies.

According to Lyon, "the ability to read and comprehend is dependent on rapid and automatic recognition and decoding of single words. Slow and inaccurate decoding are the best predictors of deficits in reading comprehension" (1996, p. 64). Additional factors impeding reading comprehension include vocabulary deficits, lack of background knowledge for understanding text information, deficient understanding of semantic and syntactic structures, insufficient knowledge of writing conventions for different purposes, lack of verbal reasoning, and inability to remember and/or retrieve verbal information. There are now proven strategies to maximize reading comprehension and develop background knowledge and vocabulary through reciprocal teaching and monitoring feedback.

Educators can make changes by intervening early with instruction that changes the way the brain learns. For example, neurobiological investigations show that there are differences in the parietal-temporal and occipital-temporal brain regions among individuals with dyslexia, compared to individuals without dyslexia. Although these differences affect the ability to read, neural systems for reading are malleable and highly responsive to effective reading instruction. In their research using fMRI to study the effects of a systematic phonics-based intervention with 6- to 9-year-old children, Shaywitz and colleagues (2004) found evidence of plasticity of neural systems for reading. The changes in the brain made these readers comparable with good readers. The children were still making gains in reading fluency and comprehension 1 year later after the intervention ended.

Shaywitz and colleagues concluded that providing "evidence-based reading intervention at an early age improves reading fluency and facilitates the development of those neural systems that underlie skilled reading. Teaching matters and can change the brain" (2004, p. 931). Many states are using research to guide their policy in reading education. With high-level pre-service preparation and professional development efforts that pay strict attention to this evidence, the impact of science should bring about changes at the school level. This book is dedicated to that goal and to teachers in the classroom.

There is still serious underpreparation among teachers regarding the theory and contents of language instruction. Teachers need to have multiple layers of expertise on how children acquire reading, the relationship between language development and reading development, the characteristics of disabilities, and the basic tenets of reading instruction methodologies. There needs to be serious reform in colleges of education and professional development programs.

The time has come to merge the evidence from the science of reading—the knowledge gained from research on what works in the classroom—with serious and sustained pre-service training and ongoing professional development so that teachers can better carry out the complex demands of reading instruction. Efforts are underway in many colleges, universities, and private training organizations to rethink and explore new ways of delivering coursework, online and in the classroom, in conjunction with innovative ways of gaining practical, hands-on experience with validated practices (Moats, 2003). The way to proceed has been explicitly described by many guides that prescribe what expert teachers should know and be able to do (Brady & Moats, 1997; Clark & Uhry, 1995; IDA, 2018; Learning First Alliance, 2000; NICHD, 2000; Snow et al., 1998). Appendix 1.2 lists college programs and training organizations that have been evaluated by accrediting associations that use scientifically based **Structured Literacy** standards to train their teachers to teach reading.

Teachers have to know how reading develops from pre-reading to reading for information and enjoyment. Detecting reading difficulties early and providing appropriate intervention in time to keep children from failing is critical. A thorough knowledge of the structure of language and how to teach it layer by layer helps teachers to monitor their students' progress and gives them the tools to pace lessons and move their students along based on consistent monitoring of progress (Moats, 1999; Moats & Brady, 1997). This ensures that special educators, who work with the students with the most serious problems, and general educators, who must reach a range of students with diverse needs on a daily basis, receive the best professional development based on what scientifically based reading research shows is effective. Good instruction can prevent a lifetime of difficulties: A good beginning has no end.

ONLINE COMPANION MATERIALS

The following Chapter 1 resources are available at http://www.brookespublishing.com/birshcarreker/materials:

- Reflect, Connect, and Respond Questions

- Appendix 1.1: Knowledge and Skill Assessment Answer Key

- Appendix 1.2: Resources

KNOWLEDGE AND SKILL ASSESSMENT

1. Research suggests that the defining characteristic of dyslexia is that a student does what?

    a. Reads letters and words backward

    b. Has difficulties with the phonology of language

    c. Has attention and motivation issues

    d. Has inadequate cognitive abilities

2. Impairments in phonemic awareness skills in kindergarteners will do which of the following?

    a. Resolve themselves over time

    b. Be remediated in later grades

    c. Persist without explicit instruction

    d. Affect decoding but not spelling

3. Research suggests that effective phonics instruction is what?

    a. Indirect

    b. Systematic

    c. Incidental

    d. Optional

4. How can academic language be described?

    a. Naturally acquired

    b. Everyday language

    c. Useful but not necessary

    d. Classroom language

5. Close reading is meant to reduce college students' challenges related to reading because of which of the following?

    a. The demands of complex text

    b. Issues with attention and motivation

    c. Lack of motivation and engagement

    d. Difficulties with decoding and fluency

REFERENCES

Aaron, P.G., Joshi, R.M., & Quatroche, D. (2008). *Becoming a professional reading teacher.* Baltimore, MD: Paul H. Brookes Publishing Co.

Adams, M.J. (1990). *Beginning to read: Thinking and learning about print.* Cambridge, MA: The MIT Press.

Berninger, V.W., & Wolf, B.J. (2009). *Teaching students with dyslexia and dysgraphia: Lessons from teaching and science.* Baltimore, MD: Paul H. Brookes Publishing Co.

Birsh, J.R. (2006, Fall). What is multisensory structured language? *Perspectives, 32*(4).

Brady, S., & Moats, L.C. (1997). *Informed instruction for reading success: Foundations for teacher preparation.* Baltimore, MD: The International Dyslexia Association.

Brozgold, A.Z. (2002, March 22). *The diagnosis of dyslexia in adults.* Paper presented at the 29th Annual Conference on Dyslexia and Related Learning Disabilities, New York Branch of the International Dyslexia Association.

Catts, H.W., Nielsen, D.C., Bridges, M.S., Liu, Y.S., & Bontempo, D.E. (2015). Early identification of reading disabilities within an RTI framework. *Journal of Learning Disabilities, 48*(3), 281–297.

Chall, J. (1967). *Learning to read: The great debate.* New York, NY: McGraw-Hill.

Cheesman, E.A., McGuire, J.M., Shankweiler, D., & Coyne, M. (2009). First-year teacher knowledge of phonemic awareness and its instruction. *Teacher Education and Special Education, 32*(3), 270–289. doi:10.1177/0888406409339685

Clark, D.B., & Uhry, J.K. (1995). *Dyslexia: Theory and practice of remedial instruction.* Timonium, MD: York Press.

Connor, C.M., Morrison, F.J., & Underwood, P. (2007). A second chance in second grade? The cumulative impact of first and second grade reading instruction on students' letter–word reading skills. *Scientific Studies of Reading, 11*(3), 199–233.

Council of Chief State School Officers (CCSSO) & National Governors Association Center for Best Practices (NGA Center). (2010). *Common Core State Standards for English language arts and literacy in history/social studies, science and technical subjects.* Retrieved from http://www.corestandards.org/the-standards

Darling-Hammond, L. (2000). *Teacher quality and student achievement: A review of state policy evidence.* Retrieved from https://epaa.asu.edu/ojs/article/view/392

de Groot, B.J., van den Bos, K.P., Minnaert, A.E., & van der Meulen, B.F. (2015). Phonological processing and word reading in typically developing and reading disabled children: Severity matters. *Scientific Studies of Reading, 19*(2), 166–181.

Dehaene, S. (2009). *Reading in the brain: The science and evolution of a human invention.* New York, NY: Viking Penguin.

Dickman, G.E., Hennessy, N.L., Moats, L.C., Rooney, K.J., & Tomey, H.A. (2002). *The nature of learning disabilities: Response to OSEP Summit on Learning Disabilities.* Baltimore, MD: The International Dyslexia Association.

Eden, G.F., & Moats, L.C. (2002). The role of neuroscience in the remediation of students with dyslexia. *Nature Neuroscience, 5*(Suppl.), 1080–1084.

Ehri, L.C. (2004). Teaching phonemic awareness and phonics: An explanation of the National Reading Panel meta-analyses. In P. McCardle & V. Chhabra (Eds.), *The voice of evidence in reading research* (pp. 153–186). Baltimore, MD: Paul H. Brookes Publishing Co.

Ehri, L.C., Nunes, S.R., Stahl, S.A., & Willows, D.M. (2001). Systematic phonics instruction helps students learn to read: Evidence from the National Reading Panel's meta-analysis. *Review of Educational Research, 71*(3), 393–447.

Farkas, S., & Duffett, A. (2010). *Cracks in the ivory tower: The views of education professors circa 2010.* Washington, DC: Thomas B. Fordham Institute.

Ferrer, E., Shaywitz, B.A., Holahan, J.M., Marchione, K., & Shaywitz, S.E. (2010). Uncoupling of reading and IQ over time: Empirical evidence of a definition of dyslexia. *Psychological Science, 21*(1), 93–101.

Fletcher, J.M., Coulter, W.A., Reschly, D.J., & Vaughn, S. (2004). Alternative approaches to the definition and identification of learning disabilities: Some questions and answers. *Annals of Dyslexia, 54*(2), 304–331.

Fletcher, J.M., & Francis, D.J. (2004). Scientifically based educational research: Questions, designs, and methods. In P. McCardle & V. Chhabra (Eds.), *The voice of evidence in reading research* (pp. 59–80). Baltimore, MD: Paul H. Brookes Publishing Co.

Francis, D.J., Shaywitz, S.E., Stuebing, K.K., Shaywitz, B.A., & Fletcher, J.M. (1996). Developmental lag versus deficit models of reading disability: A longitudinal, individual growth curve analysis. *Journal of Educational Psychology, 88*(1), 3–17.

Gersten, R., Compton, D., Connor, C.M., Dimino, J., Santoro, I., Linan-Thompson, S., & Tilly, W.D. (2008). *Assisting students struggling with reading: Response to intervention and multi-tier intervention for reading in the primary grades.* A practice guide (NCEE, 2009-4045). Washington, DC: U.S. Department of Education, National Center for Educational Evaluation and Regional Assistance, Institute of Educational Sciences. Retrieved from https://ies.ed.gov/ncee/wwc/PracticeGuides

Gillis, M.B. (2017, Summer). How RTI supports early identification of students with different reading profiles. *Perspectives on Language and Literacy, 43*(3), 41–45.

Hasbrouck, J., & Tindal, G. (2006). Oral reading fluency norms: A valuable assessment tool for reading teachers. *The Reading Teacher, 59*, 636–634.

Individuals with Disabilities Education Improvement Act (IDEA) of 2004, PL 108-446, 20 U.S.C. §§ 1400 *et seq.*

International Dyslexia Association, The. (2010). *Knowledge and practice standards for teachers of reading: With commentary for dyslexia specialists.* Baltimore, MD: Author.

International Dyslexia Association, The. (2018, March). *Knowledge and practice standards for teachers of reading.* Retrieved from https://dyslexiaida.org/knowledge-and-practices/

International Multisensory Structured Language Education Council. (2010). *IMSLEC directory: MSL training courses and graduates.* Dallas, TX: Author.

Juel, C. (1988). Learning to read and write: A longitudinal study of 54 children from first to fourth grades. *Journal of Educational Psychology, 80*, 437–447.

Keller-Allen, C. (2004). *The National Reading Panel: The accuracy of concerns about the report.* Unpublished manuscript.

Kilpatrick, D.A. (2015). *Essentials of assessing, preventing, and overcoming reading difficulties.* Hoboken, NJ: John Wiley & Sons.

Klingner, J.K., Morrison, A., & Eppolito, A. (2011). Metacognition to improve reading comprehension. In R.E. O'Connor & P.F. Vadasy (Eds.), *Handbook of reading interventions* (pp. 220–253). New York, NY: Guilford.

Kratochwill, T.R., Hitchcock, J., Horner, R.H., Levin, J.R., Odom, S.L., Rindskopf, D.M., & Shadish, W.R. (2010). *Single-case designs technical documentation.* Retrieved from http://files.eric.ed.gov/fulltext/ED510743.pdf

Learning First Alliance. (2000). *Every child reading: A professional development guide.* Washington, DC: Author.

Lerner, J. (1989). Educational interventions in learning disabilities. *Journal of the American Academy of Child and Adolescent Psychiatry, 28*, 326–331.

Lyon, G.R. (Ed.). (1994). *Frames of reference for the assessment of learning disabilities: New view of measurement issues.* Baltimore, MD: Paul H. Brookes Publishing Co.

Lyon, G.R. (1996, Spring). Learning disabilities. *The Future of Children, 6*(4), 54–76.

Lyon, G.R. (1999). The NICHD research program in reading development, reading disorders, and reading instruction: A summary of research findings. In *Keys to successful learning: A national summit on research in learning disabilities.* New York, NY: National Center for Learning Disabilities.

Lyon, G.R. (2004). *The NICHD research program in reading development, reading disorders, and treading instruction initiated: 1965.* Paper presented at the 31st annual conference of the New York Branch of the International Dyslexia Association.

Lyon, G.R., & Chhabra, V. (2004). The science of reading research. *Educational Leadership, 61*(6), 13–17.

Lyon, G.R., Shaywitz, S.E., & Shaywitz, B.A. (2003). A definition of dyslexia. *Annals of Dyslexia, 53*, 1–14.

McCardle, P., Chhabra, V., & Kapinus, B. (2008). *Reading research in action: A teacher's guide for student success.* Baltimore, MD: Paul H. Brookes Publishing Co.

McIntyre, C.W., & Pickering, J.S. (1995). *Clinical studies of multisensory structured language education for students with dyslexia and related disorders.* Salem, OR: International Mulitsensory Structured Language Education Council.

Moats, L.C. (1999). *Teaching reading is rocket science: What expert teachers of reading should know and be able to do* (No. 372). Washington, DC: American Federation of Teachers.

Moats, L.C. (2003). *Language Essentials for Teachers of Reading and Spelling (LETRS).* Longmont, CO: Sopris West Educational Services.

Moats, L.C., & Brady, S. (1997). *Informed instruction for reading success: Foundations for teacher preparation.* Baltimore, MD: The International Dyslexia Association.

Moats, L.C., & Foorman, B.R. (2003). Measuring teachers' content knowledge of language and reading. *Annals of Dyslexia, 53*, 23–45.

Morris, R.D., Stuebing, K.K., Fletcher, J.M., Shaywitz, S.E., Lyon, G.R., Shankweiler, D.P., . . . Shaywitz, B.A. (1998). Subtypes of reading disability: Variability around a phonological core. *Journal of Educational Psychology, 90*, 347–373.

National Center for Education Statistics. (2017). *The nation's report card: Reading 2017.* Washington, DC: U.S. Department of Education.

National Institute of Child Health and Human Development (NICHD). (2000). *Report of the National Reading Panel: Reports of the subgroups. Teaching children to read: An evidence-based assessment of the scientific research literature on reading and its implications for reading instruction* (NIH Pub No. 00-4754). Washington, DC: Government Printing Office.

No Child Left Behind Act of 2001, PL 107-110, 115 Stat. 1425, 20 U.S.C. §§ 6301 *et seq.*

Olson, R.K. (2004). Environment and genes. *Scientific Studies of Reading, 8*(2), 111–124.

Partnership for Reading. (2003, June). *Put reading first: The research building blocks for teaching children to read. Kindergarten through grade 3* (2nd ed.). Washington, DC: Author.

Piasta, S.B., Connor, C.M., Fishman, B.J., & Morrison, F.J. (2009). Teachers' knowledge of literary concepts, classroom practices, and student reading growth. *Scientific Studies of Reading, 13*(3), 224–248.

Pressley, M. (2002). *Reading instruction that works* (2nd ed.). New York, NY: Guilford.

Ramus, F., Rosen, S., Dakin, S.C., Day, B.L., Castellote, J.M., White, S., & Frith, U. (2003). Theories of developmental dyslexia: Insights from a multiple case study of dyslexic adults. *Brain, 126*, 841–865.

Rasinski, T. (2017). Readers who struggle: Why many struggle and a modest proposal for improving their reading. *The Reading Teacher, 70*(5), 519–524.

Reyna, V.F. (2004). Why scientific research? The importance of evidence in changing educational practice. In P. McCardle & V. Chhabra (Eds.), *The voice of evidence in reading research* (pp. 47–58). Baltimore, MD: Paul H. Brookes Publishing Co.

Schochet, P., Cook, T., Deke, J., Imbens, G., Lockwood, J.R., Porter, J., & Smith, J. (2010). *Standards for regression discontinuity designs.* Retrieved from https://ies.ed.gov/ncee/wwc/Docs/ReferenceResources/wwc_rd.pdf

Seidenberg, M. (2017). *Language at the speed of sight: How we read, why so many can't, and what can be done about it.* New York, NY: Basic Books.

Shaywitz, B.A., Shaywitz, S.E., Blachman, B.A., Pugh, K.R., Fulbright, R.K., Skudlarski, P., . . . Gore, J.C. (2004). Development of left occipitotemporal systems for skilled reading in children after a phonologically-based intervention. *Biological Psychiatry, 55*(9), 926–933.

Shaywitz, S.E. (1998). Current concepts: Dyslexia. *New England Journal of Medicine, 338*(5), 307–312.

Shaywitz, S. (2003). *Overcoming dyslexia: A new and complete science-based program for reading problems at any level.* New York, NY: Alfred A. Knopf.

Shaywitz, S.E., & Shaywitz, B.A. (2004). Neurobiologic basis for reading and reading disability. In P. McCardle & V. Chhabra (Eds.), *The voice of evidence in reading research* (pp. 417–442). Baltimore, MD: Paul H. Brookes Publishing Co.

Shaywitz, S.E., Shaywitz, B.A., Fletcher, J.M., & Escobar, M.D. (1990). Prevalence of reading disability of boys and girls: Results of the Connecticut Longitudinal Study. *Journal of the American Medical Association, 264*(8), 998–1002.

Snow, C.E. (2004). Foreword. In P. McCardle & V. Chhabra (Eds.), *The voice of evidence in reading research* (pp. xix–xxv). Baltimore, MD: Paul H. Brookes Publishing Co.

Snow, C.E., Burns, M.S., & Griffin, P. (Eds.). (1998). *Preventing reading difficulties in young children.* Washington, DC: National Academies Press.

Spear-Swerling, L., Brucker, P., & Alfano, M. (2005). Teachers' literacy-related knowledge and self-perception in relation to preparation and experience. *Annals of Dyslexia, 55*, 266–293.

Torgesen, J.K. (2004). Lessons learned from research on interventions for students who experience difficulty learning to read. In P. McCardle & V. Chhabra (Eds.), *The voice of evidence in reading research* (pp. 355–382). Baltimore, MD: Paul H. Brookes Publishing Co.

Torgesen, J.K., Houston, D.D., Rissman, L.M., Decker, S.M., Roberts, G., Vaughn, S., . . . Lesaux, B. (2007). *Academic literacy instruction for adolescents: A guidance document from the Center on Instruction.* Portsmouth, NH: RNC Research Corporation, Center on Instruction.

Torgesen, J.K., Wagner, R.K., & Rashotte, C.A. (1994). Longitudinal studies of phonological processing and reading. *Journal of Learning Disabilities, 27*, 276–286.

U.S. Department of Education, Institute of Education Sciences. (2008). *WWC procedures and standards handbook: Version 3.0.* Retrieved from https://ies.ed.gov/ncee/wwc/Docs/referenceresources/wwc_procedures_v3_0_standards_handbook.pdf

Vaughn, S., & Linan-Thompson, S. (2003). Group size and time allotted to intervention: Effects for students with reading difficulties. In B.R. Foorman (Ed.), *Preventing and remediating reading difficulties: Bringing science to scale* (pp. 299–324). Timonium, MD: York Press.

Walsh, K., Glaser, D., & Wilcox, D.D. (2006). *What education schools aren't teaching about reading and what elementary teachers aren't learning.* Washington, DC: National Council on Teacher Quality.

Williamson, G.L. (2008). A text readability continuum for postsecondary readiness. *Journal of Advanced Academics, 19*(4), 602–632.

Wolf, M., Bowers, P., & Biddle, K. (2000). Naming-speed processes, timing, and reading: A conceptual review. *Journal of Learning Disabilities, 33,* 322–324.

Woodcock, R.W., & Johnson, M.B. (1989). *The Woodcock-Johnson–Revised Tests of Achievement.* Itasca, IL: Riverside.

Chapter 2

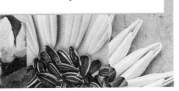

Structured Literacy Instruction

Mary L. Farrell and Nancy Cushen White

LEARNING OBJECTIVES

1. To identify the major components of language and literacy addressed within Structured Literacy content—what is taught (e.g., phonology, phonics, syllables, morphology, etymology, syntax, text reading fluency, semantics–comprehension, handwriting)

2. To define and describe each of the components of Structured Literacy content (i.e., what is taught) and explain how each is relevant to the process of learning to read and write

3. To identify Structured Literacy's core principles of instruction—how it is taught (e.g., explicit and direct; sequential, systematic, and cumulative; diagnostic; synthetic and analytic) and to explain how to apply these principles during implementation of instruction

4. To explain the purpose of simultaneous multisensory instruction for teaching language and literacy skills and to describe what this approach entails

5. To understand and be able to explain the history of the use of multisensory strategies in instruction

6. To understand and be able to summarize the research base (e.g., neurological research, research on active learning, Triple Word Form Theory) supporting the effectiveness of using multisensory instructional strategies within a Structured Literacy approach

The terms Structured Literacy instruction and Multisensory Structured Language Education have been used interchangeably. In this chapter, we use Structured Literacy instruction to represent the core content and principles of instruction to which these two terms refer. This chapter defines Structured Literacy instruction:

- Content—what is taught

- Principles of instruction—how it is taught

ACKNOWLEDGMENTS

Portions of the current chapter were written for the third edition of this book by Carolyn Cowen. Mary Farrell and Nancy Cushen White wish to thank Fumiko Hoeft for her suggestions, her responses to questions, and her wise counsel during the writing of the current chapter. Portions of the current chapter were written for the first and second editions of this book by Louisa Cook Moats. Portions of the current chapter were written for the third edition of this book by Gordon Sherman.

- **Simultaneous multisensory strategies** used in conjunction with the core content of Structured Literacy and the fundamental principles of instruction

Current findings regarding the nature of reading development, the efficacy of specific instructional practices for teaching reading, and the complexities of reading networks within the brain are leading to an increased understanding that may explain why expert teachers have remained committed to Structured Literacy approaches to instruction.

A COMMON FRAMEWORK

Research supported by the National Institute of Child Health and Human Development (NICHD) for more than 50 years has shown that, for 90%–95% of poor readers, prevention and early intervention programs combining instruction in **phoneme awareness,** phonics, fluency development, and reading comprehension strategies—provided by well-trained, linguistically informed teachers—can increase reading skills to average reading levels or above (Blachman, Schatschneider, Fletcher, & Clonan, 2003; Blachman et al., 2004; Lyon, 1997, 1998; Seidenberg, 2017; Torgesen, 2004). Converging evidence emphasizes the importance of first-rate classroom reading instruction in early grades and early intervention for at-risk students (e.g., in a small-group setting) to improve the effectiveness of remediation (Blachman et al., 2003; Blachman et al., 2004; Gaab, 2017; Torgesen, 2004).

Students want to learn, and teachers want to be successful in teaching their students. It is imperative that pre-service teacher preparation and districtwide staff development programs begin to base their curriculum content on comprehensive, evidence-based approaches to teaching reading and other written language skills.

In 2010, The International Dyslexia Association (IDA) developed professional standards for teachers who will be or are teaching students with dyslexia or related language disorders. The IDA *Knowledge and Practice Standards for Teachers of Reading* (2018) provides a comprehensive, research-based framework that articulates what all reading teachers and specialists should know and be able to demonstrate to teach reading successfully to all students. The standards focus on the structure of language and its component systems, connections of those systems to the design and delivery of instruction, and the complex nature of skilled reading. The *Knowledge and Practice Standards* points out

> Although programs that certify or support teachers, clinicians, or specialists differ in their preparation methodologies, teaching approaches, and organizational purposes, they should ascribe to a common set of professional standards for the benefit of the students they serve. Compliance with these standards should assure the public that individuals who teach in public and private schools, as well as those who teach in clinics, are prepared to implement scientifically based and clinically proven practices. (2010, p. 5)

Adherence to these standards is of particular importance for teaching students who struggle to learn to read.

Within the scientific literature, there is great overlap in the diagnostic labels used to describe subjects in studies of reading and speech and language: dyslexia, language learning disability, specific learning disability, reading disability, reading disorder, and other terms. We have chosen to use the term *reading disability* whenever possible. As Farrell and Matthews explained, "Catts and Kamhi (2005) justified the use of the term *reading disability*, stating that it is a common term used by researchers and practitioners to refer to a heterogeneous group of children who have difficulty learning to read" (2010, p. 2).

STRUCTURED LITERACY

Most Orton-Gillingham programs and approaches for teaching language-related academic skills emphasize that the core content for instruction is the carefully sequenced teaching of the structure and use of phonology; phonics, including syllable instruction; **morphology** and **etymology**; syntax; text reading fluency; vocabulary; semantics; and written expression. These approaches (e.g., Alphabetic Phonics, LANGUAGE!, Language Tool Kit, Project Read, Slingerland Approach, Sonday System, Spalding Method, Wilson Language Training) also stress the need for explicit instruction that is direct, sequential, systematic, cumulative, diagnostic, and multisensory. According to clinical consensus, the combination of this core content and these principles of instruction facilitates a student's ability to learn, recall, and apply information.

Structured Literacy: Content of Instruction

The content of Structured Literacy instruction comprises several components of language, briefly introduced in Chapter 1: phonology, phonics, syllables, morphology and etymology, syntax, fluency, semantics–comprehension, and handwriting. These language components are discussed in detail in the sections that follow.

Phonology Phonology is the study of the sound structure of spoken words within a single language (e.g., English). Within phonology are **phonemes,** the smallest units of sound contrast that create words with different meanings (e.g., *morpheme* vs. *morphine,* words whose pronunciation differs only in the final phoneme, /m/ vs. /n/). Table 2.1 illustrates how the meaning of a word changes entirely with a different phoneme in **initial, medial,** or **final** positions.

Phonemes are difficult to isolate and are altered by co-articulation (phonemes that surround them). An example can be found in different words that include the phoneme /p/: *post, spark, stop, lisp, sipped* (pronounced /sipt/). Pronounce each of these words. Focus your attention on the "feel" (tongue-lips-teeth) of pronouncing the phoneme /p/ in each word and the subtle changes you notice. Although the place and manner of articulation (pronunciation) for the /p/ in each of these different words is basically the same (and different from the unique sequence of movements for pronouncing any other phoneme), there are subtle variations.

Phonemes are not sounds processed only by listening (i.e., through the auditory system); they are articulated (spoken) sounds. It is the powerful motor system of speech (i.e., auditory to kinesthetic–motor integration) that sequences and remembers phonemes. Letters (graphemes) represent (spell) spoken sounds. Text is a way of making speech visible (Herron, 2013).

The phoneme awareness skills of blending, segmenting, and manipulation of speech sounds within words (or syllables) are a bridge to phoneme–grapheme and grapheme–phoneme associations (phonics). Phonemic awareness is the

Table 2.1. Meaning contrast based on change of a single phoneme

house	/h/ in /ʜous/	mouse	/m/ in /ṃous/	louse	/l/ in /ḷous/
street	/ē/ in /strēt/	straight	/ā/ in /strāt/	strut	/ŭ/ in /strŭt/
sheaf	/sh/ in /ṣẖēf/	beef	/b in /bēf/	thief	/th/ in /t̲ẖēf/
street	/t/ in /strēt̲/	stream	/m/ in /strēṃ/	streak	/k/ in /strēḵ/

foundation—not the whole structure—that supports reading and writing the alphabetic code. Phonemic awareness does not automatically generalize to fluency and comprehension. Discrete reading and spelling skills must be taught.

Phonics and Syllable Instruction   Phonics is not the same as phonemic awareness. Phonics requires mapping of phonemes to their spellings and mapping of spellings to their pronunciations. Phonics involves the use of grapheme–phoneme associations to read and spell familiar and unfamiliar words. English has more than 40 phonemes and more than 250 graphemes to spell them. To be able to read and spell unfamiliar words independently, students must be capable of applying decoding or encoding (spelling) strategies. Application of these strategies activates orthographic mappings in memory to retrieve the words' spellings, pronunciations, and meanings (Ehri, 2014). Herron explained:

> Perhaps we should come up with a different term to replace "sight words." The words that become "automatic" after decoding them many times could be called "acquired words" or "stored words." The "storing" of words that can be recognized automatically is a neural process that requires *many trips around the wiring* primarily between the **visual word form area (VWFA)** and **Broca's area** (speech) and **Wernicke's area** (comprehension). Once the pathways become well established, the route becomes instantaneous, and our *"impression"* is that the words are recognized "by sight." My understanding of work by Pugh, Cornellisson, Shaywitz and others is that memorizing the visual shape, contours, or appearance of a word (what teachers often do with their Dolch lists) bypasses this process and leads to LESS EFFICIENT reading. (2003)

A syllable is a unit of speech consisting of one vowel phoneme with or without surrounding consonant phonemes. The number of vowel graphemes in a word usually indicates the number of spoken syllables. Six basic syllable types, based on the type of vowel grapheme within each syllable, were regularized by Noah Webster in his 1806 dictionary. Knowledge of syllable types, based on type of vowel grapheme, allows students to systematically divide words into manageable "chunks" (syllables) for accurate pronunciation of longer, unfamiliar words. **Recognition** of the type of vowel grapheme and the vowel phoneme associated with that vowel grapheme expedites accurate pronunciation of longer unfamiliar words, especially critical content words in academic text.

Although knowledge of syllables is very useful to students when attempting to identify (read) and spell words, it is important to understand that, in English, spoken language syllable divisions often do not coincide with the conventions for dividing written words into syllables:

- In the word *little,* the spoken syllables are pronounced as /lǐ/ and /təl/. Because the first syllable, /lǐt/, has one vowel letter spoken as a short vowel sound, *it is a* **closed syllable**—and must end with a consonant. Therefore, the written syllables in the word *little* are shown as *lit* and *tle.*

- In the word *title,* the spoken syllables are pronounced as /tī/ and /təl/. Because the vowel grapheme (vowel pattern—vowel spelling) in the first syllable is one vowel letter at the end of the syllable, it is an **open syllable.** The vowel sound in this open syllable is long because the open syllable is accented (stressed). Therefore, the written syllables in the word *title* are also shown as *ti* and *tle.*

- The result of the syllable combining process leaves a doubled consonant, *tt,* in *little,* the word with a closed syllable, that is not there in *title,* the word with an open syllable. These spelling conventions were invented to help readers decide how to pronounce a word in print.

Morphology and Etymology Morphology is the study of the sequence and structure of meaningful elements (morphemes) in words. A **morpheme** is the smallest meaningful unit of language—a linguistic entity that can be a whole word (e.g., *press*), part of a word (e.g., *ject* in re*ject*, *con-* in *con*ference, and *-ed* in rest*ed*), or a single phoneme (e.g., the *e- in* e*ject* or *-y* in risk*y*). Prefixes, base elements, and suffixes are different types of morphemes:

- The **base element** within an English word is the morphological base of a word and holds the core to its meaning (e.g., *struct* is the base element in *construction*; *vide* is the base element in *evident*). A **root** is the historical source of a base element (e.g., *gregare* is the root of the base element *grege* as in *congregate*).

- **Prefixes** precede base elements within words; a single base element may have multiple prefixes (e.g., *ac-* and *com-* are different prefixes in *accommodate*).

- **Suffixes** follow base elements within words; a single base element may have multiple suffixes (e.g., *-ion* and *-al* are suffixes in *conventional*. Although there are only about 50 suffixes used in everyday English, suffixes appear in 50% of English words (Crystal, 2012).

Morphological awareness is associated with improved word identification, vocabulary, spelling, and reading comprehension (Berninger, Abbott, Nagy, & Carlisle, 2010). In a 2017 study that examined different dimensions of morphological awareness in adolescents (Goodwin, Petscher, Carlisle, & Mitchell, 2017), several factors contributed toward growth in vocabulary knowledge and improved reading comprehension: 1) ability to identify and manipulate morphemes within words, 2) use of **morphological** knowledge to determine word meanings, 3) ability to generate morphologically complex words (i.e., words with two or more morphemes, such as *abbreviate* and *brevity*), and 4) ability to think about words within morphological families.

English is a morphophonemic language in which the pronunciation of polysyllabic words is primarily determined by placement of stress. **Morphophonemics** refers to the interaction between *morph*ological and *phon*ological processes (Venezky, 1999). Table 2.2 gives examples of phonological (pronunciation) changes that occur in morphemes (minimal meaningful units) when they combine to form different words. As the number of syllables changes, the stress shifts—and the pronunciation of individual morphemes (and syllables) will change. Words with spelling connections have meaning connections. The study of spelling—with a focus on the morphophonemic nature of English—connects even unfamiliar words with a common base to their meanings.

Etymology is the study of the interrelationships of words with their own origins and with other words that share that origin—through history. **Diachronic** etymology refers to the influence that roots of words (e.g., Latin, Greek, Old English) have on the meanings and spellings of words currently in the language—how

Table 2.2. Phonological changes to morphemes when combined to form different words

Base element	Derivatives: We never know the pronunciation of a base until it lands in a word.							
sci "know"	*sci*ence	*sci*entific	con*sci*ous	uncon*sci*ous	con*sci*entious	omni*sci*ent	con*sci*ence	
fine "end"	con*fine*	in*fine*te	in*fini*ty	*fin*ish	de*fini*tion	*finite*	*fin*ality	*fin*ally

language has developed and evolved through time. **Synchronic** etymology accounts for the current spelling of a word in a language at a given time in history—interrelationships of meaning between a word (e.g., pe*o*ple) and other words (e.g., p*o*pulation) whether or not the two words share the same root.

Syntax   Syntax refers to the set of principles that dictate the sequence and function of words, phrases, and clauses in sentences to convey meaning. The study of syntax includes parts of speech, sentence structure, and language mechanics (e.g., punctuation, capitalization). Each of the eight parts of speech has a specific, meaning-based function. Working together, these eight parts of speech become the foundation for every syntactic structure that occurs in English. **Syntactic awareness** is a **metalinguistic** skill that is defined as the conscious ability to manipulate or judge word order within the context of a sentence based on the application of grammatical rules (Cain, 2007).

Parts of speech answer questions; phrases and clauses function as parts of speech in the same way that single words do. Students can be taught to consider the question each phrase or clause answers: Who? What? (noun); Where? When? Why? How? To what extent? (adverb); Which? What kind? How many? How much? (adjective). They are taught the purpose of punctuation and capitalization.

Syntactic awareness facilitates students' ability to read complex text with **prosody**—and therefore supports reading comprehension. Teaching students to chunk complex sentences into meaningful phrases provides them with a strategy for parsing sentences into manageable parts so that they are able to determine the function of words within phrases and the questions that phrases and clauses answer within sentences. Syntactic awareness is also critical for constructing sentences for both oral and written expression.

Text-Reading Fluency   Kuhn, Schwanenflugel, and Meisinger (2010) defined fluency as a combination of accuracy, automaticity, and oral reading prosody. Taken together, these fluency components support a reader's comprehension. Kuhn and colleagues reported that other researchers (Fletcher, Lyon, Fuchs, & Barnes, 2007; Hudson, Pullen, Lane, & Torgesen, 2009; Rasinski, Reutzel, Chard, & Linan-Thompson, 2010) considered appropriate pacing, along with other prosodic features, as central to their definition of fluency. Skilled readers vary reading pace depending on the difficulty of the text and the complexity of the ideas they are encountering. To become a skilled reader, it is important to learn to be flexible rather than simply fast. Fluency is about being able to mobilize as much knowledge as possible about a word fast enough to have time to think and comprehend. The role of fluency is to give the executive system sufficient time to direct attention where it is most needed: inference, understanding, and prediction (Norton & Wolf, 2012; Wolf, 2007).

Prerequisites for fluency include coordination of critical systems of language structure: orthography (spelling patterns), phonology (speech sound system), semantics (meaning), and syntax (grammar and sentence structure). Most critical are the connections between and among the systems—integration! The goal is automatic retrieval of information from each system through understanding and practice so that students are able to focus on comprehension when reading any type of text.

Slingerland noted, "Learning how to read by 'phrase units' or 'idea units' significantly increases students' understanding of what they read" (2013, p. 237).

The ability to recognize meaningful chunks of text helps develop fluency and comprehension. Though most readers chunk automatically, chunking strategies must be taught to struggling readers (Moats, 1995). Students who read complex text with prosody (i.e., in syntactically correct, meaningful phrases) comprehend what they read.

Semantics–Comprehension   Semantics refers to the meaning of words, phrases, sentences, and connected text—and the relationship of each of these to the others. Semantics is dependent on the integration of all of the other areas of core content: accurate word identification, morphology, syntax–grammar, and fluency (prosody). In addition, comprehension requires the ability to activate relevant background knowledge. Students must be able to relate what they read to what they already know. Stimulation of relevant background knowledge and reinforcement and expansion of vocabulary must be actively and systematically taught.

As Scott explained, "If a reader cannot parse the types of complex sentences that are often encountered in academic texts, no amount of comprehension strategy instruction will help" (2009, p. 189). Students must be taught to parse complex sentences into meaningful phrases, regardless of the content domain, in order to comprehend sentences and to be more fluent with complexity when talking or writing about content they have read (Scott & Balthazar, 2013). In addition, instruction must focus on unfamiliar vocabulary within phrases to clarify pronunciation and meaning.

REFLECT, CONNECT, and RESPOND

What does it mean to say a reader is fluent? What are the components of fluency? How does fluency support reading comprehension?

Handwriting   In Chapter 11, Wolf and Berninger explain how components of handwriting instruction can be **multi-modal** (i.e., **multi-motor** as well as **multisensory**). These components correspond to different modes as follows: seeing letters—visual; hearing names of letters (or phonemes represented by letters)—auditory; feeling the unique sequence of movements during speech production as each letter name (or phoneme) is pronounced—kinesthetic–motor; and feeling the unique sequence of movements as each letter is formed—kinesthetic–motor.

Integration of Written Language Content   Using students with and without learning disabilities, Alstad and colleagues (2015) studied three different types of letter production (i.e., manuscript, cursive, and keyboarding) and relationships between the type of letter production and various skills of written expression (e.g., spelling of single words, composition, copying of sentences). They emphasized the significance of understanding that letter formation is a skill of written language, not simply a motor skill, and explained that connections between "letter forms (orthographic codes) and names corresponding to letter forms (verbal codes)" support the development of "automatic retrieval" (2015, p. 227). They concluded that instruction should focus on "developing hybrid writers skilled in multiple modes of letter production for a variety of writing purposes" (2015, p. 228) and that handwriting instruction, including explicit teaching of keyboarding, should continue after fourth grade and into middle school as demands for written expression become greater.

The acts of reading and spelling are different sides of the same coin—and the reading network includes connections between functional areas specific to phonological, orthographic, and morphological information. For these reasons, instruction that integrates the teaching of reading, spelling, handwriting, and written expression through one comprehensive approach is likely to be more effective than teaching each of these aspects of written language separately (Wolf, Abbott, & Berninger, 2017).

Structured Literacy: Principles of Instruction

In addition to introducing the components of instructional content, Chapter 1 introduces core principles of instruction: the use of explicit, direct instruction; the use of a sequential, systematic, and cumulative approach; diagnostic teaching; and a combination of synthetic and analytic language instruction (e.g., working both from parts to whole and from whole to parts). These and other core principles (e.g., daily lessons that include teaching of skills as well as functional use and application of skills, introduction and consolidation of content vocabulary) are further explained in the following sections.

Explicit, Direct Instruction　Explicit instruction requires use of straightforward, consistent, and precise language for direct teaching of all skills and strategies, with continuous student–teacher interaction and provision of as much scaffolding as needed. Student responses, both correct and incorrect, are used to assess understanding.

For students experiencing difficulties, learning is never assumed. Instruction needs to make the path to academic success obvious—and accessible—by deliberately teaching essential concepts, skills, and strategies. Instead of leaving learning to chance through incidental encounters with information, the teacher explains and demonstrates—one language and print concept at a time. The teacher models, verbalizing each step, and then guides the student to demonstrate and verbalize steps with immediate corrective feedback before the student attempts the task independently (Mather & Wendling, 2012; Slingerland, 2013). Feedback is specific and directive so that the student understands what, if anything, requires a change. To optimize practice opportunities, individual students, as well as students within a group, need many opportunities to respond and receive feedback. Always, the goal is independent functional use.

Textbox 2.1 lists the procedural steps for introducing a new vowel grapheme using the Orton-Gillingham Approach.

Textbox 2.2 lists the procedural steps for introducing a new suffix using the Slingerland Approach. Suffixes are a type of morpheme (meaningful unit) added to base elements. Students automatically use suffixes in their spoken language but may need explicit instruction to understand how a suffix changes the meaning of a base element, or baseword, in print. For reading and spelling, students are taught to use suffixes through association with their prior knowledge of the suffix meanings in spoken language. Teaching "through the intellect" (Slingerland, 2013, p. 1) avoids the less reliable sole dependence on rote memorization. Teachers structure each step in the learning process to ensure that students learn a pattern for thinking about and understanding the changes in meaning that occur when a suffix is added to a base element.

TEXTBOX 2.1   Introduction of the grapheme: Vowel team *ea* (Orton-Gillingham Approach)

- *Teacher connects to prior knowledge:* The teacher shows a card with *ee* printed on it. The teacher says, "You have learned the vowel team *ee*. Today, we are going to learn another vowel team that spells the same sound."

- *Auditory introductory activity:* The teacher pronounces three words containing *ea* pattern spelling /ē/ (*bead, meat, deal*) and asks the student to identify the common sound. Next, the teacher reads these words to the student and asks the student to identify the letters representing that sound.

- *Direct instruction with visual:* The teacher presents the letters *ea* on an index card, smart board or other surface, often with a key word and related picture. The teacher says, "This vowel team spells /ē/. What does it spell?" The student says /ē/.

- *Multisensory reinforcement:* The teacher says, "Trace the letters and pronounce the sound they spell as you trace three times. Now, write the letters and pronounce the sound as you write *ea* three times." The student traces *ea* three times and then writes it three times, pronouncing the sound as he or she writes.

- *Oral reading:* The student reads a short list of words that contain the *ea* vowel pattern.

- *Spelling:* The student spells a short list of words that contain the *ea* phoneme /ē/; he or she fingerspells each word before he or she writes it; the student pronounces the sound of each phoneme as he or she writes it.

- *Reading connected text:* The student reads a controlled text featuring the *ea* vowel pattern.

- As the student works, the teacher provides corrective feedback as needed. Students are asked to trace and say letters on which they err in reading; they are asked to fingerspell letters on which they err in spelling.

REFLECT, CONNECT, and RESPOND

Why is it important to provide literacy instruction that is explicit and direct? Give an example of an instructional practice or activity that uses these principles.

Sequential, Systematic, and Cumulative Approach   A **sequential** and **systematic** approach presents material following the logical order of the English language for introducing, reviewing, and practicing concepts. **Cumulative**

TEXTBOX 2.2   Introduction of the suffix -ly (Slingerland Approach)

Auditory

C. Spelling

Baseword and Suffix

a. Verbalization of Concept -ly

Teacher develops concept of specific suffix through spoken language. Each student is given the opportunity to orally add suffix to baseword with no need to consider spelling.

Carefully choose list of words to be used to develop the concept of the new suffix.

*Wordlist: slow, loud, soft, painless, bold, calm, easy, wise, angry, brave, eager, happy, quiet

T: "*Quick* can be a describing word (adjective). When you do something in a *quick* way, how do you do it?" **A**

S: "*Quickly*" **A-Km**

T: "What do you hear at the end of *quickly*?" **A**

S: "/lē/" **A-Km**

T: "Yes." Shows *ly* card. "l-y, /lē/. It is a suffix that makes a baseword tell *how*." OR "It is a suffix that makes a baseword *into an adverb that tells how*." **V-A** "Tell me about the suffix *l-y*."

S: "*l-y*." (fwas) "/lē/. It is a suffix that makes a baseword tell *how*." **V-A-Km**

T: (Continues with a different word* for each student to take a turn verbalizing the concept of the new suffix—that is, how the suffix changes the meaning of the base element.)

b. Forming Word With Suffix—Baseword + *ly*

loud-loudly • sad-sadly • brave-bravely • soft-softly • rude-rudely

Diagram of paper with appropriate number of lines and every word to be written

1.   With Pocket Chart

2.   Without Pocket Chart

S: (Has encoded word *loud* and written on paper.) **V-A-Km**

T: "*Loud* is a describing word (adjective). When you speak in a *loud* way, how do you speak?" **A**

S: "*Loudly*" **A-Km**

T: "What will you add to *loud* to change it into a word that tells how (an adverb)?" **A**

S: "I will add the suffix *l-y*" (fwas). "/lē/. (T shows *ly* card) "It's a suffix that makes a baseword tell *how*." (Pronounces word *loudly* with *armswing* [as], spells, *fwas*, names each letter *as it is formed*.) **V-A-Km**

C: (Repeats word with *as*, spells, *fwas*, naming each letter *as it is formed*.) **V-A-Km**

C: (Repeats word *loudly,* writes on paper below baseword, naming each letter *as it is formed*.) **V-A-Km**

T: (Shows how to check baseword and suffix.) **V-A**

C: (Proofreads for spelling and letter formation.) **V-A-Km**

T: (Corrects, as needed.) **V-A-Km**

C: (Pronounces word. Traces, naming each letter *as it is formed*.) **V-A-Km**

Note: Student always pronounces whole word before beginning to write or trace.

Key: A, auditory; C, class; fwas, forms with armswing (writes in air); Km, kinesthetic–motor; S, student; T, teacher; V: visual.

---

instruction is presented in a sequence that begins with the simplest skills and concepts and progresses systematically to the more difficult. For example, single-letter vowel graphemes are taught before vowel teams, and the concept of a closed syllable is taught before the concept of an open syllable is taught, and so forth. Unknown concepts are introduced or reintroduced, usually one concept at a time, in order of difficulty. New and less familiar concepts are related to previously taught concepts, skills, and information and are always presented using consistent language in anticipation of future learning. Lessons systematically review all concepts that have been introduced in order to provide adequate practice toward the goal of mastery and to bolster memory for specific grapheme–phoneme and phoneme–grapheme associations. When a reading skill becomes what Berninger and Wolf described as "automatic (direct access without conscious awareness)," it is performed quickly in an efficient manner (2009, p. 70; 2016, p. 213). The content of cumulative lessons is controlled so that concepts unknown to the student are not included in any part of the lesson. Precise and consistent language is used for instruction at all levels.

Diagnostic Teaching to Inform Instructional Planning **Diagnostic** teaching requires continuous monitoring of a student's level of mastery and functional use of individual concepts and uses this diagnostic information to inform planning and to adjust instruction as needed. Teachers must individualize instruction, even within groups, based on careful and continuous assessment using both informal (e.g., observation) and formal (i.e., standardized) tools. Informal assessment occurs throughout Structured Literacy instruction. Teachers monitor student performance throughout every lesson for errors or even hesitation to identify already "learned" concepts that need more practice. When a Structured Literacy lesson is calibrated to the students' true level of mastery, approximately 80%–90% of student responses will be correct. Students' consistent success is a hallmark of Structured Literacy lessons that are appropriately planned and implemented.

> **REFLECT, CONNECT, and RESPOND**
> What is the purpose of diagnostic teaching? Give a specific example of how a teacher might use a diagnostic approach during reading/language arts instruction.

Synthetic and Analytic, or Deductive and Inductive, Instruction   Synthetic instruction presents parts of the language and teaches how the parts work together to form a whole; synthetic instruction is **deductive**. For example, phoneme blending, a deductive (parts-to-whole) task, requires the blending of individual speech sounds (phonemes) into a whole syllable (or word): /m/ + /a/ + /sh/ = /mash/.

Analytic instruction teaches how the whole can be broken down into its component parts; analytic instruction is **inductive.** For example, phoneme segmentation, an inductive (whole-to-parts) task, requires the segmentation of a whole syllable (or word) into individual phonemes (whole to parts): /mash/ = /m/ + /a/ + /sh/.

From Skills to Functional Use   Frequent practice of skills helps students move to functional use of these skills; as Paige, Raskinski, and Magpuri-Lavell explained, "Practice is perhaps the best way to develop fluency in any endeavor, whether that endeavor is memorizing a musical score, mastering an athletic movement, learning a dance, or reading a text" (2012, p. 72). Instruction during every lesson moves from teaching of skills to functional use and application of skills. Skills must be mastered to the level of automaticity necessary to free attention and cognitive resources for supporting higher level processes of comprehension and oral/written expression. Therefore, fluency relates to all levels of language learning.

Consistent Use of Structured Literacy Vocabulary   Consistent use of precise vocabulary for discussion of language concepts provides the exposure needed for these words to become consolidated into **long-term memory.** When needed for learning and application of strategies (e.g., decoding, spelling), teachers gradually, logically, and systematically introduce content vocabulary (e.g., *consonant, vowel, syllable, morpheme, voiced, unvoiced, before, after, final, medial, open, closed, stressed, unstressed*), thereby building the vocabulary necessary for both beginning and later learning. Precision supports explicit instruction.

MULTISENSORY INSTRUCTIONAL STRATEGIES

Within Structured Literacy programs, multisensory instructional strategies have proven to be highly effective. The sections that follow explain what multisensory strategies entail and provide a brief history of their use in instruction.

What Are Multisensory Instructional Strategies?

Language involves **intersensory** functioning (i.e., neurological organization for the automatic linkage of auditory, visual, and kinesthetic–motor impressions). The goal of simultaneous multisensory instruction is to foster automatic integration of auditory, visual, and kinesthetic–motor modalities, regardless of which **modality** carries the initial stimulus (e.g., reading begins from the visual stimulus of seeing words; spelling begins from the auditory stimulus of internally hearing words).

The term *multisensory* in this book pertains to instructional strategies used to guide students in simultaneously linking input from eye, ear, voice, and hand to bolster learning during the carefully sequenced teaching of all systems of language. For example, in learning grapheme–phoneme associations, the student receives visual reinforcement by looking at the grapheme; auditory reinforcement from listening to and hearing the phoneme identified with the grapheme; and kinesthetic reinforcement both from feeling the articulatory muscle movement (i.e., the position of the mouth, lips, and tongue) during pronunciation of the phoneme associated with the grapheme and from the unique sequence of muscle movements required for formation of each letter during handwriting. **Tactile** reinforcement occurs while tracing and/or writing the letter on a surface, sometimes roughened.

During multisensory instruction, children learn language concepts by simultaneously using all learning pathways to the brain used in performing language tasks:

1. In the example given to illustrate explicit instruction (Textbox 2.1), for introduction of the new vowel grapheme *ea* that spells the phoneme /ē/, instruction included the use of visual (V) feedback (from seeing the grapheme that represents the phoneme), auditory (A) feedback (from hearing the phoneme as it is pronounced), kinesthetic (K) feedback (from feeling the movements in the mouth as the phoneme is pronounced) and kinesthetic–tactile (Kt) feedback (from the movements of muscles as the letters are formed, i.e., written and/or traced).

2. In the example given to illustrate explicit instruction (Textbox 2.2), for introduction of the suffix -*ly*, instruction included use of the following:

   a. Auditory (A) input when developing the concept (meaning) of the suffix by connecting it to prior knowledge of spoken language

   b. Integration of auditory and kinesthetic–motor (A-Km [for speech]) input when the student listened for and pronounced the /lē/ heard at the end of the word with the suffix -*ly* added

   c. Integration of visual and auditory (V-A) input when the teacher showed the -*ly* card and gave the spelling, pronunciation, and meaning of the suffix

   d. Integration of auditory, visual, and kinesthetic–motor (A-V-Km [for speech]) when the student looked at the suffix, named each letter as it was written, pronounced the phonemes represented by the suffix, and gave the meaning of the suffix.

   In addition, when writing the word on paper, the integration of auditory, visual, and kinesthetic–motor (both speech and writing) modalities were used simultaneously.

   Additional multisensory strategies frequently used in Structured Literacy lessons include fingerspelling (segmenting a word into phonemes for spelling by tapping one phoneme per finger), tracing letters to facilitate retrieval of a phoneme from memory, tracing and/or writing letters while simultaneously pronouncing associated phonemes (or naming letters) to reinforce learning grapheme–phoneme and phoneme–grapheme associations, and using gross motor muscle movement to write with the whole arm in the air or on a desk (sometimes called forming with armswing [fwas], air writing, or writing in the air).

Simultaneous multisensory instruction purposefully integrates visual, auditory, and kinesthetic–motor (for speech and writing) pathways to support memory and learning of both oral and written language skills. The nature of every oral and written language task requires integration of at least two sensory pathways:

- *Copying:* visual to kinesthetic–motor (for writing)
- *Silent reading:* visual to auditory (inner)
- *Oral reading:* visual to auditory to kinesthetic–motor (for speech)
- *Speaking:* auditory (inner) to kinesthetic–motor (for speech)

REFLECT, CONNECT, and RESPOND
What does it mean to say instruction is multisensory? How might a teacher use a simultaneous multisensory approach to practice previously taught grapheme-phoneme relationships?

History of the Use of Multisensory Instructional Strategies

The idea that experiencing learning through multiple modalities reinforces memory has a long history in pedagogy. Educational psychologists of the late 19th century promoted the theory that all senses, including kinesthetic, are involved in learning. The second volume of *The Principles of Psychology* (James, 1890) discussed Binet's theory that all perceptions, in particular those of sight and touch, involve movements of the eyes and limbs, and because such movement is essential in seeing an object, it must be equally essential in forming a visual image of the object. This theory was illustrated through descriptions of typically developing individuals who used tracing to bolster visual memory. Consistent with this theory were observations that the loss of acquired reading ability as a result of impaired visual memory in adults with brain injury could be bypassed through the use of the kinesthetic modality (tracing letters):

> Individuals thus [injured] succeed in reading by an ingenious roundabout way which they often discover themselves: it is enough that they should trace the letters with their finger to understand their sense. . . . The motor image gives the key to the problem. If the patient can read, so to speak, with his fingers, it is because in tracing the letters he gives himself a certain number of muscular impressions which are those of writing. In one word, the patient reads by writing. (James, 1890, p. 62)

The late 19th-century medical literature also contained discussions about the use of bypass strategies in individuals who had lost their ability to read because of cerebral dysfunction (Berlin, 1887; Dejerine, 1892; Morgan, 1896). Hinshelwood (1917) was the first physician to advocate a specific instructional approach for written language disorders in children identified as word blind. On the supposition that reading failure was due to underdevelopment or injury of the brain, Hinshelwood recommended instruction using an alphabetic method in a manner that would appeal to as many cerebral centers as possible.

Orton (1925, 1928) was the first to report in the American medical literature on **word blindness.** Like Hinshelwood (1917), he advocated using all sensory pathways involved in language tasks to reinforce weak memory patterns. In *Reading, Writing and Speech Problems in Children*, Orton explained that from studies over a 10-year period, his team was able to identify one factor common to the entire group: difficulty in "repicturing or rebuilding in the order of presentation, sequences of letters, of sounds, or of units of movement" (1937, p. 145). Orton called for instructional methods based on the simultaneous association of visual, auditory, and kinesthetic fields (e.g., having a person pronounce the visually presented word and then follow the sequence of letters with the fingers during sound synthesis of syllables and words). He stressed the unity of the language system and its sensorimotor connections and stated that listening, speaking, reading, and writing were interrelated functions of language that must be taught in tandem.

Fernald and Keller (1921), Montessori (1912), and Strauss and Lehtinen (1947) developed prominent early educational approaches strongly associated with multisensory instruction; methods for teaching reading, based on their writings, are summarized in Textbox 2.3. A review of their methods reveals the multisensory nature of their instruction, and in particular, the strong role that the tactile–kinesthetic component plays in the learning process. Their rationales for kinesthetic teaching strategies reflected their belief in the tenacity of muscle memory (Montessori, 1912) or the belief that children with nonspecific, developmental neurological impairments would profit from compensatory or bypass techniques used effectively with children with brain injury (Fernald, 1943; Strauss & Lehtinen, 1947). Fernald asserted the need for tactile–kinesthetic experience in word learning and reported that learning rate increased during finger tracing, as compared with use of a stylus or pencil. She quoted the work of Husband (1928) and Miles (1928) on maze learning to support her assertion.

While the medical and psychological literature of the time influenced the use of multisensory strategies for instruction developed to serve children struggling to learn to read, using multisensory strategies also has a long history with students in the general education population. Hunt (1964) reported that motor response was considered extremely important in learning in the early 20th century. Fernald (1943) described how the kinesthetic aspect of multisensory learning, primarily used for reinforcing word recognition through writing, was incorporated into the approaches of many leading practitioners of the time (Dearborn, 1929; Gates, 1927; Hegge, Sears, & Kirk, 1932; Monroe, 1932).

Multisensory strategies are currently in frequent use as part of Orton-Gillingham–based programs and instructional approaches. Directors of Orton-Gillingham–based teacher training programs were surveyed to identify the specific sensory modality used in multisensory strategies in each section of Structured Literacy lessons as taught in their programs (e.g., phonology; phonics, which comprises phoneme–grapheme association; grapheme–phoneme association; and syllables, morphology, syntax, and semantics (Farrell, Pickering, North, & Schavio, 2004). An analysis of survey results indicates that approximately 60% of the sensory strategies were identified as ones that teachers are trained to use with at least 75% of their students.

WHY PHONICS WORKS

Research has provided evidence for why phonics instruction is necessary and effective for teaching children to read and spell an alphabetic orthography. Skilled reading requires accurate processing of the internal details of words—their

Montessori (1912)

Population: Children 3–7 years old from the tenements of Rome

Cause of disability: Economic and cultural deprivation

Method

1. Daily practice with pencil is given in nonwriting activities to develop muscles for holding and using pencil.

2. The child is prepared to write through daily use of light sandpaper. Vowels are taught, then consonants are begun.

   - The teacher presents two vowel cards and says sounds. The child traces the letters repeatedly, eventually with eyes closed.

   - The child is asked to give the teacher cards corresponding to two sounds the teacher pronounces. If the child does not recognize letters by looking, then he or she traces them.

   - The teacher asks the child to give sounds for letters that the teacher presents.

   - When the child knows some vowels and consonants, the teacher dictates familiar words that the child "spells" by selecting cardboard letters from a set containing only letters he or she knows.

3. After about 1 month (for 5-year-olds), the child spontaneously begins to write (i.e., he or she uses a pencil for composing words).

4. When the child knows all of the sounds, he or she reads slips of paper with names of objects that are well known or present.

Length of training: Two weeks is the average time for learning to read and write. The child begins reading phrases that permit the teacher and child to communicate; they play games in which the child reads directions alone and then implements them.

Curriculum control: Although Montessori reported no control for difficulty of words, there is strict control of graphemes written and read through preparatory stages. The child then reads only familiar words after learning all of the sounds.

Phonics: Within the writing program, presentation of graphemes is sequential and cumulative.

Kinesthetic component: "There develops, contemporaneously, three sensations when the teacher shows the letter to the child and has him trace it: the visual sensation, the tactile sensation, and the muscular sensation. In this way the image of the graphic sign is fixed in a much shorter space of time than when it was, according to ordinary methods, acquired only through the visual image. It will be found that the muscular memory is in the young child the most tenacious and, at the same time, the most ready. Indeed, he sometimes recognizes the letters by touching them, when he cannot do so by looking at them. These images are, besides all this, contemporaneously associated with the alphabetical sound" (Montessori, 1912, p. 277).

Strauss and Lehtinen (1947)

Population: Children with brain injury (i.e., organic impairment resulting in neuromotor disturbances in perception, thinking, and/or emotional behavior)

Cause of disability: Disturbances caused by accidental damage to the brain before, during, or after birth

Method

1. According to Strauss & Lehtinen, readiness exercises "emphasize perception and integration of wholes; visual discrimination of forms, letters, and words; organization of space; [and] constructing a figure against a background" (1947, p. 176) as well as "ear training" (p. 177).

2. The child learns to discriminate and reproduce sounds and to blend orally. Next, the child learns to associate visual symbols and writing with sounds. The child learns to articulate sound(s) while writing single letters and then pairs. The child attends to auditory components and visual words, makes words on cards or paper with a stamping set, copies them with crayons emphasizing significant features with color, writes them on the blackboard, and builds them with letter cards.

3. Before the child reads a story, he or she will have learned approximately 10 words in the story as single words, simple sentences, or phrases. The words are later presented in varying contexts or exercises to check comprehension. The child is not expected to conform to absolute standards of accuracy while reading words.

4. The child composes a short story to be dictated to the teacher. The stories are then written or typed with a primer typewriter to be read again.

Length of training: Not specified

Curriculum control: "The child's study of phonics is systematically enlarged. He prepares study materials for himself in the form of lists, cards, sliding devices, booklets, etc. using the phonograms [graphemes] which he encounters in his reading lesson. The work is extrinsic, i.e., the phonic study is supplemental to the reading lesson but closely correlated with it" (Strauss & Lehtinen, 1947, p. 180).

(continued)

TEXTBOX 2.3 *(continued)*

Phonics: No phonics training given

Kinesthetic component: "The reading instruction emphasizes accurate per-ception of words and very early attempts to make the relationship between visual and auditory perception a functioning one. In as many ways as pos-sible, his attention should be drawn to the components of a word, both visual and auditory. He should build words from copy, making them on cards or paper with a stamping set; he should copy them with crayons, emphasizing significant features with color, write them on the blackboard, and build them with letter cards" (Strauss & Lehtinen, 1947, p. 179).

Fernald and Keller (1921)

Population: Nonreaders (i.e., children of typical intelligence who failed to read after individual instruction by other recognized methods in Fer-nald's clinic)

Cause of disability: "Certain variations" (Fernald, 1943, p. 164) in the inte-grated brain functioning of the same region in which lesions are found in acquired alexia

Method

1. A word that the child requests is written in large script. The child repeatedly traces the word with index and middle fingers, saying it over to him- or herself until he or she can write it from memory. The word is erased, and the child writes it, saying the syllables to him- or herself while writing. If the word is incorrect, the process is repeated until the word can be written without the script copy. After a few words are learned, the child is asked to read the word in manuscript print as well as in cursive and then in print only. If the word is incorrect, then it is retaught as in the first presentation.

2. The child starts writing stories initially on subjects of interest to him or her and then, as the child's skill increases, on projects in various school subjects. The child asks for any word he or she does not know how to write, and it is taught as described before he or she uses it. After the story is finished, the child files new words under the proper letters in his or her word file.

Length of training: Average tracing period is about 2 months, with a range of 1–8 months. After a period of tracing, the child develops the ability to learn any new word by simply looking at it in script, copying it, and say-ing each part of the word while writing it.

Curriculum control: Because the child usually is able to recognize words after having written them, this provides a reading vocabulary that usually makes it unnecessary to simplify the content of the first reading.

Phonics: The sound of each letter is never given separately, yet the child is instructed to segment the word into syllables while writing.

Kinesthetic component: "Individuals who have failed to learn to read by visual and auditory methods show a spurt of learning as soon as the kinesthetic method is used. The end product is a skill equal to that of individuals who learn by ordinary methods" (Fernald, 1943, p. 168). Fernald and Keller (1921) reported that the learning rate is much more rapid when using tracing with finger contact than when using a stylus or a pencil.

From *Multisensory Teaching of Basic Language Skills, Third Edition* (pp. 29–30).

phonological, morphological, and orthographic features (Adams, Treiman, & Pressley, 1998; Rayner, Foorman, Perfetti, Pesetsky, & Seidenberg, 2001; Share & Stanovich, 1995; Vellutino et al., 1996). Beginning readers must be aware or must learn that words are made up of individual speech sounds (phonemes). They must be able to represent in their minds the linguistic structure of words they are learning to read—initially at the phoneme level (Ehri et al., 2001; Ehri, 2014), but also at other levels of language structure, especially morphology, or meaningful parts of words (Berninger et al., 2010; Berninger & Wolf, 2016; Henry, 2010; Seidenberg, 2017). Although it may appear that good readers guess at words or that they read whole words as units, good readers in fact process virtually every letter of the words they read (Adams, 1990) and are able, on demand, to translate print to speech rapidly and efficiently. The fluency of this translation process permits a good reader to attend to the meaning of what is read. Therefore, it is logical that effective instruction with poor readers would seek to increase their awareness of phonemes and other linguistic units and that the speech-to-print translation process would become a focus of teaching until the children read fluently enough to focus on comprehension.

Indeed, a wide range of studies has shown that poor readers are marked by weaknesses in phoneme awareness, slow and inefficient decoding skills, inaccurate spelling, and related language-processing difficulties. Poor readers' problems are linguistic in nature and are related to inaccurate and inefficient linguistic coding at basic levels of word and subword processes. Comprehension is impaired when readers cannot decode print accurately or when too much mental energy is being used to recode the message and too little is available for making meaning. Effective instruction addresses these issues as directly and systematically as possible (Berninger & Wolf, 2016; Blachman et al., 2003; Brady, Braze, & Fowler, 2011; Lyon, Fletcher, & Barnes, 2003; Seidenberg, 2017; Torgesen et al., 2001; Vellutino et al., 1996).

Efficacy of Structured Literacy Instruction

Methods for teaching reading in an **alphabetic language,** beginning with the methods used by teachers in ancient Greece, have traditionally included direct teaching of the links between speech sounds and symbols and symbols and speech sounds (graphemes and phonemes) (Matthews, 1966). Prior to 2000, several comprehensive reviews concluded that direct, systematic teaching of phonics for beginning and remedial readers, along with practice in text reading and direct instruction in various comprehension skills, were necessary components of effective instruction if all students were to become successful readers (Adams, 1990; Anderson, Hiebert, Scott, & Wilkinson, 1985; Chall, 1967, 1983). The studies reflected a variety of research methodologies, including small, well-controlled laboratory experiments and large-scale, multiple-classroom research. All of these comprehensive evaluations of research in reading instructional methods concluded that phonics is necessary for elementary reading instruction.

In 2000, the National Reading Panel (National Institute of Child Health and Human Development, 2000) reported on a meta-analysis of research experiments, undertaken between 1970 and 2000, that studied the following components of reading: phonemic awareness, phonics, vocabulary, fluency, comprehension, teacher education, and technology. Although results of the NRP study indicated that systematic phonics instruction produced better growth in reading than all types of nonsystematic or nonphonics instruction, the NRP report indicated no significant difference in results between different methods of systematic phonics instruction (Brady et al., 2011).

In a review of post-2000 studies exploring the effect of various types of phonics instruction, Brady and colleagues (2011) found that developments in research had confirmed and extended the findings of the NRP. The sizeable body of research conducted in the intervening decade indicated that how phonics is taught matters. Brady and colleagues stated that these "findings build the case for the benefits of teaching phonics systematically and explicitly, with advantages evident for complete analysis of the grapheme–phoneme composition of one-syllable words" (Brady et al., 2011, p. 80). Furthermore, these advantages were found "beyond the beginning of first grade and not just for struggling readers" (Brady et al., 2011, p. 80). In the research that has accrued, normally achieving students, students at risk, and readers with severe disabilities all have been shown to benefit from systematic, explicit instruction, with variations in the intensity required (e.g., variations in sessions per week, minutes per session, or size of instructional group). Brady and colleagues (2011) also emphasized the positive effects of classroom instruction that integrates phonics with other aspects of language structure (e.g., morphology, syntax) and language arts activities.

Galuschka, Ise, Krick, and Schulte-Körne (2014) conducted a meta-analysis, involving 22 randomized controlled trials with 49 comparisons of experimental and control groups, to determine the impact of different types of instruction on the word-reading and spelling performance of elementary school students and adolescents. Their results showed that phonics instruction is not only the intervention most frequently investigated but also the only approach (in the 2014 meta-analysis) with a statistically significant impact on reading and spelling performance in children and adolescents with reading disabilities. Adding strength to their findings, Galuschka and colleagues noted the consistency of their results with those reported in previous meta-analyses (Ehri, Nunes, Stahl, & Willows, 2001; McArthur et al., 2012). They concluded,

> At the current state of knowledge, it is adequate to conclude that the systematic instruction of letter–sound correspondences and decoding strategies, and the application of these skills in reading and writing activities, is the most effective method for improving literacy skills of children and adolescents with reading disabilities. (2014, p. 8, online version)

In conclusion, the consensus of educational researchers is that systematic phonics approaches with a focus on grapheme–phoneme associations generally result in better reading skills (i.e., word identification, passage comprehension, and spelling) than instruction that does not teach phonics at all or instruction that does not teach phonics systematically. The effects are even more positive when systematic phonics approaches are integrated with instruction focused on other systems of language structure (e.g., phonology, morphology). These results were found when studying children who do not struggle with learning to read and children who do struggle—as well as children learning to read in languages with either opaque (Ehri et al., 2001) or more transparent (deGraaff, Bosman, Hasselman, & Verhoeven, 2009) orthographies. An orthography is a set of conventions for writing a language, including spelling, hyphenation, capitalization, and punctuation. A **transparent,** or **shallow,** orthography has a one-to-one relationship between its graphemes and phonemes, so both word identification and spelling of words are very consistent. In contrast, an **opaque,** or **deep,** orthography is one that has a more complex system of phoneme–grapheme and phoneme–grapheme correspondences. There are multiple pronunciations (phonemes) associated with a single grapheme (e.g., *oo* is pronounced differently in *moon*, *book*, and *blood*); likewise, there are multiple spellings (graphemes) that represent a single phoneme (e.g., *ai*, *ay*, *a_e*, and *a* are all common spellings, or graphemes, that represent /ā/). English is one of the most opaque languages.

Evidence From Neuroscience

Studies of neuroscience also support the efficacy of using Structured Literacy approaches to teach reading. Results of meta-analyses of behavioral cognitive psychology studies indicated that strategies focusing on **sublexical** units (i.e., grapheme–phoneme associations) yield reading acquisition outcomes superior to approaches that promote memorization of whole words (Rayner et al., 2001; Taylor, Davis, & Rastle, 2017; Yoncheva, Wise, & McCandliss, 2015). Despite strong consensus across the reading research community that instruction focusing on grapheme–phoneme relationships is essential for learning to read alphabetic languages, reading instruction continues to vary across and within English-speaking countries, as Taylor and colleagues described, "from intensive phonic training to multicuing environments that teach sound- and meaning-based strategies" (2017, p. 1).

Taylor and colleagues investigated what they described as the "behavioral and neural consequences of different methods of reading instruction for learning to read single words in alphabetic writing systems" (2017, p. 22) with known oral vocabulary. After all subjects received pretraining to teach meanings of oral vocabulary, they were taught to read novel words over a period of 8 days. Training in one language was biased toward print-to-sound mappings, whereas training in the other language was biased toward print-to-meaning mappings. Results of the study demonstrated that use of systematic print–sound instruction produced marked advantages in accuracy and rate of oral reading, generalization (application) of learned print–sound associations to accurate and faster reading of untrained words, and more accurate comprehension of single vocabulary words earlier in the training cycle. Taylor and colleagues noted,

> These data therefore imply that learning focusing on arbitrary associations between print and meaning may not promote use of direct print-to-meaning associations, and instead hinders use of print-to-sound relationships. . . . Alongside broader oral language teaching, this means embracing phonics-based methods of reading instruction,

and rejecting multicuing or balanced literacy approaches which, our results suggest, may hinder the discovery of spelling–sound relationships essential for reading aloud and comprehension. (2017, p. 22)

Wong (2015) reported in the *Stanford News Service* about a study by Yoncheva, Wise, and McCandliss (2015). Results of the investigation confirmed that instruction designed to explicitly teach students to focus on grapheme–phoneme associations during learning to read unfamiliar words "can impact the circuitry subsequently recruited during reading" (Yoncheva et al., 2015, p. 23). Wong wrote that that words learned through explicit grapheme–phoneme instruction "elicited neural activity biased toward the left side of the brain" (2015, p. 30)—primary regions for visual and language processes. Wong also reported, "In contrast, words learned via whole-word association showed activity biased toward right hemisphere processing" (2015, p. 30). Dominant left-hemisphere activity during acquisition of early word recognition skills is a hallmark of skilled readers and is frequently absent in those who struggle with learning to read (Yoncheva et al., 2015). This 2015 study by Yoncheva and colleagues trained literate adults to read scripts made up of words written with "glyph" (i.e., an artificial orthography). In one condition, learners linked letters to corresponding sounds, and in another condition entire words had to be memorized. After training, **event-related potential (ERP)** responses were recorded as subjects from both conditions read the words— both the words they had been "taught" and the words that were decodable but had not been "taught." An ERP is the measured brain response that is the direct result of a specific sensory, cognitive, or motor event. Reported reaction-time patterns suggested that both trained and transfer words were accessed via sublexical units, yet a left-lateralized, late ERP response showed an enhanced left lateralization for transfer words relative to trained words, potentially reflecting effortful decoding. These findings collectively show that selective attention to grapheme–phoneme associations during learning drives the "lateralization of circuitry" (Yoncheva et al., p. 23) that supports later word recognition. In other words, brain responses to the newly learned words, and the transfer words, were influenced by how subjects learned the words—based on how the words had been taught to them.

McCandliss explained the implications of this study and emphasized how brain functioning can be affected by the instructional choices a teacher makes (as cited in Wong, 2015).

The results underscore the idea that the way a learner focuses their attention during learning has a profound impact on what is learned. It also highlights the *importance of skilled teachers* [emphasis added] in helping children focus their attention on precisely the most useful information. (Wong, 2015, p. 30)

> **REFLECT, CONNECT, and RESPOND**
> What evidence from neuroscience supports the idea that students who learn reading strategies focusing on grapheme-phoneme associations are more likely to become successful readers than students who focus on memorizing whole words?

EFFICACY OF SIMULTANEOUS MULTISENSORY INSTRUCTIONAL STRATEGIES

Clinicians and teachers have long embraced and effectively used multisensory teaching techniques (e.g., Fernald, 1943; Gillingham & Stillman, 1960; Montessori, 1912; Strauss & Lehtinen, 1947). Indeed, Bryant (1979) reported that until the 1970s, special education teachers firmly believed in the value of kinesthetic reinforcement and cited a number of well-known names in the fields of reading and learning disabilities who stressed the importance of multisensory approaches (Ayres, 1972; Cruickshank, Betzen, Ratzeburg, & Tannhauser, 1961; Dearborn, 1940; Frostig, 1965; Gates, 1935; Hegge, Kirk, & Kirk, 1940; Johnson, 1966; Kephart, 1960; Money, 1966; Monroe, 1932; Strauss & Lehtinen, 1947; Wepman, 1964). She also reported that textbooks used to train teachers of students with learning disabilities typically recommended using multisensory techniques for word-recognition instruction and other domains of symbolic and conceptual learning.

Bryant (1979), however, was unable to find any scientific evidence to support the then-current theories for why multisensory instruction was needed for students with learning disabilities (e.g., the theory of deficient **cross-modal integration,** or the ability to link visual and auditory input, such as a letter and the sound it represents). She noted that the popularity of both generic and reading-specific multisensory practices was attributable primarily to reports of success rather than to empirical evidence supporting either the theory or the practice of multisensory teaching. Bryant's (1979) review, as well as subsequent reviews of the research literature in learning disabilities (e.g., Clark, 1988; Clark & Uhry, 1995; Lyon & Moats, 1988; Moats & Lyon, 1993; Torgesen, 1991), failed to find research evidence to support the rationale for multisensory strategies.

At present, most practitioners of Structured Literacy strongly favor the use of multisensory strategies. However, the specific contribution of the multisensory component to the overall success of those programs has not yet been thoroughly documented or explained through rigorous manipulation of instructional conditions and subsequent measurement of outcomes. Likewise, although numerous studies have found the explicit teaching of language structure to be effective for teaching reading and spelling to students with reading disability (Brady et al., 2011; Henry, 2010; Moats, 2010; Washburn, Joshi, & Binks-Cantrell, 2011; see also Chapter 11), no controlled experiments have compared instructional approaches with and without a multisensory component.

Empirical evidence for the specific importance of the multisensory component to the success of Structured Literacy instruction may be explored in studies of cognition and in studies of neuroscience.

Efficacy of Multisensory Strategies: Studies of Cognition

In studies of cognition, research findings within two particular areas help to strengthen the case for using multisensory instructional strategies: research on active learning and research on Triple Word Form Theory (TWFT) (Richards et al., 2006).

Active Learning   Research in cognition demonstrating the need for **active learning** lends support to the rationale for use of simultaneous multisensory teaching strategies. Even before much was known about the nature of linguistic processing in reading disability, there was substantial evidence that successful instructional practices with students who had learning disabilities included deliberate provision of reinforcement and conscious employment of responsive, strategic learning (Brady et al., 2011; Lyon & Moats, 1988; Seidenberg, 2017; Swanson, 1999; Wong, 1991). Berninger and Wolf described how multisensory teaching approaches may make it easier for students to sustain their focus on instruction: Instruction that maintains active interactions between teacher and student(s) is likely to "increase academic engagement in learning" (2016, p. 192) in students with dyslexia and other related learning disabilities (reading disabilities).

As cognitive psychologists have demonstrated, learning is an active, constructive process in which new information is linked with established schemata (Wittrock, 1992). The brain transforms new information in accordance with stored information activated during the learning process. Active learning is learning that causes the learner to mentally search for connections between new and existing information. Instruction that includes teaching metacognition—the deliberate rearrangement, regrouping, or modal transfer of information and the conscious choice of, and evaluation of, the strategies used to accomplish a task—is more effective than rote or passive memorization approaches in almost every domain of learning. Students who must actively do something as they learn attend better to the details of a stimulus and are likely to remember more. For example, students who create their own mnemonic strategies tend to learn from those more readily than students who are provided with a **mnemonic strategy.** Students who think aloud while working remember more and make fewer errors.

Adams and colleagues (1998) completed an extensive review of the research literature on reading comprehension instruction. They concluded that the active (vocal) modeling and rehearsal of basic comprehension functions such as summarizing, questioning, and predicting during an interaction among a teacher and group of students was much more effective in improving comprehension than was structured seatwork or independent silent reading. The high rate of active response on the part of students, the combination of reading and **verbalization** of ideas, and the emphasis on deliberate employment of learning strategies characterized instructional conditions that resulted in retention and generalization of reading comprehension skills.

REFLECT, CONNECT, and RESPOND

How does cognition research demonstrating the need for active learning support the use of simultaneous multisensory teaching strategies in literacy instruction?

Triple Word Form Theory   Another area of study that supports the effectiveness of multisensory instructional strategies is the research on **Triple Word Form Theory (TWFT),** based on the need for phonology–orthography–morphology integration. Learning to read and write words is a process of increasing awareness and coordination (integration) of three different types of word forms and their parts: phonemes, graphemes, and morphemes (Richards et al., 2006). In their review of interdisciplinary research studies and literature that continues to accumulate, Richards and colleagues found compelling empirical support for TWFT: instructional (Bahr, Silliman, Berninger, & Dow, 2012; Berninger et al., 2003); brain imaging (Richards et al., 2006; Richards & Berninger, 2008); behavioral (Garcia, Abbott, & Berninger, 2010; Nagy, Berninger, & Abbott, 2006); cross-sectional (Nagy et al., 2006); longitudinal (Garcia et al., 2010); family genetics (Berninger, Raskind, Richards, Abbott, & Stock, 2008); and reviews of cross-linguistic evidence (Bahr et al., 2012; Berninger & Fayol, 2008; Nunes, Bryant, & Bindman, 2006).

Evidence demonstrates that cross-code integration (i.e., concurrent access of information from all three systems) is critical during the earliest ages and grades (Richards et al., 2006) during which children learn to spell and read—but its role increases as students move up through the grades and are expected to learn to read and spell longer, more complex words in written expression (Garcia et al., 2010). In order to develop greater efficiency and automaticity, teaching based on TWFT principles intentionally includes activities requiring integration of phonological, orthographic, and morphological processing, which requires integration of auditory and kinesthetic motor regions (phonological system), visual regions (orthographic system), and Wernicke's area of the brain (where language comprehension occurs).

Efficacy of instruction that purposefully integrates the teaching of phonology, orthography, and morphology, such as instruction based on TWFT principles, is consistent with research demonstrating that reading disability is almost always the result of deficits in multiple processes (Peterson, Pennington, & Olson, 2013). The relative contribution of each neurocognitive process to difficulty with reading and spelling varies among individuals, and even within individuals, over time (Cox, Seidenberg, & Rogers, 2015; Manis et al., 1999; Seidenberg, 2017). Simultaneous multisensory instruction purposefully integrates visual, auditory, and kinesthetic–motor (for speech and writing) pathways to support memory and learning of both oral and written language skills. Comprehensive instructional approaches that integrate the teaching of listening, speaking, reading, and written expression are incorporating simultaneous multisensory strategies that strengthen connections and enhance memory.

Decades of clinical results support the efficacy of instruction that simultaneously associates auditory, visual, and kinesthetic–motor (for speech and handwriting) modalities for supporting memory and learning both oral and written language skills. More recent studies have demonstrated that TWFT predicts development of reading and spelling (Bahr et al., 2012; Berninger, Garcia, & Abbott, 2009; Garcia et al., 2010) and vocabulary (Verhoeven & Perfetti, 2011) based on coordination of the three word forms and their parts: phonemes, graphemes, and morphemes.

Neuroscience Offers Insights Into Reading and Multisensory Processing

The efficacy of structured, systematic, explicit teaching of all language-based skills is no longer questioned by leading researchers (Adams, 1990; Berninger & Wolf, 2016; Lyon, Fletcher, Fuchs & Chhabra, 2005; Moats, 2010; Seidenberg, 2017; Wolf, 2007). However, empirical support for the efficacy of multisensory instructional strategies remains elusive in studies of reading instruction (Bryant, 1979; Clark, 1988; Clark & Uhry, 1995; Lyon & Moats, 1988; Torgesen, 1991). Nevertheless, theoretical support for the added benefit of multisensory techniques can be sought from neuroscience studies.

For example, Dehaene explained the critical role of associations between the visual and phonological systems during reading:

> Reading instruction capitalizes on the prior presence of efficient connections between visual and phonological processors. I therefore think it very likely that dyslexia arises from a joint deficit of vision and language. The weakness itself probably rests somewhere at the crossroads between invariant visual recognition and phonemic processing… brain imaging supports the claim that the crux of the problem often lies at the interface between vision and speech, inside the web of connections found in the left temporal lobe. (2009, pp. 242–243)

Although acknowledging the importance of integrating visual symbols with auditory speech signals during reading, Dehaene pointed out the additional need for visual–spatial attention:

> Good decoding skills do not arise from associations between letters and speech sounds alone—letters must also be perceived in their proper orientation at the appropriate spatial locations, and in their correct left–right order. In the young reader's brain, collaboration must take place between the **ventral visual pathway,** which recognizes the identity of letters and words, and the **dorsal pathway,** which codes for their location in space and programs eye movements and attention. When any one of these actors stumbles, reading falls flat on its face (2009, p. 298)

Dehaene attributes the success of teaching methods, such as Montessori, to their emphasis on motor gestures. He suggests, "Multisensory studies open up a whole new line of future research. Brain imaging may perhaps be able to show that the tactile method improves the functional connections linking the dorsal and ventral pathways" (2009, p. 299).

Imaging the Reading Brain: Window Into Structure and Function   In Part II of their comprehensive review of the neurobiological bases of reading disability, with particular attention to developmental considerations, Black, Xia, and Hoeft (2017) emphasized the role that rapid advances in technology, greater accessibility to modern neuroimaging techniques, and enhanced precision in methods for analysis of data have played in creation of opportunities for significant advances in understanding of the **neural correlates of typical reading and reading disability** (i.e., brain activity that corresponds with, and is necessary to produce, typical reading or reading disability).

Modern imaging techniques are yielding new insights into the structure and function of the human brain, advancing understanding of reading and reading disabilities, and elevating knowledge of the multisensory nature of the brain. In particular, **neuroimaging** research provides insights into the reading brain, whereas another body of work is generating findings about the brain's holistic multisensory design. Both are promising avenues of research for investigating the contribution of the multisensory component to the effectiveness of Structured Literacy instruction.

Structural neuroimaging (magnetic resonance imaging [MRI]) allows researchers to examine the brain's physical characteristics, or structure. **Functional neuroimaging (fMRI),** in which images are constructed showing brain activity while individuals perform specific activities, provides a glimpse of how the brain is organized to allow individuals to perform complex cognitive tasks (e.g., reading). These powerful imaging technologies explore the inner workings and architecture of living brains and have changed the landscape of neuroscience.

Studies of Normal Reading   Cognitive (Taylor, Rastle, & Davis, 2013) and computational (Seidenberg & McClelland, 1989) models of reading are working in parallel with neuroimaging research to define more precisely the multiple areas and complex brain networks involved in typical reading (Price, 2012). Figure 2.1 (Black et al., 2017) illustrates the integration of multiple brain networks required by every reading task. Research consensus (reported by Black et al., 2017, p. 5) indicates that typical reading requires the integration of orthographic, phonological, and semantic processes:

> These networks include primarily the left ventral system (including the occipito-temporal region—posterior fusiform gyrus [FG] and the inferior temporal gyrus [ITG]) for **orthographic processing,** the left dorsal system (including the temporo-parietal region—supramarginal gyrus [SMG] and posterior superior temporal gyrus [STG], as well as dorsal inferior frontal gyrus [IFG]) for phonological processing,

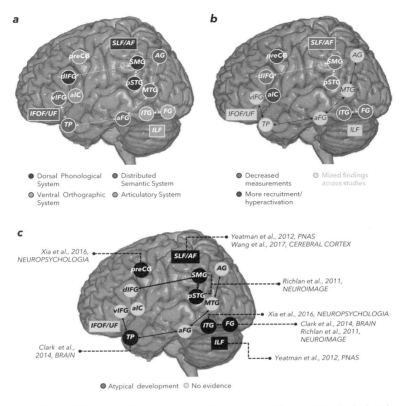

Figure 2.1. a) Neural circuits important for skilled reading; b) findings in individuals with decoding-based reading disorder; and c) atypical ontogenesis of reading-related circuits in reading disorder. A full-color version of this figure is available in the Online Companion Materials at http://www.brookespublishing.com/birshcarreker/materials. (From Black, J.M., Xia, J., & Hoeft, F. [2017]. Neurobiological bases of reading disorder, part II: The importance of developmental considerations in typical and atypical reading. *Language and Linguistics Compass, 11*[10]. Reprinted by permission.)

and a more distributed system across the brain for semantic and sentence/**syntactic processing** (including the angular gyrus, anterior FG, temporal pole, middle temporal gyrus and ventral IFG) (Graves, Desai, Humphries, Seidenberg, & Binder, 2010; Martin, Schurz, Kronbichler, & Richlan, 2015; McNorgan, Chabal, O'Young, Lukic, & Booth, 2015; Price, 2012; Taylor et al., 2013; Vigneau et al., 2006; Vigneau et al., 2011).

Black and colleagues' (2017) analysis of studies by Franceschini, Gori, Ruffino, Pedrolli, and Facoetti (2012) and Segers, Damhuis, van de Sande, and Verhoeven (2016) revealed that more generalized cognitive abilities (e.g., visual attention, executive function) not specific to the reading domain may also be associated with individual differences in reading and that early (or late) acquisition of these cognitive skills can aid, or interfere with, learning to read at later ages (Pugh et al., 2013).

Studies of Reading Disabilities (Dyslexia) A number of imaging studies documenting anatomical differences in dyslexia (reading disability) converge with the seminal neuropathological studies that found neuronal migration differences, including polymicrogyria (a severe type of neuronal migration abnormality), in the cerebral cortex of people with dyslexia (e.g., Galaburda, Sherman, Rosen, Aboitiz, & Geschwind, 1985). Additional current converging evidence suggests that dyslexia (i.e., reading disability) has multiple components.

In their 2017 review of the neurobiological bases of reading disorder, Black and colleagues acknowledged the ways that greater accessibility to neuroimaging technologies has contributed to increased understanding of language-based reading disabilities, their biological bases, and their responsiveness—or lack of responsiveness—to intervention (Maisog, Einbinder, Flowers, Turkeltaub, & Eden, 2008; Martin, Kronbichler, & Richlan, 2016).

Although there is much still to be discovered about reading disability, the consensus of researchers is that atypical brain maturation is a factor. The brain undergoes significant changes in structure and connectivity on the path from childhood to adulthood. The developmental trajectory of these changes (e.g., disruptions in structure or disruptions in connectivity) is a consideration in understanding the brain and neurodevelopmental disorders (Dennis & Thompson, 2013). Understanding the developmental trajectory in greater detail should contribute to discovery of more efficient and effective interventions.

Black and colleagues (2017) presented a summary of their findings on neural deficits in individuals with reading disability. Consensus is that reduced activation and atypical structure in brain areas associated with phonological processing is the most frequently occurring deficit for students with reading disability (Melby-Lervåg, Lyster, & Hulme, 2012) followed by anomalies in regions important for orthographic processing (Linkersdorfer et al., 2015; Richlan, 2014). When compared to both age-matched and reading-marched controls (Hoeft et al., 2006; Xia, Hoeft, Zhang, & Shu, 2016), reduced activation and atypical structure in brain areas associated with phonological processing were noted, which indicates persistent anomalies instead of maturational delay or lack of reading experience.

Hyperactivation, volume increase, and increased connectivity may indicate use of compensatory mechanisms. Hyperactivation during reading has been reported relatively consistently in students with dyslexia (reading disability) within brain region networks involved in both articulation and naming (Lopez-Barroso et al., 2013; Lopez-Barroso et al., 2015). This finding suggests the possibility that individuals with dyslexia (reading disability) can compensate for their phonological-related impairments by using an articulatory strategy (Hancock, Richlan, & Hoeft, 2017).

Sometimes brain anomalies (in structure and/or function) have been observed in brain areas not associated with phonological or orthographic processing. Consistent with a multiple deficit model of reading disability (Pennington, 2006), there may be a variety of risk factors and anomalous neural pathways (e.g., visual attention, attention shifting, procedural learning)—other than phonological or orthographic processing deficits—that are contributing to reading disability.

Developmental changes occurring throughout the life span, especially during the first 20 years of life, are determined by complex interactions between genetics and environment (Giedd & Rapoport, 2010; Richmond, Johnson, Seal, Allen, & Whittle, 2016) that vary between typical readers and those with reading disability (Bishop, 2015). In addition, it is possible that differences throughout development, between those with and without reading disability, may continue to change based on experience (i.e., before learning to read, during learning to read, and/or after reading skills has been acquired) (Goswami, Power, Lallier, & Facoetti, 2014). Studying how developmental trajectories change over time should help to clarify whether these changes are the result of poor reading over time, whether they are due to "innate vs. learning protective factors," or whether there is another causal relationship (Black et al., 2017, p. 5).

Mounting evidence has shown that poor readers, regardless of their IQ score (e.g., below-average readers with average IQ scores; average readers with high IQ scores), show similar difficulties in phonological processing and respond to reading intervention services equally well. Two studies focused on different types of identification criteria for reading disabilities: low reading achievement versus discrepancy between IQ score and reading achievement (Hancock, Gabrieli, & Hoeft, 2016; Tanaka et al., 2011). When compared to typical readers, the brains of individuals with poor single-word reading ability, including those with both low IQ scores and average IQ scores, showed similar characteristics—left temporo-parietal dysfunction believed to be associated with phonological processing (Tanaka et al., 2011). Furthermore, and more interesting, the brains of children with high IQ scores and discrepant single-word reading ability (i.e., much lower, albeit "normal to age-appropriate") showed some of the same characteristics—left temporo-parietal dysfunction—as those of poor readers with average IQ scores (Hancock et al., 2016). Children with high IQ scores and average word-reading ability showed less brain activation in these critical areas than both children with high IQ scores and high reading ability and children with normal IQ scores and normal reading ability. *The Diagnostic and Statistical Manual of Mental Disorders, Fifth Edition* explained that these high-IQ, or intellectually gifted, students "may be able to sustain apparently adequate academic functioning by using compensatory strategies, extraordinarily high effort, or support, until the learning demands or assessment procedures (e.g., timed tests) pose barriers to their demonstrating their learning or accomplishing required tasks" (American Psychiatric Association, 2013, p. 69).

Despite the challenges, deep understanding of the "neural mechanisms" at the foundation of reading disability will be necessary for accurate determination of optimal instruction and intervention.

Intervention Studies: Individuals With Dyslexia (Reading Disability) Intervention studies have focused more on the brain mechanisms of normalization and compensation than causes (Barquero, Davis, & Cutting, 2014). Several studies on the effect of intensive, systematic, structured language instruction on children with reading disabilities have shown that functional brain patterns may become more normalized as a consequence of instruction (Berninger et al., 2003; Blachman et al., 2003; Meyler, Keller, Cherkassky, Gabrieli, & Just, 2008; Shaywitz, 2003; Simos et al., 2002). Increased activation of left hemisphere parietal-temporal and occipital-temporal regions was seen in response to structured language teaching approaches. After structured language instruction, these brain areas might be better able to handle the complicated task of automatic word recognition. In addition, functional connectivity differences in children with reading disability, in comparison with controls, were eliminated after a 3-week treatment program consisting of explicit instruction in the alphabetic principle and linguistic awareness training (Richards & Berninger, 2008).

Thus, one possibility is that individuals with reading disability who have weak phonological processing must establish stronger and/or alternative circuits for word recognition to compensate for disruption of the circuitry normally relied on for reading. Also, it is possible that activation of sensorimotor pathways through the use of remedial instruction strategies involving the fingertips, hand, arm, and/or vocal speech apparatus during symbolic learning can change the circuits necessary for word recognition that are more easily established and accessed. The neurobiological mechanisms through which brain changes may be influenced by multisensory instruction are largely unknown, although there are hints from understanding the multisensory nature of the organization of the human brain.

The Multisensory Brain: A Powerful Design   For years, students of neuroscience were taught that the neocortex is subdivided into three functional areas: sensory, motor, and association. As it turns out, this traditional view of cerebral cortex organization is wrong. Science has discovered that the brain's multisensory processing capabilities are more elaborate and less compartmentalized than previously believed. Old models of cerebral cortex organization, with neatly compartmentalized regions specializing in specific modalities, are giving way to a greater appreciation of the holistic multisensory nature of the brain. For example, the learning of new vocabulary words involves integration of auditory and speech areas within the brain (Lopez-Barroso et al., 2013). The human brain does not have a single, simple language system, but instead, complex language networks. Multiple brain imaging studies have demonstrated that both common and unique brain regions activate during oral language tasks (i.e., listening, speaking) and written language tasks (i.e., reading, writing) (Berninger & Wolf, 2016).

The clinical wisdom of Structured Literacy practitioners has long capitalized on the bases that much of the brain is responsive to multiple senses and that the large portion of the human brain is dedicated to association areas, areas that have evolved more recently than other brain regions.

Research on Multisensory Integration   Basic research in neuroscience has demonstrated the facilitative effect that occurs when information is received through more than one sensory modality (Murray, Lewkowicz, Amedi, & Wallace, 2016). Evidence suggesting that these simultaneous cues from multiple senses can enhance the precision and robustness of information, and improve memory, continues to accumulate (Talsma, Senkowski, Soto-Faraco, & Woldorff, 2010; Stein, Stanford, & Rowland, 2014). However, some current studies have shown that individuals with reading disability may have particular difficulty with integrating information through multiple senses (i.e., **multisensory integration**) (Murray et al., 2016). It would be reasonable to hypothesize that use of systematic strategies to purposefully associate multisensory stimuli should particularly benefit individuals with reading disability because these strategies are likely to help compensate for this deficit in multisensory integration. To address this hypothesis, it is critically necessary that pure scientists and educational practitioners collaborate—using true-to-life instructional variables to the extent possible. Without this collaboration, scientists may design solutions based on tasks or situations that are not germane to learning to read in the real world of classrooms and clinics. As a result, teachers and clinicians will be left without evidence to support instructional strategies they find essential to teaching individuals with reading disability.

Background   Multisensory processes are essential for perception, cognition, learning, and behavior. Input to the senses is continuous, and the brain must combine (or bind) the unisensory perceptual inputs that refer to the same object (often referred to as crossmodal binding) while "tuning out" inputs that belong to different objects. Studies have revealed a general developmental pattern—multisensory perceptual narrowing and the parallel gradual emergence and growth of increasingly more discriminating multisensory associations—that exists between and among all types of pairings, such as vision and audition, as well as tactile-to-visual transfer of shape information (Murray et al., 2016). The wiring of the brain, which facilitates the integration of multisensory information, supports the binding process. For example, Murray and colleagues (2016) reported that individuals can better comprehend a speaker in a noisy room when they can see the speaker's mouth. Furthermore, Murray and colleagues (2016) reported that initially presenting a stimulus in a multisensory context (e.g., a bird together with the sound that it makes) affects the ability to recall the same stimulus when it is presented through only one modality.

A variety of studies have investigated how and when stimuli from different sensory modalities are integrated and what factors enhance binding. Studies focused on the roles that spatial and temporal factors play in crossmodal binding traditionally have shown that the closer in space and time the stimuli from different modalities are presented, the more likely multisensory integration is to occur (Spence, 2011). For example, babies attend better to multisensory events that are spatially and temporally congruent and thus associated with a common source. Another characteristic is crossmodal correspondence. Spence reported a large body of research indicating that individuals show consistent crossmodal correspondences between stimulus characteristics in different sensory modalities. He gave the following example: "People consistently match high-pitched sounds with small bright objects that are located high up in space" (Spence, 2011, p. 971). Semantic congruency, situations in which pairs of auditory and visual stimuli match in terms of their identity or meaning, is another factor that influences multisensory integration. Spence reviewed studies indicating the possibility of "several qualitatively different kinds of crossmodal correspondence—statistical, structural, and semantically mediated—and that they may have different developmental trajectories as well as different consequences for human perception and behaviour" (2011, p. 972). He reported that crossmodal associations between many different pairs of sensory modalities (e.g., vision and touch, audition and touch, auditory pitch and smell) have now been documented. He concluded that it appears likely that crossmodal correspondences exist between all possible pairings of sensory modalities.

Research on Multisensory Integration and Dyslexia (Reading Disability)
Hahn, Foxe, and Molholm (2014) reported that learning to read requires formation of cross-sensory associations between speech sounds and the letters that spell those sounds (graphemes). For most individuals, these correspondences begin to become automated; seeing graphemes eventually activates the phonological representation. They cited evidence that there is reduced integration of grapheme–phoneme inputs in individuals with reading disability. However, it is not clear if the reduced grapheme–phoneme integration is a specific deficit or if it is a consequence of a more fundamental and thus far-reaching impairment in auditory–visual multisensory integration. Hahn and colleagues (2014) proposed that the impairment could be accounted for by an insult to the regions involved in the processing and integration of graphemes and phonemes, or it may represent a more general deficit in the integration of multisensory information.

A variety of theories have been proposed to explain the problem that individuals with reading disability have with multisensory integration. Hahn and colleagues (2014) postulated that there is a temporal window of integration (TWIN) within which inputs are integrated into one perceptual unit—and that anomalies in the size of the TWIN contribute to reading difficulty. They reported that there is an indication that the multisensory TWIN (too large, or overly variable) differs in those with reading disability and may be the cause of the difficulties individuals with reading disability experience with learning grapheme–phoneme associations. They look to advances in structural neuroimaging methods, such as diffusion-weighted imaging (DWI), which has identified potential weaknesses in anatomical connectivity in reading disability. Hahn and colleagues (2014) pointed out

> These data reveal potential weaknesses in key nodes of the reading network in reading disability and the pathways that connect them. The temporo–parietal focus of reduced connectivity is consistent with deficits in the neural architecture involved in integrating multisensory inputs. (p. 12 [online manuscript])

They listed a number of studies suggesting that multisensory instruction significantly improves reading in individuals with reading disability (Ecalle, Magnan, Bouchafa, & Gombert, 2009; Kast, Baschera, Gross, Jäncke, & Meyer, 2011; Veuillet, Magnan, Ecalle, Thai-Van, & Collet, 2007).

Harrar and colleagues identified "sluggish attention shifting" (2014, p. 533) between modalities as a possible cause of difficulty that individuals with reading disability have with multisensory integration. The authors described a redundant effect in which individuals' reaction times to combined sensory stimuli were faster than to either visual or auditory alone. This is called the redundant target effect because individuals respond more rapidly when there are multiple (redundant) signals. They reported that adults with reading disability responded significantly more slowly, compared to matched controls with a motor response to either visual, auditory, or auditory–visual stimuli; the delayed response was similar across modalities. However, compared with controls, those with reading disability showed differences (i.e., difficulty shifting their attention between modalities) in auditory–visual integration. Such "sluggish attention shifting" (Harrar et al., 2014, p. 533) appeared only when individuals with reading disability shifted their attention from the visual to the auditory modality. Controls demonstrated what they considered to be typical results: Reaction times to auditory targets were faster than to visual targets. Individuals with reading disability found it harder to shift their attention away from visual stimuli or toward auditory stimuli. They concluded that 1) those with reading disability "benefit less" than controls from integrating the two senses due to a number of factors, and 2) limited attention resources are unevenly distributed in favor of vision. They hypothesized that subjects with reading disability might learn auditory–visual phonological associations faster if they first hear the sound and then see the corresponding letter/word (grapheme) because crossmodal shifts from audition to vision were not sluggish. They speculated that perceptual learning to train low-level, basic neurological processes could lead to benefits in upstream functions such as attentional networks (e.g., cross modal attention and spatial attention) and eventually reading.

Hancock, Pugh, and Hoeft suggested that neural noise (i.e., "sources of random variability in the firing activity of neural networks and membrane voltage of single neurons" [2017, p. 435]) can affect cognition and brain function, especially sensory processing in individuals with reading disability. Learning to read requires integration of multiple component processes, including sensory processing (often under perceptually noisy conditions), intact phonological awareness, orthographic processing, and the ability to map graphemes to their corresponding speech sounds. Hancock and colleagues (2017) suggested that, although effects may differ between individual students, neural noise is likely to cause disruption of multisensory integration (e.g., grapheme–phoneme mappings) for students with reading disability and perhaps disruption to some subprocesses of reading (e.g., orthographic or phonological processing).

Berninger and Wolf (2016) discussed ways that multisensory instruction can support students' learning. They emphasized the role of simultaneous multisensory instruction for supporting integration: "multimodal teaching may be necessary to help students with reading disability integrate information across sensory input modalities and link these modalities with motor output and internal language systems" (Berninger & Wolf, 2016, p. 192). In addition, instruction that involves multiple systems and input modalities for language provides students opportunities to create new "cognitive connections" (Berninger & Wolf, 2016).

REFLECT, CONNECT, and RESPOND

What research evidence suggests that individuals with reading disability have difficulties with multisensory integration? What implications does this problem have for teaching reading to students with reading disabilities?

Summary of Neuroscience Research on Multisensory Integration For in-depth information related to the findings on multisensory integration listed next, refer to Berninger and colleagues (2002); Berninger and Wolf (2016); Black and colleagues (2017); Calvert and Lewis (2004); Harrar and colleagues (2014); Lachs (2017); Macaluso and Driver (2004); Murray and colleagues (2016); Spence (2011); Stein and colleagues (2014); Talsma and colleagues (2010); Taylor, Davis, and Rastle (2017); and Wallace (2004). Key findings can be summed up as follows:

1. Multisensory processing of sensory inputs is a fundamental rule of brain structure and function. Individuals constantly use information from all of their senses. Even experiences that appear specific to one sense (e.g., vision) are modulated by activity in other senses (Calvert & Lewis, 2004; Spence, 2011).

2. The brain's multisensory design facilitates attention, perception, and learning. Reaction times are faster in reaction to multisensory stimuli (Harrar et al., 2014; Wallace, 2004).

3. Multisensory brain regions that respond to two or more sensory modalities (e.g., vision, auditory, tactile, olfactory) may exist in the human brain from infancy (Murray et al., 2016; Spence, 2011; Stein et al., 2014; Talsma et al., 2010).

4. We are not always aware of multisensory interactions. For example, there is activity in the visual cortex during tactile perception (Berninger & Wolf, 2016; Macaluso & Driver, 2004), and speech comprehension increases when a speaker is seen as well as heard (Calvert & Lewis, 2004; Lachs, 2017; Murray et al., 2016; Sumby & Pollack, 1954).

5. Voluntary motor responses link (bind) with their intended and expected perceptual effects, leading to synchronization of distant brain areas so that noise in the system is reduced and communication is improved, resulting in the "collective enhancement of precision" (Tabareau & Slotine, 2010, p. 1; see also Murray et al., 2016).

6. Speech perception is the product of multisensory networks stimulated by auditory inputs (voice) and visual inputs (observed movement of the lips and mouth), resulting in rich interpersonal interactions (Murray et al., 2016; Sumby & Pollack, 1954).

7. Not only common, but also unique, brain regions activate for listening, speaking, reading, and writing tasks (Berninger et al., 2002), so these language systems work together to some extent, but the brain does not have a single, simple language system (Berninger & Wolf, 2016; Lachs, 2017).

The human brain is a multisensory organ—with multiplicities of cross-modal convergence from the single neuron level to the cortical region level and from early to late stages of processing. The seminal work of Geschwind (1965) established relationships between the brain's structure and function. The fundamentals of these relationships have not been challenged, but converging research demonstrates that the interrelated elements and connectional patterns necessary for integrated multisensory processing are strikingly complex and intertwined (Lachs, 2017). Harnessing this powerful and encompassing cerebral design and its learning capacity should be a goal in education, particularly for children challenged by certain learning tasks (e.g., students with reading disability).

IMPLICATIONS FOR FUTURE RESEARCH AND PRACTICE: A TWO-WAY STREET

What does all this mean for educators, particularly those incorporating multisensory teaching strategies into evidence-based reading interventions for children with reading disabilities? Although studies of cognition and neuroscience have provided promising results, researchers do not yet have definitive proof of the efficacy of multisensory instructional strategies.

Three cardinal principles have emerged from scientific research to shape education policies and professional standards and practices, particularly as they relate to reading and reading disabilities:

1. Instruction should be scientifically based (NICHD, 2000).

2. Training in learning processes should be linked to the content that is to be learned. Fletcher and colleagues concluded, "Training in motor, visual, neural, or cognitive processes without academic content does not lead to better academic outcomes" (2007, p. 130). In a review that analyzed the use of cognitive tasks or "brain games" as a means to improve academic or cognitive performance on other tasks, Simons and colleagues found

    Extensive evidence that brain-training interventions improve performance on the trained tasks, less evidence that such interventions improve performance on closely related tasks, and little evidence that training enhances performance on distantly related tasks or that training improves everyday cognitive performance. (2016, p. 103)

3. Reading disabilities can be prevented in many young children (the optimal approach with the best return) and alleviated at any age. With appropriate and intensive instruction, students with all but the most severe reading disabilities can be effectively taught in the early grades so they stay on track toward academic success (Gaab, 2017; Lyon, 2016; Lyon et al., 2001; Torgesen, 2004).

All three principles are pillars of evidence-based reform and are elevating standards of knowledge and practice among educators working with children with reading disabilities or at risk for reading failure (e.g., IDA [2018] *Knowledge and Practice Standards*).

A caveat is in order regarding the first principle, however. Scientifically based instructional practices have proven value, but it does not follow that instructional practices lacking scientific evidence necessarily have no value. Sagan's controversial quote—"Absence of evidence is not evidence of absence" (1997, p. 213)—applies. As Carolyn Cowen (personal communication) has explained, "In other words, lack of scientific evidence supporting the efficacy of the multisensory strategies inherent in Structured Literacy instruction reflects lack of scientific study, the absence of which does not refute the value of these strategies." It does, however, reflect the inherent difficulties in conducting such studies. Given the brain's dynamic and holistic multisensory nature, the challenges in attempting to isolate and manipulate multisensory inputs and outputs in the context of evidence-based reading instruction cannot be overstated.

Decades of support from generations of knowledgeable and skilled practitioners certainly offer a basis for assigning value to the multisensory ingredient in Structured Literacy approaches, particularly for children with reading disabilities. However, as Cowen wrote, "In this era of evidence-based education, citing clinical support and testimony will not suffice, even when authoritative and compelling" (2004). The irony is that the community of practitioners, schools, programs, and organizations that practice and promote the principles of Structured Literacy helped lay the groundwork for research in reading and reading disability, which in turn helped pave the way for evidence-based education policies.

Still, Structured Literacy educators have a vital role to play. Cowen explained, "Just as research can inform instruction, educators' insights can inform research" (2009, p. 4). Even with all that is known, researchers do not have all the answers, and formidable challenges remain in implementing and scaling the answers they do have. An approach that partners educators and researchers tasked with generating translational research (practice-based research to achieve evidence-based practice) might lead to answers that help bridge the clinic to classroom chasm and facilitate scalable scientifically based practices (Sherman & Cowen, 2009). Clinical observations can be wellsprings for hypotheses. At the very least, knowledgeable practitioners' insights might lead researchers to important questions such as, "What is the contribution of the multisensory component to evidence-based instruction?"

Neuroscience is rapidly advancing the understanding of reading and reading disabilities and elevating knowledge of the multisensory nature of the brain. A basis of support for the multisensory strategies inherent in Structured Literacy instruction is likely to emerge from the continuing application of powerful imaging technologies to further illuminate the complexities of the brain's structure and function. Additional evidence is also likely to emerge from the unfolding of discoveries related to the brain's powerfully holistic multisensory design. Even with all the advances science and its technologies bring, fundamental points may have been overlooked. It would be a mistake to dismiss the potential value of multisensory strategies in Structured Literacy before the research has been done to validate it.

REFLECT, CONNECT, and RESPOND

A colleague mentions to you that she spends as little time as possible on phonics instruction; she herself disliked "drill-and-kill" phonics lessons as a child, so she feels phonics lessons accomplish very little and make children view reading lessons as unmotivating. What would you say to demonstrate to your colleague that phonics instruction 1) is an important component of literacy instruction, 2) has a vast base of scientific research to support its relevance, and 3) when part of a comprehensive Structured Literacy format, can be intellectually stimulating?

CLOSING THOUGHTS: MULTISENSORY STRUCTURED LITERACY

As noted in this chapter, Structured Literacy techniques have been cited (Henry, 2010; Moats, 2010; Seidenberg, 2017; Spear-Swerling & Cheesman, 2012; Washburn et al., 2011; Wolf et al., 2017; see also Chapter 11) and recommended by experts in the field of learning disorders from before and throughout the 20th century and into the 21st century. A variety of Structured Literacy approaches and programs incorporate similar content and principles of instruction. The simultaneous association of **visual, auditory, kinesthetic–motor, and tactile (VAKT)** sensory modalities used in multisensory instruction has traditionally been a staple of remedial intervention for students with reading disabilities. According to clinical reports, most practitioners of Structured Literacy strongly favor the use of multisensory strategies. Although many of the programs incorporating Structured Literacy strategies have been effective, the specific contribution of the multisensory component to the overall success of those programs has not yet been thoroughly documented or explained through rigorous manipulation of instructional conditions and subsequent measurement of outcomes.

Knowledgeable and skilled clinicians have been hoping for a scientific explanation for accepted multisensory instructional practices for years, and much progress has been made. Cognitive psychology, educational psychology, and the neurosciences may eventually provide even more definitive support for specific multisensory techniques of teaching. Although neuroscience, cognitive psychology, educational psychology, and educational intervention research continue to pave the way toward an even better understanding of the reading brain and effective instruction, the practices detailed in this book rest on both clinical experience and solid science.

ONLINE COMPANION MATERIALS

The following Chapter 2 resources are available at http://www.brookespublishing.com/birshcarreker/materials:

- Reflect, Connect, and Respond Questions
- Appendix 2.1: Knowledge and Skill Assessment Answer Key
- A full-color version of Figure 2.1 showing neural activity during reading

KNOWLEDGE AND SKILL ASSESSMENT

1. A teacher is planning a Structured Literacy lesson for her student. Initially, she used informal assessment to determine which phoneme–grapheme associations the student had mastered. For new learning, she selects the next unknown phoneme–grapheme association in order of difficulty. Which principle of Structured Literacy does this choice represent?

    a. Instruction is diagnostic.

    b. Instruction is explicit.

    c. Instruction is sequential.

    d. Instruction is multisensory.

2. A teacher is delivering a Structured Literacy lesson. Within this lesson, he presents cards with single letters printed on them and asks the student to pronounce the associated sound. He has the student read lists of single words as well as connected text. Which of the following do these activities represent?

   a. Grapheme to phoneme

   b. Phoneme to grapheme

   c. Speech to text

   d. Text to speech

3. Research studies have identified differences between the brains of individuals with and without reading disability (dyslexia). Which of the following has *not* been reported regarding students with dyslexia?

   a. Potential weaknesses in anatomical connectivity patterns have been identified.

   b. Functional brain activation patterns become more normalized after Structured Literacy intervention.

   c. During reading, there is hypoactivation within brain areas involved in articulation and naming.

   d. The process of multisensory integration occurs at a slower rate.

4. Regarding the efficacy of the use of multisensory instructional strategies, which of the following is true?

   a. Researchers have documented the efficacy of multisensory instructional strategies.

   b. Researchers have studied the efficacy of multisensory instructional strategies.

   c. The National Reading Panel recommended the use of multisensory instructional strategies.

   d. The National Reading Panel identified the best multisensory methodology for teaching phonics.

5. Which is an example that demonstrates a student's understanding English morphology?

   a. Knowing the multiple spellings for /ā/ and how to make an informed choice

   b. Knowing that *fine,* the base in the words *finish* and *definite,* means "to end"

   c. Knowing that the sentence "He the hamburger delicious ate" is grammatically incorrect

   d. Knowing that the definition of the word *left* varies depending on context

6. The Triple Word Form Theory relates to the integration of which three components of language?

   a. Phonology, orthography, and morphology

   b. Phonology, orthography, and syntax

   c. Orthography, morphology, and semantics

   d. Phonology, morphology, and syntax

7. Which statement best describes how different regions of the brain activate during various kinds of language tasks (listening, speaking, reading, writing)?

   a. Different kinds of tasks involve activation in essentially the same regions.

   b. Different kinds of tasks involve activation in different regions.

   c. Different kinds of tasks involve activation in some of the same regions as well as some regions unique to the specific task.

   d. Neurological research has so far yielded little insight into how different regions of the brain activate during different kinds of tasks.

8. Results of the National Reading Panel study indicated which of the following?

   a. Systematic phonics instruction produced better growth in reading than all types of nonsystematic or nonphonics instruction.

   b. Balanced literacy instruction produced better growth in reading than all types of phonics instruction.

   c. Direct meaning-based word identification instruction produced better growth in reading than all types of phonics instruction.

   d. Use of the three-cueing systems produced better growth in reading than all other types of instruction.

9. Which is an example of synthetic instruction?

   a. Teaching how to segment the word *sheep* into phonemes:
   /shēp/ ➔ /sh/ /ē/ /p/

   b. Teaching how to determine the morphemes in *incredible:*
   incredible ➔ *in-* + *crede* + *-ible*

   c. Teaching how to blend phonemes together to pronounce a word:
   /b/ + /l/ + /ĕ/ + /n/ + /d/ ➔ /blend/

   d. Teaching how to pronounce the word *cucumber* in syllables:
   cucumber ➔ /cū/ /kŭm/ /bər/

REFERENCES

Adams, M.J. (1990). *Beginning to read: Thinking and learning about print.* Cambridge, MA: The MIT Press.

Adams, M.J., Treiman, R., & Pressley, M. (1998). Reading, writing, and literacy. In I. Sigel & A. Renninger (Eds.), *Handbook of child psychology: Vol. 4. Child psychology in practice* (5th ed., pp. 275–355). New York, NY: Wiley.

Alstad, Z., Sanders, E., Abbott, R.D., Barnett, A.L., Henderson, S.E., Connelly, V., & Berninger, V.W. (2015). Modes of alphabet letter production during middle childhood and adolescence: Interrelationships with each other and other writing skills. *Journal of Writing Research, 6*(3), 199–231. http://doi.org/10.17239/jowr-2015.06.03.1

American Psychiatric Association. (2013). *Diagnostic and statistical manual of mental disorders* (5th ed.). Arlington, VA: Author.

Anderson, R.C., Hiebert, E.H., Scott, J.A., & Wilkinson, I.A.G. (1985). *Becoming a nation of readers: The report of the commission on reading.* Washington, DC: U.S. Department of Education, The National Institute of Education.

Ayres, J. (1972). Improving academic scores through sensory integration. *Journal of Learning Disabilities, 5*(6), 338–343.

Bahr, R.H., Silliman, E.R., Berninger, V.W., & Dow, M. (2012). Linguistic pattern analysis of misspellings of typically developing writers in grades 1 to 9. *Journal of Speech, Language, and Hearing Research: JSLHR, 55*(6), 1587–1599. http://doi.org/10.1044/1092-4388(2012/10-0335)

Barquero, L.A., Davis, N., & Cutting, L.E. (2014). Neuroimaging of reading intervention: A systematic review and activation likelihood estimate meta-analysis. *PloS One, 9*(1), e83668. https://doi.org/10.1371/journal.pone.0083668

Berlin, R. (1887). *Eine besondere art der wortblindheit: Dyslexia* [A special kind of word blindness: Dyslexia]. Wiesbaden, Germany: J.F. Bergmann.

Berninger, V.W., Abbott, R.D., Abbott, S.P., Graham, S., & Richards T. (2002). Writing and reading: Connections between language by hand and language by eye. *Journal of Learning Disabilities, 35*(1), 39–56.

Berninger, V.W., Abbott, R.D., Nagy, W., & Carlisle, J. (2010). Growth in phonological, orthographic, and morphological awareness in grades 1 to 6. *Journal of Psycholinguistic Research, 39*(2), 141–163. doi:10.1007/s10936-009-9130-6

Berninger, V.W., & Fayol, M. (2008). Why spelling is important and how to teach it effectively. In *Encyclopedia of Language and Literacy Development* (pp. 1–13). London, Canada: Canadian Language and Literacy Research Network.

Berninger, V.W., Garcia, N.P., & Abbott, R.D. (2009). Multiple processes that matter in writing instruction and assessment. In G. Troia (Ed.), *Instruction and assessment for struggling writers evidence-based practices* (pp. 15–50). New York, NY: Guilford.

Berninger, V.W., Nagy, W.E., Carlisle, J., Thomson, J., Hoffer, D., Abbott, S., . . . Aylward, E. (2003). Effective treatment for children with dyslexia in grades 4–6: Behavioral and brain evidence. In B.R. Foorman (Ed.), *Preventing and remediating reading difficulties: Bringing science to scale* (pp. 381–417). Timonium, MD: York Press.

Berninger, V.W., Raskind, W., Richards, T., Abbott, R., & Stock, P. (2008). A multidisciplinary approach to understanding developmental dyslexia within working-memory architecture: Genotypes, phenotypes, brain, and instruction. *Developmental Neuropsychology, 33*(6), 707–744. doi:10.1080/87565640802418662

Berninger, V.W., & Wolf, B.J. (2009). *Teaching students with dyslexia and dysgraphia: Lessons from teaching and science.* Baltimore, MD: Paul H. Brookes Publishing Co.

Berninger, V.W., & Wolf, B.J. (2016). *Dyslexia, dysgraphia, OWL LD, and dyscalculia: Lessons from science and teaching* (2nd ed.). Baltimore, MD: Paul H. Brookes Publishing Co.

Bishop, D.V.M. (2015). *The interface between genetics and psychology: Lessons from developmental dyslexia.* Paper presented at the Proceedings of the Royal Society B: Biological Sciences, *282*(1806), 20143139. http://doi.org/10.1098/rspb.2014.3139

Blachman, B.A., Schatschneider, C., Fletcher, J.M., & Clonan, S.M. (2003). Early reading intervention: A classroom prevention study and a remediation study. In B.R. Foorman (Ed.), *Preventing and remediating reading difficulties: Bringing science to scale* (pp. 253–271). Timonium, MD: York Press.

Blachman, B.A., Schatschneider, C., Fletcher, J.M., Francis, D.J., Clonan, S.M., Shaywitz, B.A., & Shaywitz, S.E. (2004). Effects of intensive reading remediation for second and third graders and a 1-year follow-up. *Journal of Educational Psychology, 96*, 444–461.

Black, J.M., Xia, Z., & Hoeft, F. (2017). Neurobiological bases of reading disorder, part II: The importance of developmental considerations in typical and atypical reading. *Language and Linguistic Compass, 11*(10): e12252. doi:10.1111/lnc3.12252

Brady, S.A., Braze, D., & Fowler, C.A. (2011). *Explaining individual differences in reading: theory and evidence.* New York, NY: Psychology Press.

Bryant, S. (1979). *Relative effectiveness of visual-auditory vs. visual-auditory-kinesthetic-tactile procedures for teaching sight words and letter sounds to young disabled readers.* Unpublished doctoral dissertation, Teachers College, Columbia University, New York, NY.

Cain, K. (2007). Syntactic awareness and reading ability: Is there any evidence for a special relationship? *Applied Psycholinguistics: 28*(4), 679–694. doi:https://doi.org/10.1017/S0142716407070361

Calvert, G.A., & Lewis, J.W. (2004). Hemodynamic studies of audiovisual interactions. In G. Calvert, C. Spence, & G.C. Stein (Eds.), *The handbook of multisensory processes* (pp. 483–502). Cambridge, MA: The MIT Press.

Catts, H., & Kamhi, A. (2005). *Language and reading disabilities* (2nd ed.). Boston, MA: Pearson.

Chall, J.S. (1967). *Learning to read: The great debate.* New York, NY: McGraw-Hill.

Chall, J.S. (1983). *Stages of reading development.* New York, NY: McGraw-Hill.

Clark, D.B. (1988). *Dyslexia: Theory and practice of remedial instruction.* Timonium, MD: York Press.

Clark, D.B., & Uhry, J. (1995). *Dyslexia: Theory and practice of remedial instruction* (2nd ed.). Timonium, MD: York Press.

Cowen, C.D. (2004). *International Dyslexia Association's Multisensory Research Grant Program Initiative: A bold and challenging initiative.* Retrieved from http://www.interdys.org/ResearchMSIGrantProgramandDonors.htm

Cowen, C.D. (2009). *Independent LD schools: Catalysts for change and valuable research partners.* Retrieved from http://leadershipsummit.ning.com

Cox, C.R., Seidenberg, M.S., & Rogers, T.T. (2015). Connecting functional brain imaging and parallel distributed processing. *Language, Cognition and Neuroscience, 30,* 380–394.

Cruickshank, W.M., Betzen, F.A., Ratzeburg, F.H., & Tannhauser, M.T. (1961). *A teaching method for brain-injured and hyperactive children: A demonstration-pilot study.* Syracuse, NY: Syracuse University Press.

Crystal, D. (2012). *Spell it out: The curious, enthralling, and extraordinary story of English spelling.* New York, NY: Picador.

Dehaene, S.D. (2009). *Reading in the brain: The science and evolution of a human invention.* New York, NY: Viking Adult.

Dearborn, W.F. (1929). Unpublished paper presented at the Ninth International Congress of Psychology, Yale University. New Haven, CT.

Dearborn, W.F. (1940). On the possible relations of visual fatigue to reading disabilities. *School and Society, 52,* 532–536.

deGraaff, S., Bosman, A.M.T., Hasselman, F., & Verhoeven, L. (2009). Benefits of systematic phonics instruction. *Scientific Studies of Reading, 13*(4), 318–333.

Dejerine, J. (1892, Feb. 27). Contribution a l'étude anatomo-pathologigue et clinique des différentes variétés de cécité verbale [Contribution to the anatomo-pathological and clinical studies of different types of word blindness]. *Mémoriale Société Biologigue, 61.*

Dennis, E.L., & Thompson, P.M. (2013). Typical and atypical brain development: A review of neuroimaging studies. *Dialogues in Clinical Neuroscience, 15*(3), 359–384.

Ecalle, J., Magnan, A., Bouchafa, H., & Gombert, J.E. (2009, Aug. 15). Computer-based training with ortho-phonological units in dyslexic children: New investigations. *Dyslexia, 15*(3), 218–238. doi:10.1002/dys.373

Ehri, L.C. (2014). Orthographic mapping in the acquisition of sight word reading, spelling, memory, and vocabulary learning. *Scientific Studies of Reading, 18,* 5–21. doi:10.1080/10888438.2013.819356

Ehri, L.C., Nunes, S.R., Stahl, S.A., & Willows, D.M. (2001, Autumn). Systematic phonics instruction helps students learn to read: Evidence from the National Reading Panel's meta-analysis. *Review of Educational Research, 71*(3), 393–447.

Ehri, L.C., Nunes, S.R., Willows, D.M., Schuster, B.V., Yaghoub-Zadeh, Z., & Shanahan, T. (2001). Phonemic awareness instruction helps children learn to read: Evidence from the National Reading Panel's meta-analysis. *Reading Research Quarterly, 36,* 250–287.

Farrell, M., & Matthews, F. (2010). *Ready to read: A multisensory approach to language-based comprehension instruction.* Baltimore, MD: Paul H. Brookes Publishing Co.

Farrell, M., Pickering, J., North, N., & Schavio, C. (2004, Fall). What is multisensory instruction? *The IMSLEC Record, 8*(3). Retrieved from http://www.imslec.org

Fernald, G.M. (1943). *Remedial techniques in basic school subjects.* New York, NY: McGraw-Hill.

Fernald, G.M., & Keller, H. (1921). The effect of kinesthetic factors in development of word recognition in the case of non-readers. *Journal of Educational Research, 4,* 355–377.

Finn, E.S., Shen, X., Holahan, J.M., Scheinost, D., Lacadie, C., Papademetris, X., . . . Constable, R.T. (2014). Disruption of functional networks in dyslexia: A whole-brain, data-driven analysis of connectivity. *Biology and Psychiatry, 76*(5), 397–404.

Fletcher, J.M., Lyon, G.R., Fuchs, L.S., & Barnes, M.A. (2007). *Learning disabilities: From identification to intervention.* New York, NY: Guilford.

Franceschini, S., Gori, S., Ruffino, M., Pedrolli, K., & Facoetti, A. (2012). A causal link between visual spatial attention and reading acquisition. *Current Biology, 22*(9), 814–819. doi:10.1016/j.cub.2012.03.013

Frostig, M. (1965). Corrective reading in the classroom. *The Reading Teacher, 18,* 573–580.

Gaab, N. (2017, Feb.). It's a myth that young children cannot be screened for dyslexia! *The Examiner* [International Dyslexia Association online newsletter]. Retrieved from https://dyslexiaida.org/its-a-myth-that-young-children-cannot-be-screened-for-dyslexia/

Galaburda, A.M., Sherman, G.F., Rosen, G.D., Aboitiz, F., & Geschwind, N. (1985). Developmental dyslexia: Four consecutive cases with cortical anomalies. *Annals of Neurology, 18,* 222–233.

Galuschka, K., Ise, E., Krick, K., & Schulte-Koerne, G. (2014). Effectiveness of treatment approaches for children and adolescents with reading disabilities: A meta-analysis of randomized controlled trials. *PLoS ONE, 9*(8), e105843. doi:10.1371/journal.pone.0105843

Garcia, N., Abbott, R., & Berninger, V. (2010). Predicting poor, average, and superior spellers in grades 1 to 6 from phonological, orthographic, and morphological, spelling, or reading composites. *Written Language & Literacy, 13*(1), 61–98.

Gates, A.I. (1927). Studies of phonetic training in beginning reading. *Journal of Educational Psychology, 18,* 217–226.

Gates, A. (1935). *The improvement of reading: A program of diagnostic and remedial methods.* New York, NY: Macmillan.

Geschwind, N. (1965). Disconnexion syndromes in animals and man: I–II. *Brain, 88,* 237–294, 585–644.

Giedd, J.N., & Rapoport, J.L. (2010). Structural MRI of pediatric brain development: What have we learned and where are we going? *Neuron, 67*(5), 728–734. https://doi.org/10.1016/j.neuron.2010.08.040

Gillingham, A., & Stillman, B. (1960). *Remedial training for children with specific disability in reading, spelling, and penmanship* (6th ed.). Cambridge, MA: Educators Publishing Service.

Goodwin, A.P., Petscher, Y., Carlisle, J.F., & Mitchell, A.M. (2017). Exploring the dimensionality of morphological knowledge for adolescent readers. *Journal of Research in Reading, 40*(1), 91–117. doi:10.1111/1467-9817.12064

Goswami, U., Power, A.J., Lallier, M., & Facoetti, A. (2014). Oscillatory "temporal sampling" and developmental dyslexia: Toward an over-arching theoretical framework. *Frontiers in Human Neuroscience, 8,* 904. doi:10.3389/fnhum.2014.00904

Graves, W.W., Desai, R., Humphries, C., Seidenberg, M.S., & Binder, J.R. (2010). Neural systems for reading aloud: A multiparametric approach. *Cerebral Cortex, 20*(8), 1799–815.

Hahn, N., Foxe, J.J., & Molholm, S. (2014). Impairments of multisensory integration and cross-sensory learning as pathways to dyslexia. *Neuroscience and Biobehavioral Reviews, 47,* 384–392. http://doi.org/10.1016/j.neubiorev.2014.09.007

Hancock, R., Gabrieli, J.D.E., & Hoeft, F. (2016). Shared temporoparietal dysfunction in dyslexia and typical readers with discrepantly high IQ. *Trends in Neuroscience and Education, 5*(4), 173–177. doi:10.1016/j.tine.2016.10.001

Hancock, R., Pugh, K.R., & Hoeft, F. (2017, June). Neural noise hypothesis of developmental dyslexia. *Trends in Cognitive Sciences, 21*(6). http://dx.doi.org/10.1016/j.tics.2017.03.008

Hancock, R., Richlan, F., & Hoeft, F. (2017). Possible roles for fronto-striatal circuits in reading disorder. *Neuroscience & Biobehavioral Reviews, 72,* 243–260. doi:10.1016/j.neubiorev.2016.10.025

Harrar, V., Tammam, J., Perez-Bellido, A., Pitt, A., Stein, J., & Spence, C. (2014). Multisensory integration and attention in developmental dyslexia. *Current Biology, 24*(5), 531–535.

Hegge, T.G., Kirk, S.A., & Kirk, W.D. (1940). *Remedial reading drills.* Ann Arbor, MI: George Wahr.

Hegge, T.G., Sears, R., & Kirk, S.A. (1932). Reading cases in an institution for mentally retarded problem children. *Proceedings and addresses of the fifty-sixth annual session of the American Association for the Study of Feebleminded, 15,* 149–212.

Henry, M.K. (2010). *Unlocking literacy: Effective decoding and spelling instruction* (2nd ed.). Baltimore, MD: Paul H. Brookes Publishing Co.

Herron, J. (2013). *SpellTalk Discussion Group.* Retrieved from spelltalk@listserve.com

Hinshelwood, J. (1917). *Congenital word blindness.* London, United Kingdom: H.K. Lewis.

Hoeft, F., Hernandez, A., McMillon, G., Taylor-Hill, H., Martindale, J.L., Meyler, A., . . . Gabrieli, J.D. (2006). Neural basis of dyslexia: A comparison between dyslexic and non-dyslexic children equated for reading ability. *Journal of Neuroscience, 26*(42), 10700–10708. doi:26/42/10700 [pii] 10.1523/JNEUROSCI.4931-05.2006

Hudson, R.F., Pullen, P.C., Lane, H.B., & Torgesen, J.K. (2009). The complex nature of reading fluency: A multidimensional view. *Reading & Writing Quarterly, 25*(1), 4–32. doi:10.1080/10573560802491208

Hunt, J.M. (1964). Introduction: Revisiting Montessori. In M. Montessori (Ed.), *The Montessori Method* (A.E. George, Trans.). New York, NY: Schocken Books.

Husband, R.W. (1928). Human learning on a four-section elevated finger maze. *Journal of General Psychology, 1,* 15–28.

International Dyslexia Association, The. (2010). *Knowledge and Practice Standards for Teachers of Reading.* Baltimore, MD: Author.

International Dyslexia Association, The. (2018, March). *Knowledge and practice standards for teachers of reading.* Retrieved from https://dyslexiaida.org/knowledge-and-practices/

James, W. (1890). *The principles of psychology* (Vol. 2). New York, NY: Henry Holt & Co.

Johnson, M. (1966). Tracing and kinesthetic techniques. In J. Money (Ed.), *The disabled reader: Education of the dyslexic child* (pp. 147–160). Baltimore, MD: The Johns Hopkins University Press.

Kast, M., Baschera, G.M., Gross, M., Jäncke, L., & Meyer, M. (2011, May 12). Computer-based learning of spelling skills in children with and without dyslexia. *Annals of Dyslexia, 61*(2), 177–200. doi:10.1007/s11881-011-0052-2

Kephart, N.C. (1960). *The slow learner in the classroom.* Columbus, OH: Charles E. Merrill.

Kuhn, M.R., Schwanenflugel, P.J., & Meisinger, E.B. (2010). Aligning theory and assessment of reading fluency: Automaticity, prosody, and definitions of fluency. *Reading Research Quarterly, 45*(2), 230–251.

Lachs, L. (2017). Multi-modal perception. In R. Biswas-Diener & E. Diener (Eds.), *NOBA textbook series: Psychology.* Champaign, IL: DEF Publishers. Retrieved from http://nobaproject.com/modules/multi-modal-perception

Linkersdorfer, J., Jurcoane, A., Lindberg, S., Kaiser, J., Hasselhorn, M., Fiebach, C.J., & Lonnemann, J. (2015). The association between gray matter volume and reading proficiency: A longitudinal study of beginning readers. *Journal of Cognitive Neuroscience, 27*(2), 308–318. doi:10.1162/jocn_a_00710

Lopez-Barroso, D., Catani, M., Ripolles, P., Dell'Acqua, F., Rodriguez-Fornells, A., & de Diego-Balaguer, R. (2013, Aug. 6). Word learning is mediated by the left arcuate fasciculus. *PNAS-Proceedings of the National Academy of Sciences, 110*(32), 13168–13173. doi:10.1073/pnas.1301696110

Lopez-Barroso, D., Ripolles, P., Marco-Pallares, J., Mohammadi, B., Munte, T.F., Bachoud-Levi, A.C., . . . de Diego-Balaguer, R. (2015). Multiple brain networks underpinning word learning from fluent speech revealed by independent component analysis. *Neuroimage, 110,* 182–193. doi:10.1016/j.neuroimage.2014.12.085

Lyon, G.R. (1997, July 10). *Hearing on literacy: Why kids can't read.* Testimony given to the Committee on Education and the Workforce in the United States House of Representatives.

Lyon, G.R. (1998, April 28). *Report on overview of reading and literacy initiatives.* Testimony given to the Committee on Labor and Human Resources in the United States House of Representatives.

Lyon, G.R. (2016, April 16). *Evidence-based reading instruction: The critical role of scientific research in teaching children, empowering teachers, and moving beyond the "either-or box.* Oral presentation at Annual Conference of Academic Language Therapy Association, Dallas, TX.

Lyon, G.R., Fletcher, J.M., & Barnes, M.C. (2003). Learning disabilities. In E.J. Mash & R.A. Barkley (Eds.), *Child psychopathology* (2nd ed., pp. 520–586). New York, NY: Guilford.

Lyon, G.R., Fletcher, J.M., Fuchs, L.S., & Chhabra, V. (2005). Learning disabilities. In E. Mash & R. Barkley (Eds.), *Treatment of childhood disorders* (3rd ed., pp. 512–594). New York, NY: Guilford.

Lyon, G.R., Fletcher, J.M., Shaywitz, S.E., Shaywitz, B.A., Torgesen, J.K., Wood, F.B., . . . Olson, R. (2001). Rethinking learning disabilities. In C.E. Finn, Jr., R.A. Rotherham, & C.R. Hokansom, Jr. (Eds.), *Rethinking special education for a new century* (pp. 259–287). Washington, DC: Thomas B. Fordham Foundation and Progressive Policy Institute.

Lyon, G.R., & Moats, L.C. (1988). Critical issues in the instruction of the learning disabled. *Journal of Consulting and Clinical Psychology, 56*, 830–835.

Macaluso, E., & Driver, J. (2004). Functional imaging evidence for multisensory spatial representation and cross-modal attentional interactions in the human brain. In G. Calvert, C. Spence, & G.C. Stein (Eds.), *The handbook of multisensory processes* (pp. 529–548). Cambridge, MA: The MIT Press.

Maisog, J.M., Einbinder, E.R., Flowers, D.L., Turkeltaub, P.E., & Eden, G.F. (2008). A meta-analysis of functional neuroimaging studies of dyslexia. *Annals of the New York Academy of Sciences, 1145*, 237–259. doi:NYAS1145024 [pii]

Manis, F.R., Seidenberg, M.S., Stallings, L., Joanisse, M., Bailey, C., Freedman, L., . . . Keating, P. (1999). Development of dyslexic subgroups. *Annals of Dyslexia, 49*(1), 105–134.

Martin, A., Kronbichler, M., & Richlan, F. (2016). Dyslexic brain activation abnormalities in deep and shallow orthographies: A meta-analysis of 28 functional neuroimaging studies. *Human Brain Mapp.* doi:10.1002/hbm.23202

Martin, A., Schurz, M., Kronbichler, M., & Richlan, F. (2015). Reading in the brain of children and adults: A meta-analysis of 40 functional magnetic resonance imaging studies. *Human Brain Mapp, 36*(5), 1963–1981. doi:10.1002/hbm.22749

Mather, N., & Wendling, B.J. (2012). *Essentials of dyslexia assessment and intervention.* Hoboken, NJ: John Wiley & Sons.

Matthews, M.M. (1966). *Teaching to read: Historically considered.* Chicago, IL: University of Chicago Press.

McArthur, G., Eve, P.M., Jones, K., Banales, E., Kohnen, S., Anandakumar, T, . . . Castles, A. (2012). Phonics training for English-speaking poor readers. *Cochrane Database of Systematic Reviews, 12*, CD009115.

McNorgan, C., Chabal, S., O'Young, D., Lukic, S., & Booth, J.R. (2015). Task dependent lexicality effects support interactive models of reading: A meta-analytic neuroimaging review. *Neuropsychologia, 67*, 148–158. https://doi.org/10.1016/j.neuropsychologia.2014.12.014

Melby-Lervåg, M., Lyster, S.A.H., & Hulme, C. (2012). *Phonological skills and their role in learning to read: A meta-analytic review.* Washington, DC: American Psychological Association.

Meyler, A., Keller, T.A., Cherkassky, V.L., Gabrieli, J.D., & Just, M.A. (2008). Modifying the brain activation of poor readers during sentence comprehension with extended remedial instruction: A longitudinal study of neuroplasticity. *Neuropsychologia, 46*, 2580–2592.

Miles, W. (1928). The high finger relief maze for human learning. *Journal of General Psychology, 1*, 3–14.

Moats, L.C. (1995). *Spelling: Development, disability, and instruction.* Baltimore, MD: York Press.

Moats, L.C. (2010). *Speech to print: Language essentials for teachers* (2nd ed.). Baltimore, MD: Paul H. Brookes Publishing Co.

Moats, L.C., & Lyon, G.R. (1993). Learning disabilities in the United States: Advocacy, science, and the future of the field. *Journal of Learning Disabilities, 26*, 282–294.

Money, J. (Ed.). (1966). *The disabled reader: Education of the dyslexic child.* Baltimore, MD: The Johns Hopkins University Press.

Monroe, M. (1932). *Children who cannot read.* Chicago, IL: University of Chicago Press.

Montessori, M. (1912). *The Montessori method.* New York, NY: Frederick Stokes.

Morgan, W.P. (1896, Nov. 7). Word blindness. *British Medical Journal, 2*, 1378.

Morken, F., Helland, T., Hugdahl, K., & Specht, K. (2017). Reading in dyslexia across literacy development: A longitudinal study of effective connectivity. *NeuroImage, 144*, 92–100.

Murray, M.M., Lewkowicz, D.J., Amedi, A., & Wallace, M.T. (2016, Aug.). Multisensory processes: A balancing act across the lifespan. *Trends in Neuroscience, 39*(8), 567–579. http://dx.doi.org/10.1016/j.tins.2016.05.003

Nagy, W., Berninger, V., & Abbott, R. (2006). Contributions of morphology beyond phonology to literacy outcomes of upper elementary and middle school students. *Journal of Educational Psychology, 98*(1), 134–147.

National Institute of Child Health and Human Development (NICHD). (2000). *Report of the National Reading Panel. Teaching children to read: An evidence-based assessment of the scientific research literature on reading and its implications for reading instruction. Reports of the subgroups*

(NIH Publication No. 00-4754). Washington, DC: U.S. Government Printing Office. Retrieved from https://www1.nichd.nih.gov/publications/pubs/nrp/Pages/smallbook.aspx

Norton, E.S., & Wolf, M. (2012). Rapid automatized naming (RAN) and reading fluency: Implications for understanding and treatment of reading disabilities. *Annual Review of Psychology, 63,* 427–52.

Nunes, T., Bryant, P., & Bindman, M. (2006). The effects of learning to spell on children's awareness of morphology. *Reading and Writing, 19,* 767. doi:10.1007/s11145-006-9025-y

Orton, S.T. (1925). "Word-blindness" in school children. *Archives of Neurology and Psychiatry, 14,* 581–615.

Orton, S.T. (1928). Specific reading disability—strephosymbolia. *JAMA: Journal of the American Medical Association, 90,* 1095–1099.

Orton, S.T. (1937). *Reading, writing and speech problems in children.* New York, NY: W.W. Norton & Co.

Paige, D.D., Raskinski, T.V., & Magpuri-Lavell, T. (2012). Is fluent, expressive reading important for high school readers? *Journal of Adolescent and Adult Literacy, 56*(1), 67–76.

Pennington, B.F. (2006). From single to multiple deficit models of developmental disorders. *Cognition, 101*(2), 385–413. https://doi.org/10.1016/j.cognition.2006.04.008

Peterson, R.L., Pennington, B.F., & Olson, R.K. (2013). Subtypes of developmental dyslexia: Testing the predictions of the dual-route and connectionist frameworks. *Cognition, 126*(1), 20–38. doi:10.1016/j.cognition.2012.08.007

Price, C.J. (2012). A review and synthesis of the first 20 years of PET and fMRI studies of heard speech, spoken language and reading. *Neuroimage, 62*(2), 816–847. doi:10.1016/j.neuroimage.2012.04.062

Pugh, K.R., Landi, N., Preston, J.L., Mencl, W.E., Austin, A.C., Sibley, D., . . . Frost, S.J. (2013). The relationship between phonological and auditory processing and brain organization in beginning readers. *Brain and Language, 125*(2), 173–183. http://doi.org/10.1016/j.bandl.2012.04.004

Rasinski, T.V., Reutzel, R., Chard, D., & Linan-Thompson, S. (2010). Reading fluency. In M.L. Kamil, P.D. Pearson, E.B. Moje, & P. Afflerbach (Eds.), *Handbook of reading research* (Vol. 4). Mahwah, NJ: Lawrence Erlbaum Associates.

Rayner, K., Foorman, B., Perfetti, C., Pesetsky, D., & Seidenberg, M.S. (2001). How psychological science informs the teaching of reading. *Psychological Science in the Public Interest, 2*(2), 31–74.

Richards, T.L., Aylward, E.H., Field, K.M., Grimme, A.C., Raskind, W., Richards, A.L., . . . Berninger, V.W. (2006). Converging evidence for Triple Word Form Theory in children with dyslexia. *Developmental Neuropsychology, 30*(1), 547–89.

Richards, T.L., & Berninger, V.W. (2008). Abnormal fMRI connectivity in children with dyslexia during a task: Before but not after treatment. *Journal of Neurolinguistics, 21,* 294–304.

Richlan, F. (2014). Functional neuroanatomy of developmental dyslexia: The role of orthographic depth. *Frontiers in Human Neuroscience, 8,* 347. doi:10.3389/fnhum.2014.00347

Richlan, F., Kronbichler, M., & Wimmer, H. (2011). Meta-analyzing brain dysfunctions in dyslexic children and adults. *Neuroimage, 56*(3), 1735–1742.

Richlan, F., Kronbichler, M., & Wimmer, H. (2013, Nov.). Structural abnormalities in the dyslexic brain: A meta-analysis of vowel-based morphometry studies. *Human Brain Mapp, 34*(11), 3055–3065. doi:10.1002/hbm.22127

Richmond, S., Johnson, K.A., Seal, M.L., Allen, N.B., & Whittle, S. (2016). Development of brain networks and relevance of environmental and genetic factors: A systematic review. *Neuroscience & Biobehavioral Reviews, 71,* 215–239.

Sagan, C. (1997). *The demon-haunted world: Science as a candle in the dark.* New York, NY: Ballantine.

Scott, C.M. (2009, April). A case for the sentence in reading comprehension. *Language, Speech, and Hearing Services in Schools, 40,* 184–191.

Scott, C.M., & Balthazar, C. (2013, Summer). The role of complex sentence knowledge in children with reading and writing difficulties. *Perspectives on Language and Literacy, 39*(3), 18–26.

Segers, E., Damhuis, C.M.P., van de Sande, E., & Verhoeven, L. (2016). Role of executive functioning and home environment in early reading development. *Learning and Individual Differences, 49,* 251–259.

Seidenberg, M. (2017). *Language at the speed of sight: How we read, why so many can't, and what can be done about it.* New York, NY: Basic Books.

Seidenberg, M.S., & McClelland, J.L. (1989). A distributed, developmental model of word recognition and naming. *Psychological Review, 96*(4), 523–568.

Share, D., & Stanovich, K.E. (1995). Cognitive processes in early reading development: Accommodating individual differences into a mode of acquisition. *Issues in Education: Contributions from Educational Psychology, 1,* 1–57.

Shaywitz, S. (2003). *Overcoming dyslexia: A new and complete science-based program for reading problems at any level.* New York, NY: Alfred A. Knopf.

Sherman, G.F., & Cowen, C.D. (2009). A road less traveled: From dyslexia research lab to school front lines. How bridging the researcher-educator chasm, applying lessons of cerebrodiversity, and exploring talent can advance understanding of dyslexia. In K. Pugh & P. McCardle (Eds.), *How children learn to read: Current issues and new directions in the integration of cognition, neurobiology, and genetics of reading and dyslexia research and practice* (pp. 43–64). New York, NY: Psychology Press.

Simons, D.J., Boot, W.R., Charness, N., Gathercole, S.E., Chabris, C.F., Hambrick, D.Z., & Stine-Morrow, E. (2016). Do "brain-training" programs work? *Psychological Science in the Public Interest, 17*(3), 103–186.

Simos, P.G., Fletcher, J.M., Bergman, E., Breier, J.I., Foorman, B.R., Castillo, E.M., . . . Papanicolaou, A.C. (2002). Dyslexia-specific brain activation profile becomes normal following successful remedial training. *Neurology, 58,* 1203–1213.

Slingerland, B.H. (2013). (Combined and Edited by N. King). *A practical guide to teaching reading, writing and spelling* (2nd ed.). Bellevue, WA: Slingerland Institute for Literacy.

Spear-Swerling, L., & Cheesman, E. (2012). Teachers' knowledge base for implementing response-to-intervention models in reading. *Reading and Writing, 25,* 1691–1723. doi:10.1007/s11145-011-9338-3

Spence, C. (2011). Crossmodal correspondences: Tutorial review. *Attention, Perception, & Psychophysics, 73*(4), 971–995. doi:10.3758/s13414-010-0073-7

Stein, B.E., Stanford, T.R., & Rowland, B.A. (2014). Development of multisensory integration from the perspective of the individual neuron. *Nature Reviews. Neuroscience, 15*(8), 520–535.

Strauss, A., & Lehtinen, L.E. (1947). *Psychopathology and education of the brain-injured child.* New York, NY: Grune & Stratton.

Sumby, W.H., & Pollack, I. (1954). Visual contribution to speech intelligibility in noise. *The Journal of the Acoustical Society of America, 26,* 212–215.

Swanson, H.L. (1999). Reading research for students with LD: A meta-analysis of intervention outcomes. *Journal of Learning Disabilities, 32,* 504–532.

Tabareau, N., & Slotine, J.J. (2010). How synchronization protects from noise. *PLoS Computational Biology, 6,* e1000637.

Talsma, D., Senkowski, D., Soto-Faraco, S., & Woldorff, M.G. (2010). The multifaceted interplay between attention and multisensory integration. *Trends in Cognitive Sciences, 14*(9), 400–410. http://doi.org/10.1016/j.tics.2010.06.008

Tanaka, H., Black, J.M., Hulme, C., Stanley, L.M., Kesler, S.R., Whitfield-Gabrieli, S., . . . Hoeft, F. (2011). The brain basis of the phonological deficit in dyslexia is independent of IQ. *Psychological Science, 22*(11), 1442–1451. doi:10.1177/0956797611419521

Taylor, J.S.H., Davis, M.H., & Rastle, K. (2017, April). Comparing and validating methods of reading instruction using behavioural and neural findings in an artificial orthography. *Journal of Experimental Psychology: General.* http://dx.doi.org/10.1037/xge0000301

Taylor, J.S.H., Rastle, K., & Davis, M.H. (2013). Can cognitive models explain brain activation during word and pseudoword reading? A meta-analysis of 36 neuroimaging studies. *Psychological Bulletin, 139,* 766–791. http://dx.doi.org/10.1037/a0030266

Torgesen, J. (1991). Learning disabilities: Historical and conceptual issues. In B. Wong (Ed.), *Learning about learning disabilities* (pp. 3–37). San Diego, CA: Academic Press.

Torgesen, J.K. (2004). Avoiding the devastating downward spiral: The Evidence that early intervention prevents reading failure. *American Educator, 28,* 6–19.

Torgesen, J., Alexander, A.W., Wagner, R., Rashotte, C.A., Voeller, K., & Conway, T. (2001). Intensive remedial instruction for children with severe reading disabilities: Immediate and long-term outcomes from two instructional approaches. *Journal of Learning Disabilities, 34,* 33–58.

Vellutino, F.R., Scanlon, D.M., Sipay, E.R., Small, S.G., Chen, R., Pratt, A., & Denckla, M.B. (1996). Cognitive profiles of difficult-to-remediate and readily remediated poor readers: Early intervention as a vehicle for distinguishing between cognitive and experiential deficits as basic causes of specific reading disability. *Journal of Educational Psychology, 88,* 601–638.

Venezky, R.L. (1999). *The American way of spelling.* New York, NY: Guilford.

Verhoeven, L., & Perfetti, C.A. (2011). Introduction to this special issue: Vocabulary growth and reading skill. *Scientific Studies of Reading, 15,* 1–7.

Veuillet, E., Magnan, A., Ecalle, J., Thai-Van, H., & Collet, L. (2007, Nov.). Auditory processing disorder in children with reading disabilities: Effect of audiovisual training. *Brain, 130*(Pt 11), 2915–2928.

Vigneau, M., Beaucousin, V., Herve, P.Y., Duffau, H., Crivello, F., Houde, O., . . . Tzourio-Mazoyer, N. (2006). Meta-analyzing left hemisphere language areas: Phonology, semantics, and sentence processing. *NeuroImage, 30*(4), 1414–1432. https://doi.org/10.1016/j.neuroimage.2005.11.002

Vigneau, M., Beaucousin, V., Herve, P.Y., Jobard, G., Petit, L., Crivello, F., . . . Tzourio-Mazoyer, N. (2011). What is right-hemisphere contribution to phonological, lexico-semantic, and sentence processing? Insights from a meta-analysis. *NeuroImage, 54*(1), 577–593. https://doi.org/10.1016/j.neuroimage.2010.07.036

Wallace, M.T. (2004). The development of multisensory integration. In G. Calvert, C. Spence, & G.C. Stein (Eds.), *The handbook of multisensory processes* (pp. 625–642). Cambridge: The MIT Press.

Washburn, E.K., Joshi, R.M., & Binks-Cantrell, E. (2011, June). *Annals of Dyslexia, 61*(1), 21–43. doi:10.1007/s11881-010-0040-y

Webster, N. (1806). *Compendious dictionary of the English language.* Hartford, CT: Hudson and Goodwin.

Wepman, J.M. (1964). The perceptual basis for learning. In H. Robinson (Ed.), *Meeting individual differences in reading.* Chicago, IL: University of Chicago Press.

Wittrock, M.C. (1992). Generative learning processes of the brain. *Educational Psychologist, 27,* 531–541.

Wolf, B., Abbott, R.D., & Berninger, V.W. (2017, Feb.). Effective beginning handwriting instruction: Multimodal, consistent format for 2 years, and linked to spelling and composing. *Reading and Writing, 30* (2), 299–317. doi:10.1007/s11145-016-9674-4

Wolf, M. (2007). *Proust and the squid.* New York, NY: Harper Collins Publishers.

Wong, B.Y.L. (1991). Assessment of metacognitive research in learning disabilities: Theory, research, and practice. In H.L. Swanson (Ed.), *Handbook on the assessment of learning disabilities: Theory, research, and practice* (pp. 265–283). Austin, TX: PRO-ED.

Wong, M. (2015, May 28). Stanford study on brain waves shows how different teaching methods affect reading development. *Stanford Report-Stanford News.* Retrieved from http://news.stanford.edu/2015/05/28/reading-brain-phonics-052815/

Xia, Z., Hancock, R., & Hoeft, F. (2017). Neurobiological bases of reading disorder, part I: Etiological investigations. *Language and Linguistics Compass, 11,* e12239. https://doi.org/10.1111/lnc3.12239

Xia, Z., Hoeft, F., Zhang, L., & Shu, H. (2016). Neuroanatomical anomalies of dyslexia: Disambiguating the effects of disorder, performance, and maturation. *Neuropsychologia, 81,* 68–78.

Yoncheva, Y.N., Wise, J., & McCandliss, B.D. (2015, June–July). Hemispheric specialization for visual words is shaped by attention to sublexical units during initial learning. *Brain and Language, 145–146,* 23–33. http://dx.doi.org/10.1016/j.bandl.2015.04.001

Section II

Pre-reading/ Literacy Skills

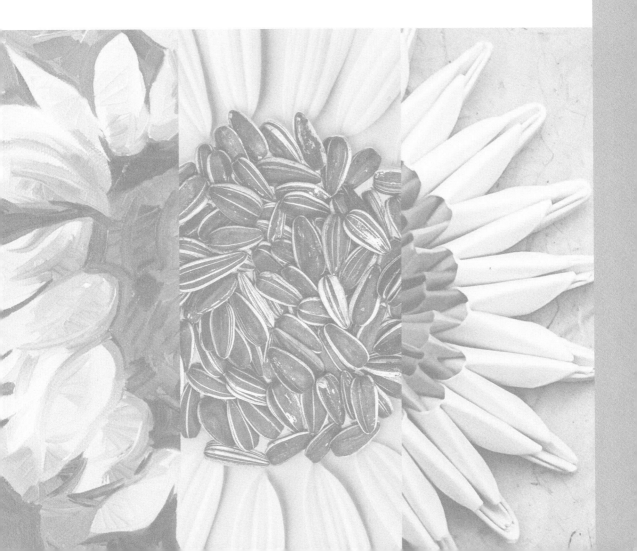

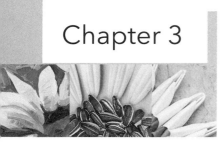

Chapter 3

Oral Language Development and Its Relationship to Literacy

Lydia H. Soifer

LEARNING OBJECTIVES

1. To understand the relationship between aspects of oral language and literacy

2. To appreciate the similarities and differences between oral and print language

3. To acquire an understanding of the role of various aspects of language impairment to literacy acquisition and performance

4. To understand the dynamic interaction between aspects of language, working memory, executive function, and academic performance

5. To appreciate the meaning of the statement "Talking is not teaching"

Imagine the elegant intricacies of Beethoven's "Ode to Joy" or Mozart's "Serenade in G Major" (*Eine Kleine Nachtmusik*) played captivatingly by an artist. It is as beguiling to the experienced listener as to the naïve ear. Now imagine pages of musical notation, an array of dots and lines splayed across a page, interrupted by assorted squiggles and swirls. If you can read music, then you may sense the beauty in your mind's ear, much the way Beethoven did. Can't read music? Then what remains is a morass of dots, lines, squiggles, and swirls. The same is true with language, an amazing latticework of interrelated complexities in which the oral (spoken) and aural (heard)—in combination with memory, sensory, and motor function; environment; and culture—form the basis from which literacy evolves. The challenge of teaching about language is that the language itself is the vehicle for learning. Thus, in large part, the very thing that you are attempting to learn about consciously in this chapter is exactly what you are experiencing spontaneously as you comprehend or generate language. Learning about language is a **metalinguistic** task in which language is analyzed and considered as an entity and behavior. When a person speaks or listens, reads or writes, and effectively communicates or understands a particular purpose or intention, the language system has performed efficiently.

Mattingly suggested that there was something "devious" (1972, p. 133) about the relationship between the processes of speaking and listening and the process of reading. Listening and reading both are linguistic processes but are not really as parallel or analogous as many people assume. The differences are

- In the form of information being presented (complex auditory signals vs. more static visual symbols)

- In the linguistic content (additional information available from the intonational and speech patterns that can be perceived in listening vs. the many possible pieces of phonological information contained in one symbol)

- In the relationship of the form to the content (enormous variation in what can be produced by voice vs. alphabets with limited information carried by any single symbol).

Listening and speaking are automatic and natural ways of perceiving and using language, acquired as part of a developmental process. In contrast, the written form of a language must generally be taught, and not all individuals are able to learn it with ease. In addition, not all spoken languages have a written form.

Researchers agree that reading is a language-based skill (Kamhi & Catts, 2012; Moats, 2010b; Perfetti, 2010; Wagner, Torgesen, & Rashotte, 1994) and that the relationship between oral language and reading is reciprocal (Kamhi & Catts, 1989; Stanovich, 1986; Wallach & Miller, 1988), with each influencing the other at different points in development (Menyuk & Chesnick, 1997; Snyder & Downey, 1991, 1997).

Oral and written language, although intimately and intricately related, are not the same. Teachers need to be aware of the similarities and differences (Moats, 1994, 2010b; Moats & Lyon, 1996) so that they can facilitate students' language learning and academic success (Bashir & Scavuzzo, 1992). This chapter helps foster an awareness of the inextricable role of language in learning to decode and comprehend. The processes of language learning (on which reading is based) begin before children receive reading instruction. This chapter provides an insight into each component of the language system, including patterns of typical and disordered development and their analogous relationships to the higher level language skills of reading and writing. In this chapter, oral and written language are viewed as a continuum, and the varying influences of oral language knowledge and use in developing early decoding processes and subsequent comprehension processes are considered. Furthermore, this chapter offers a discussion of the oral–written language connection and the different levels of language processing, intended to enhance teachers' ability to be informed observers and, as a result, to be more effective in planning instruction.

It is impossible not to recognize the advancement of our knowledge base as educators as a result of the wealth of research being done in neuroscience (Raver & Blair, 2014; Sousa, 2010; Tokuhama-Espinosa, 2011). In particular, the focus has been on executive function, identified as cognitive flexibility, inhibitory control, and working memory (Kaushanskaya, Park, Gangopadhyay, Davidson, & Ellis Weismer, 2017; Vandenbroucke, Versuchueren, & Baeyens, 2017), with a particular focus on the relationship between working memory and language functioning (Fung & Swanson, 2017; Gathercole & Holmes, 2014; Gordon-Pershey, 2014). This chapter addresses the impact of this knowledge on teaching and learning. Furthermore, given that every aspect of reading is founded in oral/aural language, this chapter is consistent with the International Dyslexia Association's (2018) *Knowledge and Practice Standards for Teachers of Reading*. Finally, it is unquestioned that in any educational setting, there exist particular Classroom Language Dynamics © (Soifer, 2013), in which teachers' awareness of what language they choose to use, how they choose to use it, and why they make those decisions is based on their active awareness of the students they are teaching. Thus, teachers must be constantly alert to answering the question, "Who is this child?" and as a result, "How must

I teach?" These needs and skills will be the integration and culmination of the information in this chapter, designed to create real-world applications for teachers.

REFLECT, CONNECT, and RESPOND

Explain the meaning of the statement "Language is the vehicle for learning."

LANGUAGE: A DYNAMIC, RULE-GOVERNED PROCESS

Learning to talk appears easy but, in fact, is enormously complex. The marvel is that most children learn to talk so well and so quickly (Hart & Risley, 1999). The enormity of the task is confounded because most children are not taught to use language but rather discover the rules that govern language in the context of social interaction as they strive to understand and convey meaning.

What is language? Decades ago, Bloom and Lahey offered a superb definition of language that is still relevant for today's classrooms: "Language is a code whereby ideas about the world are represented through a conventional system of arbitrary signals for communication" (1978, p. 4). The key concepts to consider are communication, ideas, code, system, and conventionality. The purpose of language is communication. We use language for a variety of purposes in vastly different ways according to our needs, the needs of the listener, and the circumstances surrounding us. Language enables us to express an array of ideas. We have ideas about objects, events, and relationships. Our ability to express those ideas through language is different from the objects, events, or relationships themselves.

Think about the page you are reading and the words you have available to represent your ideas about the page, what is on it, what you are doing with it, and your relationship to it. Each is different from the page itself, the writing on it, the act of reading, and how you are relating to the page by viewing it or touching it. In this way, language is a code, a means of representing one thing with another in a predictable and organized system. There are many different codes, from maps, to computer code, to words spelled in a book. Sounds may be combined into words, words into sentences, and sentences into conversation. The rule-governed predictability of the system enables us to understand it and learn how to use it. Consider the following:

'Twas brillig, and the slithy toves
Did gyre and gimble in the wabe:
All mimsy were the borogoves,
And the mome raths outgrabe.
(Carroll, 1865/1960, p. 134)

If asked, one could identify the parts of speech, such as noun (*toves, raths*), verb (*gyre, gimble*), adjective (*outgrabe*), or adverb (*brillig*); identify the subject, predicate, and object; have a reasonable idea of how to pronounce these novel words; and answer comprehension questions ("Were the borogoves mimsy?"). All of these tasks are possible because Carroll used the predictable, rule-governed nature of the sounds and grammar of English to create "Jabberwocky."

The code of language is also conventional. It consists of a socially based, tacitly agreed-on set of symbols and rules that govern their permissible combinations. The conventions of language allow users to share their ideas. A person's implicit knowledge about the rules of the language is linguistic competence. Possessed of linguistic competence, a child or an adult has the knowledge to be a competent language user. In general, unless called on to do so specifically, a language user need not state the rules of language explicitly. The ability to generate an infinite number of sentences and understand varying forms of language across a plenitude of environments demonstrates knowledge of the rules.

REFLECT, CONNECT, and RESPOND
In what ways is language a code?

ORAL-WRITTEN LANGUAGE CONNECTION

Literacy is much like a great pyramid. It is built on a broad foundation that is linguistic, sociological, cognitive, and pedagogic. Literacy evolves from well-developed oral language abilities; exposure to written language that gives rise to a child's notions of how print works and what it can do, called **emergent literacy** (Sulzby & Teale, 1991; Van Kleeck, 1990); a level of cognitive maturation that allows for metalinguistic awareness that permits a child to view language as an entity, something to be considered and analyzed; and a reasonable quality of instruction that can provide varying degrees of facilitation and support.

Language is the vehicle that drives curriculum. Although one may study aspects of the language in discrete ways (e.g., phonics, grammar, vocabulary), even then the very language being studied is the one that is employed to learn. In no instance does this resonate with greater truth than in the process of acquiring literacy skills—reading and writing. As Wallach and Butler explained, "Learning to read and write is part of, not separate from, learning to speak and comprehend language" (1994, p. 11). Despite **whole language** arguments to the contrary, however, Wallach asserted that "learning to read is not the same as learning to speak" (1990, p. 64).

Indeed, Van Kleeck (1990) allowed that the foundations of literacy are created at birth and are interrelated with the evolution and fullness of a child's oral language because reading is a language-based skill dependent on a set of well-developed oral language abilities. Language learning and literacy learning are actually reciprocal. That is to say, the relationship between the two is dynamic and changes over time, with each influencing the other at different developmental stages (Kamhi & Catts, 1989; Sawyer, 1991). Nonetheless, there are considerable differences between language learning and literacy learning (Scott, 1994) because reading is not just speech written down (Liberman, Shankweiler, Camp, Blachman, & Werfelman, 1990).

Understanding oral language requires a well-integrated knowledge of the form, content, and use of the language. Each of the following enables a listener to understand: recognizing word patterns, word structure, and sentence forms; knowing the meanings of words, how words relate to one another, and how they are influenced by their position in the sentence; and interpreting the intent of the speaker with the context and in relationship to one's own knowledge base. Understanding written text requires the same linguistic knowledge that is necessary for understanding spoken language. An analogy that serves quite well is to compare hearing spoken language to decoding print. When we hear someone tell us, "I heard what you said, but I don't know what you mean," it is similar to the phenomenon of asking a child to tell about what he or she has just read and being met with a look of noncomprehension that implies, "I know that I read [decoded] it, but

I don't know what it means!" As described throughout this chapter, deficits in oral language, syntax, morphology, **semantics** (word meaning and relationships), **pragmatics,** and narrative structure have a negative effect on reading comprehension.

In addition to oral language skills, emergent literacy is a foundation for literacy development (see Van Kleeck, 1990, for an extended discussion of emergent literacy; this topic is also discussed in depth in Chapter 4). Emergent literacy is an outgrowth of **"literacy socialization"** (Snow & Dickinson, 1991). When children are exposed to print by being read to, whether from books, signs, instructions, or birthday cards, they begin to develop a sense that the marks on the page, box, or card are related to the words being said (Linder, 1999). They also begin to develop an awareness of how books are manipulated, literally which way is up and in which direction the text flows and the pages turn. Children who have been exposed to print in early caregiver–child interactions also benefit from the positive emotional connection between reading and nurturing experiences. Provided with literacy socialization experiences and, as a result, the emergent literacy skills that precede learning to decode, children who have been read to as preschoolers unquestionably find the process of learning to read an easier experience (Dickinson & McCabe, 1991; Wolf & Dickinson, 1993). (For more information about this, see Chapter 4.)

Layzer and Goodson (2006) found that children raised in low-income families who are in child care up to 13 hours each day while their parents are working have far less exposure to enriched language, fewer play experiences designed for cognitive stimulation, and fewer literacy experiences. In child care settings in homes, fewer than half had at least 10 books appropriate for each age group cared for within that home. Furthermore, fewer than half the home care providers read even one book to children within any 13-hour day. Play activities that comprised approximately one third of the day were directed at reading or being read to less than 10% of the time. The effect on oral language development, socialization skills, and early literacy cannot be underestimated given the present-day expectations for preschool and kindergarten.

Metalinguistic ability, as discussed later in this chapter, permits a child to focus on language from a distance; to view language as an object of consideration; and to reflect on its discrete, particular aspects and characteristics. It is metalinguistically that children recognize word boundaries; make letter–sound correspondences; consider which printed sequences of letters represent which words and meanings; and analyze, blend, and reconstruct words. Little, if anything, in the oral language experience prepares children to view words as discrete units (e.g., *sit*) to isolate the parts of each unit (e.g., $s - i - t$) in order to reformulate and orally produce them (e.g., "sit"). Phonological awareness activities certainly are dependent on metalinguistic skills. Beyond the task of decoding, conscious use of linguistic knowledge strongly influences reading comprehension. Oral language development, however, does not require these metalinguistic abilities. The speech stream is continuous, with boundaries that are not discrete, and the context is immediate and supported environmentally by the situation in which the talking is occurring. In oral language development, reflection on linguistic knowledge is not part of the process until a fair degree of cognitive maturity and linguistic sophistication has been attained.

Literacy is also built on good teaching. As early as 1996, Moats and Lyon strongly urged changes in teacher education related to reading instruction to place a greater emphasis on knowledge of language structure. They cited disturbing findings in a survey of 103 teachers in which fewer than one third were proficient in the basic knowledge of language structure, such as identifying an inflected ending (*-ed* in *instructed*) or determining the number of phonemes in words such as *ox, precious,* or *thank*. Teaching children to read requires teaching them language at a higher and more conscious level. Successful teaching, particularly of those children who bring linguistic, experiential, cognitive, or environmental vulnerabilities to the task, requires a powerful, integrated knowledge of the language that is being taught. To this end, teacher training programs such as Language Essentials for Teachers of Reading and Spelling, known as LETRS (Moats, 2010a), and the certification programs of the International Multisensory Structured Language Education Council (IMSLEC) provide direct teacher training in the oral language underpinnings of literacy as well as in the application of Orton-Gillingham–based instructional methodology.

ORAL-WRITTEN LANGUAGE DIFFERENCES

There is no doubt that reading is a language-based skill, yet there are numerous and obvious differences between oral and written language. These differences have been considered from a variety of different vantage points, either as parallels or continua (Horowitz & Samuels, 1987; Kamhi & Catts, 1989; Rubin, 1987; Scott, 1994; Wallach, 1990; Westby, 1985). In the course of human development, literacy is recent (Wolf & Dickinson, 1993). Learning to read and write does not come naturally to everyone, and these skills are not a requirement in every society. Writing, as anyone who has ever struggled with a blank page or experienced writer's block well knows, requires a much greater effort than producing oral language. Rubin highlighted his difficulty when he wrote that "no one is a native speaker of writing" (1987, p. 3). Human beings are socialized to communicate, and they have a biological predisposition to oral language that enables societal groups to have and pass on oral language systems. Reading and writing are acquired deliberately, rather than spontaneously and more naturally. The differences are in the aspects of production, influences of context, grammar, and vocabulary and in the degree of explicitness.

Oral language is transient and ephemeral. It exists only at the moment when it is spoken. It can be repeated or clarified, but that occurs at the request of the listener. Written language is permanent and more enduring than oral language, except when the latter is recorded. Print allows the reader multiple opportunities for exposure and decision-making authority regarding the rate and depth of analysis with which the text is read. In oral language, the rate of presentation is at the discretion of the speaker. In oral language, temporal sequencing is crucial, whereas in print, spatial sequencing is important. Print can be revisited more readily. A word, sentence, or paragraph can be reread or rewritten. It is a different experience to have someone attempt to repeat, exactly, the sentence just uttered.

Most oral language occurs face to face. Reciprocity exists between the speaker and listener. Interpersonal context and situational support exist in the form of vocal, facial, and physical gestures. When people are engaged in conversation or discussion, less needs to be explicitly stated, and sentence structures can be more fragmentary. Vocabulary and syntax can be more familiar and less sophisticated. To appreciate the lack of explicitness, as well as the fragmentary, familiar, and contextually and physically supported nature of oral language, request a transcript of a television talk show that you have watched. While watching and listening to the discussion, you probably had little difficulty understanding the ebb and flow, intent, and effect of the exchanges among the participants. Reading the transcript of the same exchange will provide an immediate insight into the significant differences in the explicitness of a written text and the literate, grammatically dense nature of written language versus oral language that has been written down. In oral language, cohesion between sentences and ideas can be established grammatically or paralinguistically through physical signals, such as the shrug of a shoulder or a pregnant pause. In a written text, the cohesive devices and transitional markers that bind ideas or shift focus must be conveyed concretely and explicitly through a careful choice of words. The conventions of punctuating written language that are communicated orally through intonational gestures must be taught specifically; however, written text does provide other cues to organization and meaning through the structure of paragraphs and the use of boldface, italics, underlining, and other **typography.**

Although written language contains the intent to communicate with another or others or to interpret another person's message, the experience is generally more solitary and involves only the reader and the book, page, or computer screen. The interaction between writer and reader is limited and is decontextualized—writer and reader are separated by time and distance. It is necessary for the communicator to be more explicit and succinct in print.

Written language relies on the **lexicon** to create the melody and meaning provided by the **intonation, stress, pause,** and **juncture** patterns of spoken language as well as the vocal characteristics of the speaker. In oral language, an anxious tone, a sinister laugh, or a lascivious lilt can be heard, recognized, and interpreted without being explicitly named by the speaker as such. What is said and meant can be potently influenced by how it is said, and thus the message and intent of the speaker and the response of the listener may vary. The most literate of writers attain a level of mastery that enables them to arrange, adapt, maneuver, integrate, and entwine words and sentences in ways that communicate so effectively that it seems as though these writers are talking to the reader. With that level of written language mastery, it is possible to write the same thing in many ways, ranging from the most informal to the most deliberately formal tone.

After considering the oral–written continuum, it is important to look at writing itself. Writing is the most sophisticated, complex, and formal aspect of language. Even the most well-read and literate individuals may not have equivalent skill in expressing thoughts on paper. Writing is a dynamic interaction among cognitive and linguistic factors, motor skills, and emotional considerations. The most sophisticated language act, writing involves the simultaneous convergence of many complex factors:

- Cognitive factors—abstracting, generating, and ordering ideas

- Linguistic factors—arriving at semantic production (word meaning and choice) and syntactic production (grammar) appropriate to the nature of what is being written, such as a thank-you note versus an expository paragraph

- Narrative considerations—structuring information for varied purposes

- **Graphomotor** skills—recalling, planning, and executing complex motor acts

- Visual ability—recalling sequences of letters with phonetic rules for spelling

- Temporal factors—writing legibly and appropriately under specific time constraints

Furthermore, these factors converge while the writer is simultaneously controlling for the emotional factors involved in risk, exposure, and evaluation of the final product. It is readily apparent why many children (and adults) might prefer to speak rather than to write. The teaching of writing can be an art form. (See Chapter 17 for information about evidence-based composition instruction.)

COMPONENTS OF LANGUAGE

Bloom and Lahey (1978) conceptualized three major interactive components of language: form, content, and use (see Figure 3.1). Each component is governed by a complex set of rules that together compose language.

Language Form

Language form consists of the observable features of language. It includes the rules for combining sounds (phonology), structuring words (morphology), and ordering words in sentences (syntax). These features, their development, and the relationship of disorders in these elements of language form are described in the following sections.

Phonology   Phonology is the sound system of a language. It comprises **supra-segmental** aspects (intonation, stress, loudness, pitch level, juncture, and speaking rate) and **segmental** aspects (**vowels, consonants,** and phonemes).

The suprasegmental aspects of phonology provide the melody of speech. They are related to speech because they are produced by the vocal tract but are concerned with larger units of production: syllables, words, phrases, and sentences. They are significant in the ability to communicate emotions and attitudes. These suprasegmental features help distinguish different sentence types—declarative (e.g., *Joshua eats pizza*), interrogative (e.g., *Does Russell like ice cream?*), or imperative (e.g., *Sit down now!*). Awareness of phrase structure helps us understand where a comma might be placed in a sentence. These aspects of phonology also permit us to say the same sentence and communicate markedly different meanings. Varied aspects of the suprasegmental features of language are used in talking to different

LANGUAGE

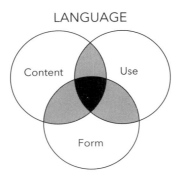

Figure 3.1. Venn diagram illustrating language form, content, and use. (Adapted from Bloom, L., & Lahey, M. [1978]. *Language development and disorders* [p. 22]. Hoboken, NJ: John Wiley & Sons.)

people of different ages and status. Consider the number of ways to say "Don't be silly" to an infant, a spouse, or an employer. At a conversational level, the suprasegmental characteristics of language also may be used to convey sarcasm, to tease, and to mock.

The suprasegmental aspects of phonology are influential in reading. When reading aloud, fluent readers read with full intonation, communicating an understanding of the author's intent. Early readers or those who struggle to decode may read each word individually, and then, having derived meaning, reread with appropriate inflection.

Inefficient readers may pause with a downward intonation at the end of a printed line of words rather than at the end of the sentence. Thus, the suprasegmental features of language play an essential role in comprehension.

Vowels and consonants compose the segmental features of language. Each language has a set of vowels, consonants, or phonemes that may be combined to form words. A phoneme is the smallest linguistic unit of sound that can change meaning in a word. Consider the word family of *bat*. Changing any of the phonemes could produce a variety of new words (e.g., *sat, bit, ban*).

Standard English orthography has only 26 letters with which to represent the approximately 44 phonemes of English. Still more strikingly, only 5 vowel letters are available to represent the approximately 15 vowel sounds. Knowledge of phonemes and their role in language and reading is essential for teachers. Long before children are able to recognize, read, and write the letters that represent the sounds of English, they must begin to master the elaborate task of making those speech sounds correctly so that they are able to clearly produce the sounds of the language. Children learn each of those 44 sounds and their possible variations by being exposed to them, hearing others speak, and storing information about the qualities that make up each sound. It is an unconscious and intricate task.

Speech production is the complex coordination of respiration (breathing), phonation (the vibration of the vocal folds), resonation (the quality of voice affected by the shape and density of the neck and cavities of the head), and **articulation** (the rapid, alternating movements of the jaw, tongue, lips, teeth, and soft palate). When we speak, the flow of speech is generally uninterrupted. Speech is produced in breath groups ("Whenneryagoin?") rather than in individual words ("When are you going?"). Yet, early readers decode word by word and, at times, sound by sound. Liberman noted that "if speech were like spelling, learning to read would be trivially easy" (as cited in Brady & Shankweiler, 1991, p. xv). Awareness that the flow of coarticulated, overlapping phonemes can be segmented into sounds, syllables, and words is a precursor to cracking the code of language in print (see Chapter 6 for information about teaching phonemic awareness). Although speech and reading are clearly related, they are not equal.

Oral language, of which speech is the observable form, is learned naturally. Reading is not (Liberman & Liberman, 1990). A bounty of literature, however, has emphasized the role of phonological awareness (the ability to attend to and recognize the sound structure of language) in acquiring early reading (Adams, 1990; Blachman, 1989, 1991; Blachman, Ball, Black, & Tangel, 2000; Ehri, Nunes, Willow, Schuster, Yaghoub-Zadeh, & Zaffiro, 2001; Stanovich, 1987; Storch & Whitehurst, 2002; Wagner & Torgesen, 1987).

The speech sound segments, vowels and consonants, may vary in their productions (variations known as **allophones**) and are guided by a set of rules for their production and placement in words. From the earliest moments of life, infants are acquiring information about the sounds of their language (Eimas, Siqueland, Jusczyk, & Vigorito, 1971). Through continuous exposure, babies acquire the set of acoustic features that define the sounds of their language. Over time, the speakers of a given language come to recognize the possible variations in phoneme production while still recognizing the specific phoneme. For example, the phoneme /p/ is a **voiceless** stop plosive (i.e., there is no vocal fold vibration when producing this sound, it is not produced in a long stream as /s/ is, and it produces a puff of air). Yet, the production of /p/ varies by the amount of **aspiration** (puff of air) produced, depending on where it appears in a word. Pronounce *pot* and *spot* aloud to feel the different amount of aspiration. Nonetheless, speakers of English recognize both variations as the phoneme /p/. Moreover, any of the plosive sounds (i.e., /p/, /b/, /t/, /d/, /k/, and /g/), when said in isolation or as a segmented phoneme, must be produced with an accompanying vowel sound, the **schwa** (/ə/), typically produced as "uh." This is particularly relevant for teachers; as Liberman noted, "The word is 'bag,' not 'buh-a-guh'" (as cited in Brady & Shankweiler, 1991, p. xv). The distortion can be so great that some children are unable to recombine the sounds into the word *bag*. Combining /b/ and /ə/ in a smooth, connected production eliminates the /ə/. In addition, by not producing the /g/ with an overemphasis, the /ə/ is once again reduced, thus allowing the word being analyzed and synthesized to sound more like its real-world production. This enables the young reader to use language knowledge of the word to recognize it as a phonological/phonemic phenomenon.

Other phonetic distinctions may be made by limitations of the vocal tract. These distinctions may become important for spelling, particularly for children with vulnerabilities in phonological awareness. Plurals, possessives, and the third-person singular marking of the verb all are accomplished by the addition of *-s* (or *-es* for certain plurals) when being spelled. The sounds produced, however, may be /z/ or /s/. This is determined by the nature of the preceding phoneme. **Coarticulation** with a **voiced** consonant (one produced with the vocal folds closed) or a vowel will create /z/ or /ĭz/. Say *hugs, kisses,* and *hits* aloud to hear and feel the distinctions. A similar pattern emerges for creating the regular past tense, typically created in print as *-ed*. In speech, however, it may be produced as /d/, /t/, or /ĭd/, as in *hugged, kissed,* or *lifted*.

Vowels and consonants, which combine to form syllable structures, are separated into distinct classes by the nature of their production. Bernthal and Bankson explained, a vowel is typically "formed as sound energy from the vibrating folds escapes through a relatively open vocal tract of a particular shape" (1998, p. 12).

The tongue, jaw, and lips serve to create the shape of the vocal tract. Because the jaw and tongue work together, vowels are classified by identifying the position of the tongue during articulation (front, mid, or back; high or low) and the lips (rounded or unrounded). Vowels may also be tense or lax. **Tense vowels** (e.g., /ē/ in *bee*) are longer in duration; **lax vowels** (e.g., /ĭ/ in *bin*) are shorter in duration. Figure 3.2 demonstrates the position in the mouth of each vowel's production. Table 3.1 shows the spellings of different vowels. Moats' (2010b) view of sound production in its relationship to spelling gives an accompanying image of the appearance of vowels (see Figure 3.3).

Consonants are created by either a complete or a partial constriction of the air stream along the vocal tract. The closure is affected by the position of the lips and the placement of the tongue in relation to the teeth and its position in the mouth. Consonants are classified as **stops** (e.g., /t/, /k/), **nasals** (e.g., /n/, /m/, /ng/), **fricatives** (e.g., /f/, /z/), **affricates** (/ch/, /j/), **glides** (e.g., /w/, /y/), or **liquids** (/l/, /r/).

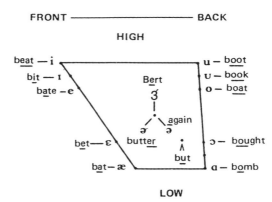

Figure 3.2. Vowel chart. (From Bernthal, J.E. [1998]. *Articulation and phonological disorders* [4th ed., p. 16]. Published by Allyn & Bacon; Boston, MA.)

Table 3.2 provides a clear view of where consonants are produced in the vocal tract. In addition, consonants may be described as voiced (caused by vibrations of the vocals folds when closed) or voiceless (open vocal folds). Several sets of phonemes, called **voiced-voiceless cognates,** are produced in the same place in the mouth, in the same manner, but vary only in the voicing characteristic. They are /p/ and /b/, /f/ and /v/, /t/ and /d/, /s/ and /z/, /k/ and /g/, /th/ (*think*) and /th/ (*this*), /sh/ and /zh/, and /ch/ and /j/. (The distinction between a voiceless and voiced phoneme can be felt as well as heard by placing the fingers gently against the throat. Start to say /s/, then without altering the position of the tongue and jaw, say /z/.) In addition, the environment in which a consonant or vowel exists (i.e., the other phonemes near it) may vary the production of that consonant or vowel.

Table 3.1.   American English vowels

Phonetic symbol	Phonic symbol	Spellings
/i/	ē	beet
/ɪ/	ĭ	bit
/e/	ā	bait
/ɛ/	ĕ	bet
/æ/	ă	bat
/ɑj/	ī	bite
/ɑ/	ŏ	bottle
/ʌ/	ŭ	butt
/ɔ/	aw	bought
/o/	ō	boat
/ʊ/	oŏ	put
/u/	ū	boot
/ə/	ə	be<u>tween</u>
/ɔj/	oi, oy	boy
/æw/	ou, ow	bough

From Moats, L.C. (2010). *Speech to print: Language essentials for teachers* (2nd ed., p. 35). Baltimore, MD: Paul H. Brookes Publishing Co.; reprinted by permission.

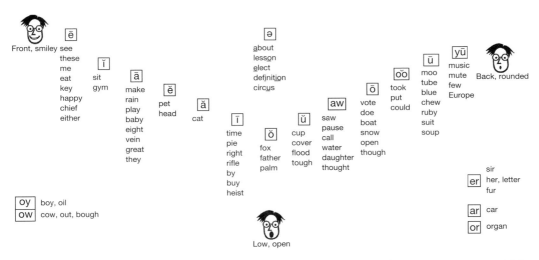

Figure 3.3.   Vowels (phonic symbols) by mouth position. (From Moats, L.C. [2010]. *Speech to print: Language essentials for teachers* [2nd ed., p. 96]. Baltimore, MD: Paul H. Brookes Publishing, Co.; adapted by permission.)

The relationship of vowel, consonant, and syllable production and **discrimination** and phonological awareness leading to more effective reading and spelling is significant. In addition to rules for the production and perception of phonemes, there are rules that apply to how phonemes may be combined into meaningful words. These rules allow some sounds to appear in certain positions in a word but not in others. For example, in English, /ng/ may appear in the **middle** or at the end of a word but never at the beginning.

Table 3.2.   American English consonants (phonic symbols)

Class of consonant	Lips	Lips/teeth	Tongue between teeth	Tongue behind teeth	Roof of mouth	Back of mouth	Throat
Stop							
voiceless	/p/			/t/		/k/	
voiced	/b/			/d/		/g/	
Nasal	/m/			/n/		/ng/	
Fricative							
voiceless		/f/	/th/	/s/	/sh/		
voiced		/v/	/th/	/z/	/zh/		
Affricate							
voiceless					/ch/		
voiced					/j/		
Glide							
voiceless						/wh/	/h/
voiced					/y/	/w/	
Liquid				/l/	/r/		

From Moats, L.C. (2010). Speech to print: Language essentials for teachers (2nd ed., p. 28). Baltimore, MD: Paul H. Brookes Publishing Co.; reprinted by permission.

Phonological Development   Speech sound development traditionally was thought to occur through unit-by-unit learning of each phoneme in a developmental sequence. In fact, phonological development is integrally related to the language system as a whole. Phonological development progresses with physical maturation, the mastery of sound features and phonological processes that reflect the linking of sounds to words and meaning, and the growth of syntactic and semantic rule knowledge and ability. Children employ phonological or natural processes to master adult-level speech productions.

Children typically produce their first recognizable words by 12–18 months of age. The ability of toddlers to make themselves fully understood (without available **context clues**) is often limited by inadequate production of sounds. However, 3-year-olds are generally intelligible and by age 4 have suppressed or eliminated the remaining phonological processes that hinder their intelligibility (Hodson, 1994). Typically developing children are able to produce speech sounds adequately by age 4 and require additional time (until age 7) for complete mastery, including the elimination of lisps and the production of **multisyllabic** words (see Table 3.3).

Relationship of Phonological Disorders to Literacy   When preparing to teach early reading skills, teachers should be aware of two areas of consideration: intelligibility of speech production and its relationship to phonological awareness. Children who have problems with speech sound production at the time they are being introduced to reading instruction or who have a history of such difficulties have been shown to be less adept at tasks of phonological awareness than their typically developing peers (Webster & Plante, 1992). Webster and Plante explained that "productive phonological impairment may hinder performance in phonological awareness because it precludes efficient phonological coding in working memory" (1992, p. 176). In the same vein, Fowler (1991) suggested that articulation ability may be an important prerequisite for acquiring an awareness of phoneme structures. Furthermore, contemporary research has demonstrated a correlation between speech sound disorders and literacy outcomes with clear indication of negative impact of severe and persistent speech sound production deficits (Peterson, Pennington, Shriberg, & Boada, 2009; Preston & Edwards, 2010; White-Canales & McElroy-Bratcher, 2015).

Table 3.3. Phonemic acquisition–age at which 75% of children tested correctly articulated consonant sounds

Age	Sounds
2.0	/m/, /n/, /h/, /p/, /n/, /r/ (*ring*)
2.4	f, j, k, d
2.8	w, b, t
3.0	g, s
3.4	r, l
3.8	/sh/ (*shy*), /ch/ (*chin*)
4.0	/th/ (*father*), /zh/ (*measure*)
4.01	/j/ (*jar*), /th/ (*thin*), v, z

From Prather, E., Hedrick, D., & Kern, C. (1975). Articulation development in children aged two to four years. *Journal of Speech and Hearing Disorders, 40*(2), 179-191; reprinted by permission.

Consider the dilemma of a child who does not have a stable speech production system. Certain speech production problems may be caused by neurological oral–motor dysfunction, including weaknesses of the musculature necessary for making the coordinated movements to produce speech (**dysarthria**). Other speech problems may be caused by sensorimotor disruptions in which the signals to the muscles necessary for speech production are not consistently or efficiently received (**dyspraxia**). When children encounter a new word, they must be able to store it in phonological short-term (working) memory as part of the process of creating a phonological representation for it. Children who have speech articulation difficulties, however, are at a disadvantage:

> What they are able to say may not match what they have heard. In the phonological awareness tasks of rhyme, segmentation, and blending and in spelling tasks, being able to rehearse a word with proper production plays a contributing role in the successful completion of those tasks. Thus, for some children, speech disorders are a hidden contributor to the apparent phonological processing and spelling difficulties. (Stackhouse & Wells, 1997)

Children with reading disabilities have been found to make more speech production errors than their typical peers (Catts, 1986; Gillon, 2004; Rvachew, 2007; Snowling, 1981). There are similar findings documented for college students with dyslexia (Catts, 1989). The college students with dyslexia had greater difficulty in repeating complex phrases rapidly and made significantly more errors than their typical peers. It is hypothesized that children and adults with reading difficulties have greater challenges in encoding phonological information and in planning (for articulation) of complex sequences of sounds (Catts, 1989).

Phonological processing difficulties may manifest differently across the developmental continuum. They may stem from a variety of causes and vary in severity (Spear-Swerling & Sternberg, 1994). In the preschool years, developing oral language may be related to slower vocabulary growth (Catts, Hu, Larrivee, & Swank, 1994), and children may be less sensitive to rhyme, **alliteration,** and **nonsense words** (Fey, Catts, & Larrivee, 1995; Pennington & Lefly, 2001; Snowling, Gallagher, & Firth, 2003). During the elementary school years, children with phonological processing difficulties may be weaker in using segmentation strategies to analyze phonemic structure and slower in word recognition, secondary to having reduced awareness of the relationship between phonemes and the alphabet (Catts, 1989; Ehri, 1989). If a child persists in having significant speech production difficulties, then spelling ability may be affected (Clark-Klein & Hodson, 1995). Reduced rate of vocabulary acquisition and difficulty acquiring words with **multiple meanings** and **figurative language** as well as word-retrieval difficulties may become obvious (Catts et al., 1994; Milosky, 1994; Snyder & Godley, 1992). Comprehension problems may begin to emerge both orally and in print (Catts, 1996; Snyder & Downey, 1991).

Phonological awareness abilities are critical to the development of early reading (see Chapter 6 for information about teaching phonemic awareness). The evidence is so strong that commercial materials have appeared with increasing regularity to aid educators in identifying weaknesses in phonological awareness abilities (Robertson & Salter, 1997) and developing these skills (Adams, Foorman, Lundberg, & Beeler, 1998; Catts & Vartiainen, 1997). The main point of the research is not only that phonological skills underlie early reading but also that they can be taught. Catts (1997) developed a checklist to aid in the early identification of language-based reading difficulties. The value of the checklist is twofold. First, its structure identifies six significant areas of observation for the teacher: speech sound awareness, word retrieval, verbal memory, speech production and perception, comprehension, and expressive language. Second, when used in collaboration with a speech-language pathologist, it can be of enormous value in targeting students who may be vulnerable to reading difficulty and pinpointing their particular areas of need. This checklist is shown in Figure 3.4. (A similar tool created subsequently combined Catts's list with one developed and published by Justice, Invernizzi, & Meier, 2002.)

Phonology is too often simplified to its superficial relationship to speech or phonics instruction. In reality, it has far-reaching significance for the rate of language acquisition (Paul & Jennings, 1992), vocabulary size (Stoel-Gammon, 1991), working memory (Adams & Gathercole, 1995), word retrieval (Katz, 1986; McGregor, 1994), and phonological awareness skills (segmentation, **sound deletion,** blending, and counting), which are believed to underlie early literacy (Catts, 1993). Expressive phonological disorders have negative effects on early literacy (Bird & Bishop, 1992; Bird, Bishop, & Freeman, 1995) and spelling (Moats, 1995). The relationship between speech and print is anchored by an understanding of phonology and phonological processes. Making this connection is a vital step for children in developing literacy. For teachers, understanding this connection brings power of knowledge to teaching.

Teachers are faced with a daunting challenge in the increasingly multicultural society as the expectations of the Every Student Succeeds Act of 2015 (PL 114-95) mandate universal literacy. As researchers work to understand the impact on literacy acquisition of variations in the language and cultural literacy of African American (Craig, Connor, & Washington, 2003; Laing & Kamhi, 2003) and **Hispanic** children (Gottardo, 2002; Hammer, Miccio, & Wagstaff, 2003), teachers must support the learning needs of culturally and linguistically diverse populations. A particular challenge facing teachers is the impact of variation in vowel and consonant production in the oral language of populations of linguistically diverse speakers. The relationship between phonology and decoding is affected at a fundamental level by these variations. For teachers to be fully effective in meeting the needs of struggling readers of cultural and linguistic backgrounds different than their own, they must know the structure of the linguistic knowledge that the children bring to school (Labov, 2003). Research is being devoted to the specific needs of Spanish-speaking **English language learners (ELLs),** who make up the largest population of children who require literacy instruction. Several findings are of importance to teachers. It is crucial to differentiate between language impairment, which would be apparent in both languages, and bilingualism. Language impairment and bilingualism represent a different status for the learner (August et al., 2006). Establishing the level of language ability in the first language is essential as well. Children who have not been exposed to English prior to school entry must be given additional time to learn English—2–3 years for conversational purposes and 5–7 years for academic functioning. Furthermore, children who have been exposed to both languages will have different knowledge and abilities than monolingual learners (Hammer & Miccio, 2006). In a study of Spanish-speaking preschool children who were acquiring English, Lopez and Greenfield (2004) established that English phonological awareness skills were predicted by English oral proficiency, Spanish oral proficiency, and Spanish phonological awareness skills. The role of oral language proficiency as a foundation for literacy development for ELLs parallels the essential role of oral

---

Early Identification of Language-Based Reading Disabilities: A Checklist

Child's name: _____   Birthday: _____

Date completed: _____   Age: _____

This checklist is designed to identify children who are at risk for language-based reading disabilities. It is intended for use with children at the end of kindergarten or beginning of first grade. Each of the descriptors listed below should be carefully considered and those that characterize the child's behavior/history should be checked. A child receiving a large number of checks should be referred for a more in-depth evaluation.

Speech sound awareness
____ Doesn't understand and enjoy rhymes
____ Doesn't easily recognize that words begin with the same sound
____ Has difficulty counting the syllables in spoken words
____ Has problem clapping hands or tapping feet in rhythm with songs and/or rhymes
____ Demonstrates problems learning sound–letter correspondences

Word retrieval
____ Has difficulty retrieving a specific word (e.g., calls a sheep a "goat" or says, "you know, a woolly animal")
____ Shows poor memory for classmates' names
____ Speech is hesitant, filled with pauses or vocalizations (e.g., "um," "you know")
____ Frequently uses words lacking specificity (e.g., "stuff," "thing," "what you call it")
____ Has a problem remembering/retrieving verbal sequences (e.g., days of the week, alphabet)

Verbal memory
____ Has difficulty remembering instructions or directions
____ Shows problems learning names of people or places
____ Has difficulty remembering the words to songs or poems
____ Has problems learning a second language

Speech production/perception
____ Has problems saying common words with difficult sound patterns (e.g., *animal, cinnamon, specific*)
____ Mishears and subsequently mispronounces words or names
____ Confuses a similar sounding word with another word (e.g., saying, "The Entire State Building is in New York")
____ Combines sound patterns of similar words (e.g., saying "escavator" for *escalator*)
____ Shows frequent slips of the tongue (e.g., saying "brue blush" for *blue brush*)
____ Has difficulty with tongue twisters (e.g., *she sells seashells*)

Comprehension
____ Only responds to part of a multiple element request or instruction
____ Requests multiple repetitions of instructions/directions with little improvement in comprehension
____ Relies too much on context to understand what is said
____ Has difficulty understanding questions
____ Fails to understand age-appropriate stories
____ Has difficulty making inferences, predicting outcomes, drawing conclusions
____ Lacks understanding of spatial terms such as left/right, front/back

Expressive language
____ Talks in short sentences
____ Makes errors in grammar (e.g., "he goed to the store" or "me want that")
____ Lacks variety in vocabulary (e.g., uses "good" to mean *happy, kind, polite*)
____ Has difficulty giving directions or explanations (e.g., may show multiple revisions or dead ends)
____ Relates stories or events in a disorganized or incomplete manner
____ May have much to say, but provides little specific detail
____ Has difficulty with the rules of conversation, such as turn taking, staying on topic, indicating when he/she does not understand

_____
(continued)

Figure 3.4.   Checklist for early identification of language-based reading disabilities. (From Catts, H.W. [1997]. Appendix A: Early identification of language-based reading disabilities. A checklist. *Language, Speech, and Hearing Services in Schools, 28,* 88–89. Reproduced with permission of American Speech-Language-Hearing Association in the format Book via Copyright Clearance Center. Some descriptors have been taken from *Language for learning: A checklist for language difficulties,* Melbourne, Australia: OZ Student.)

Figure 3.4. *(continued)*

Other important factors
____ Has a prior history of problems in language comprehension and/or production
____ Has a family history of spoken or written language problems
____ Has limited exposure to literacy in the home
____ Lacks interest in books and shared reading activities
____ Does not engage readily in pretend play
Comments

_____

_____

_____

---

language for monolingual learners. Thus, intervention designed to prevent reading difficulties among students acquiring English must carefully attend to oral language development with an emphasis on vocabulary and phonological awareness (August & Shanahan, 2006; Vaughn, Mathes, Linan-Thompson, & Francis, 2005). Indeed, the task is daunting but not insurmountable for creative, devoted educators. (See Chapter 19 for more information about language and literacy development among ELLs.)

Morphology Language form, one of the three major components of language (Bloom & Lahey, 1978), also includes a set of rules for forming words. Morphology is the study of word formation, or how morphemes (the smallest units of meaning in language) combine to form words. Morphemes (unlike phonemes) are endowed with meaning. Words are made up of one or more morphemes. A morpheme that can stand alone, such as *smile, book,* or *cute,* is called an **unbound morpheme** (or **free morpheme**). Another group of morphemes, called bound morphemes, must be attached to other morphemes. **Bound morphemes** are typically the **affixes** of a language, such as *un-* and *-ing* for the word *unsmiling, -s* in the plural *books,* and *-est* in the superlative *cutest.* Unbound morphemes have **lexical** (word) meanings of their own. They are the content words of the language: nouns, main verbs, adjectives, and adverbs. Other morphemes, called *function words* or *grammatical morphemes,* such as prepositions, articles, **conjunctions,** and auxiliary verbs, serve grammatical functions in a sentence by creating the connection between lexical morphemes. Bound morphemes may be either inflectional or derivational. **Inflectional morphemes** modify tense (*-ed* in *played*), possession (*-'s* in *Vicki's*), or number (*-s* in *dollars*). Acquiring inflectional morphemes is a hallmark of early language development and reflects a child's increasing analysis of the structure and meaning of words. **Derivational morphemes** change one part of speech to another; for example, the verb *argue* plus *-ment* becomes the noun *argument,* and the adjective *happy* plus *-ness* becomes the noun *happiness.*

The resulting changes in spelling are another indication of the underlying complexity of the relationship between speech and print. Morphemic structure allows the language user to extend and modify meaning. Young language learners making their way through the dense forest of sounds, words, and meanings learn to mark the differences in tense, number, or possession by attending to the ends of words. Older children learn to recognize the relationships among words (e.g., *nation, national, nationality, nationalism, nationalistic*). Indeed, prefixes and suffixes, which are most commonly derived from Greek and Latin, permit a learner to extend lexical knowledge (White, Power, & White, 1989). (See Chapter 14 for an in-depth discussion of influences on English morphology.)

A further intrigue exists in the **morphophonemic relationship**—change in pronunciation caused by change in the morphological structure in a word, such as the changes that occur when the following words are said aloud: *sign, signature; medicine, medical.* Although phonemically such pronunciation changes may seem irregular, from a morphological view many of these changes are predictable.

Morphological Development   In the earliest stages of language development, morphological development is measured by acquiring the first 14 morphemes that emerge in children's language (Brown, 1973). As morphemes may either be words (unbound) or affixes (bound), the first 14 morphemes range from the present progressive marker -*ing*, to the use of the irregular third-person singular verb form *has,* to the contracted copula (*to be*) such as -*'m* in *I'm going.* These acquisitions generally occur between the ages of 2 or 2½ years and 4 years. Brown identified this initial phase of acquisition as occurring across five stages of development that span the period of approximately 1½–5½ years of age. During early language development, children acquire pronouns, articles, and adjective and noun suffixes. At a certain point in early development, morphological and syntactic development merge when *no* and *not* become part of the evolution of negative sentence structures.

Later morphological development involves acquiring comparatives (-*er*) and superlatives (-*est*), irregular forms (*children*), and advanced prefixes and suffixes (*un-, dis-, -ness, -ment*), including those that mark noun and adverb **derivation** (-*er* in *baker,* -*ly* in *slowly*). Spelling and pronunciation are affected by the structure of more advanced morphological development (e.g., *child/children, happy/happiness*). Wiig and Semel provided a sequence of acquisition of morphological or word formation rules:

> 1) Regular noun plurals, 2) noun–verb agreement for singular and plural forms of irregular nouns and verbs in the present tense, 3) regular noun possessives in the singular and plural form, 4) irregular noun plurals, 5) irregular noun possessives, 6) regular past tense verbs, 7) irregular past tense verbs, 8) adjectival inflections for the comparative and superlative forms, 9) noun and adverb derivation, 10) prefixing. (1980, p. 50)

Morphology plays an essential role in language development and growth. From their earliest role in the emergence of grammar as a child passes beyond the single-word stage, to the adolescent's urgent need to master Greek and Latin roots and affixes in preparation for the SAT, morphological knowledge and mastery contribute to vocabulary growth, spelling, comprehension, and the richness of a student's written language. Across the school years, morphological knowledge is crucial to developing literacy. From early decoding to increasingly frequent exposure to lengthier, more complex words in the middle and high school years, students' morphological knowledge is an essential component of successful decoding, comprehension, spelling, and writing.

Green (2009) aptly summarized the importance of morphological awareness in developing literacy skills crucial to academic success, word decoding, fluency, comprehension, and spelling. Morphological awareness can facilitate a young reader's approach to decoding while improving linguistic comprehension and fluency. Siegel (2008) gave the example of the long, and therefore potentially intimidating, word *sleeplessness*: if the word is recognized as three morphemes, *sleep, -less, -ness*, then it becomes less of a challenge to a reader. In a similar way, when direct instruction about roots and affixes is available, it facilitates readers' pronunciation (e.g., *-tion* is pronounced *shun*) as well as their fluency. Knowledge of morphemic and **structural analysis** also enhances both vocabulary and comprehension skills. Teachers could readily improve students' awareness of word structure and word meaning and provide a metacognitive tool by teaching, creating, and displaying a derivational morphology chart that summarizes common suffixes (e.g., nouns identifying people end in *-er, -or, -cian, -ist*; nouns identifying things end in *-tion, -sion*; nouns can be formed by adding *-ment, -ity*; verbs are created by adding *-ize, -ify*). Thus, systematically teaching children about word structure (roots and affixes) provides them with both structural and strategic knowledge to be used for word reading (Carlisle, 2000; Carlisle & Stone, 2005), vocabulary growth (Baumann et al., 2002; Nagy & Anderson, 1984; Nagy & Scott, 2000), reading fluency (Bashir & Hook, 2009; Snow, Griffin, & Burns, 2005; Troia, 2004), comprehension (Katz, 2004; Nagy, Berninger, & Abbott, 2006), and spelling (Apel, Masterson, & Hart, 2004; Green et al., 2003). Morphological knowledge is influential in helping children recognize spelling changes as a result of morphological additions as well as facilitating their recall of, and access to, words. Facilitating access reduces the burden on working memory.

Morphological awareness becomes even more crucial in later elementary and middle school when textbooks are introduced and used. A majority of words encountered in informational text are **derivative** in nature (e.g., *constitute, constitution, constitutional, constitutionally*). Morphological awareness empowers a reader to analyze the internal and derivative structure of unfamiliar words by analogy to words already within his or her repertoire.

Carlisle (1988), in her studies of fourth-, sixth-, and eighth-grade students, demonstrated that children know more about derivational morphology than they use in their spelling. She recommended direct instruction of words that undergo both phonological and orthographic changes (e.g., *deep/depth*) as opposed to those that undergo only phonological change (e.g., *equal/equality*). Further indications for the merit of direct instruction appear across the literature from the benefits to early first-grade readers (Wolter, Wood, & D'zatko, 2009) to fifth- and eighth-grade students (McCutchen, Logan, & Biangardi-Orpe, 2009). Moreover, late elementary and middle school students were studied, and their performance on measures of explicit morphological production was a significant predictor of both word identification and reading comprehension.

The value of instruction in morphological awareness has become the increasing focus of more recent research (Apel, Diehm, & Apel, 2013; Goodwin & Ahn, 2013). It has become eminently clear that all students benefit from morphological instruction (Wolter & Dilworth, 2014) and that the impact of direct instruction in morphological structure and use extends beyond reading and spelling. McCutcheon and colleagues (2014) reported on the benefit of morphologically focused instruction via a fifth-grade science curriculum. Compared to the students in the control group, the students who participated in the morphological intervention program used more morphologically complex words in their written work related to the science topics being studied.

Relationship of Morphological Disorders to Literacy   Children with language learning disabilities often present with impairments in reading as their primary academic problem. The rate of morphological acquisition is slower for these children than for their typically developing peers. Although morphological acquisition has not been widely studied, several investigations have pointed to the relationship between morphological awareness and literacy. Mahoney and Mann (1992) found positive correlations between second graders' ability to appreciate phonologically and morphologically based puns and their reading ability. Ruben, Patterson, and Kantor (1991) reported a relationship between morphological knowledge and spelling ability in typically developing second graders, children with learning disabilities, and adults with literacy problems. Ruben and colleagues demonstrated that the morphemic errors made in writing reflected impairments in both the implicit and explicit levels of morphological knowledge. What was most striking, however, was their evidence that these impairments do not resolve simply by maturation and increased exposure to written language. Furthermore, underlying phonological weakness may contribute to the difficulty poor readers have with certain morphological relationships. Fowler and Liberman (1995) found that poor readers have greater difficulty in producing morphological forms that involve a phonological change (e.g., *courage/courageous*) than they do when there is no phonological change (e.g., *danger/dangerous*).

Morphology is relevant to both reading and spelling for several reasons. Among those reasons concerning English morphology, Elbro and Arnbak (1996, p. 212) identified the following:

- The role morphology plays in orthography

- The value of morphemes as indicators of meaning

- The economical nature of storing words in written lexicon as morphemes rather than as wholes (because of the relative unpredictability of sound to letter accuracy)

- Morpheme analysis and recognition as a reading strategy may provide a more direct route to the lexicon of the spoken word; certain reading and spelling errors are morphologically based (e.g., *procedure/proceed*)

Morphological awareness has been shown to be a strong indicator of reading comprehension (Carlisle, 1995), and morphological awareness training has been shown to have a positive effect on comprehension (Elbro & Arnbak, 1996). Children with dyslexia have weaker morphological awareness ability than their typical reading peers (Casalis, Cole, & Sopo, 2004; Elbro & Arnbak, 1996; Siegel, 2008). Morphological awareness training with students with dyslexia (Arnbak & Elbro, 2000) and other reading disabilities (Berninger et al., 2003; Katz & Carlisle, 2009) has been effective in improving decoding, comprehension, and spelling skills across age and grade levels (Kirk & Gillon, 2009).

Morphological awareness, however, is not seen as fully independent from phonological awareness (Fowler & Liberman, 1995). Phonological awareness skills are essential in early literacy acquisition before word structure becomes increasingly complex. Then, in concert with phonological knowledge, awareness of morphological structure and meaning plays an increasingly important role in decoding, comprehension, vocabulary, and spelling. Although researchers continue to determine the specific nature and interrelatedness of the systems of language that influence reading, teachers must remain conscious of the constant reciprocity among language components.

REFLECT, CONNECT, and RESPOND
How are phonology and morphology related to decoding?

Syntax   Syntax is a third aspect of language form. Syntax is the system of rules that directs the comprehension and production of sentences. Syntax (sometimes referred to as grammar) specifies the order of words and the organization of words within a variety of sentence types. Syntactic rules allow the user to combine words into meaningful sentences and to alter the form of a sentence (e.g., "The boy is walking" may be transposed into "Is the boy walking?") Despite a finite set of sentence types, an infinite number of sentences can be generated. In addition, syntactic knowledge allows a language user to decide whether sentences are grammatical.

Syntactic Development   Typically developing children acquire the rudiments of syntax early in the language acquisition process. As they progress beyond the basic form of noun phrase and verb phrase, children master the variety of sentence types common in preschool language: negative, interrogative, and imperative forms. They subsequently begin to develop the earliest complex sentence structures of coordination, demonstrated by the use of *and* ("Joshua went to Grandma's house *and* had a good time"); complementation, indicated by using a clause structure that modifies the verb ("Tell me *what he is eating*"); and relativization, in which a clause restricts or modifies the meaning of another portion of the sentence ("The boy *who ate the cake* has a tummy ache"). Complex structures emerge in children's language quite early. In typical language development, complex syntax begins to appear shortly after children begin to combine words between 2 and 3 years of age. Similarly, proficiency with more complex structures is observable by the start of kindergarten (Arndt & Schuele, 2013). Complex sentence development continues through the school years. Additional syntactic development skills continue to emerge across the school years, with mastery of some forms as late as 11 years old: embedding of clauses, either parallel ("She gave him a toy *that he did not like*") or nonparallel ("He called the man *who walked away*"); using **gerunds** (verbs with -*ing* that function as nouns; e.g., "*Cooking* is fun"); and using passive structures ("The cookie *was* eaten by the boy"). Other, more mature grammatical structures also evolve with the mastery of new forms such as more sophisticated conjunctions (e.g., *although, nonetheless*), mass nouns and their quantifiers ("*How much* water do you want?" rather than "*How many* water do you want?"), and using reflexive pronouns (e.g., *himself, herself*). The mature language user can use sentence complexity to convey numerous relationships among actions, ideas, and locations. Complex syntax is essential for academic development and success and is a crucial foundation for subsequent reading comprehension and written language.

As summarized by Scott (2004), several factors contribute to sentence complexity and, therefore, to the ability to comprehend complex sentences. First is the meaning relationship of words within a sentence, especially nouns and verbs. The passive structure is typically more challenging for children to process when it is in the reversible form ("The duck was chased by the goose") rather than in the nonreversible form ("The cake was baked by the girl"). Support for understanding the nonreversible form is obvious in that cakes do not bake girls. In addition, the nature of verbs themselves can influence syntactic structure. Certain verbs, for example *sit*, only require an agent that is someone to sit. Other verbs, however, such as *put*, have more complex syntactic requirements and need both an agent (someone to perform the action of putting), an object (something to put), and a location (a place to put it). Beyond the semantic–syntactic relationship (meaning to word order) are two other aspects of syntactic complexity. Sentence length, a common measure of children's language that increases with age, influences comprehension, particularly as the subject is distant from the verb as a result of dependent clauses ("Alex, a determined young man of Cuban descent who tolerated cold winters in the north so that he could reach his ultimate goal of a college education, returned to Miami for a week"); this distance places increasing demand on the listener or reader. Sentences in which pronoun referents are not transparent or relationships are ambiguous pose a challenge ("Emma hugged Nicole before *she* closed the door"; "Ellie laughed at the bookstore"). Not all sentences are equally easy to process, whether spoken or written.

Changes in the sophistication of noun and verb phrases and the development of nominal, adverbial, and relative clauses contribute to the growth in complexity of syntax. Sentence complexity continues to grow through the high school years and into adulthood, with increased maturation reflecting the development and influence of written language skills. Using expository text is the norm during the period of middle elementary school through high school. With syntax as the "vehicle even *workhorse* of meaning" (Scott, 2009, p. 185), the complexity of informational text, both for content and the syntax used to convey it, emerges as a crucial component of reading comprehension for students. Sentences written in informational text are typically longer and therefore denser than those in **narrative** text. Chaney (1992) suggested the value of good syntactic knowledge in reading comprehension and reported that readers with better awareness of grammatical structure have better paragraph comprehension, possibly because they are able to use strong grammatical knowledge to monitor comprehension.

The ability to deconstruct sentences for comprehension or to construct them either orally or in writing to convey meaning is dependent on knowledge of syntactic rules. Understanding the meaning of sentences requires knowledge of syntactic rules, word meaning, and the relationships between and among the words. It is possible to understand sentence grammar separate from meaning ("Jabberwocky") and appreciate meaning in the context of inadequate grammar ("It don't mean nothing"). In addition, to some extent, syntactic interpretation relies on the ability to maintain sentences in working memory (Adams & Gathercole, 1995) and to exploit phonological memory (Montgomery, 1996).

Whereas phonological knowledge and skills are relevant to early decoding, morphological and syntactic knowledge are significant to fluency and comprehension in later reading development. Beyond the initial stages of reading, most typically in second grade (Chall, 1983), increased fluency and comprehension become the focus of reading instruction. Knowledge of syntax enables readers to make predictions from among a set of possibilities about what type of word or words must be coming next. This can be easily demonstrated using the **cloze technique (fill-in-the-blank technique),** which is common to research designs in the study of syntax: *Sam gave Ida the* _____. Knowledge of syntactic structure helps an individual to predict the likelihood of either an adjective or a noun or both coming next. This predictive ability aids in automaticity. As a clinician and teacher trainer, I have taught many the practice of "grammatical parsing" to aid in developing fluency with appropriate-level decodable text. By teaching children to recognize phrase structure in part by their responses to a set of *wh-* questions, fluency is increased as syntactic structure is exposed ("After hearing/the dog growl/the boy/who was frightened/screamed for his mother"). Embedded in this practice is the increased transparency of word combinations based on semantic–syntactic relationships.

Relationship of Syntactic Disorders to Literacy   For children who have difficulty with expressive or receptive syntax, the effect on reading may not become obvious until later in elementary school, when the emphasis shifts from decoding to comprehension. Moreover, comprehension difficulties may not emerge until the density of text increases beyond the reader's syntactic knowledge limits. As with all aspects of language, there is a continuum that reflects both a developmental sequence and the degree of complexity (from single words to complex sentences). A parallel continuum for language difficulty involves the degree of severity and the pervasiveness of the difficulty (e.g., one particular aspect or all aspects).

Studies of early syntactic delay were predictive of subsequent reading disability (Scarborough, 1990, 2001), as were studies of children identified more globally as having language impairments in which disordered syntax was a characteristic (Aram & Hall, 1989). Moreover, research has amply documented the persistence of early identified language impairment, including syntax-specific deficits (Nippold, Mansfield, Billow, & Tomblin, 2008; Scott & Windsor, 2000) into adolescence, with academic consequences (Conte-Ramsden & Durkin, 2008; Johnson et al., 1999; Nippold, Mansfield, Billow, & Tomblin, 2009). Other research has shown that children with reading difficulties have sentence comprehension problems as well. In particular, children and adolescents have difficulty interpreting later occurring complex structures such as those that contain **embedded** or **relative clauses** (Byrne, 1981; Morice & Slaghuis, 1985; Stein, Cairns, & Zurif, 1984). For children with a history of oral language impairment, longitudinal studies document the evolution of reading disability (Catts, Adlof, & Ellis Weismer, 2006; Catts, Adlof, Hogan, & Ellis Weismer, 2005; Scarborough, 2001). The oral–written language continuum is manifested in comprehension deficits as well. Reliance on semantic (meaning) strategies and limitations in working memory that would enable the child to retain the sentence for a sufficient period of time to analyze are possible contributing factors to difficulty in sentence comprehension. Many measures of sentence comprehension are confounded by precisely this working memory factor.

Lahey and Bloom (1994) offered that sentence comprehension is far more complex than issues of working memory limitations would imply. As always, they considered a more encompassing view of sentence comprehension that includes working memory capacity, the ability to automatically retrieve the language knowledge needed to construct in mind what the sentence (and its parts) is representing, the nature of the material being processed (in or out of a context familiar to the child), and the availability and strength of any context cues. Sentence comprehension is not a simple process for anyone, but for a child with learning and language difficulties, it is an even greater task. Cain and Oakhill (2007) reviewed available research and identified the relationship between reading comprehension and syntactic awareness tasks. What remains unclear is the specific nature of the relationship between syntactic comprehension problems and reading disability, although there is sufficient evidence to suggest that they coexist. Direct instruction in the writing of complex sentences via sentence-combining techniques (Eisenberg, 2006) has been suggested by Scott (2009) as one means of improving sentence-level comprehension. Manipulating short, kernel sentences with a variety of clausal forms (e.g., adverbial, relative) allows for a range of complex sentence structures. Such activities are part of a written language program (Hochman, 2009) that uses content-area material in an integrated reading comprehension/written language program (see Chapter 17 for more on composition instruction).

Comprehension of spoken syntax is supported by the discourse (conversational) structure of the interaction as well as by the **paralinguistic** and **situational** cues. Far fewer cues are available to the reader, and thus failure to accurately analyze sentence structure can result in deficient comprehension. In addition to the differences interpreting spoken versus written sentences, genre (narrative vs. expository) influences comprehension as well (Scott, 2004, 2005).

The elements of language form (phonology, morphology, and syntax) have clear relationships to one another as one aspect of the foundation on which literacy is built. Early reading ability is strongly connected to phonological knowledge, as is the later development of spelling. Morphological knowledge adds to the skills required for spelling and comprehension. Later reading development, fluency, and comprehension have their roots in morphology and syntax while continuing to rely on efficient phonological processing.

Language Content

Language content, often referred to as semantics, is the meaning component of language. Language content reflects world knowledge and what we know about objects, events, and relationships. The study of semantics is concerned with the meanings of words and the relationship between and among words as they are used to represent knowledge of the world. As explained by Lahey (1988), language content involves both the endless number of particular topics that can be discussed and the general categories of objects, actions, and relationships. Thus, all children of different cultures or experiences talk about content in terms of the objects, events, and relationships of their world, but the topics within each of these categories are different. Children raised in Mexico City or in Brooklyn will talk about food (object), eating (action), and possession (relationship) but are likely to ask for different foods.

Language content involves not only individual word meanings, as in analyzing a child's vocabulary, but also understanding the meaning features that compose a word; how a word may (or may not) be used in a phrase, a sentence, or discourse; and the literal and figurative meanings of words. Words are composed of clusters of meaning features that allow us to define words and to differentiate among them. Most often, knowledge of these features is unconscious. Try, for example, to define the word *walk*. Although all of us know what it means, and most are able to demonstrate it, defining *walk* is quite difficult. Furthermore, when asked, "What does *draft* mean?" one could potentially supply six different responses, ranging from conscription (being drafted into the military) to an alcoholic beverage (an ice-cold draft beer). Thus, determining whether a person knows a word extends beyond checking his or her ability to point to a picture of it or even to use it in a sentence. Moreover, a person's knowledge of the world and the words used to represent that knowledge grows continuously across the life span. Over time, a person may come to associate varied meanings with each word because of increased exposure to assorted usages or varied personal experience. With exposure to print, a person may read about places, events, or people; although they are not directly experienced, the person may acquire new knowledge as well as the lexicon (vocabulary) that represents the experience. In addition, there are rules that govern how words may be used in combination.

Consider, for example, the sentence "The bachelor's wife is beautiful." Although superficially the sentence is grammatically acceptable, the relationship between *bachelor* and *wife* raises a serious question as to the meaning of the sentence. Furthermore, the varying roles that words may play in a sentence can result in ambiguity that requires the language user to consider not only word meaning but also context. Consider the sentence, "Visiting relatives can be a nuisance." The meaning varies depending on the grammatical role ascribed to *visiting* as either a gerund or an adjective. These rules for using words in combination begin to develop quite early in a child's language acquisition process and form part of the basis for later semantic knowledge.

Word meaning may be literal or figurative. Part of the richness of language is in the imagery that it can create to express the more emotional and ethereal aspects of the human experience. Whether one has *had a ball* (had a good time at a party or possessed a baseball at some time) or *opened a can of worms* (went fishing or unintentionally caused a problem), the semantic knowledge and use are reflected in the way in which meaning is colored.

Meaning in language is conveyed through using words and their combinations. Language content is the knowledge of the vast array of objects, events, and relationships and the way they are represented.

REFLECT, CONNECT, and RESPOND
How is language content culturally influenced?

Semantic Development   People talk or write to communicate meaning just as they listen or read to determine meaning. The process of learning to assign meaning begins in infancy during the preverbal stages of development. Meaning can be represented in a word, in a sentence, or across sentences, as well as in nonlinguistic ways.

Each of us has a lexicon, a mental dictionary within our semantic memory. Individual word meanings as well as how words may be used are found in the lexicon. In early development, children may ascribe different meanings to a word to represent a variety of objects or events or relationships. Thus, in the single-word stage of language development, *cup* pronounced as "kuh" may mean a request for a drink or a request that a fallen cup be returned to the tray of the highchair. In early stages of language acquisition, word meaning may be overextended so that, for example, any four-legged furry animal is called "cat." Obviously, children and adults do not use words in the same way. Although a child may use a word taken from adult lexicon (e.g., *cat*), the meaning may be different as reflected in the over-extensions of meaning that children make. Fortunately, word meanings are consistently refined over time so that speakers of the same language share common definitions for words.

In the early single-word stages of language development, children have already begun to code meaning for the words they use. They will use a word to indicate a variety of semantic categories such as existence (indicated by looking at, naming, touching, or referring to an object that exists in their world), nonexistence or disappearance (an object expected to be seen does not appear; "bye-bye"), or recurrence (the reappearance of an object or the recurrence of an event; "more").

As children progress to the two-word stage of language development, new semantic relations emerge, both individually and in combination. Between 18 and 36 months of age, children steadily acquire an increasing number of meaning relations that they can represent, such as agent-action ("Russell kiss") or attribute-entity ("big book").

With continued development, children begin to acquire vocabulary at a rapid rate and in a generally predictable order (Biemiller & Slonim, 2001; Leung, Silverman, Nandakumar, Qian, & Hines, 2010). From the toddler years through first grade, children acquire new words at a steady pace, dependent in part on the nature of the exposure to words that they experience. Bates and colleagues (1994) offered estimates of the number of words children (toddlers through age 5) have acquired and can use. They reported that expressively a 15-month-old will have 4–6 words, progressing to 20–50 words at 18 months, accelerating to 200–300 words by 24 months, 900–1000 words by age 3, 1,500–1,600 words by age 4, and over 2,000 words at 5. The rate of growth is remarkably brisk and virtually without direct instruction at this stage. Furthermore, Biemiller (2005) posited that the average 6-year-old will know more than 6,000 words. That pattern of growth once a child can decode and comprehend becomes exponential. It is a massive task and remarkable feat to acquire sufficient information from interacting with the world (with little direct instruction) to develop a lexicon of nouns, verbs, adjective, adverbs, and prepositions, as well as the words to represent a huge array of concepts such as time, space, and causality.

Learning a word is a long-term developmental process. It includes determining that a set of sounds is a word; learning the word's meaning components, privileges (where and how it is permitted to be used) and restrictions on its use (e.g., *bachelor* does not have the privilege of occurring in the phrase *the bachelor's wife* because bachelors do not have wives); and learning its syntactic properties (parts of speech, how it may be used in a sentence) and the conceptual foundations on which that word is based. Not only must children develop word meanings, but they also must learn contextual meaning. In the preschool years, words and sentence meaning expand. Later, children must learn to discern meaning from context (both linguistic and nonlinguistic) as well as to use later developing, more sophisticated cohesive devices to connect sentences into discourse.

Cohesive devices (Halliday & Hasan, 1976) include using pronouns or definite articles that refer to someone or something previously mentioned. This process is called **anaphora** (e.g., "Marsha was hungry. *She* went out to get lunch"). Another cohesive device, **ellipsis,** is the deletion of information available in a portion of the discourse immediately preceding (e.g., "Can you ice skate? I can"). Still another cohesive device, called **lexical cohesion,** involves the use of **synonyms** that refer to previously identified referents (e.g., "The *puppy* excitedly chased his tail. Our new *pet* was very entertaining").

In addition to relational meanings and contextual meaning, children must master the nonlinguistic aspects of meaning. **Deictic terms** are words that shift in meaning depending on how the nonlinguistic context changes. The meanings of words such as *I, you, here,* and *tomorrow* depend on who is speaking, where the participants are, and when the words are spoken.

Children acquire meaning of words and sentences and meaning across sentences in discourse. They must master a vast amount of information about the semantic and syntactic roles of words and about contextual and nonlinguistic aspects of meaning. It is amazing that much of this is accomplished in the preschool years. Later semantic development is concerned with continued refinement of previous content knowledge as well as with ongoing growth in vocabulary and in the mastery of **nonliteral language** such as **metaphors,** idioms, proverbs, and humor.

The power of word knowledge is seen most clearly in its impact on listening and reading comprehension, as well as writing. The strong connection between vocabulary knowledge, both breadth and depth of word meanings, and reading comprehension has a long history in research. The logic of the relationship between lexical knowledge and reading is intuitive; you will understand what you read if you know the meaning of the words. Vocabulary growth is a function of exposure, reading and problem-solving ability, and good instruction. Effective vocabulary instruction involves the creation of word-rich classroom environments, independence in word learning, development of authentic instructional strategies, and the use of realistic assessments (Blachowicz & Fisher, 2002). As children become literate, the opportunities for growth in semantic knowledge grow considerably. After children learn to read, reading becomes a vehicle for learning (see Chapter 15 for more about word learning and vocabulary instruction).

Relationship of Semantic Disorders to Literacy   There is more to reading than decoding (determining the pronunciation of words by noting the positions of vowels and consonants). The proof of a skilled, fluent reader may be the ability to read a professional manual filled with unfamiliar technical jargon. Being able to decode the words may very well be insufficient to provide the intended meaning or comprehension of the text. Once the reader has gained access to the words through decoding, the meaning of the words and sentences must be analyzed and synthesized for comprehension to occur. Comprehension in reading then is dependent on semantic, syntactic, and world knowledge. Consider *diadochokinesis,* a word unfamiliar to most. A strong decoder can syllabicate and decode the word syllable by syllable, a likely approach given the length of the word, but may not be able to guess the meaning (rapid alternating movements, such as those associated with speech articulation).

Gough and Tunmer (1986) referenced two sets of skills in reading: decoding and linguistic comprehension. Reading is not a unitary action, nor is the use of oral language. Rather, both activities reflect a complex integration of skills. When looking at different groups identified as having reading disorders, dyslexia, language disorders, or specific language impairment, it is important to consider the criteria that are selected to define the group and which skills are under investigation before generalizing the implications of research findings.

During a consideration of semantic deficits in vocabulary and word knowledge, word retrieval, and the relationship to syntax and sentence comprehension, it is necessary to be concerned with the dynamic relationship of form, content, and use. Weak phonological coding may specifically be related to establishing poorer networks of word meanings as well as poorer access to those words. Thus, facility or difficulty in one aspect of language as it relates to reading does not preclude the same ease or difficulty in the other aspects of reading. Some good decoders have poor comprehension, just as in the early stages of reading mastery, and poorer decoders may have adequate comprehension. Swank (1997) demonstrated that in addition to phonological coding, meaning and grammar are important to the decoding abilities of kindergarten and first-grade readers. Similarly, Snowling and Nation (1997) wrote that syntactic and semantic information derived from sentences allowed children to alter their inaccurate pronunciation of decoded **target**

words so that the words made sense in the context of the sentence. In older children with reading difficulties, semantic deficits may be the result of what Vellutino, Scanlon, and Spearing referred to as having "accrued" as a consequence of prolonged decoding difficulty in which poor readers are denied access to semantic information about word meaning and use (1995, p. 76). Early in their school careers, children learn to read, and for the remainder of their academic years, they read to learn (Chall, 1983). Nippold suggested a "symbiotic" relationship between literacy and learning during the later school years (1988, p. 29).

By fourth grade, reading becomes the primary means of acquiring new vocabulary. When children have inherent language deficits, semantic functions may be restricted, thus influencing learning to read as well as later reading to learn. Semantic deficits may manifest at different times in the reading process, dependent in part on the kind of reading instruction a child receives. Emphasizing phonics in a highly structured sound–symbol system in which word identification is stressed may allow comprehension difficulties based on semantic deficits to go unnoticed for longer periods of time. When text-based approaches to early reading are stressed, semantic deficits are more likely to be exposed earlier in the process of learning to read.

Semantic competence involves a high degree of organization among the concepts that are being accumulated in the semantic system. Semantic networks must be formed to provide the structure for the concepts that a child is learning. Children who are weaker at concept formation are likely to have less robust vocabulary and weaker semantic networks. Lack of exposure to concepts or difficulties in concept formation or in the organization of the concepts may result in less effective reading comprehension. So, children with ongoing oral language difficulties remain at higher risk for reading comprehension difficulties if their oral language deficits result in depressed semantic knowledge. Van Vierson and colleagues (2017) reported that early deficits in receptive and expressive vocabulary are associated with later reading difficulties. Moreover, in studying the literacy acquisition of children at risk for familial dyslexia, they noted that deficient vocabulary development in young children can be considered an additional risk factor in dyslexia.

Children with reading deficits have been shown to have difficulties in vocabulary, word categorization, and word retrieval. Many children with reading impairments have more difficulty than same-age peers in providing accurate definitions for words. Hoskins (1983) reported that children with reading impairments were more likely to offer descriptions and examples of words they were asked to define rather than to provide more formal, specific definitions. This is a frequently observed clinical behavior. It reflects one level of general comprehension of word meaning and use (e.g., "I know how to use it, but I can't really tell you what it means"). For teachers who are concerned about the reading comprehension abilities of their students, defining versus describing is a skill for which to watch.

Categorization abilities, another semantic skill reflecting a knowledge base, is also frequently deficient in children with reading difficulties. Children with reading and other learning disabilities often demonstrate restricted word meanings as well as weakly developed associations among words and classes of words. Limitations in reading comprehension may result from restricted word meanings that reduce the reader's ability to interpret sentences; reduced vocabulary knowledge so that less familiar, multisyllabic words are more difficult to decode; and poorly developed semantic networks between word meanings and categories.

Other than word meaning itself, it is necessary to consider several other important aspects of semantics. Understanding a word also requires knowledge of synonyms, **antonyms,** and multiple meanings of a word. At higher levels of abstraction, semantic knowledge includes appreciating and using humor, slang, idioms, **similes,** and metaphors (Roth & Spekman, 1989). World knowledge also plays a considerable role in how semantics functions in reading comprehension. Lack of world knowledge means that a decoding error is more likely to remain uncorrected when reading on an unfamiliar topic. Lack of an adequate knowledge base to judge the content that is being read may result in comprehension errors as well.

Word retrieval problems are another frequently observed semantic deficit that affects literacy. Word retrieval problems may be described as a person's difficulty in gaining access to a specific, intended word from his or her vocabulary. So, despite knowledge of the word, there is a disruption in recovering or retrieving the phonetic structure (sound pattern) of the word to express it in spontaneous production. Common behaviors of people with word retrieval difficulties are delay in retrieving the word; substitution of other, similar words; circumlocutions (descriptions of aspects of the word, as when a person says, "You know, the place where you swim," but means *pool*); the use of gestures or demonstration to represent the word; and the substitution of nonspecific words (e.g., *thing, stuff, the place*) for the specific word. Children with reading disabilities have been shown to have a slower rate of naming, more frequent naming errors, and longer delays before responding (Denckla & Rudel, 1976; German, 1982; Wiig, Semel, & Nystrom, 1982; see Chapter 12, on fluency, for more information about this topic).

Children with word-retrieval difficulties may read less fluently, with many hesitations and rephrasings. A child may look at a word and offer a definition but may be unable to say the specific word. Given the frequent substitution of similar or related words, comprehension may not be seriously affected; however, the dilemma may be in demonstrating comprehension when specific words are not readily accessible.

Finally, as children become more adequate decoders, they read for meaning across sentences and through extended text rather than from individual words. At this juncture, semantic knowledge must become integrated with syntactic knowledge and the more pragmatic, or discourse-related, aspects of language that include a knowledge of narrative structure and the ability to determine the writer's intent.

REFLECT, CONNECT, and RESPOND
What impact do vocabulary deficits have on reading comprehension?

Language Use, or Pragmatics

Language use is frequently referred to as pragmatics. Pragmatics involves a set of rules that dictate communicative behavior in three main areas: reasons for communication, called communicative functions or intentions; different codes or styles of communication necessary in a particular context; and conversation or discourse. Each person speaks for a variety of purposes with an assortment of intentions. These intentions refer to the speaker's goals in talking. For example, one may speak to greet, inquire, answer, request a behavior or information, negotiate, or teach, among many other possibilities.

Success in communicating intentions depends on several factors. A speaker must choose the appropriate code or style from among the variety of ways in which something can be said. To make that decision, a speaker must consider the context and the listener's needs. The words and sentences chosen to formulate the thought depend on the ages, knowledge bases, and relative status of speaker and listener. Imagine using the greeting, "Hi, sweetie!" uniformly when greeting your 3-year-old, your pharmacist, and your boss. The words chosen depend on what is occurring or what is present at the time the words are spoken. Two people standing on a train platform at 7 a.m. on a weekday would find it appropriate to hear, "Here it comes." The same utterance while standing in line at the supermarket might be met with a quizzical, "What?"

Finally, pragmatics involves rules of conversation or discourse. To communicate effectively, a speaker must be able to start a conversation, enter a conversation in process, and appropriately remain in a conversation. Moreover, competent communicators must be able to take turns within a conversation, recognize the need for clarification and provide it, change the subject appropriately, listen and respond meaningfully, and tell a coherent and cohesive story (narrative). The minutiae of competent conversation and narrative are an extensive area of study because of their significance in the social and academic lives of children (Applebee, 1978; Brinton & Fujiki, 1989, 1999; Dore, 1978; Halliday, 1975; Landa, 2005; Prutting & Kirschner, 1987; Rees, 1978).

Mastering the social uses of language is an ongoing process for young language learners. In school, classroom discourse patterns and a literate level of talking and understanding represent a level of language use that is critical for academic success.

The difference between everyday discourse and the language of the classroom and expository writing is dramatic. Although a child may have adequate linguistic ability for everyday conversational interactions, the same child may not have achieved the level of language use necessary to comprehend the language of instruction, which requires understanding more sophisticated vocabulary, words with multiple meanings, figurative usages, more varied and complex sentence structures, the distinction between what the sentence is saying and what it is intended to have the listener do, and the higher levels of understanding (those that are less direct in interpretation). Such vulnerability can be easily overlooked and is seriously deleterious to a child's learning ability.

REFLECT, CONNECT, and RESPOND
What factors influence successful communication?

Pragmatic Development The earliest observations of communicative development can be made during the period between birth and approximately 10 months of age. This stage of preverbal communication is the first of three periods identified by Bates, Camaioni, and Volterra (1975). In this earliest period, the child is not aware of the communicative effect of his or her behavior. Although a child might point or reach toward an object of interest, he or she does not do this to elicit an adult's attention or action. In the next stage of communicative development, the one-word stage, which typically occurs when children are between 10 and 15 months old, a child more definitely intends to communicate with the adults around him or her. Although these attempted communications may not involve speech, they are clearly recognized by both the infant and the adult as having intent. These attempts may be gestural and/or gestural and vocal (as differentiated from verbal attempts alone). Once an infant begins to use words to communicate, he or she is at the multiword stage, the third stage of this early period of communicative development. The infant's previous intentions were conveyed by gesture and vocalization. Now, more conventional word forms begin to serve similar purposes. As the use of words accomplishes goals for an infant or toddler, the child begins to monitor and learn from the listener's reactions. The infant begins to see the effects of his or her utterances; as such, social interaction provides the context for learning about communication.

Roth and Spekman (1984) identified three sets of categories of intentional behavior for children in preverbal, one-word, and multiword stages that reflect a developmental process:

1. Intentional behavior from preverbal attention seeking, requesting, greeting, protesting or rejecting, responding/acknowledging, and informing

2. A more advanced stage in which words are added and allow for the refinement of the original intentions and the addition of naming and commenting

3. Multiword utterance stages in which intention is more varied and refined and may now express rules and opinions

The last set is foundational for using language in a more adultlike manner for regulating and controlling conversational interactions.

As these toddlers in the multiword stage become preschoolers, they begin to learn more complex ways of using language for social purposes. Their conversational skills grow, as do their discourse skills, such as telling stories, describing with greater clarity, and recounting personal experiences. As children's language skills grow, they can use language for an increasing number of school-related skills, such as instructing or reasoning. As they progress toward the school years, children begin to use their pragmatic skills for an ever-growing number of purposes at a higher, more refined level. Now, language used to plan and organize must help to construct narratives of greater density and longer sequences of events. An increasing number of communicative intentions, more sophisticated conversational skills, and improved narrative (storytelling) skills all mark the development of language use in preschoolers.

Conversational skills develop further during the elementary school years. In the preschool years, conversation between children and adults is often supported by the adult. If a preschooler has not effectively communicated his or her intent, and a clarification is requested, then the child will typically repeat what he or she has just said. By the early elementary school years, however, a student will not only repeat but also will elaborate in an attempt to be clearer for the listener. By the middle elementary school years, a student can not only elaborate but also explain, provide additional background information, and monitor the listener's comprehension in an ongoing way (Brinton, Fujiki, Loeb, & Winkler, 1986). Conversation among school-age children also involves the mastery of slang. In addition, children speak to each other in sentence structures that are more complex, elaborate, and varied than they use when speaking to adults. This is consistent with parents' observations of the difference between the way children talk at home and how they communicate among friends (Owens, 1996). Certainly, among teenagers, using language for social purposes becomes more crucial. Also important is the ability to shift effectively from one conversational style (social) to another (academic) to meet the higher expectations of teachers for a fully literate style of language use (Larson & McKinley, 1995).

The school-age years bring with them another level of maturation and an increased demand on children's pragmatic abilities. During these years, several important changes take place in pragmatic development and use. The number of communicative functions must expand. Children have to use their language skills but must do so with increased levels of appropriateness and often more indirectly (e.g., seeing a friend in a scarf and heavy coat and commenting "Oh, you must be cold" without explicitly telling how the speaker knows this). The demands on narrative production increase steadily. Preschoolers' simple storytelling of one or two facts or events grows to fulfill the requirements of show and tell as well as book reports and essays. Children who have heard stories read and told throughout their lives come to these school-based narrative tasks better equipped than peers with fewer literacy experiences (Linder, 1999). There is a structure and pattern to the ways stories are constructed (Stein & Glenn, 1979). When children have been exposed to this pattern frequently because they have been read to on a regular basis, they come to school with a tacit knowledge of the structure of stories that becomes increasingly more available to them as it is required in the school environment.

The language of the classroom is different from the everyday language used for social interaction. In school, there is a greater degree of formality. The choice of words is often more abstract and unfamiliar; sentence structures are more complex; the interactions are planned and controlled; the topics, which are also controlled, are often related to texts; the rate of speech is faster; and, above all, the language of the classroom is decontextualized (Nelson, 1986). When classroom language is decontextualized, few contextual **clues** are available that children can use to understand this language. This is in contrast to everyday conversations when, as communicators, people are supported by context in cues such as facial expressions, gestures, intonational patterns, and the presence of the object being discussed.

Unlike conversation, instructional discourse provides less meaning and support from context. Understanding is more fully dependent on the words. The purposes of language in the classroom are more instructive, regulatory, and acknowledging and are far less individualized and supportive than in conversation. There is a communicative imbalance that is particular to the classroom. Teachers control topics and turns. They ask questions to which they already know the answers (and judge the responses) and create an environment with the language of authority. Britton (1979) wrote that in a conversation the partners are participants who have a generally equal role in the course and direction of the conversation. He described another style of conversation in which one partner is dominant and the other is more of a "spectator" (1979, p. 192). Spectators, he noted, "use language to digest experience" (p. 192). Indeed, when considering classroom discourse, students most frequently play the role of spectators. Westby (1991) provided a succinct analysis of the difference between an oral style of language use and a literate style of language use by differentiating within the categories of the function, topics, and structure of language. Considering the structure of the interaction differentiates between the social and familiar versus formal and regulatory, reflective, and non-immediate. Analysis of the topics of oral versus literate language interactions, the differences are evident in everyday, here-and-now topics versus more abstract and unfamiliar events and relationships there and then. Finally, the structure of the exchanges will be differentiated by the use of high-frequency words, with slang and jargon juxtaposed to low-frequency words, more abstract vocabulary, and more concise syntax and content.

The differences between social and instructional discourse can be highlighted by comparing a request for information and its aftermath in two different contexts: a social context and a classroom environment. A special form of instructional dialogue exists within classrooms (Cazden, 1988; Nelson, 1985), referred to as the initiation–response–evaluation interaction pattern, that consists of teacher initiation, student response, and teacher evaluation. Thus, in a classroom one might hear the following:

TEACHER: *[Initiating]* What is the capital of California?

STUDENT: *[Responding]* Sacramento.

TEACHER: *[Evaluating]* That's right. Very good.

In a social environment, a similar exchange would end somewhat differently:

SPEAKER 1:   What is the capital of California?

SPEAKER 2:   Sacramento.

SPEAKER 1:   Thanks.

In the classroom, the question is a test, although it is phrased as a request for information. In an everyday interaction, the request for information is a genuine request. (See Table 3.4 for a discussion of the differences between oral language and literate [classroom] language.)

REFLECT, CONNECT, and RESPOND
Define the differences between social and instructional discourse.

Relationship of Pragmatic Disorders to Literacy   The emphasis on the relationship between language and reading has grown stronger (Catts, 1996; Greene, 1996; Kamhi & Catts, 1986). For certain children, whose oral language skills are age appropriate when they enter school, early literacy acquisition and accommodation to school discourse may not be negatively affected. Yet, as the demands of the curriculum escalate, these same children may not have developed enough linguistically to meet expectations. Skills that were adequate in early grades when the emphasis was on decoding and when instruction was more experiential in nature are now insufficient as reading to learn becomes the expected mode (Chall, 1983). Moreover, as the curriculum expands, topics become less familiar; new vocabulary and more complex sentences, paragraphs, and texts must be analyzed and interpreted; more reading and writing are expected; and the cognitive demands become more abstract.

Reading comprehension is an enormously complex integration of high-level linguistic ability and problem-solving skills. Approaching reading with the intent to understand and gain information and with the expectation that the text will make sense are the behaviors of good readers. They recognize that the goal of reading is to comprehend, and to that end they monitor their own comprehension. Poor readers, by contrast, will often perceive the purpose of reading as sounding out and saying the words aloud. The expectation or intent to understand what has been decoded is sharply reduced or is not a concern of poorer readers (Bos & Filip, 1982; Brown, 1982; Myers & Paris, 1978; Owings, Peterson, Bransford, Morris, & Stein, 1980; see Chapter 16 for information about strategies for teaching reading comprehension).

Table 3.4. Oral/literate language differences

Oral language	Literate language
Function	
Talking to regulate social interaction— requesting, commanding, protesting, seeking interaction	Talking to reflect on the past and future— predicting, projecting into thoughts and feelings of others, reasoning, imagining
Questions generally asked by speakers to gain information they do not have	Pseudoquestions asked to get the listener to perform for the speaker who knows the answers
Used to share understanding of the concrete and practical	Used to learn and teach
Symmetrical communication—everyone has an equal right to participate in the conversation; participants collaborate on the discourse	Asymmetrical communication—one person has the floor and is responsible for organizing the entire discourse
Content	
Talk is about the here and now—the concrete	Talk is about the there and then—the past and future; the abstract
Topic-associative organization; chaining of ideas or anecdotes	Topic-centered organization; explicit, linear description of single event
Meaning is in the context (shared information or the environment)	Meaning is in the text
Structure	
Use of pronouns, slang, and jargon; expressions known only to the in-group	Use of explicit, specific vocabulary
Familiar words	Unfamiliar words
Repetitive syntax and ideas	Minimal or no repetition of syntax and ideas
Cohesion based on intonation	Cohesion based on formal linguistic markers (because, therefore, and so forth)

From Westby, C. (1995). Culture and literacy: Frameworks for understanding. *Topics in Language Disorders, 16*(1), 59; reprinted by permission.

An essential higher order linguistic ability in text comprehension is the aspect of language use called discourse, which includes both conversational and narrative ability. Numerous higher order language and cognitive skills are necessary for text comprehension, including the following (as identified by Roth & Spekman, 1989): understanding the relationship between words and word parts, grasping sentence cohesion (i.e., the relationship between two sentences or parts of a sentence as signaled by cohesive devices), identifying words based on context or familiarity, determining vocabulary meaning based on context (including multiple meaning words and figurative language), understanding at different levels from literal to inferential (identifying main ideas, summarizing, predicting, and determining character traits and emotions), determining the communicative intent of the author, identifying and retaining relevant information, and using knowledge of narrative structure.

Knowledge of narrative structure and determining the author's intent can play crucial roles in comprehension when syntax (sentence structure) and semantics (meaning aspects) are otherwise intact. Recognizing narrative structure and the intention of the writer is part of the active construction of comprehension that extends beyond the interpretations of the grammatical and meaning components of a piece of writing. Research has affirmed that the quality of narrative production of school-age children is highly relevant to educational performance. In fact, narrative analysis is more revealing of linguistic vulnerabilities than conversational analysis (Boudreau, 2008; Fey, Catts, Proctor-Williams, Tomblin, & Zhang, 2004). Narrative abilities have been shown to be highly predictive of school success (Bishop & Edmundson, 1987; Tabors, Snow, & Dickinson, 2001).

The ability to appreciate and use narrative structure in comprehension (and oral and/or written production) has been studied in children with reading problems. Using story grammars that describe a story's internal structure (both the components of the story and the rules for the order of, and relationship among, these components) has been the most common way of analyzing narratives (Mandler & Johnson, 1977; Stein & Glenn, 1979).

Stein and Glenn's (1979) story grammar consists of a setting category and a system for ordering episodes within the story. This system is easily recognizable to those with the tacit knowledge of narrative structure and familiarity with literature. They are as follows: setting statements (*Nicole looked out across the expanse of land that she knew could now be hers*), initiating events (*The matching numbers were so unexpected*), internal responses (*Nicole remained numbed by the news*), plans for obtaining a goal (*Nicole started a telephone list. There was little time to waste*), attempts at achieving the goal (*Call after call, Nicole reported the news*), direct consequences of the attempts to reach the goal (*Everyone had been reached. They would arrive within 2 days*), and reactions that describe the emotional response (*With a grin on her face, she dropped into her favorite chair, exhausted and exhilarated!*). Then, the focus on the importance of narrative development in relationship to reading comprehension and writing became more concentrated (Hedberg & Westby, 1997; Hughes, McGillivray, & Schmidek, 1997); cross-cultural (McCabe & Bliss, 2003); and related to communication development, literacy, and cognition (Stadler & Ward, 2005). From these foundational paradigms, materials and programs have been created that allow for the instruction of the concept of narrative in preschoolers. Moreau and Fidrych (1998) developed The Story Grammar Marker program. Its basic, original format can be adapted according to the age and need of the children being taught. Supported visually with icons and charts, it captures the developmental expectations and appropriate components of narrative.

Children with language and reading disabilities have less appreciation for narrative structure as defined by story grammar. Poorer understanding of temporal and causal relationships, limited detail, mistaken information, shorter retellings, and difficulty with inferential questions were also observed in children with language disorders (Gerber, 1993; Roth, 1986). Westby (1989) reported that children with language disorders tell shorter stories with fewer complete episodes, use a more restricted vocabulary, and have less well-organized stories than their peers who use language more typically.

In addition to knowing and using narrative structure, understanding the intent of the writer (or speaker, in oral discourse) is another pragmatically based aspect of comprehension. This involves appreciating information that is not presented explicitly. This grasp of suggested or implied information, called presupposition, is necessary for the message being communicated to be understood (Bates, 1976; Rees, 1978).

In order to be a successful communicator, it is necessary to have sufficient language flexibility to adjust what is being said according to the needs of the listener.

That may mean altering word choice, sentence structure, gestures, and paralinguistic features such as intonation patterns based on a variety of characteristics, including age, relative status (of speaker and listener), intellectual level, and awareness of the listener's prior knowledge of the topic. Sociolinguist Hymes offered a definition of pragmatics as "knowing what to say to whom, how and under what circumstances" (1972). A listener must monitor his or her comprehension and request clarification if necessary.

The parallels of pragmatics of oral language or discourse to reading are strong. Written language can be used for a variety of purposes with different intentions. In writing, one can request, create, solicit, inform, educate, entertain, describe, and persuade, among a lengthy list of other purposes. For the reader, the mandate is to discern the communicative intent of the author in nonfiction and of the author and characters in fiction. When children have vulnerabilities in determining a speaker's intent in oral discourse, they are clearly at risk for failing to make these determinations from print. So much emphasis is placed on the decoding process in the early school years that the functional and communicative intents of writing are often neglected (Creaghead, 1986). Children who are weaker in understanding implied meaning in conversation (e.g., the sarcasm in "Nice haircut" said with a sneer) may struggle later on when they are expected to interpret humor, sarcasm, figurative language (idioms), metaphors, and other less explicitly stated intended meanings (Bradshaw, Hoffman, & Norris, 1998; Nation, Clarke, Marshall, & Duran, 2004). Moreover, in reading, the physical and environmental cues on which speakers and listeners depend, such as an arched eyebrow, a falsetto voice, or the gape of onlookers, are absent or may be reflected in more abstract ways (should the author choose to do so) as italics or punctuation. In conversation, the speaker may recognize a listener's furrowed brow as signaling confusion and attempt to clarify before being asked to do so. No such author-given support is available to the reader. I have lost track of the number of times I have needed to help students recognize the need to actively construct their comprehension because Edgar Allan Poe, Jorge Luis Borges, and Toni Morrison are unavailable to explain themselves! Conversely, children can be motivated to consider the needs of their reader (typically a teacher) when writing an assignment via a reminder that the teacher is unlikely to call them at home and ask, "Just what did you mean in the second paragraph on page 3?"

It is crucial for teachers to recognize and remember that when children have vulnerabilities in discourse, they are at risk for comprehension difficulties with conversation and narrative despite having decoding skills. Active participation in the process of comprehending what is read involves a complex amalgam of skills among which language use or pragmatics is a subtle and often unrecognized vulnerability. When a child has adequate social language skills, the more hidden pragmatic weakness that can negatively affect comprehension may be overlooked easily. Direct instruction in narrative structure via story grammars and in identifying and interpreting the author's communicative intentions can markedly improve a student's level of reading comprehension.

Metalinguistic Development   At the most developed level of language use, beyond the basic pragmatic skills required for conversation and narrative, is another tier of language competence called metalinguistic abilities (Miller, 1990). Metalinguistic abilities permit a child to view language as an entity, something to talk and think about. Metalinguistic skills enable a child to use language to talk about language. In preschoolers, language is viewed primarily as a means of communication, not as an object of consideration. During the school-age years, however, children become increasingly able to reflect on language and make conscious decisions about their own language and how it works. This is different from having tacit, underlying knowledge that allows the generation of sentences with specific words that are appropriate to a situation. Metalinguistic skills are essential to successful school learning because they influence a number of school-based tasks and are particularly important to developing early decoding ability. Bunce (1993) identified the diverse nature of the metalinguistic skills required for literacy acquisition, comprehension, and successful school learning. At a phonological level, a child must be able to segment a word into its sounds and determine whether two words have the same sound. Another metalinguistic task is to determine whether two sentences have equal meaning or to identify a sentence by its syntactic form (e.g., declarative, interrogative). Recognizing multiple meanings, summarizing, and analyzing information are metalinguistic tasks as well.

Wallach and Miller (1988) established a sequence in the development of metalinguistic skills that evolves from 1½ to 10 years of age and older. In the earliest stages, children learn to recognize some printed symbols, such as fast-food signs or the first letter of their name. By the beginning of the later stages of metalinguistic awareness, between 5 and 8 years of age, children's metalinguistic knowledge becomes an essential part of learning to read. Among these skills are those associated with phonological awareness, such as rhyming, segmentation, and **phoneme deletion.** It is widely agreed that phonological awareness makes a major contribution to early decoding ability. Well-developed metalinguistic skills are as crucial to early reading ability as they ultimately are to classroom success in understanding the discourse patterns of the classroom and the ongoing need to analyze the language being used to teach the language that must be learned.

When children have weaker skills in language comprehension and use, they are at risk for academic difficulty at many levels. For some children, the shift from contextualized, social, familiar, adult-supported language to the decontextualized, pedagogic, novel, adult-directed, evaluative, metalinguistic language of the classroom is overwhelming. Such language difficulties can be virtually invisible in a child whose speech is clear and whose demeanor is undemanding. A common misperception is that these children lack motivation or interest; rather, their skills are not on the same level as the language and communication demands of the classroom. Language is a part of every aspect of the school day, and what appears to be inattention or lack of motivation may, in fact, be a lack of comprehension of the level of language presented and the rules of classroom discourse.

EXECUTIVE FUNCTION, WORKING MEMORY, LANGUAGE, AND LITERACY

Each day in school, a child is likely to hear the question, "What was that about?" after having read a passage. Teachers readily assume that a child will read with the intent to understand. Not all children do. Not all children can. It has been well established that reading is a language-based skill. Language is the mediator for most thinking and reasoning. As long ago as 1962, Vygotsky noted that "speech and language plays a central role in the development of self-control, self-direction, problem-solving and task performance." Moreover, language is the mediating force for an integrated set of cognitive capacities and abilities that involve storage, organization, retention, access, and manipulation of information. These capacities, identified as **executive function,** are essential to literacy development and particularly crucial to reading comprehension and writing. Executive function and self-regulation skills depend on three types of brain function: inhibitory control, working memory, and mental flexibility (Center on the Developing Child, 2012; Diamond, 2014). Chapter 8 provides an extended discussion of executive function and its role in learning. Of note, in children identified with specific language impairment (SLI), who are known to experience comprehension difficulties, there is evidence that the deficits they experience extend beyond the linguistic to specific aspects of executive function, inhibition, and cognitive flexibility (Pauls & Archibald, 2016). Of these subtypes of executive function, working memory in particular is essential to academic functioning. Working memory has been demonstrated to be an important aspect of the early development of the foundational oral/aural language skills essential for academic success. In studies of children between the ages of 2 and 4, associations were demonstrated between working memory at 2 and levels of expressive and receptive language skills at age 4 (Newbury, Klee, Stokes, & Moran, 2016). In learning, working memory and control of attention are inseparable.

Executive function is crucial to all aspects of academic learning. Teachers can appreciate the manner in which executive controls are in effect throughout the school day, particularly in reading comprehension. In order to appreciate what is being read, a student must have basic language and literacy skills, which are necessary but not sufficient to successfully comprehend. Readers must "construct" meaning from any form of text. In order to accomplish that, they must have the capacity to plan ("I am going to read this because. . ."), prioritize ("Do I need that information?"), activate prior knowledge ("What do I already know about this topic?"), hold and manipulate the information in mind (working memory), invoke strategies ("What can I do because I don't know what that word means?"), and self-monitor ("Did that make sense?"). Teachers want to avoid the experience of asking a child to read a passage, inquiring as to its meaning, being informed that the young reader has no notion of what has just been read, and hearing—in response to their incredulous question, "Well then, why did you just read that?"—the innocent but very concerning response, "Because you told me to."

Gaskins, Satlow, and Pressley (2007) identified seven executive principles that help define the relationship between reading comprehension and executive function. These principles can be explicitly taught to readers to build skills for successful engagement with text. For effective readers, such principles are a given. For those for whom reading remains a struggle (either decoding, comprehending, or both), their importance is less obvious. The seven principles underlying the reading comprehension–executive control relationship are as follows:

1. Reading must make sense.

2. Understanding is the result of planning.

3. Prioritizing leads to maximizing time and effort.

4. Gaining access to background information helps organize new information.

5. Self-checking enhances goal achievement.

6. Having a flexible mindset provides opportunities for increased understanding.

7. Understanding is improved by self-assessing.

Teaching the skills and strategies that support these principles can be done as part of the curriculum. Indeed, the curriculum itself becomes the vehicle for learning the components of executive function and the strategies that are their concrete realization.

Working memory is the capacity (as differentiated from ability) to hold information in mind for short periods of time while manipulating it. **Working memory** is essential to all aspects of learning and, therefore, academic performance; it is effectively a mental workspace (Gathercole & Alloway, 2008) where new information is temporarily stored while old information is retrieved and processed. Working memory is crucial to effective executive function. Executive function, which is metacognitive in nature, is the management function of the mind that is invoked when the challenge of a novel task is presented. Executive function plans and makes decisions in order to recognize, approach, analyze, plan, sustain involvement, tolerate obstacles, strategize, and solve a problem, along with the ability to regulate behavior, both actual and emotional ("stop, think, plan, [revise if necessary], do") (Baddeley, 2006; Denckla, 1996; Meltzer, 2007). Having sufficient working memory capacity is crucial because the "mental workspace" must be adequate for all the simultaneous mental activity. Of note, working memory is not vulnerable to socioeconomic factors (Engel, Santos, & Gathercole, 2008), whereas environmental factors have been demonstrated to have an influence on other aspects of cognitive development (e.g., language; Hart & Risley, 1999).

Richards (2003) catalogued several readily recognizable functions of working memory for a student: 1) holding an idea in mind while developing, elaborating, clarifying, or using it; 2) recalling from long-term memory while holding some information in short-term memory; 3) holding together the components of a task in memory while completing the task; 4) keeping together a series of new pieces of information so that they remain meaningful; and 5) holding a long-term plan in mind while thinking about a short-range goal. There are numerous realizations of these functions in the day-to-day activities of a classroom: 1) remembering all the components of a multistep direction; completing the steps in a multipart math problem; 2) retrieving the information necessary to answer a question while remembering the question (the failure of which can result in the often heard, "I forgot" or "Never mind"); 3) the demands of written language "mechanics" while composing; 4) decoding and blending the syllables in a multisyllabic word; and 5) rushing through a task and producing "careless" errors in the attempt to finish it before "forgetting" what was required.

Working memory is vital to language and literacy development as well as classroom learning. Limitations in working memory affect multiple aspects of language learning (Baddeley, Gathercole, & Papagno, 1998); for example, lexical and morphological (Ellis Weismer, 1996), vocabulary (Gathercole, Service, Hitch, Adams, & Martin, 1999), and comprehending complex sentences (Montgomery & Evans, 2009). The impact of limited working memory capacity (phonological and verbal) is significant in all aspects of literacy development and phonological processing, which includes phonological awareness (Kamhi & Pollack, 2005), decoding (DeJong, 2006), fluency (Swanson & O'Connor, 2009), comprehension (Cain, 2006; Cain, Oakhill, & Bryant, 2004; Cain, Oakhill, & Lemmon, 2004; Just & Carpenter, 1992; Seigneuric & Ehrlich, 2005; Seigneuric, Ehrlich, Oakhill, & Yuill, 2000; Swanson, Howard, & Saez, 2006), and writing (Kellogg, 1996; Swanson & Berninger, 1996; Swanson & Siegel, 2001). As such, the impact on classroom functioning of limited working memory capacity is far reaching and includes mathematics learning (Alloway, 2006; Bull & Espy, 2006).

> **REFLECT, CONNECT, and RESPOND**
> What is the role of working memory in comprehension?

DYNAMIC NATURE OF CLASSROOM LANGUAGE

It cannot be stressed enough that "talking is not teaching." Teachers must be empowered as communicators so that students can be successful and invigorated learners. This is particularly true when the process of understanding spoken language is a challenge, one that is directly connected to the acquisition of knowledge and appreciation of text. Crucial for teachers are two essentials. First is the knowledge of the impact that the language teachers use has on children. Second is the conscious awareness of what teachers say, how they say it, and why they must say it that way (see Figure 3.5). In order to be effective as a teacher, it is essential to note that every teacher is teaching language and that teachers must have this kind of control when teaching.

Effectively teaching children requires that teachers constantly ask and answer the question, "Who is this child?" (See Figure 3.6 for more on what this question encompasses.) Moreover, effective teaching necessitates the need to appreciate that when teaching content, the "what," "how," and "why" of doing so must be consciously considered. Simultaneously, the "what," "how," and "why" of teaching the learning skills necessary for students to learn the content is an essential part of the language of instruction. Once teachers are trained in the conscious use of this instructional framework, their control of language for thinking about teaching, and as a result the process of teaching, develop an increased power for improving any student's learning.

This image is consistent with the views expressed by the Center for Effective Reading Instruction (2016) because it expects effective reading instruction necessitates an understanding of not only the domains and structure of language but also the cognitive, behavioral, and environmental factors that influence a child's learning. Language is one aspect of the complex dynamic within each student. Teachers must have an awareness of, and sensitivity to, the invisible complexity of the learners before them. When focusing on the child's language skills as related to academic learning and life, this dynamic is invariably at play.

As teachers take into consideration the dynamic interaction of the aspects of language, content, use, and form, in the words chosen and the way in which they are

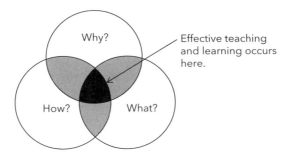

Figure 3.5.   Effective teaching. (2013 © Lydia H. Soifer)

Who Is This Child?

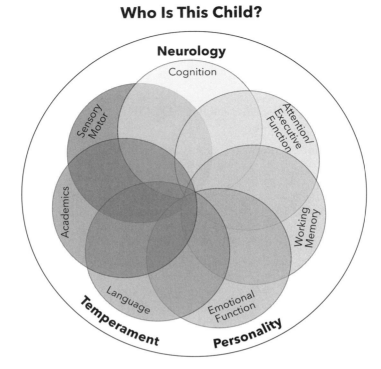

Figure 3.6.   Who is this child? (2006 © Lydia H. Soifer)

presented, several factors must be considered. Classroom Language Dynamics ©
(Soifer, 2013) identifies an array of language-based concerns regarding student
ability as well as techniques available to teachers to facilitate learning.

Common challenges faced by students can be categorized within and across
the domains of content, use, and form. Textbox 3.1 identifies some of the most frequently displayed language-based problems that will influence both oral and written comprehension, production, participation, and overall learning.

It is essential that teachers have an awareness of students' language needs.
When faced with a student or students who present with any combination of these
challenges, teachers can use several basic approaches to begin to mitigate their
impact. These include using language that is at the student's level, consciously
using their voice to make language more accessible, using synonyms deliberately and specifically, connecting language to students' direct physical experience, explicitly indicating how and under what conditions a word or its forms can
and should be used, and formulating questions with regard to students' level of
language.

For all children, it is essential that the teacher offer language at the level of the
student, regardless of the age or grade. By keeping instructions brief, chunked into
smaller parts, and repeated, the teacher provides the student with more opportunity to make sense of the information being presented. When explaining items to a
student and/or delivering an oral presentation, the teacher should use a slower rate
of speech and grammatically parse sentences (as if pausing for commas).

TEXTBOX 3.1   Common symptoms of specific language problems

Content

Word finding difficulties

Overuse of limited vocabulary

Inappropriate use of words

Narrow, more concrete meanings for words

Difficulty with multiple meaning words

Deficient comprehension of basic vocabulary and concepts

Difficulty organizing in verbal tasks

Use

Reduced ability in introducing, maintaining, and changing topics

Difficulty determining the language demands of a situation, either academic
   or social

Problems determining and adapting to listener or author expectations

Form

Difficulty determining the relationships in more complex sentences

Use of immature grammar

Difficulty understanding and using multipart verb forms

Limited understanding and use of age-appropriate conjunctions

Difficulty in activities related to phonological awareness

Content, Use, Form, and Aspects of Cognition

Trouble remembering information and repeating information presented
   orally

Difficulty following oral directions

Use of stereotyped starters (e.g., "Well, actually . . .")

Difficulty organizing thoughts and being succinct

Reduced ability to abstract and express details effectively

Difficulty making inferences

Difficulty providing information in sequence

A strong example can be drawn from an elementary school math lesson. This is important as the language of math is filled with multiple-meaning words that have very particular meaning in math (Draper, 2012; Hamilton, 2017). Consider *into*, which in math language typically signals division. However, in everyday language *into* commonly suggests "entering" as in "I'm going *into* fourth grade" or "I'll put your coat *into* the closet." Likewise, the word *family* has a common, familiar meaning (i.e., parents or guardians, children, aunts, uncles, grandparents). In math, however, the concept of *family* means something quite different. Consider the numbers 5, 3, and 2 as a number *family* in the following context. Those numbers can be converted into "number sentences," such as 3 + 2 = 5, 2 + 3 = 5, 5 – 2 = 3, 5 – 3 = 2. Thus, it behooves teachers to offer information to students with more pausing and emphasis to facilitate and allow time for processing, as follows: "Boys and girls. . . look up at the board. . . . See the numbers in the house? . . . They make a *family*. . . . Let's make some number sentences. . . with the numbers in this *family*."

One of a teacher's most powerful tools is voice. Use of vocal intonation patterns, stress, pause, and juncture, which are aspects of language *form*, can be hugely effective for emphasis and focus on key concepts. In the dynamic between *form* and *content*—that is, the words chosen and how they are formatted—it is valuable to use complex grammar that is then paraphrased into a more basic, less demanding form. In both literature and textbooks, the grammatical form called an appositive commonly appears (e.g., "Ellie, my delightful Shih Tzu, is very small"). Although it is an important form in writing for enriching vocabulary, concept development, and maturity in thinking, the appositive can pose a challenge to a student's memory. Thus, a teacher can accomplish this language-enriching exposure for his or her students while facilitating recall by offering a linguistic simplification. The following example can be readily adapted by a teacher: "The Hudson, a long and winding river, has its origin at Lake Tear of the Clouds." The modified, simplified forms would be, "The Hudson River is long and winding. It starts, has its origin, at Lake Tear . . . of the Clouds." This allows multiple exposures to the information, to the more sophisticated grammatical form as well as access to a Tier 2 word (Beck, McKeown, & Kucan, 2013)—specifically, the connection between *start* and the Tier 2 word *origin*. Moreover, it facilitates both memory and information processing for students.

Meeting students' semantic or content-related needs can be facilitated by the deliberate and specific use of synonyms. Offering a more sophisticated, Tier 2 word (Beck et al., 2013), for example, *superb* in place of *good*, in the form of a linguistic *sandwich*, exposes students to higher level vocabulary by pairing new words with familiar words. The linguistic sandwich takes this form: "He really is a *superb* skater. He's *good* at skating. Just *superb*." At the same time, the use of vocal emphasis, an aspect of *form*, highlights the connection as well as the teacher's intent (an aspect of *use*) for the student to notice the new word. Vocabulary and its complement, lexical knowledge (what you know about the words in your vocabulary) are crucial to developing listening skills, as well as laying part of the foundation for decoding and comprehension. In addition, there are any number of ways for teachers to provide students with well-planned, deliberate exposure and opportunity to retain new word meanings. There are several potent approaches to new words, consistent with the approach of deliberate, explicit formatting of the language of instruction, what, how, and why of the teacher's offering. Prior to any lesson, new words and conceptual terms must be defined with the caveat that dictionary definitions (e.g., *manifestation*—the act of manifesting) are less valuable than providing more colloquial definitions and/or synonyms, as well as visual representations of the word and examples related to the students' own experiences.

When children are first acquiring language, the adults around them label and describe in the most basic and animated manner. Such excitement activates the youngster's social-emotional and sensory systems as well as facilitating language learning. It follows that when teaching new and particularly abstract or nuanced concepts, a physical experience that taps the emotions facilitates language and memory. In science, the concept of the molecular structure of solids, liquids, and gases cannot be readily demonstrated save through illustrations. Picture a class of 10-year-olds asked to stand at their desks and then instructed to spread out all over the room, so they are dispersed and distant from each other with ample room to move about, as are the molecules in a *gas*. Then, these students are asked to move closer to the center of the room but not so near to one another as to fully limit their movements, much like the flow of a *liquid*. Finally, these same children are instructed to come to the front of the room and along with the teacher, band together into a collective hug, with arms around one another's waists. Then, everyone is instructed to move left or right as a unit or a *solid*. The students will have the memorable multisensory experience of an abstract concept and surely recall not only the events but the language and concepts they represent. (*Note:* Activity created and taught by Mr. Joseph Baynes, teacher, Eagle Hill School, Greenwich, CT.)

It cannot be overstated that language is based on experience. By connecting words (*content*) to experience, the student has a literal, personal foundation for understanding more complex terminology. In effect, teaching by analogy to personal experience establishes a basic connection while expanding knowledge. Furthermore, although at a surface level new vocabulary is content based, all aspects of language are interconnected. As such, when presenting a new word, writing it for all to view in its complete as well as syllabicated form, with a reference to root, prefix, and suffix as appropriate, is a multidimensional instructional mode. Think of the word *nation* and note the pronunciation of the first vowel, *a* (/ā/). Write it on the board in its syllabicated form, *na – tion*. Then, in a series, one at a time, add an array of suffixes (e.g., *na – tion – al, na – tion – al – ity, na – tion – al – ism*). Follow with a listing of possible prefixes (e.g., *inter – na – tion – al – ly*). By syllabicating the words to highlight the affixes, students' decoding and grammatical knowledge are enhanced. Note in particular that when the syllable structure (morphological structure) changes, so will the pronunciation from the original root word; for example, *na – tion* (*a* pronounced /ā/) becomes *na – tion – al* (*a* pronounced /ă/).

Finally, by indicating how and under what conditions a word or its forms can and should be used, teaching vocabulary is expanded into teaching language use.

The multi-faceted nature of language and the enormous array of purposes and intentions with which language are used are somewhat restricted within classroom environments. The language of instruction varies significantly from what is commonly referred to as "everyday language." This is unquestionably true for each aspect of content, use, and form. Westby (1991) differentiated between oral and literate language for both the topics and structure. In essence, the language of social interaction is more symmetric with equal rights of participation as well as a shared understanding of more concrete and practical circumstances. Questions are asked for informational purposes. As a rule, the discourse is about shared topics in the "here and now" of a shared environment. In regard to use, the topics and intentions are mutually chosen; considering content, the words chosen are more familiar and may include slang or jargon; viewing form, syntax is more repetitive and simple with a more frequent use of pronouns in the shared context of the conversation.

Alternatively, in the context of a structured learning environment, instructional discourse, a more formal and disciplined format, is the required mode of interaction. In classroom settings, the topics, aspects of use are chosen by the teacher and are likely to be about the past or the future, rather than immediacy. Moreover, discussion will lean toward the more abstract and less personal, requiring a higher level of vocabulary (content) as well as more sophisticated sentence structure (form) with an increased demand for the use of cohesive markers and more complex conjunctions. As a result, there is a topic-centered orientation, which necessitates being more explicit, linear, and event descriptive. Beyond the topic-centered nature is the asymmetry in the nature of the exchanges between speaker and listeners. One person, the teacher, holds the floor and is responsible for the flow of the exchange. Furthermore, in classroom settings, teachers ask questions to test knowledge, and language is being used to teach and learn specific topics. Classroom discourse for academic language purposes is different in content, use, and form.

Questioning is a significant part of classroom exchanges. For teachers to appreciate the discourse dynamic inherent in instruction, it is important to be conscious of facile raising and lowering the level of question according to the need of the student. Doing so takes into consideration the dynamic between language and all the aspects of cognition most crucially related to attention and executive function, including working memory. In the most basic construct regarding levels of questions, there are four levels of demand. An open-ended question, such as "Tell me what you know about bees," requires the highest degree of organization, sequencing, and language-based specificity, if it is answered efficiently. A less demanding form is a closed-end question (e.g., "What colors are bees?") that requires the location, retrieval, and formulation of language in a much more narrow and defined level of demand. When students are reluctant, unable to retrieve information or readily formulate responses, but their participation is important as they are learning how to respond to more complex questions, the use of a Yes–No form facilitates involvement without undue burden. Examples of Yes–No questions are, "Do bees fly?" and "Are bees black and yellow?" This question format limits the information that must be produced but provides the teacher with the opportunity to model a response for the child and encourage him or her to repeat. "Alex agrees that bees are black and yellow. Alex, please tell us, 'Bees are black and yellow.'" Finally, at the lowest level of cognitive and linguistic demand is the form called a tag question, in which little or no response is required but participation is made possible. A tag question takes this form: "Bees are black and yellow, aren't they?"

The complexities and nuances of language comprehension, production, purpose and intent, variations by context, and consequences are immediate and boundless. The impact of a vulnerable language system on literacy and learning cannot be underestimated. Neither should the power of the language used by educators be undervalued for its impact on Classroom Language Dynamics ©.

REFLECT, CONNECT, and RESPOND
Describe two ways in which teachers can modify presentation to facilitate the language dynamic of the classroom.

CLOSING THOUGHTS: ORAL LANGUAGE AND LITERACY

Consider once more the marvelous melodies and harmonies of *Eine Kleine Nacht-musik*. There are but seven notes in the Western musical scale, yet the combinations and permutations are endless. In a similar vein, a language system has a set of components that are conceptualized as form, content, and use. Within each of these components are an infinite number of combinations and variations that function alongside rules and regularities, permitting the language user, young or old, to communicate. No child is like every other child. Genetics, personality, experience, emotion, developmental patterns, intellect, neurology, perception, memory, and **linguistics** intertwine so that the whole is greater than the sum of its parts. Still, there are certain regularities in language development that teachers must know to enrich the understanding of how language influences a child's ability to learn. The variability from one child to another must simultaneously be kept in mind so that teachers focus on the child and not only on the task. At times, the child's knowledge and ability as well as the task itself influence performance and learning.

Throughout this chapter, four strands of research have been woven together: language and speech-language pathology, learning disabilities, reading, and education. In-depth knowledge of oral language development and language related to learning and reading comes from the discipline of speech-language pathology. Understanding the many aspects of learning and flexibility in skill and strategy development emerges from studying learning disabilities. Reading research and instruction provide an intense consideration of all aspects of the enormous task of "breaking the code" and then encoding to complete the reading process. Educational theory and practice offer a wide array of techniques for encouraging and facilitating learning. For teachers, an awareness and integration of this information offers the opportunity for greater power in teaching.

Language is omnipresent in education. It is an immutable aspect of literacy, a treasured gift that many, but not all, fully share. Teachers have a greater opportunity to share the gift by understanding and appreciating the role that language plays in learning and literacy and by thinking about the needs of one child at a time by always asking, "Who is this child?"

ONLINE COMPANION MATERIALS

The following Chapter 3 resources are available at http://www.brookespublishing.com/birshcarreker/materials:

- Reflect, Connect, and Respond Questions
- Appendix 3.1: Knowledge and Skill Assessment Answer Key

KNOWLEDGE AND SKILL ASSESSMENT

1. What are two ways in which executive function influences language performance?

   a. When planning remarks

   b. When monitoring the reaction of the listener

   c. When deciding what to say

   d. When choosing which words to use

2. How does impaired language functioning affect executive functioning?

    a. Impaired word retrieval negatively affects verbal mediation.

    b. Impaired functioning makes it harder to plan and execute responses in a timely manner.

    c. There are fewer words available to represent key ideas.

    d. All of the above

3. Which of the following are differences between speaking and decoding?

    a. Learning to speak is a "natural" process.

    b. Speaking is accompanied by suprasegmental features that influence comprehension.

    c. There are many more sounds than there are letters.

    d. Decoding rules are about phonemes and graphemes; speaking is about phonemes and inherent meaning.

    e. All of the above

4. Language pragmatics is focused on what?

    a. Practical uses of language

    b. Language for reading and writing

    c. Social communication with others

    d. The purposes and intentions with which we use and understand language orally and in print

5. How would you describe the language that teachers use?

    a. It must be consciously planned and chosen.

    b. It must be presented at the level of the learner.

    c. It must be accompanied by examples and experiences.

    d. It must have the intent of teaching content and teaching how to learn it.

    e. All of the above

6. How is vocabulary acquired by children?

    a. One word at a time

    b. Starting at birth

    c. Once they can understand many words

    d. When they are spoken or read to

REFERENCES

Adams, A., & Gathercole, S. (1995). Phonological working memory and speech production in preschool children. *Journal of Speech and Hearing Research, 38,* 403–414.

Adams, M. (1990). *Beginning to read: Thinking and learning about print.* Cambridge, MA: The MIT Press.

Adams, M.J., Foorman, B.R., Lundberg, I., & Beeler, T. (1998). *Phonemic awareness in young children: A classroom curriculum.* Baltimore, MD: Paul H. Brookes Publishing Co.

Alloway, T. (2006). How does working memory work in the classroom? *Educational Research and Reviews, 1*(4), 134–139.

Apel, K., Diehm, E., & Apel, L. (2013). Using multiple measures of morphological awareness to assess relation to reading. *Topics in Language Disorders, 33*(1), 42–56.

Apel, K., Masterson, J., & Hart, P. (2004). Integration of language components in spelling. In E. Silliman & L. Wilkinson (Eds.), *Language and literacy in schools* (pp. 292–315). New York, NY: Guilford.

Applebee, A. (1978). *The children's concept of story.* Chicago, IL: University of Chicago Press.

Aram, D., & Hall, N. (1989). Longitudinal follow-up of children with preschool communication disorders. *School Psychology Review, 18,* 487–501.

Arnbak, E., & Elbro, C. (2000). The effects of morphological awareness training on the reading and spelling skills of young dyslexics. *Scandinavian Journal of Educational Research, 44,* 229–251.

Arndt, K., & Schuele, M. (2013). Multi-clausal utterances aren't just for big kids: A framework for analysis of complex syntax production in spoken language of preschool and early school age children. *Topics in Language Disorder, 33*(2), 125–139.

August, D., & Shanahan, T. (2006). *Developing literacy in second language learners: A report on the National Literacy Panel on Language Minority Children and Youth.* Mahwah, NJ: Lawrence Erlbaum Associates.

August, D., Snow, C., Carlo, M., Proctor, C., Rolla de San Francisco, A., Duursma, E., & Szuber, A. (2006). Literacy development in elementary school second-language learners. *Topics in Language Disorder, 26*(4), 351–364.

Baddeley, A. (2006). Working memory: An overview. In S. Pickering (Ed.), *Working memory in education* (pp. 3–33). Burlington, MA: Academic Press.

Baddeley, A., Gathercole, S., & Papagno, C. (1998). The phonological loop as a language learning device. *Psychological Review, 105,* 158–173.

Bashir, A., & Hook, P. (2009). Fluency: A key link between word identification and comprehension. *Language, Speech, and Hearing Services in Schools, 40,* 196–200.

Bashir, A., & Scavuzzo, A. (1992). Children with language disorders: Natural history and academic success. *Journal of Learning Disabilities, 25,* 53–65.

Bates, E. (1976). Pragmatics and sociolinguistics in child language. In D. Morehead & A. Morehead (Eds.), *Normal and deficient child language* (pp. 411–463). Baltimore, MD: University Park Press.

Bates, E., Camaioni, L., & Volterra, V. (1975). The acquisition of performatives prior to speech. *Merrill-Palmer Quarterly, 21,* 205–226.

Bates, E., Marchman, V., Tahl, D., Fenson, L., Dale, P., Reznick, J., . . . Hartung, J. (1994). Developmental and stylistic variation in the composition of early vocabulary. *Journal of Child Language, 21,* 85–103.

Baumann, J., Edwards, E., Font, G., Tereshinski, C., Kame'enui, E., & Olejnik, S. (2002). Teaching morphemic and contextual analysis to fifth-grade students. *Reading Research Quarterly, 37*(2), 150–176.

Beck, I., McKeown, M., & Kucan, L. (2013). *Bringing words to life: Robust vocabulary instruction.* New York, NY: Guilford.

Berninger, V., Nagy, W., Carlisle, J., Thomson, J., Hoffer, D., Abbott, S., . . . Aylward, E. (2003). Effective treatment for children with dyslexia in grades 4–6: Behavioral and brain evidence. In B. Foorman (Ed.), *Preventing and remediating reading difficulties: Bringing science to scale* (pp. 381–417). Timonium, MD: York Press.

Bernthal, J.E., & Bankson, N.W. (1998). *Articulation and phonological disorders* (4th ed.). Boston, MA: Allyn & Bacon.

Biemiller, A. (2005). Size and sequence in vocabulary development: Implications for choosing words for primary grade vocabulary instruction. In E. Hiebert & M. Kamil (Eds.), *Teaching and learning vocabulary* (pp. 223–242). Mahwah, NJ: Lawrence Erlbaum Associates.

Biemiller, A., & Slonim, N. (2001). Estimating root word vocabulary growth in normative and advantaged populations: Evidence for a common sequence of vocabulary acquisition. *Journal of Educational Psychology, 93,* 498–520.

Bird, J., & Bishop, D. (1992). Perception and awareness of phonemes in phonologically impaired children. *European Journal of Disorders of Communication, 27,* 289–311.

Bird, J., Bishop, D., & Freeman, N. (1995). Phonological awareness and literacy development in children with expressive phonological impairments. *Journal of Speech and Hearing Research, 38,* 446–462.

Bishop, D., & Edmundson, A. (1987). Language impaired four-year-olds: Distinguishing transient from persistent impairment. *Journal of Speech and Hearing Disorders, 52,* 156–173.

Blachman, B. (1989). Phonological awareness and word recognition: Assessment and intervention. In A.G. Kamhi & H.W. Catts (Eds.), *Reading disabilities: A developmental language perspective* (pp. 138–158). New York, NY: Little, Brown.

Blachman, B. (1991). Early intervention for children's reading problems: Clinical applications of the research in phonological awareness. *Topics in Language Disorders, 12*(1), 51–65.

Blachman, B.A., Ball, E.W., Black, R., & Tangel, D.M. (2000). *Road to the code: A phonological awareness program for young children.* Baltimore, MD: Paul H. Brookes Publishing Co.

Blachowicz, C., & Fisher, P.J. (2002). *Teaching vocabulary in all classrooms* (2nd ed.). Upper Saddle River, NJ: Pearson Education.

Bloom, L., & Lahey, M. (1978). *Language development and language disorders.* Boston, MA: Allyn & Bacon.

Bos, C., & Filip, D. (1982). Comprehension monitoring skills in learning disabled and average readers. *Topics in Learning and Learning Disabilities, 2,* 79–85.

Boudreau, D. (2008). Narrative abilities: Advances in research and implications for clinical practice. *Topics in Language Disorders, 28,* 99–114.

Bradshaw, M., Hoffman, P., & Noris, J. (1998). Efficacy of expansions and cloze procedures in the development of interpretation by preschool children exhibiting delayed language development. *Language, Speech, and Hearing Services in the Schools, 29,* 85–95.

Brady, S., & Shankweiler, D. (Eds.). (1991). *Phonological processes in literacy: A tribute to Isabelle Y. Liberman.* Mahwah, NJ: Lawrence Erlbaum Associates.

Brinton, B., & Fujiki, M. (1989). *Conversational management with language impaired children: Pragmatic assessment and intervention.* Rockville, MD: Aspen Publishers.

Brinton, B., & Fujiki, M. (1999). Social interaction behaviors of children with specific language impairment. *Topics in Language Disorders, 19,* 49–69.

Brinton, B., Fujiki, M., Loeb, D., & Winkler, E. (1986). Development of conversational repair strategies in response to requests for clarification. *Journal of Speech and Hearing Research, 39,* 75–82.

Britton, J. (1979). Learning to use language in two modes. In N. Smith & M. Franklin (Eds.), *Symbolic functioning in childhood* (pp. 185–198). Mahwah, NJ: Lawrence Erlbaum Associates.

Brown, A. (1982). Learning how to learn from reading. In J. Langer & M. Smith-Burke (Eds.), *Reader meets author: Bridging the gap* (pp. 26–54). Newark, DE: International Reading Association.

Brown, R. (1973). *A first language: The early stages.* Cambridge, MA: Harvard University Press.

Bull, R., & Espy, K. (2006). Working memory, executive functioning and children's mathematics. In S. Pickering (Ed.), *Working memory in education.* Burlington, MA: Academic Press.

Bunce, B.H. (1993). Language of the classroom. In A. Gerber (Ed.), *Language-related learning disabilities: Their nature and treatment* (pp. 135–159). Baltimore, MD: Paul H. Brookes Publishing Co.

Byrne, B. (1981). Deficient syntactic control in poor readers: Is a weak phonetic memory code responsible? *Applied Psycholinguistics, 3,* 201–212.

Cain, K. (2006). Children's reading comprehension: The role of working memory in normal and impaired development. In S. Pickering (Ed.), *Working memory in education* (pp. 61–91). Burlington, MA: Academic Press.

Cain, K., & Oakhill, J. (2007). Reading comprehension difficulties: Causes, correlates and con- sequences. In K. Cain & J. Oakhill (Eds.), *Children's comprehension problems in oral and written language: A cognitive perspective* (pp. 41–74). New York, NY: Guilford.

Cain, K., Oakhill, J., & Bryant, P. (2004). Children's reading comprehension ability: Concurrent prediction by working memory, verbal ability, and component skills. *Journal of Educational Psychology, 96,* 31–42.

Cain, K., Oakhill, J., & Lemmon, K. (2004). Individual differences in the inference of word meaning from context: The influence of reading comprehension, vocabulary knowledge, and memory capacity. *Journal of Educational Psychology, 96*(4), 671–681.

Carlisle, J. (1988). Knowledge of derivational morphology in spelling ability in fourth, sixth and eighth graders. *Applied Psycholinguistics, 9,* 247–266.

Carlisle, J. (1995). Morphological awareness and early reading achievement. In L.B. Feldman (Ed.), *Morphological aspects of language processing* (pp. 189–210). Mahwah, NJ: Lawrence Erlbaum Associates.

Carlisle, J. (2000). Awareness of the structure and meaning of morphologically complex words: Impact on reading. *Reading and Writing: An Interdisciplinary Journal, 12*(3), 169–190.

Carlisle, J., & Stone, C. (2005). Exploring the role of morphemes in word reading. *Reading Research Quarterly, 40*(4), 428–449.

Carroll, L. (1960). *Alice's adventures in wonderland and through the looking glass.* New York, NY: The New American Library. (Original work published 1865)

Casalis, S., Cole, P., & Sopo, D. (2004). Morphological awareness in developmental dyslexia. *Annals of Dyslexia, 54*, 114–138.

Catts, H. (1986). Speech production/phonological deficits in reading disordered children. *Journal of Learning Disabilities, 19*, 504–508.

Catts, H.W. (1989). Phonological processing deficits and reading disabilities. In A.G. Kamhi & H.W. Catts (Eds.), *Reading disabilities: A developmental language perspective* (pp. 101–132). New York, NY: Little, Brown.

Catts, H. (1993). The relationship between speech and language impairments and reading disabilities. *Journal of Speech and Hearing Research, 36*(5), 948–958.

Catts, H. (1996). Defining dyslexia as a developmental language disorder: An expanded view. *Topics in Language Disorders, 16*(2), 14–25.

Catts, H. (1997). The early identification of language-based reading disabilities. *Language, Speech, and Hearing Services in Schools, 28*, 86–89.

Catts, H., Adlof, S., & Ellis Weismer, S. (2006). Language deficits in poor comprehenders: A case for the simple view of reading. *Journal of Speech, Language, Hearing Research, 49*(2), 278–293.

Catts, H., Adlof, S., Hogan, T., & Ellis Weismer, S. (2005). Are specific language impairment and dyslexia distinct disorders? *Journal of Speech, Language, and Hearing Research, 48*(6), 1378–1396.

Catts, H.W., Hu, C.F., Larrivee, L., & Swank, L. (1994). Early identification of reading disabilities in children with speech-language impairments. In S.F. Warren & J. Reichle (Series Eds.) & R.V. Watkins & M.L. Rice (Vol. Eds.), *Communication and language intervention series: Vol. 4. Specific language impairment in children* (pp. 145–160). Baltimore, MD: Paul H. Brookes Publishing Co.

Catts, H.W., & Vartiainen, T. (1997). *Sounds abound.* East Moline, IL: LinguiSystems.

Cazden, C. (1988). *Classroom discourse: The language of teaching and learning.* Portsmouth, NH: Heinemann.

Center for Effective Reading Instruction. (2016). *Knowledge and practice standards for teachers of reading.* Baltimore, MD: Author.

Center on the Developing Child. (2012). *Executive function (In brief).* Cambridge, MA: Harvard University.

Chall, J. (1983). *Stages of reading development.* New York, NY: McGraw-Hill.

Chaney, C. (1992). Language development, metalinguistic skills, and print awareness in 3-year-old children. *Applied Psycholinguistics, 13*, 485–514.

Clark-Klein, S., & Hodson, B. (1995). A phonologically based analysis of misspellings by third graders with disordered-phonology histories. *Journal of Speech and Hearing Research, 38*, 839–849.

Conte-Ramsden, G., & Durkin, K. (2008). Language and independence in adolescents with and without a history of specific language impairment (SLI). *Journal of Speech, Language, and Hearing Research, 51*(1), 70–83.

Craig, H., Connor, C., & Washington, J. (2003). Early positive predictors of later reading comprehension for African-American students: A preliminary investigation. *Language, Speech, and Hearing Services in Schools, 34*, 31–43.

Creaghead, N. (1986). Comprehension of meaning in written language. *Topics in Language Disorders, 6*(4), 73–82.

DeJong, P. (2006). Understanding normal and impaired reading: A working memory perspective. In S. Pickering (Ed.), *Working memory and education* (pp. 33–60). Burlington, MA: Academic Press.

Denckla, M.B. (1996). A theory and model of executive function: A neuropsychological perspective. In G.R. Lyon & N.A. Krasnegor (Eds.), *Attention, memory and executive function* (pp. 263–278). Baltimore, MD: Paul H. Brookes Publishing Co.

Denckla, M., & Rudel, R. (1976). Rapid "automatized" naming (RAN): Dyslexia differentiated from other learning disabilities. *Neuropsychologia, 14,* 471–479.

Diamond, A. (2014). Understanding executive functions: What helps or hinders them and how executive functions and language development mutually support each other. *Perspectives on Language and Literacy, 40*(2), 7–11.

Dickinson, D., & McCabe, A. (1991). The acquisition and development of language: A social interactionist account of language and literacy development. In J. Kavanagh (Ed.), *The language continuum: From infancy to literacy* (pp. 1–40). Timonium, MD: York Press.

Dore, J. (1978). Requestive systems in nursery school conversations: Analysis of talk in its social context. In R. Campbell & P. Smith (Eds.), *Recent advances in the psychology of language: Language development and mother–child interaction* (pp. 271–292). New York, NY: Plenum.

Draper, D. (2012). *Comprehension strategies: Comprehension strategies applied to mathematics.* Retrieved from https://www.scribd.com/doc/237559428/comprehension-and-mathematics-debbie-draper

Ehri, L. (1989). Movement into word reading and spelling: How spelling contributes to reading. In J. Mason (Ed.), *Reading and writing connections* (pp. 65–81). Boston, MA: Allyn & Bacon.

Ehri, L., Nunes, S., Willows, D., Schuster, B., Yaghoub-Zadeh, Z., & Shanahan, T. (2001). Phonemic awareness instruction helps children learn to read: Evidence from the National Reading Panel's meta-analysis. *Reading Research Quarterly, 36,* 250–287.

Eimas, P., Siqueland, E., Jusczyk, P., & Vigorito, J. (1971). Speech perception in infants. *Science, 171,* 303–306.

Eisenberg, S. (2006). Grammar: How can I say that better? In T. Ukrainetz (Ed.), *Contextualized language intervention* (pp.145–194). Eau Claire, WI: Thinking Publications.

Elbro, C., & Arnbak, A. (1996). The role of morpheme recognition and morphological awareness in dyslexia. *Annals of Dyslexia, 46,* 209–240.

Ellis Weismer, S. (1996). Capacity limitations in working memory: The impact on lexical and morphological learning by children with language impairment. *Topics in Language Disorders, 17,* 33–44.

Engel, P., Santos, F., & Gathercole, S. (2008). Are working memory measures free of socioeconomic influence? *Journal of Speech, Language, and Hearing Research, 51,* 1580–1587.

Every Student Succeeds Act of 2015, PL 114-95 [SS], 114 Stat. 1177 (2015-2016)

Fey, M.E., Catts, H.W., & Larrivee, L.S. (1995). Preparing preschoolers for the academic and social challenges of school. In S.F. Warren & J. Reichle (Series Eds.) & M.E. Fey, J. Windsor, & S.F. Warren (Vol. Eds.), *Communication and language intervention series: Vol. 5. Language intervention: Preschool through elementary years* (pp. 3–37). Baltimore, MD: Paul H. Brookes Publishing Co.

Fey, M., Catts, H., Proctor-Williams, K., Tomblin, J., & Zhang, X. (2004). Oral and written story composition skills of children with language impairment. *Journal of Speech, Language, and Hearing Research, 36,* 1301–1318.

Fowler, A. (1991). How early phonological development might set the stage for phoneme awareness. In S. Brady & D. Shankweiler (Eds.), *Phonological processes in literacy: A tribute to Isabelle Y. Liberman* (pp. 97–117). Mahwah, NJ: Lawrence Erlbaum Associates.

Fowler, A., & Liberman, I. (1995). Morphological awareness as related to early reading and spelling ability. In L. Feldman (Ed.), *Morphological aspects of language processing* (pp. 157–188). Mahwah, NJ: Lawrence Erlbaum Associates.

Fung, W., & Swanson, H. (2017). Working memory components that predict word problem solving: Is it merely a function of reading, calculation and fluid intelligence? *Memory and Cognition, 45*(5), 804–823. doi:10.3758/s13421-017-0697-0

Gaskins, I., Satlow, E., & Pressley, M. (2007). Executive control of reading comprehension in the elementary school. In L. Meltzer (Ed.), *Executive function in education: From theory to practice* (pp. 194–215). New York, NY: Guilford.

Gathercole, S., & Alloway, T. (2008). *Working memory and learning: A practical guide for teachers.* Los Angeles, CA: SAGE.

Gathercole, S., & Holmes, J. (2014). Developmental impairments in working memory: Profiles and interventions. *Perspectives on Language and Literacy, 40*(2), 36–39.

Gathercole, S., Service, E., Hitch, G., Adams, A., & Martin, A. (1999). Phonological short-term memory and vocabulary development: Further evidence on the nature of the relationship. *Applied Cognitive Psychology, 13,* 65–77.

Gerber, A. (1993). *Language-related learning disabilities: Their nature and treatment.* Baltimore, MD: Paul H. Brookes Publishing Co.

German, D. (1982). Word-finding substitution in children with learning disabilities. *Language, Speech, and Hearing Services in Schools, 13,* 223–230.

Gillon, G. (2004). *Phonological awareness: From research to practice.* New York, NY: Guilford.

Goodwin, A., & Ahn, S. (2013). A meta-analysis of morphological interventions in English: Effects on literacy outcomes for school-age children. *Scientific Studies of Reading, 17*(4), 257–285.

Gordon-Pershey, M. (2014). Executive function and language: A complementary relationship that supports learning. *Perspectives on Language and Learning, 40*(2), 23–26.

Gottardo, A. (2002). The relationship between language and reading skills in bilingual Spanish– English speakers. *Topics in Language Disorders, 22*(5), 46–70.

Gough, P., & Tunmer, W. (1986). Decoding reading and reading disability. *Remedial and Special Education, 7,* 6–10.

Green, L. (2009). Morphology and literacy: Getting our heads in the game. *Language, Speech, and Hearing Services in Schools, 40*(3), 283–285.

Green, L., McCutchen, D., Schwiebert, C., Quinlan, T., Eva-Wood, A., & Juelis, J. (2003). Morphological development in children's writing. *Journal of Educational Psychology, 95*(4), 752–761.

Greene, J. (1996). Psycholinguistic assessment: The clinical base for identification of dyslexia. *Topics in Language Disorders, 16*(2), 45–72.

Halliday, M.A.K. (1975). *Learning how to mean: Explorations in the development of language.* London, United Kingdom: Edward Arnold.

Halliday, M.A.K., & Hasan, R. (1976). *Cohesion in English.* London, United Kingdom: Longman Group.

Hamilton, J. (2017). The language of math: Finding common ground. *Perspectives in Language and Literacy, 43*(1), 47–52.

Hammer, C., & Miccio, A. (2006). Early language and reading development of bilingual preschoolers from low-income families. *Topics in Language Disorders, 26*(4), 322–337.

Hammer, C., Miccio, A., & Wagstaff, D. (2003). Home literacy experiences and their relationship to bilingual preschoolers' developing English literacy abilities: An initial investigation. *Language, Speech, and Hearing Services in Schools, 34,* 20–30.

Hart, B., & Risley, T.R. (1999). *The social world of children learning to talk.* Baltimore, MD: Paul H. Brookes Publishing Co.

Hedberg, N., & Westby, C. (1997) *Analyzing Storytelling Skills: Theory to practice.* Tucson, AZ: Communication Skill Builders.

Hochman, J. (2009). *Teaching basic writing skills: Strategies for effective expository writing instruction.* Longmont, CO: Sopris West Educational Services.

Hodson, B. (1994). Helping individuals become intelligible, literate and articulate: The role of phonology. *Topics in Language Disorders, 14*(2), 1–16.

Horowitz, R., & Samuels, J. (1987). Comprehending oral and written language: Critical contrasts for literacy and schooling. In R. Horowitz & J. Samuels (Eds.), *Comprehending oral and written language* (pp. 1–52). San Diego, CA: Academic Press.

Hoskins, B. (1983). Semantics. In C. Wren (Ed.), *Language learning disabilities* (pp. 85–111). New York, NY: Aspen Publishers.

Hughes, D., McGillivray, L., & Schmidek, M. (1997). *Guide to narrative language: Procedures for assessment.* Eau Claire, WI: Thinking Publications.

Hymes, D. (1972). On communicative competence. In J.B. Pride & J. Holmes (Eds.), *Sociolinguistics* (pp. 269–293). London, United Kingdom: Penguin Books.

International Dyslexia Association, The. (2018, March). *Knowledge and practice standards for teachers of reading.* Retrieved from https://dyslexiaida.org/knowledge-and-practices/

Johnson, C., Beitchman, J., Young, A., Escobar, M., Atkinson, L., Wilson, B., . . . Wang, M. (1999). Fourteen-year follow-up study of children with and without speech-language impairments: Speech/language stability and outcomes. *Journal of Speech, Language, and Hearing Research, 42*(3), 74–76.

Just, M., & Carpenter, A. (1992). A capacity theory of comprehension: Individual differences in working memory. *Psychological Review, 99,* 122–149.

Justice, L., Invernizzi, M., & Meier, J. (2002). Designing and implementing an early literacy screening protocol: Suggestions for the speech-language pathologist. *Language, Speech, and Hearing Services in Schools, 33,* 84–101.

Kamhi, A.G., & Catts, H.W. (1986). Toward an understanding of developmental language and reading disorders. *Journal of Speech and Hearing Disorders, 51,* 337–347.

Kamhi, A.G., & Catts, H.W. (1989). Language and reading: Convergences, divergences and development. In A.G. Kamhi & H.W. Catts (Eds.), *Reading disabilities: A developmental language perspective* (pp. 1–34). New York, NY: Little, Brown.

Kamhi, A.G., & Catts, H.W. (2012). Language and reading: Convergences, divergences and development. In A.G. Kamhi & H.W. Catts (Eds.), *Language and reading disabilities* (3rd ed., pp. 1–23). Boston, MA: Pearson.

Kamhi, A.G., & Pollack, K.E. (2005). *Phonological disorders in children: Clinical decision making in assessment and intervention.* Baltimore, MD: Paul H. Brookes Publishing Co.

Katz, L. (2004). An investigation of the relationship of morphological awareness to reading comprehension in fourth and sixth graders. (Doctoral dissertation, University of Michigan, 2004). *Dissertation Abstracts International, 65,* 2138.

Katz, L., & Carlisle, J. (2009). Teaching students with reading difficulties to be close readers: A feasibility study. *Language, Speech, and Hearing Services in Schools, 40*(3), 325–340.

Katz, R. (1986). Phonological deficiencies in children with reading disability: Evidence from an object-naming task. *Cognition, 22,* 225–257.

Kaushanskaya, M., Park, J.S., Gangopadhyay, I., Davidson, M.M., & Ellis Weismer, S. (2017). The relationship between executive functions and language abilities in children: A latent variables approach. *Journal of Speech, Language, and Hearing Research, 60*(4), 912–923.

Kellogg, R. (1996). A model of working memory in writing. In C. Levy & S. Randell (Eds.), *The science of writing* (pp. 57–71). Mahwah, NJ: Lawrence Erlbaum Associates.

Kirk, C., & Gillon, G. (2009). Integrated morphological awareness intervention as a tool for improving literacy. *Language, Speech, and Hearing Services in Schools, 40*(3), 341–351.

Labov, W. (2003). When ordinary children fail to read. *Reading Research Quarterly, 38,* 128–131.

Lahey, M. (1988). *Language disorders and language development.* New York, NY: Wiley.

Lahey, M., & Bloom, L. (1994). Variability and language learning disabilities. In G. Wallach & K. Butler (Eds.), *Language learning disabilities in school-age children and adolescents: Some principles and applications* (pp. 354–372). Boston, MA: Allyn & Bacon.

Laing, S., & Kamhi, A. (2003). Alternative assessment of language and literacy in culturally and linguistically diverse populations. *Language, Speech, and Hearing Services in Schools, 34,* 44–55.

Landa, R. (2005). Assessment of social communication in preschoolers. *Developmental Disabilities Research, 11*(3), 247–252.

Larson, V., & McKinley, N. (1995). *Language disorders in older students, preadolescents and adolescents.* Eau Claire, WI: Thinking Publications.

Layzer, J., & Goodson, B. (2006). *Care in the home: A description of family child care and the experiences of the families and children who use it. National Study of Child Care for Low Income Families.* Washington, DC: U.S. Department of Health and Human Services, Administration for Children and Families.

Leung, C., Silverman, R., Nandakumar, R., Qian, X., & Hines, S. (2011). A comparison of difficulty of levels of vocabulary in first grade basal readers for preschool dual language learners and monolingual English learners. *American Educational Research Journal, 48,* 421–461.

Liberman, I., & Liberman, A. (1990). Whole language vs. code emphasis: Underlying assumptions and their implications for reading instruction. *Annals of Dyslexia, 40,* 51–76.

Liberman, I., Shankweiler, D., Camp, L., Blachman, G., & Werfelman, M. (1990). Steps toward literacy. In P. Levinson & C. Sloan (Eds.), *Auditory processing and language: Clinical and research perspectives* (pp. 189–215). New York, NY: Grune & Stratton.

Linder, T.W. (1999). *Read, play, and learn! Storybook activities for young children. Teacher's guide.* Baltimore, MD: Paul H. Brookes Publishing Co.

Lopez, L., & Greenfield, D. (2004). The cross-language transfer of phonological skills of Hispanic Head Start children. *Bilingual Research Journal, 28,* 1–18.

Mahoney, D., & Mann, V. (1992). Using children's humor to clarify the relationship between linguistic awareness and early reading ability. *Cognition, 45,* 163–186.

Mandler, J., & Johnson, N. (1977). Remembrance of things parsed: Story structure and recall. *Cognitive Psychology, 9,* 111–151.

Mattingly, I. (1972). Reading, the linguistic process and linguistic awareness. In J. Kavanagh & I. Mattingly (Eds.), *Language by ear and by eye: The relationship between speech and reading* (pp. 133–144). Cambridge, MA: The MIT Press.

McCabe, M., & Bliss, L. (2003). *Patterns of narrative discourse: A multicultural lifespan approach.* Boston, MA: Allyn & Bacon.

McCutchen, D., Logan, B., & Biangardi-Orpe, U. (2009). Making meaning: Children's sensitivity to morphological information during word reading. *Reading Research Quarterly, 44*(4), 360–376.

McCutchen, D., Stull, S., Herrera, B., Lotas, S., & Evans, S. (2014). Putting words to work: Effects of morphological instruction on children's writing. *Journal of Learning Disabilities, 47*(1), 86–97.

McGregor, K. (1994). Use of phonological information in word-finding treatment of children. *Journal of Speech and Hearing Research, 37,* 1381–1393.

Meltzer, L. (2007). *Executive function in education: From theory to practice.* New York, NY: Guilford.

Menyuk, P., & Chesnick, M. (1997). Metalinguistic skills, oral language knowledge and reading. *Topics in Language Disorders, 17*(3), 75–87.

Miller, L. (1990). The roles of language and learning in the development of literacy. *Topics in Language Disorders, 10,* 1–24.

Milosky, L. (1994). Nonliteral language abilities: Seeing the forest for the trees. In G. Wallach & K. Butler (Eds.), *Language learning disabilities in school-aged children and adolescents: Some principles and applications* (pp. 275–303). Boston, MA: Allyn & Bacon.

Moats, L.C. (1994). Honing the concepts of listening and speaking: A prerequisite to the valid measurement of language behavior in children. In G.R. Lyon (Ed.), *Frames of reference for the assessment of learning disabilities: New views on measurement issues* (pp. 229–241). Baltimore, MD: Paul H. Brookes Publishing Co.

Moats, L.C. (1995). *Spelling: Development, disability, and instruction.* Timonium, MD: York Press.

Moats, L.C. (2010a). *Language Essentials for Teachers of Reading and Spelling (LETRS).* Dallas, TX: Sopris West.

Moats, L.C. (2010b). *Speech to print: Language essentials for teachers* (2nd ed.). Baltimore, MD: Paul H. Brookes Publishing Co.

Moats, L.C., & Lyon, G.R. (1996). Wanted: Teachers with a knowledge of language. *Topics in Language Disorders, 16*(2), 73–86.

Montgomery, J. (1996). Sentence comprehension and working memory in children with specific language impairment. *Topics in Language Disorders, 17*(1), 19–32.

Montgomery, J., & Evans, J. (2009). Complex sentence comprehension and working memory in children with specific language impairment. *Journal of Speech, Language, and Hearing Research, 52*(2), 269–288.

Moreau, M., & Fidrych, M. (1998). *The Story Grammar Marker.* Easthampton, MA: SGM.

Morice, R., & Slaghuis, W. (1985). Language performance and reading ability at 8 years of age. *Applied Psycholinguistics, 6,* 141–160.

Myers, M., & Paris, S. (1978). Children's metacognitive knowledge about reading. *Journal of Educational Psychology, 70,* 680–690.

Nagy, W., & Anderson, R. (1984). How many words are there in printed school English? *Reading Research Quarterly, 19,* 304–329.

Nagy, W., Berninger, V., & Abbott, R. (2006). Contributions of morphology beyond phonology to literacy outcomes of upper elementary and middle-school students. *Journal of Educational Psychology, 98*(1), 134–147.

Nagy, W., & Scott, C. (2000). Vocabulary processes. In M. Kamil, P. Mosenthal, P. Pearson, & R. Barr (Eds.), *Handbook of reading research* (Vol. 3, pp. 269–284). Mahwah, NJ: Lawrence Erlbaum Associates.

Nation, K., Clarke, P., Marshall, C., & Durand, M. (2004). Hidden language impairments in children: Parallels between poor reading comprehension and specific language impairment. *Journal of Speech, Language, and Hearing Research, 47,* 199–211.

Nelson, N.W. (1985). Teacher talk and child listening: Fostering a better match. In C. Simon (Ed.), *Communication skills and classroom success: Assessment of language-learning disabled students* (pp. 65–102). San Diego, CA: College-Hill Press.

Nelson, N.W. (1986). Individualized processing in classroom settings. *Topics in Language Disorders, 6*(2), 13–27.

Newbury, J., Klee, T., Stokes, S., & Moran, C. (2016). Interrelationships between working memory, processing speed, and language development in the age range 2–4 years. *Journal of Speech, Language, and Hearing Research, 59,* 1146–1158.

Nippold, M. (1988). The literate lexicon. In M. Nippold (Ed.), *Later language development: Ages nine through nineteen* (pp. 29–47). San Diego, CA: College-Hill Press.

Nippold, M., Mansfield, T., Billow, J., & Tomblin, J. (2008). Expository discourse in adolescents with language impairment: Examining syntactic development. *American Journal of Speech-Language Pathology, 17*(4), 356–366.

Nippold, M., Mansfield, T., Billow, J., & Tomblin, J. (2009). Syntactic development in adolescents with a history of language impairments: A follow-up study. *American Journal of Speech-Language Pathology, 18*(3), 241–251.

Owens, R. (1996). *Language development: An introduction* (3rd ed.). New York, NY: Merrill/Macmillan.

Owings, R., Peterson, G., Bransford, J., Morris, C., & Stein, B. (1980). Spontaneous monitoring and regulation of learning: A comparison of successful and less successful fifth graders. *Journal of Educational Psychology, 72,* 250–256.

Paul, R., & Jennings, P. (1992). Phonological behavior in toddlers with slow expressive language development. *Journal of Speech and Hearing Research, 35,* 99–107.

Pauls, J., & Archibald, L. (2016). Executive functions in children with specific language impairment: A meta-analysis. *Journal of Speech, Language, and Hearing Research, 59,* 1074–1086.

Pennington, B., & Lefly, D. (2001). Early reading development in children at family risk for dyslexia. *Child Development, 72,* 816–832.

Perfetti, C.A. (2010). Decoding, vocabulary, and comprehension: The golden triangle of reading skill. In M.G. McKeown & L. Kucan (Eds.), *Bringing reading research to life.* (pp. 291–303). New York, NY: Guilford.

Peterson, R., Pennington, B., Shriberg, L., & Boada, R. (2009). What influences literacy outcomes in children with speech sound disorder? *Journal Speech, Language, and Hearing Research, 52,* 1175–1188.

Prather, E., Hedrick, D., & Kern, C. (1975). Articulation development in children aged two to four years. *Journal of Speech and Hearing Disorders, 40,* 179–191.

Preston, J., & Edwards, M. (2010). Phonological awareness and types of sound errors in preschoolers with speech sound disorders. *Journal of Speech, Language, and Hearing Research, 53,* 44–60.

Prutting, C., & Kirschner, D. (1987). A clinical appraisal of the pragmatic aspects of language. *Journal of Speech and Hearing Disorders, 52,* 105–119.

Raver, C., & Blair, C. (2014). At the crossroads of education and developmental neuroscience: Perspectives on executive function. *Perspectives on Language and Literacy, 40*(2), 36–39.

Rees, N. (1978). Pragmatics of language: Applications to normal and disordered language development. In R. Schiefelbusch (Ed.), *Bases of language intervention* (pp. 191–268). Baltimore, MD: University Park Press.

Richards, G. (2003). *The source for learning and memory strategies.* East Moline, IL: LinguiSystems.

Robertson, C., & Salter, W. (1997). *The Phonological Awareness Test.* East Moline, IL: LinguiSystems.

Roth, F. (1986). Oral narratives of learning disabled students. *Topics in Language Disorders, 7*(1), 21–30.

Roth, F., & Spekman, N. (1984). Assessing the pragmatic abilities of children: Part I. Organizational framework and assessment parameters. *Journal of Speech and Hearing Disorders, 49,* 2–11.

Roth, F., & Spekman, N. (1989). Higher order language processes and reading disabilities. In A.G. Kamhi & H.W. Catts (Eds.), *Reading disabilities: A developmental language perspective* (pp. 159–98). New York, NY: Little, Brown.

Ruben, H., Patterson, P., & Kantor, M. (1991). Morphological development and writing ability in children and adults. *Language, Speech, and Hearing Services in Schools, 22,* 228–235.

Rubin, D. (1987). Divergence and convergence between oral and written communication. *Topics in Language Disorders, 7*(4), 1–18.

Rvachew, S. (2007). Phonological processing and reading in children with speech sound disorders. *American Journal of Speech-Language Pathology, 16,* 260–270.

Sawyer, D. (1991). Whole language in context: Insights into the great debate. *Topics in Language Disorders, 11*(3), 1–13.

Scarborough, H. (1990). Very early language deficits in dyslexic children. *Child Development, 61,* 1728–743.

Scarborough, H. (2001). Connecting early language and literacy to later reading (dis)abilities: Evidence, theory and practice. In S. Neuman & D. Dickinson (Eds.), *Handbook of early literacy research* (pp. 97–110). New York, NY: Guilford.

Scott, C. (1994). A discourse continuum for school-age students: Impact of modality and genre. In G. Wallach & K. Butler (Eds.), *Language learning disabilities in school-age children and adolescents: Some principles and applications* (pp. 219–52). Boston, MA: Allyn & Bacon.

Scott, C. (2004). Syntactic contributions to literacy learning. In A. Stone, E. Silliman, B. Ehren, & K. Apel (Eds.), *Handbook of language and literacy: Development and disorder* (pp. 340–362). New York, NY: Guilford.

Scott, C. (2005). Learning to write. In H. Catts & A. Kamhi (Eds.), *Language and reading disabilities* (2nd ed., pp. 233–273). Boston, MA: Pearson.

Scott, C. (2009). A case for the sentence in reading comprehension. *Language, Speech, and Hearing Services in Schools, 40*(2), 185–191.

Scott, C., & Windsor, J. (2000). General language performance measures in spoken and written narrative and expository discourse of school-age children with language learning disabilities. *Journal of Speech, Language, and Hearing Research, 43*(2), 329–339.

Seigneuric, A., & Ehrlich, M. (2005). Contributions of working memory capacity to children's reading comprehension: A longitudinal investigation. *Reading and Writing, 18,* 617–656.

Seigneuric, A., Ehrlich, M., Oakhill, J., & Yuill, N. (2000). Working memory resources and children's reading comprehension. *Reading and Writing: An Interdisciplinary Journal, 13,* 81–103.

Siegel, L. (2008). Morphological awareness skills of English language learners and children with dyslexia. *Topics in Language Disorders, 28*(1), 15–27.

Snow, C., & Dickinson, D. (1991). Skills that aren't basic in a new conception of literacy. In A. Purves & E. Jennings (Eds.), *Literate systems and individual lives: Perspectives on literacy and schooling* (pp. 179–192). Albany, NY: SUNY Press.

Snow, C., Griffin, P., & Burns, S. (Eds.). (2005). *Knowledge to support the teaching of reading: Preparing teachers for a changing world.* San Francisco, CA: Jossey-Bass.

Snowling, M. (1981). Phonemic deficits in developmental dyslexia. *Psychological Research, 43,* 219–234.

Snowling, M., Gallagher, A., & Firth, U. (2003). Family risk of dyslexia is continuous: Individual differences in precursors of reading skill. *Child Development, 74,* 358–373.

Snowling, M., & Nation, K. (1997). Language phonology and learning to read. In M. Snowling & C. Hulme (Eds.), *Dyslexia: Biology, cognition and remediation* (pp. 153–166). San Diego, CA: Singular Publishing Group.

Snyder, L., & Downey, D. (1991). The language of reading relationship in normal and reading disabled children. *Journal of Speech and Hearing Research, 34,* 129–140.

Snyder, L., & Downey, D. (1997). Developmental differences in the relationship between oral language deficits and reading. *Topics in Language Disorders, 17*(3), 27–40.

Snyder, L., & Godley, D. (1992). Assessment of word finding in children and adolescents. *Topics in Language Disorders, 12*(1), 15–32.

Soifer, L. (2013). *Classroom Language Dynamics: Smuggling neuroscience into your classroom.* Unpublished manuscript.

Sousa, D. (2010). *Mind, brain, and education: Neuroscience implications for the classroom.* Bloomington, IN: Solution Tree Press.

Spear-Swerling, L., & Sternberg, R. (1994). The road not taken: An integrative theoretical model of reading disability. *Journal of Learning Disabilities, 27,* 91–103.

Stackhouse, J., & Wells, B. (1997). How do speech and language problems affect literacy development? In M. Snowling & C. Hulme (Eds.), *Dyslexia: Biology, Cognition and Intervention* (pp. 182–211). San Diego, CA: Singular Publishing Group.

Stadler, M., & Ward, G. (2005). Supporting narrative development of young children. *Early Childhood Education Journal, 33*(2), 73–80.

Stanovich, K. (1986). Matthew effects in reading: Some consequences of individual differences in the acquisition of literacy. *Reading Research Quarterly, 21,* 360–407.

Stanovich, K. (Ed.). (1987). Introduction: Children's reading and the development of phonological awareness [Special issue]. *Merrill-Palmer Quarterly, 33*(3).

Stein, C., Cairns, H., & Zurif, E. (1984). Sentence comprehension limitation related to syntactic deficits in reading disabled children. *Applied Psychology, 5,* 305–322.

Stein, N., & Glenn, C. (1979). An analysis of story comprehension in elementary school children. In R. Freedle (Ed.), *New directions in discourse processing* (pp. 53–120). Greenwich, CT: Ablex.

Stoel-Gammon, C. (1991). Normal and disordered phonology in two year olds. *Topics in Language Disorders, 11*(4), 21–32.

Storch, S., & Whitehurst, G. (2002). Oral language and code-related precursors to reading: Evidence from a longitudinal structural model. *Developmental Psychology, 38*(6), 934–947.

Sulzby, E., & Teale, W. (1991). Emergent literacy. In R. Barr, M. Kamil, P. Mosenthal, & P.D. Pearson (Eds.), *Handbook of reading research* (Vol. 2, pp. 727–757). New York, NY: Longman.

Swank, L. (1997). Linguistic influences in the emergence of written word decoding in first grade. *American Journal of Speech-Language Pathology, 6*(4), 62–66.

Swanson, H., & Berninger, V. (1996). Individual differences in children's working memory and writing skill. *Journal of Educational Psychology, 63,* 358–385.

Swanson, H., Howard, C., & Saez, L. (2006). Do different components of working memory underlie different subgroups of reading disabilities? *Journal of Learning Disabilities, 39,* 252–269.

Swanson, H., & O'Connor, R. (2009). The role of working memory and fluency practice on the reading comprehension of students who are dysfluent readers. *Journal of Learning Disabilities, 47*(6), 548–575.

Swanson, H., & Siegel, L. (2001). Learning disabilities as a working memory deficit. *Issues in Education: Contributions from Educational Psychology, 7,* 1–48.

Tabors, P.O., Snow, C.E., & Dickinson, D.K. (2001). Homes and schools together: Supporting language and literacy development. In D.K. Dickinson & P.O. Tabors (Eds.), *Beginning literacy with language: Young children learning at home and school* (pp. 313–334). Baltimore, MD: Paul H. Brookes Publishing Co.

Tokuhama-Espinosa, T. (2011). *Mind, brain, and education science: A comprehensive guide to the new brain-based teaching.* New York, NY: Norton Books.

Troia, G. (2004). Building word recognition skills through empirically validated instructional practices: Collaborative efforts of speech-language pathologists and teachers. In E. Silliman & L. Wilkinson (Eds.), *Language and literacy learning in schools* (pp. 98–129). New York, NY: Guilford.

Van Kleeck, A. (1990). Emergent literacy: Learning about print before learning to read. *Topics in Language Disorders, 10*(2), 25–45.

Van Vierson, S., deBree, E., Verdan, M., Krikhaar, E., Maassen, B., van der Leij, A., & de Jong, P. (2017). Delayed early vocabulary development in children at family risk of dyslexia. *Journal of Speech, Language, and Hearing Research, 96*(4), 937–949.

Vandenbroucke, L., Versuchueren, K., & Baeyens, D. (2017). The classroom as a developmental context for cognitive development: A meta-analysis on the importance of teacher–student interactions for children's executive functions. *Review of Educational Research, 88*(1), 125–164.

Vaughn, S., Mathes, P., Linan-Thompson, S., & Francis, D. (2005). Teaching English language learners at risk for reading disabilities to read: Putting research into practice. *Learning Disabilities Research and Practice, 20,* 58–67.

Vellutino, F., Scanlon, D., & Spearing, D. (1995). Semantic and phonological coding in poor and normal readers. *Journal of Experimental Child Psychology, 59,* 76–123.

Vygotsky, L. (1962). *Thought and language.* Cambridge, MA: The MIT Press.

Wagner, R., & Torgesen, J. (1987). The nature of phonological processing and its causal roles in the equation of reading skills. *Psychological Bulletin, 101,* 192–212.

Wagner, R.K., Torgesen, J.K., & Rashotte, C.A. (1994). The development of reading-related phonological processing abilities: New evidence of bidirectional causality from a latent variable longitudinal study. *Developmental Psychology, 30,* 73–78.

Wallach, G. (1990). Magic buries Celtics: Looking for broader interpretations of language learning in literacy. *Topics in Language Disorders, 10*(2), 63–80.

Wallach, G., & Butler, K. (1994). Creating communication, literacy and academic success. In G. Wallach & K. Butler (Eds.), *Language learning disabilities in school-age children and adolescents: Some principals and applications* (pp. 2–26). Boston, MA: Allyn & Bacon.

Wallach, G., & Miller, L. (1988). *Language intervention and academic success.* New York, NY: Little, Brown.

Webster, P., & Plante, A. (1992). Effects of phonological impairment on word, syllable and phoneme segmentation and reading. *Language, Speech, and Hearing Services in Schools, 23*, 176–182.

Westby, C. (1985). Learning to talk—talking to learn: Oral literate language differences. In C. Simon (Ed.), *Communication skills and classroom success: Therapy methodologies for language learning disabled students* (pp. 181–213). San Diego, CA: College-Hill Press.

Westby, C. (1989). Assessing and remediating text comprehension problems. In A.G. Kamhi & H.W. Catts (Eds.), *Reading disabilities: A developmental language perspective* (pp. 199–260). New York, NY: Little, Brown.

Westby, C. (1991). Learning to talk—talking to learn: Oral-literate language differences. In C.S. Simon (Ed.), *Communication skills and classroom success: Assessment and therapy methodologies for language learning disabled students* (pp. 334–357). Eau Claire, WI: Thinking Publications.

Westby, C. (1995). Culture and literacy: Frameworks for understanding. *Topics in Language Disorders, 16*(1), 50–66.

White, T., Power, M., & White, S. (1989). Morphological analysis: Implications for teaching and understanding of vocabulary growth. *Reading Research Quarterly, 24*, 283–304.

White-Canales, E., & McElroy-Bratcher, A. (2015). The effect of speech sound disorders on literacy outcomes of school-age children. *American Journal of Educational Research, 3*(10), 1270–1278.

Wiig, E., & Semel, E. (1980). *Language assessment and intervention for the learning disabled.* Columbus, OH: Charles E. Merrill.

Wiig, E., Semel, E., & Nystrom, L. (1982). Comparison of rapid naming abilities in language-learning-disabled and academically achieving eight-year-olds. *Language, Speech, and Hearing Services in Schools, 12*, 11–23.

Wolf, M., & Dickinson, D. (1993). From oral to written language: Transitions in the school years. In J. Gleason (Ed.), *The development of language.* Columbus, OH: Charles E. Merrill.

Wolter, J., & Dilworth, V. (2014). The effects of multilinguistic morphological awareness approach for improving language and literacy. *Journal of Learning Disabilities, 47*(1), 76–85.

Wolter, J., Wood, A., & D'zatko, K. (2009). The influence of morphological awareness on the literacy development of first-grade children. *Language, Speech, and Hearing Services in Schools, 40*(3), 286–298.

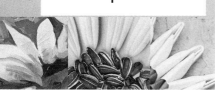

Chapter 4

Pre-Kindergarten Literacy

Eve Robinson, Carolyn DeVito, and Gloria Trabucco

LEARNING OBJECTIVES

1. To articulate the purpose of high-quality early childhood education and its relationship to acquiring preliteracy skills

2. To describe how each learning center in a preschool classroom specifically relates to preliteracy

3. To demonstrate activities that promote all of the foundational literary skills: oral language, concepts of print, phonological awareness, letter and sound awareness, and writing development

The critical role of a child's earliest experiences has been recognized by educators as a key indicator of later intellectual, social, and emotional development (Barnett, 2008). Brain development research shows conclusively that the imprint of these earliest experiences can alter brain development and influence how a child may access learning, particularly reading and phonic awareness (National Scientific Council on the Developing Child, 2004). Stressful, toxic, and neglectful experiences can permanently alter brain development and slow abilities in young children. (**Toxic stress** is defined as what happens when children experience severe, prolonged adversity without adult support; significant adversity early in life can alter a child's capacity to learn.) Therefore, to adequately assist children in acquiring literacy skills, all children can benefit from the experiences offered in high-quality early childhood classroom environments with highly knowledgeable and skilled teachers.

This chapter discusses the impact of teacher and student interactions, the strategic use of classroom design and curriculum in the development of language skills, and the assessment of early preliteracy skills. If **literacy** is defined as the ability to read and write, emergent literacy is the period when infants are beginning to attend to environmental sounds and when toddlers are pointing to pictures and scribbling on paper; **preliteracy** refers to the period when children begin to put sounds together in order to read and write words. We recommend a two-teacher model, which has great potential for early assessment that can identify developmental challenges and warning signs of poor preliteracy skills (Barnett, 2011). Two teachers in the classroom afford an opportunity for directed time with individual children without sacrificing time with the other children; this setup offers short intervals wherein assessments can be performed accurately. However, all of the discussion and examples in the chapter are appropriate for classrooms with a single teacher.

EMERGENT LITERACY

Literacy in the study and implementation of early childhood education is unique. It cannot be approached in the same way that literacy is approached in the elementary, middle, or high school levels. Weitzman and Greenberg explained, "Literacy—the ability to read and write—is an emerging skill that begins at birth" (2002, p. 2).

The term *emergent literacy* includes the period when infants are beginning to attend to environmental sounds and toddlers are pointing to pictures and scribbling on paper, until the time when children "break the code" and can put sounds together to read and write words (Chall, 1983). It is a critical time and requires skilled educators as well as the child's family to be involved with the integration of these early paths to speaking and reading. There are many components to emergent literacy. It consists of conversational skills, vocabulary, story comprehension, language knowledge, print knowledge, phonological awareness, and writing development. These pieces come together to define a child's emergent literacy development and skill level.

In the early childhood classroom, emergent literacy develops during social interactions with adults. It is important to involve children in real-life situations, such as making grocery lists, writing invitations and thank-you cards, and writing notes to friends and loved ones. When children arrive at school, the teacher should provide opportunities for the children to work on these types of tasks, which create opportunities for interactions throughout the day that offer children time to interact with letters and practice writing, both of which are emergent literacy tasks. During these windows, the teacher can enrich children's literacy development.

Why Emergent Literacy Matters

Young children who learn to read early have more exposure to print, which solidifies reading and writing skills. Children who lag behind in reading skill development have less exposure to print, fewer opportunities to practice reading, and fewer opportunities to develop vocabulary and reading comprehension strategies (Stanovich, 1986). They are more likely to develop negative attitudes about reading and school. This does not mean formally teaching preschoolers to read. It means teaching the precursors of reading, which is the essence of emergent literacy. Adults can foster emergent literacy at home and at school.

Emergent Literacy and the Home Environment

Before children enter school, there are many opportunities to develop their emergent literacy skills. Families need to speak to their children using everyday, conversational words and sentences. Families also need to read to children daily and expose them to print in as many ways as possible. The more words that children are exposed to, the stronger their language skills are and hence the stronger their literacy skills will become. A seminal study conducted by researchers Hart and Risley (1999) on infants and children's early exposures to language showed that children who were exposed to literacy in a variety of ways and with greater frequency had a better chance of developing strong oral language skills. A strong start and more exposure lead to greater success in language and literacy development, especially when there is a strong adult–child mentoring relationship.

Emergent Literacy and the Early Childhood Educator

What early childhood educators know and do greatly affects the emergent literacy skills of the children in their classrooms. Educators promote language development and literacy skills by engaging in high-quality conversations with children through frequent, intentional exchanges and by speaking with them in a pleasant, positive voice rather than giving orders or commands. It is also important to ask open-ended questions that seek to increase children's vocabularies, extend their knowledge, and encourage them to experiment with words. These educators also promote language development and literacy skills in the classroom by (NAEYC, 1998)

- Sharing books with children and modeling reading behaviors

- Talking about letters by name and sounds

- Establishing a literacy-rich environment

- Re-reading favorite stories

- Engaging children in language games

- Promoting literacy-related play activities

- Encouraging children to experiment with writing

- Assessing early literacy skills

- Teaching early literacy skills

These practices are linked to the International Dyslexia Association's (IDA; 2018) *Knowledge and Practice Standards for Teachers of Reading* and align with many of the standard practices supported by IDA. For example, the *Knowledge and Practice Standards* suggest that it is important for teachers to understand 1) early language foundation and development, 2) social and cultural factors that affect literacy development, and 3) the importance of setting appropriate goals for literacy development according to developmental expectations.

THE IMPORTANCE OF THE CLASSROOM ENVIRONMENT

Developmentally appropriate practice (DAP) is an approach to teaching grounded in the research on how young children develop and learn and in what is known about effective early education. Its framework is designed to promote young children's optimal learning and development through interaction with both adults and the environment. It has three elements: knowing about child development and learning, knowing the individual child, and knowing the cultural context of the child.

The principles of DAP in early childhood education speak directly to the importance of the classroom environment and teacher interaction to the overall growth of children. Preliteracy activities play a significant role in that environment. In a joint position statement describing DAP for young children who are learning to read and write, the National Association for the Education of Young Children (NAEYC) and The International Reading Association stated:

> Children explore their environment and build the foundations for learning to read and write. Children can
>
> - Enjoy listening to and enjoying storybooks
> - Understand that print carries a message
> - Engage in reading and writing attempts
> - Identify labels and signs in their environment
> - Participate in rhyming games
> - Identify some letters and make some letter–sound matches
> - Use known letters to represent written language. (1998, p. 44)

The Physical Space

A properly planned preschool classroom environment is considered to be a third teacher. An effective classroom environment can increase a child's ability to learn and feel comfortable as a member of the class. Moreover, the physical arrangement of a space and the organization of materials can give children clues about the types of play expected and increase the likelihood of appropriate behavior.

In contrast, a poorly arranged physical setting can send messages that may trigger behaviors such as aggressive play, running around the classroom, or superficial interactions with toys and materials (Commonwealth of Massachusetts, Department of Early Education and Care, 2015). Although it sounds contrary, the space in a classroom must be very controlled for children to move around freely. Very little productive learning is likely to occur in a classroom if the physical environment is not carefully planned and arranged. Learning centers must be clearly defined using signs with words and pictures, floor coverings, and furniture or low partitions of some kind. When considering furniture placement, traffic patterns (the ways the children move around the room) should permit safe play and prevent children from having to interrupt one another or step around one another or a work in progress. All materials and equipment need to be in good condition and readily accessible to children, and shelves need to be neat and uncluttered. The number of toys and activities must be sufficient for the size of the group but carefully planned and regulated. There should be a clearly defined place for everything so that when a child is finished working with an object or material, he or she knows where it belongs. A well-planned space allows teachers to facilitate children's play and anticipate situations where learning can be extended. It allows time for the informal give-and-take between teachers and students that helps children advance their knowledge as much as the planned curriculum. In these ways, the environment becomes a third teacher, allowing space and time to attend to those elusive teachable moments, or unplanned learning opportunities.

Learning Centers: The Foundation of Preschool Classrooms

A learning center is an area of a preschool classroom devoted to a specific set of skills. There are several reasons for subdividing the physical space into learning centers: the division gives children opportunities to explore along areas of their own interest; it promotes small-group interaction, which preschool children prefer; and it leads to more complex and meaningful play and work by the children

(Dodge et al., 2015). High-quality early childhood classrooms will include these learning centers as the fulcrum to all activities and development for the young children in the class, and each center contributes to the development of key literacy skills. The sections that follow provide an overview of different kinds of learning centers and their connection to literacy development: discovery or science centers, dramatic play centers, art centers, library centers, centers with manipulatives or tabletop toys, and block centers.

Discovery or Science Center   Children interact with materials of all colors, shapes, sizes, and textures. Objects might include differently shaped shells, crystals, leaves of all colors, a simple balance scale to compare weights, materials that produce different sounds or smells, and other objects associated with a unit of study. Adults provide names of items and ask questions such as "How are these alike?" "How are they different?" or "What do you think this is?" These questions, along with interactions with the materials, enrich vocabulary and help develop important concepts such as same and different that will be useful later when children begin to learn about letters and sounds.

Dramatic Play Center   Children use their imaginations and try on various roles from the adult world. This center can become a school, hospital, restaurant, spaceship, or something else related to the theme the class is exploring, all with accompanying word signs. Activities in this center encourage the use of both receptive and expressive language and the exploration of nascent reading and writing skills.

Art Center   Art materials are freely accessible to children to allow them to make choices and interact with a wide variety of materials. The process of working with the materials is more important than what is created. Children have the opportunity to make choices as they select different types of paper and colors of paint or crayons or pencils and experiment with the way they are applied. Children develop a vocabulary of describing words, such as *smooth, rough, striped,* or *checkered.* This is important because well-developed vocabularies contribute to reading proficiency in later childhood (Snow, Burns, & Griffin, 1998).

Library Center   Children explore all kinds of books and reading material on their own or with friends or teachers. They develop **concepts of print.** This term refers to the way print is organized to convey meaning. Children develop the ability to know and recognize the ways in which print "works" for the purposes of reading, particularly with regard to books. For example, they notice that print goes from left to right and top to bottom, that pictures often tell a story, and that the story stays the same as it is read over and over. Listening, attending, sequencing, and thinking skills are all being used as children enjoy a story. Children also become acquainted with new vocabulary words and different styles of writing and illustration.

Manipulative or Tabletop Toy Center   Children play with small toys at tables or on the floor. Controlled movements of the fingers and hands enable children to master use of the muscles necessary for writing. As children work with color and patterns, they develop visual discrimination and memory, both of which help children to differentiate between letter-forms and to recognize and remember the shapes and lines used to form letters. When children pretend, using things they have built, they are taking their first steps in the use of symbols, which are important as they begin to read and write.

Block Center   As children work with blocks they develop control of the muscles in fingers and hands and arms. Perceptions of size, weight, and shape are developing, and children's language skills are growing as they discuss what they are building.

> ### REFLECT, CONNECT, and RESPOND
> How does the physical environment of the preschool classroom affect learning and preliteracy in children?

EVIDENCE-BASED MULTISENSORY ACTIVITIES THAT DEVELOP FOUNDATIONAL LITERACY SKILLS

Long before children learn to read, they need exposure to a wide variety of language and literacy experiences that will support them in learning to read and write. Teachers must understand the developmental framework for learning in the areas of oral language, phonological awareness, concepts of print, letters and words, and writing. They must also provide young children with an environment that encourages exploration in these areas and that supports and values all reading and writing behaviors.

Oral Language

Oral language is a spoken system of words with rules for their use that includes listening to words and speaking them (see Chapter 3 for further discussion). Oral language can be receptive or expressive. **Receptive language** includes the words a child hears and (later) reads. **Expressive language** refers to the words a child speaks and (later) writes. Long before children learn to read, they need a great many language and literacy experiences that will support them later in acquiring linguistic skills necessary for reading. In the preschool years, these skills are best acquired through language-play that includes rhymes, finger-plays, songs, exploring literature of all kinds including books and poetry, writing messages, expanding oral vocabulary, and learning that reading has many purposes.

When adults engage in purposeful and high-quality conversation with children, children develop larger vocabularies (Hart & Risley, 1999; Hoff & Naigles, 2002). Research has shown that children with larger vocabularies become more proficient readers in later childhood (Snow et al., 1998). *High-quality language* means teachers ask questions that seek to extend children's knowledge; speak frequently with children, using a positive tone of voice rather than giving commands; and respond in a sensitive manner to children's words and sounds (Test, Cunningham, & Lee, 2010). When teachers ask open-ended questions, children are encouraged to think and use higher-level skills such as inference, prediction, and interpretation (Weitzman & Greenberg, 2002). In addition, conversations with children that use descriptive, complex sentences; that involve familiar topics; and that provide meaningful opportunities to use and experiment with words will allow children to enter school with the best preparation for later stages of literacy development (Test et al., 2010). Finally, reading literature aloud helps expand children's vocabulary by teaching them the meanings of unfamiliar words used in proper context (Robbins & Ehri, 1994).

The sections that follow describe how to promote oral language through classroom read-alouds, through children's play activities at classroom learning centers, and in other activities and interactions throughout the day.

Promote Oral Language Development Through Read-Alouds   Children should be exposed to good literature read aloud as often as possible. This includes books of all types and poetry. The books can be informational texts or storybooks, and the poetry need not be confined to children's verses. Adult poems such as "Who Has Seen the Wind?" by Christina Rossetti, "Poem" and "Winter Moon" by Langston Hughes, "Until I Saw the Sea" by Lillian Moore, "A Bird" by Emily Dickinson, and some of the haiku poetry of Yosa Buson and Kobayashi Issa can all be used to good effect. Listening to adult poems allows children to hear something very rare—beautiful language beautifully written. They are exposed to new and interesting vocabulary and learn that words can be used to convey ideas and images. Storybooks need to be chosen with an eye for thematic richness, carefully constructed language, and engaging illustrations that add dimension to the text. An excellent example of these concepts is *Owl Moon,* a book by Jane Yolen (1987), illustrated by John Schoenherr.

Owl Moon is a beautiful story about a young child who goes owling with her father on a cold, late autumn night. This tale about a shared experience between an adult and a child is appealing to children and easy to relate to their own lives. To make the read-aloud experience a valuable one and to support children's language skills, teachers should consider implementing the following practices:

- Showing the book before it is read and asking children to make predictions about the story based on the cover and title

- Talking about what it means to be an author and illustrator and always using those words when speaking about books and written material

- Reading the book from beginning to end with as much expression as possible; using gestures and even props such as a hat or scarf if it enhances the story and helps children to attend (Preschool teachers are actors, and their performances should always be Oscar worthy.)

- Using open-ended questions that encourage thought and expression of ideas, such as the following: "Why do you think this book is called Owl Moon?" "Why are the father and child pictured so small in the illustrations?" "Why does the picture of the owl take up the whole page near the end of the story?"

- Calling attention to the expressive language, such as the following: "What does the author mean by the phrase 'And when their voices faded away it was *as quiet as a dream*?' What might *as quiet as a dream* mean?"

- Encouraging language that goes beyond the immediate to a past or future event by asking what special moments children may have shared or would like to share with a grown-up in their lives (Language that goes beyond the immediate to past or future events is called *decontextualized* language. Decontextualized language encourages a higher order of thinking and will eventually help children to write stories and essays; Dickinson & Tabors, 2001.)

- Allowing children to "read" more and more of the story after they have heard it several times and encouraging them to notice things they may not have during the initial reading, such as new words and the character's actions and facial expressions

- Placing the book in the library center where it is available for the children to read on their own or in small groups

- Reading an informational book about owls or owling or farms during and after the harvest as a follow-up if the children express interest

Promote Oral Language Through Classroom Learning Centers Previously this chapter described the types of learning centers typically found in a preschool classroom and touched on how children's activities at these centers contribute to early literacy skills. These centers also provide opportunities for teachers to promote **oral language.** Teachers support language development in these centers by allowing sufficient time and space for children's activities—time and space for children to learn new words, experiment with new materials, ask questions, and process the answers by incorporating new knowledge into their understanding of things—and by stocking the centers with creative, interesting materials. Some (but not all) of the materials should reflect the current classroom project. The harvest project, for example (discussed later in this chapter), might include a simple word and picture recipe for apple pie, along with baking equipment, or a display of apples, cranberries, and an ear of corn with husk (all with labels) in the discovery center.

In the blocks and manipulatives center, for instance, children use language to solve problems with their constructions and to negotiate use of the materials. Teachers can encourage children to talk about their structures by asking open-ended questions: "Who lives in that building?" "How did you make that structure?" or "Where does that road go?" The use of rich vocabulary, supplying children with alternate descriptive words, also expands oral language: "Tell me about your building. It looks like a very interesting *structure*," or "The street you've built is very busy with *vehicles* going every which way." Teachers can extend conversations by expanding on what children say: "You said you wanted to do this puzzle. How should we *organize* the pieces so you can see them?" or "I know you like the whale puzzle. Do you think it's as big as an actual whale?"

In the dramatic play center, children use language to negotiate relationships and interact with other children as they explore roles and ideas both real and make-believe. Teachers can serve as good language models by using complete sentences and expanding on what children say. For example, if a child says, "Baby is going to sleep," the teacher could respond with, "The baby is going to sleep because she's tired. What do you think she did to make her so tired?"

In the science or discovery center, the intriguing materials on display should promote many interesting conversations about how objects are used, how they are made, and what properties they have. For example, commenting on a display of harvest plants or seed pods, a teacher might ask questions such as, "What do you think this is?" "Where do you think it came from?" "How would you describe the *texture*, what it feels like?" or "What colors do you see when you look at it?" Teachers can also introduce words that describe size (*large, tiny*), shape (*flat, triangular, oval*), and form (*long, thick, elongated*) into conversations.

Promote Oral Language Throughout the Day Teachers can use songs, chants, and finger-plays in circle time and throughout the day. Songs, finger-plays, and silly rhymes allow children to play with language and develop an awareness of cadence, rhythm, and different patterns of speech. These can be introduced formally at circle time and then used informally throughout the day when it's time to clean up or go outdoors or get ready for lunch. Some examples follow.

A Gathering Song (Tune: "Short'nin' Bread")
Everybody sit down, sit down, sit down.
Everybody sit down on the floor.
Not on the ceiling, not on the door!
Everybody sit down on the floor.

A Hand-Washing Song (Tune: "Yankee Doodle")
Wash your hands before you eat.
Wash those germs away.
Rinse with water, pat them dry.
You'll have clean hands today.

A Harvest Finger-Play
(Children can help to create actions to match words.)
The leaves are falling softly down.
They make a carpet on the ground.
Then SWISH! The wind comes whistling by
And sends them dancing to the sky.

Although some of these examples are connected to specific routines in the classroom, songs and chants can also be used for their own sake simply to help children experience the pleasure of singing and saying words. A chant is a rhythmic song with a strong beat that children sing in unison. Children usually get really involved in the experience, and chants are great fun for everyone, teachers included.

A Sailor Went to Sea
A sailor went to sea, sea, sea.
To see what he could see, see, see.
But all that he could see, see, see.
Was the bottom of the deep blue sea, sea, sea.

Promote Oral Language Through Games   Language games are a fun, informal way to promote oral language skills. They can be used in a small or large group or at any time during the day. Some examples are described next, the classroom guessing game and the "If You Are Wearing. . ." game, which also employs song.

Classroom Guessing Game   In the classroom guessing game, a child gives clues about an object in the classroom, and other children take turns guessing what it is. This is very challenging when children are not in the classroom. It works best when the child giving the clues whispers the name of the object to the teacher beforehand so the teacher can intervene with suggestions if the game begins to lag. This can also go in the opposite direction with children giving clues to the teacher and the teacher being the guesser. This is a good listening game that can be adjusted for a variety of purposes.

If You Are Wearing   The "If You Are Wearing" game is another good listening game that can be adjusted for a variety of purposes. For example, a teacher might say, "If you are wearing blue today, you may wash your hands now. . ." or "If your name starts with *B*, you may get your coat now. . ." or anything else teachers or children can invent. The game can suit all occasions.

Phonological Awareness

Phonological awareness is the ability to segment and manipulate the sounds of oral language (see Chapter 6 for further discussion). It is auditory and does not involve working with words in print. In preschool children, this skill develops as a progression from listening to sounds in the environment, to being able to identify rhymes in word endings (*sad, mad, bad*) and alliteration in the initial sounds of words (*purple, porky, pigs*), to being able to discern syllables in a word (*mar–ket, win–dow*). Another step in this continuum is being able to segment syllables into onset and rime. Onset is the part of the syllable before the vowel, and rime is the rest of the syllable, that is, the first vowel and everything following it. In the word *desk,* for example, /d/ is the onset and /ĕsk/ is the rime.

The terms *phonological awareness* and *phonemic awareness* are not synonymous; rather, phonemic awareness is a **sub-skill** that falls under the larger umbrella of phonological awareness skills. A phoneme is the smallest unit of sound in language. The word *desk,* for example, consists of four phonemes, /d/ - /ĕ/ - /s/ - /k/, and the word *paper* consists of four also, /p/ - /ā/ - /p/ - /er/. The ability to blend phonemes into words or segment words into phonemes, or to substitute one phoneme for another, is phonemic awareness. When children play with silly songs and sing "Nead, noulders, nees and noes" instead of "Head, shoulders, knees and toes," they are playing with phonemes. The ability to hear the sounds in words and to isolate the sounds from one another will aid children in learning to read and spell. Teachers can encourage phonological awareness skills, including phonemic awareness skills, in the classroom with songs, chants, poetry, rhymes, finger-plays, stories, and games that play with language.

Being able to manipulate the sounds of spoken language—phonological awareness—is highly related to later success in reading and spelling (Ehri et al., 2001). Research has found phonological awareness skills in preschool to be one of the most robust predictors of early reading success in a child's first few years of formal schooling (Callaghan & Alison, 2012). Phonological awareness skills are less likely to develop through incidental exposure (Sulzby & Teale, 1991); rather, they develop through intentional introduction to words and word sounds. Young children are typically able to detect words that rhyme, even when other phonological skills have not developed (Whitehurst & Lonigan, 1998), which makes the early childhood classroom an ideal environment for building skills.

Although instruction should generally progress from larger to smaller units of sound, phonological awareness is not a lockstep progression of skills, and children need not master one level before being exposed to other levels of phonological awareness (Yopp & Yopp, 2009). Children can develop a sense of the sound structure of language by saying rhymes, singing, and reciting finger-plays (Jenkins & Bowen, 1994). Alliteration requires children to pay attention to parts of words that are smaller than a syllable (Ball, 1993), and many songs and rhymes use alliteration and repetition.

Because phonological awareness is central in learning to read and spell (Ehri, 1984), it is important to be aware of how it is achieved. Although some young students will pick up (phonological) skills with relative ease—especially if the curriculum includes explicit activities—other students must be taught these met-alinguistic skills directly and systematically (Moats & Tolman, 2009). Achieving phonological awareness is not easy for many children. Without direct instructional support, roughly 25% of middle class children—and substantially more children from less economically advantaged homes—fail to develop this crucial under-standing (Abouzeid, 2010).

To promote phonological awareness in the classroom, children should be sur-rounded by the sounds of language through songs, chants, poetry, books, and games that play with the manipulation of sounds. Specific activities for promoting phonological awareness are described next.

Promote Phonological Awareness Through Nursery Rhymes That Play With Sounds   Nursery rhymes are excellent for promoting phonological aware-ness. In addition to including rhyming words, many nursery rhymes include other poetic devices, such as alliteration, that draw children's attention to the sounds in words. A good example is *Sing a Song of Sixpence,* an old English rhyme that also has alliteration.

Sing a Song of Sixpence
Sing a song of sixpence,
A pocket full of rye;
Four and twenty blackbirds
Baked in a pie.

When the pie was opened
The birds began to sing;
Wasn't that a dainty dish
To set before the king?

The king was in the counting house
Counting out his money;
The queen was in the parlor
Eating bread and honey;

The maid was in the garden
Hanging out the clothes;
Along came a blackbird,
And pecked at her nose.

To use this nursery rhyme to build children's phonological awareness, first read the rhyme and comment on the language play. Next, have children repeat the line, "Sing a song of sixpence." Then, call attention to the alliteration in the repeated sound /s/ by asking, "What sound do you hear at the beginning of each word?

Children who are able to manipulate phonemes, the smallest units of speech sounds in words, can experiment with changing the initial sound in a word or words. For example, after saying the line "Sing a song of sixpence," ask, "How does the phrase sound if the /f/ sound is substituted for the /s/ sound?"

In addition to providing opportunities to work with alliteration, the poem can be read at another time for the rhymes. Ask the children which words sound alike and substitute other words (silly or real) for the words that rhyme.

Promote Phonological Awareness Through Phonological Awareness Poems

Another way to promote phonological awareness is to introduce silly poems that play with sounds. A good example is the poem/nursery rhyme *What They Said*. A few verses of this old German rhyme are reprinted next.

What They Said
It's four o'clock,
Said the cock.
It's still dark,
Said the lark.

What's that,
Said the cat.

I want to sleep,
Said the sheep.

To use this poem for developing phonological awareness, first read the poem with expression several times, accentuating the rhymes. After one or two readings, encourage children to supply the second rhyming word in the couplet by giving clues such as saying "cock-a-doodle-doo" for the cock or "meow" for the cat. Call attention to the rhyming words and encourage substitutions for those words—*sock* for *cock* or *park* for *lark,* for instance. Revisit the poem many times and enjoy the fun along with the children.

Promote Phonological Awareness Through Songs That Play With Sounds

Songs are still another way to promote phonological awareness. Most songs have a rhyme structure, of course. In addition, songs such as *The Name Game* let children sing about their own names by changing the onset (first sound) in each verse. They can begin with the onset sounds in their own names; then, when the activity is done with a group of children, the onset sound changes as you proceed around the group and use every child's name, as in the following examples.

Madison
Madison Madison Bo Badison
Banana Fana Fo Fadison
Me My Mo Madison
Madison!

The onset would change for the name *Jonah.*

Jonah
Jonah Jonah Bo Bonah
Banana Fana Fo Fonah
Me My Mo Monah
Jonah!

Songs like *Willoughby Wallaby Woo* or *Skinamarinky Dinky Dink* are also fun songs that help children to focus on the sounds of language. It's also interesting to sing familiar songs and change the first sound (onset) of the words. Change *Head, Shoulders, Knees, and Toes,* for instance, to *Bead, Boulders, Bees, and Boes* or leave off the onset in each word and just sing the rime: *Ead, oulders, ees and oes.* Assist children who enjoy playing with the words, but do not insist that everyone do so. For some children, just listening and enjoying is enough. As with poetry, the songs should be repeated many times throughout the year at informal times.

Promote Phonological Awareness Through Playing Games With Language
Throughout the day, teachers can promote phonological awareness by playing games with language; these games can be worked into various parts of the classroom routine. The games should be fun, and teachers should support all attempts at participation. Here are just a few examples of how to incorporate language-based games into daily routines:

- Refer to the first sound in children's names when you dismiss them to get their coats or direct them to wash hands or line up. For example, say, "If your name begins with the /k/ sound, go get your coat."

- During circle time, tap out the syllables in children's names using rhythm sticks: for example, *Ta–mi–ka* or *Al–ex–an–der.* This can also be done with simple poems like nursery rhymes or with objects in the room. Instead of rhythm sticks, children can clap out syllables or tap their knees or the floor.

- Hold up two objects whose names begin with different sounds. Name the objects with the children—for example, *ball* and *cup.* Tell them that you are going to give them clues about one of the objects and have them guess which one you mean. Then, tell them the first sound of the word you are thinking about—for example, by saying, "I am thinking about the thing whose name begins with the /b/ sound." As an alternative, remove the initial sound and tell them the rime—for example, by saying, "I am thinking about the thing whose name sounds like *up.*" Celebrate all participation, and offer children the opportunity to be the clue giver.

Concepts of Print

The term concepts of print refers to the way print is organized to convey meaning. Children who are beginning to understand the concepts of print learn that written language is related to oral language and that printed language carries messages and is a source of information and enjoyment. They learn about the many functions of print, such as supplying directions, communicating information, and expressing ideas. In a **print-rich environment**—one that encourages reading, writing, and conversation through the use of many varieties of printed materials for multiple purposes, including nonacademic purposes—children learn that print has many forms, including sign-in sheets, books, cards, signs, labels charts, journals, and e-mails. Finally, children need an understanding of the rules of print. Letters and words are not placed haphazardly on a page: Books are organized from front cover to back, print is read from left to right and top to bottom, letters form words and words form sentences, and there are spaces between words and sentences.

In the early childhood classroom, awareness of print concepts provides the backdrop against which reading and writing are best learned (Texas Education Agency, 2002). These concepts of print are extremely important because they teach children how reading "works" (Holdgreve-Resendez, 2010). Children learn about print from a variety of sources, and in the process, they learn that print differs from speech but carries messages just like speech (Morrow, 1990). In the classroom, offering materials and activities throughout the room that encourage reading, writing, and talking can provide support for children's literacy development (Pool & Carter, 2016). Research has shown that knowledge of print concepts develops through direct contact with books and explicit modeling by skilled readers, as well as through exposure to environmental print (Adams, 1990). These elements are present in a high-quality early childhood environment and assist in developing important early literacy skills for children.

Promote Concepts of Print by Labeling Classroom Objects and Centers

One way to promote concepts of print in the preschool classroom is to label objects and learning centers. Words and signs should be clearly written and displayed at children's eye level. Attach word signs to the actual objects, or use pictures to help identify words. The word *door*, for instance, can be attached to the actual door, but a sign for the library center should include pictures of books as well as being posted near the center. Signs that say "open" or "closed" have practical applications such as indicating when a center is open or closed for play. Likewise, a "stop" sign affixed to the floor can indicate the end of a designated line-up area, or an "exit" sign can be used to signal the door through which children leave the classroom. (In addition, post any charts you have created with the children, and have children use sign-in sheets when they arrive and when they want to use equipment such as the computer or a favorite toy.)

Using labels and signs this way helps to promote concepts of print. Remember, however, that too much of a good thing is not a good thing. The amount of print in the environment should not be overwhelming. Signs that scream in large letters, dropping from the ceiling and affixed to every surface in the room, are counter productive and defeat the purpose of a print-rich environment.

Use all types of books in learning centers to reinforce print awareness. Teachers should review with children ahead of time whatever written material is placed in learning centers because students are likely to be at different levels of print awareness and the material needs to be meaningful for everyone.

The library center should be stocked with fiction and nonfiction books and magazines, including recorded books that allow children to follow text while listening to a recording. The books should be displayed on low shelves with the covers facing out.

The dramatic play center can include a variety of writing tools and written material. If this center is being developed as a farmer's market, for example, children can make picture or word signs for fruits and vegetables, make "open" and "closed" signs, and generate all kinds of lists and sign-ups on clipboards, as well as deciding what to name the market and making a sign. Real (empty) boxes of cereals that are familiar to children can also be a part of this center. Books and magazines about markets or with pictures and names of produce might also be placed here to assist children with their reading and writing efforts.

The discovery center is an excellent place for informational and nonfiction books related to whatever topic the class is exploring. A discovery center for a harvest project might include word signs for whatever is on display—leaves, seed pods, fruits, and vegetables—as well as charts and posters.

Promote Concepts of Print by Modeling Literate Behavior

In addition to providing the kind of print-rich environment described previously, promote concepts of print by consciously modeling literate behavior—things that readers do. Be very intentional about looking up the weather report in a newspaper or seeking the meaning of a word in the dictionary. Using an actual dictionary or newspaper is more dramatic than using a computer or a tablet. Label children's work with their own words, and do so in the children's presence so they can witness the connection between speaking and writing. Create "experience charts" with children by asking a question such as, "What is your favorite thing to do in the fall?" and recording their answers. As you write, talk about the way a sentence begins with an uppercase letter, the spaces between words, the end punctuation of sentences, and the directionality of writing.

Finally, model literate behavior by talking about books and reading them. Bring in some of your favorite childhood books, read them to the class, and explain why they were your favorites. Big books are excellent for reading to large groups. Draw attention to the name of the author and illustrator on the front cover and the dedication within, or the table of contents for a nonfiction book. Talk about the letters, words, and punctuation marks within the story as well as frequently used words. Sweep your hand from left to right as you read each sentence. Place regular-size copies of the book in the library center.

Letters, Sounds, and the Alphabetic Principle

Awareness of letters and sounds can also be supported in the preschool classroom; this includes understanding of the alphabetic principle. The alphabetic principle refers to the concept that letters and letter patterns represent the sounds of spoken language. Children acquire alphabetic knowledge through a progression of skills that begins with their learning letter names, progresses to learning letter shapes, and then advances to learning letter sounds and putting those sounds together to make words. (See Chapter 5 for further discussion on letter knowledge.)

For developing literacy, letter–sound knowledge is the prerequisite to effective word identification. A primary difference between good and poor readers is the ability to use letter–sound correspondence to identify words (Juel, 1991). Learning this skill is promoted in the early childhood classroom through interaction with the print-rich environment of the room as well as with adults who are reading and speaking during class time. The combination of instruction in phonological awareness and letter sounds appears to be the most favorable for successful early reading (Haskell, Foorman, & Swank, 1992). In addition, knowledge of the alphabet, both sounds and print, can be a strong predictor of later reading, writing, and spelling ability. Once children can identify and name letters with ease, they can begin to learn letter sounds and spelling (Texas Education Agency, 2002).

Promote Knowledge of Letters Through the Alphabet Song   To promote children's emerging knowledge of letters, sing the *Alphabet Song*. Help children to sing it clearly by using an alphabet chart and pointing to each letter as it is pronounced. Sing it slowly; sing it while standing; sing it in a high voice, a low voice, or a silly voice. Post the alphabet chart at children's eye level so they can sing this song to themselves or in small groups. Try singing the alphabet to other tunes as well, such as *Here We Go 'Round the Mulberry Bush, Mary Had a Little Lamb,* or *Happy Birthday to You*. (Note that singing the alphabet to other tunes breaks up L-M-N-O, so it does not sound like one letter.)

Promote Knowledge of Letters Through Alphabet Rhymes   Another way to promote knowledge of letters and sounds is to work with alphabet rhymes—short poems that include a focus on words beginning with one particular letter.

Write the rhymes on chart paper, emphasizing the dominant letter in the poem, and read them several times in circle time, emphasizing the dominant letter sound. For example, the following poem might be used to teach the letter *f*.

A fly and a flea in a flue
Were imprisoned, so what could they do?
Said the fly, "Let us flee!"
"Let us fly!" said the flea,
And they flew through a flaw in the flue.
(Anonymous)

Post the rhyme charts at children's eye level to allow individual or small group review.

Promote Knowledge of Letters by Planning Multisensory Alphabet Activities
Children understand concepts more easily when multiple senses are involved. Offer children a variety of ways to explore the alphabet by using felt or sandpaper letters, making letters with playdough or clay, using magnetic letters, doing alphabet puzzles large and small, using salt trays to trace or form letters, using blocks to form letters in the block area, making letters with pretzel dough or stick pretzels, and forming letters with their bodies.

Make name signs for each child and teacher. These signs can assist children with morning sign-in and are useful for many classroom activities. Teachers, for example, can hold up a name sign and say the first letter in that name as a signal that it is time for that child to get his or her coat or time to wash hands or line up. Teachers should also consider placing clipboards in each learning center, with photocopied lists of all the children in the class because the first letters children identify are usually the letters in their own names and in the names of important people in their lives such as caregivers and classmates. These lists can be used as a quick reference when children need to write their names or those of their classmates and will become the focus of many invented games.

Promote Knowledge of Letters Through Alphabet Books   Finally, the library or other learning centers can include books that focus on the letters of the alphabet. Books such as *The Construction Alphabet Book* by Jerry Pallotta and Ray Bolster (2016) are suitable for reading to a large group because they have one large letter on each page. Books such as *Animalia* by Graeme Base (1986), however, are better suited to individual or small-group reading because children must examine each page closely.

Writing Development

Emergent writing includes three main components: the manual act of producing physical marks (mechanics); the meaning children attribute to these markings (composition); and understanding how written language works (orthographic knowledge; Berninger, 2009). Because children in a preschool classroom are probably at diverse skill levels, teachers need to scaffold efforts in early writing. When learning to write, children exhibit six stages: Drawing, Wavy Scribbles, Letter-Like Scribbles, Random Letters in a Line, Patterned Letter Strings, and Conventional Writing (Sulzby & Teale, 1985; see Chapter 11 for further discussion).

Each stage helps develop the next in the sequence. For instance, if a teacher labels a drawing or painting with the child's own words, that child is given the opportunity to express in words what has previously only been expressed through a painting or drawing. With these consistent experiences, children will attempt to imitate the writing of adults by using wavy and letterlike scribbles. Once they have practiced these scribbles and continue watching adults write sentences, they will begin to use invented letterlike scribbles across a page to represent words. Once children have learned how to form a few actual letter shapes, using random letters in a line assists children in practicing writing until they are ready to move toward writing patterned strings of letters that are recognizable. This often begins with the letters in a child's name. Last, a connection between the sounds children are trying to write and the letters on the page develops. At this stage, the writing can be read by others, though there are misspellings and backward letters. The environment in a high-quality early childhood center will create opportunities for children to practice writing and develop skills through each of these six stages.

In the classroom, the writing center should be filled with the tools of writing: pads, pencils, colored pencils, markers, envelopes (save the ones that come with advertisements in the mail), stickers, tape, rubber stamps and stamp pads, paper punches, paper clips, cards, and erasers. This is also a good place to keep name cards. Children will use these materials in ways that correlate with their skill level. Specific ways to promote emergent writing skills are described in the sections that follow.

Promote Emergent Writing Skills by Encouraging Children to Write Messages   Regardless of their skill level, have children write messages. They can write to their caregivers inviting them to visit the classroom, or write a sign telling people not to knock over their block structure, or write a message saying the class is outdoors. Involve children in writing instructions, such as "Please flush" or "Do not touch." Collaborate with children in writing a list of class rules with accompanying pictures, and refer to the list often. Follow a simple cooking activity and write the recipe on chart paper (cooking activities are best done in small groups). Read and follow the recipe steps one at a time. When children write messages or instructions, they learn that writing can tell people how to do something.

Promote Emergent Writing Skills by Setting Up Mailboxes   Another way to promote writing is to set up a mailbox for each child or set up a class mailbox. Through writing cards and notes, children learn that writing enables people to communicate with one another. Have children write thank-you notes to classroom volunteers or guests. Make cards for classroom birthdays or get-well cards if someone is ill. Make cards for family members and caregivers for special occasions. Enlist another class in a pen-pal program and write letters and notes to one another.

Promote Emergent Writing Skills by Making Lists   List-making promotes emergent writing skills and can easily be incorporated into daily activities. Make lists of things children would like to learn about or supplies needed for the classroom. Use sign-up lists to use a popular toy or piece of equipment. Make a list of favorite books or where children would like to go for a pretend vacation or favorite colors or food. Children can use these lists to recall information.

Promote Emergent Writing Skills by Creating a Word Wall or a Collection of Word Cards The class can use the word wall for reference when writing independently. Add to the list of reference words throughout the year.

Promote Emergent Writing Skills by Creating Journals Individual journals can be used to promote writing skills. Give each child a personal journal to draw or write about anything they choose. Through journal writing, children can express thoughts and ideas. Journal work is also a good indicator of a child's skill development throughout the year. Having children dictate captions for their artwork is another good way for children to associate writing with expression of ideas.

Promote Emergent Writing Skills by Making Experience Charts Experience charts can be related to a unit of study or a class trip or an interesting event. Teachers write a question at the top of a large paper and then write the children's individual answers. Children who are able to do so can write their own answers or draw a picture or decorate the chart. For example, a teacher might create a class experience chart based on questions such as "What is your favorite thing to do in the fall?" or "What was your favorite part of our trip to the farmer's market?"

Promote Emergent Writing Skills by Creating Literature Working with students to create stories supports their writing skill development. In a small group, encourage children to create stories about their favorite book or television characters or about an experience. Creating group stories allows children with less well-developed skills to learn from their peers. Write some or all the words and have children supply the illustrations. Another approach is to have individual children supply words to go with their artwork. Placing blank books in the writing center also encourages story creation through words or pictures or a combination of both. Celebrating all levels of participation allows children to feel empowered and to see themselves as readers and writers.

REFLECT, CONNECT, and RESPOND
What is the impact of adult-child interactions in a preschool setting? How can these interactions set the stage for later word and print awareness?

A PROJECT-BASED APPROACH TO DEVELOPING EMERGENT LITERACY

One of the most recognized ways to engage young children in learning is through a project-based approach. This approach supports a child's disposition to analyze, question, and hypothesize (Allen, 2001). A project is an in-depth study of a content-rich topic. The time frame depends on the children's level of interest, so it can last a week, a month, or several months, and it involves activities of all types, including linguistic, scientific, musical, and mathematical activities. The project encourages children to identify what they know about a topic and helps them use literacy and word development skills as well all their senses to extend their knowledge. The ideas for projects should spring from the children's interests. A step-by-step example of a preschool project is provided next.

Autumn or The Harvest

Autumn or the Harvest is a topic about which children are always interested because it happens outdoors and involves things they can see, hear, and touch.

Step 1: The Beginning: What Children Know   A good project begins with what children know and then helps them use their everyday experiences to extend their knowledge. Teachers can begin creating a list of what children know about a topic during large-group time when children are all together and continue adding to the list informally for several days. For example, a teacher might talk with children about what they know about autumn or the harvest and then write the following list using the words of the children.

What We Know About Autumn or the Harvest

- It's getting colder.

- We need our jackets in the morning.

- The leaves are changing colors.

- The colors of the leaves in our play area are red, yellow, and orange.

- Some leaves are on the ground.

- The squirrels are very busy burying things outdoors.

- Outdoors, we see large groups of birds flying overhead.

- There are lots of apples in the supermarket.

- There are lots of pumpkins around.

- It's getting dark when we eat supper.

Step 2: What Children Would Like to Explore   The list of *What We Know* focuses thought and attention on a topic and can serve as the basis for another important activity: determining what children would like to learn about the topic. Again, teachers can create a list to capture children's responses in their own words, as in the following example.

What We Would Like to Learn About Autumn or The Harvest.

- Why is it getting colder? When will it be warm again?

- Do leaves turn pink? Why are they falling from the trees?

- What happens to the leaves after they've fallen?

- Why are apples different colors? Do they all taste the same?

- What happened to the flowers in our garden?

- Where are the birds going?

- What are the squirrels in our play area eating?

- What are the things falling from the maple and horse chestnut trees in our playground?

- Do pumpkins grow from trees?

- What are some things we can do with our pumpkin?

- What is the harvest? How is it celebrated? Does everyone celebrate the same way?

As with the *What We Know* list, the teacher can continue adding to this list for several days, and it can become the framework for the project's activities, experiences, and lesson plans. Both lists can help teachers plan activities that extend children's knowledge and answer their questions. In addition, this type of activity supports language development and emergent literacy by allowing children to practice listening and speaking skills, such as listening to enter into a dialogue, describing previous experiences and relating them to new ideas, using language to communicate ideas, and listening and responding appropriately in group interactions (New Jersey Department of Education, 2004). Some other project ideas that might develop from the "Autumn or The Harvest" study are listed in Table 4.1.

Following are two examples that show how the questions in the table can be used to develop activities that support emergent literacy skills.

1. Where are the birds going that fly in big groups? Write the poem "Fly Away, Fly Away Over the Sea" by Christina Rossetti on large chart paper with small illustrations of important words. Read the poem to students, moving the hand from left to right under each line (every time you read the poem) and calling attention to the imagery and the rhyming words at the end of each line. Then, read the poem together with the group and dramatize (act out) the poem with the children, suggesting movements to go with the words. Post the poem chart in a prominent place at the children's level. Use the poem as an introduction to learning about the migratory patterns of a few common birds. Take a "bird walk" outdoors and look for birds flying in groups and birds that seem to be sticking around for the winter. Try to identify birds with a nature guide (or a bird identification app).

This activity supports literacy in several ways through building these skills:

- Phonological awareness—listening to and identifying rhyming words

- Concepts of print—understanding that individuals read from left to right and top to bottom

- Oral language—learning that words can be used to describe things and to convey information and can be connected to real experiences

- Letters and sounds—learning that letters form words and words represent the sounds of spoken language

- Learning to connect spoken words with print

- Learning that reading is an important way to acquire information

Table 4.1. Alternate project ideas

Subject	What children know	What they would like to explore
Squirrels	Squirrels are grey.	Where do squirrels live?
	They hop.	Can we find baby squirrels?
	They're good jumpers	When they jump from tree to tree do they ever fall?
	They eat acorns.	Why are their tails so big?
Birds	Birds have feathers.	Do all birds have feathers?
	They make different sounds.	What birds live near our playground?
	They have two wings.	Can all birds fly?
	Birds fly in the air.	Where are the birds going that fly in big groups?

2. What are some things we can do with our pumpkin? Cut open a pumpkin with small groups of children. Encourage children to touch and smell and try to describe what the inside looks and smells and feels like. Record descriptive words, read them with the group, and post them next to the pumpkin when the activity is completed. Collect some seeds to roast and taste. Seeds that have dried for a few days can be planted by allowing each child to "plant" some between damp paper towels placed in individual plastic bags. Hang the bags on a clothesline to make a "hanging garden." Children can make and decorate signs for the garden using words and pictures. In addition, make a simple graph that allows children to predict whether their seed experiment will be successful by having them write their names or place marks under the words *yes* or *no*. Post the completed graph at children's level, and refer to it often as the experiment progresses.

This activity supports literacy in several ways through building these skills:

- Oral language—using language to express and communicate feelings and ideas

- Oral language—listening and responding to directions

- Oral language—increasing vocabulary and using words to engage in higher-level skills such as prediction

- Concepts of print—using print to label objects

- Learning to connect spoken words with print

- Exercising hand muscles that are important for writing

As teachers use these lists to brainstorm possible activities and experiments, the framework for a unit of study begins to emerge. It is important to note that project activities are in addition to ongoing daily routines that are in place in all areas of the classroom schedule. Children are people, and any unit of study will elicit varying degrees of interest. A good preschool classroom allows children the opportunity to choose from a wide variety of interesting, developmentally appropriate activities. As with grown-ups, one size does not fit all.

REFLECT, CONNECT, and RESPOND
John Dewey, the American educator, said: "Give the pupils something to do, not something to learn; and the doing is of such a nature as to demand thinking; learning naturally results." How does this statement apply to the development of early literacy?

ASSESSMENT OF LEARNING IN PRESCHOOL: FORMAL AND INFORMAL SYSTEMS

One of the essential elements of a high-quality early childhood program is the assessment of each child's individual growth and development. Formal and informal assessment systems help teachers and parents to understand how a child is developing as well as helping them to develop activities to address each child's strengths and limitations. (See Chapter 7 for further discussion of the role of assessment in literacy instruction.) To help a child to grow and learn, the teacher needs to determine where the child is and how to move him or her forward. The early childhood teacher must have the ability to utilize assessment methods to help measure developmental progress in each child.

The early childhood teacher has at his or her disposal many different types of formal and informal assessment strategies. Formal measures, such as checklists, standardized testing, developmental profiles, and/or language batteries, may help to pinpoint specific areas where children may need assistance and are most often used to compare a student's progress in a specific content area against specific norms. Informal assessment, often known as authentic assessment, refers to systematic observations as well as a collection of each child's work. In both cases, early delays can be documented through assessment and appropriate developmental interventions planned during the school year, including evaluation for learning disabilities, if warranted.

Formal Assessment Tools

When choosing a formal assessment tool for preschool, it is important that it meets the following qualifications: 1) it should be reliable (tested), meaning it yields consistent results, 2) it should have validity, meaning it is a meaningful measure of the skills it is intended to measure, and 3) it should be developmentally appropriate to the age group of 3- to 5-year-olds. The NAEYC and National Association of Early Childhood Specialists in State Departments of Education (NAECS/SDE; 2003) published guidelines for using formal assessments and resources for making choices of tools. Many of the tools are part of a research-based curriculum, and the assessment is a way to document the steps of progress children have made in each objective area that the curriculum offers. In other instances, the measurement is related to the social-emotional development areas. In still other instances, the tools focus on the domain of oral language and literacy skills in particular (Dickinson, McCabe, & Sprague, 2003).

A teacher may use anecdotal notes from his or her observations to assess a child's language development, making comparisons in the areas of the child's use of expressive language and his or her receptive language ability to answer questions posed or even pose a question. The child's ability to recall a story can also give the teacher information regarding the child's language development. Using a flannel board representation of the story and characters of the story will allow the teacher the opportunity to observe a child's understanding of the story as well as the child's knowledge of the concepts of a story the plot and his or her ability to sequence of the details of the story. Teachers can include index cards or blank books in centers to collect writing samples and have a space in the classroom for children to display the work being written. Audio and video recordings are another way by which teacher can assess a child's language in order to understand if it is developing "normally."

Many different types of **formal assessment** have been used in the preschool classroom. **Criterion-referenced tests** are one type. These tests compare a child's progress, as indicated by the child's score(s), to an established criterion as the child masters very specific content. With these types of tests, even in the preschool classroom there may be a cut-off score that each child must reach to show mastery of the skill. There are also **norm-referenced assessments** that can be used to compare one group of students to another group, marking progress of groups on specific tasks and comparing the groups. Norm-referenced means that, when these types of tests are developed, **norms** are set that indicate the average performance of children within a specific age group.

The most common formal assessment, used widely with older children, is the standardized test. When administering this type of test, the conditions and directions are read verbatim and the directions are always the same no matter where the test is administered. These tests are prepared by publishing houses and are norm referenced. One of the most utilized standardized tests for preschoolers is the Head Start National Reporting System, administered at the beginning and end of each school year. It measures a wide variety of skills in expressive and receptive language as well as development of letter and number recognition and identification. This test is used to indicate the overall progress of children in Head Start and not to assess the development of individual children.

Each of the norm-referenced standardized tests are measured for validity and will show results in measurement of critical areas of development. Public preschool programs as well as Head Start programs rely on research-based assessments to measure progress of both individual students and overall programs as well.

Formal assessment in the field of early childhood education, however, is an area of concern and controversy. There is a growing concern that testing in the early years may not be developmentally appropriate and therefore not truly valid or useable, particularly because preschool children may have trouble following the directions being given. Very young children may not possess the attention span needed to concentrate as long as may be necessary to complete the assessment. In addition, some argue that, as with later uses of standardized testing, there may be an element of cultural insensitivity to the experience of the child that may invalidate results. For example, a child living in an urban area may never have seen a barn, yet a photo may be included on a standardized test asking for the initial consonant sound. If a child's life or cultural experiences do not include a contextual reference to the question being asked, should the child be penalized for not having the information? A child whose primary language is one other than English may not be familiar with a specific word and may then answer incorrectly. Standardized testing does not take into account children's individual learning styles or children's varied linguistic and cultural backgrounds.

Informal Assessment Processes

In contrast to formal assessments that take place less frequently, informal assessment is part of the daily routine in early childhood settings. Teachers must be observing and analyzing the children while they are engaged in daily activities and measure the progress they may be achieving in various developmental domains through these interactions with the environment, including interactions with adults as well as peers. The anecdotal notes taken during these observations inform the teachers by helping them to develop activities that address not only the children's interests but also their abilities. The notes are collected, analyzed, and then interpreted so that the teachers can make decisions about their instruction. With informal assessment happening more frequently, instruction can be changed to meet the changing needs of each child. When children are assessed only once or twice a year, it is more difficult to know where they are and what they need. The most wide-ranging picture of the child comes from observing and recording the child's actual behaviors.

Maintaining a portfolio is an excellent way to conduct ongoing informal assessment of an individual child's progress. A portfolio system started early in the school year assists teachers in documenting this progress through the use of photos, samples of the child's writing and artwork, as well as documentation of other milestones during the classroom experience. A portfolio is a good way to help both the teacher and parent mark this progress together and in partnership.

By gathering these samples of a child's actual work, a portfolio truly illustrates what each child knows, what he or she can do, and how he or she has progressed over time.

Portfolios need to contain a few core elements, collected three or more times throughout the year for all children in the classroom, that serve as evidence to reflect very specific skills that are acquired during the preschool years. Collecting these items throughout the year provides evidence of the child's individual growth. Some examples of core elements would be samples of the child's ability to write his or her name, to draw a self-portrait, to use scissors, and to create a representational drawing, just to name a few. Other elements in the portfolio would be items specific to the individual child. For example, if an individual child demonstrates strength in science, the teacher might collect evidence of this intelligence, such as weather charts or graphs the child has used, the child's drawings of the outside environment, or documentation of the experiments in which the child has explored science topics.

It is important to understand that no single measure should be the sole resource used for evaluating a child's progress and development. Using multiple assessment tools will give the teacher the clearest, most complete picture of each child's development in all domains and of the child's disposition toward learning.

REFLECT, CONNECT, and RESPOND
What insights did you gain from this chapter regarding preschool education and its value to later development of academic skills such as reading?

CLOSING THOUGHTS: EMERGENT LITERACY IN THE PRE-KINDERGARTEN YEARS

The knowledge and application of recent brain research on early development as well as a fundamental understanding of early childhood best practices contribute to the development of language and literacy in preschool-age children. It is vital that early childhood classrooms (infant, toddler, and preschool) reflect these understandings through the physical environment as well as the intentional teaching practices of the teacher in the classroom. In addition, for teachers in later grades to be prepared to introduce the concepts of letter and sound mastery, they must understand how children's brains develop early on to be able to learn these concepts as well as optimal educational settings that can prepare children when they are ready to advance their language and literacy development.

ONLINE COMPANION MATERIALS

The following Chapter 4 resources are available at http://www.brookespublishing .com/birshcarreker/materials:

- Reflect, Connect, and Respond Questions

- Appendix 4.1: Technology Resources

- Appendix 4.2: Knowledge and Skill Assessment Answer Key

- Appendix 4.3: Formal Assessment Tools and Resources

- Appendix 4.4: Autumn or The Harvest

KNOWLEDGE AND SKILL ASSESSMENT

1. Which is *not* a component of early literacy skills?

    a. Spelling correctly

    b. Phonological awareness

    c. Storytelling

    d. Writing development

2. Which is *not* a purpose of learning centers in the early childhood classroom?

    a. Learning centers give teachers a chance to step away from the activities in the class.

    b. Learning centers give children opportunities to explore areas of their own interest.

    c. Learning centers promote small-group interaction.

    d. Learning centers lead to more complex and meaningful play and work by the children.

3. Which is an example of an open-ended question that promotes oral awareness?

    a. Point to the building.

    b. Where do you think it came from?

    c. Did you have fun building that?

    d. Where are the petals on this flower?

4. Which is a true statement about print awareness?

    a. It helps children distinguish oral and printed messages.

    b. It is not needed in early childhood because children don't read.

    c. It does not occur until after age 6.

    d. It should be delayed until first grade.

5. Which is a true statement about assessments in early childhood?

    a. They include both formal and informal tools for teachers to use.

    b. They are unreliable and do not give useful information.

    c. They keep children from succeeding.

    d. They take valuable time away from the class.

REFERENCES

Abouzeid, M. (2010). *Reading first: A guide to phonemic awareness instruction*. Retrieved from Reading First in Virginia's online forum: http://www.readingfirst.virginia.edu/prof_dev/phonemic_awareness/introduction_p.html

Adams, M.J. (1990). *Beginning to read: Thinking and learning about print*. Cambridge, MA: MIT Press.

Allen, R. (2001, Spring). The project approach to learning. *Early Childhood Learning Curriculum Update.*

Ball, E. (1993). Assessing phoneme awareness. *Language, Speech and Hearing Services in Schools, 24*(3), 130–139

Barnett, W.S. (2008). *Preschool education and its lasting effects: Research and policy implications.* Boulder, CO: Education and Public Interest Center & Education Policy Research Unit.

Barnett, W.S. (2011). Effectiveness of early educational intervention. *Science, 333,* 975–978.

Base, G. (1986). *Animalia.* New York, NY: Harry N. Abrams.

Berninger, V.W. (2009). Highlights of programmatic, interdisciplinary research on writing. *Learning Disabilities Research and Practice, 24*(2), 69–80. Retrieved from http://www.readingrockets.org/article/how-do-i-write-scaffolding-preschoolers-early-writing-skills

Callaghan, G., & Alison, M. (2012). Levelling the playing field for kindergarten entry: Research implications for preschool early literacy instruction. *Australasian Journal of Early Childhood, 37*(1), 13–23.

Chall, J.S. (1983). *Stages of reading development.* New York, NY: McGraw-Hill.

Commonwealth of Massachusetts, Department of Early Education and Care. (2015). *Classroom physical environment* (pp. 1–12). Retrieved from http://www.mass.gov/edu/docs/eec/licensing/technical-assisstance/classroom-physical-environment

Dickinson, D.K., McCabe, A., & Sprague, K. (2003). Teacher Rating of Oral Language and Literacy (TROLL): Individualizing early literacy instruction with a standards-based rating tool. *The Reading Teacher, 56*(6), 554–564.

Dickinson, D.K., & Tabors, P.O. (Eds.). (2001). *Beginning literacy with language* (pp. 223–255). Baltimore, MD: Paul H. Brookes Publishing Co.

Dodge, D.T., Berke, K., Rudick, S., Baker, H., Sparling, J., Lewis, I., & Teaching Strategies. (2015). *The Creative Curriculum for Pre-School* (6th ed.). [Kit]. Bethesda, MD: Teaching Strategies.

Ehri, L.C. (1984). How orthography alters spoken language competencies in children learning to read and spell. *Language awareness and learning to read.* New York, NY: Springer Verlag.

Ehri, L.C., Nunes, S.R., Willows, D.M., Schuster, B.V., Yaghoub-Zadeh, Z., & Shanahan, T. (2001). Phonemic awareness instruction helps children learn to read: Evidence from the National Reading Panel's meta-analysis. *Reading Research Quarterly, 36*(3), 250–287.

Hart, B., & Risley, T.R. (1999). *The social world of children learning to talk.* Baltimore, MD: Paul H. Brookes Publishing Co.

Haskell, D.W., Foorman, B.R., & Swank, P.R. (1992). Effects of three orthographic/phonological units on first-grade reading. *Remedial and Special Education, 13*(2), 40–49.

Hoff, E., & Naigles, L. (2002). How children use input to acquire a lexicon. *Child Development, 73*(2), 418–433.

Holdgreve-Resendez, R.T. (2010). *Concepts of print and genre.* Retrieved from http://legitliteracy.weebly.com/concepts-of-print.html

International Dyslexia Association, The. (2018, March). *Knowledge and practice standards for teachers of reading.* Retrieved from https://dyslexiaida.org/knowledge-and-practices/

Jenkins, R., & Bowen, L. (1994). Facilitating development of preliterate children's phonological abilities. *Topics in Language Disorders, 14*(2), 26–39.

Juel, C. (1991). Beginning reading. In R. Barr, M.L. Kamil, P.B. Mosental, & P.D. Pearson (Eds.), *Handbook of reading research.* (Vol. 2, pp. 759–788). Reading, MA: Addison Wesley Longman.

Moats, L., & Tolman, C. (2009). *Language essentials for teachers of reading and spelling: The speech sounds of English: Phonetics, phonology, and phoneme awareness* (Module 2). Boston, MA/Longmont, CO: Sopris West.

Morrow, L.M. (1990). Preparing the classroom environment to promote literacy during play. *Early Childhood Research Quarterly, 5*(4), 537–554.

National Association for the Education of Young Children (NAEYC). (1998). Learning to read and write: Developmentally appropriate practices for young children. *Young Children, 53*(4), 30–46.

National Association for the Education of Young Children (NAEYC) & National Association of Early Childhood Specialists in State Departments of Education (NAECS/SDE) (2003). *Early childhood curriculum, assessment and program evaluation: A joint position statement of the NAEYC and NAECS/SDE.* Retrieved from https://www.naeyc.org/sites/default/files/globally-shared/downloads/PDFs/resources/position-statements/pscape.pdf

National Scientific Council on the Developing Child. (2004). *Young children develop in an environment of relationships: Working paper No. 1.* Retrieved from http://www.developingchild.harvard.edu

New Jersey Department of Education. (2004, July). Language arts literacy. In *Preschool teaching & learning expectations: Standards of quality* (pp. 36–41). Retrieved from http://www.state.nj.us/education/ece/archives/code/expectations/expectations.pdf

Pallotta, J., & Bolster, R. (2016). *The construction alphabet book.* Watertown, MA: Charlesbridge.

Pool, J.L., & Carter, D.R. (2016). Creating print-rich learning centers. *Teaching Young Children, 4*(4), 18–20.

Robbins, C., & Ehri, L.C. (1994). Reading storybooks to kindergarteners help them learn new vocabulary words. *Journal of Educational Psychology, 86*(1), 4–64.

Snow, C., Burns, M.S., & Griffin, P. (Eds.). (1998). *Preventing reading difficulties in young children.* Washington, DC: National Academy Press.

Stanovich, K.E. (1986). Matthew effects in reading: Some consequences of individual differences in the acquisition of literacy. *Reading Research Quarterly, 21*(4), 360–407.

Sulzby, E., & Teale, W.H. (1985). Writing development in early childhood. *Educational Horizons, 64*(1), 8–12.

Sulzby, E., & Teale, W.H. (1991). Emergent literacy. In R. Barr, M.L. Kamil, P.B. Mosenthal, & P.D. Pearson (Eds.), *Handbook of reading research* (Vol. 2, pp. 727–757). New York, NY: Longman.

Test, J.E., Cunningham, D.D., & Lees, A.C. (2010). Talking with young children: How teachers encourage learning. *Dimensions of Early Childhood, 38*(3), 3–14.

Texas Education Agency. (2002). *Guidelines for examining phonics and word recognition programs: Texas Reading Initiative.* Retrieved from http://www.readingrockets.org/article/alphabetic-principle

Weitzman, E., & Greenberg, J. (2002). *Learning language and loving it: A guide to promoting a child's social, language, and literacy development in early childhood settings* (2nd ed.). Toronto, Canada: The Hanen Center.

Whitehurst, G.T., & Lonigan, C.J. (1998). Child development and emergent literacy. *Child Development, 69*(3), 848–872.

Yolen, J. (1987). *Owl moon.* New York, NY: Philomel Books.

Yopp, H.K., & Yopp, R.H. (2009). Phonological awareness is child's play! *Young Children. 64*(1), 12–18, 21.

Technology Resources

Elaine A. Cheesman

PROGRAMS/APPS FOR ORAL LANGUAGE

Effective programs/apps have the following features:

- They encourage language interactions among adults and children.

- They promote vocabulary development.

Beginning with Babble   http://leapempowers.org

> This is a free app for parents and teachers who work with children from birth to 5. It provides brief, useful, and research-based tips about interacting with children through age-appropriate language and play.

Comparative Adjectives   http://www.alligatorapps.com

> In this program, the user touches the picture that matches the oral word (tallest man).

PROGRAMS/APPS FOR PHONOLOGICAL AND PHONEMIC AWARENESS

Effective programs/apps have the following features:

- They do not require knowledge of letter names.

- They emphasize sounds of spoken language.

Beginning Sounds Interactive Game   http://www.lakeshorelearning.com

> In this game, the user categorizes first sounds in words using three picture prompts in an arcade-format game; it provides clear enunciation using an adult voice.

Partners in Rhyme   http://www.preschoolu.com

> This program provides practice in recognizing rhyme in spoken words using four interactive games; it has clear enunciation using an adult voice.

PROGRAMS/APPS FOR CONCEPTS OF PRINT

Effective programs/apps have the following features:

- They explicitly connect oral and written language through highlighted narrated text.

- They include highlighted narration.

- They facilitate exposure to print.

- They broaden background knowledge.

- They have simulated page turning.

Loudcrow Interactive Books   http://loudcrow.com/apps

This company has a growing list of award-winning interactive book apps of familiar children's literature, including Peanuts characters, Sandra Boynton books, and classics such as Peter Rabbit. Highlighted narration and simulated page turning promote concepts of print.

Oceanhouse Media   http://www.oceanhousemedia.com

This company adapts classic children's literature and informational texts into interactive book apps featuring highlighted narration, tap-and-learn vocabulary, and interactive games. Titles include books by Dr. Seuss and The Berenstain Bears series. Informational books created by the Smithsonian Institution include "Alphabet of Space" and "Alphabet of Dinosaurs." These alphabet books feature rhyming verses for each letter of the alphabet that provide interesting information about the topics. Problems include letters that correspond to something other than the most common sound (e.g., *E* is for earth, *I* is for ISS space station, *U* is for U.S. Moon landing, *X* is for X-15).

PROGRAMS/APPS FOR KNOWLEDGE OF LETTERS

Effective programs/apps have the following features:

- They link the shape of the letter with the name of the letter.

- They provide explicit oral instructions on letter formation.

- They include adjustable speed options.

- They have adjustable tolerance for straying off the mark.

- They match upper- and lowercase forms.

- They challenge the user to form the letter independently without tracing.

- They provide oral formation prompts.

- They provide immediate, explicit corrective feedback for poorly formed letters or incorrect starting points.

- They record user progress and errors.

- They are adjustable for left- or right-handed users.

- They link the most common and accurate sounds for printed letters.

Alphabet Dots Game: Build Letter Confidence   http://elliesgames.com

This game provides opportunities to practice alphabet sequence using lower-case letters.

DotToDot   http://www.appsinmypocket.com

This app orally pronounces names of letters and numbers in alphabetical and numerical order. The user can adjust settings for older students.

Handwriting Without Tears: Wet Dry Try   http://wetdrytry.com

This program provides instruction and practice with manuscript letters and numeral writing. It has clear verbal instructions and models of each stroke and optional settings for stroke-error tolerance and left- or right-handed users. Oral feedback is prompt and specific ("Don't go outside the line!). The program supports unlimited users with progress monitoring data and computer reports. Educators can view online reports, graphs, and data for individuals or the whole class.

Letter Case   http://elliesgames.com

This game provides practice in matching upper and lower-case letters in various fonts.

Letter Find   http://rubberchickenapps.com

This app provides opportunities to identify the target letter from among many other letters in random order.

Teachnology   http://www.teach-nology.com/worksheets/language_arts/handwriting/

This site provides free, downloadable PDFs of letter formation practice sheets featuring single letters on one sheet, with guiding arrows and lined practice area. Worksheets are available in different styles of manuscript and cursive.

PROGRAMS/APPS FOR LINKING LETTERS TO SOUNDS

Effective programs/apps have the following features:

- They connect the name, shape, and most common sound of the letter through hearing, tracing, and pronunciation (recording the user's voice).

ABC Reading Magic series   http://www.preschoolu.com

This series of apps includes both phonemic awareness activities (blends, oral words presented as photographs) and decoding (decoding letters to form words shown as photographs). The mature narration and photographs makes this app suitable for all ages. In a few two-syllable words, vowels in open syllables are pronounced with the short, not long, sound.

Reading 1: CVC words

Reading 2: CCVC, CCCVC, CVCC, CVCCC

Reading 3: Two-syllable words

Reading 4: Vowel-Consonant-Silent-e words

ABC Magic series   http://www.preschoolu.com

This site matches picture prompts to initial sounds and letters.

Alpha-read   http://alpha-read.com

This site links letters, key word pictures, and the most common sound. Spelling–sound correspondences are sequenced, not in alphabetical order but according to their utility for spelling words (e.g., *a, t, m, s*). Review mode allows the teacher or user to select letters to review.

Blending SE Student Edition and TE (Teacher Edition)
http://www.95percentgroup.com

This app helps students practice blending skills after receiving instruction from their teacher. It helps them recognize spoken words that are pronounced as blended words and sound by sound. It is an excellent and effective app for students who have difficulty blending sounds.

CVC words   http://www.alligatorapps.com

This app allows the child to practice reading and spelling phonetically regular words. It is organized by word family, or rime (*hop, pop, mop*). Children can practice reading and spelling words using 14 engaging games. The optional text-to-speech feature reads sentences.

I Can Alphabetics

This program provides systematic, explicit instruction and practice in the given letter's name, shape, and most common sound. The practice games are very repetitive and good for at-risk children.

Starfall ABCs/Starfall Learn to Read   http://www.starfall.com

Starfall provides an identical free and ad-free web site and mobile app. It has engaging animations and games for learning letter–sound correspondences. The letter name, not its sound, is used in the key word for *x* (x-ray). A better key word is *box* for /k-s/.

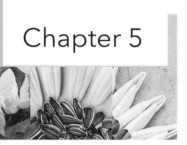

Chapter 5

Alphabet Knowledge

Letter Recognition, Letter Naming, and Letter Sequencing

Kay A. Allen and Graham F. Neuhaus

LEARNING OBJECTIVES

1. To describe how students' letter knowledge underpins their learning to read and spell

2. To list and discuss at least three principles of successful multisensory, structured teaching

3. To become familiar with structured, sequenced activities for teaching letter names and basic terminology related to reading instruction

Letters make reading possible. Letters are those abstract visual symbols that bridge the gap between oral language and written alphabetic languages. Awareness of the alphabetic principle, the idea that letters represent the sounds of spoken language, is essential for learning to read in any alphabetic language: Letters represent the sounds of spoken language (Liberman & Liberman, 1990; Perfetti & Bolger, 2004; Snow, Burns, & Griffin, 1998). When children can recognize and name the letters of the alphabet accurately and automatically, they have a foundation for learning the alphabetic principle and learning to read (Adams, 1994; Ehri, 2005).

As described in the International Dyslexia Association's (IDA; 2018) *Knowledge and Practice Standards for Teachers of Reading*, orthographic print—in which the sounds of a language are represented by written symbols—is an important underpinning to proficient reading and writing. Orthographic print begins with the recognition of letters, or graphemes. With knowledge of this aspect of language, students are able to map phonemes to graphemes and establish the understanding of the alphabetic principle.

Alphabet knowledge is a term that refers to a student's ability to identify and name the letters of the alphabet. In addition to letter names, many researchers include students' knowledge of the sounds (phonemes) associated with those letters in the definition of alphabet knowledge. Although the two skills are closely interrelated, they are separate skills, as several research studies have indicated (Lonigan & Shanahan, 2009; Schatschneider, Fletcher, Francis, Carlson, & Foorman, 2004; Snowling, Gallagher, & Frith, 2003). The instruction and activities in this chapter specifically address letter recognition and letter naming.

The first section of this chapter discusses the importance of alphabet knowledge within the reading process. The next section provides some considerations for teaching these skills, including principles of effective Structured Literacy teaching, and the final section provides the instruction, guided practice, and review that all students, especially those with dyslexia, require to fully develop accurate and automatic letter recognition and letter naming skills.

ROLE OF LETTER RECOGNITION IN THE READING PROCESS

Expert Structured Literacy instruction includes the explicit, systematic teaching of letter names and letter recognition.

Letters—The Building Blocks of Literacy

Letters are the written symbols that are cognitively processed to make reading possible (Adams, 2002).

Adams succinctly identified just how essential letter recognition is in learning to read:

> Unless and until a child can reliably recognize the letters, the memorability of printed words is limited and phonics and spelling instruction are out of reach, because unless and until a child can reliably recognize the letters, the mind cannot possibly build stable connections between them. (2002, p. 74).

Skilled readers usually are not aware of the role that letters play in the reading process. As unlikely as it may seem, "Skillful readers visually process virtually every individual letter of every word as they read, and this is true whether they are reading isolated words or meaningful, connected text" (Adams, 1990, p. 18). Although processing is not perceived on a conscious level, studies show that misprints of even familiar words (e.g., omitting the *h* in *the*) cause eye-fixation times to increase by milliseconds and thus slow down reading (Adams, 1990).

Letter recognition is one of the three parallel processes that take place simultaneously rather than sequentially when expert readers read: the reader recognizes letters in print, recodes them into auditory data (what the word sounds like), and connects them to the correct meaning of the word in light of the context (e.g., *rose* as flower or action) (Ehri, 2005). If readers have fast, accurate recognition of individual letters, then they can identify and learn familiar letter sequences. As letters become recognized faster and more accurately, frequently occurring letter patterns are recognized as whole letter sequences, or words. This multi-letter recognition is known as unitization and occurs through **repeated reading** of words (Ehri, 2005; Ehri & McCormick, 2013). This advanced phase of reading development is built on the foundation of accurate, automatic letter recognition.

Letter Names—The Stable Property

Letter names are the only property of a letter that does not change.

A letter's name is its only stable property (Cox, 1992), as the shape may change (e.g., upper- and lowercase forms, cursive and printed forms, different fonts), and the speech sounds represented by letters may change (e.g., long and **short vowel** sounds). Letter names anchor the varying properties of letters. According to Adams (1994), it is particularly important to have an unchanging, distinctive label for concepts whose expression changes. Also, letter names provide a common referent for symbols, a way for students and teachers to refer to the same symbol, which is particularly important in discussing spelling.

Some reading programs begin by teaching students to associate a letter shape with the sound it represents rather than with the letter's name. Because students will eventually need to associate symbols with sounds, some educators ask, "Why not go directly to sound–symbol association and bypass letter names?" According to Adams (1994), there are drawbacks to teaching only sound–symbol associations without teaching the names of the symbols:

- Several graphemes in English regularly represent more than one phoneme (e.g., *c* can be pronounced as /k/ as in *cat* or /s/ as in *city*).

- When trying to identify unknown words, new readers without letter-name knowledge are limited to the number of letter–sound correspondences that have been taught; however, students with more complete letter-name knowledge may be able to use it to help retrieve the sounds of the letters that they are still learning.

- Labeling an item helps consolidate information about that item in long-term memory so that its memory can be recalled quickly and accurately.

Letter Names—Catalysts for Learning Letter Sounds

Knowing letter names provides a springboard for learning and remembering letter–sound relationships—the alphabetic principle—a foundational skill for learning to read (Ehri, 2005; Foulin, 2005; National Institute of Child Health & Human Development [NICHD], 2000).

A student must learn that in an alphabetic language such as English, letters represent sounds and then learn which sound or sounds are associated with each letter and letter group (e.g., *ea, ou, tch, wh*). When students have reliable knowledge of phoneme–grapheme correspondences, they understand the alphabetic principle—the phonemes of language correspond to (or map onto) the letters that represent them. Liberman and Liberman explained that to translate spoken language to the written code, children must acquire the explicit awareness "that all words are specified by an internal phonological structure, the shortest elements of which are the phonemes that the letters of the alphabet represent" (1990, p. 60). Even beginning readers must learn that words do not differ "holistically, one from another, but only in the particulars of their internal structure" (Liberman & Liberman, 1990, p. 61) such that *time* and *tame* differ in one letter and the phoneme it represents.

A significant way in which letter-name knowledge helps students make the **sound–symbol association** is that the sounds represented by letters are often embedded within the letters' names (Ehri, 2005, Treiman, 2006). For example, the sound /m/ is found within the letter name *m*. Likewise, the names of vowels represent phonemes—the **long vowel** sounds—that are identical to their names. The spellings of young children (**invented spelling,** or transitional spelling) reflect their assimilation of this knowledge: *tm* represents *team*; *bkm* represents *became*. When writing a word the way it sounds, students begin to use sound–symbol correspondences and develop an appreciation of the sequencing of the sounds and letters in words. These are essential skills both for reading and spelling.

Some letter names are more helpful than others in providing a clue to the phonemes they represent (McBride-Chang, 1999; Treiman, Tincoff, Rodriguez, Mouzaki, & Francis, 1998). Some researchers have found that the letter names that are most helpful to children learning to read and write are those that contain the phoneme at the beginning of the letter name (i.e., *b, d, k, p, t, v*; /bē/, /dē/, /kā/, /pē/, /tē/, /vē/) (Bowman & Treiman, 2002). The next most helpful are the letter names, such as *l, m, n,* and *s,* that have the phoneme they represent at the end of their letter names (/ĕl/, /ĕm/, /ĕn/, and /ĕs/). Letter names such as *h* and *w* provide no clue to the sounds they represent. Even though teachers and parents do not usually point out these existing cues to students, a wide variety of students instinctively use letter name cues in their beginning reading and writing.

> ### REFLECT, CONNECT, and RESPOND
> What are three of the compelling reasons for teaching letter recognition and naming? Are your own experiences with developing literacy (as a teacher or as a learner) consistent with extant research findings on the importance of these skills? Why or why not?

From Individual Letters to Letter Sequences

Beginning readers who automatically recognize individual letters can begin to see familiar letter sequences as units that belong together (e.g., ea, tch, ite, ing), an essential step in automatic word recognition (Ehri & McCormick, 2013; Neuhaus, Roldan, Boulware-Gooden, & Swank, 2006).

In order to understand the importance of progressing from reading individual letters to recognizing familiar letter sequences within words, an overview of researcher Ehri's theory of reading phases may be helpful (Ehri 1983, 1995, 2005; Ehri & McCormick, 2013). Ehri's phase theory, perhaps the best known of several theories centered on graphophonemic connections, posits four phases in the process of learning to read.

In the first phase, the **pre-alphabetic** phase, a student begins to recognize words in connection with the images with which they are associated (e.g., McDonald's, Wendy's, traffic stop signs). Children are not associating sounds with the letters in the word, but there may be a salient feature, such as *oo* in *look* that students associate with two eyes (Gough, Juel, & Griffith, 1992). In Ehri's second phase, **partial alphabetic**—later referred to by others as early alphabetic—children know some sound–symbol relationships but not enough to process an entire word phonetically. Boundary letters (first and last letters of a word) are often the ones used to read a word in this phase (e.g., *moon* may be read as *men*). Ehri (2005) pointed out that older students with reading difficulties are often functioning at this level—partial knowledge of sound–symbol relationships, with many errors involving medial letters in words.

It is in the third, or **full alphabetic,** phase that the reader has full knowledge of sound–symbol relationships and can use that information to decode unknown words. For words with regular spellings, there is a one-to-one match between grapheme and phoneme—the letters *m–e–n–d* translate to the word /mĕnd/. Even for irregularly spelled words, such as *island,* Ehri (2005) illustrated that there is letter–sound correspondence for all of the letters except for the *s.* The exceptional letter may be noted in memory as silent or as an extra letter, or a spelling pronunciation may be given because some students use it to help remember (e.g., *Wed–nes–day*).

Letters help the reader form the mental bond between the pronunciation of the word, its representation, and its meaning. Ehri (2005) referred to letters as the mnemonic device that assists the reader in connecting a word with its sound and meaning. In a similar way, when trying to learn a person's name, many individuals want to see how it is spelled so that the letters help bond it in memory.

The reader in the third phase eventually begins to see familiar sequences of letters as units that belong together rather than individual letters that represent individual sounds. Examples include seeing the sequence *ink* (known as the rime) in *blink* as a unit, as well as seeing *bl* (the onset) as a unit; recognizing word parts such as prefixes, suffixes, and root words; and seeing familiar syllable patterns, such as *ite* in which the final *e* is silent and the vowel *i* represents its long sound.

In the fourth, or **consolidated alphabetic** phase, readers can instantly recognize entire words (rather than sequences of letters). Instant word recognition—gained through repeated bonding of letters, sounds, and meaning—frees the reader to attend to comprehending the text (Perfetti, Landis, & Oakhill, 2005), the ultimate goal in reading.

Ehri refers to the reading in this phase as sight word reading, but that term should not be confused with a common definition of sight words as those that do not follow usual sound–symbol correspondences. Rather, in Ehri's phase theory, sight word reading applies to all words that the reader recognizes instantly as units because of repeated exposures forming bonds between the letter sequences, their auditory equivalent, and meaning.

Even though Ehri's phase theory ends with instant reading of words from memory as units, Ehri wrote, "The process of accessing them in memory is still phonological in that graphophonemic connections are rapidly activated to retrieve pronunciations and meanings in memory" (2005, pp. 182–183). That is, the letters still have a role to play in reading. Ehri and Wilce explained that even sight word reading involves recognizing each individual letter within a word because ultimately letters are the "distinctive cues that make one word different from all the others" (1983, p. 13). For example, the *t* and *d* are the only two letters that differentiate the words *time* and *dime*.

REFLECT, CONNECT, and RESPOND
What role do letters play in the reading process, according to Ehri's phases of reading theory?

Letter-Name Knowledge Predicts Reading Achievement

Research shows and has consistently shown for decades that letter-name knowledge is one of the most powerful predictors of learning to read and of later reading achievement (Caravolas, Hulme, & Snowling, 2001; Leppanen, Aunola, Niemi, & Nurmi, 2008; Schatschneider et al., 2004).

Letter-name knowledge in preschool and kindergarten is one of the strongest predictors of reading in first grade, and Scarborough (1998) found that a letter naming test (a student names the letters of the alphabet when shown the written letters) "appears to be nearly as successful at predicting future reading as is giving a more comprehensive readiness battery" (cited in Foulin, 2005, pp. 130–131). Alphabet letter knowledge in preschool and kindergarten strongly predicts later decoding, comprehension, and spelling skills, even when IQ score and socioeconomic status are controlled, as found in the meta-analysis of literacy research done by the National Literacy Panel (Lonigan & Shanahan, 2009).

Preschool and kindergarten letter naming predicts word recognition because of the underlying similarity of the two skills. Reading both letters and words requires the ability to encode, store, and retrieve lexical labels for abstract symbols. Although letter naming has often been assumed to be a pre-reading skill

(Badian, 1995), it has been recognized as a simple form of reading (Neuhaus & Swank, 2002).

Accurate letter recognition forms the basis for developing decoding skills. On the contrary, Berninger and colleagues wrote that imperfect knowledge of single letters and **letter clusters** has been shown to "compromise early reading development for at-risk beginning readers in general, not just the slow responders, especially in application of the alphabetic principle to unfamiliar words" (2002, p. 63). Moreover, inaccurate or inconsistent letter recognition prevents the developing reader from unitizing letters into whole words that he or she can recognize within one second (Ehri & Wilce, 1983). Students who struggle with gaining alphabet knowledge tend to be the students later diagnosed as having reading disabilities (Gallagher, Frith, & Snowling, 2000; O'Malley, Francis, Foorman, Fletcher, & Swank, 2002). In addition, children with a family history of dyslexia often have lower or more slowly developing alphabet knowledge than their peers (Snowling et al., 2003).

Letter-name knowledge before first grade has been found to predict reading comprehension, reading vocabulary, and spelling achievement in sixth grade (Badian, 1995). Accurate letter-name knowledge is foundational for developing decoding skills and leads to recognizing words instantly, which in turn frees up the reader's attention to focus on comprehending the text, developing new vocabulary, and understanding more complex syntax. Stanovich (1986) named this sequence (and its opposite) the **Matthew effect** (i.e., the rich get richer and the poor get poorer). The student in the lower reading group reads fewer words during reading group time and is therefore exposed to many fewer words in text than the student with on-target decoding skills, finds reading difficult and avoids it, does not develop automaticity in word recognition, and must use mental resources for word recognition rather than developing vocabulary, understanding the syntax, and comprehending the text. Its opposite, the successful reading sequence, begins with accurate alphabet knowledge.

The importance of alphabet knowledge is acknowledged by national education initiatives, including Head Start, whose 2015 guidelines stated that by 5 years of age, a child in the program should be able to name 18 upper- and 15 lowercase letters and know the sounds associated with several letters (Head Start Program Performance Standards, 2015). The Common Core Standards for Kindergarten (Council of Chief State School Officers [CCSSO] & National Governors Association Center for Best Practices [NGA Center], 2010) included the goals of recognizing and naming all upper- and lowercase letters of the alphabet, being able to produce the primary sound or many of the most frequent sounds for each consonant, and being able to associate the long and short sounds with the common spellings for the five major vowels.

Letter Recognition and Naming—The Need for Automaticity

Research supports not only that letter naming must be accurate, but it must also be fast. (Neuhaus & Swank, 2002).

Rapid letter naming is the basis for accurate word reading (Neuhaus, Carlson, Jeng, Post, & Swank, 2001; Neuhaus, Foorman, Francis, & Carlson, 2001; Neuhaus & Swank, 2002; Wolf, 1997; Wolf, Bowers, & Biddle, 2000; Wolf & Obregón, 1997). Wolf and Obregón noted succinctly, "The need to develop automatic letter and word recognition skills is critical" (1997, p. 200). Automatic single-letter recognition is essential if students are to benefit from further reading instruction (Berninger et al., 2002; Vellutino, Scanlon, & Jaccard, 2003).

Letter-naming speed has been identified as the single largest predictor of word-reading ability for first-grade students (Neuhaus & Swank, 2002). The goal of all letter identification is to be able to recognize each letter automatically. Letters, letter clusters, and words are recognized automatically when they are processed accurately, rapidly, and unconsciously. Automaticity is thought to be achieved when 1) letter identification is very quick; 2) letter identification is effortless; and 3) it occurs without willful initiation, and it cannot be willfully stopped. To better understand automatic letter recognition, complete this 30-second exercise. Cover this page with your hand, and then move your hand to expose a few words. Now, do *not* read the words. Can you stop the reading process, or do you unconsciously or automatically read and understand the words you see? For clarity, automaticity is reached when reading occurs without any conscious awareness that any effort is expended to accomplish the task. It is literally easier to recognize and read a letter or word than it is *not* to read it.

The importance of automatic letter reading cannot be overstated. Fast and accurate letter reading is not the end goal, however; rather, it is the stepping-off point to automatic word reading that frees cognitive attention to focus on higher level skills, fluency, and reading comprehension (Schwanenflugel, Hamilton, Kuhn, Wisenbaker, & Stahl, 2004).

Letter Recognition and Naming—The Need for Differentiated Instruction

"Provide instruction that is aligned with current emphases on assessment-driven decision making… and differentiated instruction" (Piasta, 2014, p. 203).

Although the goal of fast, automatic letter recognition sounds easy, it may be one of the most difficult tasks for the reading educator to teach, and likewise, one of the most formidable goals for beginning students to master. There are two important factors influencing automatic letter recognition: 1) Students process information at different rates, and 2) letter automaticity assumes that all 26 letters must become equally automatic, but not all letters are equally familiar to every student. We will address automaticity first.

For readers to become successful, recognizing each of the 26 letters must become automatic. There are clearly no unimportant letters. Students are more familiar with some letters than others. Beginning readers often are familiar with the letters in their names, even if the letters are used infrequently in other words. The goal for the instructor is to identify which letters each child is familiar with and which letters require greater familiarization and more practice for the child. All letters must be read automatically because when an unfamiliar letter appears in a word, it stops the reader from identifying the word readily, and it disrupts the attention needed to comprehend the text. As a consequence, all letters must become automatically recognized before fluent reading and reading comprehension can be achieved.

The time and practice needed to reach automatic letter reading varies dramatically among students. Berninger (2000) found that students identified with dyslexia needed more than 20 times the practice than students without dyslexia to learn letter sequences. For example, good readers may learn to rapidly spell a word with 20 repetitions; however, poor readers may be challenged to reach automaticity with 400 repetitions, or 20 times the amount of practice the good readers require. In addition, Neuhaus, Carlson, and colleagues (2001) found that even second-, third-, and fourth-grade students still have significant variation in their letter-naming speed, meaning that letter knowledge for many students is not fully automatic by first grade, and secure letter knowledge requires more extensive exposure and practice for some students. Therefore, allowing each student sufficient time and practice to solidify knowledge of letter names, shapes, and sounds is time-consuming and challenging but imperative.

Furthermore, letter-naming speed is influenced by a number of learned skills and cognitive abilities: specifically, phonological awareness, orthographic recognition, general naming speed, and visual attention skills. These are the same skills and abilities needed to read words, demonstrating that letter reading, such as word reading, requires multiple sources of knowledge and exact coordination of cognitive systems.

REFLECT, CONNECT, and RESPOND
Why is letter knowledge in preschool and kindergarten one of the strongest predictors of later reading ability?

Letter Recognition and Naming—Reversals

"Contrary to popular belief, impaired readers do not see letters and words in reverse, nor do they suffer from inherent spatial confusion or other visual anomalies of the types proposed in the early literature" (Vellutino, Fletcher, Snowling, & Scanlon, 2004, p. 31).

Research shows that letter reversals may be more a function of the orientation of written letters rather than a characteristic of the students who make them. More of the alphabet letters face right, as in the letters *b, c, f, h, p,* and *r,* in contrast to left-facing letters such as *j, d,* and *z.* Treiman, Gordon, Boada, Peterson, and Pennington (2014) hypothesized that when students cannot remember which way a letter faces, they choose to orient the letter to the right, as most letters face, using statistical learning—use of common patterns. Treiman and colleagues worked with a group of 132 students, ages 5–6, 92 of whom had a history of speech sound disorder (SSD) and 20 of the 92 having been diagnosed as language impaired. The study found that 1) the students made a significantly greater number of reversal errors on left-facing letters, and 2) letter reversals were not statistically significant in regard to the students' reading ability tested 2 ¾ years later. The number of letter errors (e.g., letter formation) was significant, but the number of reversal errors was not.

Letter reversals in reading and writing (*b* and *d*), rotations (*p, d, b*), and sequencing errors (*was* for *saw* or *flet* for *felt*) have historically been thought to be symptoms of dyslexia by experts in the field (Collette, 1979; Hermann, 1959; Orton, 1937) as well as the general public. Reading deficits were thought to be a result of visual deficits such as visual perception, visual discrimination, and visual memory, but research since the 1970s has demonstrated the linguistic basis of reading as well as the difficulties associated with it.

Students, even students with dyslexia, do not visually perceive letters and words differently. Rather, research indicates that poor readers often have degraded reading performance on tasks that require associating linguistic labels with letters (Vellutino, Smith, Steger, & Kaman, 1975), such as associating a letter's name with the letter (the name *b* with the symbol *b*), mapping sounds onto symbols (the letter *b* represents the phoneme /b/), and bonding a letter group with the sound it represents (*igh* = /ī/). When a student misidentifies *b* as *d* or *p*, the student has most likely not made a reliable association between the letter name or sound and the shape or spatial orientation of the letter (Vellutino, 1979). For many students, it is only through extensive practice that secure associations are formed between the visual form and its verbal label.

> ### REFLECT, CONNECT, and RESPOND
> What accounts for the misidentification of letters such as *b* and *d* by students with dyslexia?

CONSIDERATIONS FOR INSTRUCTION

Students come to school with varying degrees of preexisting letter knowledge. Although many students come to school with literally years of exposure to letters, others do not. In addition, students have individual differences in their ability to create and store visual as well as verbal memories. Simply stated, there are innate and environmental differences that influence students' letter knowledge, including 1) visual memory ability, 2) verbal memory ability, 3) the ability to connect visual to verbal memories, 4) general letter familiarity, and 5) exposure to specific letters, such as those in their names.

When entering kindergarten, children ideally have the opportunity to develop or consolidate letter identification with uppercase letters before lowercase letters are formally introduced because they contain fewer confusing letter shapes and are more graphically distinct. Much confusion among kindergarten and first-grade students can be avoided if letter names are secure.

Writing plays an influential role in the beginning reader's ability to recognize letters. Letter writing practice focuses students' attention on the particular features of letters' shapes and thus reinforces letter recognition.

Although the letter learning process is the same for all students, Foorman and Torgesen (2001) and Berninger and colleagues (2002) found that some students will become literate only when the instruction is more intense, more explicit, more comprehensive, and more supportive. In other words, the same effective pedagogy for all students is required, but for some students, more practice or repetitions; greater clarification of concepts; and additional reteaching of letters, letter names, and sounds is necessary to reach the same level of proficiency that others reach with less intensity, practice, reteaching, and support (Berninger, 2000).

Implementing response to intervention (RTI) should prevent many students from reaching upper grades without adequate letter knowledge, but a child without secure letter knowledge may somehow slip through and reach third or fourth grade without well-developed letter knowledge. This means that most students in the class have already been instructed in both upper- and lowercase letters and perhaps in both print and cursive handwriting. Use of the multisensory, structured alphabet letter activities that follow can remediate even students well beyond the optimal age of letter learning.

In Structured Literacy lesson plans developed especially for students struggling with reading, students learn to recognize uppercase block letters accurately and speedily during the Alphabet segment of a lesson. They are introduced to lowercase printed letters through the "linking procedure" presented in Chapter 9. The letter names and sounds they represent are reviewed using a Reading Deck. During the Alphabet segment of the lesson, students progress from working with the uppercase alphabet letter strips and 3-D letters to the lowercase letter strips and 3-D letters.

PRINCIPLES OF EFFECTIVE INSTRUCTION

Teachers should keep in mind several general principles of effective instruction for developing students' alphabet knowledge: the importance of multisensory teaching and sequential presentation; the need for early identification of difficulties and early intervention; the effectiveness of **guided discovery teaching** and brief segments of instruction; and the need to teach skills to automaticity and teach proofreading. These principles are discussed next.

1. Multisensory teaching. The purpose of multisensory teaching is to provide instruction that simultaneously engages and encodes the information in different forms. This provides an opportunity for knowledge to be retained in multiple domain-specific memory stores, especially those associated with visual, verbal, kinesthetic, and tactile experiences. Multisensory instruction is consistent with connectionist theory that suggests that reading ability is optimized when both phonological and orthographic representations are simultaneously engaged and interactive (Harm & Seidenberg, 2004; Plaut, McClelland, Seidenberg, & Patterson, 1996). More important, multisensory reading instruction has been found to be significantly more effective than traditional instruction for teaching phonological awareness, decoding skills, and reading comprehension (Carreker et al., 2005; Carreker et al., 2007; Foorman, Francis, Shaywitz, Shaywitz, & Fletcher, 1997; Joshi, Dahlgren, & Boulware-Gooden, 2002).

This instruction may be more effective because it allows the storage of information in multiple sensory-specific memory systems (Gardner, 1985) and allows students with limitations in one storage system to gain access to information from other memory modules (Hallahan & Kauffman, 1976). It appears that children's visual attention is focused by their manual tasks (Thorpe & Borden, 1985), so physical manipulation of stimuli such as letter forms increases the likelihood that the letter shapes are remembered.

Students with reading difficulty often have trouble storing and retrieving lexical labels (including letter names) and need the opportunity to learn and practice, especially through simultaneously engaging at least two or three learning modalities: visual, auditory, and tactile/kinesthetic (involving muscle memory). For example, students can say the names of letters as they see and touch 3-D plastic letters and arrange them in alphabetical order. Simply put, using multisensory instruction seems to help build visual, verbal, and tactile/kinesthetic memories associated with letters.

2. Sequential presentation. Information must be presented in a sequence that builds logically on previously taught material.

3. Early identification and intervention. Any reading dysfunction, including slow or inaccurate letter recognition, should be identified as early as possible so that children's reading-related difficulties can be remediated before they experience years of frustration and school failure. Vellutino and colleagues (1996, 2003) suggested that the majority of students who are ultimately identified with reading difficulties have instructional deprivation rather than basic cognitive deficits. Therefore, deficient achievement levels of letter recognition or any skill known to predict later difficulty with word reading and reading comprehension must be identified and remediated early in a child's academic career.

4. Guided discovery teaching. The **Socratic method** leads learners to discover information through carefully guided questioning based on information they already possess. For example, rather than stating that all words must contain at least one vowel sound that opens the mouth, the teacher can invite students to create a word composed of only consonants, such as /k/ – /t/ for the word *cat*, or /d/ – /g/ for *dog*. This method builds interest and aids memory. Also, when the teacher reviews by starting a sentence and then pauses for students to complete it, students are encouraged to participate rather than being placed on the defensive by a direct question (e.g., "The initial letter of the alphabet is _____," rather than, "What is the initial letter of the alphabet?").

5. *Brief instructional segments.* Frequent and brief instructional segments are more effective than less frequent segments lasting longer periods of time. Extensive guided practice is required for letter-reading automaticity, and more intense practice will be needed when a student does not easily make memories of letters and connect them to names and sounds.

6. *Teaching to automaticity.* After presenting the letters through guided discovery, the teacher models and provides ample practice activities, reviews the material on a regular basis, and assesses whether students can accurately name the letters previously taught. The rate at which students will reach letter automaticity will vary according to their ability to store, coordinate, and reconstruct the visual and verbal memories associated with each letter. The teacher should ensure success for all students by reviewing the procedure or concept before asking students to apply it. For example, a quick warm-up of touching and naming the letters on an alphabet strip is strongly encouraged before students work on sequencing or alphabetizing. This review sets up the student for success, an underlying tenet of all informed instruction.

7. *Teaching proofreading.* The teacher guides students through the process of proofreading by which they discover and correct their own errors instead of relying on an outside source (teacher or computer). For example, after students place the plastic letters in alphabetical order, they check their accuracy by touching and naming the letters. Although proofreading seems old-fashioned, its greatest benefit, the do over, is current. Inform students that making mistakes is a large part of reading and writing, but when they catch their own mistakes, they get a do over, even if the mistake is just incorrectly reading or writing a single letter.

> ### REFLECT, CONNECT, and RESPOND
> What is your opinion of Vellutino's finding that the source of dysfunctional reading is more often experiential or instructional deprivation rather than an innate learning disability?

ACTIVITIES FOR TEACHING LETTER RECOGNITION

The following activities and recommended materials are based on the work and writings of Cox (1992); Gillingham and Stillman (1960); Hogan and Smith (1987); Neuhaus Education Center (2006); and the Luke Waites Center for Dyslexia and Learning Disorders of the Scottish Rite Hospital in Dallas, Texas.

Materials for Instruction

The following materials are needed to implement the activities:

- A small, round mirror for each student, approximately 2" in diameter, with plastic encasing the edges.

- Classroom uppercase alphabet strip, a minimum of 3" × 48", with block letters, without pictures or graphics, which can be visually distracting to students, mounted at students' eye level

- Set of 3-D plastic uppercase block letters for each student and for the teacher

- Individual uppercase alphabet strip for each student, made of laminated strip of cardstock, approximately 2" × 17", with block letters

- Class set of instant letter recognition charts, seven with uppercase letters and seven with lowercase letters (see Figure 5.1); each chart has five rows of six letters

- For each student, 8 sets of 10 word cards, approximately 1" × 2", with words printed in lowercase, to be used for alphabetization by 1) first letter; 2) second letter; 3) first and second letters; 4) third letters; 5) second and third letters; 6) fourth letter; 7) third and fourth letters; and 8) first, second, third, and fourth letters. The card sets should be identical across the class. Use different colors of cards for the eight sets of cards. Word sets can be stored in small plastic sandwich bags. These card sets are described in further detail in the section on alphabetizing activities.

- For the teacher, 8 sets of word cards, approximately 5" × 7", with words printed in lowercase. The words used in the teacher's sets should not be identical to

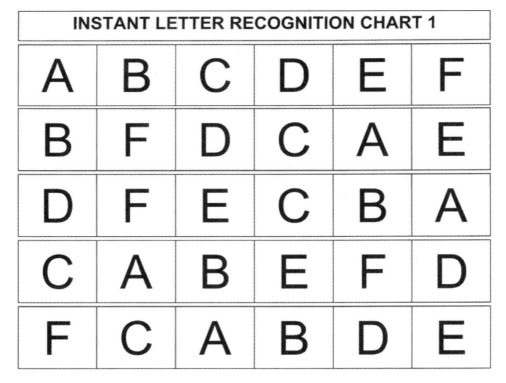

Figure 5.1. Instant letter recognition chart. (From Carreker, S. [2002]. *Reading readiness*. Bellaire, TX: Neuhaus Education Center; reprinted by permission.)

those in the students' sets. The teacher's cards are larger than the students' cards so that all students can see them.

- Container for each student in which to store the individual alphabet strip(s), plastic letters, and word cards to be alphabetized

For younger students:

- Alphabet matching mat made of poster board or heavy laminated paper, approximately 24" × 18", with the outlines of uppercase block letter shapes arranged alphabetically in an arc (see Figure 5.2). Students can practice matching by placing plastic letters on the mat.

For students who do not need to start with a matching activity:

- Alphabet sequencing mat made of poster board or heavy laminated paper, approximately 24" × 18", with uppercase block letters in alphabetical order printed across the top and the letters *A, M, N,* and *Z* forming an arc (or rainbow) beneath. *M* and *N* are printed at the top of the arc, *A* and *Z* are in the initial and final positions, and space is left for the missing letters to be placed within the arc (see Figure 5.3).

For students who have learned uppercase letters:

- Individual lowercase alphabet strip for each student, made of a 2" × 17" strip of laminated cardstock

- Classroom lowercase alphabet strip, minimum of 3" × 48", with block letters, without pictures or graphics, mounted at students' eye level

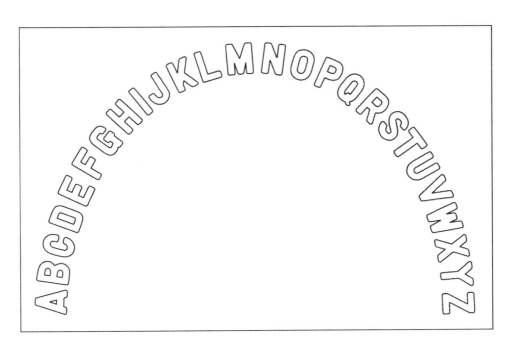

Figure 5.2. Alphabet matching mat. (From *Multisensory Teaching of Basic Language Skills, Third Edition* [p. 156].)

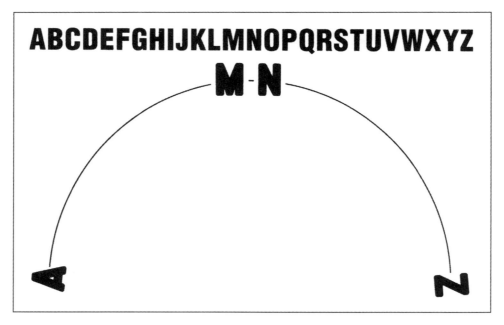

Figure 5.3. Alphabet sequencing mat. (From *Multisensory Teaching of Basic Language Skills, Third Edition* [p. 157].)

Activities for Developing Letter Identification, Naming, and Sequencing Skills

The schedule and activities described in this section can be used to build letter identification, rapid naming, and sequencing skills.

Schedule　Allot 5 minutes within a 50- to 60-minute lesson for letter identification, rapid naming, and sequencing activities. Continue using uppercase letters in these activities until students can rapidly and accurately identify all uppercase letters in sequence and at random.

Lowercase letters (and letter clusters) should be taught individually through a multisensory letter-introduction procedure often referred to as *linking* in which the letter's name, shape, and sound(s) it represents are concurrently linked in memory. Lowercase letter names should be reviewed daily by using a reading deck. (See Chapter 11, on teaching handwriting, for more information about linking and about using a reading deck.)

Students may need to reinforce speed and accuracy of lowercase letter recognition through the same activities and materials discussed for uppercase letters. Use the lowercase instant letter recognition charts to increase students' speed of letter naming even after accuracy has been established.

The activities that follow can be rotated within a weekly lesson plan. Students should touch and name letters on an alphabet strip as a warm-up before each activity. The strip remains in place during the activity as a reference.

Matching and Naming　The following materials are needed for this activity:

- 3-D uppercase letter sets
- Alphabet matching mats (see Figure 5.2)

Students who cannot match 3-D uppercase letters with the outlines of uppercase letters printed on paper should begin with this activity. First, the teacher has students turn the 3-D plastic letters right side up and facing the correct direction inside the arc on the alphabet matching mat. The teacher tells students that these are the letters found in the words we read and write. He or she points out the alphabet on the classroom alphabet strip and leads students to discover that an alphabet contains these same letters in a fixed order. The teacher then asks students to name each letter before they place the plastic letter on top of the printed form on their individual alphabet matching mats. If all of the letters are not matched within 5 minutes, then the activity is repeated the next day, starting with the letters matched the day before and continuing with additional letters until students can place all of the letters on the mat. The teacher also has students check their work each time by touching and naming the letters they have just placed (e.g., students say "A" and touch the plastic letter sitting on top of the printed letter). The teacher leads students to discover the number of letters in the alphabet by pointing to each letter and counting. The teacher leads students in completing the sentence, "The number of letters in the alphabet is [26]."

Students progress from 1) placing the plastic letters on top of the printed forms on the mat for matching, to 2) placing the letters beneath the printed letters on an alphabet strip, to 3) placing the letters in an arc on the mat for sequencing (see Figure 5.3). When students can accurately place plastic letters beneath the letters on an alphabet strip, they are ready for the following activity.

Naming, Sequencing, and Discovery of Middle   The following materials are needed for this activity:

- Classroom uppercase alphabet strip

- Individual uppercase alphabet strips

Students who do not need to start with a matching activity will start here. To begin, the teacher leads students to discover the number of letters in the alphabet (see description in Matching and Naming).

The teacher asks students to name each letter as he or she points to it in sequential order on the classroom uppercase alphabet strip. The teacher asks students to touch and name each letter on their individual uppercase alphabet strips as he or she leads them in naming the letters together.

The teacher asks students to discover the middle of the alphabet by putting one index finger on the first letter of the alphabet and one index finger on the last letter and moving in toward the middle. Students discover that the exact middle is between the letters M and N. The teacher leads students in completing the sentence, "The two middle letters of the alphabet are [M and N]."

After students can accurately perform this touching and naming activity, any daily alphabet activity should begin with a warm-up in which students touch and name the letters of the alphabet on their strips. This warm-up activity provides the repetition that many students require to develop automaticity.

Discovery of Vowel and Consonant Sounds   The following materials are needed for this activity:

- Mirror for each student

Before students learn that there are two kinds of letters in the alphabet (conso-nants and vowels), the teacher introduces the concept of two kinds of sounds. The teacher leads students to discover that we use only two kinds of sounds when we talk: the sounds we form when the mouth is open (vowels) and the sounds we form when the mouth is closed or partially closed (consonants). The teacher illus-trates that when we say words, we open and close our mouths. First the students try to talk by putting together only closed-mouth sounds, such as /m/, /l/, or /p/. Then, students try to talk using only open-mouth sounds, such as /ă/, /ĕ/, or /ŭ/. The teacher explains that to form words, we must both open and close our mouths. The teacher illustrates by slowly saying a word, such as *map*, and letting the students see the mouth closing for the consonant, opening for the vowel, and closing for the consonant.

Following this demonstration, the teacher asks students to look into a mir-ror as they say /ă/, /ĕ/, /ĭ/, /ŏ/, and /ŭ/ and leads them to discover that their mouths are open when they say these sounds. The shape of the mouth changes, but noth-ing blocks the air that comes out of the mouth to form these sounds. The teacher explains that vowel sounds open our mouths. Next, the teacher directs students to look in a mirror to see what happens when they say the sound /s/. The teacher explains that their teeth and tongue partially close their mouths. Then, the teacher has the students say /l/ and notice that the tongue partially closes their mouths. Students then say /m/ and notice that their lips close their mouths. These are con-sonant sounds. The teacher says that consonant sounds close or partially close our mouths. The teeth, tongue, and/or lips block the air used in making these sounds. The teacher leads the students in saying, "Vowel sounds open our mouths, and consonant sounds close or partially close our mouths with our teeth, tongue, or lips." The teacher and students use gestures for open (hands open like a crocodile mouth) and closed (palms together) and point to their teeth, tongue, and lips.

To reinforce the distinction, the teacher provides practice for the students in differentiating between consonant and vowel sounds by having students look into their mirror, repeat sounds, and discover whether their mouth is open or closed (or partially closed) when they say the sound. The teacher starts with consonant sounds for which the mouth is obviously closed or partially closed, such as /s/, /l/, /m/, or /n/, interspersed with both long and short vowel sounds. After students are aware of the difference between consonant and vowel sounds, they are ready to discover that the letters that represent these sounds are classified as consonant letters and vowel letters.

Discovery of Vowel and Consonant Letters   The following materials are needed for this activity:

- Individual uppercase alphabet strips (for reference)

- Mirrors

The teacher begins by telling the students that they are going to discover the two kinds of letters in the alphabet. The teacher explains that just as there are two kinds of sounds (vowels and consonants) in spoken words, there are two kinds of letters in the alphabet. The teacher and students review together, "Vowel sounds open our mouths, and consonant sounds close or partially close our mouths." The names of the letters give clues as to which letters will be called vowels and which will be called consonants. To illustrate this idea, the teacher directs the students to look in a mirror to see what happens to their mouths when they say the names of the letters *a, e, i, o,* and *u*. Their mouths stay open when they say these letter names. The teacher tells students that these letters represent vowel sounds.

Next, students use their mirror to discover that when they say the name of the letter *s*, the mouth is partially closed by the teeth and tongue. When they say the name of the letter *l*, the mouth is partially closed, with the tongue closing against the roof of the mouth. When they say the name of the letter *m*, the lips close the mouth.

After students are aware that the alphabet is made up of vowel and consonant letters that represent vowel and consonant sounds, the teacher can vary the daily warm-up activity of touching and naming the letters by having students whisper or cheer for the vowel letters.

Discovery of Initial, Medial, and Final   The following materials are needed for this activity:

- Classroom uppercase alphabet strip

- Individual uppercase alphabet strips

The alphabet can be used to teach students terminology that will be used in other aspects of written language training. For example, in phonemic awareness training, students will be asked whether they hear a specific sound in the initial, medial, or final position in a word. Students can understand the meaning of the abstract spatial terms *initial, medial,* and *final* by learning them in relation to the alphabet strip. The terms *initial, medial,* and *final* can be introduced by teaching the initial, medial, and final letters of the alphabet.

To begin introducing these terms, the teacher writes the initials of his or her name on the board and leads students to discover that these letters are the first letters of his or her name. The teacher writes several students' initials on the board and helps students discover that initials are the first letters of names. The teacher explains that *initial* means first and that the alphabet also has an initial letter, *A*. The teacher points to the *A* on the classroom alphabet strip, asks students to touch the letter *A* on their alphabet strips, and leads them in saying, "*A* is the [initial] letter of the alphabet."

Next, the teacher touches *Z* on the classroom alphabet strip and asks students to touch *Z* on their strips. The teacher tells students that the last letter of the alphabet is *Z* and that another way of saying *last* is *final*. The teacher leads students in saying, "*Z* is the [final] letter of the alphabet." Then the teacher tells students that all of the letters between *A* and *Z* are medial letters and that there is a difference between *medial* and *middle*. The teacher explains that the exact *middle* of the alphabet is found between the letters *M* and *N*; however, *medial* means anything between initial or final. Therefore, a medial letter is any letter occurring between *A* and *Z*. The teacher asks students to name some of the medial alphabet letters (any letter that is not *A* or *Z*) and identify initial, medial, and final letters within other words written on the board, such as their own names or the teacher's name.

Throughout the activity, the teacher provides kinesthetic reinforcement for this information through gestures. The teacher stands with his or her back to the students, facing the classroom alphabet strip, and raises both arms, fingers pointing above his or her head. The teacher drops his or her left arm horizontally to the left (parallel to the floor) while saying, "Initial means *first*." The teacher drops his or her right arm horizontally to the right while saying, "Final means *last*." The teacher brings both arms back above his or her head and says, "Medial means anything between initial (dropping left arm to horizontal) and final (dropping right arm to horizontal)."

Sequencing With 3-D Letters   The following materials are needed for this activity:

- Individual uppercase alphabet strips (for reference)

- 3-D uppercase letter sets

- Alphabet sequencing mats (most older students will place the letters on their desks rather than using mats)

First, the teacher writes *A, M, N,* and *Z* in an arc on the board, with *M* and *N* at the top of the arc. The teacher directs students to name and place the initial letter of the alphabet on their alphabet sequencing mats (or desks). They name and place *A* and say, "*A* is the initial letter of the alphabet." Then, students name and place *Z* and say, "*Z* is the final letter of the alphabet." Then, students name and place *M* and *N* and say, "*M* and *N* are the two middle letters of the alphabet." Next, the teacher directs students, "Name it, find it, place it," as they fill in the arc with missing letters in alphabetical order. Students say a letter, find it, and place it in the arc, repeating this process until the alphabet is complete. Students then proofread their work by touching and naming each letter from *A* to *Z*, using the index finger of their writing hand.

Soon after beginning this activity, the teacher begins timing the students and charting results. The initial goal is accurate naming and placement of all letters in less than 5 minutes, with an ultimate goal of 2 minutes or less. The reason that students place letters in an arc is that often there is not enough space on a desk or a tabletop to place all of the letters in a straight line.

Note for Working With Younger Students   Some young students may have difficulty crossing the mid-line (moving the right hand and arm into the space to the left of the mid-line of their body or vice versa for left-handed students). These students will want to place the first half of the alphabet letters with their left hand and the second half with their right hand rather than place all of the letters with their writing hand. This is a function of motor skill development; the teacher will encourage them to work toward the time when they can place all of the letters with their writing hand.

Note for Working With Older Students   Older students may enjoy a variation of this activity. For sequencing, have students use plastic poker chips labeled with block capital letters. Older students particularly enjoy the challenge of being timed and having their progress charted.

Other variations include the following:

- Students proofread by returning letters to the storage container in sequence and naming each letter, rather than just touching and naming letters to check.

- After students are able to place the plastic letters in alphabetical order, students may place *A, M, N,* and *Z* as usual and then randomly select letters and place them one by one in the approximate place in the semicircle.

Discovery of Before and After   The following materials are needed for this activity:

• Classroom uppercase alphabet strip

• Individual uppercase alphabet strips

Students often have difficulty with abstract spatial terms such as *before* and *after* and may be confused by directions such as, "Look at the consonant after the vowel" or "Listen for the sound before the /k/ sound." To make the abstract terms *before* and *after* more concrete, the teacher directs students to place both hands below their alphabet strips and then models for students with the classroom alphabet strip. First, the teacher asks students to raise the hand that is closer to *A* and tells them that this is their *before* hand. Then, the teacher asks students to raise the hand closer to *Z,* which is their *after* hand. Next, the teacher names a letter, such as *E,* and places both index fingers under that letter on the classroom alphabet strip. The teacher moves the index finger of the *after* hand to the letter after *E* and says, "*F* is after *E.*" Students then echo and place their index finger under the chosen letter (*E*) on their individual alphabet strips. With the index finger of their *after* hand, students touch and name the letter that comes after the named letter. Students say, "*F* is after *E.*" The teacher then names several other letters, and students respond appropriately.

The concept *after* is taught first because it reflects the left-to-right progression of the alphabet. The concept *after* should be practiced in several sessions until it is mastered. Then, the teacher has students work with the concept *before.* The teacher names a letter, such as *T,* and asks students to tell which letter is before it. Students place both index fingers under *T,* point to *S* with the index finger of their *before* hand, and say, "*S* is before *T.*" Finally, the teacher provides practice with both *before* and *after:* "Find *W.* Tell me what is before and after *W.*"

Instant Letter Recognition Charts   The following materials are needed for this activity:

• Class set of seven uppercase instant letter recognition charts and seven with lowercase letters (see Figure 5.1)

Each chart is a grid of five rows of six letters. Chart 1 has *A, B, C, D, E,* and *F* in the first row. In Rows 2–5, those letters are randomly distributed with six letters in each row. To begin this activity, the teacher displays Chart 1 to the class and names the six letters in the first row. The teacher points to each letter in the first row as students name the letters. Students then name the letters as the teacher points to them in Rows 2–5. Later, students are timed, and the number of letters read in 1 minute is charted and compared with later timed readings. Students progress from Charts 1–7 with all uppercase letters to Charts 8–14 with all lowercase letters. This exercise provides vital practice in developing accuracy and speed in letter naming.

Missing Letter Decks   The following materials are needed for this activity:

• Individual uppercase alphabet strips (for reference)

• Missing letter decks (teacher-made uppercase decks and commercially available lowercase deck)

In advance of the activity, the teacher will need to make missing letter decks. To make a missing letter deck with uppercase block letters, the teacher prints the alphabet on cards, with two letters and a blank on each card. In the first deck or set, the third letter is missing and is represented by a blank line (AB_, BC_). In the second set, the alphabet is printed in groups of three letters with the middle letter missing (A_C, B_D, C_E). In the third set, the first letter is missing (_DE). In the fourth set, the first and third letters are missing. (_B_, _C_, _D_).

After students can place all 26 3-D letters of the alphabet in correct sequence within 3 minutes, the teacher introduces the uppercase missing letter deck. (Only after students have been introduced to all lowercase letters should the commercially available missing letter deck with lowercase block letters be used.) While engaged in this activity, students keep their alphabet strips in front of them to refer to if needed. The teacher makes sure the missing letter deck is in alphabetical order and holds up the first card in the first set of cards. Students then name the two letters on each card and the missing letter: AB_[C], BC_[D], and so forth. When students can rapidly and accurately name all three letters on each card with the cards in alphabetical sequence (after many practice sessions), the teacher shuffles the cards and presents them in random order. The students then progress to the second, third, and fourth teacher-made sets of the missing letter decks. As with the first set, these are practiced first in sequence, then shuffled. Students should be fluent at each level before progressing to the next level. Note that students do not need to master all four levels before the teacher introduces the additional activities that follow. The teacher intersperses the missing letter deck activity within a weekly lesson plan with more advanced activities for developing alphabetizing and dictionary skills.

Accent and Rhythm   The following materials are needed for this activity:

• Mirrors

Many students have difficulty hearing the rhythm or the accented syllable in a word. This difficulty has consequences for developing reading and spelling skills. The following activity provides practice in hearing accented syllables while also reinforcing alphabetic sequence. The teacher begins by saying the names of several students, overemphasizing the accented syllable in their names (*Ja – mal′, Sta′ – cy, Ta – ke′ – sha, Ja′ – son, Jo – sé′*). The teacher asks students whether they hear a difference in the way one part of the name is said. The teacher then models "robot talk" in which there is no **accent.** In this way, the students discover that we say some parts of spoken words louder than other parts. Next, the teacher explains that when we accent one part of a word, the mouth opens wider, the voice is louder, and the tone is higher. The teacher reinforces each part of the definition with gestures: Mouth opens wider (hands open like a crocodile mouth), voice is louder (cupped hand behind ear), and tone is higher (flattened hand, palm to floor, is raised above head to designate higher).

Some students can learn to "see" accented syllables by using a mirror to notice when their mouths open wider. For students who find perceiving accent particularly difficult, the teacher models laying both hands along the jaw line so that students can feel the jaw opening wider on the accented syllable. Students may be better able to discern the change in pitch that occurs with accent if they place their hands over their ears and hum a word rather than say it.

Next, the teacher recites the letters of the alphabet in pairs and accents the first letter of each pair: "*A′ B, C′ D, E′ F, G′ H,*" and so forth. The teacher asks students whether the first or the second letter is being accented. The teacher encourages students to use a mirror to see their mouths opening wider and to cup their jaws in their hands to feel their mouth opening wider. Using block letters and accenting the first letter in each pair, the teacher writes the first eight letters of the alphabet on the board in pairs: *A B, C D, E F, G H*. Stressing the first letter in each pair, the teacher reads the list. With their alphabet strips in view, students say the alphabet and accent the first letter in each pair. Variations include having students clap on the accented letter. After students are able to accent the first letter of each pair (after many practice sessions), the teacher writes on the board and leads students in accenting the second letter: *"A B′, C D′, E F′, G H′,"* and so forth. Students eventually practice accenting the first of a group of three letters (*"A′ BC, D′ EF"*), then the second letter (*"A B′ C, D E′ F"*), and finally, the third letter (*"AB C′, DE F′"*). Students will need to apply their knowledge of accenting patterns when reading unfamiliar longer words. In English, multisyllabic words are accented more often on the first syllable (e.g., *bas′ – ket*), and second most often on the second syllable (*pa – rade′, con – ven′ –tion*).

Naming of Lowercase Letters The following materials are needed for this activity:

- Individual lowercase alphabet strips

Chapter 9 describes introducing lowercase letters through multisensory letter introduction. If students need additional practice in naming the lowercase letters accurately and rapidly, then many of the previous activities for uppercase letters may be used. The daily warm-up of touching and naming letters can be done with an alphabet strip of lowercase letters, as can activities such as the instant letter recognition charts, missing letter decks, accent and rhythm, and the game Don't Say *Z*.

Games to Reinforce Letter Identification, Naming, and Sequencing Skills

The activities described in this section can be used to build letter identification, rapid naming, and sequencing skills.

Alphabet Battle The following materials are needed for this activity:

- Individual alphabet strip and 3-D letter set for each pair of students

   Begin by having students form pairs. Both players simultaneously draw a letter from the set of 3-D letters without looking at the letters. Each player places his or her letter on the desk and says the name of the letter. The player whose letter is closer in alphabetical order to *Z* wins both letters. The student must say, for example, *"U* is after *G."* The winner is the player with the most letters at the end of the game.

   Variation: The player whose letter is closer to *A* wins the letters (e.g., *"J* is before *T"*).

Alphabet Bingo The following materials are needed for this activity:

- Individual alphabet strip (for reference) and 3-D letter set for each student
- 3-D letter set for the teacher

To begin the activity, each student selects any seven letters from his or her container of letters and places them on the desk in a vertical column on the *before* (left-hand) side. The other letters are put away. The teacher then selects one letter from another container, shows it to the students, and names it. Students repeat the name. If they have the letter on their desk, then they move it to the *after* (right-hand) side of the desk to form a second vertical column. The first person to move all seven letters to the *after* side of the desk is the winner. Finally, the teacher checks for accuracy by having the winner name the seven letters.

Alphabet Dominoes   The following materials are needed for this activity:

- Individual alphabet strip (for reference) and 3-D letter set for each pair of students

Before engaging in this activity, students should be proficient in *before* and *after* activities. To begin, have students form pairs. Each pair of students places the letters *M* and *N* on the desk. Next, each student draws five letters without looking. The remaining letters become the "bone yard" and are placed inside the storage container on top of the desk.

The teacher then designates which student in each pair goes first. That student tries to play a letter immediately before *M* or after *N*. The student must have *L* or *O* to play initially. If not, then he or she draws a letter from the bone yard without looking. The letters are to be played in alphabetical order to the right of *N* and in reverse alphabetical order to the left of *M*. For example, if the letters *JKLMNOPQ* have been placed, then the next player may play *I* or *R*. If a player draws a letter from the bone yard that can be played, then he or she must wait until the next turn to play it. Each player plays only one letter at a time. As each student places a letter, he or she says, "[Letter] is before (or after) [letter]." The winner is the first student to play all of his or her letters (even if there are letters remaining in the bone yard).

Guess What?   The following materials are needed for this activity:

- 3-D letter set for each pair of students

Have students form pairs. To begin, one student closes his or her eyes and draws a letter from a container. The student then tries to identify the letter by its shape. If successful, the student keeps the letter and his or her opponent takes a turn. If unsuccessful, the student returns the letter to the container and his or her opponent takes a turn. Play continues until all 26 letters have been named or time runs out. The student with the most letters at the end of play is the winner.

Don't Say Z   The following materials are needed for this activity:

- Individual alphabet strip for each pair of students

Have students form pairs. In each pair, the two players alternate saying letters of the alphabet in sequence. Each player may choose to say two or three letters in one turn. For example, if Player 1 says *"AB"* and Player 2 says *"CDE,"* then Player 1 can say *"FG"* or *"FGH,"* and so forth. The object is to avoid saying *Z*.

Variation: The game can be changed to "Catch the *Z*" in which the object is to be the player who does say *Z*. An additional challenge is added when an object such as a stuffed animal is tossed between teacher and student while saying two or three letter sequences. This kinesthetic reinforcement of alphabet sequence also provides a way to wake up a tired or distracted student about to begin a one-to-one remedial session.

Twenty Questions   For this activity, no materials are needed apart from a writing surface and writing utensil. To begin, the teacher prints the alphabet on the board (or on a sheet of paper, if working with one or two students). The teacher then says, "I am thinking of a letter. I want you to try to guess the letter. You can ask me questions about the letter. I can only answer 'yes' or 'no.' See if you can guess the letter in fewer than 20 questions." Students begin to ask questions about the letter. The teacher encourages students to ask questions that eliminate several letters at a time. Questions such as "Is it a vowel?" or "Is it made of only straight lines?" will eliminate several letters at a time. The teacher helps students to rephrase questions that require more than an answer of "yes" or "no."

As students eliminate letters, the teacher crosses the letters off the alphabet. The teacher records the number of questions required for students to guess the letter. The teacher can chart the number of questions. Students can compare the number of questions they ask each time the game is played.

Super Sleuth   The following materials are needed for this activity:

- One individual alphabet strip (for reference) and 3-D letter set for each pair of students

- Pencil and paper

First, the students work together in pairs to arrange the 3-D letters in an arc. Then, the first student closes his or her eyes while the second student removes one letter and closes the gap in the arc. The first student must discover the missing letter by sight or by looking at the arc. After the missing letter has been identified, it is replaced in the arc and the other student gets the chance to identify a missing letter. Students may keep track of correct guesses to determine the winner. The game continues until time runs out.

REFLECT, CONNECT, and RESPOND

Review the suggested teacher-led activities for teaching accurate and efficient letter recognition. Choose one activity you could implement with a student or group of students with whom you currently work. Explain why you chose this activity based on the student or students' current level of alphabet knowledge. If possible, implement the activity with students and reflect on what went well and what you might do differently next time.

Activities for Developing Alphabetizing Skills

The alphabet provides a systematic approach to organizing, classifying, and codifying information in myriad fields, such as science, law, engineering, the social sciences, business, education, communication, and entertainment. The order of the alphabet provides the order of words for every kind of information in libraries, books, newspapers, and on the Internet. The following schedule and activities can be used to develop alphabetizing skills.

Schedule   Students are ready to learn to alphabetize words when they show competence with letter recognition, naming, and sequencing. They should be able to place the 3-D plastic letters in an arc within 2 minutes, be fluent with at least the first set of the uppercase missing letter deck, and be accurate with random naming of upper- and lowercase letters. Have students begin by alphabetizing word cards rather than lists of words. Mistakes can be easily corrected by rearranging a card rather than erasing a word in a list. As they develop alphabetizing skills, students move from alphabetizing word cards, to alphabetizing lists of words, and then to locating words in the dictionary and other reference materials. The missing letter decks activity should be interspersed among the following activities within the weekly schedule to provide review for letter sequencing.

Have students touch and name letters on an alphabet strip as a warm-up before any sequencing-related activity. The strip remains in place as a reference.

Alphabetizing Word Cards by the First Letter   The following materials are needed for this activity:

- Pocket chart

- For the teacher, a set of 10 cards, each of which has a word beginning with a different lowercase letter

- For each student, a set of 10 cards, each of which has a word beginning with a different lowercase letter

- Individual alphabet strips (for warm-up activity and reference)

To begin the activity, the teacher places 10 cards in a vertical column on the *before* side of the pocket chart (or desk, if working with one or two students), ensuring that the words are not in alphabetical order. (Note that in keeping with the principle of having one focus, the words on these cards are for alphabetizing, not for reading.) The teacher then asks students whether the first letter of each word is the same as or different from the first letters of the other words. Students respond that they are different. Next, the teacher asks the students which letter will guide them in putting these words into alphabetical order. The teacher explains that the letter used for alphabetizing is called the **guide letter.** The answer to the question is always an ordinal number (e.g., "The first letter is the guide letter").

Next, the teacher points to the first letter of each word as the students recite the alphabet. For example, as students say, "*A*," the teacher points to the first letter of each word. If the students see a word beginning with the letter *A* as they are saying, "*A*," then they say, "Stop!" The teacher then forms a second column by placing the word card at the top of the pocket chart on the right side. To continue, the teacher points to the first word in the first column as the students say "*B*" and look at the first letter of each of the remaining words. The students continue reciting the alphabet and saying, "Stop!" as the cards are aligned in alphabetical order. The students should finish saying the alphabet even after all of the cards are placed. Students proofread by saying the alphabet again, as the teacher touches the first letter of each card when the students say that letter. The teacher taps the space to the left of the words when students say letters not found at the beginning of one of the words.

To continue the activity, students should have sets of word cards that are the same as each other for ease in checking. Students line up their set of word cards vertically on the *before* side of their desks. The teacher then asks students which letter is their guide letter. The students reply, "The first letter is my guide letter."

The students recite the alphabet while pointing to the first letter of each word. If students find a word beginning with *A*, then they place it in a vertical column on the *after* side of the desk. They follow the same procedures for saying the entire alphabet and then proofread.

Have several different sets of word cards to be alphabetized by the first letter so that the students work with different sets over a period of time. When students can perform this activity easily and efficiently, they are ready to progress to the next level—alphabetizing word cards by the second letter.

Alphabetizing Word Cards by the Second Letter   The following materials are needed for this activity:

- Pocket chart

- For the teacher, a set of 10 cards with words that begin with the same first letter followed by a different letter, such as *set, sun, street, six, sled, sand, scout, show, sip,* and *snake*

- For each student, a set of 10 smaller cards with words that begin with the same first letter but are followed by different second letters

- Individual alphabet strips (for warm-up activity and reference)

To begin, the teacher places 10 cards in a vertical column on the *before* side of the pocket chart, ensuring that the words are not in alphabetical order. The teacher asks students whether the first letter of each word is the same as or different from the first letters of the other words. Students respond that they are the same. The teacher asks if the second letters are the same. The students respond that the second letters are different. Next, the teacher asks the students which letter will guide them in putting these words into alphabetical order. The students respond that the second letter will guide them.

The teacher points to the second letter of each of the words as students follow the procedures detailed in the previous activity for reciting the alphabet, forming a new column on the *after* side, and proofreading. Students follow the same procedures as they practice with their word cards in columns on their desks.

Alphabetizing Word Cards by the First and Second Letters   The following materials are needed for this activity:

- Pocket chart

- For the teacher, a set of 10 cards with words, some of which have the same first letter and some of which have a different first letter

- For each student, a set of 10 cards with words, some of which have the same first letter and some of which have a different first letter

- Individual alphabet strips (for warm-up activity and reference)

To begin, the teacher places 10 cards in a vertical column on the *before* side of the pocket chart, ensuring that the words are not in alphabetical order. The teacher asks students whether the first letter of each word is the same as or different from the first letters of the other words. The students discover that some of the first letters are the same and some are different. Students respond to "What is your guide letter?" by saying, "For most of the words, the first letter is the guide letter; for some, the second letter is the guide letter." Next students recite the alphabet, saying "Stop!" when they see a word beginning with the letter they are saying. For example, in a list of words that contains *tent* and *trunk,* when students say "*T,*" they say, "Stop!" The teacher moves both *tent* and *trunk* to the column on the right and aligns them side by side, with a space beneath the two words. Students continue reciting the alphabet through *Z* as the teacher places the words in order in the column to the right. Students then come back to the two words beginning with *T* and say, "*Te* comes before *tr.*" The teacher places *trunk* in the empty space below *tent.* Students recite the alphabet again to proofread their work as usual. After saying, "*T,*" students say, "*Te* comes before *tr, U, V, W, X, Y, Z.*" Students follow the same procedures as they practice with their word cards on their desks.

After students are proficient at this level, the teacher introduces and students practice the following skills: alphabetizing by the third letter; by the second and third letters; by the fourth letter; by third and fourth letters; and finally, by first, second, third, and fourth letters. In typical classrooms, students can apply this procedure by alphabetizing their spelling or vocabulary words written on index cards. After students can efficiently alphabetize a group of word cards with mixed guide letters, students are ready to alphabetize word lists.

Alphabetizing Words in Lists by the First Letter   The following materials are needed for this activity:

- Individual alphabet strips (for warm-up activity and reference)

To begin, the teacher writes a list of words on the board to be alphabetized by the first letter. Students discover that the initial letter is their guide letter, and the teacher underlines each initial letter. Students then recite the alphabet as the teacher points to the initial letter of each word. Students say, "Stop!" when they say a letter that matches the letter to which the teacher is pointing. The teacher numbers the words to the left of the word list to indicate alphabetical order. The teacher then gives students a list of words on paper to be alphabetized by first letter, and students follow the same procedure in numbering the words. As always, students check their work by reciting the alphabet again.

Alphabetizing a List of Words by the First and Second Letters   The following materials are needed for this activity:

- Individual alphabet strips (for warm-up activity and reference)

To begin, the teacher writes a list of words on the board to be alphabetized by first and second letters. Some words have the same first letters, and some do not. Next, the teacher draws a column of lines to the right of the list labeled *Letter* and a second column of lines labeled *Number.* An example follows.

Word	Letter	Number
track	_____	_____
den	_____	_____
tag	_____	_____
cube	_____	_____
bland	_____	_____

vote   _____   _____

same   _____   _____

gloss   _____   _____

camp   _____   _____

again   _____   _____

The students discover that the first and sometimes second letters are their guide letters. The teacher then asks the students to name the initial letter of each word and writes the letter on the *Letter* line. If a letter is a duplicate, then the students name and the teacher writes the second letter of the word beside the initial letter. An example follows:

Word	Letter	Number
track	_tr_	_____
den	_d_	_____
tag	_ta_	_____

Students then recite the alphabet as the teacher points to the letters in the *Letter* column. The teacher numbers the words when the students say the guide letter(s). When the second letter is the guide letter, as with *track* and *tag,* students say, "*Ta* comes before *tr.*" *Tag* is given the next number and *track* the next.

Next, the teacher gives students a list of words on paper with *Letter* and *Number* columns to the right of the list. Students follow the same procedures for numbering their list of words and checking their work. Students may then progress to the following skills: alphabetizing word lists by the third letter; by the second and third letters; by the fourth letter; by the third and fourth letters; and by the first, second, third, and fourth letters. Students will eventually number mixed word lists without the *Letter* column.

REFLECT, CONNECT, and RESPOND

What are four of the principles of effective letter recognition and naming instruction? How might you apply these principles in your own teaching?

CLOSING THOUGHTS: BUILDING ALPHABET KNOWLEDGE

Complete letter knowledge is essential for reading success. Knowledge of letters' shapes, names, and the phonemes they represent provides students with a solid foundation for using the alphabetic principle in learning to read. Moreover, this foundation needs to be strongly formed early in a child's academic career because word knowledge is built on letter knowledge. Inaccurate, incomplete, or inconsistent letter knowledge jeopardizes a student's ability to unitize letter sequences that can be automatically recognized by sight.

The ability to learn letter knowledge is dependent on multiple factors. First, some children have an advantage because they come to school with knowledge of letters' shapes, names, and sounds. Still other children begin school without any real letter knowledge and are already at an academic disadvantage when they begin formal schooling (Vellutino et al., 2003; Vellutino et al., 1996). Moreover, students learn about letters at inherently different rates. Regardless of each child's innate ability or preschool learning history, every child must know the shapes, names, and sounds of all the letters to be a good reader.

This presents a challenge to teachers because they must provide adequate letter learning experiences for each child regardless of his or her prior letter knowledge or inherent ability to remember letters. As a consequence, instruction must be individualized to meet the specific needs of every child in the class. Although some children may need only 10–20 exposures to a letter to recognize it automatically, other children may need 20 times that amount of exposure to overlearn the letters to the point of automaticity.

The National Reading Panel's meta-analysis (NICHD, 2000) stressed that letter knowledge enhances the effectiveness of both phonemic awareness and systematic phonics instruction for reading and spelling. In other words, students benefit more from instruction when the sound structure of words is linked to letters. Multisensory instruction directly and concretely links sounds and letter names to letter shapes to build a solid foundation of letter knowledge in the beginning reader. This type of instruction introduces letter knowledge and reinforces that knowledge by providing concrete mnemonic strategies and varied exercises designed to provide opportunities for letter mastery. Multisensory instruction is also paced so that prior knowledge is well established before new knowledge is introduced.

Beginning readers must also learn to sequentially process the letters they see in words, as well as the phonemes the letters represent. Repeated exposure to letters in the alphabet and practice in sequencing the alphabet provide reinforcement of sequential processing of letters.

In review, good word-reading ability starts with well-established letter reading. Letter reading may seem simple, but learning the alphabet is challenging for many young readers. Vellutino and colleagues (1996, 2003) have found that dysfunctional readers more often have experiential or instructional deprivation rather than an innate learning disability. Intensive, systematic, and cumulative instruction has been validated as instruction that enhances children's ability to develop well-established letter knowledge. Over time, teaching practice has shown that multisensory, structured, sequential instruction provides the strong foundation of letter knowledge that is required to support good word reading.

ONLINE COMPANION MATERIALS

The following Chapter 5 resources are available at http://www.brookespublishing.com/birshcarreker/materials:

- Reflect, Connect, and Respond Questions

- Appendix 5.1: Technology Resources

- Appendix 5.2: Knowledge and Skill Assessment Answer Key

- Appendix 5.3: Additional Resources

- Appendix 5.4: Activities for Developing Dictionary Skills

KNOWLEDGE AND SKILL ASSESSMENT

1. Letter-name knowledge in beginning grades is one of the most reliable predictors of what in middle and high school?

    a. Reading achievement

    b. Comprehension

    c. Spelling ability

    d. Decoding ability

    e. All of the above

2. Students learn letter names at different rates. Which of the following is true?

    a. Students who are significantly slower in learning letter names may later be diagnosed as having a reading disability.

    b. Most beginning students who have significant difficulty with letter names catch up in reading by fourth grade.

    c. Students with dyslexia may require as much as 20 times more repetition and practice in order to acquire letter-name knowledge.

    d. Both b and c

    e. Both a and c

3. What is a major source of reading difficulty for students with dyslexia?

    a. Difficulty with visual memory

    b. Difficulty associating a letter's name with the sound it represents.

    c. Visual perception—seeing letters backward

    d. Difficulty with motor skills

    e. All of the above

4. Guided discovery learning involves which of the following?

    a. Leading students to discover the information through Socratic questioning

    b. The student becoming the teacher for other students

    c. Using motor skills to develop learning

    d. Using multisensory learning

    e. None of the above

5. Alphabet activities can be used to teach which of the following skills?

    a. Recognizing and producing an accented syllable in a word

    b. Knowing the difference between vowel and consonant sounds (phonemes)

    c.   Alphabetizing words

    d.   All of the above

    e.   None of the above

6.   Unitization in Ehri's stages of reading theory refers to what?

    a.   Categorizing concepts for increased comprehension

    b.   Seeing individual letters as distinct units

    c.   Seeing familiar letter sequences as belonging together

    d.   Dividing the 26 letters of the alphabet into designated groups

    e.   Knowing if a word follows regular patterns for decoding

REFERENCES

Adams, M.J. (1990). *Beginning to read: Thinking and learning about print [A summary]*. (Prepared by S.A. Stahl, J. Osborn, & F. Lehr). Cambridge, MA: The MIT Press.

Adams, M.J. (1994). *Beginning to read: Thinking and learning about print*. Cambridge, MA: The MIT Press.

Adams, M.J. (2002). Alphabetic anxiety and explicit, systematic phonics instruction: A cognitive science perspective. In S.B.N. Neuman & D.K. Dickinson (Eds.), *Handbook of early literacy research, 1*, 66–80. New York, NY: Guilford.

Badian, N.A. (1995). Predicting reading ability over the long term: The changing roles of letter naming, phonological awareness and orthographic processing. *Annals of Dyslexia, 45*, 79–96.

Berninger, V.B. (2000, Nov.). *Language based reading and writing intervention: Findings of the University of Washington Multi-Disciplinary Disability Center*. Paper presented at the meeting of the International Dyslexia Association, Washington, DC.

Berninger, V.B., Abbott, R.D., Vermeulen, K., Ogier, S., Brooksher, L., Zook, D., & Lemos, L. (2002). The comparison of faster and slower responders to early intervention in reading: Differentiating features of their language profiles. *Learning Disability Quarterly, 25*(1), 59–76.

Bowman, M., & Treiman, R. (2002). Relating print and speech: The effects of letter names and word position on reading and spelling performance. *Journal of Experimental Child Psychology, 82*, 305–340.

Caravolas, M., Hulme, C., & Snowling, M.J. (2001). The foundations of spelling ability: Evidence from a 3-year longitudinal study. *Journal of Memory and Language, 45*(4), 751–774. doi:10.1006/jmla.2000.2785

Carreker, S. (2002). *Reading readiness*. Bellaire, TX: Neuhaus Education Center.

Carreker, S.H., Neuhaus, G.F., Swank, P.R., Johnson, P., Monfils, M.J., & Montemayor, M.L., (2007). Teachers with linguistically informed knowledge of reading subskills are associated with a Matthew effect in reading comprehension for monolingual and bilingual students. *Reading Psychology, 28*, 187–212.

Carreker, S.H., Swank, P.R., Tillman-Dowdy, L., Neuhaus, G.F., Monfils, M.J., Montemayor, M.L., & Johnson, P. (2005). Language enrichment teacher preparation and practice predicts third grade reading comprehension. *Reading Psychology, 26*, 401–432.

Collette, M.A. (1979). Dyslexia and classic pathognomic signs. *Perceptual and Motor Skills, 48*(3 Suppl), 1055–1062. doi:10.2466/pms.1979.48.3c.1055

Council of Chief State School Officers (CCSSO) & National Governors Association Center for Best Practices (NGA Center). (2010). *Common Core State Standards for English language arts and literacy in history/social studies, science and technical subjects*. Retrieved from http://www.corestandards.org/the-standards

Cox, A.R. (1992). *Foundations for literacy: Structures and techniques for multisensory teaching of basic written English language skills*. Cambridge, MA: Educators Publishing Service.

Ehri, L.C. (1983). A critique of five studies related to letter-name knowledge and learning to read. In L.M. Gentile, M.L. Kamil, & J.S. Blanchard (Eds.), *Reading research revisited* (pp. 143–153). Columbus, OH: Charles E. Merrill.

Ehri, L.C. (1995). Phases of development in learning to read words by sight. *Journal of Research in Reading, 18*(2), 116–125. doi:10.1111/j.1467-9817.1995.tb00077.x

Ehri. L.C. (2005). Learning to read words: Theory, findings, and issues. *Scientific Studies of Reading, 9*(2), 167–188.

Ehri, L.C., & McCormick, S. (2013). Phases of word learning: Implications for instruction with delayed and disabled readers. *Theoretical Models and Processes of Reading,* 339–361. doi:10.1598/0710.12

Ehri, L.C., & Wilce, L.S. (1983). Development of word identification speed in skilled and less skilled beginning readers. *Journal of Educational Psychology, 75,* 3–18.

Foorman, B.R., Francis, D.J., Shaywitz, S.E., Shaywitz, B.A., & Fletcher, J.M. (1997). The case for early reading intervention. In B. Blachman (Ed.), *Foundations of reading acquisition and dyslexia* (pp. 243–264). Mahwah, NJ: Lawrence Erlbaum Associates.

Foorman, B.R., & Torgesen, J. (2001). Critical elements of classroom and small-group instruction promote reading success in all children. *Learning Disabilities Research and Practice, 16*(4), 203–212.

Foulin, J.N. (2005). Why is letter-name knowledge such a good predictor of learning to read? *Reading and Writing, 18*(2), 129–155. doi:10.1007/s11145-004-5892-2

Gallagher, A., Frith, U., & Snowling, M.J. (2000). Precursors of literacy delay among children at genetic risk of dyslexia. *Journal of Child Psychology and Psychiatry, and Allied Disciplines, 41*(2), 203–213. doi:10.1017/S0021963099005284

Gardner, H. (1985). *Frames of mind: The theory of multiple intelligences.* New York, NY: Basic Books.

Gillingham, A., & Stillman, B.W. (1960). *Remedial training for children with specific disability in reading, spelling, and penmanship* (6th ed.). Cambridge, MA: Educators Publishing Service.

Gough, P.B., Juel, C., & Griffith, P.L. (1992). *Reading, spelling, and the orthographic cipher.* Hillsdale, NJ: Lawrence Erlbaum Associates.

Hallahan, D.P., & Kauffman, J.M. (1976). *Introduction to learning disabilities: A psychobehavioral approach.* Upper Saddle River, NJ: Prentice Hall.

Harm, M.W., & Seidenberg, M.S. (2004). Computing the meanings of words in reading: Cooperative division of labor between visual and phonological processes. *Psychological Review, 111*(3), 662–720.

Head Start Program Performance Standards. (2015). *Early learning outcomes framework: Ages birth to five.* Washington, DC: U.S. Department of Health and Human Services. Retrieved from https://eclkc.ohs.acf.hhs.gov/policy

Hermann, K. (1959). *Reading disability: A medical study of word-blindness and related handicaps.* Copenhagen, Denmark: Munksgaard.

Hogan, E.A., & Smith, M.T. (1987). *Alphabet and dictionary skills guide.* Forney, TX: MTS Publications.

International Dyslexia Association, The. (2018, March). *Knowledge and practice standards for teachers of reading.* Retrieved from https://dyslexiaida.org/knowledge-and-practices/

Joshi, R.M., Dahlgren, M., & Boulware-Gooden, R. (2002). Teaching reading in an inner city school through a multisensory teaching approach. *Annals of Dyslexia, 52,* 229–242.

Leppanen, U., Aunola, K., Niemi, P., & Nurmi, J.-E. (2008). Letter knowledge predicts grade 4 reading fluency and reading comprehension. *Learning and Instruction, 18,* 548–564.

Liberman, I.Y., & Liberman, A.M. (1990). Whole language vs. code emphasis: Underlying assumptions and their implications for reading instruction. *Annals of Dyslexia, 40*(1), 51–76. doi:10.1007/bf02648140

Lonigan, C.J., & Shanahan, T. (2009). Developing early literacy: Report of the National Early Literacy Panel. Executive summary. A scientific synthesis of early literacy development and implications for intervention. National Institute for Literacy. Retrieved from http://www.nifl.gov

McBride-Chang, C. (1999). The abc's of the abc's: The development of letter-name and letter-sound knowledge. *Merrill-Palmer Quarterly, 45*(2), 285–308.

National Institute of Child Health & Human Development (NICHD). (2000). *Report of the National Reading Panel: Teaching children to read: An evidence-based assessment of the scientific research literature on reading and its implications for reading instruction: Reports of the subgroups* (NIH Publication No. 00-4754). Washington, DC: U.S. Government Printing Office.

Neuhaus Education Center. (2006). *Basic language skills: Book 1.* Bellaire, TX: Suzanne Carreker.

Neuhaus, G.F., Carlson, C., Jeng, M.W., Post, Y., & Swank, P.R. (2001). The reliability and validity of rapid automatized naming (RAN) scoring software for the determination of pause and articulation component durations. *Educational and Psychological Measurement, 61*(3), 490–504.

Neuhaus, G.F., Foorman, B.R., Francis, D.J., & Carlson, C. (2001). Measures of information processing in rapid automatized naming (RAN) and their relation to reading. *Journal of Experimental Child Psychology, 78*(4), 359–373.

Neuhaus, G.F., Roldan, L.W., Bouware-Gooden, R., & Swank, P.R. (2006). Parsimonious reading models: Identifying teachable subskills. *Reading Psychology, 27*, 37–58.

Neuhaus, G.F., & Swank, P.R. (2002). Understanding the relations between RAN letters subtest components and word reading in first grade students. *Journal of Learning Disabilities, 35*(2), 158–174.

O'Malley, K.J., Francis, D.J., Foorman, B.R., Fletcher, J.M., & Swank, P.R. (2002). Growth in precursor and reading-related skills: Do low-achieving and IQ-discrepant readers develop differently? *Learning Disabilities Research & Practice, 17*(1), 19–34.

Orton S.T. (1937). *Reading, writing, and speech problems in children.* New York, NY: Norton.

Perfetti, C.A., & Bolger, D.J. (2004). The brain might read that way. *Scientific Studies of Reading, 8*(3), 293–304. doi:10.1207/s1532799xssr0803_7

Perfetti, C.A., Landis, N., & Oakhill, J. (2005). The acquisition of reading comprehension skill. In M.J. Snowling & C.H. Hulme (Eds.), *The science of reading: A handbook* (pp. 227–247). Oxford, United Kingdom: Blackwell Publishing. Retrieved from http://www.blackwellreference.com/public/book

Piasta, S.B. (2014). Moving to assessment-guided differentiated instruction to support young children's alphabet knowledge. *The Reading Teacher, 68*(3), 202–211. doi:10.1002/trtr.1316

Plaut, D.C., McClelland, J.L., Seidenberg, M., & Patterson, K.E. (1996). Understanding normal and impaired word reading: Computational principles in quasi-regular domains. *Psychological Review, 103*, 56–115.

Scarborough, H.S. (1998). Early identification of children at risk for reading disabilities: Phonological awareness and some other promising predictors. In B.K. Shapiro, P.J. Accardo, & A.J. Capute (Eds.), *Specific reading disability: A view of the spectrum* (75–119). Timonium, MD: York Press.

Schatschneider, C., Fletcher, J.M., Francis, D.J., Carlson, C.D., & Foorman, B.R. (2004). Kindergarten prediction of reading skills: A longitudinal comparative analysis. *Journal of Educational Psychology, 96*(2), 265–282. doi:10.1037/0022-0663.96.2.265

Schwanenflugel, P.J., Hamilton, A.M., Kuhn, M.R., Wisenbaker, J.M., & Stahl, S.A. (2004). Becoming a fluent reader: Reading skill and prosodic features in the oral reading of young readers. *Journal of Educational Psychology, 96*(1), 119.

Snow, C.E., Burns, M.S., & Griffin, P. (1998). *Preventing reading difficulties in young children.* Washington, DC: National Research Council, Committee on the Prevention of Reading Difficulties in Young Children.

Snowling, M.J., Gallagher, A., & Frith, U. (2003). Family risk of dyslexia is continuous: Individual differences in the precursors of reading skill. *Child Development, 74*(2), 358–373.

Stanovich, K.E. (1986). Matthew effects in reading: Some consequences of individual differences in the acquisition of literacy. *Reading Research Quarterly, 21*(4), 360–407. doi:10.1598/rrq.21.4.1

Thorpe, H.W., & Borden, K.S. (1985). The effect of multisensory instruction upon the on-task behaviors and word reading accuracy of learning disabled children. *Journal of Learning Disabilities, 18*, 279–286.

Treiman, R. (2006). Knowledge about letters as a foundation for reading and spelling. In R.M. Joshi, & P.G. Aaron (Eds.), *Handbook of orthography and literacy* (pp. 581–599). Mahwah, NJ: Lawrence Erlbaum Associates.

Treiman, R., Gordon, J., Boada, R., Peterson, R.L., & Pennington, B.F. (2014). Statistical learning, letter reversals, and reading. *Scientific Studies of Reading, 18*(6), 383–394. http://doi.org/10.1080/10888438.2013.873937

Treiman, R., Tincoff, R., Rodriguez, K., Mouzaki, A., & Francis, D. (1998). The foundations of literacy: Learning the sounds of letters. *Child Development, 69*(6), 1524–1540.

Vellutino, F.R. (1979). *Dyslexia: Theory and research.* Cambridge, MA: The MIT Press.

Vellutino, F.R., Fletcher, J.M., Snowling, M.J., & Scanlon, D.M. (2004). Specific reading disability (dyslexia): What have we learned in the past four decades? *Journal of Child Psychology and Psychiatry, 45*(1), 2–40. doi:10.1046/j.0021-9630.2003.00305.x

Vellutino, F.R., Scanlon, D.M., & Jaccard, J. (2003). Toward distinguishing between cognitive and experiential deficits as primary sources of difficulty in learning to read: A two year follow-up of difficult to remediate and readily remediated poor readers. In B. Foorman (Ed.), *Preventing and remediating reading difficulties: Bringing science to scale* (pp. 73–120). Timonium, MD: York Press.

Vellutino, F.R., Scanlon, D.M., Sipay, E.R., Small, S.G., Pratt, A., Chen, R., & Denckla, M.B. (1996). Cognitive profiles of difficult to remediate and readily remediated poor readers: Early intervention as a vehicle for distinguishing between cognitive and experiential deficits as basic causes of specific reading disability. *Journal of Educational Psychology, 88*(4), 601–638.

Vellutino, F.R., Smith, H., Steger, J.A., & Kaman, M. (1975). Reading disability: Age differences and the perceptual deficit hypothesis. *Child Development, 46,* 487–493.

Wolf, M. (1997). A provisional, integrative account of phonological and naming-speed deficits in dyslexia: Implications for diagnosis and intervention. In B. Blachman (Ed.), *Foundation of reading acquisition and dyslexia: Implications for early intervention* (pp. 67–92). Mahwah, NJ: Lawrence Erlbaum Associates.

Wolf, M., Bowers, P.G., & Biddle, K. (2000). Naming-speed processes, timing, and reading: A conceptual review. *Journal of Learning Disabilities, 33,* 387–407.

Wolf, M., & Obregón, M. (1997). The "double-deficit" hypothesis: Implications for diagnosis and practice in reading disabilities. In L. Putnam (Ed.), *Readings on language and literacy* (pp. 177–209). Cambridge, MA: Brookline Books.

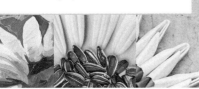

Appendix 5.1

Technology Resources

Elaine A. Cheesman

Effective programs/apps have the following features:

- They link the shape of the letter with the name of the letter.
- They include upper- and lowercase forms.
- They provide alphabetizing practice.

Alphabet Dots Game: Build Letter Confidence   http://elliesgames.com

This game provides opportunities to practice alphabet sequence using lower-case letters.

DotToDot   http://www.appsinmypocket.com

This app orally pronounces names of letters and numbers in alphabetical and numerical order. The user can adjust settings for older students.

Letter Case   http://elliesgames.com

This game provides practice in matching upper- and lowercase letters in various fonts. It is designed for young children.

Letter Quiz   http://tantrumapps.com

This engaging app helps the child identify and form the letters of the alphabet, match upper- and lowercase forms, and learn the associated sound. Some associated sounds are not the most common sounds (e.g., *X* is for x-ray).

SpellingCity   http://www.spellingcity.com

This game has the student alphabetize lists of words. The teacher or parent can import lists from other users or published programs or create original lists. The game is good for learners of all ages.

Chapter 6

Teaching Phonemic Awareness

Lucy Hart Paulson

LEARNING OBJECTIVES

1. To understand the interactions of phonemic awareness within the components, functions, and connections of the phonological processing system

2. To describe and interpret assessment data based on phonemic awareness developmental sequences and grade expectations

3. To design and implement activities for teaching phonemic awareness skills in the early grades and intervention activities as needed for students who struggle with learning these skills

Phonemic awareness, the ability to manipulate the speech sounds in words, is a vital foundation in learning to read and write. Students with well-developed phonemic awareness skills are likely to be successful readers and writers. Basic phonemic awareness skills in preschool and kindergarten are highly predictive of later literacy learning in the primary grades. For students who experience difficulty with literacy learning, underdeveloped phonemic awareness is most often at the core of this challenge.

This chapter describes the definitions and interrelated connections of phonemic awareness within the phonological processing system, important for all the skills of listening, speaking, reading, and writing. Developmental sequences are described, with age and grade expectations in preschool through the elementary grades linked to assessment considerations. Finally, instruction strategies are discussed across grade levels within a tiered system of support for prevention, instruction, and intervention.

The content of this chapter is based on scientific literacy research and provides the reader with background knowledge supported by the Center for Effective Reading Instruction (CERI) and the International Dyslexia Association's (IDA; 2018) *Knowledge and Practice Standards for Teachers of Reading*. These standards require a deep level of understanding of the phonological system and the sequences of development vital for planning and implementing literacy instruction. This rigorous level of knowledge is important so teachers are qualified to teach all students effectively, especially those who may struggle with the processes of learning to read and write.

PHONEMIC AWARENESS WITHIN PHONOLOGICAL PROCESSING ABILITIES

In the seminal report of the National Reading Panel (National Institute of Child Health and Human Development [NICHD], 2000), phonemic awareness was well-established as a required component in the process of learning to read. It is first in the list of the big five components of reading, followed by phonics, vocabulary, fluency, and comprehension (NICHD, 2000). These components are highly inter-related, and phonemic awareness ability contributes to growth and competency in each of them.

In order to understand phonemic awareness, one must look at encompass-ing phonological processing abilities. There are a number of related and inter-connected terms, and all of them have a *ph* spelling pattern representing the /f/ sound. Phonemes are the speech sounds of oral language, the consonant and vowel sounds in spoken words. A phoneme is the smallest unit of speech that makes one word distinguishable from another in a phonetic language such as English (e.g., the /k/ sound in *cap* distinguishes this word from *tap*). Phonemes are represented in print between two slash marks / /, called **virgules.** The *phone* in phonemic is Greek for "sound, voice," referring to the speech sounds used to hear and say words as well as the speech sounds represented by letters used to read and write. Consider the list of terms with the *ph* spelling pattern in Figure 6.1. All of these terms are connected to phonemic awareness in some manner. As you review them, rate your familiarity with each term on a con-tinuum of 1 to 4.

Some of these terms may be quite familiar. A number of them sound very much the same. Each one has an important connection to literacy. An under-standing of these terms' definitions, relationships, and contributions to literacy is important in being able to assess and to teach students learning to read and write.

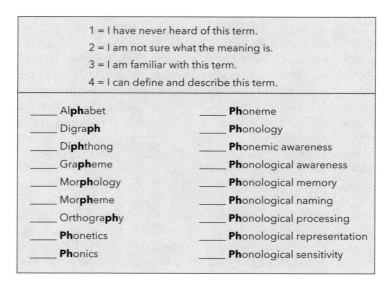

Figure 6.1. Rating understanding of *ph* terms.

Phonological Processing

Phonological processing is the ability to perceive, understand, and use the sound structures of words in both oral and written language. Skills include remembering words accurately, recalling known words, and differentiating between similar sounding words (Anthony & Francis, 2005; Wagner & Torgesen, 1987; Wagner, Torgesen, & Rashotte, 1994). Every word heard, said, read, and written is processed phonologically. Three components of phonological processing, as illustrated in Figure 6.2, include **phonological memory, phonological naming,** and phonological awareness. **Phonological representation** is a related and highly connected skill as well. These component skills are important foundations of literacy acquisition (Anthony & Francis, 2005; Lonigan, 2006; Troia, 2014; Wagner et al., 1994; Whitehurst & Lonigan, 2002).

Phonological Memory   Phonological memory is the ability to immediately process and recall sound-based information (i.e., something you have heard) in **short-term memory** for temporary storage (Anthony & Francis, 2005; Whitehurst & Lonigan, 2002). A key aspect of this storage is short-term. When you hear a novel word or sentence, you need to do something with it or the sound image disappears. For instance, think of a time when you were introduced to a new friend. You heard the person's name and then joined in some small talk. After a short time (seconds), when you wanted to recall the new friend's name, it seemed to have evaporated from your short-term memory. If, however, you repeated the person's name, or if the name was familiar to you already, you would be more likely to remember it. These elements of rehearsal (repeating the name) and familiarity with an already known word help you learn and recall new words (Gathercole & Adams, 1993). Here is another example. Think of the situation of a first-grader working arduously to sound out a string of words in a sentence. She slowly decodes the words, and by the time she gets to the last word of the sentence, the first words may have disappeared from her phonological memory, affecting her understanding of what she just tried to read.

From a cognitive perspective, working memory capacity develops over time. Preschool children are able to hold onto 1–2 items or chunks of information at the same time; elementary students extend the number to 3–4 elements; and memory capacity expands in adults to 5 or so pieces of information (Sousa, 2011). Students' phonological memory capacity affects their ability to retain what they hear and read, which influences their ability to process the meaning.

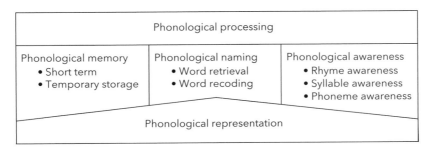

Figure 6.2.   Connections of *ph* processing terms.

Phonological Naming Phonological naming is the ability to efficiently retrieve words stored in **long-term memory** using phonological information (Lonigan, 2006; Whitehurst & Lonigan, 2002). This term is also called **phonological retrieval.** Think of a time when you wanted to say a word and it seemed to be on the tip of your tongue. Your phonological naming got a bit stuck. In trying to say the word, if you were able to think of the beginning sound or other phonological structure of the word (syllable pattern or rhythm), then you might be more likely to retrieve and say it.

Saying and reading words requires phonological naming skills. Students who are able to retrieve words in a fluent manner are better able to say them. One kind of assessment task, called **rapid automatic naming (RAN),** requires a student to look at a series of repeated random letters, numerals, common objects, geometric shapes, or colored dots and say the names of the items as quickly as possible. Figure 6.3 displays examples of RAN tasks used to measure how rapidly a student is able to retrieve and say the names of the items. RAN is important for the development of **reading fluency** and affects reading comprehension (de Groot, van den Bos, Minnaert, & van der Meulen, 2015; Vandewalle, Boets, Ghesquière, & Zink, 2012).

Certain RAN assessment tasks are more relevant at different ages and instructional levels. Before receiving reading instruction, RAN tasks of naming objects, colors, and shapes are more predictive of literacy development for younger students. After the onset of reading instruction for older students, letter and numeral naming tasks are better predictors of further reading development (de Jong, 2011; Lervåg & Hulme, 2009).

Think of a kindergarten child engaged in a letter-naming task. He looks at the letter shape and has to retrieve the label for the letter's name. If his phonological naming skill is fluent, the naming will happen more readily. If, however, he is still unsure of the difference between the letters with similar sounding names and shapes, such as *b* and *d,* he may have more difficulty retrieving the labels. These letter names may not have a solid representation in his long-term memory yet.

Phonological and Phonemic Awareness The third phonological processing component, phonological awareness, is the ability to consciously manipulate (play with) rhymes, syllables, and phonemes (speech sounds) in words. Phonemic

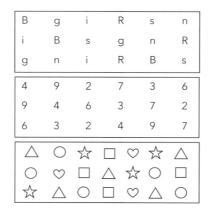

Figure 6.3. Examples of rapid automatic naming (RAN) tasks.

awareness, a more sophisticated sub-skill within phonological awareness, is ability to reflect on and consciously manipulate the phonemes in words. Phonological and phonemic awareness are metalinguistic (*meta*—intentionally thinking about; *linguistic*—language) skills. Examples of phonological awareness skills and corresponding tasks are as follows:

- *Rhyme awareness:* Say three words that rhyme with the word *train.*

- *Syllable awareness:* Clap the syllables in the word *watermelon.*

- *Phonemic awareness:* Identify the sounds in the word *crab.*

Of the phonological processing components, phonological and phonemic awareness are the most strongly related to literacy development (Anthony & Francis, 2005; Lonigan, 2006). These skills can be taught, and skill development is predictive of later literacy learning (Catts, Nielsen, Bridges, Liu, & Bontempo, 2015; de Groot et al., 2015; Melby-Lervåg, Lyster, & Hulme, 2012; Lonigan & Shanahan, 2008; NICHD, 2000). On the other hand, phonological memory and word retrieval skills are important skills to measure in the assessment process. Research has not established the efficacy of intentionally teaching phonological memory or phonological naming. However, enhanced phonological awareness skills result in positive impacts on phonological memory and naming (Kerins, 2006; Krafnick, Flowers, Napoliello, & Eden, 2011; Torgesen, Wagner, Rashotte, Herron, & Lindamood, 2010; Vaughn, Linan-Thompson, & Hickman, 2003; Vukovic & Siegel, 2006; Wolff, 2014). A range of early, basic, and complex phonological awareness skills are important to literacy learning at various ages and stages (Kilpatrick, 2015). The development, assessment, and instruction of phonological and phonemic awareness are discussed in detail later in this chapter.

Phonological Representation

Phonological representation is the quality or distinctness of how well words are stored in long-term memory and the ability to access word representations in a conscious manner (Sutherland & Gillon, 2005). When you learn a new word, you develop a sense of inner speech or a phonological representation of what a word sounds like in your mind. All familiar words and word parts (e.g., *-ing, -tion, un-*) are stored with phonological representations (Kilpatrick, 2015).

Phonological representation has a strong connection to phonological naming in retrieving words to say them. Here is an example: Recall the name of the last thing you ate. You most likely are able to hear the word for the food item in your mind even though you did not say the word aloud. Because the word has a strong phonological representation stored in your long-term memory, you were able to access it. Saying the word aloud taps your phonological naming skills.

Phonological memory is influenced by phonological representation. When you are hearing something that already is represented in long-term memory, it is easier to hold in working memory.

Learning new words requires making a connection to their meaning and developing phonological distinctions from other words that sound similar (Metsala & Walley, 1998). A young child learning the difference between the words *elevator* and *escalator* must develop an understanding of the word meanings as well as their pronunciations, with a distinct phonological representation of each word.

Having distinct phonological representations of spoken words contributes to one's accessing the phonological segments (syllables and phonemes) needed for phonological awareness (Gillon, 2004; Metsala & Walley, 1998). The quality of the underlying phonological representation and the ability to access this representation in a conscious manner is critical for reading and spelling development (Elbro, Borstrøm, & Peterson, 1998; Sutherland & Gillon, 2005). How well words are stored and accessed makes a significant contribution to **sight-word** recognition and reading development (Kilpatrick, 2015).

Here is an illustration of how phonological processing skills contribute to completing phonemic awareness tasks. Say the word *paper*. Then, say it again without saying the second /p/ sound. In order to complete this task, you needed to hold the word *paper* in your phonological memory, use phonemic awareness skills to remove the second /p/ sound, and then come up with a new word, *payer*. Both words have stored phonological representations.

PHONEMIC AWARENESS FOUNDATIONS FOR DECODING, SPELLING, VOCABULARY, AND FLUENCY

Framed within the component skills of phonological processing, phonemic awareness is a required foundation for phonics, spelling, vocabulary, fluency, and ultimately reading comprehension and writing composition. Here are more *ph* terms related to language study! An understanding of the interconnections is included in both the CERI and IDA knowledge standards.

Phonics

Phonics describes the study of the relationships between graphemes (letter patterns) and phonemes (speech sounds). Grapheme patterns are related to orthography, the conventional spelling system of a language, including print conventions such as punctuation, capitalization, and word breaks. A specific type of grapheme with two letters representing one sound is called a **digraph.** Common digraphs are *sh, ch,* and *th.* Here is a simple example: The word *fish* has four letters, three graphemes (*f – i – sh*), and three phonemes (/f/ - /ĭ/ - /sh/).

Phonemic awareness is not phonics but is a required component, along with alphabet knowledge, for phonics skills to develop. (Notice the *ph* in the middle of the word *alphabet*.) An **alphabet** is an invention of a group of written symbols created to represent speech sounds. Reading a word (**decoding**) uses grapheme-to-phoneme knowledge, and spelling a word (**encoding**) requires phoneme-to-grapheme understanding.

When decoding a printed word, beginning readers need to identify the graphemes and convert the letters to their corresponding phonemes, then blend the sounds together to say the word (Baddeley, Gathercole, & Papagno, 1998; NICHD, 2000; Troia, 2014). A young reader looks at the written word *hat,* and breaks or segments the letters apart saying the phonemes (/h/ - /ă/ - /t/) representing the letters and blends the sounds together to read/say "hat." The phonological representation is accessed in stored memory and retrieved to determine the spoken form of the word. The phonemic awareness skill of blending (putting segments together to say a word) is centrally involved in phonic decoding in the early stages of learning to read.

Sight-word reading is also dependent on phonemic awareness skills. Most written words have some phonemic connection to the word's spelling. The sounds in the word represented in long-term storage act as anchoring points for remembering the spelling sequences, which is key for sight-word learning (Kilpatrick, 2015). Young students who are still developing phonemic awareness skills will have difficulty learning sight words until their letter knowledge is in place and their phonemic awareness skills have progressed to a level sufficient to support letter–sound learning (Adams, 2013; Ehri, 2014).

Spelling

Spelling requires making phoneme-to-grapheme connections by isolating or segmenting the phonemes in a word and identifying the grapheme pattern(s). To spell a word, a student segments the phonemes in the word (/h/ - /ă/ - /t/), identifies the grapheme patterns (*h, a, t*) and writes the letters to form the word *hat*. The phonemic awareness skill of segmenting (pulling word segments apart) is required for spelling.

In kindergarten and first grade, students often spell words in a phonetic manner by matching up speech sounds in words with the corresponding letters. At this stage, young students have not been taught more intricate spelling patterns. A young student may write the word *once* as *wuns,* making a phonetic connection to the sounds in the word and his or her letter–sound knowledge. He or she may also sound out the word *walked* and write it as *yokt* using the sound cue in the letter *y* (pronounced /wī/), short /ŏ/, /k/, and /t/, based on the pronunciation as he or she said the word.

In the later grades and into middle school, older students' phonemic awareness skills contribute to proficient decoding skills (Roman, Kirby, Parrila, Wade-Woolley, & Deacon, 2009). Spelling continues to require phonemic awareness, along with a developing understanding of morphology, the study of the forms of words, and morphemes, meaningful units of words including **base words,** prefixes, and suffixes. An older student, who has learned more about morphemes and spelling conventions, will be able to spell the word *walked* correctly, knowing that there is a silent letter *l* and that the past tense verb ending is spelled with *-ed,* even though it is pronounced with a /t/ phoneme.

Vocabulary

Learning vocabulary requires gaining an understanding of a word's meaning as well as a phonological representation that involves developing and storing the word's pronunciation (Baddeley et al., 1998). The depth of a student's word knowledge is critical to overall comprehension. Think of the potential confusion of a young student learning about pedestrians and Presbyterians, both words with some connection to people and similar-sounding word structures.

Fluency

Fluency is defined as reading words at an adequate rate, with a high level of accuracy, and with appropriate expression. Reading fluency is considered the bridge between lower level skills of phonemic awareness, phonics, and vocabulary to reading comprehension. Phonological naming is required to fluidly or fluently retrieve the pronunciations (phonological form) of words being read.

Causal Connections of Phonemic Awareness

With all of these relationships, it is easy to see the connections between phonemic awareness and other language skills, and the importance of phonemic awareness as a foundation skill to phonics, spelling, vocabulary, and fluency. These skills are necessary for reading comprehension as well as writing composition. Well-developed phonemic awareness facilitates literacy learning, while underdeveloped phonemic awareness makes literacy learning a challenge.

Phonemic awareness appears to have a causal role in the acquisition of basic literacy skills (Melby-Lervåg et al., 2012; Perfetti, Beck, Bell, & Hughes, 1987; Sauval, Perre, & Casalis, 2016; Torgesen, Wagner, & Rashotte, 1994). Phonemic awareness contributes to learning grapheme–phoneme connections needed for decoding and fluent, accurate word recognition, which in turn leads to comprehending what was read. Advances in reading proficiency reciprocally promote further development of phonemic awareness.

> ### REFLECT, CONNECT, and RESPOND
> What challenges might a third-grade student with weak phonemic awareness skills have with decoding, reading fluency, spelling, and vocabulary?

WHAT IS A PHONEME?

As described, a phoneme is a speech sound, not an alphabet letter, although there is an important connection between the two entities. Remember that speech sounds in print are designated by using virgules / /. (For example, /m/ represents the first sound in the word *me,* which is spelled with the letter *m*). Educators' own phonemic awareness skills will affect their ability to competently assess and teach these skills to students. Check your own phonemic awareness skills for accuracy by identifying how many sounds are in each of the words in Figure 6.4.

Of note, identifying and segmenting phonemes in words may be challenging for adults because the reading process has become so automatic that isolating the phonemes in words does not need to be a conscious task (Ehri, 2014). However, teachers, who are responsible for helping students develop and refine phonemic awareness skills, need to be able to accurately and fluidly complete and teach phonemic awareness tasks.

PHONOLOGICAL AND PHONEMIC AWARENESS COMPONENTS AND DEVELOPMENTAL SEQUENCES

Of the phonological processing abilities, phonological and phonemic awareness are skills that can most readily be taught. Recall the definition of phonological awareness as the ability to consciously identify and manipulate the syllable, **onset** and

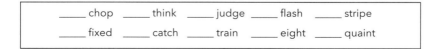

_____ chop   _____ think   _____ judge   _____ flash   _____ stripe

_____ fixed   _____ catch   _____ train   _____ eight   _____ quaint

Figure 6.4.   Phonemic awareness skill check. (*Answers:* chop, 3, ch – o – p; think, 4, th – i – n – k; judge, 3, j – u – dge; flash, 4, f – l – a – sh; stripe, 5, s – t – r – i – pe; fixed, 5, f – i – /k/ – /s/ – /t/; catch, 3, c – a – tch; train, 4, t – r – ai – n; eight, 2, eigh – t; quaint, 5, /k/ – /w/ – ai – n – t.)

rime, and phoneme segments of words. Phonemic awareness specifically attends to the sound structures, not letters, and can be done in the dark! Being able to describe the component skills and developmental sequences are important elements in both the CERI and IDA standards.

Phonological Awareness Components on the Linguistic Hierarchy

Phonological awareness includes aspects of rhyme awareness, syllable awareness, and phoneme awareness. Rhyme awareness is one phonological awareness construct, whereas syllable and phoneme awareness can be combined into a second construct (Anthony et al., 2002). Rhyme awareness begins to develop across the toddler and preschool years, with detection of words that rhyme, and progresses into the early elementary grades, with the ability to produce words that rhyme.

Syllable and phoneme awareness focus on blending and segmenting tasks. Blending (also called synthesizing) is the ability to combine or synthesize a sequence of isolated word segments of syllables, onsets (initial sounds), or phonemes to produce a recognizable word (e.g., hearing *kan – ga – roo* and saying "kangaroo"; hearing *p – op* and saying "pop"; or hearing *j – a – ck* and saying "jack"). Segmentation (also called analysis) requires the ability to analyze the segments of a word and isolate them by syllables, onsets, and individual phonemes (e.g., saying *kangaroo* as "kan – ga – roo," saying *pop* as "p – op," or saying *jack* as "j – a – ck"). These examples illustrate the progression of syllable and phoneme awareness development along the **linguistic hierarchy** (see Figure 6.5), which includes segmental levels of 1) word boundaries within sentences, 2) syllables in words, 3) onset/rime units, and 4) phonemes in words.

Starting at the bottom and moving up the hierarchy, blending and segmenting skills develop first with larger segments of syllables, progressing to smaller units of onsets, then individual phonemes (Adams, 1990; Anthony et al., 2002; Lonigan & Shanahan, 2008; NICHD, 2000). Another layer to the linguistic hierarchy is a series of more complex manipulation skills of adding, deleting, substituting, and reversing word segments.

Word Boundaries   The lowest level on the linguistic hierarchy is word awareness. This skill focuses on determining word boundaries, where they begin and end, within the flow of speech. In the early stages of learning language, babies and toddlers develop a sensitivity to the structures of words and determine word boundaries. Their understanding focuses mainly on word meanings, with little awareness of word structures (Gombert, 1992; Metsala & Walley, 1998; Morais, 1991). As their vocabulary grows and they begin saying longer words, children need to become sensitive to differences in word pronunciations to distinguish

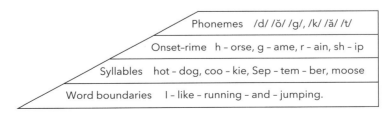

Figure 6.5.   Linguistic hierarchy of words.

similar sounding words. This sensitivity, in a sense, forces them to begin to attend to word structures.

On another level, an understanding of word boundaries affects one's ability to learn another language. In the process of acquiring a second language, a learner listening to a native speaker of the language often considers the speaker's rate of speech to be quite fast. This sense of rapidity occurs because the learner is not yet familiar with the word boundaries within the flow of speech. More practice and experience learning the new language helps the learner determine the word boundaries as a phonologic sensitivity develops for the words in the new language.

Syllables   The next step on the hierarchy involves attending to syllable segments in words. On this step at the syllable level, a skill progression begins with segmenting and blending **compound words** (e.g., *cup – cake, hot – dog, snow – man*), then multisyllabic words (e.g., *kan – ga – roo, ba – na – na, mo – tor – cy – cle*), and a recognition that some words have one syllable (e.g., *moose, chair, run*).

The rhythmic nature of syllables helps with children's word awareness (Goswami et al., 2013). Many activities designed for young children have an implicit focus on syllables. Singing songs and saying nursery rhymes have a rhythmic component and an element of playing with the syllable structures of words. For example, in singing the song "Twinkle, Twinkle Little Star," one naturally segments the words' syllables saying, "Twin – kle, twin – kle, li – ttle star." Experiences such as these help young children learn that words have a structure in addition to a meaning.

Onset-Rime   The next step up on the linguistic hierarchy is onset–rime, with a focus on beginning sounds in words. The onset–rime step on the linguistic hierarchy is a transition from syllable awareness to phonemic phonological awareness skill levels. By definition, a word onset is the beginning consonant sound or consonant **blend** of a single-syllable word or syllable, and the rime is the vowel and rest of the word or syllable. These words are divided by onset–rime: *f – un, p – art, v – ase, z – est, st – op, cl – ock, dr – ink, pl –ane.*

Another literacy concept associated at the onset–rime level is alliteration, the occurrence of the same sound at the beginning of words. Examples are *fish/phone, cent/sun, jar/gent*. Notice that the word pairs begin with the same phonemes; however, the graphemes are different. This illustrates again that phonological awareness is about sounds, not letters.

Attention to the term *onset* as related to phonological awareness is important at this step on the linguistic hierarchy. Consider these consonant blends, which are word onsets: **tr** – ain, **sm** – oke, **bl** – ue, **gr** – eat. An important phonemic awareness skill is to isolate and identify the beginning *sound* in words. So, the initial phonemes in these words actually are: /t/ – rain, /s/ –moke, /b/ – lue, and /g/ – reat. In completing phonemic awareness tasks with a focus on initial sounds, students should learn to isolate the first consonant sound in words beginning with consonant blends.

Phonemes   The top step on the linguistic hierarchy involves attending to the smallest segments in words, the individual phonemes. Skill development at this level is indeed a metalinguistic skill with a conscious focus on isolating, identifying, and, in some way, manipulating the phonemes in words. Common tasks at the phoneme level are blending individual sounds together to make a word and segmenting a whole word into its individual phonemes.

Complex Manipulation Skills Older students learn to complete complex phonemic awareness manipulation skills that include adding, deleting, substituting, and reversing phonemes in words. These tasks require higher levels of cognitive development and abstract thinking as well as more well-developed phonological memory and naming skills.

Adding phonemes is a manipulation task that requires inclusion of another syllable or phoneme to a given word. This skill requires holding a word in memory, adding an element, and saying the new word. Attending to the linguistic hierarchy, a segment is added to a word at the syllable level. These examples use prefixes and suffixes (e.g., add *un-* to *happy* to get "unhappy"; add *re-* to *turn* to get "return"; add *-ing* to the end and *dis-* to the beginning of *miss*). At the phoneme level, a sound can be added to the beginning, middle, or end of a word (e.g., add /s/ to the beginning of *top* to get *stop*; add /s/ before /t/ in *wet* to get *west*; add /t/ to the end of *ten* to get *tent*).

A focus on morphemes in oral language pronunciations provides a connection to how those patterns are spelled in written language. For example, have students say and spell *miss* and add a past tense *-ed* ending to say *missed*, then have them say the initial word again and add a /t/ sound, then spell the word, which results in *mist*. Compare the pronunciations. Both words sound the same but have different meanings and spellings. This example illustrates the phonological connections with other linguistic elements of morphology, vocabulary, and syntax (sentence structure) in oral language with impacts on written language.

Deletion, also called **elision,** tasks remove a word segment. To complete a deletion task, one must hold the word in memory, identify the segment to be removed, mentally remove it, and then say the new word, requiring each phonological processing ability. For older preschool children, this task may include compound words. An example might be to have a 5-year-old say the word *snowman* and say it again without saying *man* (i.e. with a correct response of *snow*). In first grade, deletion might entail having a student say the word *stop* and say it again without saying /s/, responding with *top*. Harder tasks involve deleting the second phoneme in a consonant blend (e.g., say *blank* and say it again without saying /l/) or deleting a consonant in the middle of a word (e.g., say *best*, and say it again without saying /s/; or say *window*, and say it again without saying /n/).

Another higher level manipulation task is **substitution,** which requires both deleting and adding skills by removing a syllable or phoneme from a word and adding a new one to say a different word. These syllable-level examples use morphemes by changing prefixes in words. Say *disappear* and change *dis-* to *re-*; or say *inform* and change the *in-* to *re-*, then *con-*. At the phoneme level, sounds at the beginning, middle, and end of words can be substituted. For example, say *sun*, change the /s/ to /t/ (to get *ton*); say *ton*, change the /ŭ/ to /ă/ (to get *tan*); say *tan*, change the /n/ to /p/ (to get *tap*).

An even harder manipulation task is **reversing** or switching sounds within a word. This skill requires one to hold the word in memory, identify the sounds to reverse, remove and replace them, and say the new word. An example of this task may be to say the word *tab* and switch the beginning and ending sounds to come up with *bat*, or to reverse the last two sounds in the word *mats* to say *mast*.

> **REFLECT, CONNECT, and RESPOND**
> Describe the contribution of the phonological processing components of memory, naming, and representation when a student is completing a phoneme deletion task by removing the /s/ sound from the word *mast*.

Development Along the Hierarchy

The linguistic hierarchy provides a sequential way to think about the progression of how children develop phonological awareness skills, beginning at the word level and progressing to the phonemic level and onto more complex manipulation skills. Young children most often are able to interact with larger linguistic units of syllables in words before the smaller units of phonemes. However, phonological skills do not develop in discrete steps or in isolation of each other (Papadopoulos, Kendeou, & Spanoudis, 2012). Younger students may successfully segment words into syllables most of the time and also be learning to identify beginning sounds. More familiar words may be manipulated at higher levels, are less taxing on phonological memory, and may be easier to retrieve. A young student may be able to segment all the sounds in the word *cat* but not in the word *jazz*. The word *cat* may be more familiar, making it easier to focus on manipulating the sounds. Older students, with better developed cognition and language, learn to manipulate words at higher levels. The next consideration is determining at what ages and stages these skills should be taught and expected.

DEVELOPMENT OF SIMPLE TO COMPLEX PHONOLOGICAL AND PHONEMIC AWARENESS

The foundations for phonemic awareness begin to develop before babies are even born. In utero, infants become sensitive to the rhythm and patterns of speech, and they develop the capacity to discriminate among different syllables in human speech (Mahmoudzadeh et al., 2013). During their first year, babies listen to the language they hear around them and become sensitive to the phonemes in those words. This attention to the syllables and phonemes of language is **phonological sensitivity** (Morais, 1991), also called **speech decoding** (van Goch, McQueen, & Verhoeven, 2014). As their sensitivity to phonemes expands, babies between 6 and 8 months of age begin to babble the sounds of the language they have heard. During this stage, they become sensitive to word boundaries in the flow of language. Even at this early age, these developing phonological skills are predictive of later literacy acquisition (Guttorm et al., 2005).

As babies grow into toddlers, their oral language develops from babbling to saying simple words, demonstrating their sensitivity to and understanding of word boundaries. Their early words have a phonological structure that resembles the adult form of the words. A toddler might say "Dere a doddy an a too too tain" for *There is a doggy and a choo choo train*. This young child is saying words with a semblance to the standard pronunciation. However, he is still developing his phonological system and learning to say all of the speech sounds. Learning to say many words requires young children to enhance their phonological sensitivity by attending to words at the phoneme level, particularly those that sound similar. For example, a young child learns to differentiate similar sounding words, such as *baba* (bottle) and *baby, no* and *nose, bye* and *bite* with an understanding of the differences in meaning as well as differences in the phoneme structure in how the words sound.

To accommodate a rapidly growing expressive vocabulary, toddlers expand their phonological processing skills to be able to say distinctly many new and different words. They also begin to play with words and word structures before they are consciously aware of what they are doing. A good example is to listen to a toddler sing songs by following the rhythm and syllable structure in the song pattern. The pattern they use in singing words differs from the way they say words when talking.

As they grow into preschoolers, children develop an awareness of word structure, which is the beginning of phonological awareness. In the earliest stages of word play, young children have an implicit sensitivity to word structure known as **epilinguistic** awareness (Gombert, 1992; Morais, 1991; Savage, Blair & Rvachew, 2006). They develop the ability to detect aspects of word structure such as rhyme, syllables, and initial sounds implicitly rather than with conscious or metalinguistic awareness (Goswami, 2000). A preschooler may say "daddy, baddy, maddy," playing with the word *daddy*. Another child may stomp her feet while saying *"di* (stomp) – *no* (stomp) – *saur* (stomp)." Young Molly may excitedly explain, "Mom and Molly start the same!" In these examples, children are playing with word structures, but they do not yet consciously understand what they are doing to manipulate the syllables and sounds.

Older preschoolers, with bigger vocabularies and higher levels of cognition, develop a conscious and intentional ability to play with and manipulate the syllables and phonemes of language, which is now metalinguistic awareness. They easily segment and blend words at the syllable level and intentionally identify beginning sounds in words.

During kindergarten and first grade, children hone their phonemic awareness skills, learning to identify, isolate, blend, and segment phonemes in simple words. In subsequent grades, these basic skills become more complex with manipulation by adding, deleting, substituting, and/or reversing phonemes in words. Figure 6.6

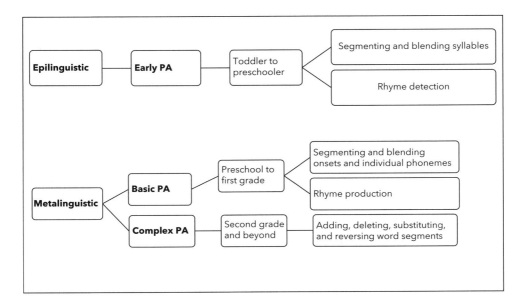

Figure 6.6.   Progression of phonological and phonemic awareness (PA) development.

illustrates the progression from easy, epilinguistic to basic and complex metalinguistic skill development and related tasks.

Rhyme Awareness Development

Sensitivity to rhyme is an epilinguistic skill and is one of the first phonological awareness skills observed as young children learn to say the words in finger-plays, songs, and nursery rhymes. At 2–3 years of age, children may be able to detect words that rhyme when other phonological skills are too difficult (MacLean, Bryant, & Bradley, 1987; Whitehurst & Lonigan, 2002). Rhyme sensitivity emerges as young children develop articulation skills and learn to accurately say speech sounds (Rvachew & Grawburg, 2006).

Following rhyme sensitivity is rhyme detection, which typically occurs in 3- to 4-year-old children as they learn to match words that sound the same at the end (Anthony et al., 2002). Earlier in this phase, rhyme detection is implicit, not intentional. As children become more experienced with word play, their skills develop into a metalinguistic focus on rhyming words. They may hear a phrase such as *bug in a rug* and excitedly exclaim, "Those words rhyme!" This familiarity leads to an ability to produce rhyming words, expected in 4- and 5-year-olds (Anthony et al., 2002) and then generate a string of words that rhyme with a particular word, expected in kindergarten into first grade. Table 6.1 outlines the progression and age expectations for rhyming abilities.

Consider the level of rhyming displayed by this first grader who was experiencing difficulty with reading. The examiner was administering a phonological awareness test to determine this girl's phonological awareness skills. In a rhyme detection task, she was asked to determine if a series of word pairs rhymed as the examiner said them (e.g., "Do these words rhyme: *rain – cane*?"). This girl scored within the expected range for her grade level on this task. On the rhyme production task, she was asked to say a word that rhymed with a given word. Her responses followed this pattern. For the word *hug,* she said "bug"; for *coat,* she said "boat"; for *sack,* she said "back"; for *white,* she said "bite"; for *ball,* she hesitated and said "bat." She had a fairly high level of success providing rhyming words. However, did she have well-developed rhyming skills? The answer is no. She had one strategy for producing rhyming words and that was to start her rhyming word with a /b/ sound. When she needed to provide a rhyming word for the word *ball,* her strategy did not work. Her overall phonological and phonemic awareness skills were underdeveloped, making her literacy learning difficult.

Rhyming develops first with a sensitivity to how words sound. Then, a receptive ability to detect rhyme in words is followed by an expressive level of producing words that rhyme. These steps progress from an early level to a basic level

Table 6.1.   Rhyming development and age expectations

Task	Age expectations
Say some words in songs, finger-plays, or nursery rhymes	2–3 years of age
Detect and match words that rhyme (receptive)	3–4 years of age
Produce words that rhyme (expressive)	4–5 years of age
Produce a string of words with the same rhyme (expressive)	5–6 years of age

of phonological awareness. For some children, rhyming seems to develop fairly naturally, and for others, it is a difficult task that continues to be challenging in the elementary grades. Difficulty with rhyming may be an indicator of underdeveloped phonological processing skills, although, from an assessment perspective, rhyming in the early grades is not as strong of a predictor of literacy learning as other phonological awareness skills (Lonigan & Shanahan, 2008).

Syllable to Phoneme Awareness With Blending and Segmenting

In general, 3- to 4-year-old children learn to blend and segment words at the syllable level (Anthony et al., 2002). Young children enjoy segmenting their names into syllables in an opening circle or morning meeting to see who is present for the day (e.g., *Ja – son, Ste – pha – nie, Hec – tor, Ja – den*). Then, 4- to 5-year-old preschoolers learn to blend the beginning sounds to the rest of the word. For example, when children line up, the teacher may segment the initial sound in their names for them to blend (e.g., "I need P – olly, now S – am, now N – athan"). Also at this age, children typically learn to blend all the sounds in simple **consonant-vowel-consonant (CVC)** words. They may play a game in which the teacher hides a small object in his or her hand and segments the phonemes saying "/f/ - /i/ - /sh/" for the children to blend together to say *fish*, naming the item in his or her hand; then the teacher continues with other items such as /p/ - /ĭ/ - /g/ *(pig)*, and /g/ - /ō/ - /t/ *(goat)*.

Blending sounds into words tends to be an easier task than segmenting words into phonemes for young children. Segmenting of phonemes occurs during the 4- to 5-year range as children learn to identify and sort words or find the objects beginning with the same sound, which is an alliteration task. A subsequent and related step is focusing on words with the same *ending* sound. Blending and segmenting skills progress from the epilinguistic (early) level with syllables to the metalinguistic (basic) level with the ability to intentionally think about phonemes in words.

In the transition from pre-kindergarten to kindergarten, children learn to identify and isolate the beginning sound in words. In kindergarten, children learn to segment phonemes in simple CVC words. This skill progresses in first grade to the ability to segment words with consonant blends (e.g., CCVC as in /s/ - /t/ - /ŏ/ - /p/ and CVCC as in /b/ - /ĕ/ - /s/ - /t/). Basic phoneme blending and phoneme segmentation are generally mastered by the end of first grade (Kilpatrick, 2012; Swank & Catts, 1994; Wagner et al., 1997). Both blending and segmenting skills are needed for competent reading development (Fox & Routh, 1976, 1983). Table 6.2 outlines the progression of early to basic blending and segmenting skills.

Table 6.2. Developmental progression of blending and segmenting

	Blending	Segmenting
3–4 years	Blend syllables to produce words.	Segment syllables in words.
4–5 years	Blend initial sound/rime and sounds to produce words.	Sort words and identify initial sound.
5–6 years	Blend sounds to produce longer words.	Segment sounds in simple CVC words.
6–7 years	Blend sounds to produce longer words.	Segment sounds in CCVC or CVCC words.

Key: CVC, consonant-vowel-consonant; *CCVC,* consonant-consonant-vowel-consonant; *CVCC,* consonant-vowel-consonant-consonant

During preschool and the early grades, phonological awareness skills follow a general trend in development through the linguistic hierarchy from larger segments (syllables) to smaller ones (phonemes). Other influencing factors include developing cognition, which affects memory and other linguistic characteristics (Anthony et al., 2003; Sousa, 2011). More familiar words are linguistically easier to manipulate than less familiar ones. A preschooler may be able to blend the syllables in familiar words such as *rhinoceros* or *hippopotamus* more readily than in words such as *multiplication* or *geography*. Familiar words are easier to hold in memory because they have stronger phonological representations (Lonigan, Burgess, Anthony, & Barker, 1998; Wagner et al., 1994).

Complex Phonemic Awareness Skills

Much of the research and description on phonemic awareness development, assessment, and instruction is related to the early and basic phonological awareness skills of young children in preschool through first grade. These skills are indeed important and vital for early reading and writing stages. For students in the subsequent grades who are experiencing difficulty learning to read and write, attention to complex phonological awareness is particularly important. The next step in the progression of phonemic awareness is development of higher level manipulation skills of adding, deleting, substituting, and reversing phonemes.

More complex phonemic awareness skills continue to develop in typical readers until about third or fourth grade and level off by fifth grade (Kilpatrick, 2015; Vaessen & Blomert, 2010). These higher level manipulation skills appear to develop with growth in reading and writing skills through the grades, and enhanced phonemic awareness growth appears to affect reading development (Ashby, Dix, Bontrager, Dey, & Archer, 2013; de Jong & van der Leij, 2002, Kilpatrick, 2015; Wagner, Torgesen, & Rashotte, 1999; Wagner, Torgesen, Rashotte, & Pearson, 2013). This relationship highlights the reciprocal nature between phonemic awareness and literacy learning. Students with developing orthographic skills are able to "visualize" the orthographic or written word form and may rely on this skill to complete the task. Typical readers at this level are able to complete these phonemic awareness tasks automatically, within 2 seconds (Kilpatrick, 2015). The level of automaticity in completing these tasks helps to determine phonemic awareness skill development. Older students requiring more than 3 seconds to complete tasks such as these may have underdeveloped phonemic awareness skills (Kilpatrick, 2015), which may then affect their literacy learning.

REFLECT, CONNECT, and RESPOND
Describe epilinguistic and metalinguistic phonological awareness in terms of early, basic, and complex skill development.

PHONEMIC AWARENESS SKILL EXPECTATIONS ACCORDING TO STATE STANDARDS

Standards have been developed to guide skill-level expectations that students should achieve through their educational career. Early learning standards describe what young children (infants, toddlers, and preschoolers) should be learning across those years. Many states have adopted the standards that address phonological awareness on some level in the early grades.

Early Learning Standards

Each U.S. state has developed its own set of early learning standards (also called early learning and development standards). The early learning standards may be broad and general, covering wide age ranges (e.g., 3- to 5-year-olds) or may have more specificity detailing particular age-level expectations (e.g., skills for 3-year-olds, 4-year-olds, and 5-year-olds). There is, however, a good deal of consistency, including consistency of phonological awareness expectations, within states' early learning standards. The early developing phonological skill descriptions most often include

- *Phonological awareness:* hear, identify, and make oral rhymes and manipulate syllables in spoken words

- *Phonemic awareness:* discriminate and identify phonemes in spoken words

There are varying levels of detail and skill expectation across the states' early learning standards (DeBruin-Parecki & Slutzky, 2016).

State Standards

English language arts standards have been adopted for kindergarten through Grade 12. Many states have adopted the Common Core State Standards, or CCSS (National Governors Association Center for Best Practices, Council of Chief State School Officers, 2010) or an adapted version. Other states have created their own set of standards. In any case, there is consistency in the description of basic phonological and phonemic awareness skill expectations. In the CCSS, these skills are listed in the Reading Standards: Foundational Skills section, Item 2. Textbox 6.1 lists the skill expectations by the end of kindergarten and the end of first grade. The listed anchor standards reflect early to basic phonemic awareness skills.

Standards for complex phonemic awareness skills most often are not included or addressed in the subsequent grades. However, these skills are still important to develop from second to fifth grade and beyond (Kilpatrick, 2015).

Compare the descriptions of the standards for preschool, kindergarten, and first grade. There is a fair amount of overlap in skill expectations from preschool into kindergarten and onto first grade and some specificity in the expectations across the age and grade levels. A general guideline to follow for skill expectations includes the following:

- Isolating initial sounds of words in pre-kindergarten

- Isolating sounds in CVC words by the end of kindergarten

- Isolating sounds in CCVC words by the end of first grade

Understanding the developmental sequences and the range of typical development for students at various stages is important for educators to be able to make informed decisions for assessment and instruction.

Phonemic Awareness as a Predictive Indicator of Literacy Development

So far in this chapter, phonemic awareness has been defined, described, developmentally detailed, and discussed. The causal relationship between phonemic awareness and literacy development is well-established in the research, and phonemic awareness skills can be taught with positive effects on literacy achievement

TEXTBOX 6.1   **Common Core State Standards for phonological and phonemic awareness in kindergarten and first grade**

Kindergarten Reading Standards: Foundational Skills

1. Phonological awareness: Demonstrates understanding of spoken words, syllables, sounds.

   - Recognize and produce rhyming words.

   - Count, pronounce, blend, segment syllables in spoken words.

   - Blend and segment onsets and rimes of single syllable spoken words.

   - Isolate and pronounce initial, medial vowel, and final sounds (phonemes) in CVC words.

   - Add or substitute individual sounds (phonemes) in simple, one-syllable words to make new words.

Grade 1 Reading Standards: Foundational Skills

2. Phonological awareness: Demonstrates understanding of spoken words, syllables, sounds.

   - Distinguish long from short vowel sounds (phonemes) in spoken single-syllable words.

   - Orally produce single-syllable words by blending sounds (phonemes) including consonant blends.

   - Isolate and pronounce initial, medial vowel, and final sounds (phonemes) in spoken single-syllable words.

   - Segment spoken single-syllable words into their complete sequence of individual sounds (phonemes).

(see Troia, 2014). Research has established specific phonemic awareness skills as predictive indicators of future literacy learning. There are significant connections to deficits in phonemic awareness ability in struggling readers.

The reports of the National Reading Panel (NICHD, 2000) and the National Early Literacy Panel (Lonigan & Shanahan, 2008), both meta-analyses of the scientific research, describe the skill development in phonemic awareness at different stages as predictive of future literacy learning. At the transition between pre-kindergarten and kindergarten, a student's ability to isolate and identify the beginning sounds in words is a strong predictive indicator of how well that student should be reading at the end of second grade (Lonigan & Shanahan, 2008; NICHD, 2000). At the end of kindergarten, a student's ability to segment all of the sounds in a single syllable word becomes a better indicator of later literacy learning

(Lonigan & Shanahan, 2008; NICHD, 2000). This research finding is reflected in the CCSS standards describing phonological awareness at the kindergarten level. Beyond the early grades, complex phonemic awareness skill development continues to predict competency in learning to read and write (Kilpatrick, 2015).

Students who display difficulty learning to read and write most often have a core phonological deficit and demonstrate underdeveloped phonological processing skills. The causes of this impairment may be genetic and/or environmental. A student who has a family member who also struggles or struggled learning to read has a 60% increased risk of also experiencing difficulty with literacy learning, whereas environmental experiences and exposures contribute 20%–40% of the risk (Plomin, 2013).

Students with a core phonological deficit are often diagnosed as having dyslexia. In her seminal book, *Overcoming Dyslexia*, Shaywitz (2003) reported that 88% of struggling readers displayed a weakness in the phonological processing system, based on neurologic testing. Difficulty attending to the phonological aspects of words interferes with decoding words (Lyon, 1995; Share & Stanovich, 1995; Stanovich & Siegel, 1994), which interferes with fluent reading, which then affects comprehension (Birch, 2016; Juel, Griffith, & Gough, 1986). Studies also indicated that phonological representations may be less specified for students with a core phonological deficit. Individuals with dyslexia or a language-based learning disability displayed inaccurate word pronunciations and difficulty repeating long, familiar words (Elbro & Jensen, 2005; Swan & Goswami, 1997), and this manifestation then affected phonological and phonemic awareness abilities.

Research has shown that phonological deficits separate good readers from poor ones, that deficits do not go away on their own, and that they can be identified early (Dehaene, 2009; Shaywitz, 2003; Wolf & Stoodley, 2008). These phonological processing deficits continue to afflict most adults who struggle with reading (Greenberg, Ehri, & Perin, 1997; Wilson & Lesaux, 2001).

The good news is that phonological and phonemic awareness skills can be assessed and taught to young children to help them build a strong phonological foundation before learning to read and write. For students of any age displaying difficulty with literacy learning, phonemic awareness skills can be strengthened, which will help to improve decoding of words, leading to better fluency and, ultimately, better comprehension. Enhanced skill development has a positive impact on literacy learning and results in improved literacy, which can be maintained after the intervention ends (Kilpatrick, 2015; Shaywitz et al., 2004). Any time phonemic awareness is negatively affecting literacy, progress will be limited unless these skills are developed (Bruck, 1992; Truch, 1994). It is never too late to teach phonemic awareness skills.

REFLECT, CONNECT, and RESPOND
Should the CCSS include phonemic awareness skills beyond first grade? If so, which grades should be included and what should the benchmarks be for each grade?

PHONEME CHARACTERISTICS

A deeper understanding of how and where phonemes are produced in one's mouth may be valuable for honing one's own phonemic awareness skills as well as developing the background knowledge on phonology, as referenced in the CERI and IDA standards. Each vowel and consonant phoneme has characteristics that make the pronunciation unique, based on placement, manner, and voicing. This classification of speech sounds is called **phonetics.**

Vowel Phonemes of Standard American English

Vowel phonemes, in contrast to consonants, are open, with little constriction of the mouth and articulators (tongue, lips, jaw). Each vowel sound is produced by tongue placement in the mouth, from high to low and front to back, with either lip rounding or spreading. A short vowel mark is called a **breve** (e.g., /ĭ/), and a long vowel mark is called a **macron** (e.g., /ē/). Long vowels are not "longer" in pronunciation than short vowel sounds; that is, they do not take a longer time to say. They are pronounced with more muscle tension or stress. Short vowels are produced with less tension. Short vowels are simple vowels, meaning there is no mouth movement needed when saying a short vowel sound. Some long vowels are simple, and some are complex, requiring mouth movement for production. Some vowels use lip rounding (e.g., /ō/, /ū/) and others use lip spreading (e.g., /ē/, /ā/). The phonetic symbol /ə/, which looks like an upside-down *e*, is a schwa and is the same sound as the short /ŭ/ but is always used in unstressed or unaccented syllables. See Table 6.3 for a listing of the simple Standard American English (SAE) vowel sounds with word examples.

Look in a mirror while saying each vowel sound. Observe the shape of your mouth, and feel where your tongue is in your mouth, high to low and front to back. Notice if your lips are spread or rounded. Listen to how the vowels sound as you say them. Each of these sensory inputs adds information by helping a speaker be able to discern and discriminate vowel sounds. These elements may be helpful to students learning the vowel sounds and the corresponding alphabet letters.

As mentioned, some long vowel sounds are complex; so are **diphthongs,** which are combinations of simple vowels glided together into one vowel phoneme and produced with mouth movement. The diphthongs in SAE include /ow/ as in the word *cow*, /oi/ as in the word *boy*, and /ī/ as in the word *high*. Another vowel sound with mouth movement is the /yū/ sound as in the word *few* or *unit*. For this sound, the /y/ functions as a vowel sound glided to /ū/, with more lip movement than the simple /ū/ vowel. The word *few* has this vowel whereas the first syllable in the word *futon* has the /ū/ vowel.

The remaining vowels are /r/-controlled. These include /er/ as in the words *bird, her,* and *fir; /ŏr/* as in the words *car* and *star;* /ĕr/ as in the words *bear* and *hair;* /ĭr/ as in the words *deer* and *hear;* and /ōr/ as in the words *for* and *more.*

The complex vowels are listed in Table 6.4. Say each of these words containing complex vowels while looking into a mirror. Notice the movement of your tongue, jaw, and lips.

Table 6.3.   Simple Standard American English vowel placements

Tongue placement	Front of mouth	Middle of mouth	Back of mouth
High	/ē/ meet, beat, seat		/ū/* moot, boot, shoot
	/ĭ/ mitt, bit, sit		/oo/* book, look, shook
Mid	/ā/ mate, bait, state	/ə/ **a**muck, **a**bout, **a**ssure	/ō/* moat, boat, spoke
	/ĕ/ met, bet, set	/ŭ/ mutt, but, shut	
Low	/ă/ mat, bat, sat		/ŏ/ mop, bought, sock

*Indicates vowel sounds with rounded lips.

Table 6.4. Listing of complex Standard American English vowels

Complex vowels types	Symbol	Word examples
Diphthongs	/ow/	cow, how, mouse
	/oi/	boy, coin, oink
	/ī/	bye, sigh, tie
"U"nique	/yū/	cue, few, Ute
R-controlled vowels	/er/	bird, her, fir, sure
	/ŏr/	car, jar, star
	/ĕr/	bear, care, hair
	/ĭr/	deer, hear, tier
	/ōr/	door, core, for

The SAE vowel structure is complex in relation to other languages. A good comparison is with the Spanish language. Spoken English has 19 vowel sounds (Bauman-Waengler, 2009) in contrast to 5 vowels in Spanish. In addition, the English spelling patterns of vowel sounds in written language have a lot of variability (see Table 6.4 for a few written word examples). There are many more English vowel phonemes than alphabet letters to represent them. Think of how many graphemes (letters or letter patterns) may be used to spell the /ā/ phoneme in words. There are more than 10 spellings of this vowel sound, such as *a, ai, ay,* and *eigh,* to name a few.

In speech development, vowel production begins in infancy and is a relatively simple task. In literacy, learning to decode and spell vowel patterns takes time and may be challenging for a range of literacy learners and users.

Consonant Phonemes of Standard American English

Consonant sounds are considered to be closed and produced with some type of constriction in the mouth, with a variety of movements of the articulators (tongue, lips, teeth, jaw, roof, and back and way back of the mouth). In contrast to vowels, consonant sounds have more distinction in their production. Consonant phonemes of any spoken language are described with three characteristics: place, manner, and voicing. Consider the characteristics of the 25 SAE consonant phonemes.

Place Characteristic of Consonant Phonemes The place characteristic describes where in the mouth consonant sounds are produced from front to back and what articulators are used in saying them (see Table 6.5). Say each sound

Table 6.5. Place characteristic of Standard American English consonants

Place	Phonemes
Lips	/p/, /b/, /m/, /f/, /v/, /w/, /wh/
Between teeth	/th/ (as in *thing*), /<u>th</u>/ (as in *there*)
Behind front teeth	/t/, /d/, /n/, /l/, /s/, /z/
Roof of mouth	/sh/, /zh/, /ch/, /j/, /r/, /y/
Back of mouth	/k/, /g/, /ng/
Way in back of mouth	/h/

while looking in a mirror, and feel where the sound is produced. Make sure to say the consonant sound only (e.g., say /p/ and not /puh/ or /m/ and not /muh/).

The lip sounds are produced by closing both lips (/b/, /p/, /m/), using the bottom lip and top teeth (/f/, /v/), or by using lip rounding and movement (/w/, /wh/). The /th/ sounds (/th/ is voiceless, and /<u>th</u>/ is voiced) are produced by placing the tongue tip between the teeth. Placing the tongue tip behind the front teeth and tapping (/t/, /d/), dropping (/l/), or holding (/n/, /s/, /z/) produces the sounds noted in the parentheses. Placing the tongue on the roof of the mouth creates a range of sounds (/sh/, /zh/, /ch/, /j/, /r/, /y/). Tongue placement on the back part of the mouth makes three phonemes (/k/, /g/, /ng/). Opening the vocal folds in the larynx (voice box) and pushing air out makes the /h/ sound.

Consonant sounds produced in the front of the mouth provide a visual advantage when it comes to developing phonemic awareness because the speaker has the ability to see the articulators used in producing these phonemes. Having students see and feel mouth movements may make an important difference when helping students develop phonemic awareness skills as well as letter name and sound knowledge.

Manner Characteristic of Consonant Phonemes   The manner characteristic describes how consonant phonemes are produced. The six categories (listed in Table 6.6) each have particular movement and air flow. Look in the mirror, and say the consonant sounds in each category. Notice the articulatory movement creating the consonant sounds.

Stop sounds are produced by first stopping the airflow somewhere in your mouth, then letting the air puff out making a sound with a short duration. Say the stop sounds, and determine where the airflow stopped in your mouth. Refer to Table 6.3 to verify the placement. Stop phonemes are used in all positions of words (initial, middle, and final), which is not the case for all manner types. These words have a stop in the initial and final positions: *big, pat,* and *kid.* These words have stop sounds in all three positions: *docket, puppet, ticket.*

Fricative phonemes may be produced for as long as your breath allows. Fricative sounds use friction when air is forced through a constricted area some place in your mouth. Look in a mirror, say the fricative sounds, and observe and feel where the constriction happens. Fricative sounds can be used in all word positions, for the most part. Here are word examples with fricatives in word positions: *cheese, vest, scissors, fusions,* and *jester.* The /zh/ sound mostly occurs in the middle and ends of words, as in *vision* and *beige*; but this sound is not often used at the beginning of words in SAE.

Table 6.6.   Manner characteristic of Standard American English consonants

Manner type	Phonemes
Stops	/p/, /b/, /t/, /d/, /k/, /g/
Fricatives	/f/, /v/, /th/, /<u>th</u>/, /s/, /z/, /sh/, /zh/, /h/
Affricates	/ch/, /j/
Nasals	/m/, /n/, /ng/
Glides	/w/, /y/, /wh/
Liquids	/l/, /r/

The /h/ sound only exists before vowels as in *hand* and *behave* but not at the end of a word. Words with a letter *h* spelling at the end are part of a vowel grapheme, such as *weigh* or *high*; or the *h* spelling is part of a digraph (*sh, ch,* and *th*). Sometimes *h* is part of a **trigraph** (a three-letter pattern representing one sound) as in the word *watch* and *light*. Digraphs are spelling patterns needed to represent the 40-some speech sounds with an alphabet of 26 letters.

Affricates (/ch/ and /j/) are a combination of stop and fricative sounds. The /ch/ sound actually starts with a /t/ tongue placement and continues with a /sh/, and /j/ starts with a /d/ and continues with a /zh/ sound. Watch and feel your mouth as you say these sounds. Affricates sounds occur in all positions within a word, as in the words *church, catcher, judge,* and *major*.

Nasal sounds are produced with airflow going through the nose instead of the mouth. Put your finger on the bridge of your nose while saying the words *man* and *name*. You should feel your nose vibrate. Nasal sounds /m/ and /n/ occur in all word positions (initial, middle, and final). The /ng/ sound only occurs after a vowel, as in the word *ring, donkey,* and *jingle*. You can say nasal sounds for as long as your breath lasts.

The consonant glides /w/, /y/, and /wh/ only exist before vowels, as in the words *wait, yes,* and *which*. For words with spelling patterns such as *ow* in *snow* and *oy* in *boy*, the letters *w* and *y* are part of a vowel spelling. The /wh/ consonant glide sound is actually a /hw/ pronunciation. Try saying the word *whether* and *which* (by beginning these words with a /wh/ sound) differently from *weather* and *witch* (by beginning these words with /w/). These words may be said distinctly, and they can also be pronounced the same depending on "wh"–ether the /wh/ sound is used in contrast to /w/. The /wh/ sound is used more consistently in British English. In SAE, /wh/ is disappearing and may not be considered to be a phoneme in the future. This shift demonstrates the dynamic nature of oral language.

Liquid sounds, /l/ and /r/, are unique in that they are produced differently depending on their position in a word. These sounds are consonants at the beginning of a word or syllable and are vowel or vowel-like sounds at the end. To accommodate this difference, they are produced differently as consonants and vowels.

Look in the mirror and say the words *lob* and *ball*. Observe and feel your tongue movement. The /l/ in *lob* is produced with the tongue starting up behind the top front teeth and dropping down. The /l/ sound in *ball* is produced with the tongue starting down and moving up. The same movement pattern occurs with the /r/ sound in word beginnings as in *raw* and word endings as in *are*. The /r/ sound in *raw* is a consonant, produced with the tongue starting at the top of the mouth and dropping down. At the end of a word, /r/ is produced as a vowel with your tongue starting down and moving up. Beginning /l/ and /r/ sounds in a word or syllable are consonants. Word- or syllable-ending /l/ and /r/ sounds become vowels (e.g., *table, car, per, door*).

Another manner contrast is between short sounds and **continuant** sounds. Stop sounds and affricates are produced for a brief period of time. Continuant sounds, including fricatives, nasals, liquids, and glides, can be made in an extended manner. See how long you can say the consonant sounds in the following words: *sun, fish, lathe, swim*. Now see how long you can say the consonant sounds in these words: *bag, pick, get, chip*. The consonant sounds in the first group can be said for an extended time whereas those in the second group of words are short. Because continuant sounds can be held for a longer time, these sounds may be easier for young students to attend to and process, which is particularly important for phonemic awareness development.

Voicing Characteristic of Consonant Phonemes   The third consonant characteristic contrasts phonemes that are voiced (voice-on sounds) or voiceless (voice-off sounds). Voicing occurs in the larynx (voice box) as air from the lungs passes through the vocal folds, which open and close at a very rapid rate. This movement causes vibration resulting in voicing. Voiceless consonants are produced with air from the lungs passing through the larynx with the vocal folds open. Place your hand on your larynx in the front of your neck, say, and extend "aaaaah." Your voice is on, so you should feel vibration. All vowels are voiced. Say the vowel sounds, and feel your neck for the vibration caused by voicing.

Now, feel your larynx while you make the sound /sssssss/ for an extended time. When you say this sound, you should not feel any vibration because your voice is off. Table 6.7 lists the voiced and voiceless consonant sounds. Look at the columns in the shaded area and say the consonant phoneme pairs in each column. What pattern do you notice?

The pairs of consonant sounds (in the shaded area) are produced in the same place and in the same manner but differ in voicing. Say the /f/ sound while feeling your larynx and concentrating on where your lip is. Now say the /v/ sound. You should feel your lip do the same movement for both sounds, but the vibration is different. Try this with each voiced/voiceless pair. These pairs include stops, fricatives, and affricates. The consonant sounds in the unshaded area do not have the same voiced/voiceless pairing. The /h/ and /wh/ sounds are voiceless; and liquids, glides, and nasal phonemes are voiced.

These phoneme characteristics describe the properties of vowel and consonant sounds of SAE. The phonemes are the building blocks of words in oral language as well as of words in written language. Whether words are heard, said, read, or written, they are processed phonologically, every time. Having a deeper understanding of phoneme characteristics helps educators hone their own phonemic awareness. This knowledge facilitates assessment and instruction of literacy skills.

Phonemes in Written Language

The 44 phonemes of SAE are represented by 26 alphabet letters, creating an unbalanced match between sounds and letters. There are an estimated 250 graphemes for the English phonemes. Think of the different spellings for the /f/ sound (e.g., in the words *fish, phone, stuff,* and *rough*) or the /ī/ sound (e.g., in the words *hi, high, bye, my, bite, height, tie,* and *chai*). English has a deep orthographic written language system, using a variety of spelling or orthographic patterns to represent the phonemes of oral language. In contrast, Spanish has a transparent orthographic written language system, which has a much closer match for the number of phonemes and the letters used to represent the Spanish phonemes.

At the beginning of this section, you were asked to identify the number of phonemes in a series of words. Identify the number of phonemes in the words

Table 6.7.   Voicing characteristic of Standard American English consonants

Voiced	/b/	/v/	/<u>th</u>/	/d/	/z/	/zh/	/j/	/g/	/y/, /w/, /l/, /r/, /m/, /n/, /ng/
Voiceless	/p/	/f/	/th/	/t/	/s/	/sh/	/ch/	/k/	/h/, /wh/

Word	Phonemes	Number of sounds
mouse		
tacked		
knock		
taxed		
straw		
weigh		
dream		
notched		
brother		
quench		

Figure 6.7. Phonemic awareness skill recheck. (*Answers: mouse,* m – ou – se, 3; *tacked,* t – a – ck – /t/, 4; *knock,* kn – o – ck, 3; *taxed,* t – a -/k/ – /s/ – /t/, 5; *straw,* s – t – r – aw, 4; *weigh,* w – eigh, 2; *dream,* d – r – ea – m, 4; *notched,* n – o – tch – /t/, 4; *brother,* b – r – o – th – er, 5; *quench,* /k/ – /w/ – e – n – ch, 5.)

in Figure 6.7, and see if your understanding or ability to segment phonemes has changed as a result of this phoneme knowledge. Kudos to you if the task is easy. If the task is difficult, consider more practice opportunities to enhance your own skill development.

ASSESSING PHONEMIC AWARENESS

Important to the assessment process is an understanding of the developmental stages and age/grade expectations. Assessment of phonological and phonemic awareness entails a range of tasks and procedures, including the other phonological processing abilities of memory and naming. The skills being measured need to be predictive of literacy learning. An assessment procedure should include screening and progress monitoring, to ensure adequate growth of phonemic awareness skills, as well as a diagnostic component for students who are not developing at the expected rate. (For more on assessment in literacy instruction and **formative** and **summative data collection,** see Chapter 7.)

Screening and Progress Monitoring Procedures

The purpose of screening is to identify students who have developed expected skills to an established benchmark and, more important, those who have not. Students not meeting benchmark expectations may be at risk for experiencing difficulties in learning to read and write. Screening processes should be universal, in that all students are screened. These measures (**screeners**) should obtain relevant data in an efficient manner to provide an estimate of what students have learned related to an identified benchmark or expectation. The collected data needs to be useful for planning and implementing instruction based on what students need to learn.

Because of the predictive nature of early phonemic awareness, it is clear how important it is to screen for skill development in preschool and the early grades. Screening for higher level phonemic awareness manipulation skills in the later grades is also important to identify students who have not met expected literacy learning outcomes and then to plan and implement appropriate instruction and intervention.

Pre-Kindergarten to Kindergarten   The phonemic awareness and phonological processing skills that are strong predictors of later literacy learning should be included in the assessment process. At the end of preschool and beginning of kindergarten, initial-sound awareness is a strong predictor of later literacy learning (Catts et al., 2015; Foulin, 2005; Lonigan & Shanahan, 2008; NICHD, 2000). Along with phoneme segmentation, other skills to include early in kindergarten are the phonological processing skills of rapid automatic naming and nonword repetition tasks, as they are predictive of literacy at the end of first grade (Catts et al., 2015; Lonigan & Shanahan, 2008). As the kindergarten year progresses, the initial-sound task should expand to phoneme segmentation of simple CVC words and continued monitoring of RAN (Catts et al., 2015; Lonigan & Shanahan, 2008).

Kindergarten to First Grade   At the end of kindergarten and beginning of first grade, a screening procedure should include, at a minimum, phoneme segmentation of single-syllable words with consonant blends (e.g., words such as *black* and *rest*). This task is a common measure on many available screening tools. However, by the end of first grade, most students have achieved mastery of this skill.

The results of a screening task that is mastered by most students do not provide information about how students are learning more advanced skills and do not provide predictive information for the next level of development (Kilpatrick, 2015). For these reasons, screening during first grade should include higher level phoneme manipulation tasks (i.e., phoneme addition, deletion, and substitution), which have displayed a higher correlation with word-level reading than phoneme segmentation (Caravolas, Kessler, Hulme, & Snowling, 2005; Kilpatrick, 2015; Swank & Catts, 1994).

Young students who have had stimulating language environments and also have mild phonological core deficits may develop early and basic phonemic awareness skills and perform at an adequate level on screening measures in kindergarten and first grade. Often these students do not develop the advanced skills needed for continued literacy development, which will affect their continued growth in literacy learning. Including higher level manipulation tasks in a screening procedure will help to provide early identification so those students can be identified early and participate in appropriate instruction to help them build the foundation skills they need. This is a prevention strategy, helping students learn the skills that will facilitate their learning to read and write instead of waiting until they begin to struggle and experience failure.

Second Grade On   As a preventive measure, students in second grade should be screened for higher level phonemic awareness abilities (Kilpatrick, 2015). Measures should include deletion tasks (e.g., say *stop* without saying /s/) and substitution tasks (e.g., say *hat* but instead of /h/ say /ch/.) In addition, processing speed is an important indicator. Kilpatrick (2015) recommended that these tasks need to be timed informally and completed within 2 seconds to measure automaticity. These measures would not need to be re-administered for students who do well on an initial screening. However, any student displaying difficulty with reading or spelling should be screened for complex phonemic skills as well as other phonological processing abilities. For older students in middle and high school, a phoneme reversal task (e.g., switch the beginning and ending sounds in the word *cash* to get *shack,* or in the word *much* to get *chum*) appears to be more sensitive to reading challenges than a deletion task (Kilpatrick, 2015).

Progress Monitoring

Screening tools may serve to track growth of student learning using the same procedure at different points through the academic year (e.g., September, January, May). In addition, **progress monitoring assessment** is needed for students identified as not meeting learning expectations and who participate in specialized instruction to help them develop needed skills. Progress monitoring tasks are used after short intervals of instruction to measure students' learning and to determine the impact of the provided instruction. For example, suppose a small group of first-grade students were identified in the screening process as having underdeveloped phonemic awareness skills. They were not able to identify or isolate sounds in words to the expected level. So, their teacher had them participate in a specific phoneme awareness instruction program to teach them this task. After 2 weeks of instruction, their skill level was reassessed, using the same assessment procedure but with different words. The results provide data to see if their skills are improving and if the instruction is working. If their skills are improving, then instruction may be needed until their skill ability has developed to the expected level. If their skills are not improving, then a different type of instruction and further assessment may be needed.

Many schools, districts, and programs have an identified assessment process and schedule for obtaining student learning data. Ensuring that the predictive indicators, described previously, are included in the process is important.

Screening and Progress Monitoring Tools

A number of screening and progress monitoring tools are published and available. Some are for purchase, and others are open-source. The following is a partial listing of commonly used screening and progress monitoring tools that measure phonemic awareness development.

AIMSweb AIMSweb (Shinn & Shinn, 2002) is a universal screening, progress monitoring, and data management system for kindergarten through Grade 12. Specific to phonemic awareness is a phoneme segmentation task designed to be given in kindergarten (in winter and spring) and in first grade (in fall and winter). More information is available on the AIMSweb site at http://www.aimsweb.com.

Dynamic Indicators of Basic Early Literacy Skills Next Dynamic Indicators of Basic Early Literacy Skills (DIBELS) Next (Good & Kaminski, 2011) is a screening and progress monitoring assessment measuring literacy skills from kindergarten through sixth grade. The specific phonemic awareness measures include First Sound Fluency in kindergarten and Phoneme Segmentation Fluency in kindergarten and first grade. More information is available online on the DIBELS web site at https://dibels.org/dibelsnext.html.

My IGDIS (Individual Growth and Development Indicators) My IGDIS (McConnell, Bradfield, Wackerle-Hollman, & Rodriguez, 2013) is a screening and progress monitoring tool designed to measure early literacy skills in preschool-age children on their way to kindergarten. The indicators include a rhyming task, initial sound task, word-naming task, and letter–sound task. More information is available online on the MY IGDIS web site at https://www.myigdis.com/preschool-assessments/early-literacy-assessments/.

Phonological Awareness Literacy Screening   Phonological Awareness Literacy Screening (PALS) (Invernizzi, Meier, Swank, & Juel, 2004) includes a screening, progress monitoring, and diagnostic tool for measuring the fundamental components of literacy using three instruments, PALS-PreK, PALS-K and PALS 1–3 (used in Grades 1–8). The PALS-Pre-K measures beginning sound awareness, rhyme awareness and nursery rhyme awareness skills. The PALS-K continues with rhyme awareness and beginning sound awareness. The PALS 1–3 and an additional component, PALS Plus, are leveled instruments used in Grades 1–8 as a screener to identify students at risk of reading difficulties. Information about these tools is on the PALS web site at https://pals.virginia.edu/tools-1-3.html.

Phonological Awareness Screening Test   The Phonological Awareness Screening Test (PAST) (see Kilpatrick, 2015) is a screening tool that assesses basic phonological awareness skills at pre-kindergarten and kindergarten levels and advanced phonemic awareness skills in kindergarten, first, second, and late second grade to adult levels. This tool is adapted from the Rosner and Simon (1971) Auditory Analysis Test and based on the subsequent research. Information about obtaining this tool is in *Essentials of Assessing, Preventing, and Overcoming Reading Difficulties* (Kilpatrick, 2015).

Diagnostic Procedures and Available Tools

Any student demonstrating difficulty with word-level reading should have his or her phonological skills assessed, including phonological memory and phonological naming abilities. The following is a partial listing of available diagnostic tests specific to phonological and phonemic awareness development.

Assessment of Literacy and Language   The Assessment of Literacy and Language ALL (Lombardino, Lieberman, & Brown, 2005) is used to assess spoken and written language skills in pre-kindergarten through first grade. Subtests include listening comprehension, language comprehension, semantics, syntax, phonological awareness, alphabetic principle/phonics, and concepts about print.

Test of Preschool Early Literacy   The Test of Preschool Early Literacy (TOPEL) (Lonigan, Wagner, Torgesen, & Rashotte, 2007) is designed to identify 3- to 5-year-old preschoolers who are at risk for challenges with literacy learning. The Print Knowledge subtest includes alphabet knowledge and early knowledge about written language conventions and form. The Definitional Vocabulary subtest measures single-word oral vocabulary and definitional vocabulary (assessing both surface and deep vocabulary knowledge).

Phonological Awareness Test-2   The Phonological Awareness Test-2 (PAT-2) (Robinson & Salter, 2007) is a standardized assessment measuring a range of phonological awareness skills along with phoneme–grapheme correspondences and nonword phonetic decoding for students in kindergarten up to Grade 4. The phonological awareness measures include rhyming, segmentation, and blending (at syllable and phoneme levels); initial, medial, and final sound isolation within words; and sound substitution.

Comprehensive Test of Phonological Processing–2   The Comprehensive Test of Phonological Processing–2 (CTOPP-2) (Wagner, Torgesen, Rashotte, & Pearson, 2013) is used to identify phonological abilities of students ages 7–24 years in phonological memory, phonological naming, and phonological awareness. It may be used to document progress in phonological processing skills as a result of special intervention services over time.

Lindamood-Bell Auditory Conceptualization Test-3   The Lindamood-Bell Auditory Conceptualization Test–3 (LAC-3) (Lindamood & Lindamood, 2004) tasks include isolating phonemes, tracking (manipulating) phonemes, counting syllables, tracking syllables, and tracking syllables and phonemes.

Test of Integrated Language and Literacy Skills   The Test of Integrated Language and Literacy Skills (TILLS) (Nelson, Plante, Helm-Estabrooks, & Hotz, 2015) includes 15 measures to measure oral and written language skills in students ages 6–18 years. Specific to phonemic awareness, the tasks include isolation of single sounds within real and nonsense words and initial sound deletion in words. To measure phonological memory, forward and backward digit span tasks are used.

Other tools are available that assess other areas of the reading and writing processes. Inclusion of phonological processing abilities, especially phonological and phonemic tasks, is important to the diagnostic assessment process because the majority of struggling readers have a core phonological deficit.

INSTRUCTION IN PHONEMIC AWARENESS FOR PREVENTION AND INTERVENTION

Teaching phonemic awareness helps many students improve their reading ability, including those who have typically developing skills, those who are at risk of experiencing literacy difficulties, those who are diagnosed with a learning disability with impacts on reading and writing, and those learning English as another language, no matter the socioeconomic level (Kilpatrick, 2015; Lonigan & Shanahan, 2008; Melby-Lervåg et al., 2012; NICHD, 2000; Troia, 2014). Teaching phonemic awareness in combination with phonics instruction is proven to be the most effective instructional approach in helping students learn to read (Ball & Blachman, 1988; Kilpatrick, 2015; Lonigan & Shanahan, 2008; NICHD, 2000; Russell, Ukoumunne, Ryder, Golding, & Norwich, 2016; Shapiro & Solity, 2008; Shaywitz et al., 2004; Szabo, 2010). This type of improved phonemic awareness also enhances phonological memory and naming skills, which reciprocally contributes to phonemic awareness (Kerins, 2006; Krafnick et al., 2011; Torgesen et al., 2010; Vaughn et al., 2003; Vukovic & Siegel, 2006; Wolff, 2014).

Students will not benefit from phonics instruction until they have developed phonemic awareness skills; and some children, particularly those from households at lower socioeconomic levels and those learning English as another language, may need more intensive instruction in phonemic awareness (Juel, 1988). Teaching these skills early and sufficiently is important to prevent reading failure. Instruction should always be based on good assessment data. For older students who find reading and writing a challenge, teach phonemic awareness skills to more competent levels.

Tier 1 to Tier 2 Instruction and on to Tier 3 Intervention

Students in any classroom will possess differing levels of phonological skill development, so differentiated instruction will be needed. Framed within the response to instruction (RTI) approach, also called multi-tiered systems of supports (MTSS), Tier 1 core instruction includes prevention strategies used for all students. Students showing some difficulty in learning to read and write may need Tier 2 level instruction. Strategies used at this level may include more practice with phonemic awareness tasks, more explicit instruction, and instruction within a smaller group. Students who display a significant delay, or who have been diagnosed with a disability in the literacy area, may need intensive Tier 3 level intervention. This most intense level of instruction involves even smaller group sizes, increased time of instruction, and use of specially designed programs that provide more explicit, systematic, and sequenced instruction in the foundation skills within contextual activities, not isolated skill practice. Elements need to include integrated instruction in phonemic awareness, letter and word recognition and spelling, text comprehension and writing composition strategies. Compensation strategies, such as rehearsal and chunking of information, and self-regulation monitoring of learning are often also needed (Dehn, 2011).

Phonemic awareness in the early grades should be a regular Tier 1 instructional component in pre-kindergarten through first grade to ensure all students are developing these important foundation skills to support literacy learning. Students who are not meeting learning expectations at this level should be identified early and be provided with Tier 2 instruction and potentially Tier 3 intervention before these students experience further failure in learning to read and write.

Shapiro and Solity (2008) provided explicit and systematic phonemic awareness along with letter–sound instruction with kindergarten students from low socioeconomic status (SES) conditions and compared learning outcomes to students matched for SES and beginning skills in classrooms without explicit phonemic awareness instruction. They measured student literacy learning at the end of first grade and found that the number of students from the experimental group struggling with learning to read was 75% lower than the number of students in the comparison school. These findings illustrate the importance of providing phonemic instruction early to prevent or at least minimize the difficulty some students may have with literacy learning.

Letter name learning, when combined with letter–sound instruction, may causally affect students' letter–sound acquisition (Piasta & Wagner, 2010b). In the earliest grades, teaching phonemic awareness in an integrated manner with letter learning has the greatest impact on young students' literacy learning. Phonemic skills need to be taught in an explicit and systematic manner as an oral skill (without letters) and integrated with written language (with letters).

A concern in the early grades is young students' tendency to reverse letters or letter sequences when reading words or writing them. This difficulty is often attributed to visual processing. However, the underlying challenge is with the phoneme sequence, accurate phonological memory, and/or retrieval of words being read or written (Kilpatrick, 2015). Students with poor phonemic awareness do not have a clear recognition of the phonemes in spoken words, or their memory for sound sequences may not be well-established. As a result, they may read and/or spell words with sounds that are not present or that are in an incorrect sequence. From a prevention perspective, young students displaying these behaviors may need more instruction in phonemic awareness to help build these skills so their literacy is not further affected.

It is considerably more efficient and effective to deliver intervention earlier in elementary school rather than later. Later intervention is less effective and takes longer to obtain the desired learning outcomes. It takes four times as long to remediate a student with poor reading skills in fourth grade, compared to remediating in kindergarten or early first grade (Lyon & Fletcher, 2001).

Using planned activities to intentionally help children develop phonemic awareness skills in small group settings is an evidence-based strategy (Piasta & Wagner, 2010a). Children can be grouped by skill level so the teacher can provide the appropriate level and amount of instruction. Activities can absolutely be engaging, developmentally appropriate, and effective in helping young children develop the phonological foundations needed for successful literacy learning.

For students in need of Tier 2 or Tier 3 instruction, phonemic awareness and other phonological processing abilities need to be part of a comprehensive evaluation to determine strengths and areas of need. Students with core phonological deficits almost never develop complex phonemic awareness skills on their own (Kilpatrick, 2015). Students with working memory or naming deficits may need a more intensive level of instruction than students who do not display difficulty in these areas (Al Otaiba & Fuchs, 2006; Stage, Abbott, Jenkins, & Berninger, 2003). Students with phonological processing deficits in memory and naming are often "treatment resistors" (Torgesen, 2000) and in need of more intensive intervention, often at a Tier 3 level. They can learn to sound out words accurately, but they do not develop a large sight-word vocabulary for instant access. Fluent reading becomes a major struggle for them, which then affects comprehension (Perfetti & Hart, 2002; Seymour, 2008; Staels & Van den Broeck, 2015; Van den Broeck & Geuden, 2012; Ziegler & Goswami, 2005).

Curriculum Supports   A scope and sequence of phonological and phonemic awareness skill development and instruction are included in many early learning and literacy curricula. Most programs have a focus on early and basic levels of phonological and phonemic awareness skill development. However, programs guiding instruction of complex phonemic awareness skills are not as prevalent.

Some programs have more explicit instructional strategies than others, and some attend to skill development in a more sequential manner than others. Teachers' strong background knowledge of these sequences helps in determining which curriculum is appropriate for their students. Enhanced background knowledge and understanding contributes to more skillful assessing, planning, and implementing of evidence-based instruction for students in their care, particularly when a program is less sequential, less systematic, or less explicit. Instruction should be based on children's skill level and focus on the next steps in their learning sequence.

A number of resources are available to teachers who need to supplement a program that is already in place. These may provide an evidence-based approach and guidance for teachers as needed. Examples of available programs are listed at the end of this section.

A casual search on the Internet will provide a plethora of resources for phonemic awareness descriptions and activities to develop these skills. A word of caution is to vet sites for appropriateness and accuracy within the evidence provided by the scientific research. Here are a few valuable web site links. The Florida Center for Reading Research has a wide range of phonological and phonemic awareness activities and resources for teachers. The activities are organized by task and grade level. The web site link is http://www.fcrr.org/FAIR_Search_Tool. The PALS web site (described in the assessment section) also has a variety of basic phonemic aware-ness activities across a range of grade levels. These are available on the PALS Activi-ties page at https://pals.virginia.edu/tools-activities.html. Another general site with valuable information is the Reading Rockets site: http://www.readingrockets.org. This web site in particular is designed for educators as well as families.

Instructional Considerations   In planning focused phonemic awareness les-sons at any tier, one must consider a number of factors such as the task difficulty (e. g., segmenting, blending, deletion, substitution, reversals), the linguistic level (e.g., syllables, onsets, phonemes), and the linguistic characteristics of the stimulus words (e.g., word length, words with consonant blends, phoneme types such as continuant sounds vs. stop sounds). Tasks within an activity may be modified and made simpler to increase student success rate, and they can be more complex to extend student learning. Here are a few hints:

- Say each syllable or sound in 1-second intervals. Decrease the time interval to make the task easier as needed, and use longer pauses to create more of a challenge.

- Say consonant sounds in words in isolation (without adding /uh/). For exam-ple, say /h/ - /ă/ - /t/, not /huh/ - /ă/ - /tuh/, which is actually "huhatuh").

- Initial sounds are easier to isolate than final sounds, and middle sounds are the hardest.

- Words with consonant blends are more difficult than those with single consonants.

Teaching of phonemic skills should include initial teacher modeling (I Do), followed by guided and prompted practice (We Do), and then opportunities for independent task performance with teacher monitoring (You Do). Practice oppor-tunities should include high levels of accuracy (minimum of 90%–95%) for strong skill development. This routine provides opportunity to monitor student growth and progress as well as for accommodations to instruction.

Including multisensory components (auditory, kinesthetic, and visual) in instructional routines helps students make deeper connections and contribute to their accuracy and success. Here are some of the ways to include these multisen-sory components.

Auditory   Have students repeat the words, syllables, or phonemes that are part of an activity or instruction. For example, when having students segment the syllables or sounds in a word, have them say the whole word first, segment the parts, then say the whole word again. When matching or producing rhymes, have students repeat the word or words. This approach helps students to hold the word in their phonological memory and taps into the phonological representation (inner speech) of the words.

Kinesthetic   When participating in segmenting activities of any type, pro-vide a consistent kinesthetic movement for the task. For syllables, tap the left hand on the right arm, moving upward in a sequence of wrist, elbow, shoulder, head—depending on how many syllables are in a particular word. For example, in segmenting the word *table,* tap one hand on the other wrist and elbow for the two syllables; for the word *utensil,* tap one hand on the other wrist, elbow, and shoulder for three syllables; and for the name *Elizabeth,* tap one hand on the other wrist, elbow, and shoulder and then the head. For longer words, continue across to the other shoulder and on down to the hip and knee, as needed. Another strategy is to place your fingers under your chin to feel your jaw movement made when saying the syllables in multisyllabic words.

For phonemes, tap an index finger of one hand on the fingers of the other hand—pointer, middle, ring, pinkie, and thumb (depending on the number of phonemes in the word) while segmenting the sounds in a word. Another strategy is to move an arm in an up/down motion while extending a finger on the same hand for each phoneme in the word, beginning with the pointer for the first sound, middle finger for the second sound, and ring finger for the third sound, followed by the pinkie and thumb, as needed. For longer words, the fingerspelling gestures of sign language or fingers on the other hand can be used. Both of these strategies provide clues to the number of sounds in a particular word.

Visual When appropriate, provide picture supports for words to reduce the burden on phonological memory, leaving more brain energy available for the phonological or phonemic task. For example, having pictures for matching or producing rhyming words helps support phonologic memory. When segmenting words, a picture may help to keep the word active and present. When having students blend words, the teacher may hold a picture out of sight from the students while segmenting the word parts; then, following the students' blended response, the teacher shows them the picture to confirm the word.

REFLECT, CONNECT, and RESPOND

Why is including a multisensory approach when teaching phonemic awareness a valuable strategy to support students' learning? Select a phonemic awareness task, and provide an example of an auditory, kinesthetic, and visual cue that could be used in teaching this skill.

Sequences of Instruction Phonemic awareness instruction needs to be a core element of Tier 1 instruction in preschool and kindergarten and continuing into first grade (NICHD, 2000). Instruction should include rhyming and word play with syllables and phonemes embedded into everyday routines and planned activities. Embedded word play is a valuable strategy; however, this approach should be supplemental to, and not replace, intentional instruction. Any student displaying difficulty with letter learning and/or word reading may need Tier 2 and possibly Tier 3 instruction.

In the later grades, the instant and effortless access to the phonological aspects of reading unfamiliar words in connected text requires a greater degree of phonemic proficiency (Kilpatrick, 2015). Tier 1 instruction may include a short routine with quick high-level manipulation tasks. Tier 2 instruction and Tier 3 intervention are needed for students not making adequate progress. Just as in the early stages of learning to read, phonemic awareness facilitates skill development. Growth in reading proficiency is facilitated by complex phonemic awareness. There is a reciprocal effect, with improved skill in one area facilitating development in the other. Teaching advanced phonemic awareness skills has a positive impact on literacy development (Kilpatrick, 2015).

Rhyming Instruction

Instruction in rhyming can be provided from preschool through second grade and beyond as follows.

Preschool and Kindergarten Rhyming has been a long-standing component in early childhood education. General activities include singing songs, reciting finger-plays, and reading books with a focus on rhyming. During these routines, intentionally point out words that sound the same at the end. In small groups, have children participate in rhyming games and activities. These experiences provide opportunities for young children to learn about rhyme as well as providing occasions to monitor their developing skills.

In planned activities, model, by thinking aloud, how to produce rhyming words. When having students think of a word that rhymes, you might follow this sequence:

- **I Do:** Say, "I wonder what rhymes with *boat*. Let's try *coat*. *Boat–coat*, do those rhyme, sound the same at the end?" In this way, you provide an opportunity for students to detect if words rhyme and also guide them in producing rhyming words.

- **We Do:** Say, "Your turn, what word rhymes with *sock*?" Provide guidance and support as needed along with feedback for student performance.

- **You Do:** Provide students with opportunities to create rhymes while you monitor their performance.

Include nonsense words when producing words that rhyme, and talk about whether a nonsense word has a meaning or not. This strategy has a focus on rhyme as well as a focus on vocabulary knowledge. It creates a metalinguistic focus on word meaning and structure.

Embedding rhyme into everyday routines is also valuable. Here are some examples:

- Change the beginning sound in students' names to create a rhyme (e.g., *Terry–Berry, Chris–Fris, Jaylon–Chaylon*).

- When giving directions, change familiar words with a rhyming one. Tell the children to line up at the door to go to the "bribary" instead of library or to put on their "zoat" and "pittens" to get ready for "decess."

- Play an I Spy game having the children find an object that rhymes with a rhyming word you provide. Say, "I see something that rhymes with *bear*"; the children can find hair or a chair.

These examples provide opportunities for students to detect and produce rhymes. They also provide an opportunity to meet students at their level of learning.

Kindergarten to First Grade At this level, students should be able to produce a string of rhyming words. Provide opportunities to practice producing rhyming words. Here are some examples:

- Change words to begin with a particular sound corresponding to letter patterns being taught (e.g., *Merry, Mris, Maylon*).

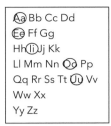

Figure 6.8. ABC eye chart for rhyming words.

- Use an alphabet chart (see Figure 6.8) with the vowels signaled (circled, covered, or somehow designated) and have students give a rhyming word as you point to a particular letter. This example uses the "ABC Eye Chart" activity (Paulson, Noble, Jepson, & van den Pol, 2001) in which the letters are arranged in the pattern of the alphabet song.

- Make a chart using word patterns that are part of the phonics lessons being learned. Create a string of rhyming words based on the letter pattern. The example in Figure 6.9 creates words and nonwords for the -*at* family progressing through the alphabet.

It is easy to see how activities building phonemic awareness and word reading support each other.

Second Grade and Beyond As students continue to progress in their literacy learning, rhyming can be incorporated into writing tasks using poetry and other literary structures. Spelling patterns for rhyming words can be compared to help students see the similarities and differences among the many grapheme patterns in English (e.g., *boat, coat, note, vote* or *play, they, weigh*).

REFLECT, CONNECT, and RESPOND
Why is intentionally teaching phonemic awareness in the early grades a strategy for preventing and/or minimizing literacy learning difficulties?

-at	
bat	nat
cat	pat
dat	rat
fat	sat
gat	tat
hat	vat
jat	wat
kat	yat
lat	zat
mat	

Figure 6.9. Word family rhyming.

Segmenting and Blending Instruction

Instruction in segmenting and blending can be provided from preschool through second grade and beyond as follows.

Preschool and Kindergarten   Along with intentional lessons teaching phonological and phonemic awareness in explicit, sequenced, and systematic manner, teachers have many ways to embed syllable and sound play in everyday routines and activities. All of these strategies need to be developmentally appropriate. Remember to consider children's level of development along the linguistic hierarchy. For preschool children to succeed in playing with phonemes, they may need more teacher support and so will children displaying difficulty with phonemic awareness learning. Here are some examples of helpful instructional activities:

- Segment and blend students' names while taking attendance, first by the syllables, then with a focus on initial sounds, followed by a focus on ending sounds.

- Have children say new vocabulary words by segmenting and blending the syllables to help them establish a phonological representation for the words and make more connections to deepen their learning.

- When giving directions, use "robot reporting" (e.g., "To – day – we – are – go – ing – to – the – li – bra – ry.") (Paulson et al., 2001).

- Compare picture pairs, using a balance scale and counters, to see which word "weighs more" according to its number of syllables or phonemes (Paulson et al., 2001). For example, a picture of a kangaroo will have three counters (representing its three syllables), in contrast to a picture of a donkey with two counters (for two syllables). The word *kangaroo* "weighs" more than *donkey*.

- Play an I Spy game by segmenting the word for an object or picture for children to identify by blending the word segments at their developmental level. For example, say, "I spy a *blan – ket*." Then, have them take turns segmenting a word for a partner to blend.

- Sort objects by beginning sounds. Have children think of words that begin with a particular sound.

- Segment the onset–rime in CVC words for children to blend together while holding a picture of an object from their view. Do the same activity with a focus on the final sounds in single-syllable words. When children are successful at this level, try the middle sound of CVC words. As their skills progress, go to the next level by including CCVC and CVCC words.

- Find pictures and cut them into "picture puzzles" (see Figure 6.10) based in syllables, initial sound, and individual phonemes (Paulson et al., 2001). Have the students find the pieces for the puzzle pictures and segment and blend the word segments. Letters on the pictures provide a connection to the spelling patterns for the sounds and syllables in the words.

- Use **Elkonin boxes** to tap a finger or place chips in designated boxes to match the number of syllables in words. Figure 6.11 depicts an example for the words *arrow, triangle,* and *diamond.*

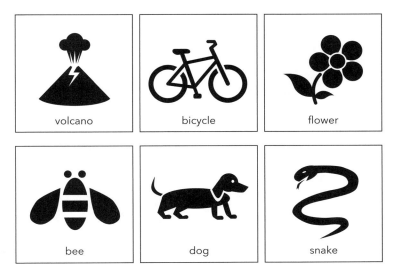

Figure 6.10. Picture puzzles.

Many of these activities may or may not also include corresponding letters, depending on the learning outcome. For students at this developmental level, including letters leads to better overall literacy learning (Ball & Blachman, 1988). A good balance of activities focusing on phonemes and others that combine letters and sounds helps young children make important learning connections.

Kindergarten to First Grade   At this level, learning outcomes focus on phonemes in progressively more complex words. Early developing syllable awareness skills should be in place. There are many activities to provide opportunities for students to deepen their phonemic awareness skills.

- Have students sort a series of pictures with single-syllable words into piles with the same number of sounds (e.g., 2: *b − ee, c − ow*; 3: *p − i − g, g − oa − t*; 4: *f − r − o − g, w − o − l − f*).

- Use Elkonin boxes to match the number of phonemes in single-syllable words (see Figure 6.12). Here is an example for the words *moon, sun,* and *cloud.* Students may use their finger to tap the boxes or place chips in boxes appropriate for the segment length.

- Use a string of boxes for a variety of word lengths for a say-it-move-it activity (see Figure 6.13). Provide a word for students. Have them say the word,

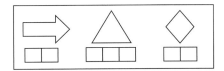

Figure 6.11.   Elkonin boxes for syllables.

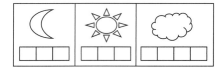

Figure 6.12. Elkonin boxes for phonemes.

segment the phonemes and move a chip into a box for each sound, then blend the sounds together to say the complete word again. As an extended and connected activity to print, students also may write the word in a row below the chips for a say-it-move-it-write-it activity.

As with the preschool and kindergarten levels, students should be provided with activities that include letters and, more importantly, activities that do not include letters. Phoneme-to-grapheme as well as grapheme-to-phoneme sequences are important competencies for students. Including letters helps young students see the connection between sounds and print. However, students need to be able to isolate sounds in words without the use or support of letters.

Second Grade and Beyond By the beginning of second grade, students should have well-developed basic phonemic awareness skills. If not, they should absolutely receive a comprehensive phonological processing assessment to determine the areas of need. Phonemic awareness activities for these students should not include letters. The letter cues may provide a context for the phonemes in words and hinder students' ability to identify and isolate the phonemes, apart from the letters, needed to develop more competent phonemic awareness skills. Techniques for teaching older students basic skills need to be appropriate for their age in word choice and context. Using adult terminology, such as *phoneme deletion* and *morphemic structure,* is an example of a suitable adaptation.

Higher Level Manipulation Tasks

Instruction in higher level phonemic manipulation tasks can be provided from preschool through second grade and beyond as follows.

Preschool and Kindergarten These tasks in the earliest grades will need teacher support for student success. Activities may be embedded into everyday routines as well. Have children complete a word said without a sound. A teacher might say, "Help me finish this word. You can ride a bi___" (/k/, *bike*) or "Meow, says the ca ___" (/t/, *cat*) or "The apple is ___ ed" (/r/, *red*). Focus on a structured

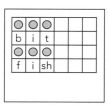

Figure 6.13. Say-it-move-it-write-it activity.

rhyme production activity by having the children provide a rhyming word that begins with a particular sound (e.g. "Tell me a word that rhymes with *kite* that begins with /s/.")

Kindergarten to First Grade Students in these grades should develop basic phoneme segmenting and blending skills and progress to more complex tasks. Here are some teaching examples.

- Extend a say-it-move-it activity into a sound substitution task. This task may involve an activity called **chaining** in which a phoneme in a word changes in a string of words. Provide a few colored chips (in a minimum of four different colors) for each student and give them a CVC word. Have them select a different colored chip for each sound in the word. Then, have them change the colored chip to represent a new word. For example, a chain at the initial word position might be, "Say *hat* and change the /h/ to /k/ to get *cat*, change the /k/ to /p/ to get *pat*, change the /p/ to /r/ to get *rat*," or, "Say *rake* and change the /r/ to /t/ to get *take*, change the /t/ to /l/ to get *lake*, change /l/ to /b/ to get *bake*." Chains with a beginning-sound focus look a lot like rhyming and illustrate how producing rhyming words is actually a higher level manipulation task. Chains with a focus on beginning sounds are easier than those with a focus on sounds in other word positions.

- Complete ending sound chains, which are a bit more difficult than beginning sounds (e.g., "Say *mat* and change the /t/ to /n/ to get *man*; change the /n/ to /s/; change the /s/ to /p/; change /p/ to /d/"; this chain results in *mass–map–mad*).

- Continue to medial-position chains, which most often change the vowel sound (e.g., "Say *bet* and change /ĕ/ to /ē/ to /ă/ to /ĭ/ to /ŭ/"; this chain results in *beet–bat–bit–but*). This position tends to be more difficult than final word positions.

- Chains with phonemic changes in a variety of positions are the most challenging. Figure 6.14 shows an example of such a chain beginning with the word *tap*.

- Extend this activity and have students write the letters that represent each word.

- Focus on morphemes being learned in a reading and spelling context by adding them to words (e.g., see how many words students can make by adding *un-* to get *unhappy*, *undo*, and *unless*).

Second Grade and Beyond Complex phonemic awareness can be developed to help students develop deeper literacy skills. These skills may be useful

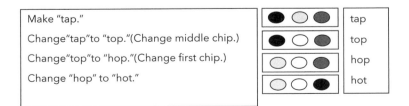

Figure 6.14. Word chain activity.

in learning spelling patterns and for reading longer multisyllabic words. Here are some examples:

- Emphasize morphemes, prefixes, roots, and suffixes in words like *fine, define, refine, confine, finest, fines,* and *fined.* Morpheme addition and substitution combines areas within word study and helps make connections for students.

- For short phoneme tune-ups using reversal tasks, have students say a single-syllable CVC word and switch the first and last consonant sounds (e.g., *tap* becomes *pat, sub* becomes *bus, tick* becomes *kit, teach* becomes *cheat*). Have students think of words that follow the pattern of reversing the beginning and ending consonant sounds to make other words.

- Teach a Pig Latin task requiring students to remove a beginning sound, move it to the end of the word and add the *-ay* syllable (e.g., *lock* becomes /ŏk/ - /lā/, *job* becomes /ŏb/ - /jā/).

Activities for older students may be purely phonological (able to be done with one's eyes closed) and may be tied to print as well, depending on the learning goal. Activities to create words and write them can be very effective in honing phonemic awareness skills, resulting in better literacy learning.

Programs for Teaching Phonemic Awareness

Educational researchers now have an unequivocal understanding of how phonemic awareness and other phonological processing abilities contribute to children's learning to read and write. This understanding has led to a proliferation of published programs and online resources with a focus on phonemic awareness. Many of the programs are designed to provide explicit, sequenced, and systematic instruction facilitating phonemic awareness learning. The following is a listing of some of these programs organized for younger to older students, for instruction ranging from general classroom instruction to intensive intervention.

Tier 1 Programs   *Ladders to Literacy: A Kindergarten Activity Book* (O'Connor, Notari-Syverson, & Vadasy, 2005) is an activity-based curriculum designed to teach print awareness, phonological awareness skills, and oral language skills across the kindergarten year.

Phonemic Awareness (Heggerty, 2004) is a program with levels for pre-kindergarten, kindergarten, Grades 1–3, and English learners, designed for whole-group instruction with daily lessons. Each lesson includes 10 skills: letter naming, rhyming, onset fluency, blending, identifying final and/or medial sounds, segmenting, adding phonemes, deleting phonemes, substituting phonemes, and language awareness.

Phonemic Awareness in Young Children: A Classroom Curriculum (Adams, Foorman, Lundberg, & Beeler, 1998) is a pre-reading program of simple to more advanced activities in rhyming, alliteration, and segmentation, organized in a developmental sequence in 15- to 20- minute lessons through the school year to boost young students' phonemic awareness skills.

Reading Readiness (Neuhaus Education Center, 1992) is a literacy instructional framework designed for kindergarten and may also be used for targeted instruction in first and second grade. Explicit routines focus on phonological awareness, letter recognition, the alphabetic principle, sight-word recognition, oral language, and listening comprehension. More information is available at the Neuhaus Education Center at https://www.neuhaus.org.

Road to the Code: A Phonological Awareness Program for Young Children (Blachman, Ball, Black, & Tangel, 2000) is a teacher's guide for a series of 44 activities in an 11-week sequence for small-group or individual instruction in kindergarten and first grade. Although the program was designed for students in need of extra instruction, it can be used in any classroom of beginning readers. Each lesson includes three activities, including phoneme segmentation, letter name and sound instruction, and phonological awareness practice, using a variety of games, songs, and read-alouds.

Tier 1 to Tier 2 Programs *Phonological Awareness Training for Reading, Second Edition* (Torgesen & Bryant, 2013), is designed to increase the level of phonological awareness in at-risk students in kindergarten and first or second grade having difficulties learning to read. The program teaches rhyming with a focused attention to sounds in words, blending individual sounds to make words, segmenting sounds in words, followed by using letters to represent phonemes in reading and spelling. The program is appropriate for small groups or individuals with lessons three to four times a week over a 12- to 14-week period.

Fundations: Wilson Language Basics for K–3, a component of the Wilson Language Training programs, is a series of multisensory and structured language programs designed for Tier 1 and early intervention in Tier 2 with explicit and systematic instruction for kindergarten through Grade 3. A range of interconnected skills, including phonemic blending and segmenting, phonics and word study, reading fluency, vocabulary, comprehension, handwriting, and spelling, are emphasized.

SPELL-Links to Reading & Writing (Wasowicz, Apel, Masterson, & Whitney, 2004) is a word-study curriculum designed to teach all aspects of literacy in reading, writing, spelling, speaking, listening, and vocabulary for students at all grade levels. Instruction may be used for Tier 1 core instruction as well as at Tier 2 and 3 levels for students with identified learning challenges affecting literacy, including speech-language impairment and dyslexia, as well as students learning English.

Tier 2 and Tier 3 Programs The *Lindamood Phoneme Sequencing Program (LiPS)* (Lindamood & Lindamood, 1998) is designed to develop oral-motor, visual, and auditory feedback that helps students learn to identify, count, and sequence phonemes in syllables and words. This program provides more intensive instruction than a traditional phonics program and has been used in Tiers 2 and 3 effectively for students struggling with learning to read and write.

Wilson Reading System (Wilson, 1996) is a Tier 3 program designed for students in Grades 2–12 and adults who are not making sufficient progress or who require more intensive instruction due to a language-based learning disability or dyslexia. The lessons are 45–90 minutes in length, taught 2–5 times per week for individuals or in small-group settings.

REFLECT, CONNECT, and RESPOND

Reflect on your own phonemic awareness skills. What insights have you made about your phonological processing skills and your ability to manipulate phonemes in words?

CLOSING THOUGHTS: PHONEMIC AWARENESS AND LITERACY

Phonemic awareness, along with phonological memory and phonological naming, provides access to sound structures in words needed for listening, speaking, reading, and writing. Phonological skills begin to develop in infancy and continue well into the elementary grades. Skill progression follows the linguistic hierarchy with early and basic phonemic awareness and develops into complex manipulation.

Because of the predictive nature of phonological skills and phonemic awareness across the early childhood years, screening and progress monitoring of phonemic awareness skill attainment and growth is an important aspect of an assessment procedure in preschool into the primary grades. Learning standards provide a guide for skill expectations up to first grade, and continued skill development of complex phonemic awareness furthers literacy learning. Students who are able to play with and manipulate the sounds and syllables of words are generally successful literacy learners. Some students do not develop these skills. For them, the leading cause of difficulty learning to read and write is a core deficit in the phonological system.

Teaching early and basic phonemic awareness in the earliest grades is effective in helping all young students build a strong foundation to prevent learning challenges with reading and writing. When literacy learning is a challenge, instruction and intervention is most likely needed to help students develop a better ability to play with and manipulate the sound structures of words. Explicit, sequenced, and systematic instruction has proven to be the most effective in helping students develop these skills—at any age. It is also never too late to learn phonemic awareness skills.

A strong understanding of the *ph* terms and interconnections as well as being able to accurately complete phonemic awareness tasks are important competencies for effective instruction. At the beginning of this chapter, you rated your understanding of the terms connected to phonemic awareness. Return to Figure 6.1, and see how your understanding has deepened. Consider your own phonemic awareness skill ability. This knowledge and enhanced skills will make an important difference for the students in your care.

ONLINE COMPANION MATERIALS

The following Chapter 6 resources are available at http://www.brookespublishing .com/birshcarreker/materials:

- Reflect, Connect, and Respond Questions

- Appendix 6.1: Technology Resources

- Appendix 6.2: Knowledge and Skill Assessment Answer Key

KNOWLEDGE AND SKILL ASSESSMENT

1. What is a typical developmental sequence of phonological awareness?

   a. Syllable segmentation, initial sound isolation, sound segmentation of single-syllable words, and sound deletion.

b. Sound deletion, sound segmentation of single-syllable words, syllable segmentation, and initial sound isolation.

c. Initial sound isolation, sound segmentation of single-syllable words, sound deletion, and syllable segmentation.

d. Syllable segmentation, sound deletion, initial sound isolation, and sound segmentation of single-syllable words.

2. What is the phonemic awareness skill expectation for students leaving first grade, according to state standards?

a. Isolate and identify the phonemes in CCVC words

b. Produce a string of three rhyming words

c. Decode single-syllable words

d. Identify final consonant sounds

3. For children entering kindergarten, what phonemic awareness skill is a strong predictive indicator of later literacy learning in the primary grades?

a. Phoneme segmentation of single-syllable words

b. Deletion of phonemes

c. Production of rhyming words

d. Initial phoneme isolation and identification

4. Alliteration can be connected to which step on the linguistic hierarchy?

a. Words in sentences

b. Onset–rime

c. Phonemes

d. Syllables

5. Which pair of words has four sounds each?

a. Fish, chat

b. Eight, though

c. Box, queen

d. Comb, talk

6. Which phonemic awareness task should be included in a screening assessment for kindergarten students?

a. A phoneme-reversal task of two-syllable words

b. A syllable-blending task of familiar words

c. A phoneme-segmenting task of single-syllable words

d. A deletion task of final consonant sounds

7.   A screening tool for older students should measure which phonemic aware-
      ness skills?

      a.   Syllable segmenting and blending

      b.   Rhyme matching and production

      c.   Phoneme segmenting and blending

      d.   Phoneme deletion and substitution

8.   What is the impact on student learning when phonemic awareness instruction
      is included in the early grades?

      a.   More students experience success learning to read and write.

      b.   Fewer students will need higher levels of literacy instruction.

      c.   More students will achieve expected literacy learning outcomes.

      d.   All of the above.

REFERENCES

Adams, M.J. (1990). *Beginning to read, thinking and learning about print*. Cambridge, MA: MIT
   Press.
Adams, M.J. (2013). *ABC foundations for young children: A classroom curriculum*. Baltimore, MD:
   Paul H. Brookes Publishing Co.
Adams, M.J., Foorman, B.R., Lundberg, I., & Beeler, T. (1998). *Phonemic awareness in young
   children: A classroom curriculum*. Baltimore, MD: Paul H. Brookes Publishing Co.
Al Otaiba, S., & Fuchs, D. (2006). Who are the young children for whom best practices in
   reading are ineffective? An experimental and longitudinal study. *Journal of Learning Dis-
   abilities, 39*(5), 414–431.
Anthony, J.L., & Francis, D.J. (2005). Development of phonological awareness. *Current Directions in Psychological Science, 14*(5), 255–259.
Anthony, J.L., Lonigan, C.J., Burgess, S.R., Driscoll, K., Phillips, B.M., & Cantor, B.G. (2002).
   Structure of preschool phonological sensitivity: Overlapping sensitivity to rhyme, words,
   syllables, and phonemes. *Journal of Experimental Child Psychology, 82*(1), 65–92.
Anthony, J.L., Lonigan, C.J., Driscoll, K., Phillips, B.M., & Burgess, S.R. (2003). Phonological sensitivity: A quasi-parallel progression of word structure units and cognitive operations. *Reading Research Quarterly, 38*(4), 470–487.
Ashby, J., Dix, H., Bontrager, M., Dey, R., & Archer, A. (2013). Phonemic awareness contributes to text reading fluency: Evidence from eye movements. *School Psychology Review,
   42*(2), 157.
Baddeley, A., Gathercole, S., & Papagno, C. (1998). The phonological loop as a language
   learning device. *Psychological Review, 105*(1), 158.
Ball, E.W., & Blachman, B.A. (1988). Phoneme segmentation training: Effect on reading readiness. *Annals of Dyslexia, 38*(1), 208–225.
Bauman-Waengler, J. (2009). *Introduction to phonetics and phonology: From concepts to transcription*. Boston, MA: Pearson.
Birch, S.L. (2016). Prevalence and profile of phonological and surface subgroups in college
   students with a history of reading disability. *Journal of Learning Disabilities, 49*(4), 339–353.
Blachman, B.A., Ball, E.W., Black, R., & Tangel, D.M. (2000). *Road to the code: A phonological
   awareness program for young children*. Baltimore, MD: Paul H. Brookes Publishing Co.
Bruck, M. (1992). Persistence of dyslexics' phonological awareness deficits. *Developmental
   Psychology, 28*(5), 874.
Caravolas, M., Kessler, B., Hulme, C., & Snowling, M. (2005). Effects of orthographic consistency, frequency, and letter knowledge on children's vowel spelling development. *Journal
   of Experimental Child Psychology, 92*(4), 307–321.
Catts, H.W., Nielsen, D.C., Bridges, M.S., Liu, Y.S., & Bontempo, D.E. (2015). Early identification of reading disabilities within an RTI framework. *Journal of Learning Disabilities, 48*(3),
   281–297.

de Groot, B.J., van den Bos, K.P., Minnaert, A.E., & van der Meulen, B.F. (2015). Phonological processing and word reading in typically developing and reading disabled children: Severity matters. *Scientific Studies of Reading, 19*(2), 166–181.

de Jong, P.F. (2011). What discrete and serial rapid automatized naming can reveal about reading. *Scientific Studies of Reading, 15*(4), 314–337.

de Jong, P.F., & van der Leij, A. (2002). Effects of phonological abilities and linguistic comprehension on the development of reading. *Scientific Studies of Reading, 6*(1), 51–77.

DeBruin-Parecki, A., & Slutzky, C. (2016). Exploring pre-k age 4 learning standards and their role in early childhood education: research and policy implications. *ETS Research Report Series*.

Dehaene, S. (2009). *Reading in the brain: The new science of how we read.* New York, NY: Penguin.

Dehn, M.J. (2011). *Working memory and academic learning: Assessment and intervention.* Hoboken, NJ: John Wiley & Sons.

Ehri, L.C. (2014). Orthographic mapping in the acquisition of sight word reading, spelling memory, and vocabulary learning. *Scientific Studies of Reading, 18*(1), 5–21.

Elbro, C., Borstrøm, I., & Petersen, D.K. (1998). Predicting dyslexia from kindergarten: The importance of distinctness of phonological representations of lexical items. *Reading Research Quarterly, 33*(1), 36–60.

Elbro, C., & Jensen, M.N. (2005). Quality of phonological representations, verbal learning, and phoneme awareness in dyslexic and normal readers. *Scandinavian Journal of Psychology, 46*(4), 375–384.

Foulin, J.N. (2005). Why is letter-name knowledge such a good predictor of learning to read? *Reading and Writing, 18*(2), 129–155.

Fox, B., & Routh, D.K. (1976). Phonemic analysis and synthesis as word-attack skills. *Journal of Educational Psychology, 68*(1), 70.

Fox, B., & Routh, D.K. (1983). Reading disability, phonemic analysis, and dysphonetic spelling: A follow-up study. *Journal of Clinical Child & Adolescent Psychology, 12*(1), 28–32.

Gathercole, S.E., & Adams, A.M. (1993). Phonological working memory in very young children. *Developmental Psychology, 29*(4), 770.

Gillon, G.T. (2004). *Phonological awareness: From research to practice.* New York, NY: Guilford.

Gombert, J.E. (1992). *Metalinguistic development.* Chicago, IL: University of Chicago Press.

Good, R.H., & Kaminski, R.A. (2011). *DIBELS next assessment manual.* Eugene, OR: Dynamic Measurement Group.

Goswami, U. (2000). Phonological representations, reading development and dyslexia: Towards a cross-linguistic theoretical framework. *Dyslexia, 6*(2), 133–151.

Goswami, U., Mead, N., Fosker, T., Huss, M., Barnes, L., & Leong, V. (2013). Impaired perception of syllable stress in children with dyslexia: a longitudinal study. *Journal of Memory and Language, 69*(1), 1–17.

Greenberg, D., Ehri, L.C., & Perin, D. (1997). Are word-reading processes the same or different in adult literacy students and third–fifth graders matched for reading level? *Journal of Educational Psychology, 89*(2), 262.

Guttorm, T.K., Leppänen, P.H., Poikkeus, A.M., Eklund, K.M., Lyytinen, P., & Lyytinen, H. (2005). Brain event-related potentials (ERPs) measured at birth predict later language development in children with and without familial risk for dyslexia. *Cortex, 41*(3), 291–303.

Heggerty, M. (2004). *Phonemic awareness: The skills that they need to help them succeed.* River Forest, IL: Literacy Resources.

International Dyslexia Association, The. (2018, March). *Knowledge and practice standards for teachers of reading.* Retrieved from https://dyslexiaida.org/knowledge-and-practices/

Invernizzi, M., Meier, J., Swank, L., & Juel, C. (2004). *PALS: Phonological awareness literacy screening.* Charlottesville: University of Virginia.

Juel, C. (1988). Learning to read and write: A longitudinal study of 54 children from first through fourth grades. *Journal of Educational Psychology, 80*(4), 437.

Juel, C., Griffith, P.L., & Gough, P.B. (1986). Acquisition of literacy: A longitudinal study of children in first and second grade. *Journal of Educational Psychology, 78*(4), 243.

Kerins, M. (2006). The effects of systematic reading instruction on three classifications of readers. *Literacy Research and Instruction, 45*(3), 243–260.

Kilpatrick, D.A. (2012). Phonological segmentation assessment is not enough: A comparison of three phonological awareness tests with first and second graders. *Canadian Journal of School Psychology, 27*(2), 150–165.

Kilpatrick, D.A. (2015). *Essentials of assessing, preventing, and overcoming reading difficulties.* Hoboken, NJ: John Wiley & Sons.

Krafnick, A.J., Flowers, D.L., Napoliello, E.M., & Eden, G.F. (2011). Gray matter volume changes following reading intervention in dyslexic children. *Neuroimage, 57*(3), 733–741.

Lervåg, A., & Hulme, C. (2009). Rapid automatized naming (RAN) taps a mechanism that places constraints on the development of early reading fluency. *Psychological Science, 20*(8), 1040–1048.

Lindamood, P.C., & Lindamood, P. (1998). *The Lindamood phoneme sequencing program for reading, spelling, and speech: lips: Teacher's manual for the classroom and clinic.* Austin, TX: PRO-ED.

Lindamood, P.C., & Lindamood, P. (2004). *Lindamood Auditory Conceptualization Test: Examiner's manual.* Austin, TX: PRO-ED.

Lombardino, L.J., Lieberman, R.J., & Brown, J.J. (2005). *ALL: Assessment of literacy and language.* New York, NY: PsychCorp.

Lonigan, C.J. (2006). Development, assessment, and promotion of preliteracy skills. *Early Education and Development, 17*(1), 91–114.

Lonigan, C.J., Burgess, S.R., Anthony, J.L., & Barker, T.A. (1998). Development of phonological sensitivity in 2-to 5-year-old children. *Journal of Educational Psychology, 90*(2), 294.

Lonigan, C.J., & Shanahan, T. (2008). Developing early literacy: Report of the national early literacy panel. Executive summary. A scientific synthesis of early literacy development and implications for intervention. *National Institute for Literacy.*

Lonigan, C.J., Wagner, R.K., Torgesen, J.K., & Rashotte, C.A. (2007). *Test of Preschool Early Literacy.* Austin, TX: PRO-ED.

Lyon, G.R. (1995). Toward a definition of dyslexia. *Annals of Dyslexia, 45*(1), 1–27.

Lyon, G.R., & Fletcher, J.M. (2001). Early identification, prevention and early intervention for children at-risk for reading failure. *Publication of the Council for Basic Education.*

MacLean, M., Bryant, P., & Bradley, L. (1987). Rhymes, nursery rhymes, and reading in early childhood. *Merrill-Palmer Quarterly, 33,* 255–282.

Mahmoudzadeh, M., Dehaene-Lambertz, G., Fournier, M., Kongolo, G., Goudjil, S., Dubois, J. & Wallois, F. (2013). Syllabic discrimination in premature human infants prior to complete formation of cortical layers. *Proceedings of the National Academy of Sciences, 110*(12), 4846–4851.

McConnell, S., Bradfield, T., Wackerle-Hollman, A., & Rodriguez, M. (2013). *My IGDIs of Early Literacy.* Minneapolis: Regents of the University of Minnesota, Early Learning Labs.

Melby-Lervåg, M., Lyster, S.A.H., & Hulme, C. (2012). Phonological skills and their role in learning to read: A meta-analytic review. *Psychological Bulletin, 138*(2), 322–352.

Metsala, J.L., & Walley, A.C. (1998). Spoken vocabulary growth and the segmental restructuring of lexical representations: Precursors to phonemic awareness and early reading ability. In J.L. Metsala & L.C. Ehri (Eds.), *Word recognition in beginning literacy* (pp. 89–120). Mahwah, NJ: Lawrence Erlbaum Associates.

Morais, J. (1991). Constraints on the development of phonemic awareness. *Phonological Processes in Literacy: A Tribute to Isabelle Y. Liberman,* 5–27.

National Governors Association Center for Best Practices, Council of Chief State School Officers (2010). *Common Core State Standards for English language arts and literacy in history/social studies, science, and technical subjects.* Washington, DC: Author.

National Institute of Child Health and Human Development (NICHD). (2000). *Report of the National Reading Panel: Reports of the subgroups. Teaching children to read: An evidence-based assessment of the scientific research literature on reading and its implications for reading instruction* (NIH Publication No. 00-4754). Washington, DC: Government Printing Office.

Nelson, N., Plante, E., Helm-Estabrooks, N., & Hotz, G. (2015). *Test of Integrated Language and Literacy Skills™ (TILLS™).* Baltimore, MD: Paul H. Brookes Publishing Co.

Neuhaus Education Center (1992). *Reading readiness.* Bellaire, TX: Author.

O'Connor, R.E., Notari-Syverson, A., & Vadasy, P.F. (2005). *Ladders to literacy: A kindergarten activity book.* Baltimore, MD: Paul H. Brookes Publishing Co.

Papadopoulos, T.C., Kendeou, P., & Spanoudis, G. (2012). Investigating the factor structure and measurement invariance of phonological abilities in a sufficiently transparent language. *Journal of Educational Psychology, 104*(2), 321.

Paulson, L.H., Noble, L.A., Jepson, S., & van den Pol, R. (2001). *Building early literacy and language skills: A resource and activity guide for preschool and kindergarten.* Longmont, CO: Sopris West.

Perfetti, C.A., Beck, I., Bell, L.C., & Hughes, C. (1987). Phonemic knowledge and learning to read are reciprocal: A longitudinal study of first grade children. *Merrill-Palmer Quarterly, 1982,* 283–319.

Perfetti, C.A., & Hart, L. (2002). The lexical quality hypothesis. In L. Verhoeven. C. Elbro, & P. Reitsma (Eds.), *Precursors of functional literacy* (pp. 189–213). Philadelphia, PA: John Benjamins.

Piasta, S.B., & Wagner, R.K. (2010a). Developing early literacy skills: A meta-analysis of alphabet learning and instruction. *Reading Research Quarterly, 45*(1), 8–38.

Piasta, S.B., & Wagner, R.K. (2010b). Learning letter names and sounds: Effects of instruction, letter type, and phonological processing skill. *Journal of Experimental Child Psychology, 105*(4), 324–344.

Plomin, R. (2013). Child development and molecular genetics: 14 years later. *Child Development, 84*(1), 104–120.

Robinson, C., & Salter, W. (2007). *Phonological Awareness Test 2 (PAT-2).* Austin, TX: Linguisystems.

Roman, A.A., Kirby, J.R., Parrila, R.K., Wade-Woolley, L., & Deacon, S.H. (2009). Toward a comprehensive view of the skills involved in word reading in Grades 4, 6, and 8. *Journal of Experimental Child Psychology, 102*(1), 96–113.

Rosner, J., & Simon, D.P. (1971). The auditory analysis test: An initial report. *Journal of Learning disabilities, 4*(7), 384–392.

Russell, G., Ukoumunne, O.C., Ryder, D., Golding, J., & Norwich, B. (2016). Predictors of word-reading ability in 7-year-olds: Analysis of data from a UK cohort study. *Journal of Research in Reading.* doi:10.1111/1467-9817.12087

Rvachew, S., & Grawburg, M. (2006). Correlates of phonological awareness in preschoolers with speech sound disorders. *Journal of Speech, Language, and Hearing Research, 49*(1), 74–87.

Sauval, K., Perre, L., & Casalis, S. (2016). Phonological contribution during visual word recognition in child readers. An intermodal priming study in grades 3 and 5. *Journal of Research in Reading.*

Savage, R., Blair, R., & Rvachew, S. (2006). Rimes are not necessarily favored by prereaders: Evidence from meta-and epilinguistic phonological tasks. *Journal of Experimental Child Psychology, 94*(3), 183–205.

Seymour, P.H. (2008). Continuity and discontinuity in the development of single-word reading: theoretical speculations. In E.L. Grigorenko & A.J. Waples (Eds.), *Single-word reading: Behavioral and biological perspectives* (pp. 1–24). Florence, KY: Psychology Press.

Shapiro, L.R., & Solity, J. (2008). Delivering phonological and phonics training within whole-class teaching. *British Journal of Educational Psychology, 78*(4), 597–620.

Share, D.L., & Stanovich, K.E. (1995). Cognitive processes in early reading development: Accommodating individual differences into a model of acquisition. *Issues in Education, 1*(1), 1–57.

Shaywitz, S.E. (2003). *Overcoming dyslexia: A new and complete science-based program for reading problems at any level.* New York, NY: Alfred A. Knoff.

Shaywitz, B.A., Shaywitz, S.E., Blachman, B.A., Pugh, K.R., Fulbright, R.K., Skudlarski, P., . . . Fletcher, J.M. (2004). Development of left occipitotemporal systems for skilled reading in children after a phonologically-based intervention. *Biological Psychiatry, 55*(9), 926–933.

Shinn, M.M., & Shinn, M.R. (2002). *AIMSweb training workbook: Administration and scoring of reading curriculum-based measurement (R-CBM) for use in general outcome measurement.* Eden Prairie, MN: Edformation.

Sousa, D.A. (2011). *How the brain learns.* Thousand Oaks, CA: Corwin.

Staels, E., & Van den Broeck, W. (2015). Orthographic learning and the role of text-to-speech software in Dutch disabled readers. *Journal of Learning Disabilities, 48*(1), 39–50.

Stage, S.A., Abbott, R.D., Jenkins, J.R., & Berninger, V.W. (2003). Predicting response to early reading intervention from verbal IQ, reading-related language abilities, attention ratings, and verbal IQ—word reading discrepancy: Failure to validate discrepancy method. *Journal of Learning Disabilities, 36*(1), 24–33.

Stanovich, K.E., & Siegel, L.S. (1994). Phenotypic performance profile of children with reading disabilities: A regression-based test of the phonological-core variable-difference model. *Journal of Educational Psychology, 86*(1), 24.

Sutherland, D., & Gillon, G.T. (2005). Assessment of phonological representations in children with speech impairment. *Language, Speech, and Hearing Services in Schools, 36*(4), 294–307.

Swan, D., & Goswami, U. (1997). Phonological awareness deficits in developmental dyslexia and the phonological representations hypothesis. *Journal of Experimental Child Psychology, 66*(1), 18–41.

Swank, L.K., & Catts, H.W. (1994). Phonological awareness and written word decoding. *Language, Speech, and Hearing Services in Schools, 25*(1), 9–14.

Szabo, S. (2010). Older children need phonemic awareness instruction, too. *TESOL Journal, 1*(1), 130–141.

Torgesen, J.K. (2000). Individual differences in response to early interventions in reading: The lingering problem of treatment resisters. *Learning Disabilities Research & Practice, 15*(1), 55–64.

Torgesen, J.K., & Bryant, B.R. (2013). *Phonological awareness training for reading* (2nd ed.). Austin, TX: PRO-ED.

Torgesen, J.K., Wagner, R.K., & Rashotte, C.A. (1994). Longitudinal studies of phonological processing and reading. *Journal of Learning Disabilities*.

Torgesen, J.K., Wagner, R.K., Rashotte, C.A., Herron, J., & Lindamood, P. (2010). Computer-assisted instruction to prevent early reading difficulties in students at risk for dyslexia: Outcomes from two instructional approaches. *Annals of Dyslexia, 60*(1), 40–56.

Troia, G. (2014). Current evidence and future directions. In *Handbook of language and literacy: Development and disorders* (2nd ed.). New York, NY: Guilford.

Truch, S. (1994). Stimulating basic reading processes using auditory discrimination in depth. *Annals of Dyslexia, 44*(1), 60–80.

Vaessen, A., & Blomert, L. (2010). Long-term cognitive dynamics of fluent reading development. *Journal of Experimental Child Psychology, 105*(3), 213–231.

Van den Broeck, W., & Geudens, A. (2012). Old and new ways to study characteristics of reading disability: The case of the nonword-reading deficit. *Cognitive Psychology, 65*(3), 414–456.

van Goch, M.M., McQueen, J.M., & Verhoeven, L. (2014). Learning phonologically specific new words fosters rhyme awareness in Dutch preliterate children. *Scientific Studies of Reading, 18*(3), 155–172.

Vandewalle, E., Boets, B., Ghesquière, P., & Zink, I. (2012). Development of phonological processing skills in children with specific language impairment with and without literacy delay: A 3-year longitudinal study. *Journal of Speech, Language, and Hearing Research, 55*(4), 1053–1067.

Vaughn, S., Linan-Thompson, S., & Hickman, P. (2003). Response to instruction as a means of identifying students with reading/learning disabilities. *Exceptional Children, 69*(4), 391–409.

Vukovic, R.K., & Siegel, L.S. (2006). The double-deficit hypothesis: A comprehensive analysis of the evidence. *Journal of Learning Disabilities, 39*(1), 25–47.

Wagner, R.K., & Torgesen, J.K. (1987). The nature of phonological processing and its causal role in the acquisition of reading skills. *Psychological Bulletin, 101*(2), 192.

Wagner, R.K., Torgesen, J.K., & Rashotte, C.A. (1994). Development of reading-related phonological processing abilities: New evidence of bidirectional causality from a latent variable longitudinal study. *Developmental Psychology, 30*(1), 73.

Wagner, R.K., Torgesen, J.K., & Rashotte, C.A. (1999). *CTOPP: Comprehensive test of phonological processing*. Austin, TX: PRO-ED.

Wagner, R.K., Torgesen, J.K., Rashotte, C.A., Hecht, S.A., Barker, T.A., Burgess, S.R., . . . Garon, T. (1997). Changing relations between phonological processing abilities and word-level reading as children develop from beginning to skilled readers: A 5-year longitudinal study. *Developmental Psychology, 33*(3), 468.

Wagner, R.K., Torgesen, J.K., Rashotte, C.A., & Pearson, N.A. (2013). *Comprehensive Test of Phonological Processing: CTOPP2*. Austin, TX: PRO-ED.

Wasowicz, J., Apel, K., Masterson, J.J., & Whitney, A. (2004). *SPELL-Links to reading and writing*. Evanston, IL: Learning By Design.

Whitehurst, G.J., & Lonigan, C.J. (2002). Emergent literacy: Development from prereaders to readers. In S.B. Neuman & D.K. Dickinson (Eds.), *Handbook of early literacy research* (pp. 11–29). New York, NY: Guilford.

Wilson, A.M., & Lesaux, N.K. (2001). Persistence of phonological processing deficits in college students with dyslexia who have age-appropriate reading skills. *Journal of Learning Disabilities, 34*(5), 394–400.

Wilson, B.A. (1996). *Wilson Reading System.* Oxford, MA: Wilson Language Training Corp.

Wolf, M., & Stoodley, C.J. (2008). *Proust and the squid: The story and science of the reading brain.* Cambridge, United Kingdom: Icon.

Wolff, U. (2014). RAN as a predictor of reading skills, and vice versa: Results from a randomized reading intervention. *Annals of Dyslexia, 64*(2), 151–165.

Ziegler, J.C., & Goswami, U. (2005). Reading acquisition, developmental dyslexia, and skilled reading across languages: A psycholinguistic grain size theory. *Psychological Bulletin, 131*(1), 3.

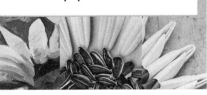

Appendix 6.1

Technology Resources

Elaine A. Cheesman

Effective programs/apps have the following features:

- They emphasize the sounds of spoken language (syllables, onset–rime, phonemes).

- They provide practice in blending phonemes to make words (supports reading) or segmenting oral words into phonemes (supports spelling).

- They do not require knowledge of letter names but can incorporate some letters into the activities.

PROGRAMS/APPS

ABC Reading Magic series   http://www.preschoolu.com

This program provides practice blending oral words presented as photographs. It has four levels:

Reading 1: CVC words

Reading 2: CCVC and CVCC

Reading 3: Two-syllable words

Reading 4: "Phonograms" Digraphs, Vowel-r, and vowel team syllables in one- and two-syllable words

Reading 5: Vowel-Consonant-Silent-e words

ABC Spelling Magic series   http://www.preschoolu.com

This program provides practice segmenting oral words presented as photographs. It has five levels:

Spelling 1: CVC words

Spelling 2: CCVC and CVCC

Spelling 3: Two-syllable words

Spelling 4: Vowel-Consonant-Silent-e words

Blending SE and TE (Student/Teacher Edition)   http://store.95percentgroup
.com

> This program provides oral, explicit, step-by-step sound-blending instruction
> and practice and systematic practice to distinguish between spoken words that
> are pronounced with pauses between sounds—/f/ /i/ /g/—or sounds together—
> /fig/—to reading several whole words. It reinforces concepts taught by the par-
> ent or teacher using 95% Group Teacher's Guidebook, "Teaching Blending from
> /k/ /ă/ /t/ to /cat/ in 8 Stages."

Beginning Sounds Interactive Game   http://www.lakeshorelearning.com

> This program helps children categorize first sounds using three picture prompts.
> It has an engaging arcade game format.

Partners in Rhyme   http://www.preschoolu.com

> This program helps children practice recognizing rhyme in spoken words using
> four interactive games. The use of an adult voice makes this appropriate for
> learners of all ages.

WEB SITES: MATERIALS AND
ACTIVITIES FOR TEACHERS AND LEARNERS

Florida Center for Reading Research   http://www.fcrr.org

> This web site has thousands of downloadable "Center" activities in all five com-
> ponents of reading: phonemic awareness, phonics, fluency, vocabulary, and
> comprehension. It also has research and resources for teachers.

Beginning Reading/Literacy Skills

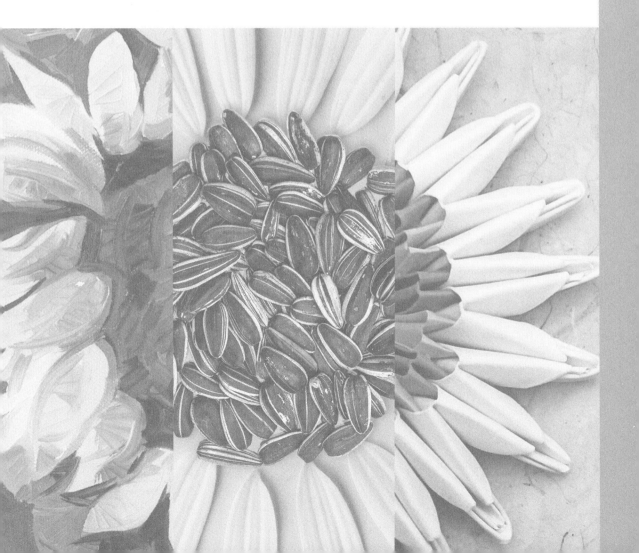

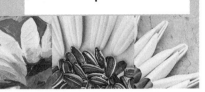

Chapter 7

Assessment of Reading Skills

A Review of Select Key Ideas and Best Practices

Larry E. Hess and Eileen S. Marzola

LEARNING OBJECTIVES

1. To understand foundational concepts underlying effective design and use of assessments (e.g., reliability, validity, norms and norming procedures, ethics, limitations of assessments)

2. To describe and distinguish among different types of assessments and the purposes thereof (e.g., formative and summative, screeners and progress monitoring tests), including their uses within a response to intervention framework

3. To identify specific standardized assessments used to measure component literacy skills (e.g., phonological processing, word identification, comprehension) and choose assessments appropriate to a given instructional purpose

4. To identify common pitfalls in interpreting assessment data and apply this knowledge when interpreting test results and communicating about these results to others

5. To describe the purposes of nonstandardized and formative assessments in literacy instruction, including multisensory language programs

Assessment involves an organized and methodical way of obtaining samples of a student's learning, thinking, and achieving. The obtained data can be used to guide decisions about appropriate placement as well as specific interventions. Assessments can inform in various ways both the teaching of reading and the related educational planning for students with reading difficulties, including those with co-morbid problems such as language disorders, weak self- esteem, or attention-deficit/hyperactivity disorder (ADHD). This chapter reviews some important considerations for teachers to keep in mind regarding best practices in the assessment of reading skills, and it includes much of the information recommended in the International Dyslexia Association's (2018) *Knowledge and Practice Standards for Teachers of Reading*. The chapter focuses on some basic concepts that pre-service teachers and students of teaching, as well as practicing teachers, clinicians, and administrators, should know about the assessment of reading, especially as it pertains to best practices for teaching. Throughout, we highlight

The authors wish to thank David Kilpatrick, Ph.D., for his comments on an earlier version of this chapter. The views expressed herein remain solely those of the authors.

recommendations for best practices in assessment. Given the scope of the chapter, and the complexity of the topic, we do not delve into the normal and pathological development of reading. For solid reviews, please see Kilpatrick (2015) and Seidenberg (2017).

BASIC MEASUREMENT CONCEPTS AND STATISTICS FOR STANDARDIZED ASSESSMENT

Much of this chapter is devoted to discussion of best practices for standardized assessment in reading. To understand fully these best practices and their underlying rationales, it is important to grasp fundamental theoretical concepts pertaining to assessment: reliability, validity, norms and norming procedures, and ethics.

Reliability and Validity

Assessment often results in numerical scores, and the production of accurate and meaningful numbers requires careful test construction. The creation of a test involves specific mathematical procedures and use of certain concepts, such as reliability and validity. Our overview does not review such concepts in depth, but interested readers can refer to Anastasi and Urbina, 1997; Overton, 2011; Sattler and Hoge, 2006; or Strauss, Sherman, and Spreen, 2006.

Assessments come in various forms. **Standardized assessment** involves the use of reliable and valid tests, which are created painstakingly over long periods, with much study and by using established methods. **Reliability** refers to the consistencies of the following: 1) the test results across individuals administering it; 2) results between various forms of the test; 3) the test items to each other; and, 4) results on retesting (usually for a short period, to avoid changes in what is being measured). Such consistency is important because a poorly constructed test may have scores that vary wildly between test administrations for no reason (e.g., low test–retest reliability). With low reliability, it becomes less clear that a test result changed due to growth in the student, as opposed to reflecting a quality of the test itself.

Reliability places a cap on validity in that a test must be reliable to be valid. Test results that vary randomly across raters or between administrations of the measure cannot be meaningful. **Validity** refers to the meaning that can be assigned to a test result. Validity can be explored by various research methods by the test manufacturer and by others who study the test after its publication. For example, researchers can see whether individuals with certain difficulties, such as dyslexia, tend to perform less well on the test and whether the test scores correlate with previous, relatively established tests. It is important to keep in mind that some measures may have just **face validity.** This type of validity is merely the appearance of measuring an aspect or of having meaning: the test looks as if it must be measuring reading comprehension, for example, so one assumes that is what it is doing. However, it is possible for a test to appear valid without being reliable or valid. Unreliable and invalid tests are published, or mislabeled, not necessarily intentionally, as reliable and valid. Strictly speaking, only a specific administration of a test can be considered valid or invalid (meaningful or not meaningful) because something may occur during the test session that invalidates the administration at that time. For example, the test might have been administered in a noisy environment or with an observer present, when the test was designed for use in quiet environments with only the examiner and student in the room. Test instructions may have been paraphrased; doing so can change test results (Lee, Reynolds, & Willson, 2003).

Norms

When standardized tests are made, they are administered to groups of carefully selected individuals. For the best-made tests for use in the United States, the characteristics of the subjects in the normative sample will usually match the U.S. Census, and the subjects will be selected from throughout the country, from a mix of public, parochial, and independent schools. The results of these tests then lead to tables or software wherein one can convert the raw scores into standardized scores and percentile ranks. Standardized scores measure qualities, such as decoding ability, in equally spaced units.

Norms for frequently used standardized tests, such as the Woodcock-Johnson IV (Mather & Jaffe, 2016), are usually national, which allows for comparison to a stable reference base. Some standardized group-administered tests, such as those frequently used annually in schools, provide both public and independent school norms. Interested school staff, with help from a statistician, could create their own local norms for some of these measures. These local norms would not allow disability determination, which should be based on national norms (see Strauss et al., 2006). Local norms could provide valuable comparisons to other students within the same program. For local results, school staff could also just rank the raw scores from highest to lowest, or determine the mean or most common (modal) performances. Some schools with difficult curricula might be tempted to use grade-based norms for students older than the ones taking the test, but this practice is not advisable because it produces misleading numbers. Local norms or measures of central tendency would be better in such a case.

Some tests are **co-normed**. This means that when the test was created, it was administered to the same students along with one or more other tests so that results can be more productively compared without the variability that is introduced by using different samples. When comparing results across samples used in different tests, one must wonder if the score differences are due to differences between the students' skills or between the samples. Frequently used examples of co-normed tests include the Woodcock-Johnson IV (WJ-IV) Tests of Cognitive Abilities (Schrank, McGrew, & Mather, 2014) co-normed with the WJ-IV Tests of Achievement (Schrank, Mather, & McGrew, 2014a) and the WJ-IV Tests of Oral Language (Schrank, Mather, & McGrew, 2014b), or the Wechsler Intelligence Scale for Children–Fifth Edition (WISC-V; Wechsler, 2014) co-normed with the WIAT-III (Wechsler, 2009). One can, with co-normed measures, see how frequently discrepancies occurred based on actual performances of students who were administered the test during its construction. For example, with the Woodcock-Johnson IV, one could determine how students with a certain level of functioning with oral language tended to perform on academic measures. This information can help examiners see whether a child is achieving at a level that other children with similar levels of oral language functioning were able to achieve. If the child is not achieving to that level, then perhaps the teaching approach needs to be strategically altered. In our opinion, comparisons between Full Scale IQ and reading achievement also can be informative to see whether a student with reading comprehension problems, for instance, might have generally weaker cognitive skills.

Ethics

Evaluators should be familiar with standards in the field for the ethical use of assessments, such as the *Standards for Educational and Psychological Testing* (2014), developed jointly by the American Educational Research Association (AERA), the American Psychological Association (APA), and the National Council on Measurement in Education (NCME; 2014). Among other aspects, ethical practice includes the use of nondiscriminatory tests, confidentiality of test materials and of students' results, familiarity with states' laws and guidelines regarding who can use which tests for which purposes in which settings, and the use of valid and reliable measures. There is tremendous variability across states in terms of laws and regulations that apply to assessment. Most test manuals present a section on user qualifications. For full details, please see the standards (AERA, APA, & NCME, 2014).

> ### REFLECT, CONNECT, and RESPOND
> Explain in your own words what it means to say a given assessment has validity. What is the difference between face validity and validity? Give an example of a test that has validity and one that has face validity.

OVERVIEW: TYPES OF ASSESSMENT

Assessments come in many forms, varying with the types of scores and information they produce, as well as the purposes to which they are put and the settings in which they are commonly used. For example, standardized tests involve the same test being given to everyone in a set manner, with very specific directions, format, scoring, and interpretation, usually delineated in a test manual (Overton, 2011). An example might be a driving test. All who take this test undergo the same procedure (unless they are receiving test accommodations). Nonstandardized measures, in contrast, involve different tests being given to different students. The students receive different conditions and essentially different evaluations. Standardized tests can be used for high-stakes purposes, as with the ACT or SAT. However, nonstandardized assessments can be used for high-stakes purposes as well, such as an oral exam to defend one's dissertation. Both standardized and nonstandardized (but usually standardized) measures can be used to screen students for various purposes. Their basic purpose is to sort students efficiently but accurately into different groups. For example, all students may not take a comprehensive assessment that lasts hours and hours, but they might receive screening to determine if further assessment is necessary. Another form of assessment involves progress monitoring and serial assessment to investigate mathematically or not how a student has progressed. Finally, assessment tools play an important role (along with history taking, clinical judgment, and so forth) in the diagnosis of learning disorders such as dyslexia. All of these types of assessments and their subtypes are detailed next. First, however, it is important to note the possible misuse of assessment by warning against common pitfalls that appear too regularly in practice.

INTERPRETING RESULTS: SOME COMMON PITFALLS TO AVOID

Caldwell and Leslie (2009), Kilpatrick (2015), Reutzel and Cooter (2011), Mascolo, Alfonso, and Flanagan (2014), Mather and Jaffe (2016), and Vannest, Stroud, and Reynolds (2011) presented (mostly empirically based) recommendations related to comprehension, fluency, rate, prosody, and reading motivation. For example, one might find that a student has a sparse vocabulary, which affects his or her reading comprehension, so strategies for development of lexicon may be performed. A student might be weak with making inferences, which implies the need for modeling of inferential thinking. As Kilpatrick pointed out,

> Because the available tests are not always ideally suited for assessing the various components of reading, the best reading assessment tool is the evaluator's knowledge of research on reading acquisition and reading difficulties. The commercially available assessments are simply tools. (2015, p. 151)

There are some myths and pitfalls to avoid when using these tools. One myth states that a 22-point difference between two standard scores (e.g., Full Scale IQ score and a reading score) is significant, but this is not true. The significance of the difference between standard scores should be determined by using the statistical tables provided by the test manufacturer, not by this 22-point rule of thumb (McGrew, 2011).

Speaking of difference, it is also common to look for scatter in the scores that one receives, particularly a large test battery. **Scatter** refers to the range and uneven alignment of scores, and it is actually very common, especially in large test batteries (Palmer, Boone, Less, & Wohl, 1998; Sattler & Hoge, 2006). Scatter also can come from using tests that were created in different years that use different normative samples (Sattler & Hoge, 2006). It is important to consider the possible sources of the scatter or of low scores and whether associated weaknesses appear in daily life. In other words, assessment is not just a statistical approach using test scores but a process that links together the student's history and other sources of information with the obtained test scores. Whenever possible, scores of interest should be followed up with further examination using related tests. For example, a student might obtain a high or low score on a reading assessment due to chance factors such as fatigue, recent contact with some of the background knowledge for a reading comprehension test, coincidental familiarity with some of the words because they were just on a spelling test, or lack of rapport with the examiner.

For reasons such as these, important decisions should not be made based on one score, although measures of similar constructs can still result in different scores, for reasons that need to be considered (Bracken, 1988). This is a vital point in assessment that too often becomes overlooked. A low score for an important cause should be followed up with a similar test, to make sure the low score is not a statistical fluke due to something besides weak ability in the measured area, and a composite score with greater reliability could be made. Different reading comprehension measures can produce different results (Keenan & Meenan, 2014). The same applies to phonemic processing measures such as the Comprehensive Test of Phonological Processing, Second Edition (CTOPP-2; Wagner, Torgesen, Rashotte, & Pearson, 2013). A weak result on a part of the CTOPP-2 (or any test) does not necessarily imply difficulty with the skill the test measures. The weak score could come from other results. Thus, a similar test should be given on a different day to confirm the result, which also should be checked against the student's history.

Subtest scores can vary widely, and composite scores vary less so. It is a best practice, when the individual assessed receives a low score to follow up on a different day with a similar test from a different battery (Kilpatrick, 2015; Sattler & Hoge, 2006). This method helps to make sure that the result was not just due to measurement error. If the correlation between the tests is known, then one can create a more reliable composite score based on the two tests (Schneider, 2013). Software is available to make such composites and to determine the significance of score differences, such as the Cross-Battery Assessment Software System, also known as X-BASS (available at http://www.wiley.com/WileyCDA/Section/id-829676.html and described in Flanagan, Ortiz, & Alfonso, 2013). The psychologist Joel Schneider, Ph.D., also has free spreadsheets and software available online for various **psychometric assessment** purposes at http://my.ilstu.edu/~wjschne/AssessingPsyche/AssessingPsycheSoftware.html. Use of such systems usually requires advanced training in psychometrics.

The likelihood of scores being similar depends largely on the correlation between the tests. Tests with higher correlations between them will more often be similar than ones with lower correlations. For well-made tests with similar normative samples and tasks, as well as strong correlations between them, the scores are often impressively close. The correlations between tests are often very high. For example, the WJ-IV Reading composite score correlates with the WIAT-III (Wechsler, 2009) Total Reading composite at 0.93.

The individual giving a test and the individual teaching the student should be different to avoid teaching toward the test, even unconsciously. For example, a reading teacher who also gives the Dynamic Indicators of Basic Early Literacy Skills (DIBELS; Good & Kaminski, 2002) might emphasize word endings that will appear on the next administration, even without fully intending to do so. Teaching to the test interferes with the interpretation of its scores (its validity).

Percentile ranks are commonly misunderstood. There are different spaces between them, so scores closer to the mean will require a greater distance between them for significance, as opposed to ones further from the mean. Percentile ranks close to the mean can look far apart but be close. Percentile ranks far from the mean can look close but in fact remain far apart. For example, going from a standard score of 138 to 148 could be a meaningful difference, but the percentile rank increases from only 99.0 to 99.9. Closer to the mean, going from a standard score of 102 to 103 is meaningless, but the percentile ranks jump from 55 to 58. Percentile ranks can help parents in particular to grasp basic ideas in that one can say that a student scored better than a certain percentage of other students of the same age or grade.

Also worth noting is that a certain observed result does not always imply a particular problem (Lezak, Howieson, Bigler, & Tranel, 2012). Technically stated, there are no pathognomonic signs in psychology. This means that, for example, weak reading does not necessarily mean that the individual has dyslexia because the person might have lack of opportunities, generally weak language, or intellectual disability.

Another potential pitfall is that although grade and age equivalents may seem intuitive, they are misleading, and many experts advise against even reporting them. Sattler and Hoge (2006) listed several difficulties associated with them. These included unequal spaces between the scores, an uneven correspondence to norm-referenced scores, and that fact that a minor change in raw scores can lead to large movements in the grade-equivalence scores. Grade- and age-equivalent scores can make it appear that a student has improved by, say, two grade levels in 12 months when in fact he or she is falling further behind peers when standardized scores are used. For older students, grade-equivalent scores start to lose their meaning. A school's curriculum for a grade may be easier or harder than the grade-equivalent score implies. Because grade-equivalent scores do not have even spaces between them, they cannot be subtracted. For example, it might seem intuitively appealing to say that a student's reading skill jumped two grade levels, given grade equivalent scores going from 2.2 to 4.4 on the WIAT-III. Despite the intuitive appeal, this is not a meaningful statement. For more about grade equivalents, see Reynolds (1981).

The final pitfall to avoid involves using too few sources of data. Assessments with individuals who struggle with reading, spelling, and writing can and should, depending on the context and purpose of the assessment, use several sources for data, including the following: 1) family, developmental, medical, and educational histories; 2) school records and examples of schoolwork; 3) interviews; 4) observations; 5) formal and informal tests; 6) rating scales; and 7) structured presentations of reading, spelling, and writing tasks. Data collection for a comprehensive assessment may include examinations by physicians and speech-language pathologists as well as neuropsychologists and occupational therapists.

REFLECT, CONNECT, and RESPOND

In your own words, describe two to three potential pitfalls teachers should be aware of when interpreting students' standardized test scores.

STANDARDIZED ASSESSMENT WITHIN THE RESPONSE TO INTERVENTION MODEL

Once tests are made, they are used in a variety of settings and for various purposes, including response to intervention (RTI; e.g., movement between tiers; for more on tiers, see Chapter 6), serial assessment, classification and diagnosis, and screening. Some of the possible purposes are explored next.

Inconsistent Results in the Real World

RTI is a service-delivery model that has become widely used, although doing so is not required by the federal government. The basic ideas involve providing students with valid and reliable interventions while tracking their progress and changing the interventions as needed in response to progress or lack thereof. The Individuals with Disabilities Education Improvement Act (IDEA) of 2004 (PL 108-446) includes RTI as one of several possible procedures for identifying a specific learning disability (SLD). This authorization of the law neither requires nor prohibits discrepancy between IQ score and achievement to determine SLD. IDEA 2004 permits school teams to use an individual's response to research-based intervention as part of the evaluation used to determine SLD. IDEA 2004 emphasized underachievement; per its specifications, the learning problem cannot result primarily from issues such as emotional disturbance; cultural factors; limited English proficiency; environmental or economic disadvantage; intellectual disability; or a disability of vision, hearing, or motor skills.

It is usually best practice to consider carefully whether the student has received research-based reading instruction that includes phonemic awareness, phonics, reading fluency, vocabulary, and comprehension as recommended by the National Reading Panel (NRP, National Institute on Child Health and Human Development [NICHD]) and incorporated into the No Child Left Behind (NCLB) Act of 2001 (PL 107-110). Individuals who conduct RTI research and those who implement RTI in schools tend to describe it in different ways. Those engaged in early reading research might explain RTI as a program designed to prevent reading failure (Gersten et al., 2009). School administrators might say that it is a means for controlling the flow of students into special education. As one learns more about it within this frame of reference, one might conclude that it is an effort to improve the pre-referral practices that many states require before a teacher can refer a child for a special education evaluation (Batsche et al., 2005), even though a comprehensive assessment can be requested by a parent at any time (see Learning Disabilities Association of America, 2013). If one asks a school psychologist serving as head of a child study team in a public school, he or she might say that RTI is an alternate and better way to identify students who have a specific learning disability in reading, which seems to be the intent of some RTI researchers (Fuchs, Fuchs, & Compton, 2004; Speece, Case, & Molloy, 2003; Vaughn & Fuchs, 2003).

Issues with scaling RTI up to larger settings, and the unfortunate choices that some school staff make regarding the types of interventions and assessments, have limited the success in the real world for schools that claim they are performing RTI (Balu, Zhu, Doolittle, Schiller, Jenkins, & Gersten, 2015; Noll, 2013). Unfortunate choices can include the utilization of reading strategies that have not been empirically shown to work or sloppy ways of tracking progress. The negative results of the Balu and colleagues' (2015) study indicate that schools often require more support in making RTI work up to its potential. (The negative results include how first-grade students assigned to interventions ended up with lower reading scores than those just above the intervention threshold, and the lack of significant impacts from interventions for second- and third-grade students just below the intervention threshold.) What follows are some thoughts about assessment that may pertain especially to RTI (but also remain relevant to environments in which RTI is not being used).

Serial Assessment and Score Changes Over Time

RTI involves serial assessment. According to Strauss, Sherman, and Spreen (2006) and Heilbronner and colleagues (2010), test scores can change over time due to various factors. These include the states of the examiner or examinee, the identity of the examiner, environmental conditions, such as level of noise or distractions, and practice with the items or with a similar format. A mathematical way to examine change over the time, though it is rarely used for various reasons, such as the lack of the appropriate information to plug into the formula, is the Reliable Change Index (Strauss et al., 2006). With progress monitoring, one has first to ask exactly what is being compared to what and how. There are many different types of scores, and they all track different constructs and can result in different classifications of responsiveness (Fuchs et al., 2004; Reynolds, 2009; Reynolds & Shaywitz, 2009).

Measuring a Response to an Intervention

Reynolds and Shaywitz (2009) recommended that age- or grade-corrected deviation standard scores be used to measure a response to an intervention. Tests such as the Woodcock Johnson IV or the WIAT-III provide these types of scores. According to

Reynolds (2009), evaluating the *R* in RTI is an important practical issue that may seem intuitive on the surface, even though it is actually complex. Reynolds (2009) noted that **raw scores,** equal interval growth scores, criterion-referenced scores, or grade-corrected or age-correct deviation scores answer different questions. Growth scores would reflect whether a student's spelling performance, say, has increased in relation to the starting point of the intervention. By contrast, raw scores remain difficult to interpret for such a purpose of tracking growth from a starting point. **Criterion-referenced scores** examine whether the student has met a goal, such as reading a certain number of words per minute with a text. **Standard scores** address a student's change in performance relative to the mean rate of change for other students of his or her age or grade. Reynolds recommended using standard scores in tracking progress, to see "whether the student is progressing at a lesser rate, the same pace, or more quickly than other students of the same age." (2009, p. 20). We note that this practice would be ideal, but it is not always possible, given the practical challenge of how difficult it is to make valid and reliable tests. They thus remain relatively rare. Such well-made tests are often best reserved for annual or semi-annual formal measurement, not for weekly **formative** and **summative assessment** in the classroom or small reading group. The use of arbitrary measures dilutes the effectiveness of tracking and of a tiered system. Also, other types of assessments can be used by teachers to guide daily teaching goals, as opposed to making placement decisions. However, informal tests that the teacher creates, or draws on from other sources, can certainly serve as daily sources of important qualitative data (for sources of numerous thoughtfully constructed informal tests, see McKenna & Stahl, 2015, and Reutzel & Cooter, 2011).

Difficulties can and do occur when invalid and unreliable tests are used to measure something, including progress, so for important decisions, one should avoid what are called arbitrary measures. Kazdin wrote, "It is possible that evidence-based treatments with effects demonstrated on arbitrary metrics do not actually help people, that is, reduce their symptoms and improve their functioning" (2006, p. 42). An arbitrary measure might be an informal test designed on the fly based on face validity, where the test looks like it must measure something. For example, a cloze reading comprehension test might actually be measuring word decoding more than reading comprehension. Arbitrary assessments should not be relied on to make important academic decisions.

The types of scores matter because Fuchs, Fuchs, and Compton concluded

> As demonstrated in our analyses . . . different measurement systems using different criteria [all with reference to RTI] result in identification of different groups of students. The critical question is which combination of assessment components is most accurate for identifying children who will experience serious and chronic reading problems that prevent reading for meaning in the upper grades and impair their capacity to function successfully as adults. At this point, relatively little is known to answer this question when RTI is the assessment framework. (2004, p. 226)

The use of standard score comparison over time is mathematically difficult because the test manufacturers generally do not provide the information required to examine this comparison quantitatively. Dramatic effects and very clear-cut cases do exist, of course. Many children show growth in gray areas, however, which can lead to the use of (subjective) judgment when mathematical methods are lacking. For example, a child's decoding skills may be improving but just slightly slower than those of peers, without drastic, extremely obvious growth. Judges of the progress may disagree, leading to minimal reliability between them and thus capping validity.

Moving Between Tiers

Based on assessment results in RTI, it is also not entirely clear how long to wait before moving between tiers. As Mather and Kaufman pointed out, paraphrasing Foorman and Ciancio (2005),

> No established standards presently exist for how to operationalize response adequacy. Thus, how RTI is implemented will be a localized, contextualized decision that will vary depending on human and material resources as well as a district's commitment to high expectations for all students. (2006, p. 831)

Kilpatrick (2015) recommended Tier 2 for those scoring in the bottom 25%. Having cutoff points assumes in a way that each student has average potential (Reynolds & Shaywitz, 2009), which is not necessarily the case either because some students' skills will remain weak. Measures such as DIBELS 6th Edition (discussed later) offer benchmarks. For some students, progress will be clear, but for some, it will not be. Further research is needed about when to move to another tier.

IMPORTANCE OF EARLY SCREENING AND INTERVENTION

The following sections discuss the purposes of screeners, provide examples, and discuss how screeners are used in the primary grades and in Grades 4–12.

Using Screeners in School Settings

Valid and reliable tests can also be screeners. Screeners generally (but not necessarily) are shorter, less expensive tests to predict whether individuals will have a particular condition on a "gold standard" test (or group of tests). The idea is that screeners can be administered more easily to large groups of people than the costlier gold standard. For example, a screener for dyslexia can be used to sort students into groups of those who need further assessment and those who do not. One difficulty with screeners for learning disorders is that the gold standard arguably does not objectively exist because the definition of dyslexia or other learning disorders involves the use of arbitrarily chosen cutoff points. Will the definition include the bottom 5%, 7%, or another percent? It is usually better to err in the direction of overidentification, given that the monitoring in Tier 2 should be able to resolve quickly the identification of false positives (i.e., students identified as having a problem when they do not). The choice of the cutoff point influences the reference point of the screener, which is supposed to substitute for the gold standard. The base rate of the condition in the general population, such as how many individuals have reading difficulties, also affects interpretation (see Strauss et al., 2006, for details).

Screening Instruments

A substantial number of screening instruments may be used as early as kindergarten or even pre-kindergarten to identify children who are at high risk for reading failure and who may require more intense, systematic reading instruction (Smartt & Glaser, 2010). The International Dyslexia Association (https://dyslexiaida.org/universal-screening-k-2-reading/) recommends the following screeners: Shaywitz DyslexicScreen (Shaywitz, 2016), Colorado Learning Disabilities Questionnaire–Reading Subscale (CLDQ-R) School Age Screener (https://dyslexiaida.org/screening-for-dyslexia/dyslexia-screener-for-school-age-children/), DIBELS Next, AIMSweb, Predictive Assessment of Reading (PAR; http://onlinepar.net/), and Texas Primary Reading Inventory (TPRI; https://www.tpri.org/index.html). Additional screeners are also listed at http://www.rti4success.org, although this web site reviews materials only available before May 2014. An example is the Phonological Awareness Literacy Screening (PALS; Invernizzi, Juel, Swank, & Meier, 2003; Invernizzi, Meier, & Juel, 2002; Invernizzi, Sullivan, & Meier, 2001). Note that the reviews at sources such as the rti4success web site may be positive for some aspects of the measure but weaker for others.

DIBELS is widely used in the United States. See the http:///www.rti4success .org web site for a handy review of evidence of reliability and validity for various versions and components of DIBELS. Careful instructors will regularly check available resources, such as this web site, to determine if there are updates to the empirical basis of a test. The DIBELS measures are standardized and designed as indicators of the basic early literacy skills of phonemic awareness, the alphabetic principle and phonics, accurate and fluent reading of connected text, and reading comprehension. Benchmark target goals are set for each skill and based on the likelihood of a student reaching later reading outcome goals. DIBELS universal screening is called benchmark assessment and occurs three times per year (typically September, January, and May for schools on a September to June calendar). Sets of alternate forms for each of these standardized, 1-minute fluency measures are available to conduct more frequent progress monitoring for students who are not meeting the benchmark goals so that instructional interventions can be adjusted based on progress. Several data management services are available that allow schools to enter DIBELS data and generate automated reports, including the DIBELS Data System from the University of Oregon (http://dibels.uoregon.edu/) and VPORT from Sopris West (https://vport.voyagersopris.com/).

Consequences of Delaying Intervention

Prompt assessment is important because of the dangers of waiting to intervene. As Torgesen advised, "The best solution to the problem of reading failure is to allocate resources for early identification and prevention" (1998, p. 1). The research is clear. As Lyon and Chhabra explained, the majority of young children entering kindergarten and elementary school at risk for reading failure have the potential to learn to read at average or above-average levels if they are identified early and given appropriate "systematic, intensive instruction in phonemic awareness, phonics, reading fluency, vocabulary, and reading comprehension strategies" (2004, p. 16). The consequences of delaying identification and intervention are ominous. As Shaywitz (2003) reported, at least 70% of students who do not learn to read by age 9 will never catch up to their typically developing peers. Even the youngest children who may be at risk for reading problems can be identified. For example, Adams (1990) cited rapid identification of upper- and lowercase letters of the alphabet as the single best predictor of early reading achievement. That, coupled with an assessment of phonemic awareness, which is shown to be directly related to the growth of early word-reading skills (Torgesen, 1998), can be helpful in identifying young children at risk for reading failure.

Although common signs of reading difficulties may be apparent before a child even begins formal schooling, reviews of early identification research (Scarborough, 1998) have revealed substantial levels of false positives; an average of 45% of children identified during kindergarten as at risk for reading problems turn out not to be among the readers with the most serious problems by the end of first grade. The flip side is that about a quarter of children who are later judged to have serious reading difficulties are not identified through kindergarten screenings. Some frequently used screening measures, with reviews as of May 2014, appear at the rti4success web site at http://www.rti4success.org/resources/tools-charts/screening-tools-chart. For more recent recommendations, please see https://dyslexiaida.org/universal-screening-k-2-reading/. Some screening measures focus on the child's skills per direct assessment, whereas others, such as the Shaywitz DyslexiaScreen (Shaywitz, 2016; http://dyslexia.yale.edu/EDU_ShaywitzDyslexiaScreen.html), focus on teacher observations. Screeners can be examined by factors such as how well they predict future reading performance or by their accuracy in sorting students into categories, given the caveats listed previously.

Focus of Early Identification in Kindergarten Through Grade 3

It is important for users to review and understand the purposes of screeners and what their results imply. Torgesen (2006) reflected on the "pillars of reading" when recommending the areas to be focused on in screening students in kindergarten through third grade. It is important to remember, however, that although phonemic awareness, phonics, fluency, vocabulary, and reading comprehension should all be addressed, assessing each area must be conducted in a manner that is appropriate to the grade level of the child. In addition, issues of cultural and linguistic differences in this population must be kept in mind. The National Early Childhood Technical Assistance Center cautioned that appropriate nonbiased assessment instruments and procedures should be used and that one must ensure that important results do not simply stem from cultural and linguistic differences. The center's web site (http://www.nectac.org/) provides a bibliography of articles and guidelines that can help practitioners employ culturally sensitive practices.

For kindergarten students, screenings should involve phonemic awareness and phonics skills (as reflected by knowledge of letters and of beginning decoding skills), as well as vocabulary. Fluency and reading comprehension, however, rarely are sufficiently developed for assessment at this level. Instead, listening comprehension is often assessed instead of reading comprehension to tap into the language processing skills that will be part of the necessary skill set for comprehending text once word reading accuracy and fluency are established. (Numerous other skills affect reading comprehension as well, such as fluid reasoning, attention, working memory, knowledge base, and so forth.)

Although phonemic awareness and decoding skills should continue to be monitored in first-grade students, oral reading fluency increases in its significance with the appearance of the ability to read connected text with reasonable accuracy. Growth in vocabulary should also be assessed regularly at this age, and reading comprehension can be evaluated by the end of first grade for most children.

As second- and third-grade students progress to decoding multisyllabic words, they need continued monitoring of their phonemic decoding ability. The close monitoring of reading fluency is critical at this stage to determine grade-level reading proficiency. The roles of vocabulary and comprehension assume even greater focus during this time.

> ## REFLECT, CONNECT, and RESPOND
> Why is it important to use screeners to assess literacy skills in the primary grades? What skills should be assessed in kindergarten, Grade 1, and Grades 2-3?

Screening Through the Grades: Grades 4–12

If early identification and early intervention are carried out carefully with strong, effective tools, then it can be assumed that the numbers of children who will need services after third grade will diminish (Biancarosa & Snow, 2006). Under the best of circumstances, however, it is doubtful that screening to identify struggling readers beyond early elementary grades and into middle and high school grades will be implemented. Students at these levels typically are no longer being taught basic decoding skills. Instead, they are expected to read to learn content. Yet, millions of students between 4th and 12th grade struggle to read at grade level (Biancarosa & Snow, 2006). *The Condition of Education 2016* from the U.S. Department of Education (Kena et al., 2016) indicates little recent improvement in reading abilities.

Torgesen and Miller (2009) called for **universal screening** as one component of a comprehensive literacy assessment. Universal screening involves the use of screeners with all students. Although universal screening may seem to be an overwhelming task in secondary school settings, Torgesen and Miller suggested using the data that have already been collected on students to identify those who may need targeted reading interventions. They advised using general screening information from the previous year's summative, or comprehensive, assessments to identify which students did not meet grade-level benchmarks. Schools may also use benchmark assessments in the fall that are designed to predict end-of-year state test results. After these data have been analyzed and used to determine an initial pool of students in need, additional assessments should be conducted to determine the nature and severity of reading problems.

The reasons behind poor performance on these summative assessments are not always clear. Some students may perform poorly because they simply cannot read the words on the page. Others are not fluent readers even if they are relatively accurate, so they may not be able to complete the test in a timely manner. A substantial number of students at this level have deficient banks of prior knowledge and relevant vocabulary required to comprehend content-area text. Still others have generally weak active comprehension strategies available to them. There is a subgroup who may be classified as students with disabilities who are late-emergent readers. These students may have been relatively successful in school with or without early intervention, but their competence crumbles once they must master more sophisticated content (Compton, Fuchs, Fuchs, Elleman, & Gilbert, 2008).

Torgesen and Miller (2009) suggested that screening tests at this point should be targeted at word-level reading skills, fluency, and comprehension so that interventions can be matched with specific areas of need. Resources are available to fulfill this mission. Johnson and Pool (2009) provided a list of screening measures for students in 4th through 12th grade as well as tools such as informal, or nonstandardized, reading and interest inventories plus decoding, comprehension, and fluency measures to identify specific reading problems of students struggling at this level. Morsy, Kieffer, and Snow (2010) targeted reading comprehension assessments appropriate for adolescents that can be used to inform interventions.

Finally, AIMSweb and the Florida Assessments for Instruction in Reading (FAIR) are computer-assisted screening measures that can be used for screening and formative assessment. Both measures are discussed later in the chapter.

REFLECT, CONNECT, and RESPOND
A colleague of yours tells you she added a new student, Neal, to her second-grade class 3 weeks ago. Neal's family has moved around a great deal, so she does not yet have all of his K–1 records; so far, she has had little contact with his family. Although Neal seems engaged and responsive during language arts lessons, he scored well below benchmark on a recently administered literacy screener. What advice would you give your colleague about how to use these test results to make decisions about Neal's reading instruction?

Underlying Deficits Associated With Reading Difficulties

Often children's reading difficulties are related to problems with specific skills or processes. The following sections discuss the potential impact of deficits in two specific areas: phonological processing and working memory.

    Phonological Processing Most children with dyslexia have phonological processing issues, and building advanced phonological processing skills is an important part of treatment (that also includes opportunities to read connected text and to become skilled with phonics, per Kilpatrick, 2015). However, the skills related to reading are multifactorial. With reading, it is important to keep in mind that phonological awareness does not explain everything; it would be impossible for one deficit to do so, unless there were a correlation of 1.0. Deficits in phonological awareness do nevertheless remain the most common factor associated with weak reading of words (Ahmed, Wagner, & Kantor, 2012). However, Peterson and Pennington (2012) pointed out,

> Mounting evidence shows that, although phonological deficits are standard in individuals with dyslexia, a single phonological deficit is probably not sufficient to cause the disorder. . . . Consistent with a multiple deficit hypothesis, we noted that a lot of children with a history of speech sound disorder developed normal literacy despite persistent deficits in phonological awareness. Furthermore, phonological awareness alone predicted literacy outcome less well than did a model that also included syntax and nonverbal IQ. (p. 2000)

    Peterson and Pennington (2012) also pointed out that reading fluency is also predicted by nonverbal measures of processing speed.

    Working Memory Working memory is defined differently by various researchers but basically involves moving pieces of information in and out of short-term awareness while performing an action related to this information, such as considering one's next move in a chess game while considering the opponent's possible moves. Weaknesses with working memory tend to be associated with problems in word reading (Gathercole, Alloway, Willis, & Adams, 2006; see Chapter 8 for more about the role of working memory and executive function in literacy instruction). Working memory is best assessed using a comprehensive assessment, as it can be hard to tease out from other areas, such as inattention. In terms of teaching strategies, a student with weak working memory may need tasks broken down into smaller units, along with visual cues, such as blocks for phonological manipulation training (Kilpatrick, 2015).

Swanson, Zheng, and Jerman wrote

Clearly, children with RD [reading disabilities] do not suffer deficits in all aspects of the phonological loop (e.g., several studies have shown they have relatively normal abilities in producing spontaneous speech and have few difficulties in oral language comprehension; see, e.g., Siegel, 1993, for a review) or the executive system (e.g., they have normal abilities in planning and sustaining attention across time; Swanson, 1981). Those aspects of the phonological system that appear problematic for children with RD were related to the accurate access to speech codes, and those aspects of the executive system that appear faulty were related to the concurrent monitoring of processing and storage demands. (2009, p. 279)

TECHNOLOGY-ENHANCED SCREENING AND PROGRESS MONITORING SYSTEMS

Since 2000, assessment systems that rely on technology have been developed to help teachers collect and use assessment data to refine instruction. Many of these assessment systems are not tied to a specific curriculum or textbook series (Salvia, Ysseldyke, & Bolt, 2017). Electronic data collection, management, and reporting systems are key to resolving teachers' concerns about the practicality of formative assessment of learning.

AIMSweb (http://www.aimsweb.com; see the review at http://www.rti4success .org) is an example of a commonly used direct, frequent, and continuous benchmark and progress monitoring system. AIMSweb has curriculum-based measures, with probes in reading, math, spelling, writing, and behavior for students in kindergarten through eighth grade. The AIMSweb system can generate graphs, tables, and reports to help teachers manage instruction. The system can also set goals and calculate learning rates for individual students in response to changes in instruction. Different versions of AIMSweb have received varying levels of empirical support (for details, see the data provided in the Screening Tools Chart available at the rti4success web site at http://www.rti4success.org/resources/tools-charts/ screening-tools-chart). Florida Assessments for Instruction in Reading (FAIR, http://www.fcrr.org/fair/index.shtm), which was developed by the Florida Center for Reading Research in collaboration with Just Read, Florida, is an assessment system that offers teachers screening, diagnostic, and progress monitoring information for students in kindergarten through 12th grade. As mentioned previously, the National Center on Response to Intervention maintains a Progress Monitoring Tools Chart and a Screening Tools Chart on its web site (http://www.rti4success .org). The Progress Monitoring Tools Chart evaluates progress monitoring tools on 10 dimensions, including reliability and validity of performance-level scores and of slopes. (See Salvia et. al., 2017 for more information about technology tools that support screening and progress monitoring.) Table 7.1 presents a comprehensive list of assessment resources available online.

ROLE OF COMPREHENSIVE ASSESSMENTS

Federal law requires a full individual evaluation before the initial provision of special education and related services. The evaluation must be conducted by a qualified multidisciplinary team with technically sound evaluation procedures. Parents must be informed of the purpose of the evaluation and each evaluation procedure and give written consent. Emphasis is placed on the functional nature of the evaluation, meaning that results from the evaluation will inform instruction and determine if the student needs services in addition to special education, such as

Table 7.1.   Commonly used assessments

Tests	Publisher/web site	Ages	Grades
Tests of academic achievement and intelligence			
Achievement tests			
Diagnostic Achievement Battery–Fourth Edition (DAB-4; Newcomer, 2014)	PRO-ED (http://www.proedinc.com)	6:0–14:11 years	–
Stanford Achievement Test– Tenth Edition (Harcourt Assessment, 2003)	Pearson Assessments (http://www.pearsonassessments.com)	–	K–12
Terra Nova–III (2008)	CTB/McGraw-Hill (http://www.mheducation.com)	–	K–12
Wechsler Individual Achievement Test–Third Edition (WIAT-III; Wechsler, 2009)	Pearson Assessments (http://www.pearsonassessments.com)	4:0–50:11 years	–
Wide Range Achievement Test–Fourth Edition (WRAT-4; Wilkinson & Robertson, 2006)	PRO-ED (http://www.proedinc.com)	5–94 years	–
Woodcock-Johnson IV Tests of Achievement (WJ-IV-ACH; Schrank, Mather, & McGrew, 2014)	Houghton Mifflin Harcourt (http://www.hmhco.com)	2 years to adult	–
Intelligence tests			
Kaufman Assessment Battery for Children, Second Edition (KABC-II; Kaufman & Kaufman, 2004)	Psychcorp/Pearson Assessments (http://www.pearsonclinical.com)	3–18 years	–
Stanford-Binet Intelligence Scales–Fifth Edition (Roid, 2003)	Houghton Mifflin Harcourt (http://www.hmco.com)	2–85 years	–
Wechsler Intelligence Scale for Children–Fifth Edition Integrated (WISC-V; Wechsler, 2014)	Psychcorp/Pearson Assessments (http://www.pearsonclinical.com)	6:0–16:11 years	–
Wechsler Adult Intelligence Scale for Adults–Fourth Edition (WAIS-IV; Wechsler, 2008a)	Psychcorp/Pearson Assessments (http://www.pearsonclinical.com)	16:0–90:11 years	–
Wechsler Preschool and Primary Scale of Intelligence– Fourth Edition (WPPSI-IV; Wechsler, 2008b)	Psychcorp/Pearson Assessments (http://www.pearsonclinical.com)	2:6–7:7 years	–
Woodcock-Johnson IV: Tests of Cognitive Abilities (Schrank, McGrew, & Mather, 2014)	Houghton Mifflin Harcourt (http://www.hmhco.com)	2–19 years	–
Diagnostic assessments of reading, spelling, and writing			
Analytical Reading Inventory– Tenth Edition (Woods & Moe, 2015)	Pearson Higher Education (http://www.Pearsonhighered.com)	–	K–12
Basic Reading Inventory– Eleventh Edition (BRI; Johns, 2012)	Kendall Hunt Publishing (http://www.kendallhunt.com)	–	Preprimer through 12th grade

(continued)

Table 7.1. *(continued)*

Tests	Publisher/web site	Ages	Grades
Phonics Surveys in CORE Assessing Reading Multiple Measures, 2nd ed. (Diamond & Thorsnes, 2008)	Arena Press Books/Academic Therapy (http://www.AcademicTherapy.com)	–	K–3+
Degrees of Reading Power (Questar Assessment, 2015)	Questar Assessment (http://www.questarai.com)	–	2–12
Developmental Reading Assessment, Second Edition (Beaver & Carter, 2006)	Pearson School (http://www.pearsonschool.com)	–	K–8
Early Reading Diagnostic Assessment, Second Edition (ERDA-2; Jordan, Kirk, & King, 2005)	Pearson Clinical (http://www.pearsonclinical.com)	–	K–3
Gates-MacGinitie Reading Tests–Fourth Edition (2006 norms) (MacGinitie, MacGinitie, Maria, & Dreyer, 2006)	Houghton Mifflin Harcourt (http://www.hmhco.com)	–	K through adult
Gray Oral Reading Test–Fifth Edition (GORT-5; Wiederholt & Bryant, 2012)	PRO-ED (http://www.proedinc.com)	6:0–18:11 years	–
Group Reading Assessment and Diagnostic Evaluation (GRADE; 2001)	Pearson Assessments (http://www.pearsonassessments.com)	–	Pre-K through 12th grade
Qualitative Reading Inventory–Sixth Edition (QRI-6; Leslie & Caldwell, 2016)	Pearson Higher Ed (http://www.pearsonhighered.com)	–	K–12
Renaissance STAR Reading (web based; Renaissance Learning, 1996)	Renaissance Learning (http://www.renaissance.com)	–	K–12
Shaywitz DyslexiaScreen (Shaywitz, 2016)	Pearson Assessments (http://www.pearsonassessments.com)	–	K–1
Slosson Oral Reading Test–SORT-3 (Slosson, Nicholson, & Larson, 2015)	Slosson Educational (http://www.slosson.com)	–	Preschool through adult
Spelling Performance Evaluation for Language and Literacy–Second Edition (SPELL-2; Masterson, Apel, & Wasowicz, 2006)	Learning by Design (http://www.learningbydesign.com)	–	Grade 2+
Test of Early Reading Ability–Third Edition (TERA-3; Reid, Hresko, & Hammill, 2001)	PRO-ED (http://www.proedinc.com)	3:6–8:6 years	–
Test of Integrated Language and Literacy Skills™ (TILLS™; Nelson, Plante, Helm-Estabrooks, & Hotz, 2016)	Brookes Publishing (http://www.brookespublishing.com)	6–18 years	–
Test of Reading Comprehension–Fourth Edition (TORC-4; Brown, Wiederholt, & Hammill, 2009)	PRO-ED (http://www.proedinc.com)	7:0–17:11 years	–

Tests	Publisher/web site	Ages	Grades
Test of Silent Word Reading Fluency–Second Edition (TOSWRF-2; Mather, Hammill, Allen, & Roberts, 2014)	PRO-ED (http://www.proedinc.com)	6:3–24:11 years	–
Test of Word Reading Efficiency-2 (TOWRE-2; Torgesen, Wagner, & Rashotte, 2012)	PRO-ED (http://www.proedinc.com)	6:0–24:11 years	–
Test of Written Language–Fourth Edition (TOWL-4; Hammill & Larsen, 2009)	PRO-ED (http://www.proedinc.com)	9:0–17:11 years	–
Test of Written Spelling–Fifth Edition (TWS-5; Larsen, Hammill, & Moats, 2013)	PRO-ED (http://www.proedinc.com)	–	1–12
Woodcock-Johnson III Diagnostic Reading Battery (Woodcock, Mather, & Schrank, 2004)	Houghton Mifflin Harcourt (http://www.hmhco.com)	2–90 years	–
Woodcock Reading Mastery Tests, Third Edition (WRMT III; Woodcock, 2011)	Pearson Clinical (http://www.pearsonclinical.com)	4:6–79:11 years	K–12
Word Identification and Spelling (WIST; Wilson & Felton, 2004)	PRO-ED (http://www.proedinc.com)	7:0–18:11 years	2–5; 6–12
Language tests			
Clinical Evaluation of Language Functions–Fifth Edition (CELF-5; Wiig, Semel, & Secord, 2013)	Pearson Clinical (http://www.pearsonclinical.com)	5:0–21:11 years	–
Comprehensive Assessment of Spoken Language-2 (CASL-2; Carrow-Woolfolk, 2017)	PRO-ED (http://www.proedinc.com)	3:0–21:11 years	–
Comprehensive Receptive and Expressive Vocabulary Tests–Third Edition (CREVT-3; Wallace & Hammill, 2013)	PRO-ED (http://www.proedinc.com)	5:0–89 years	–
Comprehensive Test of Phonological Processing-Second Edition (CTOPP-2; Wagner, Torgesen, Rashotte, & Pearson, 2013)	PRO-ED (http://www.proedinc.com)	4:0–24:11 years	–
Goldman-Fristoe Test of Articulation-3 (GFTA-3; Goldman & Fristoe, 2015)	PRO-ED (http://www.proedinc.com)	2–21 years	–
Lindamood Auditory Conceptualization Test–Third Edition (LAC-3; Lindamood & Lindamood, 2004)	Linguisystems (http:// www.proedinc.com)	5:0–18:11 years	K–Adult
Oral and Written Language Scales-2nd ed. (OWLS-2; Carrow-Woolfolk, 2012)	PRO-ED (http://www.proedinc.com)	3:0–21:11 years	–

(continued)

Table 7.1. *(continued)*

Tests	Publisher/web site	Ages	Grades
Peabody Picture Vocabu-lary Test–Fourth Edition (PPVT-4; Dunn & Dunn, 2007)	Pearson Clinical (http://www.pearsonclinical.com)	2-6 years to 90+ years	–
Phonological Awareness Test–Second Edition (PAT-2; Robertson & Salter, 2007)	Linguisystems (http://www.Linguisystems.com)	5-9 years	K-4
Test for Auditory Compre-hension of Language–Fourth Edition (TACL-4; Carrow-Woolfolk, 2014)	PRO-ED (http://www.proedinc.com)	3:0-12:11 years	–
Test of Language Competence–Expanded (TLC Expanded; Wiig & Secord, 1989)	Pearson Assessments (http://www.pearsonassessments.com)	L1: 5-9 years; L2: 10-18 years	–
Test of Language Develop-ment, Primary–Fourth Edi-tion (TOLD: P4; Newcomer & Hammill, 2008)	PRO-ED (http://www.proedinc.com)	4:0-8:11 years	–
Test of Language Develop-ment, Intermediate–Fourth Edition (TOLD: I4; Hammill & Newcomer, 2008)	PRO-ED (http://www.proedinc.com)	8:0-17:11 years	–
Test of Phonological Aware-ness–Second Edition: Plus (TOPA-2+; Torgesen & Bryant, 2004)	PRO-ED (http://www.proedinc.com)	5-8 years	–
Test of Word Knowledge (TOWK; Wiig & Secord, 1992)	Pearson Clinical (http://www.pearsonclinical.com)	5-17 years	–
Yopp-Singer Test of Pho-neme Segmentation (informal assessment)	(https://www.coloradoplc.org/files/archives/yopp_singer_phoneme_segmentation_test.pdf)	–	K-3

Note: This table presents some commonly used tests. Not all the tests have established validity for particular uses. Users should be aware of the pros and cons for each test and the research behind the validity of using them for particular purposes. Some are more appropriate for qualitative exploration of reading problems and should not be used for high-stakes decisions.

speech-language therapy or counseling. Parents have the right to request an out-side evaluation (paid for by the school district), after the school has performed an assessment, on a written request within 2 years of the school district's assessment (see 34 C.F.R §300.502[b][2]). Comprehensive assessments are informative and important because research shows that children with reading problems often have other difficulties. For example, 25%–40% of children whose situation meets criteria for either significant inattention/hyperactivity or for dyslexia also face the other challenge (Peterson & Pennington, 2012). Language impairments are especially common with reading disorders (Peterson & Pennington, 2012). There is also some empirical evidence that using cognitive assessment of certain skills to help design academic interventions is helpful, though more research is needed (Schneider & Kaufman, 2017). Comprehensive assessment also provides the big picture of a student (Schneider & Kaufman, 2017). For dozens of examples of case studies, please see Mather and Jaffe (2011).

SKILLS COMMONLY MEASURED ON STANDARDIZED ASSESSMENTS

Reading relates in various ways to other cognitive skills, such as general intelligence, working memory, attention, fluid reasoning, or spoken language; for good reviews please see Flanagan, Ortiz, and Alfonso (2013) or Kilpatrick (2015). A few of the most noteworthy factors appear next.

Phonemic Awareness

Kilpatrick (2015) pointed out that tasks of phoneme segmentation commonly appear on reading measures, even though segmentation tests are relatively insensitive and minimally relevant past the first grade. On the other hand, Kilpatrick continued, some of the commonly used assessments omit phonological awareness past first grade, even though such awareness continues to be important and to require enhancement. Kilpatrick wrote

> Advanced phonological awareness . . . continues to develop until about third or fourth grade. Tests that involve manipulating phonemes, such as deleting, substituting, or reversing phonemes within words, appear to tap into this advanced level of phonological awareness/proficiency. . . . Because all of the major universal screeners (DIBELS, AIMSweb and Easy CBM) only track basic phonological awareness, they are not sensitive to the advanced phonological awareness skills that are needed for efficient word learning. This is important because many children with reading problems can develop the phonological awareness needed for letter–sound knowledge and can also develop the phonological blending needed for phonic decoding. However, their phonological awareness development stalls at that point due to a mild to moderate phonological- core deficit. Such page students become slow, laborious readers (Fox & Routh, 1983). (2015, p. 119).

Students with more severe phonological-core deficits even struggle with letter–sound knowledge and basic phonic decoding.

Phonological blending (sometimes called synthesis) develops early for good readers. Synthesis is important for phonic decoding because it involves the recognition of a slowly spoken word. A student can perform well on measures of phonological blending yet remain a poor reader (Kilpatrick, 2012). Thus, one must give measures of phonological analysis, not just synthesis.

Phonological analysis features the taking apart of words. Manipulation of phonemes correlates higher with reading skills than segmentation does (Catts, Fey, Zhang, & Tomblin, 2001). Manipulation involves deleting, reversing, and substituting sounds of words, such as asking a child to say *cat* without the /k/, say *bat* backward, or say *parachute* without *para*. Kilpatrick (2015) found phonemic reversal tasks relatively useful in middle school and high school students based on clinical experience and recommended using the first version of the Comprehensive Test of Phonological Processing (CTOPP; Wagner, Torgesen, & Rashotte, (1999) because it still contains reversal tasks (which are otherwise difficult to find). Kilpatrick (2015) also recommended that phonological awareness tasks ideally should include timing because students could apply less relevant strategies (e.g., mental spelling of the word and then deleting or reversing it) to slowly, laboriously, but correctly answer items. That is, students with advanced phonemic awareness will respond immediately, but a timing element is not incorporated in many of these tests. Thus, one should record the time that a student takes in order to estimate the student's level of phonemic proficiency. The Phonological Awareness Skills Test by Kilpatrick (2015) includes a timed element. Mental spelling could also be minimized by using items that are orthographically inconsistent (Kilpatrick 2015), such as *bought*. Kilpatrick (2015) pointed out that some awareness tests, such as Phonological Processing on the WJ-IV Tests of Cognitive Abilities, combine various tasks into one subtest, which can create some diagnostic confusion.

Rapid Automatized Naming and Rapid Alternating Stimulus

Measures of rapid automatized naming (RAN) and rapid alternating stimulus (RAS) assess a "microcosm of the systems of reading" (Norton & Wolf, 2012) that is independent of phonological awareness and involves the reading of random strings of colors, letters, or numbers. Norton and Wolf noted that the CTOPP (now CTOPP-2) rapid naming tests and the RAN-RAS Tests have standardized measures. They reported that many other rapid naming tests

> Are not fully normed and only criterion scores are given (e.g., performance is categorized only as normal versus non-normal). The Dynamic Indicators of Basic Literacy Skills, 6th edition (DIBELS) contains several "fluency" subtests, including letter-naming fluency, but this test uses all the upper and lowercase letters in one array and scores the number of letters correctly identified in one minute, a procedure that differs significantly from classic RAN tasks. (2012, p. 435)

Students with difficulties in both RAN and in phonological awareness tend to have relatively severe reading problems, with exceptions (Pennington, Cardoso-Martins, Green, & Lefly, 2001; Wolf & Bowers, 1999). Training RAN is not done directly, though RAN can improve when other aspects of reading improve (Norton & Wolf, 2012). Slower RAN is also correlated with slower rates of reading and of recalling math facts (Norton & Wolf, 2012).

Nonsense Word Reading

Reading of nonsense words involves sounding out words that follow the English cipher but are not actually real words in English. Sounding out nonsense words arguably mirrors the process by which one sounds out any unfamiliar word. Nonsense word measures are commonly available. Kilpatrick (2015) recommended supplementing them with the Test of Word Reading Efficiency, Second Edition (TOWRE-2; Torgesen, Wagner, & Rashotte, 2012) or the Kaufman Test of Educational Achievement, Third Edition (KTEA-3) Decoding Fluency (Kaufman & Kaufman, 2014) because the timed aspects of these measures are important. Students who are capable with phonemic awareness but weaker with nonsense words should have interventions for phonics, and nonsense word reading is especially sensitive to future reading problems in young children (Kilpatrick, 2015). One can compare the results on nonsense word reading to those for blending real and nonsense words that the student hears and to spelling of nonsense words.

Word Identification

Kilpatrick (2015) also pointed out that a test-taker can use phonic decoding, guessing, instant word recognition, or any combination of these on word identification tests that consist of lists of words. To help know whether a student holds a certain word in memory, Kilpatrick recommended attending to factors such as pronunciations of the same word that vary over time or last more than 1 second or involve self-corrections or stresses on the wrong syllable. For such reasons, Kilpatrick recommended using timed word recognition measures, such as the TOWRE-2. Kilpatrick also pointed out that some timed measures such as sentence fluency are likely more appropriate for elementary-age students because the tests use easier words throughout, rather than the words expected of a more experienced reader. The Test of Silent Reading Efficiency and Comprehension (TOSREC; Wagner, Torgesen, Rashotte, & Pearson, 2010), the Wechsler Individual Achievement Test-III (WIAT-III; Wechsler, 2009), and the Gray Oral Reading Test-5 (GORT-5; Wiederholt & Bryant, 2012) present oral and silent reading fluency measures with words that increase in difficulty for later passages.

Reading Comprehension

Keep in mind that reading comprehension instruments measure different skills, so scores on them do not always correlate very highly (Cutting & Scarborough, 2006; Keenan, Betjemann, & Olson, 2008; Nation & Snowling, 1998). Thus, more than one measure of reading comprehension should be administered. Cloze tests tend to rely heavily on word recognition, especially for single words that provide a key to the answer (Keenan et al., 2008). Comprehension of texts involves multiple cognitive processes; see Chapter 15 as well as Flanagan and colleagues (2013) and Kilpatrick (2015). Reading comprehension tests vary in the skills they measure and in the results they give. For example, Keenan and Meenan (2012) found considerable inconsistency between results when giving the same children four different comprehension measures. Thus, it is especially important to keep in mind the nature of the reading comprehension test and its relationship to other cognitive and academic skills that the child has, such as IQ score, word retrieval, oral language, and so forth. These types of skills are assessed using comprehensive assessments.

Reed and Vaughn (2012) reviewed reading retell measures. They reported a moderate correlation between reading retell and standardized reading comprehension tools. With older students, reading retell correlated at a lower level with decoding and fluency. They described numerous factors that can influence reading retell performances, including qualities of the measures themselves, such as genre, scoring methods, or prompting rules. They recommended further research before using them as a progress monitoring tool because **interrater reliability** (the agreement in scores between different people giving the test) is sometimes low for such measures.

Kilpatrick (2015) stated that, given the several types of reading comprehension tests, it may be best to administer one test of each type (story retell, question and answer, and those with one or two sentences), though two from each category (for a total of six tests) would be preferable psychometrically. Intervention then is based on how much of the difficulty came from word-level reading and how much from other types of skills (Kilpatrick, 2015). A comprehensive assessment would be appropriate here, as many of the skills measured in this type of assessment—attention, working memory, vocabulary, background knowledge—can affect reading comprehension. Kilpatrick (2015) pointed out that longer passages may more accurately measure reading comprehension than shorter ones.

Kilpatrick (2015) described a "compensator" type of weak reader, who often is strong with spoken language but relatively weak (though often still average) with comprehension of texts, with low average to average word-reading ability. Compensators perform less well with timed nonsense word reading and timed phonemic awareness. Their stronger skills with language can mask the efforts that compensators need to put into decoding words, which can undermine their reading comprehension (which one would expect to be stronger given their excellent oral language skills).

> **REFLECT, CONNECT, and RESPOND**
> Name two areas of literacy skill that are commonly measured on standardized assessments. Explain why it is important to assess a student's skills in each area.

ROLE OF NONSTANDARDIZED ASSESSMENTS IN READING INSTRUCTION

Informal assessments primarily provide opportunities for a teacher to observe qualitatively a student's responses. Informal assessments are not necessarily created by research or by the application of statistics in test creation. This quality makes it harder to show that the informal test measures what its developer intended. Only well-constructed tests should be used with placement decisions and for diagnosis of a learning disorder, in conjunction, of course, with a good history, rule-outs of alternate conditions, and so forth. However, other types of assessment, summative and formative, as well as curriculum-based, can inform weekly teaching goals. With informal assessments, it can be helpful to use the same ones habitually over time, to obtain familiarity with the instrument and to gain experience with how students in one's school tend to respond. One thus internalizes a sense of how students should perform, and vagaries stand out more noticeably than they would with unfamiliar measures.

Formative and Summative Assessment

Formative assessment guides daily or weekly instruction, in effect helping to "form" or "inform" the teaching. Formative assessments are generally administered on a regular basis to decide issues such as what letter–sound relationships need to be taught. Examples include homework, quizzes, discussions, and self-assessments. A major difference between standardized (formal) and formative tests can be the level of information about specific "micro-skills" to work on during a specific time. Formative assessments usually have not been assessed for reliability and validity, and thus it is not clear whether they are consistent internally or across raters or what exact meaning to assign to them with confidence. However, formative assessments provide more and ongoing opportunities to observe, especially when those observations are informed by a solid knowledge of reading skills.

Summative assessment summarizes what has been learned. An example might be a mid-term or final exam. Salvia, Ysseldyke and Bolt (2017) warned against using only one summative assessment because doing so can magnify a measure's inadequacies.

Curriculum-Based Measures

One way to measure progress is to use **curriculum-based measures (CBMs),** such as DIBELS, with many materials available for free at http://www.dibels.uoregon.edu. (CBMs assess how well a student performs for the standards of a particular curriculum, such as a particular school's reading program.) Similar measures include AIMSweb or F.A.S.T. CBMs look closely at goals and the progress towards them (see Overton, 2011, for an overview). CBMs are a prime example of formative assessment used during instruction (Overton, 2011). Per Deno (1985, summarized in Overton, 2011), some of the important considerations when selecting CBMs include reliability and validity, convenience of use and of explanation to others, and pricing.

Overton (2011) provided a technique for creating CBMs for reading, by selecting a large number of grade-level passages and having the student read them aloud for 1 minute. The baseline score of errors is graphed, along with progress over time. Overton (2011), along with Deno, Fuchs, Marston, and Shinn (2001), provided some information on what to expect for progress with the creation of aim lines and trend lines. Silberglitt and Hintze (2007) showed that students' rates of growth vary per initial level of performance because the weakest and strongest students grow more slowly than ones toward the middle of the distribution. Thus, one might use goals geared toward a student's initial decile, or use a criterion reference goal. Mehrens and Clarizio (1993) indicated that CBM supplement the assessment and remediation of academic problems. However, it needs to be used with a more encompassing systematic psycho-educational assessment program, instead of replacing it.

Measures such as DIBELS include benchmark goals, and they also estimate a student's risk with cutoff scores. Related issues include the assumption that each child will have at least average potential and consideration of which children to use for comparison (see Reynolds & Shaywitz, 2009). For reasons such as these, CBM measures alone should not be used for diagnosis of dyslexia (Reynolds & Shaywitz, 2009). Valid and reliable tests must be used in the diagnosis of a reading disorder such as dyslexia, which also involves a review of presenting symptoms, history taking, and behavioral observations (Pennington, 2009). Diagnosis of a mental disorder should be performed by those authorized in their states to do so in a setting; regulations and practices vary across states. There is not one test used to diagnose a reading disorder, but the DSM-5 merely recommends the use of "administered standardized achievement measures" (American Psychiatric Association, 2013, p. 67). Definitions of learning disorders vary widely between researchers, regulatory bodies and other authorities, although some features remain common between them (Flanagan, Ortiz, Alfonso, & Dynda, 2006).

SOURCES FOR TESTS

Table 7.1 presents commonly used reading tests. For further reading, summaries of the validity and reliability of standardized tests, along with numerous curriculum-based and formative and summative measures are provided in the following resources: Buros Center for Testing, Carlson, Geisinger, & Jonson (2014); Diamond and Thorsnes (2008); Kilpatrick (2015); McKenna and Stahl (2015); and Reutzel and Cooter (2011) as well as http://www.understood.org.

FORMATIVE ASSESSMENT IN MULTISENSORY LANGUAGE PROGRAMS

There are options for creating informal progress monitoring tools, keeping in mind the caveats mentioned elsewhere. Some multisensory programs include information on how to make formative assessments of progress. For example, Alphabetic Phonics (Cox, 1992) uses curriculum-referenced tasks called benchmark measures (Cox, 1986) and progress measurements (Rumsey, 1992), respectively, to assess progress in letter-knowledge acquisition and alphabetizing skills and to assess reading, spelling, and handwriting. Teachers who use Road to Reading (Blachman & Tangel, 2008) administer the levels assessments to each student, which includes a record of regular and high-frequency words the student has learned to read. Notes from the daily lesson plans are put in a folder, dated, and arranged chronologically to facilitate evaluation of progress. The Basic Language Skills program (Carreker, 2008) has a series of mastery checks given after concepts have been introduced and practiced. The Wilson Reading System (http://www.wilsonlanguage.com) and other multisensory structured language education programs include pre- and posttesting along with tests to get a sense of mastery of knowledge taught in one curriculum unit before a student moves to the next curriculum unit. Assessing progress in these programs focuses on students' mastery of word-recognition and spelling skills.

Building on Multisensory Language Instruction Benchmarks

To build on this tradition of assessing progress in multisensory programs, educators can identify the classes of data needed to assess progress and identify some methods of data collection. The following skills should be tracked: phoneme segmentation, letter identification, graphophonemic knowledge (letter–sound associations), word recognition fluency, spelling, oral vocabulary, comprehension, and composition. Although it is useful to assess children's knowledge of letter–sound associations using checklists of phonics knowledge (e.g., Blachowicz, 1980), children's spellings also provide a window on their knowledge of letter–sound relationships. By examining children's spellings, teachers can gain insight into children's skills with phonics (Treiman, 1998). Using spelling to assess phonics knowledge requires a spelling curriculum that includes a systematic outline of English spelling, knowledge of the developmental sequence for acquiring English spellings, and a method for scoring spellings that evaluates spelling elements within words rather than simply marking words as correct or incorrect. Reading and spelling are usually taught as separate subjects; as a consequence, teachers might not think to use spelling to assess reading.

Although not intended for this purpose, the Spelling Performance Evaluation for Language and Literacy–Second Edition (SPELL-2) assessment tool, which includes a cross-platform CD-ROM and a manual (Masterson, Apel, & Wasowicz, 2006), is a criterion-referenced instrument that is organized to allow the simultaneous assessment of spelling and phonics knowledge. (See Moats, 1995, and Mosely, 1997, for more information about spelling assessment.) SPELL-2 is composed of tests that assess knowledge of phonological awareness and alphabetic letter–sound relationships, letter patterns and vocabulary word parts (prefixes, suffixes, base words), and mental images of words. The Word Identification and Spelling Test (WIST; Wilson & Felton, 2004) is another spelling assessment for qualitative data with normative information as well as diagnostic cues for instruction. The spelling subtest assesses a student's ability to spell words correctly from dictation, ability to recall correct letter sequences from familiar words, and ability to apply sound–symbol relationships of English orthography. Regular and irregular words are assessed separately for comparison. Error analysis leads to an appropriate intervention plan to improve spelling. (See Chapter 10 for an example of an error analysis rubric.) Preventing Academic Failure also has the Single Word Reading Test (available at the Preventing Academic Failure program web site at http://www .pafprogram.com/free-downloads/). This measure is frequently used in multisensory programs. The Gallistel-Ellis Test of Coding Skills is available at the Montage Press web site at http://www.montagepress.net/products-test-of-coding-skills .html. The Gallistel-Ellis assesses a student's knowledge of the sounds for letters and units or clusters, as well as recognition and spelling of words created from the sounds.

Informal Reading Inventories

Informal reading inventories (see Leslie & Caldwell, 2016; Woods & Moe, 2015) can be used to obtain some of the data needed to plan remedial programs. The structure of these inventories is used to establish reading levels for individual students based on accuracy in reading single words, words in text, and answering comprehension questions. These inventories include conventions for marking reading errors (insertions, hesitations, mispronunciations, omissions, regressions, substitutions, self-corrections, pauses, and repetitions) and, more important, provide classification systems for word-reading errors, which are commonly called **miscues.**

Mispronounced words (words read incorrectly) are classified as graphically similar, semantically acceptable, or syntactically correct. This classification allows the teacher to make some inferences about the word-recognition strategies students are using. Some informal reading inventories (e.g., Leslie & Caldwell, 2016) provide procedures for assessing reading rate for words and text and give standards for evaluating a student's fluency with word lists and texts. In most informal reading inventories, comprehension is assessed by observing students thinking aloud as they read, retelling stories they have read, and answering questions about the text. Background knowledge is assessed by observing students making predictions about the text before they read based on the title and the first few sentences of the text. Vocabulary is assessed by observing students defining words encountered in the text.

The Developmental Reading Assessment, Second Edition (DRA-2, also available as an app for smartphone, tablet or computer) is another informal reading inventory (Beaver & Carter, 2006). It is a criterion-measured assessment used to measure accuracy, fluency, and comprehension for students in kindergarten through third grade (Beaver & Carter, 2006). Reviewers wrote, "Developers report convincing evidence for face validity and construct validity to identify reading difficulties; however, there is no evidence to support some of the recommended applications, such as progress monitoring or identification of specific strengths or weaknesses" (McCarthy & Christ, 2010, p. 184). McCarthy and Christ (2010) recommended that the DRA-2 should not be used for high-stakes decisions, given the reliability level, but it does have a number of positive features.

Most inventories are organized to permit comparisons between a student's skills (e.g., fluency, comprehension) with narrative text and his or her skills with expository text. Comparisons can be made between a student's reading performance (e.g., accuracy, fluency) with word lists versus text. Distinctions between reading and listening comprehension may also be drawn. These inventories are criterion-referenced tests, even though the authors may not view the inventories from this perspective. As indicated previously, data obtained from these inventories are used to construct remedial programs. The rules included in these inventories for marking reading errors, classifying miscues, and assessing reading rate can be used to create **curriculum-referenced assessments** based on the texts used for instruction. These structured observations of reading of texts that students use for reading instruction can also be used to assess comprehension, vocabulary, and use of background knowledge. It is easy to imagine an assessment folder that includes records of such observations made on a regular basis. These records would resemble the running assessment records recommended by Clay (1995). The text is from the students' reading lessons; the structure for assessing reading is borrowed from informal inventories.

REFLECT, CONNECT, and RESPOND

List a few examples of formative assessments a teacher might use. What is the purpose of administering these formative assessments? What advantages do formative assessments have over formal, standardized measures? What are their potential shortcomings?

CLOSING THOUGHTS: BEST PRACTICES FOR ASSESSMENT AND RECOMMENDATIONS FOR FURTHER RESEARCH

The purpose of assessment is to inform instruction and educational planning using the best methods possible to meet specific student needs. This chapter has reviewed some key points and best practices for various forms of assessment. Future research should emphasize the creation of a greater number of reliable and valid assessment tools for everyday use. Many formative and summative assessments may have face validity, but they have little in the way of established validity. Test makers need to be clear about how they derive benchmarks and how they measure progress. It would be useful with standardized measures to see how often a score gain occurred over a particular time in the normative sample, as well as to have a larger number of alternate versions of tests. Greater use of technology, such as software and computer-administrated tests, or even virtual reality tests, will likely be the wave of the future.

ONLINE COMPANION MATERIALS

The following Chapter 7 resources are available at http://www.brookespublishing.com/birshcarreker/materials:

- Reflect, Connect, and Respond Questions

- Appendix 7.1: Online Resources for Assessment

- Appendix 7.2: Knowledge and Skill Assessment Answer Key

KNOWLEDGE AND SKILL ASSESSMENT

1. The reliability of a test refers to which of the following?

    a. The consistency of test results across evaluators administering it

    b. The consistency of the test results between various forms of the test

    c. The consistency of the test items to each other

    d. The consistency of the test results upon retesting

    e. All of the above

2. Which of these statements is true of face validity?

    a. It is always required before using a test.

    b. It is highly correlated with reliability.

    c. It is sometimes misleading because it refers simply to whether a test appears to measure something.

    d. It is more important than criterion validity.

    e. It is more important than construct validity.

3. Which of the following statements is true for the Individuals with Disabilities Education Improvement Act (IDEA) of 2004 (PL 108-446)?

    a. It requires the use of RTI to determine the presence of a specific learning disability (SLD).

    b. It neither requires nor prohibits the use of a discrepancy between IQ score and achievement to determine SLD.

    c. It requires the use of a discrepancy between IQ score and achievement to determine the presence of a SLD.

    d. It does not mention methods of identifying SLDs.

    e. It mentions only dyslexia.

4. Which of these statements is true of formative assessment?

    a. It is provided often to guide daily or weekly instruction.

    b. It summarizes the overall picture of a child and is given rarely.

    c. It always uses standardized tests.

    d. It never uses standardized tests.

    e. It is no longer used.

5. Which of these statements is true of grade-equivalent scores?

    a. They have unequal spaces between the scores.

    b. They correspond unevenly to norm-referenced scores.

    c. They can change in large ways due to small movements in the raw data.

    d. All of the above.

    e. None of the above.

REFERENCES

Adams, M.J. (1990). *Beginning to read: Thinking and learning about print.* Cambridge, MA: The MIT Press.

Ahmed, Y., Wagner, R.K., & Kantor, P.T. (2012). How visual word recognition is affected by developmental dyslexia. *Visual Word Recognition, 2,* 196–215.

American Educational Research Association (AERA), American Psychological Association (APA), & National Council on Measurement in Education (NCME). (2014). *Standards for educational and psychological testing.* Washington, DC: American Educational Research Association.

American Psychiatric Association. (2013). *Diagnostic and statistical manual of mental disorders,* (5th ed.). Arlington, VA: Author.

Anastasi, A., & Urbina, S. (1997). *Psychological testing.* Upper Saddle River, NJ: Prentice Hall.

Balu, R., Zhu, P., Doolittle, F., Schiller, E., Jenkins, J., & Gersten, R. (2015). *Evaluation of response to intervention practices for elementary school reading* (NCEE 2016–4000). Washington, DC: National Center for Education Evaluation and Regional Assistance.

Batsche, G., Elliott, J., Graden, J.L., Grimes, J., Kovaleski, J.F., Prasse, D., & Tilly, III, W.D. (2005). *Response to intervention: Policy considerations and implementation.* Alexandria, VA: National Association of State Directors of Special Education.

Beaver, J.M., & Carter, M.A. (2003). *Teacher guide: Developmental reading assessment: Grades 4–8* (2nd ed.). Parsippany, NJ: Pearson Education.

Beaver, J.M., & Carter, M.A. (2006). *Teacher guide: Developmental reading assessment: Grades K–3* (2nd ed.). Parsippany, NJ: Pearson Education.

Biancarosa, G., & Snow, C.E. (2006). *Reading next: A vision for action and research in middle and high school literacy. A report to the Carnegie Corporation of New York.* Washington, DC: Alliance for Excellent Education.

Blachman, B.A., & Tangel, D.M. (2008). *Road to reading: A program for preventing and remediating reading difficulties.* Baltimore, MD: Paul H. Brookes Publishing Co.

Blachowicz, C.L.Z. (1980). *Blachowicz informal phonics survey.* Unpublished assessment device, National College of Education, Evanston, IL. Available as a free download from http://readingportfolio.wiki.westga.edu/file/view/Blachowicz+Informal+Phonics+Survey+%28Barr%2C+2000%29.doc

Bracken, B.A. (1988). Ten psychometric reasons why similar tests produce dissimilar results. *Journal of Psychology, 26,* 155–166.

Brown, V., Wiederholt, J., & Hammill, D. (2009). *Test of Reading Comprehension–Fourth Edition (TORC-4).* Austin, TX: PRO-ED.

Buros Center for Testing, Carlson, J.F., Geisinger, K.F., & Jonson, J.L. (2014). *The nineteenth mental measurements yearbook.* Lincoln: University of Nebraska–Lincoln.

Caldwell, J., & Leslie, L. (2009). Intervention strategies to follow informal reading inventory assessment: So what do i do now? (2nd ed.). Boston, MA: Allyn & Bacon.

Carreker, S. (2008). *Basic language skills.* Bellaire, TX: Neuhaus Education Center.

Carrow-Woolfolk, E. (2012). *Oral and Written Language Scales–Second Edition (OWLS-II).* Austin, TX: PRO-ED.

Carrow-Woolfolk, E. (2014). *Test for Auditory Comprehension of Language–Fourth Edition (TACL-4).* Austin, TX: PRO-ED.

Carrow-Woolfolk, E. (2017). *Comprehensive Assessment of Spoken Language–Second Edition (CASL-2).* Austin, TX: PRO-ED.

Catts, H.W., Fey, M.E., Zhang, X., & Tomblin, J.B. (2001). Estimating the risk of future reading difficulties in kindergarten children: A research-based model and its clinical implementation. *Language, Speech, and Hearing Services in Schools, 32*(1), 38–50.

Clay, M.M. (1995). *An observation survey of early literacy attainment* (Rev. ed.). Portsmouth, NH: Heinemann.

Compton, D.L., Fuchs, D., Fuchs, L.S., Elleman, A.M., & Gilbert, J.K. (2008). Tracking children who fly below the radar: Latent transition modeling of students with late-emerging reading disability. *Learning and Individual Differences, 18,* 329–337.

Cox, A.R. (1986). *Benchmark measures.* Cambridge, MA: Educators Publishing Service.

Cox, A.R. (1992). *Foundations for literacy: Structures and techniques for multisensory teaching of basic written English language skills.* Cambridge, MA: Educators Publishing Service.

Cutting, L.E., & Scarborough, H.S. (2006). Prediction of reading comprehension: Relative contributions of word recognition, language proficiency, and other cognitive skills can depend on how comprehension is measured. *Scientific Studies of Reading, 10*(3), 277–299.

Deno, S.L., Fuchs, L.S., Marston, D., & Shin, J. (2001). Using curriculum-based measurements to establish growth standards for students with learning disabilities. *School Psychology Review, 30*(4), 507.

Diamond, L., & Thorsnes, B.J. (2008). *Assessing reading: Multiple measures for kindergarten through twelfth grade.* Berkeley, CA: Consortium on Reading Excellence.

Dunn, L.M., & Dunn, D.M. (2007). *Peabody Picture Vocabulary Test–Fourth Edition (PPVT-4).* New York, NY: Pearson Clinical.

Flanagan, D.P., Ortiz, S.O., & Alfonso, V.C. (2013). *Essentials of Cross-Battery Assessment* (3rd ed.). Hoboken, NJ: John Wiley and Sons.

Flanagan, D.P., Ortiz, S.O., Alfonso, V.C., & Dynda, A.M. (2006). Integration of response to intervention and norm-referenced tests in learning disability identification: Learning from the Tower of Babel. *Psychology in the Schools, 43*(7), 807–825.

Foorman, B.R., & Ciancio, D.J. (2005). Screening for secondary intervention: Concept and context. *Journal of Learning Disabilities, 38*(6), 494–499.

Fox, B., & Routh, D. K. (1983). Reading disability, phonemic analysis, and dysphonetic spelling: A follow-up study. *Journal of Clinical Child & Adolescent Psychology, 12*(1), 28–32.

Fuchs, D., Fuchs, L., & Compton, D. (2004). Identifying reading disabilities by responsiveness-to-instruction: Specifying measures and criteria. *Learning Disability Quarterly, 27,* 216–227.

Gathercole, S.E., Alloway, T.P., Willis, C., & Adams, A M. (2006). Working memory in children with reading disabilities. *Journal of Experimental Child Psychology, 93*(3), 265–281.

Gersten, R., Compton, D., Connor, C.M., Dimino, J., Santoro, L., Linan-Thompson, S., & Tilly, W.D. (2009). *Assisting students struggling with reading: Response to intervention for reading in the primary grades. A practice guide* (NCEE 2009–4043). Washington, DC: U.S. Department of Education, National Center for Educational Evaluation and Regional Assistance, Institute of Educational Sciences. Retrieved from http://ies.ed.gov/ncee/wwc/publications/practice guides/

Goldman, R., & Fristoe, M. (2015). *Goldman-Fristoe Test of Articulation–3 (GFTA-3).* Austin, TX: PRO-ED.

Good, R.H., & Kaminski, R.A. (Eds.). (2002). *Dynamic Indicators of Basic Early Literacy Skills* (6th ed.). Eugene, OR: Institute for Development of Educational Achievement. Available from http://dibels.uoregon.edu

Hammill, D.D., & Larsen, S.C. (2009). *Test of Written Language–Fourth Edition (TOWL-4).* Austin, TX: PRO-ED.

Hammill, D.D., & Newcomer, P.L. (2008). *Test of Language Development, Intermediate–Fourth Edition (TOLD: I4).* Austin, TX: PRO-ED.

Harcourt Assessment. (2003). *Stanford Achievement Test–Tenth Edition.* New York, NY: Pearson Assessments.

Heilbronner, R.L., Sweet, J.J., Attix, D.K., Krull, K.R., Henry, G.K., & Hart, R.P. (2010). Official position of the American Academy of Clinical Neuropsychology on serial neuropsychological assessments: The utility and challenges of repeat test administrations in clinical and forensic contexts. *The Clinical Neuropsychologist, 24*(8), 1267–1278.

Individuals with Disabilities Education Improvement Act (IDEA) of 2004, PL 108-446, 20 U.S.C. §§ 1400 *et seq.*

International Dyslexia Association, The. (2018, March). *Knowledge and practice standards for teachers of reading.* Retrieved from https://dyslexiaida.org/knowledge-and-practices/

Invernizzi, M., Juel, C., Swank, L., & Meier, C. (2003). *Phonological Awareness Literacy Screening: Kindergarten (PALS-K).* Charlottesville: University of Virginia.

Invernizzi, M., Meier, J., & Juel, C. (2002). *Phonological Awareness Literacy Screening 1–3 (PALS 1–3).* Charlottesville: University of Virginia.

Invernizzi, M., Sullivan, A., & Meier, J. (2001). *Phonological Awareness Literacy Screening: Prekindergarten (PALS-PreK).* Charlottesville: University of Virginia.

Johns, J.L. (2012). *Basic Reading Inventory–Eleventh Edition.* Dubuque, IA: Kendall Hunt.

Johnson, E.S., & Pool, J.L. (2009). *Screening for reading problems in Grades 4–12.* Retrieved from http://www.rtinetwork.org

Jordan, R.R., Kirk, D.J., & King, K. (2005). *Early Reading Diagnostic Assessment, Second Edition (ERDA-2).* New York, NY: Pearson Clinical.

Kaufman, A.S., & Kaufman, N.L. (2004). *Kaufman Assessment Battery for Children, Second Edition (KABC-II).* New York, NY: Pearson Assessments.

Kaufman, A.S., & Kaufman, N.L. (2014). *Kaufman Test of Educational Achievement, Third Edition (KTEA-3).* New York, NY: Pearson Assessments.

Kazdin, A. (2006). Arbitrary metrics: Implications for identifying evidence-based treatments. *American Psychologist, 61*(1), 42–49.

Keenan, J.M., Betjemann, R.S., & Olson, R.K. (2008). Reading comprehension tests vary in the skills they assess: Differential dependence on decoding and oral comprehension. *Scientific Studies of Reading, 12*(3), 281–300.

Keenan, J.M., & Meenan, C.E. (2012). Test differences in diagnosing reading comprehension deficits. *Journal of Learning Disabilities, 47*(2), 125–135.

Kena, G., Hussar W., McFarland, J., de Brey, C., Musu-Gillette, L., Wang, X., . . . Dunlop Velez, E. (2016). *The Condition of Education 2016* (NCES 2016–144). Washington, DC: U.S. Department of Education, National Center for Education Statistics. Retrieved from http://nces.ed.gov/pubsearch

Kilpatrick, D.A. (2012). Phonological segmentation assessment is not enough: A comparison of three phonological awareness tests with first and second graders. *Canadian Journal of School Psychology,* 0829573512438635.

Kilpatrick, D.A. (2015). *Essentials of assessing, preventing, and overcoming reading difficulties.* Hoboken, NJ: John Wiley & Sons.

Larsen, S.C., Hammill, S.C., & Moats, L. (2013). *Test of Written Spelling–Fifth Edition (TWS-5).* Austin, TX: PRO-ED.

Learning Disabilities Association of America. (2013). *Right to an evaluation of a child for special education services.* Retrieved from https://ldaamerica.org/advocacy/lda-position-papers/right-to-an-evaluation-of-a-child-for-special-education-services/

Lee, D., Reynolds, C.R., & Willson, V.L. (2003). Standardized test administration: Why bother? *Journal of Forensic Neuropsychology, 3*(3), 55–81.

Leslie, L., & Caldwell, J. (2016). *Qualitative Reading Inventory–Sixth Edition.* Parsippany, NJ: Pearson.

Lezak, M., Howieson, D., Bigler, E., & Tranel, D. (2012). *Neuropsychological assessment* (5th ed.). New York, NY: Oxford University Press.

Lindamood, P.C., & Lindamood, P. (2004). *Lindamood Auditory Conceptualization Test–Third Edition (LAC-3).* Austin, TX: Linguisystems.

Lyon, G.R. & Chhabra, V. (2004). The science of reading research. *Educational Leadership, 61*(6), 12–17.

MacGinitie, W., MacGinitie, R., Maria, K., & Dreyer, L. (2006). *Gates-MacGinitie Reading Tests–Fourth Edition.* New York, NY: Houghton Mifflin Harcourt.

Mascolo, J., Alfonso, V., & Flanagan, D. (2014). *Essentials of planning, selecting and tailoring interventions for unique learners.* New York, NY: Wiley.

Masterson, J.J., Apel, K., & Wasowicz, J. (2006). *Spelling Performance Evaluation for Language and Literacy–Second Edition* [Computer software]. Evanston, IL: Learning By Design.

Mather, N., Hammill, D.D., Allen, E.A., & Roberts, R. (2014). *Test of Silent Word Reading Fluency–Second Edition* (TOSWRF-2). Austin, TX: PRO-ED.

Mather, N., & Jaffe, L. (2011). *Comprehensive evaluations: Case reports for psychologists, diagnosticians, and special educators.* Hoboken, NJ: John Wiley and Sons.

Mather, N., & Jaffe, L. (2016). *Woodcock-Johnson IV: Reports, recommendations, and strategies.* New York, NY: Wiley.

Mather, N., & Kaufman, N. (2006). Introduction to the special issue, part two: It's about the what, the how well, and the why. *Psychology in the Schools, 43*(8), 829–834.

McCarthy, A., & Christ, T. (2010). Test review: The developmental reading assessment-second edition. *Assessment for Effective Intervention, 35*(3), 182–185

McGrew, K. (2011). *IAP 101 Psychometric Brief # 9: The problem with the 1/1.5 SD SS (15/22) subtest comparison "rule-of-thumb."* Retrieved from http://www.iqscorner.com/2011/06/iap-101-psychometric-brief-problem-with.html

McKenna, M.C., & Stahl, K.A.D. (2015). *Assessment for reading instruction.* New York, NY: Guilford.

Mehrens, W.A., & Clarizio, H.F. (1993). Curriculum-based measurement: Conceptual and psychometric considerations. *Psychology in the Schools, 30*(3), 241–254.

Moats, L.C. (1995). *Spelling: Development, disability, and instruction.* Timonium, MD: York Press.

Morsy, L., Kieffer, M., & Snow, C. (2010). *Measure for measure: A critical consumers' guide to reading comprehension assessments for adolescents. Final report from Carnegie Corporation of New York's Council on Advancing Adolescent Literacy.* New York, NY: Carnegie Corporation of New York.

Mosely, D.V. (1997). Assessment of spelling and related aspects of written expression. In J.R. Beech & C. Singleton (Eds.), *The psychological assessment of reading* (pp. 204–223). London, United Kingdom: Routledge.

Nation, K., & Snowling, M.J. (1998). Individual differences in contextual facilitation: Evidence from dyslexia and poor reading comprehension. *Child Development, 69*(4), 996–1011.

Nelson, N.N., Plante, E., Helm-Estabrooks, N., & Hotz, G., (2016). *Test of Integrated Language and Literacy Skills™ (TILLS™)*. Baltimore, MD: Paul H. Brookes Publishing Co.

Newcomer, P.L. (2014). *Diagnostic Achievement Battery–Fourth Edition (DAB-4)*. Austin, TX: PRO-ED.

Newcomer, P.L., & Hammill, D.D. (2008). *Test of Language Development, Primary–Fourth Edition (TOLD: P4)*. Austin, TX: PRO-ED.

No Child Left Behind Act (NCLB) of 2001, PL 107-110, 115 Stat. 1425, 20 U.S.C. §§ 6301 *et seq.*

Noll, B. (2013). Seven ways to kill RTI. *Phi Delta Kappan, 94*(6), 55–59.

Norton, E.S., & Wolf, M. (2012). Rapid automatized naming (RAN) and reading fluency: Implications for understanding and treatment of reading disabilities. *Annual Review of Psychology, 63*, 427–452.

Overton, T. (2011). *Assessing learners with special needs* (7th ed.). Upper Saddle River, NJ: Pearson/Merrill Prentice Hall.

Palmer, B., Boone, K., Less, I., & Wohl, M. (1998). Base rates of "impaired" neuropsychological test performance among healthy older adults. *Archives of Clinical Neuropsychology, 13*, 503–511.

Pennington, B.F. (2009). *Diagnosing learning disorders: A neuropsychological framework* (2nd ed.). New York, NY: Guilford.

Pennington, B.F., Cardoso-Martins, C., Green, P.A., & Lefly, D.L. (2001). Comparing the phonological and double deficit hypotheses for developmental dyslexia. *Reading and Writing, 14*(7–8), 707–755.

Peterson, R., & Pennington, B. (2012). Developmental dyslexia. *The Lancet, 379*(9830), 1997–2007.

Questar Assessment. (2015). *Degrees of Reading Power*. Apple Valley, MN: Author.

Reed, D.K., & Vaughn, S. (2012). Retell as an indicator of reading comprehension. *Scientific Studies of Reading, 16*(3), 187–217.

Reid, D.K., Hresko, W.P., & Hammill, D.D. (2001). *Test of Early Reading Ability–Third Edition (TERA-3)*. Austin, TX: PRO-ED.

Renaissance Learning. (1996). *Renaissance STAR Reading*. Wisconsin Rapids, WI: Author.

Reutzel, D., & Cooter Jr., R.B. (2011). *Strategies for reading assessment and instruction: Helping every child succeed*. Parsippany, NJ: Pearson.

Reynolds, C.R. (1981). The fallacy of "two years below grade level for age" as a diagnostic for reading disorders. *Journal of School Psychology, 19*(4), 350–358.

Reynolds, C.R. (2009). *Determining the r in RTI: Which score is the best score?* Workshop presented at the NASP Annual Convention, Boston, MA.

Reynolds, C., & Shaywitz, S. (2009). Response to intervention: Ready or not? or, from wait-to- fail to watch-them fail. *School Psychology Quarterly, 24*(2), 130–145.

Robertson, C., & Salter, W. (2007). *Phonological Awareness Test–Second Edition (PAT-2)*. Austin, TX: PRO-ED.

Roid, G.H. (2003). *Stanford-Binet Intelligence Scales–Fifth Edition (SB5)*. Itasca, IL: Riverside.

Rumsey, M.B. (1992). *Dyslexia training program progress measurements* (Schedules I–III). Cambridge, MA: Educators Publishing Service.

Salvia, J., Ysseldyke, J., & Bolt, S. (2017). *Assessment in special and inclusive education* (13th ed.). Boston, MA: Cengage Learning.

Sattler, J.M., & Hoge, R.D. (2006). *Assessment of children: Behavioral, social, and clinical foundations* (5th ed.). San Diego, CA: Jerome M. Sattler.

Scarborough, H. S. (1998). Predicting the future achievement of second graders with reading disabilities: Contributions of phonemic awareness, verbal memory, rapid naming, and IQ. *Annals of Dyslexia, 48*(1), 115–136.

Schneider, J., & Kaufman, A. (2017). Let's not do away with comprehensive cognitive assessments just yet. *Archives of Clinical Neuropsychology, 32*, 8–20.

Schneider, W. (2013). Principles of assessment of aptitude and achievement. *The Oxford handbook of child psychological assessment*. New York, NY: The Oxford University Press.

Schrank, F.A., Mather, N., & McGrew, K.S. (2014a). *Woodcock-Johnson IV Tests of Achievement*. Rolling Meadows, IL: Riverside.

Schrank, F.A., Mather, N., & McGrew, K.S. (2014b). *Woodcock-Johnson IV Tests of Oral Language*. Rolling Meadows, IL: Riverside.

Schrank, F.A., McGrew, K.S., & Mather, N. (2014). *Woodcock-Johnson IV Tests of Cognitive Abilities*. Rolling Meadows, IL: Riverside.

Seidenberg, M. (2017). *Language at the speed of sight: How we read, why so many cannot, and what can be done about it*. New York, NY: Basic Books.

Shaywitz, S.E. (2003). *Overcoming dyslexia: A new and complete science-based program for reading problems at any level*. New York, NY: Knopf.

Shaywitz, S.E. (2016). *Shaywitz DyslexiaScreen*. New York, NY: Pearson.

Siegel, L. S. (1993). Phonological processing deficits as a basis for reading disabilities. *Developmental Review, 13*, 246–257.

Silbergliitt, B., & Hintze, J.M. (2007). How much growth can we expect? A conditional analysis of R—CBM growth rates by level of performance. *Exceptional Children, 74*(1), 71–84.

Slosson, R., Nicholson, C., & Larson, S. (2015). *Slosson Oral Reading Test–SORT-3*. East Aurora, NY: Slosson Educational.

Smartt, S.M., & Glaser, D.R. (2010). *Next STEPS in literacy instruction: Connecting assessments to effective interventions*. Baltimore, MD: Paul H. Brookes Publishing Co.

Speece, D.L., Case, L.P., & Molloy, D.E. (2003). Responsiveness to general education instruction as the first gate to learning disabilities identification. *Learning Disabilities Research & Practice, 18*(3), 147–156.

Strauss, E., Sherman, E.M., & Spreen, O. (2006). *A compendium of neuropsychological tests: Administration, norms, and commentary*. Washington, DC: American Chemical Society.

Swanson, H.L. (1981). Vigilance deficits in learning disabled children: A signal detection analysis. *Journal of Child Psychology and Psychiatry, 22*, 393–399.

Swanson, H.L., Zheng, X., & Jerman, O. (2009). Working memory, short-term memory, and reading disabilities: A selective meta-analysis of the literature. *Journal of Learning Disabilities, 42*(3), 260–287.

Torgesen, J.K. (1998, Spring/Summer). Catch them before they fall: Identification and assessment to prevent reading failure in young children. *American Educator, 1*–8.

Torgesen, J.K. (2006). *A comprehensive K–3 reading assessment plan: Guidance for school leaders*. Portsmouth, NH. RMC Research Corporation.

Torgesen, J.K., & Bryant, B.R. (2004). *Test of Phonological Awareness–Second Edition: PLUS (TOPA-2+)*. Austin, TX: PRO-ED.

Torgesen, J.K., & Miller, D.H. (2009). *Assessments to guide adolescent literacy*. Portsmouth, NH: RMC Research Corporation.

Torgesen, J.K., Wagner, R.K., & Rashotte, C.A. (2012). *Test of Word Reading Efficiency–Second Edition (TOWRE-2)*. Austin, TX: PRO-ED.

Treiman, R. (1998). Why spelling? The benefits of incorporating spelling into beginning reading instruction. In J.L. Metsala & L.C. Ehri (Eds.), *Word recognition in beginning literacy* (pp. 289–313). Mahwah, NJ: Lawrence Erlbaum Associates.

Vannest, K., Stroud, K., & Reynolds, C. (2011). *Strategies for academic success: An instructional handbook for teaching K–12 students how to study, learn and take tests*. Torrance, CA: Western Psychological Service.

Vaughn, S., & Fuchs, L.S. (2003). Redefining learning disabilities as inadequate response to instruction: The promise and potential problems. *Learning Disabilities Research & Practice, 18*(3), 137–146.

Wagner, R.K., Torgesen, J.K., & Rashotte, C. (1999). *Comprehensive Test of Phonological Processing (CTOPP)*. Austin, TX: PRO-ED.

Wagner, R.K., Torgesen, J.K., Rashotte, C.A., & Pearson, N.A. (2010). *Test of Silent Reading Efficiency and Comprehension*. Austin, TX: PRO-ED.

Wagner, R.K., Torgesen, J.K., Rashotte, C.A., & Pearson, N.A. (2013). *Comprehensive Test of Phonological Processing–Second Edition (CTOPP-2)*. Austin, TX: PRO-ED.

Wallace, G., & Hammill, D.D. (2013). *Comprehensive Receptive and Expressive Vocabulary Tests–Third Edition (CREVT-3)*. Austin, TX: PRO-ED.

Wechsler, D. (2008a). *Wechsler Adult Intelligence Scale for Adults–Fourth Edition (WAIS-IV)*. New York, NY: Pearson Assessments.

Wechsler, D. (2008b). *Wechsler Preschool and Primary Scale of Intelligence–Fourth Edition (WPPSI-IV)*. New York, NY: Pearson Assessments.

Wechsler, D. (2009). *Wechsler Individual Achievement Test–Third Edition (WIAT-III)*. New York, NY: Pearson.

Wechsler, D. (2014). *Wechsler Intelligence Scale for Children–Fifth Edition (WISC-V)*. New York, NY: Pearson.

Wiederholt, J.L., & Bryant, B.R. (2012). *Gray Oral Reading Test–Fifth Edition (GORT-5)*. Austin, TX: PRO-ED.

Wiig, E.H., & Secord, W. (1989). *Test of Language Competence–Expanded (TLC Expanded)*. New York, NY: Pearson Assessments.

Wiig, E.H., & Secord, W. (1992). *Test of Word Knowledge (TOWK)*. New York, NY: Pearson Clinical.

Wiig, E.H., Semel, E., & Secord, W.A. (2013). *Clinical Evaluation of Language Functions–Fifth Edition (CELF-5)*. New York, NY: Pearson Clinical.

Wilkinson, G.S., & Robertson, G.J. (2006). *Wide Range Achievement Test–Fourth Edition (WRAT-4)*. Austin, TX: PRO-ED.

Wilson, B., & Felton, R. (2004). *Word Identification and Spelling Test (WIST)*. Austin, TX: PRO-ED.

Wolf, M., & Bowers, P.G. (1999). The double-deficit hypothesis for the developmental dyslexias. *Journal of educational psychology, 91*(3), 415.

Woodcock, R.W. (2011). *Woodcock Reading Mastery Tests, Third Edition (WRMT-III)*. New York, NY: Pearson Clinical.

Woodcock, R., Mather, N., & Schrank, F.A. (2004). *Woodcock-Johnson III Diagnostic Reading Battery*. New York, NY: Houghton Mifflin Harcourt.

Woods, M., & Moe, A. (2015). *Analytical Reading Inventory: Comprehensive standards-based assessment for all students including gifted and remedial* (10th ed.). Parsippany, NJ: Pearson.

Online Resources for Assessment

The following online resources provide general information and guidelines on assessment as well as specific assessment tools.

GENERAL INFORMATION AND GUIDELINES

See the following resources for general information and guidelines related to assessment.

The Florida Center for Reading Research (http://fcrr.org) has a number of online guidelines, checklists, and related materials under the "Resources" tab.

The federal government's web site for the Individuals with Disabilities Education Act (https://www2.ed.gov/about/offices/list/osers/osep/osep-idea.html) has official memos and regulations.

The International Dyslexia Association (https://dyslexiaida.org/universal-screening-k-2-reading/) provides information on universal screening in the primary grades.

The National Council on Measurement in Education (http://www.ncme.org/NCME) has a glossary of terms under the "Resource Center" tab.

The web site for the Center on Response to Intervention at the American Institutes for Research (http://www.rti4success.org) provides numerous publications, training modules, and other resources related to RTI.

The Research Methods Knowledge Base web site (http://www.socialresearch methods.net/kb/reliable.php) presents a discussion on the reliability of measures.

TIBCO Software Inc. (http://www.statsoft.com/Textbook/Basic-Statistics) provides information on basic statistics.

TEST MANUFACTURERS

See the web sites of the following test manufacturers for various specific assessment tools.

Academic Therapy Publications   http://www.AcademicTherapy.com

The Achenbach System of Empirically Based Assessment   http://www.aseba.org

Paul H. Brookes Publishing Co.   http://www.brookespublishing.com

The Data Recognition Corporation   http://www.datarecognitioncorp.com

Houghton Mifflin Harcourt   http://www.hmhco.com

Kendall Hunt Publishing   http://www.kendallhunt.com

Learning By Design   http://www.learningbydesign.com

LinguiSystems   http://www.linguisystems.com

Pearson Education—Assessment   http://www.pearsonassessments.com

Pearson Higher Education   http://www.pearsonhighered.com

PRO-ED   http://www.proedinc.com

Questar   http://www.questarai.com

Renaissance K–12 Education   http://www.renaissance.com

Slosson Educational Publications   http://www.slosson.com

Chapter 8

The Role of Executive Function in Literacy Instruction

Monica Gordon-Pershey

LEARNING OBJECTIVES

1. To describe how executive function is a cognitive process that influences literacy learning and academic success

2. To describe the importance of language skills in the development and enhancement of executive function

3. To describe the characteristics of students who require assessment of executive function

4. To describe the nature of assessments of executive function

5. To describe interventions to enhance executive function, language, literacy, and academic learning

Executive function is the mental process that allows individuals to regulate their thinking and behaviors. Parents and educators expect school-age and adolescent learners to initiate, control, and accomplish a multitude of academic learning tasks and interactional behaviors that are dependent on the use of executive function. Learners commonly need the executive control that regulates focusing attention, planning actions, reasoning, remembering, integrating past experiences with present contexts, and choice making, as well as being able to identify optimal actions, engage in social interactions, and achieve emotional **self-regulation** (Tridas, 2013).

Executive function and language skills have an ongoing and recursive relationship that supports learning. Proficient executive function provides the cognitive foundation for the growth of academic language and learning. Learners can recursively employ language to regulate their use of executive function and to learn academic concepts and skills. Language helps learners mediate and control the executive processes that underlie academic learning. This is especially important for the language-based learning involved in literacy. Then, with enhanced learning, students bring more background, knowledge, and experience to the task of using their executive function and improving their language growth. Language skill can be both a cause and a consequence of learning. This multidirectional relationship is illustrated in Figure 8.1, which depicts how executive function, language, and learning are mutually supportive capabilities. Literacy, in this conceptualization,

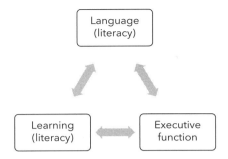

Figure 8.1.   Executive function, language, and learning.

is a language ability, and it is also a specific type of learning that involves many skills and processes.

The intent of this chapter is to describe how learners can use language to support and improve executive functioning and, reciprocally, how the growth of executive function can improve oral language, literacy, and academic learning. This chapter provides language-based strategies to help regulate students' learning and behaviors so that they can succeed in academic and interactional contexts.

EXECUTIVE FUNCTION, DEFINED AND DESCRIBED

Executive function is the mental process used to perform activities of self-regulation. Examples of everyday self-regulation skills include paying attention, planning, organizing, strategizing, prioritizing, managing time and space, and reasoning (National Center for Learning Disabilities [NCLD], 2018; for a full description see Diamond, 2013). Tridas (2013) described executive function as the "cognitive inputs" that facilitate decision making. Executive functioning refers to the thinking processes that govern how individuals choose what to do and when to do it, how to do it, and why to do it.

Diamond (2013; see also Miyake et al., 2000) identified three core subtypes of executive function. One primary subtype is **cognitive flexibility** (being able to shift attention among competing stimuli and consider alternatives). A second core subtype is **inhibitory control** (the ability to consider when to act and when to not act, that is, the ability to choose which actions to exhibit and which to inhibit). Although the ability to remember is not in itself an executive function, a third main subtype is **working memory** (Baddeley, 1996; Baddeley & Hitch, 1994; D'Esposito, 2002; Smith, 2000). Working memory is the ability to hold information in mind while thinking about it—the use of the so-called "mental sketchpad" or "on-screen memory." Working memory provides a basis for flexible thinking and self-regulation because working memory keeps the current situation in mind long enough for an individual to consider alternatives and inhibit overly quick reactions. Baddeley's (2000) model of working memory proposes that a central executive system is responsible for control of attention and is linked to three subsystems: the phonological loop, the visuo-spatial sketchpad, and the episodic buffer. The phonological loop and visuo-spatial sketchpad are responsible for temporarily storing information for processing. The episodic buffer integrates representations from long-term memory and language storage with the present contents of working memory.

Garon, Bryson, and Smith (2008) proposed a developmental integrative framework for the child's growth in executive function during the preschool years (as reported by Kapa & Plante, 2015; see also Best & Miller, 2010). Young children first develop their attentional skills then gain the working memory skill to retain and manipulate information. Next, children acquire inhibitory control to self-regulate behavior, and then they acquire the cognitive flexibility that coordinates shifting their attention and thought across stimuli and actions. This developmental model suggested that later developing skills employ the earlier capabilities. Insufficient development of the earlier abilities could have a negative effect on the later developing competencies (Kapa & Plante, 2015).

The three main subtypes, cognitive flexibility, inhibitory control, and working memory, work together to allow the mind to choose what to focus on and to hold this priority in mind long enough to think about it. At the same time, executive function inhibits involvement in other circumstances that would detract from thinking about the matter at hand. Executive function is needed to process, understand, and react to information, circumstances, and events. Executive functioning takes advantage of recall memory, which includes remembering stored information, and working memory, which integrates past experiences with present contexts. Memories that are recalled help influence decision making and identifying optimal actions (Kaufman, 2010; Tulving, 1993). If these cognitive processes are present and working appropriately, they guide individuals to know what to do.

However, this is not the entire course of the mind's actions. The human mind must then experience the cognitive processes it generates. How does the mind experience, for example, that it is remembering? In many cases, the mind uses language to think and reason. The mind makes sense of its resources of memories, cognitive and emotional choices, and intellectual strategies by putting thoughts into words. This process is known as verbalization. Verbalized thoughts help to govern actions. Verbalization occurs during speaking and writing and in self-talk, which happens when individuals silently or quietly use inner language to talk to themselves while thinking.

Verbalization is one of the most critical ways by which the mind reasons. Most of the time, language is used so that the mind can translate its cognitive resources of working memory, choice making, and past experiences into words, and these words can guide actions. The process that the mind employs to use words to consider events and information, to think about circumstances, and to solve problems by using language is known as **verbal reasoning.** This abstract mental processing of ideas contrasts with how individuals process physical events that are experienced directly through sensory and perceptual exposure and by motor actions. As Bruner (1966) proposed, learners use three modes of mental representation of information and memories: enactive representations, which are stored as information about physical actions and muscle memories; iconic representations, which are stored as visualizations or mental pictures; and symbolic representations, which are stored as language. Verbal reasoning does not replace physical or iconic representations, but verbal reasoning is necessary for learning about concepts and events that cannot be directly experienced and for advanced intellectual development, as well as for the forethought needed for inhibiting actions. Barkley (2011) stated that verbal working memory is evidenced by self-talk, and nonverbal working memory is experienced as visual imagery and the recollections of the experiences of the other senses.

REFLECT, CONNECT, and RESPOND
Describe Baddeley's (2000) model of working memory and its importance for learning to read.

Executive Function and Academic Learning

Academic learning requires students to have considerable capacity for verbal reasoning and to be able to verbalize their verbal reasoning. Students must put their thinking into words. Although the mind can reason nonverbally and individuals can think explicitly in images or in other nonverbal ways—as is the case with music, visual arts, or dance—the bulk of academic learning pertains to demonstration of verbal reasoning. Schoolwork generally requires that students verbalize aloud or in writing in order to demonstrate that they have learned concepts and skills. A fair proportion of schoolwork involves remembering and recalling verbal information that has been heard or read and that describes abstract concepts and complicated events that the students have not experienced firsthand. Students are required to reason through this verbal information in order to produce verbal products: they take tests, write papers, work in cooperative groups, give presentations, and complete other school tasks that involve considerable use of language. Demonstration of these various capabilities shows that the student has the cognitive flexibility to address this assortment of language and learning demands and perform well across alternative situations.

In the context of academic learning, with its emphasis on verbal reasoning, the relationship between executive functioning and language is ongoing and complementary throughout recursive cycles of learning, as depicted in Figure 8.2. In any academic context where information is heard or read, a learner's attention, cognitive flexibility, working memory, information storage, and integration of past experiences with present contexts are brought to bear. Studying involves repeated verbal rehearsal of the information to be learned. For students to progress academically, ongoing study involving verbalization of verbal reasoning must be maintained throughout a class period, and then retained cumulatively for days, weeks, and even years. Throughout, the student exerts the inhibitory control needed to reduce distractibility, forgetfulness, and off-task thoughts and behaviors.

To demonstrate learning, a student's underlying cognitive skills are operationalized as language output. To operationalize a skill means to show how the skill is put to use—to demonstrate by overt evidence that the skill is occurring. The cognitive act of remembering actually becomes the linguistic act of recounting; the cognitive act of understanding is evidenced by the learner's overt demonstration of verbal reasoning, in spoken or written form. Parents, educators, and other service providers can observe what the student does or does not say, but they cannot actually be certain of what the student does or does not know. Overt language provides a window on students' executive functioning and possibly serves as the best available proxy for observing how students manage their executive skills. (Other windows into what students know include their nonverbal demonstrations of enactive response, as in asking a child to demonstrate a behavior or action, point, or gesture and evidence of his or her thinking in images, e.g., "Draw a picture of your answer.") Traditional schoolwork, however, may not offer many opportunities to use nonverbal behaviors to demonstrate the learning of conceptual information.)

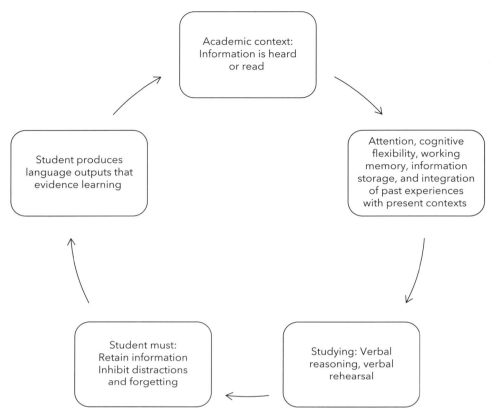

Figure 8.2.   How executive function and language are used during learning.

REFLECT, CONNECT, and RESPOND
Why are verbal reasoning abilities necessary for academic achievement?

Role of Language in Executive Function

A caveat to the recursive cycle depicted in Figure 8.2 is necessary: Language is concurrently operative during each part of the process of enacting executive function. When a learner is receiving academic input by listening or reading, this itself is a language-processing task. Working memory, information storage, and integration of past experiences with present contexts are mediated by the inner language that the learner uses to make sense of the incoming information. Cognitive flexibility (i.e., considering alternatives) and inhibitory control are also mediated by the inner language that the learner uses to regulate choices (Alarcón-Rubio, Sánchez-Medina, & Prieto-García, 2014). Studying involves repeated silent or overt verbal rehearsal of information. As such, language is a faculty that learners use before, during, and/or after speaking or taking action. Language helps learners plan what to do, govern what they do, and review what they have done.

Just as language is a window into the operation of executive function, the reciprocal process is true as well: Executive function reveals language in use, even when this is covert inner language. Language capabilities must be present and employed in the service of executive function. Language is a component of the repertoire of human faculties and behaviors, but it also can function as the governor of these repertoires.

This reveals the root of what language does for learners: Language is arguably the most important means for human thought. If executive function is the process that humans use to go about their thinking and learning, and individuals think predominantly in language, then executive function is a process that is realized by language. Executive function is enacted because it can be governed by language. Human beings must have the language that is needed to arrive at executive decisions. Executive skills would suffer if any part (or parts) of this process is limited due to language deficits.

Executive function is not just the little voice that tells individuals what to do, or tells right from wrong, like the proverbial angel on one shoulder and devil on the other. Executive functioning means that individuals can weigh options, strategize, and reason through circumstances. The point is that executive functioning allows individuals to use language to know how to "think it over." When learners are struggling, parents and educators need to be able to carefully examine whether and how the ability to use language to govern learning might be a part of the difficulty.

In sum, executive function lets individuals know what to do, when to do it, how to do it, and why to do it. For school learners, "what to do" means what to learn in an academic setting and how to show that they have learned it. Executive function accomplishes the following:

- Activates thought

- Regulates how individuals think

- Regulates how individuals learn

- Helps individuals interpret their environment and the world.

In so doing, executive function allows for decisions about several cognitive and behavioral activities, including how to do the following (Kaufman, 2010; Tridas, 2013):

- Initiate thought

- Initiate action

- Inhibit thought

- Inhibit action

In general, executive function affords the cognitive and behavioral governance of each of the following activities in which an individual engages:

- Attentional activities

- Memory-dependent activities

- Organizational activities

- Self-regulation activities

- Interactions with the environment

THE TWO DOMAINS OF EXECUTIVE
SELF-REGULATION: METACOGNITIVE AND SOCIAL EMOTIONAL

The three core subtypes of executive function, cognitive flexibility, inhibitory control, and working memory, are needed to operate the two general domains of executive self-regulation: the **metacognitive** and social-emotional domains.

Metacognitive Domain

In the metacognitive domain, executive function governs how individuals think about thinking. This includes intellectual problem solving and reflective thought. Educators often stimulate learners to achieve thinking for connections (see, e.g., the International Literacy Association/National Council of Teachers of English [2017] *ReadWriteThink* pages), higher order thinking (see Reading Rockets for "HOT" descriptions of higher order thinking [Thomas & Thorne, 2017]), or **critical thinking** (i.e., an attitude of thoughtfulness, along with knowledge of methods of logical inquiry and reasoning, and persistent effort to examine problems, evidence, conclusions, interpretations, and arguments) (Foundation for Critical Thinking, 2015). When learners develop the habit of thinking about thinking, they can be purposeful and independent thinkers. Strengths in cognitive flexibility and working memory are essential.

Social-Emotional Domain

In the social-emotional domain, executive function governs how individuals think about feeling. Cognitive flexibility, inhibitory control, and working memory team together to help individuals regulate their actions and their responses to the environment and the social field. Self-regulation of behaviors involves knowing when and how to initiate behaviors and when to exert inhibitory control over behaviors. Control of behavioral impulses arises, in part, from having the cognitive flexibility to inhibit one course of action and do something else or nothing at all. This control, in turn, arises in part from bringing working memory to bear to keep the current situation in mind while considering alternatives and inhibiting overly quick reactions (see Alderson, Rapport, Hudec, Sarver, & Kofler, 2010). Long-term recall of past learning, events, outcomes, and consequences is quickly called up by working memory so that control of behavioral impulses can occur based on past knowledge and experiences. Davis and Stone (2003) suggested that self-regulation of social behaviors is dependent on recall of long-term understandings about the minds, feelings, and emotions of others. This knowledge arises from the child's theory of mind, that is, the cognitive ability to understand that others have beliefs, desires, intentions, and perspectives that are different from one's own, and the metacognitive ability to self-examine those understandings (Baron-Cohen, 1991; Hughes, 1998; Perner, 1998).

In the same way, self-regulation of emotions draws on the inhibitory control needed to determine when an emotional response can be initiated or should be inhibited. This kind of emotional self-regulation relies on working memory to call up past experiences of the events that arose and the past feedback that was received when emotions were displayed, even if this was witnessed vicariously. Cognitive flexibility allows individuals to work in the present moment to adjust their inner emotional reactions and overt displays of emotional responses to meet the conditions of the environment and to know that their emotions can be deferred and revisited at another time when the setting is appropriate and better supports are available. This cognitive flexibility fits in with the individual's self-concept (Baumeister, 1999), that is, one's beliefs about oneself and one's attributes. In this case, the individual would have the cognitive flexibility and inhibitory control needed to bring to bear the belief that he or she is able to self-regulate emotions.

REFLECT, CONNECT, and RESPOND

Explain how executive function allows students to develop self-regulation strategies.

In sum, executive function drives the cognitive skills that help self-regulate social-emotional behaviors. **Social cognition** refers to how individuals perceive, process, and recall social information and apply their knowledge in social contexts (Cherry, 2016). Social cognitive processes are needed for social-emotional self-regulation. Hamilton (2005) noted that the cognitive processes of attention, retention, and recall provide the basis for the gatekeeping and selectivity needed for appropriate emotional reactions and social behaviors. Individuals can control emotions better when they have the cognitive flexibility to understand emotions. Emotional intelligence (Coleman, 2005) relies on acquiring social cognitions in the form of social-emotional problem-solving skills that are learned, retained, and adaptably applied so that one's emotions can be labeled, expressed, understood, interpreted, tolerated, and used constructively and effectively and so that one has resilience in the face of social-emotional adversity.

REFLECT, CONNECT, and RESPOND

Explain how executive function allows students to develop emotional intelligence.

How Language Mediates the Two Domains of Executive Function

Language mediates both of the general domains of executive self-regulation: the metacognitive and social-emotional domains. Verbalization of executive functioning is an important component of revealing how individuals get to the point of knowing what to do in both domains. From the perspective of the teacher or parent, students' executive function is evidenced by their use of language to overtly describe their self-regulation of the cognitive and social-emotional resources that govern attention, working memory, decision making, and identification of optimal actions. For instance, in the metacognitive domain, learners may be asked to perform the higher order thinking task of verbally describing how they discovered their answers during a science lab experiment. A common example of executive self-regulation in the social-emotional domain is when parents or teachers ask a child to verbalize the choices available in a given circumstance and describe the reasons why one choice would be better than the others. In so doing, the child is given the opportunity to hold both the goal and the prohibitions firmly in mind as he or she explains.

However, from the perspective of the student, using language to govern thought and action can be a conscious process or an unconscious part of his or her daily living. Children may not think to use overt language to bring their executive function into their own conscious focus or to share their realizations with others. Some learners overtly describe their self-regulation of their attention,

working memory, and decision making; some do not; and some might do so sometimes. Some children may be more adept at verbally describing their intellectual
metacognitive reflections, and some children may evidence more verbal sharing
of their social-emotional self-regulation. In the metacognitive domain, when students reflect on their own intellectual thought processes, their levels of emotional
arousal are usually not high, so metacognition is called "cold" functioning (Brock,
Rimm-Kaufman, Nathanson, & Grimm, 2009; Hongwnishkul, Happaney, Lee,
& Zelazo, 2005; Kerr & Zelazo, 2004). When students use executive function to
regulate their affect, social-emotional reactions, and related behaviors, levels of
emotional arousal are usually somewhat higher, so these functions are termed
"hot" (Brock et al., 2009; Hongwnishkul et al., 2005; Kerr & Zelazo, 2004). A consideration about language that is apparent in both the cold and hot contexts is
that learners must be able to use language reflectively and elaborately to interpret
the world, to explain their recollections, and to govern their behavioral repertoire
(see, e.g., Nippold, Mansfield, & Billow, 2007, for a discussion of the language skills
needed).

> **REFLECT, CONNECT, and RESPOND**
> What are the "hot" and "cold" aspects of executive functioning?

CHARACTERISTICS OF STUDENTS WHO REQUIRE ASSESSMENT OF EXECUTIVE FUNCTION AND LANGUAGE PERFORMANCE

A range of different children and teens will be referred to psychologists, special
education teachers, learning disabilities specialists, speech-language pathologists, and other educational and medical personnel for assessment of suspected
executive function deficits. Other students will be referred for assessment for concerns regarding language skills, literacy acquisition, and academic learning, or
for social-emotional and/or behavioral difficulties, and sometimes, in the course
of examining these capabilities, executive function deficits will be identified. For
some children, the presence of executive function deficits will be a characteristic
of a primary disorder where executive function deficits are embedded in a more
complex array of sensory, learning, and language disturbances, as in the setting of
intellectual disabilities (ID), autism spectrum disorders (ASD), or acquired brain
injury. The assessment and teaching of students with these multifaceted diagnoses
are beyond the scope of this chapter. However, there are students from several
other populations who would present for assessment and for whom the relationship between executive function and language is an important concern.

Students With Deficits in Attention

Barkley (1997, 2005, 2006, 2011, 2012) documented that deficits in executive function, notably in self-regulation and goal-directed problem solving, appear regularly in individuals who are diagnosed with **attention deficit disorder (ADD)** or
attention-deficit/hyperactivity disorder (ADHD). The core problems of inattention, distractibility, **impulsivity,** and hyperactivity that are characteristic of ADD/
ADHD (according to the American Psychiatric Association's *Diagnostic and Statistical Manual of Mental Disorders, Fifth Edition* [DSM-5; 2013]) underlie Barkley's characterization of an executive function deficit as being a difficulty with sustaining

self-directed action to achieve a future goal. Barkley observed that problems with self-regulation are a consequence of an individual with attention deficits having an array of possible weaknesses that may include decrements in inhibition, resistance to distraction, self-awareness, working memory, self-talk, emotional self-control, and motivation. Barkley claimed little difference exists between the difficulties that have typically been characterized as a deficit in attention and the symptoms that would suggest a deficit in executive function. Kasper, Alderson, and Hudec (2012) and Kofler and colleagues (2011) identified that students with attention deficits may have core difficulties with working memory. As such, examiners would expect to find executive function concerns in students who have met the criteria for diagnosis of ADD/ADHD.

Barkley (2011) characterized executive function deficits in individuals with ADD/ADHD as "not absolute," as might occur in individuals with more severe intellectual deficits, for whom the underlying cognitive capacity for acquiring the knowledge to perform self-directed tasks might be at issue. In students with deficits in attention and executive function, adequate underlying knowledge and skills are in place but are not easily utilized for the performance of tasks. These deficits in performance are often the reason why students with attention difficulties may be among those who are referred for assessment of executive function, reading, and oral and written language abilities. With appropriate diagnosis and interventions, students with ADD/ADHD are potentially responsive to teaching, environmental accommodations, and compensatory behaviors that can improve performance.

Students With Specific Learning Disabilities

The Individuals with Disabilities Improvement Act (IDEA) of 2004 (PL 108-446) defined **specific learning disability** as a disorder in one or more of the basic processes involved in understanding or producing spoken or written language, as manifested in the ability to listen, think, speak, read, write, spell, or perform mathematical calculations. The identification of the broad skill of "thinking" would indicate where the core executive deficits in cognitive flexibility, inhibitory control, and working memory would be pertinent to the struggles with language that characterize a specific learning disability. IDEA 2004 identified dyslexia as a specific learning disability.

The Learning Disabilities Association of America (LDA; 2017) report on executive function stated that deficits in executive function are not a learning disability, but weakness in executive function is often noted in the learning profiles of individuals with specific learning disabilities. Learning disabilities may involve difficulty with planning, organization, strategizing, paying attention to and remembering details, and managing time and space (LDA, 2017).

A specific learning disability may challenge the development of executive functioning. Children with learning disabilities may struggle with being disorganized and forgetful and may have lesser skills in problem solving and self-reflection. Cognitive flexibility, inhibitory control, and working memory are needed for gaining proficiency in reading, writing, and math, all of which involve complicated rule-governed skills and goal-directed behaviors. Students are faced with academic tasks that their underlying executive functioning mechanisms have difficulty supporting and that become increasingly more demanding as the academic grade levels advance. For example, using phonics to decode words requires cognitive flexibility and working memory to organize letter–sound correspondences, and purposeful reading adds in the need to divide attention flexibly between decoding and comprehension. During literacy tasks, the child may have trouble understanding which aspects of language to pay attention to and why. Lack of inhibitory control may interfere with the sustained attention and persistence that are needed to learn and study, and the learner's approach to a task may be interrupted by the child's frustration or anxiety. The student is trying to apply ineffectual perseverance to language tasks, which is compounded by the fact that language is the student's inherent area of weakness. Lesser prioritization skills may cause the student to be confused about how to use language-learning strategies effectively across academic contexts.

The problems faced by students with specific learning disabilities are compounded as time goes on. Lack of school success undermines the more sophisticated academic learning that advances the development of metacognitive executive function. Lack of experience with complex thinking exacerbates the degree of the specific learning disability itself. It is apparent that students with specific learning disabilities will be among those who present for assessment of executive function and oral and written language abilities.

Students With Language Disorders

The American Speech-Language-Hearing Association (ASHA; n.d.b) explained that a spoken language disorder, also known as an oral language disorder, involves a deficit in auditory comprehension and/or spoken production of any of the five domains of language (i.e., phonology, morphology, syntax, semantics, and pragmatics). A spoken language disorder may occur in the presence of other conditions, such as ID, ASD, or ADD/ADHD. When a spoken language disorder is not accompanied by any other disorder, disability, or medical condition, it is considered a **specific language impairment (SLI).**

A spoken language disorder may be diagnosed in a young child before the child is of an age to develop literacy. The symptoms of the language disorder may persist and change over time such that academic weaknesses in reading and written language arise in children with spoken language difficulties. Students who were diagnosed with spoken language disorders at a young age may be labeled in their academic years as having a specific learning disability (ASHA, n.d.b, n.d.c). A school-age learner may be diagnosed with a **written language disorder,** which involves impairment in reading decoding, sight-word recognition, reading comprehension, written spelling, and/or written expression (ASHA, n.d.c). Written language disorders, as with spoken language disorders, can involve any of the five language domains (phonology, morphology, syntax, semantics, and pragmatics). Deficits can affect language awareness, comprehension, and production at the sound, syllable, word, sentence, and discourse levels (ASHA, n.d.c). The criterion for a specific learning disability is that there is an impairment of one or more of the basic processes involved in understanding or producing spoken and/or written language that affect listening, speaking, reading, writing, spelling, and mathematical calculations (IDEA 2004). There is considerable symptom overlap across the diagnostic labels of language disorder (spoken and/or written) and specific learning disability.

The various diagnostic terms can lead to confusion for educational teams working with students with academic concerns. Diagnostic labeling diverges such that 1) some students with language disorders may have coexisting diagnoses of specific learning disabilities; 2) some students with language disorders may not have coexisting diagnoses of specific learning disabilities; 3) some students with specific learning disabilities may have coexisting diagnoses of language disorders; 4) some students with specific learning disabilities may not have coexisting diagnoses of language disorders; 5) language disorders may occur in the context of another disorder, disability, or condition, such as with ADD/ADHD; and 6) sometimes the learning disability is described as a **language-based learning disability (LBLD),** although this is a somewhat redundant term given that a specific learning disability is defined as a disorder in one or more of the basic processes involved in understanding or producing spoken or written language (IDEA 2004). (Still another possibility is that language disorders may be specific, that is, unitary, meaning not accompanied by any other disorder, disability, or medical condition; that might mean that a student's language deficits do not cause an adverse academic impact, so the student would not qualify for the label of specific learning disability. However, lack of impact is an unlikely possibility because even a social communication disorder [ASHA, n.d.a, n.d.b] can interfere with a student's interactions with teachers and peers in an educational setting.)

REFLECT, CONNECT, and RESPOND
What kinds of learning difficulties are seen in children who have difficulty with executive functioning?

Regardless of the diagnostic terminology, these children are in a condition where their academic growth is impeded because of deficient comprehension and/or use of language. Moving from using language as a form of communication to engaging in an intellectual, metalinguistic exploration of language as a topic of study can be quite effortful. Learners may have difficulty learning the code-based language skills needed for phonological awareness, alphabetics, phonics, decoding, and spelling, and/or the meaning-based skills needed for auditory comprehension, reading comprehension, and oral and written expression. They may toil with language-based academic tasks, such as vocabulary, word study, and grammar (Conti-Ramsden, Ullman, & Lum, 2015) and may need to exert much effort to achieve language-based organizational skills, such as using punctuation, paragraph arrangement, titles and section headers, indexes, tables, graphs, and charts. Some students may exhibit **word-finding problems,** also known as **word-retrieval problems** (Messer & Dockrell, 2011). This is the phenomenon of "the word is on the tip of my tongue," where a speaker knows the word he or she needs to say but cannot recall it at the moment. Other students may seem to be very literal communicators; they may miss the point of jokes, word play, double entendre, and figures of speech, and they may not see the hidden meanings in what other people say or in what they read. They may not appreciate song lyrics or poetry. Some students may not observe or may misread body language, facial expressions, and gestures.

Newhall noted that students may present with different profiles of language difficulties with different levels of severity:

> One student may have difficulty sounding out words for reading or spelling, but no difficulty with oral expression or listening comprehension. Another may struggle with all three. The spectrum … ranges from students who experience minor interferences that may be addressed in class to students who need specialized, individualized attention throughout the school day in order to develop fluent language skills. (2017)

The exercise of these capacities is simultaneously an arrangement of actions, reactions, and inhibitions. Tonnessen observed that "reading is a skill that requires both automatization and awareness" of sub-skills (1999, p. 386). Learners need to perform "flexible and functional combinations" of conscious judgments and automatic behaviors (1999, p. 391). Insufficient performance is indicative of insufficient awareness, insufficient automatization, or an insufficient ability to switch between the two "in a flexible and expedient manner" (1999, p. 391)

REFLECT, CONNECT, and RESPOND
What is a word-finding problem?

Language Disorders and Executive Function	Among children with language disorders, the issue at hand is whether a weakness in language contributes to inferior executive functioning. The reciprocal may be true as well: weaker executive functioning may be a factor that contributes to difficulty learning and developing language. Assessing whether the source of children's academic and/or social-emotional difficulties is due to language, executive function, or both can be challenging and inexact. The coexistence of language and executive concerns is intertwined (Singer & Bashir, 1999). Reporting on a study of 243 children, Gooch, Thompson, Nash, Snowling, and Hulme (2016) concluded that there was a strong concurrent relationship between abilities in language and executive function, and there was considerable longitudinal stability of performance in language and executive function over the preschool and early school years.

Barkley (2011, 2012) described a situation experienced by some learners. Suppose that a student's psychometric assessment ruled out difficulties with attention and concentration. The child has adequate intelligence and demonstrated knowledge of a fund of information that is reasonable for grade level; these assessments would demonstrate that the acquisition of language itself is sufficient. However, testing shows that the student's processing of language input is insufficient. Language input is not reasoned with well or employed effectively. An individual who, despite having some knowledge of the topic at hand, is not reasoning well about this topic fits the description of an individual with deficits in verbal reasoning. As illustrated by Figure 8.2, this learner's cognitive flexibility, working memory, information storage, and integration of past experiences with present contexts are not brought to bear on the language input. This an example of when metacognitive language capabilities are not being employed in the service of executive function. This child's metacognitive language is not sufficient to govern executive functioning. Performance, rather than knowledge, is deficient. The result would be academic underachievement.

Barkley's pristine hypothetical example was meant to uncover the relationship of executive function and language. However, as Barkley also stated, in terms of how students achieve day-to-day functional behaviors and successful learning outcomes, a diagnosis of diminished executive function versus a diagnosis of attention deficit yields few differences. The difficulties that students face because of deficits in attention are very much like the symptoms that would suggest deficits in executive function. Although attention deficits and executive function deficits are not synonymous (see Brown, 2006), much of the research literature identifies language and learning weaknesses in the contexts of deficits that could be attributed to attention and/or executive functioning, and the literature may not exactly differentiate the two. In an extensive review of the co-occurrence of attention deficits and language impairment, Redmond and Timler (2013) showed that there is co-occurrence, although there is an instability in the co-occurrence rates reported. Redmond (2014) identified ADHD as a context for the co-occurrence of language impairment, but the affected population is heterogeneous.

The research literature provides abundant examples of the heterogeneity of the language skill deficits that can co-occur in the presence of attention and/or executive function deficits (see, e.g., a review by Westby & Robinson, 2007). Language deficit areas that have been researched for coexistence with deficits in attention and/or executive function include the following:

- Oral language (Adams, Bourke, & Willis, 1999; Baker & Cantwell, 1992; Humphries, Koltun, Malone, & Roberts, 1994; Kim & Kaiser, 2000; Oram, Fine, Okamoto, & Tannock, 1999; Tannock & Schachar, 1996; Tirosh & Cohen, 1998)

- Listening comprehension (McInnes, Humphries, Hogg-Johnson, & Tannock, 2003)

- Language processing (Im-Bolter, Johnson, & Pascual-Leone, 2006), specifically, word- and sentence-level memory (Berninger et al., 2010)

- Regulating the self-talk needed for learning and remembering (Berk & Potts, 1991) and for self-regulation (Nippold et al., 2007; Westby & Cutler, 1994)

- **Pragmatic language** concerns, that is, language as it is used in interactional contexts (Bruce, Thernlund, & Nettelbladt, 2006; Camarata & Gibson, 1999)

- Code-based skills needed for reading, for example, phonological memory (Bolden, Rapport, Raiker, Sarver, & Kofler, 2012; Boudreau & Costanza-Smith, 2011; Gathercole & Baddeley, 1993; Gray, 2006; Swanson & Sachse-Lee, 2001); phonological processing, alphabet knowledge, morphological processing, sight words, and oral reading fluency (Dittman, 2016; Gathercole, Alloway, Willis, & Adams, 2006; McCloskey & Perkins, 2012); single word decoding (Arrington, Kulesz, Francis, Fletcher, & Barnes, 2014; Henry, Messer, & Nash, 2012)

- Language skill deficits that could affect both spoken and written language skills, such as syntactic processing (Montgomery, Magimairaj, & Finney, 2010; Redmond, 2005)

- Metaphor comprehension (Carriedo, Corral, Montoro, Herrero, Ballestrino, & Sebastián, 2016)

- Discourse organization (Westby & Cutler, 1994; Westby & Robinson, 2007)

- Narrative comprehension (oral and written) (e.g., identification of a goal-based narrative structure, causal connections; resolving difficulty with ambiguity and extraneous information) (Duinmeijer, Jong, & de Scheper, 2012; Flory, Milich, Lorch, Hayden, Strange, & Welsh, 2006; Montgomery, Polunenko, & Marinellie, 2009; Tannock, Purvis, & Schachar, 1992; Westby & Robinson, 2007)

- Written expression (Berninger et al., 2010; Reid & Lienemann, 2006; Vanderberg & Swanson, 2007)

- Reading comprehension (Arrington et al., 2014; Barkley, 2005; Berninger et al., 2010; Berninger & Richards, 2002; Brock & Knapp, 1996; Cain, Oakhill, & Bryant, 2004; De Jong, 1998; McCloskey, Perkins, & Van Divner, 2009; Purvis &

Tannock, 1997), including understanding main ideas, inferencing, and self-monitoring for comprehension (Westby & Robinson, 2007)

- Story comprehension (Lorch, Berthiaume, Milich, & van den Broek, 2007; Lorch, Milich, Astrin, & Berthiaume, 2006; Lorch et al., 2000; Renz et al., 2003).

Kapa and Plante (2015) indicated that numerous studies have shown that children with language concerns have demonstrated deficits in some or all of the three components of executive function and also proposed the possibility that language deficits might be a part of more generalized, overarching problems with the cognitive representation of information that is gained from multisensory inputs (see Bavin, Wilson, Maruff, & Sleeman, 2005). Some investigations (Vugs, Cuperus, Hendriks, & Verhoeven, 2013; Vugs, Hendriks, Cuperus, & Verhoeven, 2014) implicated the visuo-spatial aspects of working memory as interacting with language impairment to affect learners' overall performance. Moreover, children who have language disorders may actually have any number of a variety of nonlinguistic deficits (Gallinat & Spaulding, 2014), which may include motor control, slower processing of stimuli and slower response speed, and deficits in **procedural memory** (Ullman & Pierpont, 2005) and/or planning. It is possible that slower processing may disrupt children from developing the rapid, automatic linguistic facilities that are involved in literacy, such as are needed for parsing the speech stream into words, morphemes, and phonemes, and the fast-mapping of phoneme–grapheme correspondences (Gray, 2006). Weaknesses in motor control and/or procedural memory (Lum, Conti-Ramsden, Page, & Ullman, 2012) may interfere with performing rapid, routinized literacy tasks, such as decoding, fluent reading, spelling, and using written language conventions, such as punctuation.

Henry, Messer, and Nash (2012) and Vissers, Koolen, Hermans, Scheper, and Knoors, (2015) proposed that disorders of language work against cognitive flexibility, working memory (see also Leonard et al., 2007; Marton & Schwartz, 2003), and inhibitory control (see also Marton, Kelmenson, & Pinkhasova, 2007). Evidence of deficits is ongoing throughout the preschool and school years, as learning demands increase.

Specific Concerns for Language Disorders and Working Memory   Boudreau and Costanza-Smith (2011) converged on the relationship of language and working memory by noting that aspects of working memory are critical to language and academic success. Boudreau and Costanza-Smith's report stressed that working memory capabilities entail processing, storage, and retrieval. Learners with weaker working memory skills may experience significant challenges in academic settings (Alloway, 2009; Archibald & Gathercole, 2006). Decoding itself is a working memory task, as Boudreau and Costanza-Smith noted:

> Decoding a novel word requires a child to break a word into its individual sounds and hold the accompanying phonological representations in memory until each letter/letter sequence is encoded and can be blended together to form a word—a process similar to writing and spelling as a child breaks each word into its individual parts, accesses the accompanying phonological representation in memory (or letter–sound), and represents each sound with a graphic symbol. (2011, p. 154)

Beyond decoding, **phonological working memory** is important for the development and automatic use of vocabulary and underlies morphological and grammatical accuracy (Bishop, 2006; Gray, 2006). Mackie, Dockrell, and Lindsay (2013) attributed variance in writing accuracy in children with language disorders to phonological working memory in the areas of orthographic spelling errors, omissions of whole words (e.g., auxiliary verbs and subject nouns), and omissions of grammatical morphology (e.g., past tense -*ed*) that reflected oral language production errors.

Language comprehension and production require sufficient phonological working memory to process incoming verbal information and construct an appropriate response. For learners with adequate phonological working memory, language input would be processed more automatically. Weaker phonological working memory can slow down other language skills that are dependent on efficient phonological processing, such as rate of learning of new vocabulary and reading automaticity.

Archibald, Joanisse, and Edmunds explored the social, behavioral, and academic characteristics of children with difficulties with language or memory alone, and children with both difficulties present: "The children with memory impairments were found to have some language-related difficulties, and the children with language impairments, some memory-related difficulties" (2011, p. 294). Overall, these learners required assistance with schoolwork, maintaining attention, and moderating their classroom behavior. Archibald and colleagues attributed the observed difficulties more to language than to memory. Learners sometimes mediated their working memory difficulties by using verbal explanations, but the investigators did not observe that children with language impairment produced memory-related comments.

When a learner's working memory resources need to be specifically allocated to processing aspects of the language input that is heard or read, especially when there is a demand for processing complex sentences (Montgomery & Evans, 2009), this leaves fewer cognitive resources available for performance of tasks and acquiring long-term learning. Working memory may activate in a piecemeal fashion such that schoolwork may require several attempts at completion. Information may need to be repeated or reviewed in order for a learner to process and store it, and written responses may need to be drafted and revised. The result is less efficiency during all school subjects, noticeably in skills that require considerable verbal rehearsal, such as mathematics, reasoning, and problem solving. The greater amount of time that learning and performance require can lead to the potential for falling behind the student's academic peer group.

REFLECT, CONNECT, and RESPOND
What is the relationship of executive functioning to the development of language skills in an academic setting?

Specific Concerns for Language Disorders and Attention Deficits   The literature on the relationship of language skills and attention deficits includes many investigations of capacity limitations related not only to attending itself but also to the cognitive flexibility to allocate attentional resources across tasks and the inhibitory control needed to purposefully direct attention to language processing and performance (e.g., Castellanos, Sonuga-Barke, Milham, & Tannock, 2006; Ellis Weismer, Plante, Jones, & Tomblin, 2005; Hutchinson, Bavin, Efron, & Sciberras, 2011; Jonsdottir, Bouma, Sergeant, & Scherder, 2005; Marton et al., 2007). In a retrospective review of 100 students' assessment files, DaParma, Geffner, and Martin (2011) identified children with ADHD as having receptive language weaknesses in understanding spoken language, following directions, understanding concepts, and understanding grammatical relationships, and expressive language concerns in formulating sentences, recalling words rapidly, and performing word association tasks. Memory weaknesses were apparent on tasks of retaining and recalling information. DaParma, Geffner, and Martin proposed that when children with attention deficits seem not to be listening, perhaps this behavior may reflect a deficit in comprehending spoken language, and they argued that the defining characteristics of attention deficit disorders might necessarily need to include a risk of language impairment.

Addressing the complexity of attributional concerns, Redmond (2014) and Redmond and Timler (2013) reviewed numerous studies in an attempt to sort out performance deficits that can be ascribed to language disorders, versus weakness in executive function, versus ADD/ADHD. Their work alluded to four compelling possibilities that put forward why these problems sometimes can be almost inextricably intertwined, especially in assessment and intervention settings.

First, students with language impairments may obtain false positive results on tests of ADHD and executive function. Measures meant to assess attention or executive function require oral language comprehension and use and may use letters or numbers. Written language symbols may confound children with language disorders and/or specific learning disabilities. The oral and written language demands may lead to false positive scores on the tests of attention or executive function when lesser language skills are really at issue.

Second, as the DSM-5 (American Psychiatric Association, 2013) stated, children with specific learning disabilities may appear inattentive to academic work because of their frustration, lack of interest, or limited language-based abilities. For some children, their attention is not impaired outside of academic work. Academic abilities testing does not always allow for a naturalistic sampling of children's daily play and interactions, where their better attentional skills may be evident. A diagnosis of an attentional concern may not be entirely accurate, and it may detract from educators and parents focusing their interventions on the learner's language deficits.

Third, children with language disorders who have overt attentional and behavioral difficulties may actually perform better on academic abilities testing than children with language disorders without behavioral difficulties because their problematic behaviors have caused teachers and parents to request that the children be identified, referred for assessment, and provided with instruction and interventions. Although not exactly a false negative result for the presence of language deficits and specific learning disabilities if the academic skills tested are in place, the possibility exists that the effect of prior instruction and interventions makes it harder to observe the impact of behavioral difficulties on language and academic performance. It may also suggest that language disorders alone do not trigger the same degree of concern and responsiveness in parents and teachers as attentional and behavioral difficulties do and that the children with language disorders without behavioral issues may not receive the interventions they need.

Fourth, pragmatic language production difficulties in interactional contexts can be observed in children with language disorders, ADD/ADHD, or executive function deficits. These difficulties include spoken language that exhibits false starts, self-revisions, excessive talking, interruptions, little attention to detail, unnecessary or inappropriate questioning, poor turn-taking in conversation, not listening to what others say, and weak cohesion in narratives and conversations. However, parents and teachers may misidentify a child's inability to readily convey a point in conversation as inattention, distractibility, or impulsivity, which are the symptoms of ADD/ADHD, when these behaviors actually signal a pragmatic language deficit in message formulation.

> **REFLECT, CONNECT, and RESPOND**
> Explain how executive function deficits can coexist with other disorders: specific learning disabilities, language disorders, and attention deficit disorders.

Meta-Analysis of Executive Function in Children With Language Impairment Pauls and Archibald (2016) conducted a meta-analysis of 46 studies of children ages 4–14 with language impairment performing behavioral measures of cognitive flexibility and inhibitory control. These researchers found results that were somewhat contrary to most of the information available on the relationship of language and executive function. In this meta-analysis, inhibition was studied as resistance to internal distractions (sometimes called "cognitive interference") and external distractions (sometimes conceived of as **selective attention**). Cognitive flexibility was explored as set shifting or task switching. As a whole, the meta-analysis of the studies reviewed confirmed with statistical significance that children with language impairment performed more poorly than unimpaired controls on tasks of cognitive flexibility and inhibitory control. However, the severity of participants' language impairment, the linguistic demands of the studies' tasks, and the age of the children had no bearing on the results of the meta-analysis. As such, the verbal load was not found to be contributory. This would suggest that cognitive flexibility and inhibitory control were uniquely implicated in the poorer performance of children with language impairment. Although the authors did not point to verbal processes as operable in the executive function deficits they identified, they noted an executive functioning advantage for children without language impairments. The Pauls and Archibald (2016) results suggested that deficient language performance in the presence of attention deficits is a function of weaker skills in both attention and language and that better nonlinguistic inhibitory control skills appeared to facilitate better language processing. These findings suggested a domain generality of attention skills and that nonlinguistic attention skills may be in use during linguistic tasks.

ASSESSING EXECUTIVE FUNCTION IN THE CONTEXT OF ASSESSING OTHER ABILITIES

Students with known or suspected learning disabilities, attention deficits, and/or language disorders may be among those who present for assessment of their language skills, literacy skills, and/or academic abilities. The primary question is whether the executive processes of cognitive flexibility, working memory, and inhibitory control may be impaired and, if so, can these processes be implicated as reasons for the examinee's language, literacy and/or academic learning concerns. Care needs to be taken to conduct an appropriate assessment of the complex learning, attentional, and language problems that each student exhibits and arrive at an accurate differential diagnosis of when, where, and how executive function is potentially involved in the student's performance.

As McCloskey noted, executive function must be assessed in tandem with cognitive processes, learned abilities and skills, and/or retrieval of linguistic information: "Specific measures of executive functions always involve the assessment, to some degree, of a capacity other than executive functions" (n.d., p. 29). McCloskey stated that executive function cannot be tested "in a vacuum…. [i]n order to evaluate how executive functions cue and direct, they must have something (i.e., specific perceptions, emotions, thoughts, or actions) to cue and direct" (n.d., p. 28).

Psychometric Testing of Executive Function

Psychometricians have prepared a number of tests that are intended to assess the construct of executive function. When students require assessment of their language skills, literacy skills, and/or academic abilities, the educational team may include a psychologist, neuropsychologist, psychiatrist, or other service providers who perform psychometric assessment of executive function.

The team member responsible for testing executive function must exercise care to select testing that would have concurrent and/or predictive validity for school success. Many executive function tests are designed for the neuropsychological assessment of adults or children with acquired brain injuries, neurological or psychiatric disorders, or psychosocial concerns (e.g., as described by Chan, Shum, Toulopoulou, & Chen, 2008), and such tests may not be directly relevant to school-age and adolescent learners. For example, one executive function test described by Chan and colleagues asks the examinee to inhibit a predictable response to a sentence fill-in question and instead offer an unusual, irrelevant response. Inhibitory control is observed. However, students may be confused as to why inhibiting a logical response would be required, when this is essentially the opposite of what is expected at school. Although these tests may reveal an impairment of the basic properties of executive functioning, their findings may not readily translate to a description of how learners may struggle in an academic context; as such, the test's functionality and **ecological validity** (i.e., its resemblance to the contexts of everyday life) may be insufficient (Chan et al., 2008). In other types of testing, the student's limitations in language and learning might obscure a clear view of how the examinee applies the executive processes. Consider, for instance, how tests that require arithmetic, picture naming, or writing to dictation (Chan et al., 2008) might actually be measuring the application of a learner's prior language skills and academic knowledge rather than the learner's regulation of executive processes in an on-demand situation. A learner may not demonstrate the executive skill of sustained attention, for example, not because he or she cannot attend to the task long enough to complete it, but because he or she cannot enact the series of cognitive-linguistic processes required for that task. A false positive finding of an executive function disturbance might ensue.

Executive function assessment is targeted toward either the "cold" metacognitive tasks or the "hot" social-emotional tasks, and sometimes to both. The "cold" tests involve primarily recall, logic, reasoning, and planning, often in the context of choice-making or inhibiting competing stimuli. One commonly used test of "cold" executive function is a Stroop test (Stroop, 1935). In this test, an examinee looks at a word, for example, a color word such as *green*, but the word is written in another color ink, such as red. The examinee has to inhibit saying "red" and respond with "green." This task involves the cognitive flexibility to think about the word and the ink color simultaneously and the inhibitory control to suppress any response that would name the color of the ink. Stroop tests for children (e.g., Golden, Freshwater, & Golden, n.d.) may include naming of shapes or pictures, rather than reading words, in tasks that require choosing from two conflicting stimuli to respond as directed. Other tests measure a variety of self-regulatory behaviors that are dependent on cognitive flexibility and inhibitory control, such as motor reaction time, choice-making reaction time, concentration on tasks, dividing attention across two separate and unrelated tasks that have to be performed alternatively, prioritizing steps to complete a response, and suppression of habituated responses (Chan et al., 2008).

Working memory can be assessed by measuring performance following a delay, as in asking an examinee to hold words or performance tasks in short-term memory, then to complete a distractor task, then to return to the operations involving the items originally held in short-term memory. Other tests of working memory require matching visual stimuli or reciting a span of digits, numbers, letters, or words. Span testing can ask examinees to logically process the stimuli in working memory, for example, to order the numbers from smallest to largest or largest to smallest, order letters or words alphabetically, or perform some mental operation on the stimuli held in mind (Chan et al., 2008).

Testing of the "hot" social-emotional executive function involves primarily social-emotional judgments, decision making, and goal management, along with inhibition and self-control. Some tests use situational tasks that employ gambling on gain or loss as an indicator of inhibitory control. Examinees may be asked to postpone an immediate gain or satisfaction in anticipation of an even greater reward after a delay in gratification (e.g., deciding whether to eat a treat that is present or to refrain from eating the treat and to wait for a better or bigger treat promised for later). Other tests ask examinees to strategize how to avoid some future loss or negative consequence. Enacting behaviors that are advantageous and inhibiting behaviors that are disadvantageous is the test's indicator of social-emotional executive control (Chan et al., 2008).

The determination of appropriate instrumentation, however, must ultimately be made by the professionals who assess the youngster's symptomatology. The choice of testing depends on whether the purpose of the assessment is to uncover a neuropsychological or psychosocial impairment in executive function or to reveal the nature of the student's functional activity and/or the limitations to participate in school learning, and hence school progress (Chan et al., 2008; World Health Organization, 2005). If the purpose of the assessment is to ascertain how executive function may be a component of the student's functional difficulties with accomplishing academic progress, then using executive function tests that may more specifically reveal how a student approaches academic tasks might be more relevant. Tests chosen would be those that use a more **naturalistic assessment** of activities that are commonly participated in at school and would yield more ecological validity. In short, the test items and required performances would be similar to academic tasks and would have greater practical utility and user friendliness.

REFLECT, CONNECT, and RESPOND

What are the strengths and weaknesses of psychometric tests of executive functioning?

Assessing Executive Function in the Context of Language, Literacy, and Academic Testing

Consider the list of concerns that parents and teachers are apt to provide when they refer a student for testing of language, literacy, and/or academic abilities.

The reason for referral is underachievement in these areas of learning and performance, but along with the specific language, literacy, and/or academic deficits that they mention, they may characterize a student's difficulties as any of the following:

- Inconsistently paying attention

- Inconsistent persistence (the student gives up)

- Tendency not to remember information well or inconsistency in recall

- Difficulty remembering what to do; need for cues and inconsistency in acquiring skills

- Difficulty reasoning well

- Weak planning skills; difficulties with calendars, clocks, and schedules

- Tendency to be messy and disorganized

- Behavioral issues when frustrated

- Inconsistent impulse control

Psychometric testing may identify these concerns. However, apart from using specific psychometric testing of executive functioning, or in addition to those tests, assessors can interpret language, literacy, and/or academic abilities testing to uncover executive functioning. In a comprehensive assessment process, every subtest and every task can reveal something about the test taker's executive functioning skills. Tests that are designed to identify specific language, literacy, and/or academic difficulties reveal how language, literacy, and academic skills have been developed and achieved but also indirectly or incidentally reveal how these abilities and skills have been achieved given the quality of the child's executive functioning. An assessor can have a view of how executive functioning has been achieved given the quality of the child's abilities and skills. The assessor's summary report includes the scores that the student obtained along with a careful description of how the student obtained these scores, meaning how the student functioned and behaved during testing.

Interpreting Testing to Reveal Cognitive Flexibility   An examinee's behavior during testing may reveal how he or she shifts his or her attention among competing stimuli and considers alternatives. The examiner may consider these questions:

- Is the student aware of whether he or she is paying attention? (When called back to task, does the student fail to acknowledge that his or her attention shifted?)

- Does the student need breaks during testing? Does the student employ bartering to reduce the burden of sustained attention and concentration? ("Can I do half of this, then take a break?")

- Is the student's attention facilitated by the examiner's redirection cues or use of external rewards?

- Is the student procrastinating during testing?

- Is the student showing selective attention, notably as interest in and willingness to complete some tasks but not others?

- Is the student fatiguing during testing? (Is concentration tiring?)

- Does the student **perseverate** across different tasks, meaning does the student have difficulty shifting gears between different kinds of performance tasks? (The student may seem stuck or repetitive when transitions are needed.)

The examiner may include statements about cognitive flexibility in the testing report summary. Examples of such statements are as follows:

- "A's test-taking behaviors showed attentional skills to be [adequate for X minutes; adequate when given breaks every X minutes; adequate with external reinforcers; inadequate even given frequent redirection]."

- "A's demonstration of issues with attention and concentration did not compromise attaining an age-appropriate score in X."

- "Attentional issues appear to have contributed to A's attaining a lower score in X."

In academic learning, cognitive flexibility may be an underlying component of verbal reasoning. Tests may require students to demonstrate reasoning and problem solving. Text comprehension tests may have inferential questions (requiring reading between the lines to explain something alluded to in the text, e.g., explaining a character's reasons or motivations). Other sorts of questions that require flexible verbal reasoning include "what if" questions, questions that require the reader or listener to determine the meaning of a multiple meaning word in given context, and cause-and-effect questions where multiple causes and/ or effects are possible.

To delve further into performance of executive functioning than the published test questions can, examiners can extend the demands of the test questions. Of course, test administration requires following the test's instructions in order for the test to be valid and reliable. However, keeping this in mind, it is legitimate for an examiner to return to test questions later on in the testing session, once the required administration protocol has been completed, to probe verbal reasoning and problem solving. The examiner might ask the examinee to discuss a question and the examinee's prior response, with questions such as the following:

- "Tell me why you answered this way."

- "How did you know that?"

- "How did you get your answer?"

- "Why is the answer not _____?"

If a test question allowed the examinee to offer only one answer but other answers are plausible, the examiner might offer a probe such as "Was your answer only one way to solve the problem? What if it did not work—what would you do next?"

The examiner may include statements about verbal reasoning and problem solving in the testing report summary. Examples of such statements are as follows:

"B correctly answered 3 of 7 reasoning questions related to a 100-word third-grade level paragraph. B defined 2 meanings of 6 multiple meaning words among the 9 words that were asked. When asked at the end of the testing session if she could think of any multiple meaning words, she said 'Call, like I call you and what this is called.' While this is not strictly a multiple meaning word, this shows emerging reasoning about how a word can convey different meanings."

"B answered 11 problem solving questions that extended the stimuli on the test. She proposed a reasonable solution to a problem for 9 of the 11 questions."

Interpreting Testing to Reveal Inhibitory Control   Inhibitory control may be evidenced by a student's approach to a test's tasks. The test administrator may observe the student's behavioral self-regulation of inhibition. Overall, the assessor may want to take note of any behaviors that merit acknowledgment. This can include physical or bodily movements that seem uninhibited, inappropriate behaviors for a school or clinical setting, procrastination during test taking, or noncompliance or refusal during testing. A student may enact false starts or need do-overs to complete tasks because other impulses, whether exhibited or covert, interfered with performing a task.

Impulse control difficulties may be revealed by impulsivity, which means that the test taker changes his or her focus nonpurposefully, sometimes distractedly, and perhaps to something of low priority. The student seems driven by an impulse to do something different from whatever is required at the moment. The assessor may notice that the student interrupts the assessor, or blurts out remarks, or rushes to answer questions before the questions have been fully asked. The student may disregard directions, change his or her approach to a task midway through the task, or hop from topic to topic rather than discussing a topic for more than a sentence or two. Impulsivity may coincide with a lack of perseverance; the student appears to be too flexible in the way he or she thinks and performs. The student may not inhibit fatiguing or stopping during tasks; if the student experiences an impulse to quit, he or she gives in to the impulse.

Test administrators may notice that test takers who exhibit difficulty with impulse control may attempt to countermand the administrator's plans for rewards and reinforcements during the testing session. The student may contrive scenarios to bring about immediate gratification, when the administrator had planned for delayed gratification. Test takers may try to negotiate a change in tasks and thereby may influence what it takes to be rewarded (even if that reward is only to finish the testing session). In terms of the social-emotional content of behaviors and interactions, students who struggle with impulse control may make uncensored remarks or be untruthful.

The examiner may include statements about inhibitory control in the testing report summary. Examples of such statements are as follows:

"C asked to end testing three times. He tried to negotiate a change of task twice. He said that he did not like being out of class and was missing a test. (There was no test in class that day.)"

"After we began the vocabulary subtest, when we reached Item 4, C said, 'Oh, wait. Can we start over?'"

"C habituated easily to the use of a schedule for work time and break time during the assessment."

Interpreting Testing to Reveal Working Memory   All testing performance is functionally dependent on working memory. Test takers have to hold information in mind while thinking about it. The stimulus–response testing paradigm highlights how the examinee's working memory skills are operative when producing a response. For the most part, an examinee's responses allow the examiner to see what the student is thinking as he or she responds. Responses reveal what has been "on-screen" to formulate the response.

Testing behaviors can reveal difficulties with working memory. Speed of response is generally a requirement for satisfactory test performance. An immediate response means that the examinee has efficiently and readily brought to mind the information that is needed to process the question and produce a response and has the background knowledge to do so. **Latency of response** means that the examinee is responding more slowly than would be expected for the demand that was presented. The delay can reveal difficulties with processing stimuli and/or formulating a response. The time it takes for the examinee to respond may be the result of slower processing (i.e., needing a lengthier processing time) or slower response formulation (using language to reply takes a longer time).

Other test-taking behaviors that may evidence the efficiency of the examinee's working memory are delineated by the following questions:

- Does the examinee think aloud?

- Does the examinee forget stimuli and ask for a repeat of the stimuli?

- Does the examinee forget stimuli and *not* ask for a repeat of the stimuli? (This could suggest concerns with comprehending the stimuli well enough to even ask for repetition, or a lack of motivation or persistence to continue.)

- Does the examinee forget the process or procedure midway through a subtest or task?

- Does the examinee fail to build up a response pattern during subtests where a growing awareness of a patterned sort of response is an apparent strategy for success?

- Does the examinee lose track of thought? ("What was I saying?" "What was I doing?")

- Does the examinee offer a delayed response? (This may involve interjecting responses later in the session for items that were completed earlier: "Oh, I just remembered…")

- How well does the examinee return to task following distractions?

- How well does the examinee perform on tasks that require purposefully divided attention?

Working memory difficulty may be characterized by word-finding problems, also known as word-retrieval problems. Sometimes a test taker may state that he or she is having difficulty recalling a word, but word finding is also evidenced by the following:

- A slow naming rate (response latency for identifying an object by its name, including the names of letters, shapes, symbols, or numbers)

- Naming errors

- Self-rehearsal and/or rephrasing when producing a message ("Okay, this is how I am going to say it…")

- Self-cuing (which may appear to be searching for meaning: "What is the thing called that…?")

- Using place-holder words ("That thingamabob")

- Substituting words when the target word is not found ("Well, it's not a _____, but it is like a _____.")

- Creating neologisms (literally, "new words"; making up a word when a target word cannot be recalled)

Tests of language abilities may offer a particularly valuable glimpse of working memory. The subtests of standardized tests of language may reveal working memory function through a variety of tasks, including the following:

- Sentence repetition

- Verbal recall of the details of a paragraph heard read aloud

- Retelling information heard spoken

- Following verbal directions

- Pressure naming (naming items quickly, as in "Name all of the animals that you can in one minute.")

- Rapid naming of pictures of items, colors, or shapes

- Sentence formulation (listening to a group of words and arranging them into a sentence [e.g., *bag, pack, forget, don't, to, your*])

An example of a published test that was designed to tap abilities in spoken language and executive function is the Executive Functions Test–Elementary (ages 7–12, Grades 2–7) (Bowers & Huisingh, 2014). The Executive Functions Test–Elementary is a test of using language skills during tasks that involve working memory, problem solving, inferring, predicting outcomes, and shifting tasks. The test comprises four subtests, A–D.

Subtest A: Attention and Immediate Memory–Auditory presents short passages with follow-up questions to determine a student's ability to pay attention to details and remember what he or she hears. *Subtest B: Attention and Immediate Memory–Auditory and Visual* presents illustrations and short vignettes. Students answer questions that require attention to detail and a problem to be solved. *Subtest C: Working Memory and Flexible Thinking* tests working memory and cognitive flexibility by asking the student to listen to a short passage and answer two "thinking" questions. *Subtest D: Shifting* tests working memory and cognitive flexibility by asking the examinee to compare items across categories.

McCloskey suggested that identifying certain reading errors might be a window onto a student's "ineffective engagement of executive functions during task performance" (n.d., p. 36). Reading performance tests reveal orthographic, phonological, and semantic retrieval capabilities, as evidenced by the reader's reading speed and pacing. McCloskey proposed that an assessment battery include tests of rapid automatic naming and single word reading (with both sight word reading and the rapid application of decoding skills to single words and nonwords), such as are included in the Test of Word Reading Efficiency (TOWRE; Torgesen, Wagner, & Rashotte, 2012) and the Process Assessment of the Learner–Second Edition: Diagnostics for Reading and Writing (PAL-II Reading and Writing; Berninger, 2007).

In sum, working memory difficulties may result in students producing disorganized messages, appearing to not get to the point of what they are saying, appearing to not have learned certain information (when they simply cannot bring it to mind at the moment), and demonstrating deficiency in expressing transitions between ideas. The examiner may include statements about working memory in the testing report summary. Examples of such statements are as follows:

"D's working memory was taxed during the language assessment. D forgot the test question on 4 occasions and had to ask for the question to be repeated. Upon repetition, he answered the questions correctly. He was able to recall 4 details of a paragraph that had 8 prominent details. (He recalled the name of a character, where the story took place, and two elements of the action sequence.)"

REFLECT, CONNECT, and RESPOND
Describe how executive functioning can be observed in the context of language, literacy, and/or academic abilities testing.

IMPROVEMENT OF EXECUTIVE FUNCTION IN THE CONTEXT OF LEARNING LANGUAGE, LITERACY, AND/OR ACADEMICS

The International Dyslexia Association's (IDA; 2018) *Knowledge and Practice Standards for Teachers of Reading* affirmed that when educators and parents teach language and literacy skills to students, their teaching approaches should simultaneously support students' development of psychological processes, including executive functioning. According to the IDA *Knowledge and Practice Standards,* teachers are expected to "understand and explain other aspects of cognition and behavior that affect reading and writing (attention, executive function, memory, processing speed)" (2010, p. 4). Teachers are required to "understand research-based adaptations of instruction for students with weaknesses in working memory, attention, executive functioning, or processing speed" (2010, p. 9)

It is important for teachers to recognize that "dyslexia often coexists with other developmental difficulties and disabilities, including problems with attention, memory, and executive function" (2010, p. 18). The IDA *Knowledge and Practice Standards* referenced Westby (2004) as a source of additional reading for preparing educators to incorporate students' development of executive functioning during language and literacy instruction.

Newhall (2017) stressed that academic proficiency is coordinated by executive function that allows students to maintain focus, connect new learning with existing knowledge, self-monitor comprehension, and apply strategies to repair any lapses in these areas. Newhall acknowledged that executive function enables students to set goals, develop **study skills,** modulate their frustrations, and manage their time and materials, but this is all dependent on the language and literacy skills that students bring to these self-regulation tasks.

REFLECT, CONNECT, and RESPOND
Explain how executive function has a cognitive influence on reading abilities.

Language in Use During the Performance of Executive Function

It is an old adage that "talking" is one thing and "doing" is another, and this poses a quandary for educators who attempt to teach students how to self-regulate their executive skills by teaching them the language that people use to govern their executive function. Barkley recommended that interventions to improve learners' executive function involve "active intervention at the point of performance," that is, during the moments that the learner is obligated to self-regulate (2011, p. 200).

For many learners, their language appears to be well-developed enough to govern self-direction. They can verbalize the metacognitive processes that guide learning. Verbal rehearsal has led them to be able to tell adults what they would do in a performance situation. However, when the need to perform arises, these students do not do what they have said that they know how to do. The quandary is that the students have long-term verbal recall of the strategies, but their routine, self-initiated use of strategies is less easily achieved. In cases where students continually struggle with transferring learning processes from task to task, it would seem that they have difficulty initiating the cognitive flexibility and the working memory needed to bring learning strategies "on-screen" when they are needed. This is sometimes referred to as carry-over of strategies. The student's language is well-developed enough to support these metacognitive demands, but carry-over of the tasks is not readily achieved.

There may be some possible explanations for this breakdown. "Working on memory" through recitation is a verbal memory skill. Verbal memory is not the same as episodic memory (Tulving, 1993), that is, an individual's memories of the "episodes" of life that the individual has experienced. Verbal recitation, even if reviewed on many occasions, does not necessarily translate to performing a certain way when a life episode (a "point of performance" [Barkley, 2011]) calls for it. It is similarly problematic that verbal recitation of how to be organized—how to plan a performance or the sequence of steps to complete a task—does not necessarily translate into being organized in daily life. Verbal memory is not the same as procedural memory (Bullemer, Nissen, & Willingham, 1989), which is the way that memory stores and retrieves how to perform a task. In a context where a procedure is required, there is a breakdown in performance if the verbalizations that the student learned are not brought into working memory to guide performance.

This quandary would suggest that if adults want students to learn executive skills, the adults must teach executive skills within performance contexts (not simply "what-if" verbalizations about executive tasks) and students must practice executive tasks. This suggestion stems from Thorndike's (1932) educational theory (see Hergenhahn & Olson, 2005). The theory of identical elements states that the extent to which information that was learned in one situation will transfer to another situation is determined by the similarity between the two situations; if two situations have little in common, information learned in one situation will not be of much value in the other situation. Transferring responses across situations requires the two situations to be similar. In the case of verbal rehearsal leading to the performance of actions in a new setting, there may be little transfer across these situations. It seems less effective to work on the language that would go with the tasks in the absence of the tasks themselves. It would not be effective to learn the language of the tasks in isolation and then hope the student remembers that language when it comes time to do the tasks.

Simply put, hypothetical situations only go so far to stimulate how to perform; saying what to do is different from conscious, real-time regulation of what an individual is doing. "Saying it" is just language. Self-regulation is a behavior that is mediated by language. Application to contexts means using the right language to go with the tasks. This entails using the language that unlocks the tasks and performing the tasks that unlock the language.

Facilitating Students' Self-Regulated, Language-Based Learning Behaviors

As depicted in Figure 8.2, language use is evident throughout a five-component process of learning. Each component of this process is composed of instances where educators and parents expect students to employ self-regulation to achieve certain behavioral performances. Figure 8.3 reconceptualizes Figure 8.2 to offer a model of how to facilitate students' active performance of the self-regulated, language-based learning behaviors that are needed to achieve each component of the learning process.

Figure 8.3 presents suggestions designed to allow students to successfully use cognitive flexibility, inhibitory control, and working memory throughout the five-component process of learning.

As Figure 8.3 illustrates, in the first of the five components, academic context, when a learner is receiving academic input by listening or reading, teachers and parents can help students by

- Minimizing distractions

- Limiting multitasking

- Setting task goals

- Promoting internal motivation

Affording learners a "point of performance" (Barkley, 2011) with fewer distractions or multitasking demands reduces the need for shifting attention among competing stimuli and alternatives. The burden of using cognitive flexibility to shift among an array of alternatives is diminished. Setting task goals provides clear expectations so that learners are guided toward inhibitory control. Learners can choose which actions to exhibit and which to inhibit to achieve their goals. Internal motivation is aided by making learning fun and enjoyable. Suggestions include using interesting subject matter, relevant examples, engaging materials and media, facilitative tools and technologies, learning games, multisensory movement, and social interaction. Learners may be less distracted when learning is enjoyable.

In the second component in Figure 8.3, in any academic context where a learner's attention, cognitive flexibility, working memory, information storage, and integration of past experiences with present contexts are brought to bear, teachers and parents can assist learners by

- Activating learners' prior knowledge

- Offering memorable learning experiences

- Offering quality learning materials

Learners may not independently know how to activate the prior knowledge that is relevant to the "point of performance" (Barkley, 2011). Educators and parents can help students connect the new to the known by having students review familiar concepts first before it is time to introduce new concepts. One option is to use comparison charts or other graphic organizers that show the known information and leave spaces for the new information to be actively entered as it is being learned. Planned stopping points in a lesson where the established concepts and the new information are synthesized show learners how to use cognitive flexibility to shift between the two sets of information. The demands on working memory to hold information in mind are lessened when concepts are reviewed and refreshed

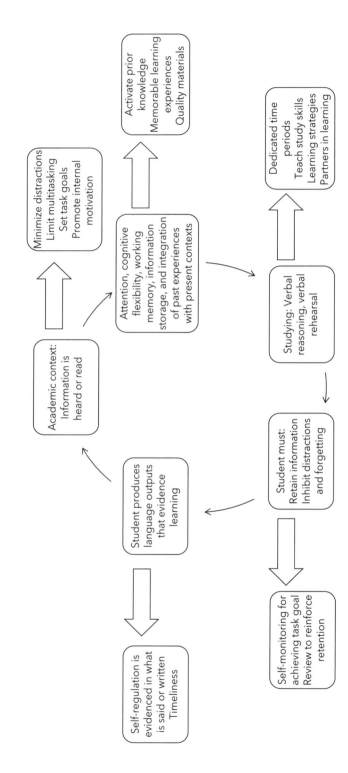

Figure 8.3. Improving executive function in the context of language and literacy learning.

and when the teacher guides the learners to write their notations on the graphic organizer. Active learning engages the learner's attention and helps the learner exert the inhibitory control needed to stay focused. At the end of a lesson, learners can make connections among ideas by answering the question, "What did you already know before that helped you learn something new today?"

Memorable learning experiences using quality materials facilitate learners' attention, working memory, and information storage and motivate learners to use language reflectively to interpret relevant new information. Materials that light a spark of curiosity and enthusiasm can bring about purposeful and independent thinkers and learners. Adults know that youngsters stay on task when they have engaging materials to use. Quality materials are clear and interesting, are of an appropriate length that allows for immersion but not an overtaxation of the learner's stamina, and are an appropriate challenge to the learner's level of language, reading, and academic background (i.e., not too difficult and not too easy). Materials should not be so difficult that students cannot ask questions about them, nor so easy that they do not need to ask any questions. Quality materials promote asking interesting questions.

The third component shown on Figure 8.3, studying, entails verbal rehearsal of the information that needs to be reasoned through and retained. Studying requires sustained focus, endurance, and vigilance so that learning and storage are solidified. The student exerts inhibitory control to reduce distractibility and must keep working memory in operation throughout the study period. Parents and teachers can facilitate effective self-regulation during studying as a "point of performance" (Barkley, 2011) by

- Having dedicated time periods for studying in dedicated study areas

- Teaching study skills

- Teaching learning strategies

- Positioning themselves as partners in learning

Having dedicated time periods for studying may be difficult to achieve in the context of busy schedules at school and at home, but the student who needs support to develop and employ executive functioning skills needs specific periods of time for studying when the student is not fatigued, distracted, or hurried. With that, students need a place to study that is quiet and free of distractions. An executive function deficit is by its nature a deficit in the cognitive processes needed to flexibly attend, inhibit distractions, and review and retain information in working memory. It is counterproductive to expect students with **executive function difficulties** to study in conditions that do not optimally reduce barriers to focusing and storing information. For some students, a headset that plays a recording of nature sounds or nondistracting music helps them focus and screens out environmental noise.

Effective studying involves having study skills and learning strategies. Parents can provide direct and explicit instructions on how to study and learn. Some study skills are generalizable across different academic subjects. Study skills such as "read all directions before beginning an assignment," "highlight key words," "highlight topic sentences," "make a list of questions that you have," "write a brief summary of main ideas," "make up some quiz questions for yourself," and "create mnemonic devices" are generalizable. Learning strategies are similar to study skills but may point more directly toward a systematized way to learn certain concepts and explain ideas. "Make up quiz questions for yourself" as a study skill becomes a learning strategy when the quiz questions ask, for example, for strategic learning by enumeration ("There are four causes for…"), or for learning by thinking in categories ("The planets are…. The moons of each planet are…"), or by going from general to specific ("Living creatures need oxygen, but specific ways for creatures to obtain oxygen are… "). Working memory is used to its best effect when information is processed in a strategic, organized fashion. Information is not only in the forefront of the learner's mind; it is being actively processed in a way that facilitates a structured plan for recalling the information. (In the previous examples, the student can plan to recall the causes, the categories, and the general and the specific.) Learners use cognitive flexibility to consider alternatives but in a methodical way.

A final consideration for effective studying is for parents and teachers to position themselves as partners in learning with the student, who is working to bring executive function skills to the task of studying. Adults might not only guide and direct, from the stance of expert helping novice, but they can also model behaviors, share tasks, and cue and assist their learners from the stance of another person who is also in the position of learning how to figure out how to succeed at a task. For example, an adult can model cognitive flexibility (e.g., "I am going to draft my ideas on paper and not even think about correct spelling and punctuation. Once I like how I have written my ideas, I will review my paper a few times. That's when I'll shift my focus to pay careful attention to correct spelling and punctuation"). Sharing a task may involve a division of labor for the adult and the student (e.g., "On this page, I will underline the signal words, and you underline the key words. On the next page, we'll switch"). An adult can cue the student to stimulate inhibitory control (e.g., "Try closing your laptop while we discuss what we have read on that web site so that the screen is not a distraction"). Assisting can involve helping only when help is needed (e.g., "Try this problem, and let me know if you need help"). Assisting in this way facilitates the self-monitoring to ask for help when help is needed. Sometimes a reflective question such as "Why do you need help now?" offers the student the chance to verbalize his or her learning needs and thus further self-monitor (e.g., "I forget what the next step should be"). Studying with a partner in learning can feel more inviting to students than performing their studying before the audience of an overseeing adult.

The fourth component shown in Figure 8.3 is for learners to retain information and inhibit distractions and forgetting. Suggestions to help facilitate this component are

- Self-monitoring for achieving task goal

- Reviewing to reinforce retention

Students can self-monitor their attention and cognitive flexibility when performing goal-directed tasks. Self-verbalizations may include "Have I read the directions?" "Have I completed every question?" "Have I read key words, as in questions that say 'not' or 'except'?" "What is the best way to tackle this job?" "How do I set up a page so I can take notes?" and "How long will it take to finish this homework assignment?" Metacognition allows learners to describe their own thought processes. Learners' metacognition is visible when parents and educators ask learners to make connections among ideas. Metacognitive questions include,

"How did you find your answer?" "What is your reason for your answer?" "What were you thinking of that helped you answer?" and "What made you say that answer?" This intensive self-monitoring brings about thoroughness and vigilance in learning and studying, which are integral to retaining information. Reviewing to reinforce retention is simply the act of bringing information into working memory on repeated occasions. Revisiting information in multisensory ways or by using different contexts and materials can bring novelty to the act of reviewing information and can give learners various experiences that will help them retain information.

The fifth component shown in Figure 8.3 is that students produce language outputs that evidence learning. Students' active performance involves

- Evidencing self-regulation in what is said or written

- Adhering to timeliness (students work within time constraints) (Barkley, 2011)

Students' spoken and written products reveal self-regulation when their outputs overtly verbalize the cognitive processes that they employed. Students can say (or write), for instance, "This is how I found my answer," or "My answer was not _____ because." Students may explain how they planned, prioritized, or organized their tasks. Working within time constraints shows self-regulation and may entail self-monitoring of how much to say or write within the time allowed in order to achieve an adequate self-expression.

Executive Function Toolbox

The following four tools can help educators and parents assemble an executive function toolbox to support learners of any age and across learning contexts in their growth of language, literacy, and academic skills.

Tools to Build Cognitive Flexibility   Two tools help build cognitive flexibility: 1) using all learning modalities and integrating students' experiences across these modalities, and 2) emphasizing "portable," generalizable, transferrable academic skills.

Tool 1: Use all learning modalities, and integrate experiences across modalities. Making use of all learning modalities helps build cognitive flexibility. For example, the VAK-POINT model (Clark, 2011; Greathead, n.d.) suggests using activities that are Visual, Auditory, Kinesthetic, Print Oriented, and Interactive.

Visual learning employs looking, watching, and observing. Learning devices include photographs, videos, posters, artwork, and PowerPoint presentations. Teachers invite learners to doodle, draw, or diagram to understand concepts; use spatial maps and concept mapping systems; and use visual imagery in their "mind's eye."

Auditory learning employs listening. Learning devices include audio sources such as speeches, music, and sound effects and even words and phrases in other languages. Auditory strategies include rhythm, rhyme, and rap to aid memorization, as well as recorded books and read alouds.

Kinesthetic learning employs sensory learning such as use of tactile materials and three-dimensional models. Learning strategies involve using the hands and body; for example, through manual tasks, motor tasks, and dance. Teachers encourage learners to build, create, disassemble, and rebuild physical items that aide learning, such as three-dimensional models.

Print-oriented learning incorporates reading and writing for pleasure. Learning materials include interactive print media online, texting, and other new literacies.

Finally, *interactive learning* uses discussion, dialogue, group work, and cooperative learning. Teachers build students' skills as leaders and followers in group dynamics.

Tool 2: Emphasize "portable," generalizable, transferrable academic skills. Another way to build cognitive flexibility is to emphasize portable skills. A number of these portable skills are involved in reading texts. For example, students can learn to recognize and analyze text structures (e.g., series of events, description, enumeration, compare and contrast, cause and effect, problem–solution) and to explore texts for point-of-view shifts (flexibility in point of reference). Readers can learn to use text features (e.g., header, tables); preview, review, and summarize text (flexibly paraphrasing); skim and scan; and looking back in text to find information or confirm what was learned. Other portable skills applicable to a variety of academic texts involve self-monitoring for comprehension breakdowns; asking clarification questions ("If I understand correctly, you said _____"); and inferencing, that is, "reading between the lines," to infer information that is not said and to predict what is going to happen in a story.

Several portable skills apply to vocabulary acquisition and use, for example, being able to explore and use lesson and text vocabulary. Another skill is vocabulary flexibility: working with words with multiple meanings (contextual or domain-specific meanings), or with literal versus nonliteral meanings. Understanding of word morphology and derivations is a portable skill as well.

Finally, skills related to academic language are portable or generalizable and thus help build cognitive flexibility. These skills include learning to understand the varied language of questions (how test questions are written): literal questions in which answers can be found in the text; the *wh-* questions (*when, where, which, what, how*); sequence questions ("What happened first [e.g., second, last, after]?"); questions about vocabulary in context ("In this story/paragraph/sentence, what does the word _____ mean?"); and other types such as summarizing questions, inferential questions, and main idea questions. Knowledge of academic task words is also generalizable. Common task words include *circle, color, copy, trace, alphabetize, match, unscramble, categorize, measure, outline, review, revise, total, compare, estimate, organize, separate, observe, analyze, generate, illustrate, solve, note, construct, diagram, differentiate, eliminate, graph,* and *rearrange* (see Harvey & Goudvis, 2007; Hasselbeck, Elledge, & Combs, 2013; Smiley & Goldstein, 1998).

Tools to Build Inhibitory Control   In addition to the tools that build cognitive flexibility, the executive toolbox includes tools to build inhibitory control—specifically, teaching students the language needed to self-regulate their actions and teaching the responses needed to build social-emotional skills.

Tool 3: Teach students the language to self-regulate their actions and responses to build social-emotional skills. The first part of this tool focuses on teaching language. This includes teaching the vocabulary of self-regulation; for example, the meaning of words such as *initiate, inhibit, impulse,* and *emotion.* It also encompasses teaching students to describe their own impulse control, adaptability, habits, responsibilities, frustrations, and distractions and teaching them to describe their own activity level. (Have students use words to describe an appropriate level, not hyper- or hypoactive for the situation.)

The second part of this tool involves teaching social problem solving using self-questioning: "Why do other people act for themselves (and not just do what I want)? How do my actions affect others? What is the right thing to say now? What is helpful when interacting with others? What is hurtful to others?" Finally, students can be taught how to incorporate feedback to adjust responses and emotions: "I will do that again—and here's why." "I will not do that again—and here's why." "I will change how I do that—and here's why."

Tools to Build Working Memory Finally, the executive toolbox includes tools to build working memory by facilitating storage; facilitating retrieval, recall, and remembering; and addressing difficulties with forgetting.

Tool 4: Facilitate memory functions. The first aspect of this tool is using strategies to facilitate storage. These include beginning a lesson by stating its purpose and objectives and previewing lesson content. Material to be learned can and should be presented in a way that will facilitate storage, with visuals, redundancy, and external memory aides, such as notes, word walls, and glossaries. Content should be presented as files of related information. Chunk ideas (for schema building), present a manageable number of details, and use concept charts (see Martinelli & Mraz, 2012). Material to be learned should be stored with efficiency, not in haste or when distractions were present. Content should be meaningful, promoting true comprehension and enjoyment. Finally, address how memorization causes anxiety; reduce anxiety when possible.

Other strategies can be used to facilitate retrieval, recall, and remembering. Experiential memories tend to be strong, so teach concepts with vivid, lived-through experiences (experiments, projects, and dramatizations).

Finally, build working memory by addressing any issues with forgetting. Discuss what is retained and why, and what is forgotten and why. Keep practicing the use of storage aids: paradoxically, the student may forget how to use the memory aid!

REFLECT, CONNECT, and RESPOND
How does effective executive functioning enhance literacy development?

CLOSING THOUGHTS:
EXECUTIVE FUNCTION IN LITERACY INSTRUCTION

Executive function is the marriage of two complementary opposites: perseverance and flexibility. Executive function allows school-age and adolescent learners to persevere so that they can learn and accomplish a multitude of academic learning tasks and social behaviors. At the same time, executive function allows learners to adjust their thinking and behaviors. Individuals who successfully employ executive functioning are able to be strategic but spontaneous, planful but also responsive. Because executive functioning allows individuals to identify optimal actions and self-regulate behaviors, this duality can coexist. Language helps learners make conscious, deliberate, and overt use of the executive processes that underlie academic learning.

Individuals with strong executive functioning, however, must ultimately rely on numerous cognitive and social-emotional competencies that are intuited and seldom overtly rehearsed. Their executive skills are seemingly unconscious and are fluidly generalized across contexts. Another paradox is that this automaticity potentially limits the number of intentional executive decisions that a person with competent executive functioning needs to make. Until these intuitive competencies are established, parents and educators are empowered to provide the guidance and supports that teach young people how to incorporate executive skills into their daily lifestyles.

ONLINE COMPANION MATERIALS

The following Chapter 8 resources are available at http://www.brookespublishing .com/birshcarreker/materials:

- Reflect, Connect, and Respond Questions

- Appendix 8.1: Technology Resources

- Appendix 8.2: Knowledge and Skill Assessment Answer Key

KNOWLEDGE AND SKILL ASSESSMENT

1. Executive function is defined by which three main components?

    a. Self-control, attention, and memory

    b. Language, literacy, and working memory

    c. Emotional intelligence, social skills, and communication skills

    d. Cognitive flexibility, inhibitory control, and working memory

2. How is working memory defined?

    a. The ability to hold information in mind while thinking about it—the so-called "mental sketchpad" or "on-screen memory"

    b. Short-term memory

    c. Rapid recall of information

    d. Efficient storage of information for later recall

3. Which learning behaviors reveal the learner's use of executive function?

    a. Learning that involves understanding and using multisensory information

    b. Learning that involves focusing attention, studying, and retaining information

    c. Learning by following the example of another person

    d. All of the above

4. Why might learners who have difficulty with executive function experience lesser motivation to read?

    a. They have few story characters with whom they can identify.

    b. They have difficulty with sustaining self-directed action to achieve a future goal.

   c. They have insufficient language skills to retell stories.

   d. They have difficulty reading at grade level.

5. Which teaching strategies enhance executive function?

   a. Visual, auditory, kinesthetic, print-oriented, and interactive experiences

   b. Strict stimulus-response teaching paradigms

   c. Drill exercises to build storage and recall of information

   d. Reducing the amount of language-based work that the students is responsible for completing

6. Which of the following statements about assessment of executive function is *not* true?

   a. Testing may identify difficulties in paying attention, being persistent, and remembering.

   b. Testing may identify difficulties with organization, impulse control, and frustration.

   c. Testing may identify the presence of a biological, physical, or organic reason for learning difficulties.

   d. Testing may identify some reasons for academic underachievement.

7. What is difficulty with executive function?

   a. A required condition for the diagnosis of dyslexia

   b. A required condition for the diagnosis of specific language impairment (SLI)

   c. A possible cognitive difference that distinguishes good readers from poor readers

   d. A form of autism spectrum disorder

8. Why is instructional intensity important for learners with executive function difficulties?

   a. Intensive instruction is designed to regulate behavioral outbursts.

   b. Repeated, consistent, and intensive practice allows learners to learn strategies to retain information and inhibit forgetting.

   c. Intensive instruction is important for learners who may have a tendency to waste time.

   d. All specialized instruction for students with learning needs is legally mandated to be intensive.

REFERENCES

Adams, A., Bourke, L., & Willis, C. (1999). Working memory and spoken language comprehension in young children. *International Journal of Psychology, 34,* 364–373.

Alarcón-Rubio, D., Sánchez-Medina, J.A., & Prieto-García, J.R. (2014). Executive function and verbal self-regulation in childhood: Developmental linkages between partially internalized private speech and cognitive flexibility. *Early Childhood Research Quarterly, 29,* 95–105.

Alderson, R.M., Rapport, M.D., Hudec, K., Sarver, D.E., & Kofler, M.J. (2010). Competing core processes in attention-deficit/hyperactivity disorder (ADHD): Do working memory deficiencies underlie behavioral inhibition deficits? *Journal of Abnormal Child Psychology, 38,* 497–507.

Alloway, T.P. (2009). Working memory, but not IQ, predicts subsequent learning in children with learning difficulties. *European Journal of Psychological Assessment, 25,* 92–98.

American Psychiatric Association. (2013). *Diagnostic and statistical manual of mental disorders* (5th ed.). Washington, DC: Author.

American Speech-Language-Hearing Association. (n.d.a). *Social communication disorders in school-age children.* Retrieved from http://www.asha.org/Practice-Portal/Clinical-Topics/Social-Communication-Disorders-in-School-Age-Children/

American Speech-Language-Hearing Association. (n.d.b). *Spoken language disorders.* Retrieved from http://www.asha.org/PRPSpecificTopic.aspx?folderid=8589935327&section=Overview

American Speech-Language-Hearing Association. (n.d.c). *Written language disorders.* Retrieved from http://www.asha.org/PRPSpecificTopic.aspx?folderid=8589942549&section=References

Archibald, L.M., & Gathercole, S.E. (2006). Short-term and working memory in specific language impairment. *International Journal of Language and Communication Disorders, 41*(6), 675–693.

Archibald, L., Joanisse, M., & Edmunds, A. (2011). Specific language or working memory impairments: A small scale observational study. *Child Language Teaching and Therapy, 27,* 294–312.

Arrington, C.N., Kulesz, P.A., Francis, D.J., Fletcher, J.M., & Barnes, M.A. (2014). The contribution of attentional control and working memory to reading comprehension and decoding. *Scientific Studies of Reading, 18,* 325–346.

Baddeley, A. (1996). Exploring the central executive. *The Quarterly Journal of Experimental Psychology, 49,* 5–28.

Baddeley, A. (2000). The episodic buffer: a new component of working memory. *Trends Cognitive Science, 4,* 417–423.

Baddeley, A.D., & Hitch, G.J. (1994). Developments in the concept of working memory. *Neuropsychology, 8*(4), 485–493.

Baker, L., & Cantwell, D.P. (1992). Attention deficit disorder and speech/language disorders. *Comprehensive Mental Health Care, 2,* 3–16.

Barkley, R.A. (1997). Behavioral inhibition, sustained attention, and executive functions: Constructing a unifying theory of ADHD. *Psychological Bulletin, 121,* 65–94.

Barkley, R.A. (2005). *ADHD and the nature of self-control.* New York, NY: Guilford.

Barkley, R.A. (2006). A theory of ADHD. In R.A. Barkley (Ed.), *Attention-deficit hyperactivity disorder* (pp. 297–334). New York, NY: Guilford.

Barkley, R. A. (2011). *The important role of executive functioning and self-regulation in ADHD.* Retrieved from http://www.russellbarkley.org/factsheets/ADHD_EF_and_SR.pdf

Barkley, R.A. (2012). *Executive functions: What they are, how they work, and why they evolved.* New York, NY: Guilford.

Baron-Cohen, S. (1991). Precursors to a theory of mind: Understanding attention in others. In A. Whiten (Ed.), *Natural theories of mind: Evolution, development and simulation of everyday mindreading* (pp. 233–251). Oxford, United Kingdom: Basil Blackwell.

Baumeister, R.F. (Ed.). (1999). *The self in social psychology.* Philadelphia, PA: Psychology Press.

Bavin, E.L., Wilson, P.H., Maruff, P., & Sleeman, F. (2005). Spatiovisual memory of children with specific language impairment: Evidence for generalized processing problems. *International Journal of Language Communication Disorders, 40,* 319–332.

Berk, L.E., & Potts, M.K. (1991). Development and functional significance of private speech among attention-deficit hyperactivity disorder and normal boys. *Journal of Abnormal Child Psychology, 19,* 357–377.

Berninger, V.W. (2007). *Process Assessment of the Learner–Second Edition: Diagnostics for Reading and Writing.* San Antonio, TX: Pearson.

Berninger, V.W., Abbott, R.D., Swanson, H.L., Lovitt, D., Trevedi, P., Lin, S., Gould, L., … Amtmann, D. (2010). Relationship of word- and sentence-level working memory to reading and writing in second, fourth, and sixth grade. *Language, Speech, and Hearing Services in Schools, 41,* 179–193.

Berninger, V., & Richards, T. (2002). *Brain literacy for educators and psychologists*. New York, NY: Academic Press.

Best, J.R., & Miller, P.H. (2010). A developmental perspective on executive function. *Child Development, 81*(6), 1641–1660.

Bishop, D.V.M. (2006). What causes specific language impairment in children? *Current Directions in Psychological Sciences, 15*, 217–221.

Bolden, J., Rapport, M.D., Raiker, J.S., Sarver, D.E., & Kofler, M.J. (2012). Understanding phonological memory deficits in boys with attention-deficit/hyperactivity disorder (ADHD): Dissociation of short-term storage and articulatory rehearsal processes. *Journal of Abnormal Child Psychology, 40*, 999–1011.

Boudreau, D., & Costanza-Smith, A. (2011). Assessment and treatment of working memory deficits in school-age children: The role of the speech-language pathologist. *Language, Speech, and Hearing Services in Schools, 42*, 152–166.

Bowers, L., & Huisingh, R. (2014). *Executive Functions Test–Elementary*. Austin, TX: PRO-ED.

Brock, L.L., Rimm-Kaufman, S.E., Nathanson, L., & Grimm, K.J. (2009). The contributions of "hot" and "cool" executive function to children's academic achievement, learning-related behaviors, and engagement in kindergarten. *Early Childhood Research Quarterly, 24*(3), 337–349.

Brock, S.W., & Knapp, P.K. (1996). Reading comprehension abilities of children with attention deficit/hyperactivity disorder. *Journal of Attention Disorders, 1*, 173–186.

Brown, T.E. (2006). Executive functions and attention deficit hyperactivity disorder: Implications of two conflicting views. *International Journal of Disability, Development and Education, 53*(1), 35–46.

Bruce, B., Thernlund, G., & Nettelbladt, U. (2006). ADHD and language impairment: A study of the parent questionnaire FTF (Five to Fifteen). *European Child and Adolescent Psychiatry, 15*, 52–60.

Bruner, J.S. (1966). *Toward a theory of instruction*. Cambridge, MA: Belkapp Press.

Bullemer, P., Nissen, M.J., & Willingham, D.B. (1989). On the development of procedural knowledge. *Journal of Experimental Psychology: Learning, Memory and Cognition, 15*(6), 1047–1060.

Cain, K., Oakhill, J., & Bryant, P. (2004). Children's reading comprehension ability: Concurrent prediction by working memory, verbal ability, and component skills. *Journal of Educational Psychology, 96*, 31–42.

Camarata, S.M., & Gibson, T. (1999). Pragmatic language deficits in attention-deficit hyperactivity disorder (ADHD). *Mental Retardation and Developmental Disabilities Research Reviews, 5*, 202–214.

Carriedo, N., Corral, A., Montoro, P.R., Herrero, L., Ballestrino, P., & Sebastián, I. (2016). The development of metaphor comprehension and its relationship with relational verbal reasoning and executive function. *Plos ONE, 11*(3), 1–20.

Castellanos, F.X., Sonuga-Barke, E.J.S., Milham, M.P., & Tannock, R. (2006). Characterizing cognition in ADHD: Beyond executive dysfunction. *Trends in Cognitive Science, 10*, 117–123.

Chan, R.C.K., Shum, D., Toulopoulou, T., & Chen, E.Y.H. (2008). Assessment of executive functions: Review of instruments and identification of critical issues. *Archives of Clinical Neuropsychology, 23*(2), 201–216.

Cherry, K. (2016). *What is social cognition?* Retrieved from http://www.verywell.com

Clark, D. (2011). Visual, auditory, and kinesthetic learning styles. Retrieved from http://www.nwlink.com/~donclark/hrd/styles/vakt.html

Coleman, D. (2005). *Emotional intelligence: Why it can matter more than IQ*. New York, NY: Bantam Books.

Conti-Ramsden, G., Ullman, M.T., and Lum, J.A.G. (2015). The relation between receptive grammar and procedural, declarative and working memory in specific language impairment. *Frontiers in Psychology, 6*, 1090.

DaParma, A., Geffner, D., & Martin, N. (2011). Prevalence and nature of language impairment in children with attention deficit/hyperactivity disorder. *Contemporary Issues in Communication Science and Disorders, 38*, 119–125.

Davis, M., & Stone, T. (2003). Synthesis: Psychological understanding and social skills. In B. Repacholi & V. Slaugher (Eds.), *Individual differences in theory of mind: Implications for typical and atypical development* (pp. 306–352). New York, NY: Psychology Press.

De Jong, P.F. (1998). Working memory deficits of reading disabled children. *Journal of Experimental Child Psychology, 70*, 75–96.

D'Esposito, M. (2002). The neural basis of working memory: Evidence from neuropsychological, pharmacological and neuroimaging studies. In L.T. Connor & L.K. Obler (Eds.), *Neurobehavior of language and cognition* (pp. 179–200). Norwell, MA: Kluwer Academic.

Diamond, A. (2013). Executive functions. *Annual Review of Psychology, 64,* 135–168.

Dittman, C. (2016). Associations between inattention, hyperactivity and pre-reading skills before and after formal reading instruction begins. *Reading and Writing, 29,* 1771–1791.

Duinmeijer, I., Jong, J., & de Scheper, A. (2012). Narrative abilities, memory and attention in children with a specific language impairment. *International Journal of Language Communication Disorders, 47,* 542–555.

Ellis Weismer, S., Plante, E., Jones, M., & Tomblin, J.B. (2005). A functional magnetic resonance imaging investigation of verbal working memory in adolescents with specific language impairment. *Journal of Speech, Language, and Hearing Research, 48,* 405–425.

Flory, K., Milich, R., Lorch, E.P., Hayden, A.N., Strange, C., & Welsh, R. (2006). Online story comprehension among children with ADHD: Which core deficits are involved? *Journal of Abnormal Child Psychology, 34,* 850–862.

Foundation for Critical Thinking. (2015). *Defining critical thinking.* Retrieved from http://www.criticalthinking.org/pages/defining-critical-thinking/766

Gallinat, E., & Spaulding, T.J. (2014). Differences in the performance of children with specific language impairment and their typically developing peers on nonverbal cognitive tests: A meta-analysis. *Journal of Speech, Language, and Hearing Research, 57,* 1363–1382.

Garon, N., Bryson, S E., & Smith, I.M. (2008). Executive function in preschoolers: A review using an integrative framework. *Psychological Bulletin, 134,* 31–60.

Gathercole, S.E., Alloway, T.P., Willis, C., & Adams, A. (2006). Working memory in children with reading disabilities. *Journal of Experimental Child Psychology, 93,* 265–281.

Gathercole, S.E., & Baddeley, A.D. (1993). Phonological working memory: A critical building block for reading development and vocabulary acquisition. *European Journal of Psychology of Education, 8,* 259–272.

Golden, C.J., Freshwater, S.M., & Golden, Z. (n.d.). *Stroop Color and Word Test: Children's Version.* Lutz, FL: PAR.

Gooch, D., Thompson, P., Nash, H., Snowling, M., & Hulme, C. (2016). The development of executive function and language skills in the early school years. *Journal of Child Psychology & Psychiatry, 57*(2), 180–187.

Gray, S. (2006). The relationship between phonological memory, receptive vocabulary, and fast mapping in young children with specific language impairment. *Journal of Speech, Language, and Hearing Research, 49,* 955–969.

Greathead, P. (n.d.). *Language disorders and attention deficit hyperactivity disorder.* Retrieved from http://addiss.co.uk/languagedisorders.htm

Hamilton, D.L. (2005). Social cognition: An introductory overview. In D.L. Hamilton (Ed.), *Social cognition* (pp. 1–26). New York, NY: Psychology Press.

Harvey, S., & Goudvis, A. (2007). *Strategies that work.* Portland, ME: Stenhouse.

Hasselbeck, E., Elledge, D., & Combs, S. (2013, March 14–16). *Empowering the SLP: Strategies for reading comprehension across the curriculum.* Presented at the Ohio Speech-Language-Hearing Convention, Columbus, OH.

Henry, L.A., Messer, D.J., & Nash, G. (2012). Executive functioning in children with specific language impairment. *Journal of Child Psychology and Psychiatry, 53,* 37–45.

Hergenhahn, B.R., & Olson, M.H. (2005). *An introduction to the theories of learning.* New York, NY: Pearson Education.

Hongwnishkul, D., Happaney, K.R., Lee, W., & Zelazo, P.D. (2005). Assessment of hot and cool executive function: Age-related changes and individual differences. *Developmental Neuropsychology, 28,* 617–644.

Hughes, C. (1998). Executive function in preschoolers: Links with theory of mind and verbal ability. *British Journal of Developmental Psychology, 16,* 233–253.

Humphries, T., Koltun, H., Malone, M., & Roberts, W. (1994). Teacher-identified oral language difficulties among boys with attention problems. *Journal of Developmental and Behavioral Pediatrics, 15,* 92–98.

Hutchinson, E., Bavin, A., Efron, D., & Sciberras, E. (2011). A comparison of working memory profiles in school-aged children with specific language impairment, attention deficit/hyperactivity disorder, comorbid SLI and ADHD and their typically developing peers. *Child Neuropsychology, 1018,* 190–207.

Im-Bolter, N., Johnson, J., & Pascual-Leone, J. (2006). Processing limitations in children with specific language impairment: The role of executive function. *Child Development, 77,* 1822–1841.

Individuals with Disabilities Education Improvement Act (IDEA) of 2004, PL 108-446, 20 U.S.C. § 1400 *et seq.*

International Dyslexia Association, The. (2010). *Knowledge and practice standards for teachers of reading.* Baltimore, MD: Author.

International Dyslexia Association, The. (2018, March). *Knowledge and practice standards for teachers of reading.* Retrieved from https://dyslexiaida.org/knowledge-and-practices/

International Literacy Association/National Council of Teachers of English. (2017). *Connection stems.* Retrieved from http://www.readwritethink.org/classroom-resources/printouts/connection-stems-30840.html

Jonsdottir, S., Bouma, A., Sergeant, J.A., & Scherder, E.J.A. (2005). The impact of specific language impairment on working memory in children with ADHD combined subtype. *Archives in Clinical Neuropsychology, 20,* 443–456.

Kapa, L.L., & Plante, E. (2015). Executive function in SLI: Recent advances and future directions. *Current Developmental Disorders Report, 2*(3), 245–252.

Kasper, L.J., Alderson, R.M., & Hudec, K.L. (2012). Moderators of working memory deficits in children with attention-deficit/hyperactivity disorder (ADHD): A meta-analytic review. *Clinical Psychology Review, 32,* 605–617.

Kaufman, C. (2010). *Executive function in the classroom: Practical strategies for improving performance and enhancing skills for all students.* Baltimore, MD: Paul H. Brookes Publishing Co.

Kerr, A., & Zelazo, P.D. (2004). Development of "hot" executive function: The children's gambling task. *Brain and Cognition, 55,* 148–157.

Kim, O.H., & Kaiser, A.P. (2000). Language characteristics of children with ADHD. *Communication Disorders Quarterly, 21*(3), 154–165.

Kofler, M.J., Rapport, M.D., Bolden, J., Sarver, D.E., Raiker, J.S., & Alderson, R.M. (2011). Working memory deficits and social problems in children with ADHD. *Journal of Abnormal Child Psychology, 39,* 805–817.

Learning Disabilities Association of America. (2017). *Executive functions development and learning disabilities.* Retrieved from https://ldaamerica.org/executive-functions-development-and-learning-disabilities/

Leonard, L.B., Ellis Weismer, S., Miller, C.A., Francis, D.J., Tomblin, J.B., & Kail, R.V. (2007). Speed of processing, working memory, and language impairment in children. *Journal of Speech, Language, and Hearing Research, 50,* 408–428.

Lorch, E.P., Berthiaume, K.S., Milich, R., & van den Broek, P. (2007). Story comprehension impairments in children with attention-deficit/hyperactivity disorder. In K. Cain & J. Oakhill (Eds.), *Children's comprehension problems in oral and written language* (pp. 128–156). New York, NY: Guilford.

Lorch, E., Milich, R., Astrin, C., & Berthiaume, K. (2006). Cognitive engagement and story comprehension in typically developing children and children with ADHD from preschool through elementary school. *Developmental Psychology, 42,* 1206–1219.

Lorch, E.P., Milich, R., Sanchez, R.P., van den Broek, P., Baer, S., Hooks, K., … Welsh, R. (2000). Comprehension of televised stories in attention deficit hyperactivity disordered and nonreferred boys. *Journal of Abnormal Psychology, 109,* 321–330.

Lum, J.A.G., Conti-Ramsden, G., Page, D., & Ullman, M.T. (2012). Working, declarative, and procedural memory in specific language impairment. *Cortex, 48,* 1138–1154.

Mackie, C.J., Dockrell, J., & Lindsay, G. (2013). An evaluation of the written texts of children with SLI: The contributions of oral language, reading and phonological short-term memory. *Reading and Writing, 26,* 865–888.

Martinelli, M., & Mraz, K. (2012). *Smarter charts K–2.* Portsmouth, NH: Heinemann.

Marton, K., Kelmenson, L., & Pinkhasova, M. (2007). Inhibition control and working memory capacity in children with SLI. *Psychologia, 50,* 110–121.

Marton, K., & Schwartz, R.G. (2003). Working memory capacity and language processes in children with specific language impairment. *Journal of Speech, Language, and Hearing Research, 46,* 1138–1153.

McCloskey, G. (n.d.). *Executive functions and Reading: A neuropsychological perspective.* Retrieved from http://images.pearsonclinical.com/images/PDF/Webinar/Ef-Reading_Webinar.pdf

McCloskey, G., & Perkins, L.A. (2012). *Essentials of executive functions assessment.* New York, NY: Wiley.

McCloskey, G., Perkins, L.A., & Van Divner, B. (2009). *Assessment and intervention for executive function difficulties*. New York, NY: Taylor & Francis.

McInnes, A., Humphries, T., Hogg-Johnson, S., & Tannock, R. (2003). Listening comprehension and working memory are impaired in attention-deficit hyperactivity disorder. *Journal of Abnormal Child Psychology, 31*(4), 427–443.

Messer, D., & Dockrell, J.D. (2011). Lexical access and literacy in children with word finding difficulties. *International Journal of Language & Communication Disorders, 46*, 473–480.

Miyake, A., Friedman, N.P., Emerson, M.J., Witzki, A.H., Howerter, A., & Wager, T. (2000). The unity and diversity of executive functions and their contributions to complex "frontal lobe" tasks: A latent variable analysis. *Cognitive Psychology, 41*, 49–100.

Montgomery, J.W., & Evans, J.L. (2009). Complex sentence comprehension and working memory in children with specific language impairment. *Journal of Speech, Language, and Hearing Research, 52*, 269–288.

Montgomery, J.W., Magimairaj, B.M., & Finney, M.C. (2010). Working memory and specific language impairment: An update on the relation and perspectives on assessment and treatment. *American Journal of Speech-Language Pathology, 19*, 78–94.

Montgomery, J.W., Polunenko, A., & Marinellie, S.A. (2009). Role of working memory in children's understanding of spoken narrative: A preliminary investigation. *Applied Psycholinguistics, 30*, 485–509.

National Center for Learning Disabilities (NCLD). (2018). *Executive function fact sheet*. Retrieved from http://www.ldonline.org/article/24880/

Newhall, P.W. (2017). *Language-based learning disability: What to know*. Retrieved from http://www.ldonline.org/article/56113/

Nippold, M.A., Mansfield, T.C., & Billow, J.L. (2007). Peer conflict explanations in children, adolescents, and adults: Examining the development of complex syntax. *American Journal of Speech-Language Pathology, 1*, 179–188.

Oram, J., Fine, J., Okamoto, C., & Tannock, R. (1999). Assessing the language of children with attention deficit hyperactivity disorder. *American Journal of Speech-Language Pathology, 8*, 72–80.

Pauls, L.J., & Archibald, L.M. (2016). Executive functions in children with specific language impairment: A meta-analysis. *Journal of Speech, Language, and Hearing Research, 59*, 1074–1086.

Perner, J. (1998). The meta-intentional nature of executive functions and theory of mind. In P. Carruthers & J. Boucher (Eds.), *Language and thought: Interdisciplinary themes* (pp. 270–316). Cambridge, United Kingdom: Cambridge University Press.

Purvis, K.L., & Tannock, R. (1997). Language abilities in children with attention deficit hyperactivity disorder, reading disabilities, and normal controls. *Journal of Abnormal Child Psychology, 25*, 133–144.

Redmond, S.M. (2005). Differentiating SLI from ADHD using children's sentence recall and production of past tense morphology. *Clinical Linguistics & Phonetics, 19*, 109–127.

Redmond, S. (2014). *Language impairment in the ADHD context*. Retrieved from http://cred.pubs.asha.org/article.aspx?articleid=2411204

Redmond, S.M., & Timler, G.R. (2013). *Language profiles associated with pediatric ADHD with & without co-occurring LI*. Retrieved from http://www.asha.org

Reid, R., & Lienemann, T.O. (2006). Self-regulated strategy development for written expression with students with attention deficit/hyperactivity disorder. *Exceptional Children, 73*, 53–68.

Renz, K., Lorch, E.P., Milich, R., Lemberger, C., Bodner, A., & Welsh, R. (2003). Online story representation in boys with attention deficit hyperactivity disorder. *Journal of Abnormal Child Psychology, 31*, 93–104.

Singer, B.D., & Bashir, A.S. (1999). What are executive functions and self-regulation and what do they have to do with language-learning disorders? *Language, Speech, and Hearing Services in Schools, 30*, 265–273.

Smiley, L., & Goldstein, P. (1998). *Language delays and disorders*. San Diego, CA: Singular Publishing Group.

Smith, E.E. (2000). Neural bases of human working memory. *Current Directions in Psychological Science, 9*, 45–49.

Stroop, J.R. (1935). Studies of interference in serial verbal reactions. *Journal of Experimental Psychology, 18*(6), 643–662.

Swanson, H.L., & Sachse-Lee, C. (2001). Mathematical problem solving and working memory in children with learning disabilities: Both executive and phonological processes are important. *Journal of Educational Psychology, 96,* 471–491.

Tannock, R., Purvis, K.L., & Schachar, R.J. (1992). Narrative abilities in children with attention deficit hyperactivity disorder and normal peers. *Journal of Abnormal Child Psychology, 21,* 103–117.

Tannock, R., & Schachar, R. (1996). Executive dysfunction as an underlying mechanism of behaviour and language problems in attention deficit hyperactivity disorders. In J.H. Beitchman, N.J. Cohen, M.M. Konstantareas, & R.R. Tannock (Eds.), *Language learning and behavior disorders: Developmental, biological, and clinical perspective* (pp. 128–155). New York, NY: Cambridge University Press.

Thomas, A., & Thorne, G. (2017). *Higher order thinking.* Retrieved from http://www.readingrockets.org/article/higher-order-thinking

Thorndike, E.L. (1932). *The fundamentals of learning.* New York, NY: Columbia University.

Tirosh, E., & Cohen, A. (1998). Language deficit with attention-deficit disorder: A prevalent comorbidity. *Journal of Child Neurology, 13,* 493–497.

Tonnessen, F.E. (1999). Options and limitations of the cognitive psychological approach to the treatment of dyslexia. *Journal of Learning Disabilities, 32*(5), 386–393.

Torgesen, J., Wagner, R., & Rashotte, C. (2012). *Test of Word Reading Efficiency, Second Edition.* (TOWRE-2). Upper Saddle River, NJ: Pearson Education.

Tridas, E. (2013, March 9). *Executive functions.* Presented at the 25th Annual Symposium of the Northern Ohio Branch of the International Dyslexia Association, Cleveland, OH.

Tulving, E. (1993). What is episodic memory? *Current Directions in Psychological Science, 2,* 67–70.

Ullman, M.T., & Pierpont, E.I. (2005). Specific language impairment is not specific to language: The procedural deficit hypothesis. *Cortex, 41,* 399–433.

Vanderberg, R., & Swanson, H.L. (2007). Which components of working memory are important in the writing process? *Reading and Writing, 20,* 721–752.

Vissers, C., Koolen, S., Hermans, D., Scheper, A., & Knoors, H. (2015). Executive functioning in preschoolers with specific language impairment. *Frontiers in Psychology, 6,* 1–8.

Vugs, B., Cuperus, J., Hendriks, M., & Verhoeven, L. (2013). Visuospatial working memory in specific language impairment: A meta-analysis. *Research in Developmental Disabilities, 34,* 2586–2597.

Vugs, B., Hendriks, M., Cuperus, J., & Verhoeven, L. (2014). Working memory performance and executive function behaviors in young children with SLI. *Research in Developmental Disabilities, 35,* 62–74.

Westby, C. (2004). A language perspective on executive functioning, metacognition, and self-regulation in reading. In C.A. Stone, E.R. Silliman, B.J. Ehren, & K. Apel (Eds.), *Handbook of language and literacy: Development and disorders* (pp. 398–427). New York, NY: Guilford.

Westby, C.E., & Cutler, S. (1994). Language and ADHD: Understanding the bases and treatment of self-regulatory behaviors. *Topics in Language Disorders, 14*(4), 58–76.

Westby, C., & Robinson, L. (2007). *Understanding language impairments in children with ADHD.* Retrieved from http://www.asha.org

World Health Organization. (2005). *International classification of diseases and health related problems: ICD-10* (2nd ed.). Geneva, Switzerland: Author.

Appendix 8.1

Technology Resources

Elaine A. Cheesman

PROGRAMS/APPS: TO-DO LISTS

Effective programs/apps have the following features:

- They have a simple interface.

- They can add notes with speech.

- They synchronize across all platforms (Android, Chrome, Apple) and all devices (desktop computers, tablets, phones and watches).

- They can easily group tasks by category.

- They provide reminders and due dates.

- They have the ability to print and/or e-mail task lists.

- They can share with others (i.e., parents and teachers).

- They can add notes to tasks.

- They are searchable.

- They can sort tasks.

- They can undo deleted tasks.

Google Keep   http://www.google.com/keep

> This free app has all but one of the features listed above—individuals cannot sort lists. Users can add pictures and audio to lists and color-code lists or categories.

Wunderlist   http://www.wunderlist.com

> This award-winning app has all the features listed above. The free version is sufficient for most users; the paid version includes many useful features (e.g., sort by due date or create a template for tasks used in more than one situation). Users can create lists for directions by numbering and sorting steps. It is appropriate for individuals ages 10 and older and requires reading skills.

PROGRAMS/APPS: FOCUS AND ATTENTION

Effective programs/apps have the following features:

- They do not require extra time to use.

- They work without undue distractions.

- They manage inhibitory control.

- They provide opportunities for breaks.

- They limit distractions.

FocusBooster   http://www.focusboosterapp.com

This desktop application helps improve focus and productivity. It divides user-labeled work sessions into customizable work and break sessions. The desktop timer shows the time spent and signals time for a break at the end of the work session. It provides a chart of time spent on specific tasks. Professionals can sign up for a free 30-day trial; students can sign up for a reduced rate. Installation includes instructional videos.

Freedom   https://freedom.to

This app blocks all of the best-known web-based distractions for a set period of time or according to a preset schedule of recurring times during specific days. Sites include Twitter, Facebook, Flickr, YouTube, Hulu, Vimeo, all standard e-mail programs, and the entire Internet. Users can customize the list of prohibited sites and the amount of time. The app works on PCs, Macs, iPhones, and iPads. Sessions can start automatically according to the schedule the user or parent sets.

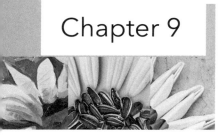

Chapter 9

Teaching Reading

Accurate Decoding

Suzanne Carreker

LEARNING OBJECTIVES

1. To describe the role decoding plays in reading proficiency

2. To explain the importance of Structured Literacy instruction in developing accurate decoding

3. To outline a structured, sequential, and cumulative progression of skills for decoding instruction

How important are a teacher's knowledge and practices to students' reading achievement? In a study of 42 first-grade teachers, Piasta, Connor, Fishman, and Morrison (2009) examined the literacy-related knowledge of the teachers and the impact of teacher knowledge on student growth in word reading. Teachers with knowledge at the 75th percentile who consistently taught decoding had students with the greatest gains in word reading. Teachers with the same knowledge who did not consistently teach decoding had students with word-reading outcomes that were equal to the outcomes made by students of teachers with much lower levels of literacy content knowledge. The students with the weakest gains were consistently taught decoding by teachers with knowledge at the 25th percentile or below. Therefore, student gains were the result of an interaction between teacher knowledge and instructional practices. Knowledge and practice count!

Reading is important for academic success, economic opportunities, and lifelong learning. In addition, Seidenberg suggested, "There is an urgent need to reduce the number of people who have read little or not at all to ensure that future generations will be sufficiently literate to thrive in the world they inhabit" (2017, p. 13). The International Dyslexia Association (IDA) is promoting the teaching of Structured Literacy, which is an umbrella term for the evidence-based instructional strategies and techniques presented in this volume that support reading and all other areas of literacy. Structured Literacy is effective for all students and is essential for students with dyslexia. The IDA (2018) *Knowledge and Practice Standards for Teachers of Reading* outlined what a highly knowledgeable and skilled teacher of reading needs to know and be able to do to teach Structured Literacy well. This chapter introduces the underlying theories and principles, terminology, concepts, and instructional practices of effective decoding instruction within a Structured Literacy program.

THE KNOWLEDGE BASE: THE ROLE OF DECODING

Decoding is not an end in itself but is a necessary step in getting to the heart of read-ing: comprehension. For a person to comprehend written language, symbols on the printed page must be translated into spoken words (i.e., decoding), and meaning must be connected to those words. According to Gough and Tunmer (1986) and Hoover and Gough (1990), reading comprehension is the product of decoding and linguistic or language comprehension. These two components work together in a delicate, interdependent balance. Inefficiency in one of the components can lead to overall reading failure. The reader who has difficulty with decoding will not be able to derive meaning from the text; on the contrary, the reader who has dif-ficulty with specific levels of spoken language will receive little reward for his or her decoding efforts.

A student may have efficient decoding and language comprehension but dem-onstrate difficulties in reading comprehension because of a slow processing rate, which results in dysfluent reading (Joshi & Aaron, 2000). Dysfluent reading diverts attention from the meaning of the text and adversely affects comprehension. For students to become fully literate, especially students with dyslexia, decoding, com-prehension, fluency, and all other elements of literacy instruction must be explic-itly or directly taught in an informed, comprehensive approach (Brady & Moats, 1997; National Institute of Child Health and Human Development [NICHD], 2000). Accurate and automatic decoding supports the development of fluent reading that leads to efficient comprehension and reading achievement.

Decoding facilitates the reader's linkage of the printed word to the spoken word (Beck & Juel, 1995). A reader sees a page full of symbols. The reader's success in making sense of these symbols depends on how well he or she understands that the symbols represent spoken language. Successfully establishing the relationship between the symbols and spoken language is dependent on the reader's sensitiv-ity to the internal sound structure of language (i.e., phonemic awareness; Adams, 1990). The reader must realize that spoken words have constituent sounds. In addi-tion to recognizing that words have sounds, the reader must realize that printed words consist of letters that correspond to those speech sounds. These insights enable the reader to establish the alphabetic principle or code that is necessary for acquiring decoding skills. The importance of phonemic awareness cannot be over-emphasized because it provides the foundation for decoding, enabling the reader to unlock the printed word (Adams, 1990; Bradley & Bryant, 1983; Carson, Gillon, & Boustead, 2013; Ehri, 2013; Goswami & Bryant, 1990; Liberman, Shankweiler, & Liberman, 1989). (See Chapter 6 for further discussion of how to teach phonemic awareness.)

> **REFLECT, CONNECT, and RESPOND**
> What are the two necessary components of reading comprehension, and how does each component contribute to proficient reading?

Decoding Strategies

Decoding requires knowledge of the phonemic, **graphophonemic,** syllabic, and morphemic structures of the language. A skilled reader uses a variety of strategies for translating the printed word into its spoken equivalent: sound–symbol corre-spondences, structural analysis, **instant word recognition,** and contextual clues.

Although the primary focuses of this chapter are decoding and fluency, the crucial role of oral language in the reading process must be stressed. (See Chapter 3 for more information about the relationship between oral language development and literacy.) Not only is oral language the foundation of comprehension, it also greatly influences and assists the reader's efficient and effective use of the various decoding strategies.

A reader's appreciation of the relationship between sounds and letters develops through phonemic awareness and instant letter recognition (i.e., print awareness; Adams, 1990). This understanding, in turn, develops sound–symbol correspondences (i.e., graphophonemic patterns) that enable the reader to sound out unfamiliar words. The beginning reader initially recognizes words by associating a word with some visually distinguishing characteristics (e.g., *dog* has a circle in the middle and a tail at the end; Gough & Hillinger, 1980). As the reader encounters more and more words, the visual characteristics that make words distinguishable diminish. The reader begins to cue recognition by selecting some of the letters in a word, usually the first and last letters (Ehri, 1991). He or she is now better able to distinguish words, but accuracy is limited because many words share the same initial and final letters. When the reader attends to all of the letters, he or she can sound out the correct pronunciation of an unfamiliar word (Gough & Hillinger, 1980).

Both phonological awareness and sound–symbol correspondences are critical requisites in reading acquisition (Share & Stanovich, 1995). The reader needs an introduction to a few sound–symbol patterns to begin sounding out words. As the reader sounds out words, he or she reinforces the sound–symbol correspondences that have been introduced and establishes new ones (Adams, 1990; Ehri, 2014). New sound–symbol correspondences are then acquired through what Share and Stanovich referred to as the "self-teaching mechanism" (1995, p. 17). By using known sound–symbol correspondences and phonological sensitivity, the reader approximates the pronunciation of the unknown word. This approximate pronunciation, combined with available contextual clues, enables the reader to determine the correct pronunciation and thereby provides the reader an opportunity to acquire knowledge of the sound–symbol correspondences within the unknown word. With repeated encounters, the reader builds an **orthographic memory** (i.e., memory for patterns of written language) of words so that eventually he or she instantly recognizes the words without having to sound them out (Adams, 1990; Ehri, 2014).

In addition to letters, printed words have syllables (i.e., speech units) and morphemes (i.e., meaning units). Structural analysis, the perception of orthographic syllables and morphemes, enables the reader to decode long, unfamiliar words and fosters a decoding process that is less cumbersome and more efficient than sounding out each letter. Once the reader can recognize different kinds of syllables, he or she can accurately predict the sound of the vowel in a syllable. With knowledge of morphemes, the reader can focus on units of letters that recur in words (e.g., the reader sees *tract* in *tractor, attractive,* and *subtraction*). The reader does not have to sound out every letter in an unknown word, only the letters that he or she does not recognize as part of a morpheme (Henry, 1988). Morphemes also give clues that allow the reader to infer the meanings of words (Henry, 1988, 2010; Moats, 1994).

Orthographic patterns established through graphophonemic, syllabic, and morphemic awareness greatly economize the learning of a reader's **lexicon** (i.e., spoken and written word knowledge). All of the words in the reader's lexicon, which may number more than 50,000 words by the time he or she reaches college, do not have to be stored in memory as separate items. The reader has a way of dealing with the words that he or she has heard and may use in speaking but has never seen in print before (Gough & Hillinger, 1980). (For example, a young child may not have seen the words *wizard* and *sorcerer* before but may be familiar with the words because he or she has seen a Harry Potter movie.)

The ease and automaticity with which a skilled reader is able to read individual words is known as instant word recognition. Instant word recognition is achieved by repeated encounters with words and by **overlearning** (i.e., learning to automaticity) the orthographic and phonological patterns of the language. The ultimate goal of decoding instruction is the immediate, facile translation of a printed word into its spoken equivalent (Ehri, 2013). Automaticity with this translation has a significant impact on the reader's attitude toward reading, comprehension, and overall reading success. Word recognition makes reading effortless, and reading becomes enjoyable. When reading is enjoyable, the reader will read more and, thereby, increase his or her word-recognition skills (Beck & Juel, 1995; Juel, 1991). Inadequate word recognition has a negative effect on fluency and comprehension (Ehri, 2013). Chall explained that the reader who does not attain automaticity in word recognition is said to be "glued" to the print (1983, p. 17). The reader must focus all of his or her attention on sounding out words and is diverted away from figuring out the meaning (Adams, 1990; Liberman & Liberman, 1990; Perfetti, 1985).

Evidence suggests that word-recognition accuracy and speed in first-grade students is predictive of later reading comprehension success (Beck & Juel, 1995; Juel, 1991). For example, Juel found that the probability of students who were good readers in first grade remaining good readers in fourth grade was .87; however, students who were poor readers in first grade had a probability of .88 of remaining poor readers in fourth grade. A study of 1,785 students in Grades 6–8 found that the majority of middle school students with deficits in reading comprehension also had deficits in word-recognition skills (Cirino et al., 2013). In a 10-year longitudinal study with more than 400 students who were followed from Grades K–10, Nippold (2017) found that the deficits in underlying word-recognition skills of kindergarteners did not go away with time and adversely impacted reading comprehension.

The skilled reader uses contextual clues to predict unfamiliar words, but evidence suggests that context is not the primary strategy used for word recognition (Juel, 1991; Share & Stanovich, 1995). First, the text may prove to be unreliable in yielding clues for accurate prediction. In most cases, context enables the reader to accurately predict only one out of every four words (Gough & Hillinger, 1980), and the content words that carry meaning are predictable only 10% of the time (Gough, 1983). Therefore, context is not useful when it is needed (Share & Stanovich, 1995). Second, eye-movement research shows that the eyes fixate on a majority of words in a text and do not skip over long words, as a heavy reliance on context as a means for predicting words would suggest.

Only the short, predictable words are skipped. The duration of fixation depends on the length, **frequency,** and predictability of the word as the reader processes its component letters (Rayner & Pollatsek, 1986). Using context facilitates recognition of an unfamiliar word only when it is coupled with the reader's orthographic knowledge. When context clues are combined with knowledge of sound–symbol correspondences, the skilled reader should be able to identify words that are part of his or her listening vocabulary (Adams, 1990; Perfetti, 1985).

The skilled reader monitors his or her decoding using syntactic (i.e., sentence structure) and semantic (i.e., word meaning) cues (Tunmer, Herriman, & Nesdale, 1988). The reader is able to detect and self-correct a misread word in a sentence using cues and sound–symbol correspondences. Knowing how to detect and self-correct errors also builds sound–symbol correspondences and word recognition as the reader deals with unfamiliar words. It is a particularly beneficial combination with the reader's discovery of more complex sound–symbol relationships.

Although the skilled reader uses sound–symbol correspondences, syntactic cues, and semantic cues, this does not endorse a **three-cueing systems** (e.g., Clay, 1993). Syntactic and semantic cues support, but are not equivalent to, the use of sound–symbol correspondences. It is not a matter of trying out one cueing system to see if it works and then trying another system if the first one does not work (Seidenberg, 2017). Syntactic and semantic cues do not subordinate the role of sound–symbol correspondences. Adams (1998) opined that the three-cueing schematic was designed to diminish the importance of teaching sound–symbol correspondences, which the skilled reader uses as the primary strategy to recognize unfamiliar words.

REFLECT, CONNECT, and RESPOND
What is the self-teaching mechanism, and how does it support the development of a student's decoding skills?

Teaching Decoding Through Structured Literacy Instruction

The English language, which has approximately 44 speech sounds and 26 letters, operates on an alphabetic principle or code. The speech sounds are represented in print by letters. About 75% of the school population will deduce the alphabetic principle regardless of how they are taught (Liberman & Liberman, 1990). The other 25% of students, including students with dyslexia, will not intuit this principle and will require explicit, systematic, and sequential instruction. Failure to receive such instruction can intensify these students' reading difficulties (Brady & Moats, 1997; Felton, 1993; Foorman, Francis, Beeler, Winikates, & Fletcher, 1997). A meta-analysis by Wanzek and Vaughn (2007) identified 18 effective or promising early literacy interventions for struggling readers. The beneficial effects of explicit teaching of the alphabetic principle, however, are not limited to students who have difficulty with reading. There is evidence that all students benefit from such instruction (Carreker et al., 2007; Carreker et al., 2005; Hattie, 2008; Joshi, Dahlgren, & Boulware-Gooden, 2002; NICHD, 2000; Prescott, Bundschuh, Kazakoff, & Macaruso, 2017; Ryder, Tunmer, & Greaney, 2007; Tunmer & Arrow, 2013).

Decoding requires knowledge of orthographic patterns of the language that is based on solid phonological processing. Key elements of decoding instruction include the following:

- Phonological awareness training, especially in phonemic awareness
- Instant letter-recognition training
- Introduction of sound–symbol correspondences
- Introduction of the six orthographic types of syllables
- Introduction of morphemes—prefixes, suffixes, roots, and combining forms

- Introduction of common syllable-division patterns

- Training in recognizing and understanding word origins (see Chapter 14)

- Teaching of a procedure for learning to read **irregular words**

- Instruction in the orthographic patterns for spelling

- Practice for accuracy and fluency

Teaching decoding is not an incidental part of reading instruction. It is not done through the use of worksheets or rote learning. Successful decoding instruction is a vital part of reading instruction that engages students in active, reflective, and inductive learning. Students learn to be analytic and scientific in their approach to learning the structure of the language. The intensity of instruction will depend on the instructional needs of the students.

Decoding instruction requires a structured presentation within a language context. The National Reading Panel (NRP; NICHD, 2000) emphasized that any decoding or phonics instruction should be explicit and incorporated with other reading instruction, such as vocabulary and comprehension instruction, to create a comprehensive reading program. Multisensory instruction implies using multiple senses or modalities—visual, auditory, tactile–kinesthetic—simultaneously or in rapid succession. The concept of multisensory instruction is embraced by many teachers and practitioners for its efficacy, but multisensory instruction has yet to garner support from the research community. As Carreker stated:

> The fundamental question is whether it is engagement of multiple senses, or the teaching of the structure of language, or the combination of the two that makes the instruction effective. . . . It may be some time before research definitively corroborates the value or the role of multisensory instruction. In the meantime, teachers and practitioners can explicitly teach the structure of the language, engage multiple senses, and promote reading success by making sure all the bases are covered. (2006, pp. 24, 28)

Although using multisensory instruction has not been documented empirically by science, the explicit teaching of language structures in this chapter is accompanied by suggestions for the multisensory teaching of those structures.

In learning to read, students must apprehend phonemes and instantly recognize letters before they are ready for careful instruction in sound–symbol correspondences, structural analysis, and other concepts. (See Chapters 5 and 6 for more information about alphabet knowledge and phonemic awareness.) There is no evidence of a best order of concept presentation. Any systematic, sequential order of presentation ensures that all important concepts are taught and maximizes the learning of these concepts.

A logically ordered presentation begins with the most basic concepts and progresses to more difficult concepts, with new learning building on prior knowledge. For example, phonemic segmentation and letter recognition are followed by the concepts of vowel and consonant sounds (i.e., vowel sounds are open; consonant sounds are **blocked** or **partially blocked** by the tongue, teeth, or lips).

The concept of blending letter sounds together to form words is introduced, and students begin to read words. Students are taught that a vowel in a syllable that ends in at least one consonant (i.e., closed syllable) is short. After a few more consonants and short vowels are taught, one-syllable words in word lists, phrases, and sentences are presented for students to read.

Success with structural analysis is dependent on students' knowledge of syllables, syllable-division patterns, prefixes, suffixes, and roots. Information about structural analysis can be introduced when students can read simple words with affixes. Common suffixes such as -s or -ing are introduced. One-syllable words and derivatives are presented for practice. Once students understand closed syllables, they are taught that two-syllable words with two medial consonants are divided between the consonants (e.g., VC|CV syllable-division pattern as in *mascot* or *napkin*), and, subsequently, one- and two-syllable words and derivatives are presented for practice. After letter clusters, such as *ck* and *sh*, are taught, along with additional syllable types such as open, consonant-*le*, and vowel-consonant-*e* syllables, words of various lengths can be read. As each concept is introduced, it is practiced to mastery, first through **homogeneous practice** and then through **heterogeneous practice**.

Difficulty With Decoding for Readers With Dyslexia

There is considerable agreement that readers who are at risk and have dyslexia are unable to decode and recognize words accurately and fluently (Adams & Bruck, 1993; Lyon, Shaywitz, & Shaywitz, 2003; Perfetti, 1985; Seidenberg, 2017; Share & Stanovich, 1995; Stanovich, 1986). Dyslexia stems from a core deficit in phonological processing, not a deficit in visual processing (Adams, 1990; Goswami & Bryant, 1990; Stanovich, 1991; Vellutino, 1980). This difficulty with phonological processing is not a developmental delay. It is a deficit that interferes with reading and spelling development (Foorman, Francis, Shaywitz, Shaywitz, & Fletcher, 1997). Students who have difficulty learning to read have difficulty discovering that spoken words are made up of units of sounds (i.e., phonemic awareness) that relate to letters (Adams, 1990; Adams & Bruck, 1995; Brady & Moats, 1997; Brady & Shankweiler, 1991; Gough, Ehri, & Treiman, 1992). Without this realization, students fail to learn the alphabetic principle and how to decode words accurately. They subsequently fail to thrive in reading (Stanovich, 1986).

Evidence suggests that in addition to deficits in phonological processing, students may also exhibit a deficit in naming speed, which can interfere with developing automatic decoding and fluent text reading (Wolf, 1997; Wolf & Bowers, 1999, 2000; Wolf & Obregón, 1992; see also Chapters 5 and 6). This deficit and intervention strategies are discussed later in this chapter.

The student with dyslexia often displays a performance in reading that is unexpected, given that the student may have strengths in other areas (e.g., verbal or spatial abilities) (Lyon et al., 2003). The results of a longitudinal study empirically documented unexpected underachievement in readers with reading disabilities (Ferrer, Shaywitz, Holahan, Marchione, & Shaywitz, 2009). In typically developing readers, IQ score and reading achievement progress together, with a reciprocal and bidirectional influence of IQ score on reading ability and reading ability on IQ score. In contrast, adults who were identified as at-risk readers in kindergarten and continued to be poor readers to adulthood showed continued growth in IQ score without commensurate growth in reading ability. This means that students with reading disabilities, such as dyslexia, have the cognitive resources to learn to read but do not learn; hence, the unexpected underachievement. The conclusion here is that early intervention is essential because future academic success is dependent on accurate and automatic word-recognition skills (Cirino et al., 2013; Nippold, 2017). The knowledgeable and skilled classroom teacher can provide the early intervention that can resolve many difficulties in learning to read or, the very least, ameliorate them. (Note, however, that the strategies discussed next for teaching decoding and word study can also be used with older students who struggle with reading; for more information, see Chapter 20.)

PRACTICE: TEACHING SOUND-SYMBOL CORRESPONDENCES

The intent of this chapter is not to provide a curriculum. If curricula are not available, then the information from Tables 9.1 and 9.2 (consonants and consonant clusters; vowels and vowel pairs) can be fashioned into an order of presentation. At first, three or four high-frequency consonants with predictable sounds, such as those in Table 9.1, along with a short vowel from Table 9.2, are taught.

Table 9.1. Consonants and consonant clusters

Consonants with one frequent, predictable sound

b = /b/ (*bat*)	j = /j/ (*jam*)	**p** = /p/ (*pig*)	w = /w/ (*wagon*)
d = /d/ (*dog*)	k = /k/ (*kite*)	r = /r/ (*rabbit*)	z = /z/ (*zipper*)
f = /f/ (*fish*)	**l** = /l/ (*leaf*)	t = /t/ (*table*)	
h = /h/ (*house*)	**m** = /m/ (*mitten*)	v = /v/ (*valentine*)	

Consonants with more than one sound

c = /k/ (*kite*)—before *a, o, u,* or any consonant   **s** = /s/ (*sock*)
     /s/ (*city*)—before *e, i,* or *y*   /z/ (*pansy*)

g = /g/ (*goat*)—before *a, o, u,* or any consonant   x = /z/ (*xylophone*)—in initial position*
     /j/ (*gem*)—before *e, i,* or *y*   /ks/ (*excite, box*)—in medial or final

n = /n/ (*nest*)   position*
     /ng/ (*sink or finger*)—before any letter that
       says /k/ or /g/

Consonant digraphs with one frequent sound

ck = /k/ (*truck*)   sh = /sh/ (*ship*)
ng = /ng/ (*king*)   wh = /hw/** (*whistle*)

Consonant digraphs with more than one sound

ch = /ch/ (*chair*)   th = /th/ (*thimble*)
     /k/ (*school*)—in words of Greek origin   /th/ (*mother*)
     /sh/ (*chef*)—in words of French origin

Trigraphs with one sound

dge = /j/ (*badge*)   tch = /ch/ (*witch*)

Special situations

y = /y/ in initial or medial position*   qu = /kw/ (*queen*)—*q* is always followed by *u*
       as a consonant

The boldface letters are frequently used consonants that are good to use when beginning to introduce sound-symbol correspondences. When these frequent consonants are combined with short *a, i,* and *o,* many simple words can be presented for reading.

*Initial refers to the first position of a syllable or word; *final* refers to the last position of a syllable or word; and *medial* refers to any position between the first and last positions of a syllable or word.

**This exaggerated pronunciation aids in establishing a strong orthographic memory of words that contain *wh.*

From *Multisensory Teaching of Basic Language Skills, Third Edition* (p. 213).

The beginning order might present concepts as follows:

1. Teach definitions of vowels and consonants.

2. Introduce *t* = /t/.

3. Introduce *i* = /ĭ/.

4. Introduce open syllable with the word *I*.

5. Introduce *p* = /p/ and closed syllable with the words *it* and *pit*.

6. Introduce *a* = /ă/ and blending.

7. Introduce *s* = /s/. (Cumulatively, students can read words such as *it, at, pit, pat, sit, sat, I, sip, tip, tap, sap*.)

8. Introduce suffix *-s*.

9. Introduce *n* = /n/.

10. Introduce *f* = /f/.

11. Introduce *l* = /l/.

12. Introduce *g* = /g/.

13. Introduce *m* = /m/.

14. Introduce *ng* = /ng/.

15. Introduce suffix *-ing*.

16. Introduce *o* = /ŏ/.

17. Introduce *k* = /k/.

18. Introduce *c* = /k/ before *a, o, u,* or any consonant. (Cumulatively, students can read words such as *flip, stamps, sang, clasp, claps, lasting, singing*.)

19. Introduce VCCV with *mascot* and *napkin*.

20. Introduce *ck* = /k/.

21. Introduce vowel-consonant-*e* syllable. (Students can read contrast words such as *not–note, back–bake, rip–ripe, cut–cute*.)

22. Introduce vowel pair *ee* = /ē/.

23. The introduction of concepts—more letters, letter clusters, syllable types, syllable division patterns, suffixes, stems, and prefixes—continues, progressing systematically from simple to complex, with each concept building on those previously mastered.

Building a Solid Foundation for Sound-Symbol Correspondences

Both phonological awareness and print awareness provide a solid foundation for students to learn sound–symbol correspondences. Phonological awareness involves a sensitivity to the sound structure of spoken language, such as rhyming, counting words in sentences, counting syllables in words, and identifying specific sounds in a word. Phonemic awareness, the ability to perceive the constituent sounds of a word, is the key component of phonological awareness (Adams, 1990;

Table 9.2. Vowels and vowel pairs

Short vowels in closed syllables

a = /ă/ (*apple*)	**i** = /ĭ/ (*it*)	u = /ŭ/ (*up*)
e = /ĕ/ (*echo*)	**o** = /ŏ/ (*octopus*)	

Long vowels in open, accented syllables

a = /ā/ (*apron*)	i = /ī/ (*iris*)	u = /ū/ (*unicorn*)
e = /ē/ (*equal*)	o = /ō/ (*open*)	y = /ī/ (*fly*)

Vowels in open, unaccented syllables

a = /ŭ/ (*alike*)	i = /ĭ/ (*divide*)	y = /ē/ (*penny*)

Long vowels in vowel-consonant-e syllables

a-consonant-e = /ā/ (*cake*)	i-consonant-e = /ī/ (*five*)	u-consonant-e = /ū/ (*cube*)
e-consonant-e = /ē/ (*athlete*)	o-consonant-e = /ō/ (*rope*)	y-consonant-e = /ī/ (*type*)

Vowels in vowel-r syllables

ar = /âr/ (*star*)–accented	or = /ôr/ (*fork*)–accented
/er/ (*dollar*)–unaccented	/er/ (*world*)–after w
er = /êr/ (*fern*)	/er/ (*doctor*)–unaccented
ir = /êr/ (*bird*)	ur = /êr/ (*turtle*)

Vowel pairs with one frequent sound

ai = /ā/ (*sail*)	ei = /ē/ (*ceiling*)	oe = /ō/ (*toe*)
au = /au/ (*August*)	eu = /ū/ (*Europe*)	oi = /oi/ (*boil*)
aw = /au/ (*saw*)	ew = /ū/ (*few*)	oy = /oi/ (*toy*)
ay = /ā/ (*play*)	ey = /ē/ (*monkey*)	ue = /ū/ (*rescue*)
ee = /ē/ (*feet*)	ie = /ē/ (*chief*)	

Vowel pairs with more than one frequent sound

ea = /ē/ (*eat*)	ou = /ou/ (*out*)	ow = /ou/ (*cow*)
/ĕ/ (*head*)	/o͞o/ (*soup*)	/ō/ (*snow*)
oo = /o͞o/ (*food*)		
/o͝o/ (*book*)		

Special situations

a = /ŏ/ (*watch*)–after w	eigh = /ā/ (*eight*)	o = /ŭ/ (*onion*)
a = /au/ (*ball*)–before l	igh = /ī/ (*light*)	

The boldface letters are good concepts and letters for beginning reading instruction.
From *Multisensory Teaching of Basic Language Skills, Third Edition* (p. 214).

Ball & Blachman, 1988; Liberman, 1987; Lundberg, Frost, & Petersen, 1988; Yopp, 1992). Print awareness involves sensitivity to the conventions of the printed page, such as top to bottom, left to right, punctuation, indentations, spaces between words, and the awareness that words consist of letters. The key component of print awareness is the ability to instantly recognize letters (Adams, 1990).

Instant Letter Recognition   A beginning reader's instant letter recognition is a strong predictor of reading success. Knowing the names of the letters can facilitate the learning of the letter sounds because many sounds are embedded in the letter names (e.g., students can hear the /m/ sound in the name of the letter *m*) (Adams, 1990; Gough & Hillinger, 1980). All letters have four properties: name, sound, shape, and feel (i.e., the sensation of muscle movements while writing the letter or while producing the sound). The name is the only property that does not change; thus, the name of the letter is an anchor to which the reader can attach its other properties. Automatic letter recognition allows the reader to see words as groups of letters instead of as individual letters that must be identified (Adams, 1990). Activities to reinforce letter recognition are easily incorporated into the classroom routine, as in the following examples:

- The teacher writes a letter on the board. All students whose names begin with that letter line up.

- The teacher writes a letter on the board and calls on a student who must name the letter before lining up.

- The teacher writes a letter on the board and calls on a student who must name the target letter and the letter that comes after (or before) the target letter before lining up.

Phonemic Awareness   A beginning reader's ability to segment a word into its phonemes (i.e., phoneme segmentation) is one of the best predictors of reading success. A phoneme is the smallest unit of speech that makes a difference in the utterance of a word. Thus, the reader's awareness of individual sounds in a word increases his or her understanding of the role of the individual letters in words and how the written letters can be mapped onto the sounds. Without these insights, the reader will not successfully learn the code of the language (Adams, 1990; Ball & Blachman, 1988; see Chapter 6). Because of the importance of phonemic awareness, activities for reinforcing phonemic awareness should be ongoing and are easily incorporated into the classroom routine, as in these examples:

- The teacher guesses what was for lunch. Students give the teacher rhyming clues so that the teacher can guess what students ate for lunch (e.g., "I had a mapple, a mandwich, and a mookie;" Rubin & Eberhardt, 1996).

- The teacher says a sound. All students whose names begin (or end) with the sound take their place in line (Rubin & Eberhardt, 1996).

- The teacher takes the class roll using blending. The teacher calls out the names slowly. Students guess the name, and the named student indicates his or her presence.

- The teacher says a word with three or four phonemes (e.g., *lap, sit, run, top, dog, jump, stop*).

- The teacher calls on a student to **unblend** the word (i.e., say the word slowly) before lining up.

- To hone their attention, students establish a word of the week. The teacher gains students' attention by saying the word. Students respond by **unblending** the word.

- After the teacher reads a book, students apply their phonological awareness skills to play with words from the book (Rubin & Eberhardt, 1996; Yopp, 1995). For example, after reading *The Wind Blew* (Hutchins, 1974), students discover that various items were blown into the air. Students can play with the names of the items. They say words that rhyme with *wig, hat,* and *flag.* They count the syllables in *balloon, letters, umbrella,* and *newspapers.* They segment the words *kite, shirt,* and *scarf* into their component sounds.

REFLECT, CONNECT, and RESPOND

Why is phonemic awareness instruction critical for a student with dyslexia?

Teaching Orthographic Patterns

As students acquire basic sound–symbol correspondences, they build their knowledge of orthographic patterns in the language and create a scaffold for refining and expanding their knowledge of the spelling–sound system (Share & Stanovich, 1995).

Some letters have one frequent sound or a one-to-one correspondence with a sound (e.g., letters such as *d, m, p,* and *v* have one sound). However, letter–sound correspondences are not always one-to-one. Two adjacent letters in a syllable that represent one speech sound are called digraphs. Digraphs that consist of two adjacent consonants are called consonant digraphs (e.g., *sh, ng, ck, th*); digraphs that consist of two adjacent vowels are called vowel digraphs (e.g., *ai, ea, ee, oa*). Some digraphs have one frequent sound (e.g., *sh* as in *ship, ng* as in *king, ck* as in *truck, oa* as in *boat*).

Other digraphs have several sounds (e.g., *th* as in *thimble* and *mother; ea* as in *each, head,* and *steak*). Three adjacent letters in a syllable that represent one speech sound are called *trigraphs* (e.g., *tch, dge*). **Quadrigraphs** consist of four adjacent letters in a syllable that represent one speech sound (e.g., *eigh*). Two adjacent vowels whose sounds blend together are called *diphthongs* (e.g., *ou, ow, oi, oy*). Considerable attention to orthography is needed for readers to deal with letters that have more than one possible sound. Pronouncing such a letter may depend on its occurrence with other letters (e.g., *c* is pronounced as /k/ before *a, o, u,* or any consonant but as /s/ before *e, i,* or *y*) and/or its position in a word (e.g., *y* is a consonant in initial position pronounced as /y/ but is a vowel in final position, pronounced as /ī/ or /ē/). Knowing these patterns of language helps the reader choose the best pronunciation of a letter with more than one possible sound. In addition, there are constraints to the orthography of English. Some letters and letter clusters may not occur in certain positions in a word (e.g., English base words do not end in *j* or *v*). Some letters may or may not occur adjacent to certain letters (e.g., *q* is almost always followed by *u; scr* occurs within a syllable, but *skr* does not). Finally, some letters never or rarely double (e.g., *h, j, k, v, w, x, y*) (Moats, 1995; Perfetti, 1985). Careful, reflective study of orthography reinforces information readers need for reading and spelling.

Introducing a Letter

Sound–symbol correspondences are established thorough instruction of letters and letter clusters. The three major learning modalities or pathways—auditory, visual, and kinesthetic—are engaged in introducing a letter or letter cluster. Students link the look of a letter (visual) with its sound (auditory) and its feel (kinesthetic) to form the letter sound and written shape. The information received through more than one sensory pathway increases the certainty of learning and retrieval. The grouping of the modalities strengthens the weaker pathway(s) as the strongest pathway assumes the lead in learning. The following terms and procedures are helpful in understanding multisensory instruction.

Use of Kinesthetic Awareness   Kinesthetic awareness involves sensitivity to muscle movement. Kinesthetic information heightens students' memory and ability to discriminate speech sounds. Students' awareness of the position of the mouth, tongue, teeth, or lips and the activity of the vocal cords during the production of a sound assists the definitive learning of speech sounds. Kinesthetic information also heightens students' visual memory and ability to discriminate letter shapes. Students' awareness of how a letter feels when written in the air (i.e., sky writing) or on paper connects kinesthetic and visual information so that the letter shapes can be thoroughly learned.

Awareness of Sounds   The exact individual sounds of letters (i.e., phonemes) are difficult to isolate. Speech sounds do not occur as single units in running speech. In spoken language, sounds in a word are blended together into units with other sounds so that when the speaker says a word, it does not sound as though he or she is spelling the word out loud sound by sound (e.g., *bag* is not pronounced /b/ - /ǎ/ - /g/ but rather /bǎ/ - /g/) (Liberman, 1987).

The blending of speech sounds into units is termed co-articulation. For students to learn the sound–symbol correspondences, it is necessary for them to be able to isolate the sounds as close approximations of the actual sounds that will be co-articulated with other sounds. The following terminology helps build the teacher's understanding of sound–symbol relationships:

- A *voiced speech* sound is a sound in which the vocal cords vibrate during its production.

- An *unvoiced speech* sound is a sound in which the vocal cords do not vibrate during its production.

- A *vowel sound* is an open speech sound, produced by the easy passage of air through a relatively open vocal tract. It is unblocked by the tongue, teeth, or lips and is voiced. (The sound /h/ opens the mouth, but because it is not voiced, it is a consonant sound.)

- A *consonant sound* is a sound that is blocked (e.g., /l/, /s/, /m/) or partially blocked (e.g., /p/, /b/) by the tongue, teeth, or lips and may be voiced (e.g., /m/, /l/, /r/) or unvoiced (e.g., /t/, /s/, /k/).

  Note: For decoding instruction, the terms *blocked* and *partially blocked* refer to the kinesthetic feel and visual display of the position of the tongue, teeth, or lips during the production of sounds in isolation. *Blocked* refers to the steady position of the tongue, teeth, or lips during the entire production of a sound (e.g., the lips stay together in a steady position as /m/ is pronounced). *Partially blocked* refers to a released position of the tongue or lips during production (e.g., the tongue is released from the ridge behind the teeth as /t/ is pronounced). These terms are used in decoding instruction because students can easily and clearly feel or see the characteristics that distinguish consonant sounds from vowel sounds.

- *Voiced and unvoiced pairs* (see Table 9.3) are sounds that have the same visual display (i.e., the same position of the tongue, teeth, and lips) and kinesthetic feel but which differ because the vocal cords vibrate during the production of one (voiced) and not the other (unvoiced).

- A *continuant speech sound* is prolonged in its production (e.g., /m/, /s/, /f/).

- A *stop consonant* is obstructed at its **place of articulation** and not prolonged in its production (e.g., /g/, /p/, /t/, /k/). These sounds must be clipped to prevent the addition of /ǔh/ at the end of the sound (e.g., /p/ not /pǔh/).

Table 9.3. Voiced and unvoiced pairs

Unvoiced	Voiced
/p/	/b/
/t/	/d/
/k/	/g/
/f/	/v/
/s/	/z/
/th/	/<u>th</u>/
/ch/	/j/
/sh/	/zh/

From *Multisensory Teaching of Basic Language Skills, Third Edition* (p. 219).

Note: The terms *continuant* and *stop consonant* are linguistic terms. In decoding instruction, the term *continuant consonant* is synonymous with *blocked consonant.* The term *stop consonant* is synonymous with *partially blocked.*

- A *fricative* is produced by forcing air from the mouth through a narrow opening (e.g., /f/, /v/, /sh/, /s/, /z/).

- A *nasal sound* is produced by forcing air out through the nose (e.g., /n/, /m/, /ng/).

Use of Key Words   Key words serve as a memory device to unlock letter sounds and as a trigger for rapid elicitation of letter sounds. A key word illustrates the sound of a letter and provides a connection of that sound to a written symbol (Cox, 1992; Ehri, 2014; Gillingham & Stillman, 1997). A letter–sound deck can be used to systematically review key words and sounds. When students are shown a letter card, they name the letter, say a key word, and produce the sound (e.g., when shown a card with the letter *a*, students respond, "*a, apple,* /ă/"). Pictures of the key words may be added to the letter cards.

Use of Coding   Using **diacritical markings** for vowels and other code marks provides students with additional visual and kinesthetic information to reinforce the letter sounds. Short vowels are coded with a *breve* (˘). Long vowels are coded with a *macron* (¯). The obscure *a*, found in the word *along* and pronounced /ŭ/, is coded with a dot: à. Vowel digraphs (e.g., *ai, ea, ee, oa*), consonant digraphs (e.g., *ch, ng, sh*), and trigraphs (e.g., *tch, dge*) that represent one speech sound are underlined. Vowel diphthongs that represent two speech sounds that are blended together are coded with an arc:

$$ou \quad ow \quad oi \quad oy$$

Silent letters are crossed out:

$$ai \text{ or } tch$$

Additional codes are introduced later in this chapter.

Use of Sky Writing   **Sky writing** involves engaging the large "learning" muscles of the upper arm and shoulder. The movement of these muscles produces a strong neurological imprint of letter shapes (Waites & Cox, 1976). For sky writing, the arm of the writing hand is fully extended and tensed. Students use the whole writing arm, with fingers extended, to write large letters in the air, with a large model in front of them, to develop muscle memory. The nonwriting hand is placed on the upper arm or shoulder of the writing arm to create tension and help students feel the individual strokes more discernibly.

Guided Discovery Teaching Guided discovery teaching is effective in ensuring that students learn sound–symbol correspondences and other patterns of language. The word *education* comes from the Latin word *educere,* which means *to lead out.* Guided discovery teaching uses the Socratic method of asking questions to lead students to discover new information. When students make a discovery, they understand and connect the new learning to prior knowledge.

Students, for example, are led to discover the difference between vowel and consonant sounds. The teacher asks students to repeat each of the following sounds one at a time while looking in a mirror: /ă/, /ĕ/, /ĭ/, /ŏ/, /ŭ/. The teacher asks, "What do you see happening to your mouth as each sound is pronounced?" (The mouth is open.)

The teacher asks students to say the sounds again while placing their fingers on the vocal cords. The teacher asks, "What do you feel?" (The vocal cords are activated, or the throat vibrates.) The teacher explains that these sounds are vowel sounds. Students verbalize what they have learned about vowel sounds through discovery: Vowel sounds are open and voiced (make the throat vibrate).

The teacher can also use guided discovery teaching to help students make discoveries about consonant sounds. When students are asked to repeat consonant sounds such as /l/, /s/, /m/, /b/, and /p/ while looking in a mirror, they discover that these sounds are blocked (/l/, /s/, /m/) or partially blocked (/b/, /p/) by the tongue, teeth, or lips. Consonant sounds can be voiced or unvoiced. Students verbalize what they have learned about consonant sounds through discovery: "Consonant sounds are blocked or partially blocked by the tongue, teeth, or lips. They may be voiced or unvoiced."

Procedure for Introducing a Letter or Letter Cluster Letter–sound relationships can be introduced through discovery teaching and a multisensory structured procedure, which can be adjusted to meet the specific learning needs of students (Cox, 1992; Gillingham & Stillman, 1997):

1. The teacher reads five or six **discovery words** that contain the new letter sound.

2. Students repeat each word while looking in a mirror and listening for the sound that is the same in all of the words.

3. While looking in the mirror, students repeat the sound and discover the position of the mouth. Is it opened or is it blocked or partially blocked by the tongue, teeth, or lips?

4. While placing their fingers on their vocal cords, students repeat the sound to discover whether the sound is voiced (i.e., the vocal cords vibrate) or unvoiced (i.e., there is no vibration).

5. Students determine whether the new sound is a vowel or a consonant sound. Vowel sounds are open and voiced. Consonant sounds are blocked or partially blocked by the tongue, teeth, or lips. They may be voiced or unvoiced.

6. Students guess the key word for the new sound by listening to a riddle or by feeling an object obscured in a container. The key word holds the new sound in memory.

7. The teacher writes the discovery words on the board.

8. Students determine the letter that is the same in all of the words and that represents the new sound.

9. The teacher shows a card with the new letter on it.

10. Students name the letter, say the key word, and give the sound.

11. The teacher names the new letter just before writing a large model of the letter on the board.

12. The teacher names the letter and then demonstrates sky writing. The teacher describes the letter strokes while sky writing the letter.

13. Students stand and sky write, naming the letter before writing.

14. The teacher distributes papers with a large model of the new letter.

15. Students trace the model three times with the pointer finger of the writing hand and three times with a pencil. Students name the letter each time before writing.

16. Students turn the model over, and the teacher dictates the name of the letter.

17. Students repeat the letter name and write the letter.

18. The teacher shows the letter card again as students name the letter, say the key word, and produce the sound.

During the various steps in this procedure, the four properties of the letter—name, sound, shape, and feel—are being connected through the use of the auditory, visual, and kinesthetic modalities. This multisensory teaching reinforces the discovery information and builds associations in memory.

Teaching Blending

Once students have identified the letter–sound relationships of a word, they must meld the sounds to produce a word. Blending sounds in a word is a critical component of learning sound–symbol correspondences. Fluid blending of letter sounds aids students in producing recognizable words. Before students begin reading words, they should have opportunities to blend sounds together orally by using manipulatives (e.g., blocks, buttons, math counters, pennies). Because of the effects of co-articulation on sounds, letter-by-letter blending in reading does not always produce a recognizable word. Several different strategies described next, best presented one-to-one or in small groups, are used to promote the skill of blending when reading words. When introducing any of the blending activities for reading, it is desirable to begin blending words that have continuant initial sounds (e.g., /f/, /l/, /m/, /n/, /s/). Continuant sounds are easier to blend than the stop consonant sounds (e.g., /d/, /p/, /k/). The continuant sounds allow students to slide into the vowel sound. Blending with initial stop consonants is introduced after students have demonstrated facility with the blending of continuant initial sounds.

Say It Slowly   Using one set of letter cards or lettered tiles, the teacher sets out *m, e,* and *t.* The teacher demonstrates how to say the word *met* by blending the sounds together in units—by saying /m/, then /mĕ/, then /mĕt/, not by saying /m/ - /ĕ/ - /t/ (Beck & Juel, 1995).

Say It Faster, Move It Closer   Using one set of letter cards or lettered tiles, the teacher sets out *s* and, separated by a wide space, *a.* The teacher points to the first letter. Students say /s/ and hold the sound until the teacher points to the second letter and students produce /ă/. The letters are moved closer together and the procedure is repeated, with students blending the sounds together faster. The letters are moved closer together and sounds are produced together faster until students can produce the two sounds as a single unit, /să/. A final consonant is added and blended with the unit to produce a word (e.g., *sat, sad, sap;* Blachman, 1987; Englemann, 1969).

Onsets and Rimes   Using letter cards or lettered tiles, the teacher sets out *a* and *t.* Students blend the letter sounds to produce /ăt/. This /ăt/ unit is the *rime,* the combination of the vowel and the consonant(s) that comes after it in a syllable. The teacher places the letter *m* before the rime. This letter is the onset, the consonant(s) of a syllable before the vowel. Students blend /m/ and /ăt/ to produce /măt/. The teacher changes the onset to create new words that students blend and read (e.g., *sat, rat, fat, bat*). Other rimes for practice include the following: *in, it, an, am, op, ang, ing,* and *ink* (Adams, 1990; Goswami & Bryant, 1990).

Playing With Sounds   Using one set of letter cards or lettered tiles, the teacher sets out *a* and *t.* The student blends the letter sounds to produce /ăt/. The teacher asks the student to change /ăt/ to /săt/. The student adds the card or tile with *s* and reads /săt/. The teacher asks the student to read new words by changing or adding new letter sounds (e.g., change *sat* to *mat, mat* to *map, map* to *mop, mop* to *top, top* to *stop*) (Beck & Juel, 1995; Blachman, 1987; Blachman, Ball, Black, & Tangel, 2000; Slingerland, 1971).

Tapping Out   The teacher lays out or displays letter cards or lettered tiles to form a word such as *mat.* Using one hand, students quickly tap the pointer finger to the thumb and say the sound of the first letter, /m/. In quick succession, they tap the middle finger to the thumb and say the sound of the second letter, /ă/. Finally, they tap the ring finger to the thumb and say the sound of the final letter, /t/. When all of the letter sounds have been tapped out, students say the word as they drag the thumb across their fingers, beginning with the index finger (Wilson, 1996).

Tapping and Sweeping   The teacher lays out letter cards or lettered tiles to form a word such as *mat.* Each student takes a turn. He or she makes a fist and taps under the *m* as he or she says the sound /m/. Next, he or she taps under the *a* and says /ă/. Finally, he or she taps under the *t* and says /t/. After the student has said each sound, he or she sweeps a fist under the letters and says the word (Greene & Enfield, 1985).

Strategies for Improving Accuracy

Accurately reading words is key to associating pronunciations with correct orthographic patterns as well as facilitating comprehension. The teacher can use the following strategies to guide a student to the accurate decoding of a word or to correct a mistake when he or she is reading:

- *When misreading or skipping letters:* If a student misreads a letter in a word (e.g., *lid* for *lip*) or omits a letter in a word (e.g., *pat* for *past*), then the teacher directs the student to name the letters in the word. Naming the letters focuses the student's attention on the letters and also strengthens the orthographic identity of the word.

- *When misreading a word:* If a student misreads a word (e.g., *pane* for *plant*), the teacher directs the student to use a backing-up procedure. The student identifies the syllable type, determines the vowel sound (short or long), and codes the vowel accordingly (i.e., marks it with a breve or a macron). The student produces the appropriate vowel sound and blends it with the consonant sound immediately after the vowel. He or she blends this unit with any remaining consonant sounds after the vowel, adding sounds one at a time. The reader then blends the vowel and all of the consonant sounds after the vowel with the consonant sound immediately before the vowel. Any remaining consonants that precede the vowel are blended on one at a time.

The backing-up procedure with the word *plant* looks like this:

Step 1: The student codes *a* with a breve and says /ă/   plănt

Step 2: The student blends /ă/ with /n/.   plănt

Step 3: The student blends /ăn/ with /t/.   plănt

Step 4: The student blends /l/ with /ănt/.   plănt

Step 5: The student blends the whole word.   plănt

Knowing sound–symbol correspondences enables a reader to successfully read one-syllable base words. Once the reader has established a few sound–symbol correspondences and can blend them together successfully to form words, information about structural analysis is taught concurrently with new sound–symbol correspondences.

PRACTICE: TEACHING MONOSYLLABIC AND MULTISYLLABIC WORDS

Knowledge of the syllabic and morphemic segments of language facilitates the accurate recognition of monosyllabic and multisyllabic words. Syllables are speech units of language that contain one vowel sound and can be represented in written language as words (e.g., *cat, mop, sad*) or parts of words (e.g., *mu, hin, ter*), with a single vowel or pair of vowels denoting the vowel sound. When a syllable is part of a word, it does not necessarily carry meaning (e.g., *mu* in *music, per* in *scamper*). Awareness of syllables helps the reader perceive the natural divisions of words to aid recognition. Six types of syllables are represented in written English (e.g., a closed syllable ends in at least one consonant; an open syllable ends in one vowel). The types of syllables are discussed in detail later in this chapter.

Awareness of **syllable types** gives the reader a way to determine how to pronounce the vowel sound in a syllable (e.g., the vowel in a closed syllable is short; the vowel in an open, accented syllable is long). *Morphemes* are meaning-carrying units of written language (Moats, 1994), such as base words (e.g., *cat, number, salamander*), prefixes (e.g., *un-, re-, mis-*), suffixes (e.g., *-ful, -ness, -ment*), combining forms (e.g., *bio, helio, polis*), and roots (e.g., *vis, struct, vert*). Awareness of morphemes aids instant word recognition as well as word meaning.

Introducing Syllables

The teacher leads students to discover the concept of a syllable. Students are asked to repeat words of varying lengths (e.g., *mop, robot, fantastic*), one at time, while looking in a mirror and observing how many times their mouths open when each word is pronounced. They are asked to repeat each word again while cupping their jaws in their hands and feeling how many times their jaws drop or their mouths open. This visual information of seeing the mouth open and kinesthetic information of feeling the mouth open reinforces students' understanding of a syllable. The teacher explains that a syllable is a word or a part of a word made with one opening of the mouth. Students are asked to think about which kind of letter sounds open the mouth. (Vowel sounds open the mouth.) The teacher explains that a syllable has one vowel sound. When students say a word, they determine the number of syllables by counting the number of times the mouth opens when pronouncing the word. This concept carries over when students look at a printed word; they determine the number of syllables in the word by counting the number of sounded vowels.

Auditory Awareness of Syllables The following activities promote awareness of syllables in words:

- Students begin to develop syllable awareness early, by identifying or generating short words (*farm, feet, fat, fork, food*) and long words (*February, firefighter, fisherman*). The chosen words might begin with a certain sound or pertain to a particular unit of study (*plants, animals, ocean, United States*; Rubin & Eberhardt, 1996).

- Students repeat words dictated by the teacher. They clap or tap out the number of syllables. The teacher starts with compound words (*playground, flashlight, cowboy*), then moves on to two-syllable words (*velvet, plastic, mascot*) and then on to words with three or more syllables (*fantastic, investment, invitation*).

- Students repeat words dictated by the teacher and move a counter (e.g., *block, button, penny*) for each syllable they hear. Using counters provides a visual and kinesthetic anchor for the sounds.

- Students repeat a word with two or more syllables dictated by the teacher. Students are asked to repeat the word again, omitting a designated syllable (Rosner, 1975), as illustrated in the following dialogue.

> TEACHER: Say *transportation.*
>
> STUDENTS: Transportation.
>
> TEACHER: Say *transportation* without *trans.*
>
> STUDENTS: Portation.
>
> TEACHER: Say *transportation* without *tion.*
>
> STUDENTS: Transporta.

This activity is effective in helping students pronounce words correctly and aids reading and spelling words of more than one syllable.

Awareness of Accent Correct placement of the accent or stress on a syllable supports students in pronouncing and recognizing words. The mouth opens wider and the voice is louder and higher when the accented syllable is pronounced. The following activities promote awareness of accent:

- Students practice accent by saying the alphabet in pairs, accenting the first letter in the pair: "A′ B, C′ D, E′ F, G′ H, I′ J."

- Students practice flexibility in accenting by saying the alphabet in pairs and shifting the accent to the second letter in the pair: "A B′, C D′, E F′, G H′, I J′."

- Students practice accenting by saying two-syllable words, first placing an exaggerated accent on the first syllable and then placing it on the second. They then choose the correct accent placement (e.g., *bas′|ket*, not *bas|ket′*; *can|teen′*, not *can′|teen*).

Some words have a noun form and a verb form, and the accent may fall on either syllable depending on the form of the word. The nouns are accented on the first syllable, and the verbs are accented on the second (e.g., *con′|duct, con|duct′; ob′|ject, ob|ject′*).

Teaching the Six Types of Syllables

The instability of vowels is a complicating factor in learning the sound–symbol correspondences of written English. They have more than one sound (e.g., short sound, long sound, unexpected sound when followed by *r* or in combination with another vowel). This instability is one reason why knowledge of syllable types is an important organizing tool for decoding unknown words. Students can group letters into known syllable types that give clues about the sounds of the vowels. Table 9.4 presents the six orthographic types of syllables: closed, open, vowel-consonant-*e*, vowel pair (vowel team), vowel-*r* (*r*-controlled), and consonant-*le* (which is one kind of **final stable syllable**; Steere, Peck, & Kahn, 1984). A high percentage of the more than 600,000 words of English can be categorized as one of these syllable types or as a composite of different syllable types.

Combining this knowledge of syllable types with known morphemes (e.g., suffixes, prefixes) simplifies decoding words with more than one syllable. The

Table 9.4. Six syllable types

Closed	Open	Vowel-consonant-*e*	Vowel pair (vowel team)	Vowel-*r*	Consonant-*le**
it	hi	name	each	fern	-dle
bed	no	five	boil	burn	-fle
and	me	slope	sweet	thirst	-gle
lost	she	these	tray	star	-ple

*A consonant-*le* syllable is a kind of final stable syllable. Other final stable syllables include *-age, -sion, -tion*, and *-ture*.

From *Multisensory Teaching of Basic Language Skills, Third Edition* (p. 226).

closed syllable is the most frequent syllable type in English (Stanback, 1992). After students have learned three or four consonants and one short vowel, they can be introduced to the closed syllable. The remaining sound–symbol correspondences and syllable types are taught sequentially and cumulatively until all have been introduced, and then students practice them until all are mastered.

Guided discovery teaching techniques for the six syllable types are discussed in the following sections. The syllable types are introduced in the order that they might be presented to students. Students are led to discover the salient characteristics of each syllable type and the effect of the syllabic pattern on the vowel sound. The teacher pauses after the questions to solicit answers from students.

Closed Syllable   Closed syllables can be taught as indicated.

TEACHER: *[Writes discovery words on the board and directs students' attention to them.]* Look at these words: *hat, got, hip, mend.* How many vowels are in each word?

STUDENTS: There is only one vowel in each word.

TEACHER: Look at the end of each word. How does each word end?

STUDENTS: The words end in at least one consonant.

TEACHER: Listen as I read the words. How are the vowels pronounced? *[Reads the words.]*

STUDENTS: The vowels are short.

TEACHER: Each of these words ends in at least one consonant after one vowel. What happens to the mouth when a consonant sound is made?

STUDENTS: The tongue, teeth, or lips close the sound.

TEACHER: Yes, a consonant closes the mouth. What would be a good name for a syllable that ends in a consonant?

STUDENTS: A good name is closed syllable.

TEACHER: A closed syllable ends in at least one consonant after one vowel. Therefore, these words are closed syllables. The vowel in a closed syllable is short; the vowel is coded with a breve that is written as (˘). *[Writes a breve over the vowel in each word.]* The word *breve* comes from the Latin word *brevis,* which means short. What other words might come from the same Latin word?

STUDENTS: *Brief, brevity,* and *abbreviate* also come from the same Latin word.

TEACHER: Let's review what you have discovered about closed syllables. A closed syllable ends in at least one consonant after one vowel. The vowel is short; code it with a breve.

Note: When reviewing the concept of a closed syllable, or any kind of syllable, a cloze procedure can be used, with students filling in the most salient characteristics of the syllable type. Pausing for students' replies, the teacher says, "A closed syllable ends in at least one [consonant] after one [vowel]. The vowel is [short]; code it with a [breve]."

Students must be sensitive to the fact that accent may affect the sound of a vowel in a syllable. Short vowel sounds in unaccented closed syllables, particularly before *m, n,* or *l,* may be distorted. The resultant vowel sound is schwa, which is denoted as /ə/ and is pronounced approximately as /ŭ/. This sound does not build a strong orthographic memory of the words because the schwa sound is not uniquely represented by one letter (Ehri, Wilce, & Taylor, 1987). Students should use an **exaggerated pronunciation,** or spelling-based pronunciation, when decoding these words (e.g., students pronounce *ribbon* as /rĭbŏn/). The teacher helps students match the printed word to a familiar word in running speech.

Short vowels before nasal sounds /m/, /n/, or /ng/ are nasalized and may seem distorted (e.g., *jam, ant, drank, thing*). Awareness of this possibility helps students better match the orthographic representation with a known word in their listening and speaking vocabularies. (See Ehri et al., 1987, for more discussion of short vowels.)

Open Syllable   Open syllables can be taught as indicated.

TEACHER: *[Writes discovery words on the board and directs students' attention to them.]* Look at these words: *he, go, hi, me.* How many vowels are in each word?

STUDENTS: There is only one vowel in each word.

TEACHER: Look at the end of each word. How does each word end?

STUDENTS: The words end in one vowel.

TEACHER: Could these words be called closed syllables?

STUDENTS: No, closed syllables end in at least one consonant after one vowel.

TEACHER: When the words are read, how are the vowels pronounced? *[Reads the words.]*

STUDENTS: The vowels are long.

TEACHER: Each of these words ends in one vowel. What position is the mouth in when a vowel sound is made?

STUDENTS: The mouth is open.

TEACHER: What would be a good name for a syllable that ends in one vowel?

STUDENTS: A good name is open syllable.

TEACHER: An open syllable ends in one vowel. The vowel in an open, accented syllable is long; the vowel is coded with a macron, which is written as (‾). *[Writes a macron on the board.]* The word *macron* comes from the Greek word *makros,* which means *long.* Let's review what you have discovered about an open syllable: An open syllable ends in one vowel. The vowel is long; code it with a macron.

Vowel-Consonant-e Syllable   **Vowel-consonant-*e* syllables (VCE)** can be taught as indicated.

TEACHER: *[Writes discovery words on the board.]* Look at these words: *cake, theme, five, rope, cube.* How many vowels are in each word?

STUDENTS: There are two vowels in each word.

TEACHER: Look at the end of each word. How does each word end?

STUDENTS: They end with an *e*.

TEACHER: What comes between the vowel and the final *e* in each word?

STUDENTS: One consonant.

TEACHER: When the words are read, what happens to the final *e*? [*Reads the words.*]

STUDENTS: The *e* in final position is silent.

TEACHER: How are the vowels pronounced?

STUDENTS: They are pronounced with their long sounds.

TEACHER: Each of these words ends in one vowel, one consonant, and a final *e*. What would be a good name for this kind of syllable?

STUDENTS: A good name is vowel-consonant-*e* syllable.

TEACHER: The vowel in a vowel-consonant-*e* syllable is long. How is a long vowel coded?

STUDENTS: A macron shows a long vowel.

TEACHER: The final *e* in this syllable is silent. How can the *e* be coded?

STUDENTS: The silent *e* can be crossed out: *e̸*.

TEACHER: Let's review what you have discovered about the vowel-consonant-*e* syllable: A vowel-consonant-*e* syllable ends in one vowel, one consonant, and a final *e*. The *e* is silent; cross it out. The vowel is long; code it with a macron.

Vowel-Pair (Vowel-Team) Syllable   **Vowel pair** or **vowel team syllables** can be taught as indicated.

TEACHER: [*Writes discovery words on the board in two columns.*] Look at these words: *sea, feet, paint, boat, zoo, book, point, head*. How many vowels are in each word?

STUDENTS: There are two vowels in each word.

TEACHER: Look at the end of each word. How does each word end?

STUDENTS: Some words end with at least one consonant.

TEACHER: Are they closed syllables?

STUDENTS: No, a closed syllable has only one vowel.

TEACHER: How about the other words?

STUDENTS: They end in a vowel.

TEACHER: Are they open syllables?

STUDENTS: No, an open syllable has only one vowel.

TEACHER: These words are called *vowel-pair syllables* or *vowel-team syllables* because they have two vowels next to each other. Each vowel pair has a different letter combination and sound. Let's review what you have discovered about the vowel-pair syllable: A vowel-pair (or vowel-team) syllable has two vowels next to each other.

Note: The generalization of "when two vowels go walking, the first one does the talking" is only reliable about 45% of the time (Adams, 1990). The first four discovery words (*see, feet, paint, boat*) in this activity follow this generalization; the last four discovery words (*zoo, book, point, head*) do not. For accuracy, each pair must be explicitly taught.

Vowel-r (r-Controlled) Syllable   **Vowel-r syllables,** also called **r-controlled syllables,** can be taught as indicated.

TEACHER: *[Writes discovery words on the board.]* Look at these words: *met, red, step, hen, her.* How many vowels are in these words?

STUDENTS: There is one vowel in each word.

TEACHER: Look at the end of each word. How does each word end?

STUDENTS: They end in at least one consonant after one vowel.

TEACHER: What kind of syllable ends in at least one consonant after one vowel?

STUDENTS: A closed syllable ends in at least one consonant after one vowel.

TEACHER: Tell me about the vowel in a closed syllable.

STUDENTS: The vowel in a closed syllable is short; code it with a breve.

TEACHER: Let's code and read these words. *[Students direct the teacher to code each word. Students read each word after it is coded. When students reach the word* her, *they discover they cannot read the word with a short e sound.]* What happened when you tried to read the word *her?*

STUDENTS: The vowel is not short in the word *her.*

TEACHER: Something unexpected happens to the vowel in this word. We expect the vowel to be short because it is in a closed syllable. What letter do you see after the vowel?

STUDENTS: The letter *r* is after the vowel.

TEACHER: In the word *her,* the *r* comes after the vowel. What would be a good name for this syllable?

STUDENTS: A good name would be vowel-*r* syllable.

TEACHER: What happens to the vowel in a vowel-*r* syllable?

STUDENTS: The vowel makes an unexpected sound.

TEACHER: When an *r* comes after a vowel, the vowel and the *r* are coded with an arc beneath them:

her

The vowel-*r* combination in an accented syllable is also coded with a circumflex:

hêr

Let's review what you have discovered about a vowel-*r* syllable: A vowel-*r* syllable has an *r* after the vowel. The vowel makes an unexpected sound; in an accented syllable, code the vowel-*r* syllable with an arc and code the vowel with a circumflex.

Note: The vowel before an *r* in an accented syllable is coded with a **circumflex** (ˆ). In an unaccented syllable, the vowel-*r* combination is coded with an arc and the vowel with a tilde (~). The vowel-*r* combinations *er, ir,* and *ur* in an accented or unaccented syllable are pronounced /er/. The vowel-*r* combination *ar* in an accented syllable is pronounced /ar/ as in *star*. In an unaccented syllable, *ar* is pronounced /er/ as in *dollar*. The vowel-*r* combination *or* in an accented syllable is pronounced /or/ as in *fork*. In an unaccented syllable, *or* is pronounced /er/ as in *doctor*.

The terms *vowel-r syllable* and *r-controlled syllable* are used interchangeably. The term *vowel-r* focuses attention on the orthographic pattern, and the term *r-controlled* focuses attention on the influence of the *r* on the vowel.

Consonant-le (Final Stable) Syllable   Consonant-*le* **syllables,** which are one kind of final stable syllable, can be taught as indicated.

TEACHER: *[Writes discovery words on the board.]* Look at these words: *ramble, uncle, candle, simple, table.* What looks the same in all of these words?

STUDENTS: They all have a consonant and *l* and *e* at the end.

TEACHER: When these words are pronounced, how many syllables do you hear or feel? *[Reads the words one at a time as students echo each word.]*

STUDENTS: There are two syllables.

TEACHER: The second syllable in these words is spelled with a consonant, an *l*, and a final *e* and is called a consonant-*le* syllable. Tell me about the sound of the *e* in final position.

STUDENTS: It is silent.

TEACHER: Because the final syllable in each of these words does not have a sounded vowel, these syllables are rule breakers. The final syllable is coded with a bracket: [. The accent falls on the syllable before the final syllable. Let's code the discovery words. *[Students verbalize coding of the final syllable and the syllable before the consonant-le syllable. Students read the words.]* Let's review what you have discovered about a consonant-*le* syllable: A consonant-*le* syllable ends in a consonant, an *l*, and a final *e*. Code the syllable with a bracket, and accent the syllable before.

Note: The consonant-*le* syllable is one of several syllables that are referred to as final stable syllables (Cox, 1992). These syllables appear in the final position in words, and their pronunciations are fairly stable. Advanced final stable syllables, which include syllables such as *ture, age, sion,* and *tion,* are also coded with a bracket. Some of the advanced final stable syllables are also identified as suffixes. The advantage of treating these units as final stable syllables is twofold (Cox & Hutcheson, 1988):

1) They serve as an early, interim bridge to reading words of more than one syllable before students know **syllable division** or advanced morphemes (e.g., *pic′*[*ture, man′*[*age, mo′*[*tion*); and 2) they provide predictable identification of the accent, which usually falls on the syllable before the final stable syllable (e.g., *va*|*ca′*[*tion, ex*|*plo′*[*sion*). In the purest linguistic terms, a word such as *vacation* comprises the root *vacate* and the suffix *-ion*. However, to make the pronunciation and spelling more transparent, *-tion, -sion, -age,* and *-ture* will be taught as final stable syllables.

REFLECT, CONNECT, and RESPOND
What is the benefit of teaching students the six syllable types?

Teaching Morphology

Morphology comes from the Greek *morphe,* meaning *form,* and *ology,* meaning *study of.* Morphemes are the smallest forms or units of language—base words, prefixes, suffixes, roots, and combining forms—that carry meaning. A word may contain several syllables but represent only one morpheme (e.g., *salamander*; Moats, 1994), or a word may contain several syllables and represent several morphemes (e.g., *instructor* contains three syllables and the morphemes *in-, struct,* and *-or*). Study of morphemes not only facilitates decoding but also provides a springboard for vocabulary development and spelling (Adams, 1990) and bridges the gap between alphabetic reading (i.e., word-level reading) and comprehension (Bowers & Kirby, 2010; Bowers, Kirby, Deacon, 2010; Foorman & Schatschneider, 1997; Nippold, 2017).

   Terms to Know   The following definitions are important to the study of morphemes.

- A *base word* is a plain word with nothing added to it.

- An *affix* is a suffix or a prefix that is added to a base word or a root.

- A *root* is an essential base of letters to which prefixes and suffixes are added (e.g., *audi, vis, struct*). Roots are primarily of Latin origin. A root that stands alone as a word is called a *free morpheme*; a root that requires the addition of an affix(es) to form a word is called a *bound morpheme* (Moats, 1995).

- A *suffix* is a letter or a group of letters added to the end of a base word or a root to change its meaning, form, or usage. A suffix that begins with a consonant is called a **consonant suffix** (e.g., *-ful, -less, -ness, -ment, -cian*). A suffix that begins with a vowel is called a **vowel suffix** (e.g., *-en, -ist, -ible*). **Derivational suffixes** are added to a base word or root and change the part of speech or the function of the base word or root (e.g., *-ful, -less, -cian, -or*; Moats, 1995, 2010). Some suffixes are grammatical endings called **inflections** or **inflectional endings** (e.g., *-s, -ed, -er, -est, -ing*), which, when added to base words, change their number, tense, voice, mood, or comparison (Moats, 1995, 2010).

Note: For the most part, the spelling of a suffix does not change. The spelling of the base word, however, may change when a vowel suffix is added. In the initial stages of introduction and practice, suffixes are added to base words. The suffix can be coded with a box. This coding visually separates the base word and the suffix, making it easier for students to attend to the base word.

- A *prefix* is a letter or a group of letters added to the beginning of a base word or a root to change its meaning (e.g., *mis-, un-, con-, re-*). A prefix that ends in a consonant is called a **consonant prefix.** The spelling of a consonant prefix may change (e.g., *in-* may be spelled *il-, im-,* or *ir-*). A prefix that ends in a vowel is called a **vowel prefix.** The spelling of a vowel prefix does not change.

- A *derivative* is a base word or root plus an affix.

- **Combining forms** are similar to roots, but they are combined with equal importance in a word (e.g., *auto* and *graph,* which are neither affixes nor base words, combine to make *autograph*; see Henry, 1990). Words that are derived from combining forms can be affixed (e.g., *autobiography, autobiographic*). Combining forms are primarily of Greek origin. (See Chapter 14 for more information about the Greek, Latin, and **Anglo-Saxon** layers of English.)

Multisensory Introduction of Affixes   Quite often, the means to reading multisyllabic words is identifying affixes (i.e., prefixes and suffixes) that are part of the word. Students may be able to recognize an unfamiliar word simply by identifying the affixes and then the remaining base word or root.

Affixes can be introduced using a multisensory guided discovery teaching approach:

1. The teacher reads a list of five or six derivatives that have a common trait as students repeat each word (e.g., *joyful, careful, helpful, graceful, cheerful*).

2. Students discover what sounds the same in each word.

3. The teacher writes the derivatives on the board.

4. Students discover which letters are the same in each word and where the letters are found.

5. Students discover whether the same letters (the affix) are a suffix or a prefix, and they discover the meaning of the affix.

6. Students verbalize what they have discovered (e.g., *-ful* is a consonant suffix that means *full of*).

7. The teacher writes the new affix on an index card and adds it to an affix deck that is systematically reviewed. During review, students identify and spell the affix, give a key word, give the pronunciation, and give the meaning of the affix (e.g., when looking at the affix card for suffix *-ful,* students say, "Consonant suffix *f-u-l, hopeful,* /fŭl/, *full of*").

Teaching Syllable Division

Even students who read monosyllabic words accurately and automatically may struggle to read multisyllabic words and require explicit instruction (Nippold, 2017; Toste, Williams, & Capin, 2016). Skilled readers are able to sense where to divide longer words because they have an awareness of syllables and have internalized the orthographic patterns of the language so well (Adams, 1990). The following activities heighten students' visual awareness of syllables and **syllable division patterns.**

Separated Syllables   Students identify syllable types of separated syllables, join them into words, and read the words aloud (Gillingham & Stillman, 1997):

cac|tus   mas|cot   ban|dit   nut|meg
mag|net   gob|let   prob|lem   nap|kin

Manipulation of Multisyllabic Words   Students identify syllables written on individual cards, arrange them into words, and read the words aloud (Gillingham & Stillman, 1997):

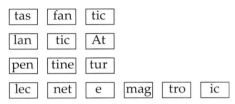

Scooping the Syllables   As students read multisyllabic words on a work-sheet, they call attention to the syllables in the words by scooping the syllables. Using a pencil, students "scoop" (i.e., draw an arc underneath) the syllables from left to right, identify the syllable type, place a syllable code under each syllable (e.g., *o* for open, *r* for *r*-controlled), and code the vowel (Wilson, 1996):

Common Patterns for Dividing Words Into Syllables   There are four major patterns in English (VCCV, VCV, VCCCV, and VV) that indicate that a word will be divided into syllables according to how it is pronounced. For each of these four patterns, there are different choices for division and accent placement. The best choices for dividing and accenting are listed here in order of frequency. Students must learn to be flexible when they make choices about dividing and accenting multisyllabic words. If the first choice of a pattern does not produce a recognizable word, then they need to try a second choice, which usually requires a change in accent placement. If necessary, they may need to try a third choice, which usually requires a change in the division of the word. Familiarity and flexibility with syllable-division patterns help students develop strategies for reading multisyllabic words; students do not have to guess or give up when they encounter unfamiliar long words.

VCCV–Two Consonants Between Two Vowels   Students try the following choices for syllable division and accent placement in words that contain the VCCV pattern:

* **VC′|CV**—When two consonants stand between two vowels, the word is usu-ally divided between the two consonants. The accent usually falls on the first syllable. Examples include the following: ***nap′****|kin,* ***vel′****|vet,* ***can′****|did,* ***cac′****|tus,* ***cam′****|pus,* ***mag′****|net,* ***bas′****|ket,* ***in′****|sect,* ***op′****|tic,* and ***mus′****|lin. Note:* Consonant digraphs such as *ch, ck, sh, ph, th,* and *wh* are treated as single consonants because they represent single speech sounds (***ath′****|lete,* ***dol′****|phin*).

- VC|**CV**'—The word may be divided between the consonants, with the accent falling on the second syllable. Examples include the following: *un*|*til*', *pas*|*tel*', *dis*|*cuss*', *can*|*teen*', *in*|*sist*'.

- **V**'|CCV—The word may be divided before both consonants with the accent falling on the first syllable. Examples include the following: *se*'|*cret*, *fra*'|*grant*, and *ma*'|*cron*.

Note: Consonant digraphs, two adjacent consonants that represent one sound (e.g., *sh, th, ck, ng*), are never divided. Some consonant clusters contain two adjacent consonants, commonly known as *consonant blends,* whose sounds flow together. It is not necessary for these clusters to be introduced as separate sound–symbol correspondences because each sound in a consonant cluster is accessible. Consonant blends may divide (e.g., *fab*|*ric*) or may not divide (e.g., *se*|*cret*).

VCV–One Consonant Between Two Vowels　　Students try the following choices for syllable division and accent placement in words that contain the VCV pattern:

- **V**'|CV—When one consonant stands between two vowels, the word is usually divided before the consonant. The accent usually falls on the first syllable. Examples include the following: *i*'|*ris*, *o*'|*pen*, *u*'|*nit*, *o*'|*ver*, *ro*'|*tate*, *a*'|*corn*, *mu*'|*sic*, *tu*'|*lip*, *va*'|*cate*, *si*'|*lent*, *su*'|*per*, and *e*'|*ven*.

- V|**CV**'—The word may be divided before the consonant, with the accent falling on the second syllable. Examples include the following: *re*|*quest*', *e*|*vent*', *o*|*mit*', *u*|*nite*', *pa*|*rade*', *a*|*like*', *a*|*lone*', *sa*|*lute*', and *di*|*vine*'.

Note: The vowels in an open, unaccented syllable require careful attention during syllable division. If students are overly sensitive to sounds in their speech, then they may not make the connection between orthography and speech (Ehri et al., 1987). For example, the *e* in the word *elect* sounds more like /ĭ/ in running speech. If students are too sensitive to the /ĭ/ sound, then they will not build an orthographic memory of *elect* spelled with *e.* The *e* in an open, unaccented syllable should be perceived as having a pronunciation that is long (e.g., *e*|*vent*') but is shorter than an *e* in an open, accented syllable (e.g., *ze*'|*ro*). In an open, unaccented syllable, *o* and *u* remain long, but their pronunciations are shortened (e.g., *o*|*mit*', *u*|*nite*'). The *e, o,* and *u* are coded with a macron. The *a* in an open, unaccented syllable is obscure and pronounced as /ŭ/ (e.g., *a*|*long*'). The *a* is coded with a dot. The *i* in an open, unaccented syllable is short (e.g., *di*|*vide*'). The *i* is coded with a breve.

- **VC**'|V—The word may be divided after the consonant, with the accent falling on the first syllable. Examples include the following: *rob*'|*in*, *riv*'|*er*, *cab*'|*in*, *trav*'|*el*, *mag*'|*ic*, *tim*'|*id*, *mod*'|*ern*, *plan*'|*et*, *sol*'|*id*, and *sev*'|*en*.

Note: As mentioned previously, consonant digraphs (i.e., two adjacent consonants that represent one sound) are treated as one consonant. Words with consonant digraphs may be divided before the digraph (e.g., *go*'|*pher*) or after the digraph (e.g., *rath*'|*er*).

VCCCV–Three Consonants Between Two Vowels Students try the following choices for syllable division and accent placement in words that contain the
VCCCV pattern:

- **VC'**|CCV—When three consonants stand between two vowels, the word is
  usually divided after the first consonant. The first syllable is usually accented.
  Examples include the following: *pil'*|*grim, chil'*|*dren, pan'*|*try, spec'*|*trum,
  mon'*|*ster, lob'*|*ster, hun'*|*dred, scoun'*|*drel, ham'*|*ster,* and *os'*|*trich.*

- VC|**CCV'**—The word may be divided after the first consonant, with the
  accent falling on the second syllable. Examples include the following: *im*|*ply',
  com*|*plete', sur*|*prise', in*|*trude', en*|*twine', em*|*blaze',* and *ex*|*treme'.*

- **VCC'**|CV—The word may be divided after the second consonant or after a
  final consonant cluster (e.g., *mp* and *nd* are consonant clusters that often occur
  in final position in one-syllable words); the accent falls on the first syllable.
  Examples include the following: *pump'*|*kin, sand'*|*wich, bank'*|*rupt, part'*|*ner,
  musk'*|*rat,* and *irk'*|*some.*

VV–Two Adjacent Vowels Students try the following choices for syllable
division and accent placement in words that contain the VV pattern:

- **V'**|V—A word with two adjacent vowels that do not form a digraph or diph-
  thong is divided between the vowels, with the accent falling on the first syllable.
  Examples include the following: *di'*|*al, cha'*|*os, tru'*|*ant, tri'*|*umph,* and *li'*|*on.*

  Note: Because the vowel pairs in these words (i.e., *ia, ao, ua, iu, io*) do not constitute digraphs or diphthongs, a reader knows immediately to divide the words
  between the two vowels.

- **V'**|V—A word with two adjacent vowels that typically form a digraph or a
  diphthong may be divided between the vowels, with the accent falling on the
  first syllable. Examples include the following: *po'*|*em, qui'*|*et, sto'*|*ic,* and *bo'*|*a.*

  Note: Adjacent vowels that frequently form digraphs or diphthongs, as in the
  word *poem*, include *ai, ay, au, aw, ea, ee, ei, ey, eu, ew, ie, oa, oe, oi, oo, ou, ow,* and *oy.*
  Although consonant digraphs are not divided, adjacent vowels that can form
  digraphs and diphthongs may be divided. A reader first tries reading an unfamiliar word with two adjacent vowels using the pronunciation of the digraph
  or diphthong that the vowels represent (e.g., reading *poem* as /pōm/). If reading
  the words in this manner does not produce a recognizable or a correct word,
  then he or she divides the words between the vowels and reads it.

- V|**V'**—The word may be divided between the vowels, with the accent falling
  on the second syllable. Examples include the following: *du*|*et', cre*|*ate',* and
  co|*erce'.*

Procedure for Dividing Words A structured procedure such as the one presented next provides readers with a systematic approach for reading long, unfamiliar words and builds an orthographic memory for syllable-division patterns.
Students with dyslexia may need additional visual and kinesthetic information
to build the memory of these patterns. Information helpful to students at risk and
with dyslexia is given in parentheses (Cox & Hutcheson, 1988).

1. Count the vowels. To determine the number of syllables in a word, students count the number of sounded vowels from left to right. Vowel pairs count as one sounded vowel. (The vowel pairs can be underlined to call attention to the fact that the two vowels make one sound.) All suffixes are boxed. By boxing suffixes, students may see a base word that requires no further division. Students place brackets before any final stable syllables. By bracketing a final stable syllable, students may see that no further division is needed.

2. Touch the vowels. Using the index fingers of both hands, students touch the sounded vowels or vowel pairs and identify them. (A line can be drawn over the word from sounded vowel to sounded vowel. The vowels can be labeled by writing a small *v* over each vowel.) For example:

v v
mascot

The word *mascot* has two syllables because it has two sounded vowels. The vowels are *a* and *o*.

3. Count the consonants. Students count the number of consonants between the two vowels or vowel pairs and identify the division pattern. (Consonant digraphs can be underlined to call attention to the fact that the two letters are treated as one consonant sound. Each consonant or consonant digraph can be labeled with *c*. Labeling the vowels and consonants expedites the orthographic memory of the syllable-division patterns.) For example:

vccv
mascot

There are two consonants between the vowels in *mascot*. The syllable-division pattern is VCCV.

4. Divide. Students draw a vertical line to divide the word according to the most frequent division of this pattern. For example, because the most common division choice for VCCV is to divide between the consonants, *mascot* is divided between *s* and *c*.

5. Accent. Students place an accent mark on the appropriate syllable according to the most frequent accent of the pattern. For example, with a VC|CV word, the accent is most frequently placed on the first syllable.

6. Code. Students identify each syllable type and code the vowels accordingly. For example, the first syllable of *mascot* is closed. The vowel is short; code it with a breve. The second syllable is closed. The vowel is short; code it with a breve.

7. Read. Students read each syllable without accenting either syllable.

8. Read again. Students read the syllables together with the appropriate accent.

9. Adjust. Students adjust the accent or division if the word is not recognizable. Adjusting the accent or the division to produce a recognizable word teaches students to be flexible with language.

Figure 9.1 is a pictorial representation of the previously delineated steps and is helpful for students with limited reading skills to use; Figure 9.2 shows the steps when dividing the word *mascot*.

Providing Reading Practice

Reading practice to reinforce a syllable-division pattern or any other decoding concepts must be focused. The teacher reviews all information that is pertinent to reinforcing the concept. For example, before reviewing a syllable-division pattern,

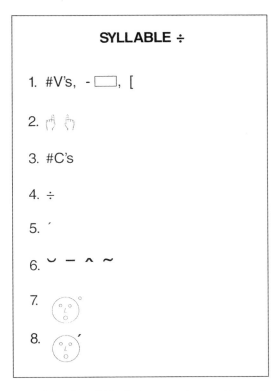

Figure 9.1. The syllable-division procedure provides ready access to multisyllabic words. Students 1) count the vowels, box suffixes, and add a bracket to mark a final stable syllable; 2) touch the vowels; 3) count the consonants; 4) draw a vertical line to divide the word; 5) mark the accent; 6) code the vowels; 7) read without accent; and 8) read with accent. (From *Multisensory Teaching of Basic Language Skills, Third Edition* [p. 237].)

the teacher might review the definition of a suffix, the syllable types that are germane to the pattern, the pattern itself, and the procedure for dividing words into syllables. After a review of relevant information, the teacher models the coding of a word while verbalizing the process and then reads the word. The teacher presents three or four additional words. Students verbalize the coding and/or division of these words and read them. The teacher then presents a list of words that contain the new concept for students to read, silently and then aloud. The teacher provides immediate feedback and leads students to self-correct errors so that students connect the correct orthographic patterns and pronunciations (Foorman, 1994). Students use words orally in complete sentences to ensure they understand the meanings of the words so that comprehension is obtained even at the word level (Foorman & Schatschneider, 1997). Students also read sentences. Spelling practice with the dictation of sounds, words, and sentences follows the reading practice. After the practice of skills, equal time is given to reading from connected text that mirrors what students have recently learned. Comprehension and fluency are addressed using this text. Irregular words that will be encountered in the text are reviewed before students read the text. Composition activities can also be incorporated at this time.

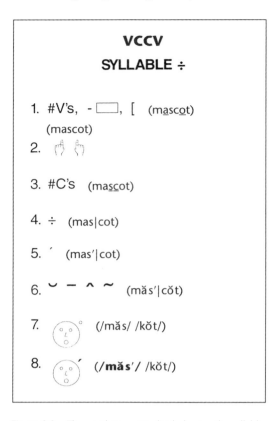

Figure 9.2. The word *mascot* is divided using the syllable-division procedures. (From *Multisensory Teaching of Basic Language Skills, Third Edition* [p. 238].)

Well-matched reading text extends and reinforces the learning of orthographic patterns and gives relevance to what is being learned (Adams, 1990). When reading in connected text, the reader should be encouraged to pause and study unknown words instead of skipping or guessing an unfamiliar word. Textbox 9.1 shows how reading practice can be incorporated into an intensive, therapeutic reading lesson, with extended reading of text.

Using Decodable Text

Decodable text is text that matches the sound–symbol correspondences and irregular words that have been systematically introduced and is a logical choice for fluency practice. Decodable text provides practice of previously introduced sound–symbol correspondences and irregular words, which builds automatic word recognition. The repeated reading of decodable text further secures those concepts in memory. A second benefit of decodable text is that it develops independence in dealing with new words. Students learn that they can sound out most unfamiliar words while reading. When selecting text to read for fluency practice, students should be able to read the text with 95% accuracy. In other words, students misread only 1 of every 20 words of text (NICHD, 2000).

Teaching Advanced Morphemes

Students benefit from learning about prefixes, suffixes, roots, and combining forms (Berninger, Abbott, Nagy, & Carlisle, 2010; Henry, 2010; Nippold, 2017; Toste et al., 2016). These morphemes are predominantly of Latin and Greek origins, respectively. The ability to instantly recognize roots and combining forms gives students a ready strategy for decoding longer words as well as insight into the meanings of the words. Once students have a core knowledge of morphemes, the first step in deciphering longer words is identifying the morphemes. For example, when students encounter a word such as *instructor*, they can identify three morphemes that aid the pronunciation of the word: *in-*, *struct*, and *-or*.

Common Latin Roots   Words of Latin origin are common in literature and academic writing. Latin words generally are characterized as having a root with affixes. The root carries the base of the meaning, as in these examples:

- *audi* (to hear)—*auditory, audience, audit, auditorium, audible, inaudible, audition*

- *dict* (to say)—*dictate, predict, dictator, edict, contradict, dictation, indict, prediction*

- *ject* (to throw)—*reject, inject, projection, interjection, eject, objection, dejection*

- *port* (to carry)—*transport, transportation, import, export, porter, portable, report, support*

- *rupt* (to break)—*rupture, erupt, eruption, interrupt, interruption, disruption*

- *scrib, script* (to write)—*scribe, describe, manuscript, inscription, transcript, descriptive, prescription*

- *spect* (to watch)—*spectator, inspect, inspector, respect, spectacle, spectacular*

- *struct* (to build)—*structure, construct, construction, instruct, destruction, reconstructionist*

- *tract* (to pull)—*tractor, traction, attract, subtraction, extract, retract, attractive*

- *vis* (to see)—*vision, visual, visit, supervisor, invisible, vista, visualize, visionary*

Common Greek Combining Forms   Words of Greek origin are most often scientific, medical, and technical terms. They are characterized as having combining forms that carry equal importance in the meaning of the word. The following Greek forms are common in English words:

- *auto* (self)—*automatic, autograph, autobiography, automobile, autocracy*

- *bio* (life)—*biology, biosphere, biography, biochemistry, biometrics, biophysics*

- *graph* (write, recording)—*graphite, geography, graphic, photograph, phonograph*

- *hydro* (water)—*anhydrous, dehydration, hydrogen, hydrant, hydrostatic, hydrophobia, hydrotherapy, hydroplane*

- *meter* (measure)—*speedometer, odometer, metronome, thermometer, chronometer, perimeter, hydrometer*

- *ology* (study of)—*geology, theology, zoology, meteorology, phonology*

- *photo* (light)—*photography, photocopy, photosynthesis, phototropism, photostat, photogenic*

- *scope* (view)—*periscope, stethoscope, telescope, microscope, microscopic*

- *tele* (at a distance)—*telephone, telepathy, telegraph, television*

- *therm* (heat)—*thermos, thermodynamics, thermostat, thermophysics*

Introduction of Roots and Combining Forms   The teacher writes a root or combining form on the board. Students generate derivatives of the word part. The teacher writes the derivatives on the board so that the new word part in each word is aligned, as shown next. Students determine the meaning of the word part (Henry, 1990).

struct

structure

destruction

instructor

reconstructionist

The teacher writes the new root or combining form on an index card and adds it to a deck that is systematically reviewed. During a review, students read the word part on each card, give the meaning, and generate derivatives of the root (e.g., students say, "*struct*; to build; *construct, structure, instructor,* and *destruction*").

REFLECT, CONNECT, and RESPOND
How does morphology instruction support both components of reading comprehension?

Dividing Words With Three or More Syllables   As previously mentioned, when students encounter longer words, students should first look for recognizable morphemes. Students may not recognize all morphemes in a longer unfamiliar word, however, or a longer word may not have recognizable morphemes that would give clues to the pronunciation of the word. The same procedure used for dividing two syllables can be used with words of three or more syllables. Students choose the most frequent division of a pattern (e.g., VCCV is usually divided between the consonants; VCV is usually divided before the consonant). Choosing accent requires the following considerations:

- Roots draw the accent; prefixes and suffixes are rarely accented (e.g., *in|vest'|ment*).

- The syllable before a final stable syllable is usually accented (e.g., *im|mi|gra'[tion*).

- A final syllable that ends in -*a* or -*ic* is not accented, and the accent usually falls on the syllable before the final syllable (e.g., *va|nil'|la, At|lan'|tic*).

- If there are no clues for accent, then try accenting the first syllable (e.g., *cu'|cum|ber*) or the second syllable (e.g., *es|tab'|lish*).

Careful attention to vowels in **polysyllabic** words is needed. The *a* in an open, unaccented syllable is obscure and is coded with a dot (e.g., *al|fal'|fa*). The *i* in an open, unaccented syllable is short and coded with a breve (e.g., *ar'|ti|choke*). The *i* before a final stable syllable is short and is coded with a breve (e.g., *ig|ni'[tion*). The *i* in an open, unaccented syllable before another vowel is pronounced as /ē/ (e.g., *sta′|di|um*).

PRACTICE: TEACHING IRREGULAR WORDS

Knowledge of the orthographic patterns of language and practice with these patterns develop instant word recognition, but how do readers learn words with irregular orthographic patterns? Despite claims to the contrary, English is a highly reliable language for reading (Gough & Hillinger, 1980). Approximately 87% of the English language is regular and can be predictably decoded using the orthographic patterns described in this chapter; this leaves only 13% of the language as irregular (Hanna, Hanna, Hodges, & Rudorf, 1966). The irregularities of written English are generally limited to the vowels and silent consonants. For most irregular words, the consonants offer sufficient support so that when the reader encounters an irregular word in everyday reading, he or she can determine the correct pronunciation of the word with partial decoding (Share & Stanovich, 1995).

Irregular words, particularly high-frequency irregular words (e.g., *the, said, have*), are learned through repeated encounters in text. Understanding word origins further assists students' orthographic memory of irregular words by giving insight into the spellings of words that do not match their pronunciations. Analyzing irregular words to determine their irregularities reinforces reliable sound–letter relationships, helps students build an orthographic memory of the words, and establishes that the irregularities in English words are not arbitrary (Gough & Hillinger, 1980). Patterns, even if infrequent, can be found in irregular words (e.g., *gh* may be silent as in *taught*, pronounced /g/ in initial position as in *ghost*, or pronounced /f/ as in *laugh*). When students discover an irregularity in a word, a resounding "Good for you! You found a word that doesn't fit the pattern!" from the teacher confirms that the students are thinking about the language and acquiring a flexible understanding of the language.

Procedure for Teaching Irregular Words

A multisensory structured procedure helps students achieve permanent memorization of irregular words (Cox, 1992; Gillingham & Stillman, 1997):

1. The teacher writes an irregular word on the board, such as *said*.

2. Students identify the syllable type and code the word according to the regular patterns of reading. Students read the word and discover it does not follow the reliable patterns of the language: /sād/.

3. The teacher erases the coded word and rewrites the word on the board: *said*. Beside the word, the teacher writes the pronunciation in parentheses: (sĕd).

4. Students compare the word and the pronunciation. They decide which part is irregular.

5. The teacher circles the irregular part:

s (ai) d

6. The teacher writes the word on the front of a 4″ × 6″ index card. On the back of the card, the teacher writes the pronunciation. The teacher cuts off the upper

left-hand corner of the front of the card. The irregular shape of the card cues students that the word printed on it is an irregular word.

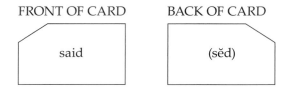

FRONT OF CARD   BACK OF CARD

said   (sĕd)

7. The teacher holds up the card so that students see the front of the card. Students read the word aloud.

8. The teacher turns the card around, and students read the pronunciation aloud.

9. The teacher slowly turns the card from front to back four or five times as students read the word and then read the pronunciation aloud.

10. The new card is added to a deck of irregular words that is reviewed daily.

Review of Irregular Words

Using a rapid word-recognition chart (RWRC; see Figure 9.3 for an example) builds instant recognition of high-frequency irregular words. The chart contains five rows of six irregular words. Each row contains the same six words in a different order. The teacher makes an RWRC that the student or students can view easily. After placing the chart in view of the students, the teacher points to 8–10 words at random as a warm-up. After the warm-up, students are timed for 1 minute. The teacher points to each square in order on the chart, starting with the top row and working across each row. Students read aloud the word in each of the squares. In

RAPID WORD RECOGNITION CHART

pretty	said	who	there	they	what
said	pretty	there	who	what	they
there	who	they	said	pretty	what
who	what	said	they	there	pretty
they	there	pretty	what	who	said

Figure 9.3. The rapid word-recognition chart (RWRC) increases instant word recognition, particularly the recognition of words with phonetically irregular orthography. (From *Multisensory Teaching of Basic Language Skills, Third Edition* [p. 242].)

the 1-minute time frame, students may read through the chart more than once. At the end of 1 minute, students count and record the number of words they have successfully read. Progress can be graphed. The practice concludes with the teacher pointing at random to any troublesome words to provide further practice and secure the recognition of those words.

Rapid Word Reading

Evidence indicates that practice that involves the rapid reading of single words can result in improved speed and comprehension of text reading (Tan & Nicholson, 1997). Using flashcards or an RWRC to preview words in a passage before reading keeps the words in memory for students to refer to as they read. In addition to using an RWRC for high-frequency, irregular words as shown in Figure 9.3, the chart can be used for repeated exposure to an orthographic pattern found in words in the planned passage (Fisher, 1999). For example, an RWRC could be filled with words that contain trigraph *tch* (e.g., *match, etch, itch, blotch, Dutch, catch*). Using the procedure described previously, students read these words and build a memory of a frequent, reliable orthographic pattern that is found in the planned passage as well as in other text.

Teaching Word Origins

A brief overview of word origins helps students develop an understanding of why some words are pronounced in an unexpected way. This understanding allows students to forgive the language for being irregular and, more important, allows them to forgive themselves for having difficulty with the language (Cox, 1992; Gillingham & Stillman, 1997; Henry, 1998). Words may be pronounced irregularly for four reasons:

1. They are borrowed from another language such as French (*hors d'oeuvre*), Dutch (*yacht*), or Greek (*ocean*).

2. They are **eponyms,** or words derived from proper names, such as the German botanist L. Fuchs (*fuchsia*) or the French statesman E. de Silhouette (*silhouette*).

3. They are words from the Anglo-Saxon language whose spellings did not keep pace with their changing pronunciations, such as *laugh, enough, said, through,* and *where.*

4. They are irregular for no easily identifiable reason or "just because," such as *curmudgeon.*

Investigating the irregularities of words raises students' **word consciousness.** Becoming more sensitive to the irregular spellings of these words builds students' memory for instant recognition.

PRACTICE: TEACHING FLUENCY

Snow referred to fluency as "both an antecedent and a consequence of comprehension" (2002, p. 13). Most successful readers seem to move from word-level reading to the fluency of phrase reading easily. Their development of fluency is due, in part, to the fact that these readers learned the alphabetic code early, had more time to read (Adams & Bruck, 1995; Juel, 1988), and received more encouragement to attend to fluency (Allington, 1983; Chall, 1983). Fluent readers can attend to meaning, which aids the prosodic flow of reading. It cannot be assumed, however, that developing accurate decoding skills guarantees application of those skills to fluency (Torgesen, 1997; Torgesen & Hudson, 2006).

Fluency development requires intentional, well-designed practice. Researchers are currently studying the brain and the time it takes the brain to process written language, and they are investigating sources for speed-related deficits that affect reading fluency. As more becomes known about the sources of speed-related deficits, the best designs for fluency interventions will be ascertained. To date, research suggests the most effective practices for improving fluency are those that involve the repeated reading of letters, words, phrases, and text and are supported by increased knowledge of the systems of oral and written language (Wolf, 2001). Textbox 9.1 delineates a daily reading lesson in which activities that improve fluency at the letter, word, phrase or sentence, and text levels are easily incorporated.

Rapid Letter Naming

Neuhaus and Swank (2002) proposed that letter naming is only slightly less complex than word reading and that automatic letter recognition is the key to automatic word recognition. Rapid letter recognition is dependent on the familiarity of the orthographic and phonological properties of letters and directly predicts rapid recognition of words. Therefore, students benefit from overlearning the associations of letter shapes, names, and sounds. The use of a letter–sound deck in a daily reading lesson firmly secures these associations (see Textbox 9.1). Chapter 5 outlines many activities that can be used for the rapid naming of letters.

Repeated Reading

The NRP (NICHD, 2000) concluded that guided oral reading, including repeated reading, is the most effective technique for improving word recognition, speed, accuracy, and fluency. **Repeated reading** involves the oral reading and re-reading

---

TEXTBOX 9.1   **Daily reading lesson plan**

1.   Review with letter-sound deck

2.   Introduction of new concept or review of previously introduced concept

3.   Reading practice: word lists and sentences

4.   Spelling practice: sound dictation, word dictation, and sentence dictation

5.   Introduction of irregular words

6.   Reading of connected text

7.   Listening to books

———

Adapted from *Multisensory Teaching of Basic Language Skills, Third Edition* (p. 239).

of the same passage of 50–200 words several times. The re-reading of the same text provides the repeated exposures of words needed for the reader to form new or access previously formed orthographic images of letter patterns and words (Torgesen, Rashotte, & Alexander, 2001; Toste et al., 2016).

Oral reading fluency is enhanced when repeated readings are proceeded by teacher modeling of fluent reading (Rose, 1984). The modeling provides a positive framework for students to strive for when they read. The teacher should provide guidance and feedback as students read and re-read the passage (NICHD, 2000; Toste et al., 2016). Background knowledge should be activated before the initial reading of the passage, and comprehension should be assessed, even informally, after the initial reading of the passage because the goal of fluency training is to aid comprehension and comprehending text aids fluency by allowing students to anticipate what is to come in the text (Wood, Flowers, & Grigorenko, 2001). Textbox 9.1 presents an example of a daily reading lesson plan. Repeated reading can be incorporated during the reading of connected text.

Prosody

Successful decoding requires the reader to translate printed words into their spoken equivalents, whereas successful fluency requires the reader to connect the flow of printed text to the flow of spoken language. Spoken language has intonation, phrasing, and stress, which are not present in written language. Early on, children rely on all of these features to understand speech (see Chapter 3 for more information). When these features are present in oral reading, there is a rhythmic flow (i.e., prosody) that makes it sound as if the reader is speaking. Although fluency practice that includes attention to prosodic features does not produce stronger gains (Torgesen et al., 2001), it is prudent to practice such features because lack of prosody results in word-by-word reading and prevents some readers from learning to group words into meaningful units that support comprehension. Oral fluency, which leads to reading fluency, can be taught to readers who do not move from the word level to the phrase level of reading. Phrasing, intonation, and stress can be applied to written language with oral practice, the study of punctuation, and the study of syntax–grammar and sentence structure. Chapter 12 provides additional information on fluency instruction.

THE KNOWLEDGE BASE:
THE SPELLING CONNECTION TO READING

Noah Webster once wrote, "Spelling is the foundation of reading and the greatest ornament of writing" (as cited in Venezky, 1980, p. 12). Spelling, by its nature, is a multisensory skill, involving translating auditory sounds into visual symbols that are reinforced with the kinesthetic act of writing. A beginning reader's use of invented spelling (Read, 1971) provides the teacher with considerable insight as to how well the reader is learning and internalizing information about the language. The beginning reader applies his or her phonological awareness and acquired knowledge of sounds and patterns to the task of spelling an unfamiliar word. Students who have a sense of how the language works become risk takers. They attempt to sound out and spell words for which they may not have a strong visual image but that are, nevertheless, the best, most appropriate words for their writing (e.g., students attempt *tremendous* or *gigantic* instead of using *big*). In their trials of spelling these unfamiliar words, students reinforce and enhance their reading skills. Using these more sophisticated words embellishes their writing and better reflects their oral vocabulary. Although it is important for students to become confident risk takers, it is also imperative for them to learn to spell words correctly because their spelling knowledge has a direct effect on their reading proficiency (Adams, 1990). Chapter 10 provides suggestions for spelling instruction and using spelling practice to reinforce reading.

CLOSING THOUGHTS: TEACHING DECODING

Reading is a complex process involving decoding, which enables a reader to translate printed symbols into words, and comprehension, which enables the reader to derive meaning from the printed page. With the insight that spoken words consist of sounds and that printed words consist of letters, the beginning reader is able to connect sounds to letters and to read words. At first, the reader is focused on sounding out words. Using other strategies depends on the reader's available knowledge about language patterns, the length and complexity of the words, the frequency of encounters with the words, and/or the availability of useful contextual clues. Practicing graphophonemic, syllabic, and morphemic patterns using word lists, phrases, sentences, and repeated readings of connected text, the reader's decoding skills become automatic, and he or she is able to give greater attention to the prosodic features of reading such as phrasing and intonation, which further aid fluency. The fluent translation of the flow of print to the flow of spoken language enables the reader to attend to the meaning rather than to the features of the printed text. Fluency is vital to comprehension, which is the main goal of reading. A student's ultimate success in reading is predicated on knowledgeable and skilled teachers who explicitly and systematically teach reliable language patterns and structures using research-based instructional practices.

ONLINE COMPANION MATERIALS

The following Chapter 9 resources are available at http://www.brookespublishing .com/birshcarreker/materials:

- Reflect, Connect, and Respond Questions

- Appendix 9.1: Technology Resources

- Appendix 9.2: Knowledge and Skill Assessment Answer Key

- Appendix 9.3: Additional Online Resources for Teachers

- Appendix 9.4a: Test Your Knowledge and Skill Quiz 1, and 9.4b: Answer Key

- Appendix 9.5a: Test Your Knowledge and Skill Quiz 2, and 9.5b: Answer Key

- Appendix 9.6: Six Syllable Types (slide presentation)

KNOWLEDGE AND SKILL ASSESSMENT

1. Partially blocked sounds do which of the following?

   a. Activate the vocal cords

   b. Release the tongue, teeth or lips during production

   c. Do not activate the vocal cords

   d. Maintain the position of the tongue, teeth or lips

2. A student misreads *splint* as *split*. What does a teacher do to build the student's accuracy?

   a. Pronounce the word for the student.

   b. Encourage the student to use syntactic cues.

   c. Ask the student to name the letters in the word.

   d. Have the student guess the word from the context.

3. Which set of words contains two types of syllables?

   a. *Shirt, sheet, short, shout*

   b. *Farm, feet, fat, fork, food*

   c. *Hand, haul, hard, hay*

   d. *Chase, sharp, thank, chart*

4. A student struggles to read the word *helpfulness*. What should the teacher ask to build the student's accuracy?

   a. Is this a short word or a long word?

   b. Are there any prefixes or suffixes?

   c. Can you guess the word from the context?

   d. What clues does the illustration give you?

5. Which set of words contains all irregular words?

   a. *Done, does, dong, dough*

   b. *Heart, their, once, been*

   c. *Enough, theme, said, give*

   d. *Would, where, went, were*

REFERENCES

Adams, M.J. (1998). The three-cueing system. In F. Lehr & J. Osborn (Eds.), *Literacy for all: Issues in teaching and learning* (pp. 73–99). New York, NY: Guilford.

Adams, M.J. (1990). *Beginning to read: Thinking and learning about print.* Cambridge, MA: The MIT Press.

Adams, M.J., & Bruck, M. (1993). Word recognition: The interface of educational policies and scientific research. *Reading and Writing: An Interdisciplinary Journal, 5,* 113–139.

Adams, M.J., & Bruck, M. (1995, Summer). Resolving the "great debate." *American Educator, 19,* 7–12.

Allington, R.L. (1983, Feb.). Fluency: The neglected reading goal. *The Reading Teacher,* 556–561.

Ball, E.W., & Blachman, B.A. (1988). Phoneme segmentation training: Effect on reading readiness. *Annals of Dyslexia, 38,* 208–225.

Beck, I., & Juel, C. (1995, Summer). The role of decoding in learning to read. *American Educator, 19,* 8–12.

Berninger, V.W., Abbott, R.D., Nagy, W., & Carlisle, J. (2010). Growth in phonological, orthographic, and morphological awareness in Grades 1 to 6. *Journal of Psycholinguistic Research, 39,* 141–163.

Blachman, B.A. (1987). An alternative classroom reading program for learning disabled and other low-achieving children. In R. Bowler (Ed.), *Intimacy with language: A forgotten basic in teacher education* (pp. 49–55). Baltimore, MD: The International Dyslexia Association.

Blachman, B.A., Ball, E.W., Black, R., & Tangel, D.M. (2000). *Road to the code: A phonological awareness program for young children.* Baltimore, MD: Paul H. Brookes Publishing Co.

Bowers, P.N, & Kirby, J.R. (2010). Effects of morphological instruction on vocabulary acquisition. *Reading and Writing, 23,* 515–597.

Bowers, P.N., Kirby, J.R., & Deacon, S.H. (2010). The effects of morphological Instruction on Literacy Skills: A systematic review of the literature. *Review of Educational Research, 80*(2), 144–179.

Bradley, L., & Bryant, P.E. (1983). Categorizing sounds and learning to read: A causal connection. *Nature, 303,* 419–421.

Brady, S., & Moats, L.C. (Eds.). (1997). *Informed instruction for reading success: Foundations for teacher preparation.* Baltimore, MD: The International Dyslexia Association.

Brady, S., & Shankweiler, D. (1991). *Phonological processes in literacy: A tribute to Isabelle Y. Liberman.* Mahwah, NJ: Lawrence Erlbaum Associates.

Carreker, S. (2006, Fall). Teaching the structure of language by seeing, hearing, and doing. *Perspectives, 32*(4), 24–28.

Carreker, S.H., Neuhaus, G.F., Swank, P.R., Johnson, P., Monfils, M.J., & Montemayor, M.L. (2007). Teachers with linguistically informed knowledge of reading subskills are associated with a Matthew effect in reading comprehension for monolingual and bilingual students. *Reading Psychology, 28,* 187–212.

Carreker, S.H., Swank, P., Tillman-Dowdy, L., Neuhaus, G., Monfils, M.J., Montemayor, M.L., & Johnson, P. (2005). Language enrichment teacher preparation and practice predicts third grade reading comprehension. *Reading Psychology, 26,* 401–432.

Carson, K.L., Gillon, G.T., & Boustead, T.M. (2013, April). Classroom phonological awareness instruction and literacy outcomes in the first year of school. *Language, Speech, and Hearing Services in Schools, 44,* 147–160. doi:10.1044/0161-1461(2012/11-0061

Chall, J.S. (1983). *Stages of reading development.* New York, NY: McGraw-Hill.

Cirino, P.T., Romain, M.A., Barth, A.E., Tolar, T.D., Fletcher, J.M., & Vaughn, S. (2013). Reading skill components and impairments in middle school struggling readers. *Reading and Writing, 26,* 1059–1086.

Clay, M.M. (1993). *An observation survey of early literacy achievement.* Portsmouth, NH: Heinemann.

Cox, A.R. (1992). *Foundations for literacy: Structures and techniques for multisensory teaching of basic written English skills.* Cambridge, MA: Educators Publishing Service.

Cox, A.R., & Hutcheson, L.M. (1988). Syllable division: A prerequisite of dyslexics' literacy. *Annals of Dyslexia, 38,* 226–242.

Ehri, L.C. (1991). Development of the ability to read words. In R. Barr, M.L. Kamil, P.B. Mosenthal, & P.D. Pearson (Eds.), *Handbook of reading research* (Vol. 2, pp. 383–417). Reading, MA: Addison Wesley Longman.

Ehri, L.C. (2013). Grapheme-phonemic knowledge is essential for learning to read words in English. In J.L. Metsala & L.C. Ehri (Eds.), *Word recognition in beginning literacy* (pp. 3–40). New York, NY: Routledge, Taylor & Francis Group

Ehri, L.C. (2014). Orthographic mapping in the acquisition of sight word reading, spelling memory, and vocabulary learning. *Scientific Studies of Reading, 18*(1), 5–21.

Ehri, L.C., Wilce, L.S., & Taylor, B.B. (1987). Children's categorization of short vowels in words and the influence of spelling. *Merrill-Palmer Quarterly, 33,* 393–421.

Englemann, S. (1969). *Preventing failure in the primary grades.* Chicago, IL: Science Research Associates.

Felton, R. (1993). Effects of instruction on decoding skills of children with phonological processing problems. *Journal of Learning Disabilities, 26,* 583–589.

Ferrer, E., Shaywitz, B.A., Holahan, J.M., Marchione, K., & Shaywitz, S.E. (2009). Uncoupling of reading and IQ over time: Empirical evidence for a definition of dyslexia. *Association for Psychological Science, 21,* 93–101.

Fisher, P. (1999). Getting up to speed. *Perspectives, 25*(2), 12–13.

Foorman, B.R. (1994). The relevance of a connectionist model for reading for "the great debate." *Educational Psychology Review, 6,* 25–47.

Foorman, B.R., Francis, D.J., Beeler, T., Winikates, D., & Fletcher, J.M. (1997). Early intervention for children with reading problems: Study designs and preliminary findings. *Learning Disabilities: A Multidisciplinary Journal, 8,* 63–71.

Foorman, B.R., Francis, D.J., Shaywitz, S.E., Shaywitz, B.A., & Fletcher, J.M. (1997). The case for early reading intervention. In B. Blachman (Ed.), *Foundations of reading acquisition and dyslexia: Implications for early intervention* (pp. 243–264). Mahwah, NJ: Lawrence Erlbaum Associates.

Foorman, B.R., & Schatschneider, C. (1997). Beyond alphabetic reading: Comments on Torgesen's prevention and intervention studies. *Journal of Academic Language Therapy, 1,* 59–65.

Gillingham, A., & Stillman, B. (1997). *The Gillingham manual: Remedial training for children with specific disability in reading, writing, and penmanship* (8th ed.). Cambridge, MA: Educators Publishing Service.

Goswami, U., & Bryant, P. (1990). *Phonological skills and learning to read.* Mahwah, NJ: Lawrence Erlbaum Associates.

Gough, P.B. (1983). Context, form and interaction. In K. Rayner (Ed.), *Eye movements in reading: Conceptual and language processes* (pp. 203–211). San Diego, CA: Academic Press.

Gough, P.B., Ehri, L., & Treiman, R. (Eds.). (1992). *Reading acquisition.* Mahwah, NJ: Lawrence Erlbaum Associates.

Gough, P.B., & Hillinger, M.L. (1980). Learning to read: An unnatural act. *Bulletin of the Orton Society, 30,* 179–196.

Gough, P.B., & Tunmer, W.E. (1986). Decoding, reading and reading disability. *Remedial and Special Education, 7,* 6–10.

Greene, V.E., & Enfield, M.L. (1985). *Project Read reading guide: Phase I.* Bloomington, MN: Bloomington Public Schools.

Hanna, P.R., Hanna, J.S., Hodges, R.E., & Rudorf, E.H. (1966). *Phoneme-grapheme correspondences as cues to spelling improvement.* Washington, DC: U.S. Government Printing Office.

Hattie, J. (2008). *Visible learning: A synthesis of 800 meta-analyses relating to achievement.* London, United Kingdom: Routledge.

Henry, M.K. (1988). Beyond phonics: Integrating decoding and spelling instruction based on word origin and structure. *Annals of Dyslexia, 38,* 259–277.

Henry, M.K. (1990). *WORDS: Integrated decoding and spelling instruction based on word origin and word structure.* Austin, TX: PRO-ED.

Henry, M.K. (2010). *Unlocking literacy: Effective decoding and spelling instruction* (2nd ed.). Baltimore, MD: Paul H. Brookes Publishing Co.

Hoover, W.A., & Gough, P.B. (1990). The simple view of reading. *Reading and Writing: An Interdisciplinary Journal, 2,* 127–160.

Hutchins, P. (1974). *The wind blew.* New York, NY: Scholastic.

International Dyslexia Association, The. (2018, March). *Knowledge and practice standards for teachers of reading.* Retrieved from https://dyslexiaida.org/knowledge-and-practices/

Joshi, R.M., & Aaron, P.G. (2000). The component model of reading: Simple view of reading made a little more complex. *Reading Psychology, 21,* 85–97.

Joshi, R.M., Dahlgren, M., & Boulware-Gooden, R. (2002). Teaching reading in an inner city school through a multisensory teaching approach. *Annals of Dyslexia, 52,* 229–242.

Juel, C. (1988). Learning to read and write: A longitudinal study of 54 children from first to fourth grades. *Journal of Educational Psychology, 80,* 437–447.

Juel, C. (1991). Beginning reading. In R. Barr, M.L. Kamil, P.B. Mosenthal, & P.D. Pearson (Eds.), *Handbook of reading research* (Vol. 2, pp. 759–788). Reading, MA: Addison Wesley Longman.

Liberman, I.Y. (1987). Language and literacy: The obligation of the schools of education. In R. Bowler (Ed.), *Intimacy with language: A forgotten basic in teacher education* (pp. 1–9). Baltimore, MD: The International Dyslexia Association.

Liberman, I.Y., & Liberman, A.M. (1990). Whole language vs. code emphasis: Underlying assumptions and their implications for reading instruction. *Annals of Dyslexia, 40,* 51–76.

Liberman, I.Y., Shankweiler, D., & Liberman, A.M. (1989). The alphabetic principle and learning to read. In D. Shankweiler & I.Y. Liberman (Eds.), *Phonology and reading disabilities: Solving the reading puzzle* (pp. 1–33). Ann Arbor: University of Michigan Press.

Lundberg, I., Frost, J., & Petersen, O.P. (1988). Effects of an extensive program for stimulating phonological awareness in preschool children. *Reading Research Quarterly, 23,* 264–284.

Lyon, G.R., Shaywitz, S.E., & Shaywitz, B.A. (2003). A definition of dyslexia. *Annals of Dyslexia, 53,* 1–14.

Moats, L.C. (1994). The missing foundation in teacher education: Knowledge of the structure of spoken and written language. *Annals of Dyslexia, 44,* 81–102.

Moats, L.C. (1995). *Spelling: Development, disabilities and instruction.* Timonium, MD: York Press.

Moats, L.C. (2010). *Speech to print: Language essentials for teachers* (2nd ed.). Baltimore, MD: Paul H. Brookes Publishing Co.

Moats, L., Carreker, S., Davis, R., Meisel, P., Spear-Swerling, L., & Wilson, B. (2010). *Knowledge and practice standards for teachers of reading.* Towson, MD: The International Dyslexia Association.

National Institute of Child Health and Human Development [NICHD]. (2000). *Report of the National Reading Panel: Reports of the subgroups. Teaching children to read: An evidence-based assessment of the scientific research literature on reading and its implications for reading instruction* (NIH Publication No. 00-4754). Washington, DC: Government Printing Office.

Neuhaus, G.F., & Swank, P.R. (2002). Understanding the relations between RAN letters subtest components and word reading in first grade students. *Journal of Learning Disabilities, 35*(2), 158–174.

Nippold, M.A. (2017). Reading comprehension deficits in adolescents: Addressing underlying language abilities. *Language, Speech, and Hearing Services in Schools, 48*(2), 125–131.

Perfetti, C.A. (1985). *Reading ability.* New York, NY: Oxford University Press.

Piasta, S.B., Connor, C.M, Fishman, B.J., & Morrison, F.J. (2009). Teachers' knowledge of literacy concepts, classroom practices and student reading growth. *Scientific Studies of Reading, 13,* 224–248.

Prescott, J. E., Bundschuh, K., Kazakoff, E.R., & Macaruso, P. (2017). Elementary school–wide implementation of a blended learning program for reading intervention. *The Journal of Educational Research.* http://dx.doi.org/10.1080/00220671.2017.1302914

Rayner, K., & Pollatsek, A. (1986). *The psychology of reading.* Upper Saddle River, NJ: Prentice Hall.

Read, C. (1971). Pre-school children's knowledge of English phonology. *Harvard Educational Review, 41,* 1–34.

Rose, T.L. (1984). The effects of two prepractice procedures on oral reading. *Journal of Learning Disabilities, 17,* 544–548.

Rosner, J. (1975). *Test of Auditory Analysis Skills: Helping children overcome learning difficulties.* New York, NY: Walker and Co.

Rubin, H., & Eberhardt, N.C. (1996). Facilitating invented spelling through language analysis instruction: An integrated model. *Reading and Writing: An Interdisciplinary Journal, 8,* 27–43.

Ryder, J.F., Tunmer, W.E., & Greaney, K.T. (2007). Explicit instruction in phonemic awareness and phonemically based decoding skills as an intervention strategy for struggling readers in whole language classrooms. *Reading and Writing: An Interdisciplinary Journal, 21,* 349–369.

Seidenberg, M. (2017). *Language at the speed of sight: How we read, why so many cannot, and what can be done about it.* New York, NY: Basic Books.

Share, D.L., & Stanovich, K.E. (1995). Cognitive processes in early reading development: Accommodating individual differences into a model of acquisition. *Issues in Education, 1*(1), 1–57.

Slingerland, B.A. (1971). *A multi-sensory approach to language arts for specific language disability children: A guide for primary teachers.* Cambridge, MA: Educators Publishing Service.

Snow, C.E. (2002). *Reading for understanding: Toward an R&D program in reading comprehension.* Santa Monica, CA: RAND Corporation.

Stanback, M.L. (1992). Analysis of frequency-based vocabulary of 17,602 words. *Annals of Dyslexia, 42,* 196–221.

Stanovich, K.E. (1986). Matthew effects in reading: Some consequences of individual differences in the acquisition of literacy. *Reading Research Quarterly, 21,* 360–407.

Stanovich, K.E. (1991). Cognitive science meets beginning reading. *Psychological Science, 2,* 70–81.

Steere, A., Peck, C.Z., & Kahn, L. (1984). *Solving language difficulties: Remedial routines.* Cambridge, MA: Educators Publishing Service.

Tan, A., & Nicholson, T. (1997). Flashcards revisited: Training poor readers to read words faster improves their comprehension of text. *Journal of Educational Psychology, 89*(2), 276–288.

Torgesen, J.K. (1997). The prevention and remediation of reading disabilities: Evaluating what we know from research. *Journal of Academic Language Therapy, 1,* 11–47.

Torgesen, J.K., & Hudson, R.F. (2006). Reading fluency: Critical issues for struggling readers. In S.J. Samuels & A.E. Farstrup (Eds.), *What research has to say about fluency instruction* (pp. 130–158). Newark, DE: International Reading Association.

Torgesen, J.K., Rashotte, C.A., & Alexander, A.W. (2001). Principles of fluency instruction in reading: Relationships with established empirical outcomes. In M. Wolf (Ed.), *Dyslexia, fluency, and the brain* (pp. 333–355). Timonium, MD: York Press.

Toste, J.R., Williams, K.J., & Capin, P. (2016, Dec. 15). Reading big words: Instructional practices to promote multisyllabic word reading fluency. *Intervention in School and Clinic* 1–9. doi:10.1177/1053451216676797

Tunmer, W.E., & Arrow, A.W. (2013). Reading: Phonics instruction. In J. Hattie & E.M. Anderman (Eds.), *International guide to student achievement.* London, United Kingdom: Routledge.

Tunmer, W.E., Herriman, M.L., & Nesdale, A.R. (1988). Metalinguistic abilities and beginning reading. *Reading Research Quarterly, 23,* 134–158.

Vellutino, F.R. (1980). Perceptual deficiency or perceptual inefficiency. In J. Kavanagh & R. Venezky (Eds.), *Orthography, reading and dyslexia* (pp. 251–270). Baltimore, MD: University Park Press.

Venezky, R.L. (1980). From Webster to rice to Roosevelt. In U. Frith (Ed.), *Cognitive processes in spelling* (pp. 9–30). London, United Kingdom: Academic Press.

Waites, L., & Cox, A.R. (1976). *Remedial training programs for developmental language disabilities.* Cambridge, MA: Educators Publishing Service.

Wanzek, J., & Vaughn, S. (2007). Research-based implications from extensive early reading interventions. *School Psychology Review, 36,* 541–561.

Wilson, B. (1996). *Wilson Reading System instructor manual* (3rd ed.). Oxford, MA: Wilson Language Training.

Wolf, M. (1997). A provisional, integrative account of phonological and naming speed deficits in dyslexia: Implications for diagnosis and intervention. In B. Blachman (Ed.), *Foundations of reading acquisition and dyslexia: Implications for early intervention* (pp. 67–92). Mahwah, NJ: Lawrence Erlbaum Associates.

Wolf, M. (Ed.). (2001). *Dyslexia, fluency, and the brain.* Timonium, MD: York Press.

Wolf, M., & Bowers, P. (1999). The "double deficit hypothesis" for the developmental dyslexias. *Journal of Educational Psychology, 91*(3), 1–24.

Wolf, M., & Bowers, P. (2000). The question of naming-speed deficits in the developmental reading disabilities: An introduction of the double-deficit hypothesis. *Journal of Learning Disabilities, 33,* 322–324.

Wolf, M., & Obregón, M. (1992). Early naming deficits, developmental dyslexia, and a specific deficit hypothesis. *Brain and Language, 42,* 219–247.

Wood, F.B., Flowers, L., & Grigorenko, E. (2001). On the functional neuroanatomy of fluency or why walking is just as important to reading as talking is. In M. Wolf (Ed.), *Dyslexia, fluency, and the brain.* Timonium, MD: York Press.

Yopp, H.K. (1992). Developing phonemic awareness in young children. *The Reading Teacher, 45*(9), 696–703.

Yopp, H.K. (1995). Read-aloud books for developing phonemic awareness: An annotated bibliography. *The Reading Teacher, 48,* 538–542.

Technology Resources

Elaine A. Cheesman

PROGRAMS/APPS FOR DECODING PHONETICALLY REGULAR WORDS

Effective programs/apps have the following features:

- Letter–sound apps match letters to the most common sound (e.g., short sounds for vowels, /ks/ for *x*, /w/ for *w*).

- Decoding apps present concepts systematically and cumulatively, progressing from easier to more difficult concepts.

- When two or more letters represent a single sound (e.g., *ll, ss, sh, ai, igh, dge*), the grapheme is shown as one unit, not separate letters.

- Narrated text pronounces the article *a* as /ə/, not long /ā/ as in *apron*.

ABC Magic series   http://www.preschoolu.com

This program matches picture prompts to initial sounds and letters.

abc PocketPhonics   http://www.appsinmypocket.com

This app combines handwriting practice and spelling graphemes (letters and letter clusters that represent one sound). It presents the alphabetic principle in a logically ordered sequence. After the graphemes are introduced, the app guides the user to apply the target spelling–sound correspondences to spell spoken words. It supports multiple users; school versions are available to enable students to work on different devices. Progress reports are available online or via a weekly e-mail. It is appropriate for learners ages 4 and older.

ABC Reading Magic series   http://www.preschoolu.com

This series of apps includes both phonemic awareness activities (blending oral words presented as photographs) and decoding (decoding letters to form words shown as photographs). The mature narration and photographs make this app series suitable for all ages. In a few two-syllable words, vowels in open syllables are pronounced with the short, not long, sound.

Reading 1: CVC words

Reading 2: CCVC, CCCVC, CVCC, CVCCC

Reading 3: Two-syllable words

*Reading 4: "Phonograms," digraphs, vowel-*r, *and vowel team syllables in one and two-syllable words*

*Reading 5: Vowel-consonant-silent-*e *words*

Alpha-read   http://alpha-read.com

This program links letters, key word pictures, and the most common sound. Spelling–sound correspondences are sequenced not in alphabetical order but according to their utility for spelling words (e.g., *a, t, m, s*). Review mode allows the teacher or user to select letters to review.

Blending SE Student Edition and TE (Teacher Edition)
http://www.95percentgroup.com

This app helps students practice blending skills after receiving instruction from their teacher. It helps them recognize spoken words that are pronounced blended and sound by sound. It is an excellent and effective app for students who have difficulty blending sounds.

Bob Books—Reading Magic   http://bobbooks.com

This program provides decodable, illustrated, interactive stories. The drag-and-drop feature provides practice for the child to spell spoken words in the story. The program orally reads the sentence after all the words are formed. Each story contains four progressively more difficult user tasks.

CVC words   http://www.alligatorapps.com

This app provides practice reading and spelling phonetically regular words. It is organized by word family, or rime (*hop, pop, mop*). It provides practice reading and spelling words using 14 engaging games. The optional text-to-speech feature reads sentences.

Lexia Core5   http://www.lexialearning.com

This program provides instruction and practice in phonemic awareness, reading, and spelling. It provides engaging, systematic, sequential practice organized by syllable type. It tracks multiple users' progress and provides comprehensive reports. It is suitable for all ages.

OG Card Deck   http://www.mayersonacademy.org

This program presents written graphemes, associated sounds, key words, and articulation video clips. A spelling drill provides sounds for users to spell. It includes multiple spellings for single sounds (e.g., /k/ = *k, c, ck, que*). It is useful for direct instruction by a teacher or independent student review.

Phonics Genius   http://www.alligatorapps.com

This app has both a teaching and practice mode. The teaching mode presents basic and advanced phoneme–grapheme associations using a flashcard format. It pronounces words and highlights vowel spellings. Users may modify word lists.

PocketPhonics Stories   http://www.appsinmypocket.com

This app contains 43 decodable books, organized by graphemes. An optional text-to-speech feature will narrate the story if activated. If a child cannot read a word, a tap will open up a pop-up picture showing the word's spelling. Phonetically irregular words are gradually introduced and are in red type. The app includes quizzes to check for comprehension, which the child must complete before moving to the next book. Progress reports are available online or via a weekly e-mail. It is appropriate for learners ages 4 and older.

Reading Ninja   http://www.alligatorapps.com

This app promotes overlearning of CVC words. The words fly up from the bottom of the screen. The user taps the word that matches the spoken word among other choices. The narration is a mature voice, which is appropriate for all ages.

Sentence Reading Magic 1 and 2   http://www.preschoolu.com

This program presents 324 two-, three-, four-, and five-word sentences with short vowels (Magic 1) or consonant blends (Magic 2). The user can match spoken and written high-frequency words (Magic 1). The program includes manuscript and cursive fonts.

SoundLiteracy   http://soundliteracy.com

For use as a teacher instructional aid, not for independent student use, this digital "tile" has virtual manipulatives for letters, graphemes, and morphemes. It includes comprehensive sets of all graphemes. It also includes a "draw" feature that can be used for syllable division teaching and practice.

Starfall ABCs/Starfall Learn to Read   http://www.starfall.com

Starfall can be accessed through an identical free (and ad-free) web site and mobile app. It has engaging animations and games for learning letter–sound correspondences. It provides the letter name, not its sound, in the key word for *x* (x-ray). A better key word is *box* for /ks/.

PROGRAMS/APPS: HIGH-FREQUENCY (SIGHT) WORDS

Effective programs/apps have the following features:

- Words are derived from the Fry "Instant Word" list of 1,000 most common words (1980) or the Dolch word list of 220 most common words for preschool through third grade.

- Words are presented in small, manageable groups.

- Practice activities develop instant word recognition.

- The article *a* is pronounced as /ə/, not long /ā/ as in *apron*.

English Words: Everyone Learns, Sight Words: Everyone Learns, and Star Speller: Kids Learn Sight Words Games
https://itunes.apple.com/us/developer/teacher-created-materials/id437178006

These three nearly identical apps have a wide variety of games to practice reading and spelling high-frequency words. The "Little Speller" is the most economical. Each contains all 300 Dolch words; users can buy separate packets for groups of 100 words. However, this set of apps costs considerably more than comparable apps. It has nine engaging practice games that involve seeing, hearing, recording, and spelling. Although more expensive than other sight word apps, the "English Words" app is appropriate for older students.

Fry Words   http://www.alligatorapps.com

This app provides systematic instruction and practice for 1,000 high-frequency words based on the Fry list. It has a "learn" mode and an engaging "game" mode that challenges users to identify high-frequency words from a choice of two to five words.

Fry Words Ninja—Reading Game   http://www.alligatorapps.com

This app promotes overlearning of 1,000 high-frequency words based on the Fry list. The words fly up from the bottom of the screen. The user taps the word that matches the spoken word among other choices. The narration is a mature voice, which is appropriate for all ages.

Sight Words   http://www.alligatorapps.com

This app provides systematic instruction and practice for 200 high-frequency words based on the Dolch list grouped by grade level, preschool to third grade. It has a "learn" mode and an engaging "game" mode that challenges users to identify high-frequency words from a choice of two to five words.

Sight Words by Little Speller   http://www.alligatorapps.com

This app helps the user learn and practice the spelling of 200 Dolch words. It uses a drag-and-drop letters format. Adjustable options are provided to scaffold task difficulty.

Sight Words by Photo Touch   http://www.grasshopperapps.com

This app builds automaticity and fluency for the 220 Dolch words. The user matches spoken and written words by selecting the correct word from a list of 3–10 words. The app automatically adjusts the number based on user success.

PROGRAMS/APPS: MORPHOLOGY (PREFIXES, SUFFIXES, ROOTS)

Effective programs/apps have the following features:

- They link the meaning with the spelling of the morpheme.

Lexia Core5   http://www.lexialearning.com

This program provides engaging, systematic, sequential practice in Latin roots and Greek combining forms. It includes vocabulary and comprehension activities as well. It tracks multiple users' progress. It is appropriate for kindergarten through adult.

Roots to Words   http://taptolearn.com

In this program, Latin roots and Greek combining forms are arranged in meaning categories (e.g., numbers, quantity, shapes). The user selects a meaning category for practice then types the spelling of the morpheme to complete a series of words. The program includes several practice activities, which apply the chosen set of morphemes within sentences.

SoundLiteracy   http://soundliteracy.com

For use as a teacher instructional aid, not for independent student use, this digital "tile" has virtual manipulatives for letters, graphemes, and morphemes. It includes comprehensive sets of all graphemes. It also includes a "draw" feature that can be used for syllable division teaching and practice.

SpellingCity   http://www.spellingcity.com

This program provides practice in spelling, handwriting, and vocabulary using customized lists of words. In the paid version, users can access and share lists with publishers and other educators. It has engaging games and practice activities for use on tablets or computers. It is appropriate for kindergarten through adult.

Voyage of Ulysses   http://elasticoapp.com

This interactive story app gives prose narration of the Voyage of Ulysses (e.g., The Cyclops, Trojan Horse). The narration provides background of word origins. The animation deepens the user's comprehension of the text.

PROGRAMS/APPS: DICTIONARIES AND THESAURI

Dictionary.com   http://www.dictionary.com

This dictionary has user-friendly definitions, synonyms, antonyms, and sample sentences; it also has illustrated language of origin.

English-Word Information   http://wordinfo.info

This is a student-friendly web site for learning the morphology and etymology of words. This is a clever and informative web site.

Longman Dictionary and Thesaurus   http://global.longmandictionaries.com

This resource provides clear definitions using only 2,000 common words. It has special features for education (e.g., flashcards, teacher resources, printable worksheets, search on idiomatic phrases, synonyms, word histories).

Online Etymology Dictionary   http://www.etymonline.com

Each entry provides the historical etymology and morphemic structure of words.

WEB SITES: MATERIALS AND ACTIVITIES FOR TEACHERS AND LEARNERS

How Many Syllables   http://www.howmanysyllables.com

This web site allows the user to type in a word to see the number of syllables, syllable division, primary and secondary stress, and oral pronunciation. The web site provides examples of how to count and divide syllables, grammar rules, and teacher resources.

Florida Center for Reading Research   http://www.fcrr.org

This web site has thousands of downloadable "Center" activities in all five components of reading—phonemic awareness, phonics, fluency, vocabulary, and comprehension. It also has research and resources for teachers.

Reading Rockets   http://www.readingrockets.org

This public broadcasting web site has a wealth of evidence-based information and resources for teachers and parents, including sections on teaching reading and helping struggling readers. For educators, "Reading 101: A Guide to Teaching Reading and Writing" is particularly valuable. This is a self-paced professional development course for K–3 teachers and special educators. It provides teachers with in-depth knowledge of reading and writing.

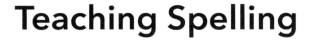

Chapter 10

Teaching Spelling

Suzanne Carreker

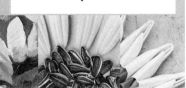

LEARNING OBJECTIVES

1. To explain how spelling is the same as and different from decoding

2. To describe the differences between good and poor spellers

3. To outline a structured, sequential, and cumulative progression of skills for spelling instruction

In many classrooms, spelling instruction is treated as an afterthought to, or as a byproduct of, reading. The assumption is that if students learn to read, they learn to spell; therefore, spelling instruction is given little importance and minimal attention during the instruction day. The subject of spelling is frequently relegated to memorization of word lists with little or no instruction (Joshi, Treiman, Carreker, & Moats, 2008/2009). This view fails to recognize the integral role spelling instruction plays in learning to read and write (Graham & Santangelo, 2014; Moats, 2005/2006).

Spelling instruction enhances reading proficiency by reinforcing sounds and letter patterns (Adams, 1990). In addition, spelling instruction facilitates learning word pronunciations and meanings and improves writing (Ehri & Rosenthal, 2007; Graham & Santangelo, 2014). Spelling, a cognitive linguistic process, is more difficult to learn than reading (Frith, 1980; Joshi et al., 2008/2009). As Ehri noted, "It is easier to read words accurately in English than to spell them. Failure to remember one or two letters dooms a perfect spelling but not necessarily an accurate reading" (2000, p. 24).

Learning to spell requires explicit instruction (Brady & Moats, 1997; Graham & Santangelo, 2014; Joshi et al., 2008/2009; McMurray & McVeigh, 2016). The International Dyslexia Association (IDA)'s (2018) *Knowledge and Practice Standards for Teachers of Reading* outlined what a knowledgeable and skilled teacher of reading should know and be able to do to teach students to spell well. This chapter discusses underlying processes of spelling, spelling development, analysis of spelling errors to inform instruction, and the explicit spelling instruction that helps students become skilled and confident spellers.

THE DISTINCTIVENESS OF SPELLING

To decode text, a reader must translate symbols on a printed page that represent spoken words (see Chapter 9). The reader must attach a speech sound to each letter in a printed word. In this manner, the reader can sound out or pronounce the spoken word that is represented by printed symbols. To spell, the speller must translate spoken words into printed symbols. That means a speller must attach a written letter or group of letters to each speech sound in a spoken word. In this manner, the speller can represent spoken words with printed symbols. It would appear from these simple descriptions that decoding and spelling are simply inverse operations that require knowledge of sound–symbol correspondences and are performed in opposite order.

Following this logic, it could be assumed that if a student can read a word, then he or she can also spell the word. Although both decoding and spelling require phonological and orthographic knowledge, the two skills are not simply inverse operations (Frith, 1980). First, sound-to-spelling translations are less dependable than spelling-to-sound translations (Adams, 1990). Second, decoding requires only recognizing words, whereas spelling requires complete, accurate recall of letter patterns and words (Frith & Frith, 1980; Fulk & Stormont-Spurgin, 1995).

Orthography refers to how spoken words are represented in written language. When the reader has mastered the decoding skills discussed in Chapter 9, English orthography becomes 87% reliable (regular) for reading (Hanna, Hanna, Hodges, & Rudorf, 1966). The reader needs to memorize or infer from the context only about 13% of the words he or she will encounter. The rest of the words that are not instantly recognized can be sounded out. To sound out an unfamiliar word, the reader assigns known sounds to known letters in the word. With the assistance of phonological awareness, approximate pronunciations, and contextual clues, the reader can accurately pronounce the unfamiliar word (Share & Stanovich, 1995). When a letter or group of letters has more than one possible pronunciation (e.g., *ea* can be pronounced /ĕ/, /ē/, or /ā/), the reader affirms his or her pronunciation choice by determining whether the chosen word makes sense in the sentence (e.g., one nods one's /hĕd/, not one's /hēd/ or /hād/). The more the reader knows about decoding, the easier it is for him or her to recognize words, but even with partial decoding, a reader can read unfamiliar words.

The 87% reliability of English orthography (Hanna et al., 1966) may make the task of spelling an unfamiliar word that one can read seem deceptively simple. The speller must rely on phonological awareness to segment the unfamiliar word into its constituent sounds and then determine how those sounds are best represented in print. However, because many speech sounds in English are represented by **multiple spellings** (e.g., initial or medial /ā/ in a one-syllable word can be spelled *a*-consonant-*e* as in *cake*, *ai* as in *rain*, *ei* as in *vein*, *eigh* as in *eight*, or *ea* as in *steak*), making the correct choice can be confusing to the speller. Contextual clues do not affirm the speller's choice of spelling (Fulk & Stormont-Spurgin, 1995). After all, the word that is pronounced /tām/ (*tame*), spelled incorrectly as *taim, teim, teighm,* or *team,* would share the same context.

The speller's only confirmation of a correct spelling is to compare the spelled word with a word held in memory. If the word is not held in memory because the speller has not seen it before or because the speller has a poor memory for letters and words (i.e., poor orthographic memory), then it is difficult for him or her to independently confirm that the spelling choice is correct. Spelling requires an awareness of and exact memory for letter patterns and words that reading does not require.

In addition to the need for exact recall and the ambiguities of sound-to-spelling translations, spelling is a complex linguistic skill that demands simultaneous integration of syntactic (see Bryant, Nunes, & Bindman, 1997, for a discussion), phonological, morphological, semantic, and orthographic knowledge (Frith, 1980; McMurray & McVeigh, 2016; Moats, 1995; Smith, 1980). This integration can be illustrated as a speller attempts to spell /jŭmpt/. Phonological awareness enables the speller to hear all of the sounds and play with the idea that /jŭmpt/ without /t/ is /jŭmp/. Syntactic awareness alerts the speller that /jŭmp/ can be used as a verb and that verbs have tenses. Morphological awareness helps the speller realize that /jŭmpt/ consists of two meaningful units—base word /jŭmp/ and suffix /t/. Semantic awareness provides the speller with the understanding that /t/ represents the past tense. Finally, using orthographic knowledge, the speller apprehends that /t/ will be spelled *ed* and not *t*.

Spelling obligates the speller to attend to multiple layers of language concurrently. Knowing how to read a word does not guarantee that a person can spell the word correctly. If this were true, then there would be no individuals who read quite well but are poor spellers, and spelling development would not lag behind reading development. Spelling instruction should be intimately integrated with the teaching of reading, but because spelling has its own distinctive characteristics and demands, it also must be distinct from reading and explicitly taught. Spellers must be taught in a manner that will increase their awareness and memory of letter patterns and words. Developing proficiency in spelling is different from developing proficiency in reading, but the English language is not chaotic (Kessler & Treiman, 2003) and hopeless, and sequential, structured instruction of language structures can lead to skilled spelling.

REFLECT, CONNECT, and RESPOND
What are the major differences between reading, a recognition skill, and spelling, a recall skill?

SPELLING DEVELOPMENT

It is important to understand how spelling develops to understand the vital role spelling plays in learning to read and the errors students make. Evidence suggests that spelling is a unitary, interactive process that requires both phonological and orthographic knowledge (Lennox & Siegel, 1998). Beginning spellers take advantage of both phonological and visual strategies (Bryant & Bradley, 1980; Treiman, Cassar, & Zukowski, 1994).

Spelling proficiency tends to develop or unfold in a fairly predictable and gradual sequence, which is often described by stages or phases; however, students will rarely move through any stages or phases in an exact and orderly progression. A young child's first writing experience is usually in the form of drawing. As the child is exposed to print, he or she begins to differentiate writing from drawing and begins to imitate the print he or she has seen, using letterlike or numberlike forms (Cassar & Treiman, 1997). In this precommunicative or **prephonetic stage** or phase (Moats, 1995), the child's writing shows a lack of understanding of the concept of a word, the alphabetic principle, or the conventions of print, such as spaces between words and the left-to-right progression of writing. Bear, Invernizzi, Templeton, and

Johnston suggested that the organization of the child's writing may be described as "willy-nilly" (1996, p. 16). Pollo, Kessler, and Treiman noted, however, "our results speak against the idea that early prephonological spellings are random and unpatterned" (2009, p. 424).

At age 3 or 4, the child may think that the length of the word reflects the size of the object it names instead of the sounds of language (e.g., *cow* should have more letters than *chicken* because a cow is bigger than a chicken) (Treiman, 1997). To the 3- or 4-year-old child, meaning takes precedence over spelling. Only when the child becomes aware that print is related to speech does he or she come to understand that letters represent speech sounds.

A grasp of the alphabetic principle emerges with the child's realization that spoken words are made of sounds that can be represented in print. He or she will first attempt to connect speech to print at the syllable level instead of at the phoneme level and will write a symbol for each syllable (e.g., *b* for *be* or *nf* for *enough*) (Ferreiro & Teberosky, 1982). As the child becomes more aware that individual letters represent individual sounds, he or she enters this **semiphonetic stage** (Moats, 1995) and uses incomplete but reasonable phonetic representations of words. The child usually uses the initial or salient consonants of a word, such as *s, c,* or *sd* for *seed* (Rubin & Eberhardt, 1996), or the child may use letter names, such as *lft* for *elephant* (Adams, 1990; Treiman, 1994). At this semiphonetic stage or phase, the child demonstrates awareness of left-to-right progression, but he or she tends to run letters together with little or no sense of word boundaries (e.g., RUDF for *Are you deaf?*) (Moats, 1995).

Further experiences with print and writing move the child to a stage of complete phonetic representations, or the **phonetic stage** (Moats, 1995). Every sound in a word is represented, but the child does not demonstrate knowledge of conventional spelling patterns. The child may spell *same* as *sam*, thus neglecting the final silent *e* (Treiman, Zukowski, & Richmond-Welty, 1995). The inflection *-ed* may be represented as *t* as in *askt* or *d* as in *hugd* (Read, 1971). At this phonetic stage, the child is aware of not only sounds but also the mouth positions used to make sounds. Moats suggested that the child may seem to be "spelling by mouth" (1995, p. 37). For example, the child may use *y* to spell /w/ because not only does the letter name contain /w/ but also the mouth position to say the letter name *y* is the same as /w/. Other odd but linguistically understandable spelling choices may be observed at this point, such as spelling /t/ before /r/ as *ch*, as in *chrie* for *try*, or /d/ before /r/ as *j*, as in *jragin* for *dragon* (Read, 1971). Phonetically, /t/ or /d/ would not be spelled with *ch* or *j*, but when /t/ or /d/ occur before /r/, the place of articulation (i.e., where the sound is obstructed in the mouth during production) matches the place of articulation for /ch/ and /j/, respectively (Treiman, 1998). Consistent spelling anomalies may occur, such as /r/ overwhelming the vowel, as in *hr* for *her*, or the omission of nasal (i.e., /m/, /n/, /ng/) and liquid sounds (i.e., /l/, /r/), as in *drik* for *drink*, *jup* for *jump*, and *od* for *old* (Treiman, 1998; Treiman et al., 1995).

In early spelling development, a child is literal in his or her spelling of words (e.g., /k/ is almost always spelled *k*). As the child begins to read more, he or she becomes more sensitive to the letter patterns in words. Without being taught, he or she may discover an orthographic pattern and sense its constraints. The child may discover that /k/ can be spelled *ck* and may sense that it does not occur in the initial position of a word. He or she is more likely to spell *cake* as *kack* than *ckak* (Treiman, 1997). In this transitional stage or phase of spelling, as the child becomes more aware of letter patterns in words, his or her spelling may seem "off-base" (Moats, 1995, p. 40). From exact phonetic representations of every sound, the child's spelling may become a mixture of phonetic components and salient visual features in words. This change in spelling usually signals a heightened awareness of letter patterns. Through their early spelling experiences, children build a foundation for reading as they begin to establish sound–symbol correspondences and develop a sensitivity to letter patterns. But just as beginning readers need explicit teaching to become good readers, beginning spellers need explicit teaching to become good spellers. Without this formal instruction, beginning spellers will not establish the awareness and memory of letter patterns that will make them good spellers.

GOOD AND POOR SPELLERS

Good spelling ability is contingent on a speller's sensitivity to letter patterns (Adams, 1990). Research has shown that good and poor spellers do not differ greatly in their visual memory abilities (Holmes, Malone, & Redenbach, 2008; Lennox & Siegel, 1996). What differs in good spellers is that they possess well-developed phonological processing skills that not only make them aware of the sounds in words but also support the learning of letter patterns in words (Lennox & Siegel, 1998; Moats, 1995). Good spellers possess an orthographic memory. This orthographic memory is a more specific memory than visual memory; it is specific to remembering letter patterns and words. Developing this memory is dependent on well-developed phonological and orthographic processing skills. Good spellers know not only how sounds are represented in language but also how words should look (Adams, 1990; McMurray & McVeigh, 2016). They are able to deal with the ambiguities of orthography (e.g., the multiple spellings of /ā/) by weighting the variable spellings by their frequency or exposure in reading (e.g., the good speller weights *a*-consonant-*e* as a more frequent or stronger connection to /ā/ than *eigh* because he or she sees it more frequently) (Adams, 1990; Foorman, 1994; McMurray & McVeigh, 2016; Seidenberg & McClelland, 1989). In addition to possessing phonological and orthographic knowledge, good spellers are able to simultaneously draw support from their awareness of syntax, morphology, and semantics. Because good spellers possess the very skills that are needed for good decoding, good spellers are good readers (i.e., decoders). It is unusual to find a good speller who is a poor reader (decoder).

The definition of dyslexia endorsed by The IDA (Lyon, Shaywitz, & Shaywitz, 2003) included reading disabilities as well as specific spelling disabilities. As noted in Chapters 6 and 9, students with dyslexia have difficulty learning to decode because of a core deficit in phonological processing (Adams, 1990; Bradley & Bryant, 1983; Goswami & Bryant, 1990). It is rare for students with dyslexia who have difficulty with decoding not to have difficulty with spelling. It is possible, however, for students to be fairly good readers but poor spellers.

Moats (1995) made these observations about poor spellers. Good readers who are poor spellers have problems with the exact recall of letter sequences and subtle difficulties with complex spelling patterns and aspects of language structure, but they do not have a deficit in phonological processing. In contrast, poor readers who are poor spellers have a deficit in phonological processing that interferes with their mastery of spelling. These readers also have a specific problem with memory of letter patterns, which is rooted in their poor phonological processing. In addition, poor spellers do not possess the ability to deal with several layers of language simultaneously. With proper instruction, poor spellers who are poor readers will improve their decoding skills, but they seldom master spelling (Moats, 1994; Oakland, Black, Stanford, Nussbaum, & Balise, 1998). McMurray and McVeigh (2016) noted that poor spellers who are poor readers continue to have difficulties with spelling into adulthood.

Roberts and Mather (1997) characterized poor spelling as the result of difficulties in both phonological and orthographic processing. Difficulties with phonological processing may include poor sequencing of sounds, omission or addition of sounds, confusion with similar-sounding phonemes (e.g., /f/ and /th/, /p/ and /b/), and limited knowledge of spelling rules. Orthographic processing difficulties are manifested as poor sequencing of nonphonetic patterns, confusion of graphemes that look similar (e.g., *b* and *d*, *n* and *u*), transposition of letters (e.g., *fro* instead of *for*), overgeneralization of rules, and overreliance on auditory features (e.g., *becuz* for *because*).

Poor spellers may be perceived as "free-spirit" spellers who spell words the way they sound without regard to conventional letter patterns. The free-spirit spellers may spell *does* as *duz, dress* as *dres,* or *girl* as *gerl.* They may spell the same word several different ways within the same paragraph, such as *thay, tha,* and *thai* for *they.* The spellers with dyslexia may be perceived as "bizarre" spellers. They struggle with the conventional letter patterns of words and use inappropriate letter sequences, such as *oridr* for *order;* transpositions, such as *gril* for *girl;* letter reversals, such as *dady* for *baby;* or incomplete letter patterns, such as *boht* for *bought.* Not only do spellers with dyslexia lack the ability to use conventional letter patterns, they also are unable to fully or correctly translate the sounds in words. They may have difficulty hearing the word correctly (e.g., hearing *fan* instead of *van*), hearing all of the sounds in a word (e.g., hearing *butful* for *beautiful*), or keeping the sounds in sequence (e.g., using *slpit* for *split*). They may have difficulty discriminating similar sounds (e.g., hearing *baf* for *bath* or *wint* for *went*).

Problems with spelling persist in adolescents and adults with dyslexia. Moats (1996) found that adolescents with dyslexia showed lingering, subtle signs of phonological difficulty, primarily in segmenting words into their phonemic and morphemic units, as evidenced by their consistent omissions, substitutions, and misrepresentations of inflected morphemes (e.g., *-ed* spelled as *t* or *d*). Their errors in spelling **high-frequency words** suggested that their underdeveloped phonological and linguistic awareness compromised the development of orthographic memory. When comparing the writing samples of adults with and without dyslexia, Sterling, Farmer, Riddick, Morgan, and Matthews (1998) found that the sentences of adults with dyslexia were no shorter or longer than those of their peers but that there was a conspicuous use of **monosyllabic** words and misuse of **homophones.** Spelling errors suggested specific phonological impairment as well as problems with the complexities of English. Adolescents and adults who are poor spellers demonstrate the tenacious nature of the phonological processing deficit and its chronic effect on spelling development. Phonological awareness, along with morphemic and orthographic awareness, must be considered significant elements of spelling instruction.

It is important to note that spelling ability and IQ scores are not related. Poor spelling does not reflect a lack of intelligence (West, 1991). Take, for example, the spelling errors of neurosurgeon Harvey Cushing: *swoolen* for *swollen, neybour* for *neighbor,* and *quire* for *choir.* Cushing was a brilliant man who was a *"mediocher"* speller.

KNOWLEDGE NEEDED FOR SPELLING PROFICIENCY

Traditional spelling instruction that involves the repetitive copying of words or the memorization of word lists does not promote active, reflective thought about language (Joshi et al., 2008/2009; McMurray & McVeigh, 2016). Informal spelling instruction that assumes that spelling will develop through writing experiences does not provide students with the necessary knowledge of language structure they need to become correct spellers. Students must be explicitly taught about language structure for spelling, and they must be actively engaged in thinking about language. The teacher must assume an active role in spelling instruction. As Moats stated, "Rather than a developmental progression characterized by distinct stages, learning to spell is more accurately described as a continual amalgamation of phonological, morphological, and orthographic knowledge" (2005, p. 14). It is imperative that the teacher have and be able to impart knowledge about the sounds of the language, the most frequent and reliable letter patterns and rules of English orthography, morphology, and word origins to help students consolidate their knowledge of language structures into correct spellings (Brady & Moats, 1997; Joshi & Carreker, 2009; see Chapter 14 for a discussion of English word origins).

Phonology

Phonetics is the study of the characteristics of individual speech sounds (i.e., phonemes) that occur in all languages (see Scarborough & Brady, 2002, for a discussion about related *phon* terms; these are also addressed in Chapter 6). There are approximately 44 speech sounds in English, with some variants of these sounds (i.e., *allophones*) that are not considered separate speech sounds (e.g., the /ă/ in the word *sank* is different from the /ă/ in *sack* but is not a separate speech sound). Phonetics involves categorizing or describing the articulation of each speech sound—where the sound is produced, the way in which air stream flows through the mouth and nose, and the activity of the vocal cords during production.

Spoken words are made up of the speech sounds. Every language has its own set of rules that governs the utterance of these sounds and the sound patterns that are allowed. This system of rules that determine how sounds are used in spoken language is called phonology (Moats, 1995). There are constraints about sound sequences in spoken language based on what humans are capable of producing easily (e.g., /np/ rarely occurs in spoken English, hence the pronunciation /ĭm|pôrt/ rather than /ĭn|pôrt/).

Pronunciation variations may occur because of a phoneme's position in a word (e.g., /p/ in *pot* is different from the /p/ in *spot* or *top*) or because of surrounding sounds (e.g., the vowel in *sank* may be perceived as a long vowel instead of a short vowel because it is nasalized before nasal /ng/). These perfunctory pronunciation differences do not affect meaning (Treiman et al., 1994). Accent, however, may vary pronunciations as well as the meanings of words (e.g., /ŏb'|jĕkt/ is a noun, and /ŏb|jĕkt'/ is a verb). It is not necessary to teach the rules that govern the use of speech sounds when a child is learning to speak (Read, 1971); the rules are unconscious rules that automatically occur in spoken language.

Phonics is an instructional method that teaches the use of written symbols to represent speech sounds for reading and spelling. Phonics provides a visual representation of the phonology of spoken language (e.g., the /ă/ in *sank* is nasalized before *n*, which is nasalized; the *n* is pronounced /ng/ instead of /n/ before any letter pronounced /k/ or /g/). In order for students to be successful with phonics, they must be aware of the sounds in spoken words.

Brady and Moats (1997) contended that knowledge of phonetics and phonology assists the teacher in understanding the reading and spelling errors of students, increases his or her ability to provide **corrective feedback,** and enables him or her to plan instruction that is linguistically informed. Knowledge of phonetics heightens the teacher's awareness of speech sounds and how they are produced so that he or she can provide correct models for students (Moats et al., 2010). Knowing phonology also gives the teacher insight into why students might have difficulty segmenting or spelling words. For example, a nasalized vowel plus a nasal consonant sound is pronounced as a unit. Therefore, students may have difficulty hearing that /jŭmp/ consists of four separate speech sounds. Students may segment it as three sounds: /j/, /ŭm/, and /p/. When spelling, students may hear /t/ before /r/ as /ch/ and spell it accordingly. As mentioned previously, /t/ before /r/ has a place of articulation in the mouth that is similar to /ch/, so using *ch* is not outrageous but instead is "reasonable and well motivated" (Treiman et al., 1994, p. 1336) and worthy of recognition (Read, 1971). The teacher need not be a linguist but rather should possess phonemic awareness skills and a working knowledge of the sound structure of English.

Correct pronunciation of speech sounds is encouraged by teaching the articulatory features of individual sounds (Ehri, 2014; Moats, 1995). Students are able to distinguish sounds better when they understand the kinesthetic feel and the visual display of the mouth as a speech sound is pronounced.

In decoding instruction, students learn that vowel sounds are open and voiced. The short vowels are most difficult to discriminate. Figure 10.1 (Cox, 1992) illustrates the mouth positions of the short vowel sounds. The teacher should study and share this figure with students. Visual awareness of the mouth positions for producing vowel sounds heightens students' ability to discriminate the vowel sounds. Awareness of the distinctive, kinesthetic feel of sounds as they are produced also assists in discriminating easily confused vowel sounds (e.g., /ĭ/ makes you grin, /ĕ/ drops your chin).

To be able to provide correct models of consonant sounds, the teacher should study the production of consonant sounds according to three properties: the

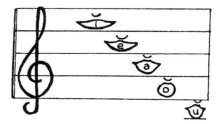

Figure 10.1. Mouth position for the short vowel sounds. (From Cox, A.R. [1992]. *Foundations for literacy: Structures and techniques for multisensory teaching of basic written English language skills* [p. 129]. Cambridge, MA: Educators Publishing Service. Used by permission of Educators Publishing Service, 625 Mt. Auburn St., Cambridge, MA, [800] 225-5750, www.epsbooks.com)

Table 10.1. Places of articulation of consonant sounds

Both lips	Teeth and lower lip	Between the teeth	Ridge behind teeth	Roof of mouth	Back of mouth	From the throat
/b/	/f/	/th/	/d/	/ch/	/g/	/h/
/m/	/v/	/<u>th</u>/	/l/	/j/	/k/	/hw/
/p/			/n/	/sh/	/ks/*	
			/r/	/y/	/kw/*	
			/s/	/zh/	/ng/	
			/t/		/w/	
			/z/			

*These combination sounds represent the most frequent sounds of *x* (/ks/) and *q* (/kw/), which is usually followed by *u*.

From *Multisensory Teaching of Basic Language Skills, Third Edition* (p. 259).

place of articulation, the flow of the air stream, and the activity of the vocal cords. Table 10.1 provides information about the place of articulation of the consonant sounds, using the phonic spellings often used in reading and spelling instruction. Table 10.2 provides information on the kinesthetic feel of the mouth and how the air stream flows from the mouth or nose during production of consonant sounds. Table 10.3 presents information about voiced and unvoiced consonant sounds.

Table 10.2. Flow of air during production of consonant sounds

Partially blocked and clipped	Blocked and continuous	Unblocked and aspirated	Through the nose, blocked, and continuous
/b/	/f/	/h/	/m/
/ch/	/hw/		/n/
/d/	/ks/		/ng/
/g/	/kw/		
/j/	/l/		
/k/	/r/		
/p/	/s/		
/t/	/sh/		
/y/	/th/		
	/<u>th</u>/		
	/v/		
	/w/		
	/z/		
	/zh/		

The terms *blocked, partially blocked,* and *unblocked* are used in spelling instruction to refer to the kinesthetic feel of the position of the tongue, teeth, or lips during the production of sounds in isolation. *Blocked* refers to the steady position of the tongue, teeth, or lips during the entire production of a sound. *Partially blocked* refers to a released position of the tongue or lips during the production of a sound. *Unblocked* refers to no obstruction of the sound by the tongue, teeth, or lips during the production of a sound. These terms are used to aid students in clearly feeling and distinguishing sounds for spelling.

From *Multisensory Teaching of Basic Language Skills, Third Edition* (p. 259).

Table 10.3. Unvoiced and voiced consonant sounds

Unvoiced	Voiced
Pairs (read across)	
/p/	/b/
/t/	/d/
/k/	/g/
/f/	/v/
/s/	/z/
/th/	/<u>th</u>/
/ch/	/j/
/sh/	/zh/
Nonpairs (read down)	
/h/	/kw/
/hw/	/l/
/ks/	/m/
	/n/
	/ng/
	/r/
	/w/
	/y/

From *Multisensory Teaching of Basic Language Skills, Third Edition* (p. 260).

Orthography

Orthography refers to the rules that govern how words are represented in writing. Chapter 9 contains information that assists the student in managing English orthography for reading. With this information, the reader knows how to translate the orthography into its spoken equivalents. The speller's task is to determine how the phonemes of oral language are transcribed into the graphemes (i.e., letters or letter clusters) of written language. There are constraints in English orthography; for example, certain letters never double (e.g., *j, y, w*), certain letters do not occur in sequence (e.g., *skr* does not occur within a syllable), and words do not end in certain letters (e.g., *v, j*). Formal spelling instruction calls attention to these constraints and helps students manage English orthography for spelling by establishing a sense of the frequency and reliability of letter patterns (Brady & Moats, 1997).

Table 10.4 presents 24 speech sounds that can be established as having a one-to-one correspondence with written letters. These sounds have only one spelling (e.g., /m/ is spelled *m*, /p/ is spelled *p*), or they have one spelling that is far more frequent than any other spelling (e.g., /f/ is spelled *f* much more often than *ph* or *gh*, /ĕ/ is spelled *e* much more often than *ea*) (Hanna et al., 1966). This information will enable students to spell more than half of the phonemes of English.

The other speech sounds of English have a more precarious link to orthography, as seen in Table 10.5. The transcription of each of these sounds depends not only on frequency but also on the position of the sound in a word, the length of the word, the accent, or the influence of surrounding sounds. To make sense

Table 10.4. Sound-to-spelling translations of speech sounds, based on frequency

Vowel sounds with one frequent spelling	Consonant sounds with one frequent spelling	Vowel sounds with more than one frequent spelling	Consonant sounds with more than one frequent spelling
/ă/ = a (*apple*)	/b/ = b (*bat*)	/ŏ/ = o (*octopus*)	/ch/ = ch (*cheek*)
/ĕ/ = e (*echo*)	/f/ = f (*fish*)	a (*watch*)	ch (*lunch, speech*)
/ĭ/ = i (*itch*)	/g/ = g (*goat*)	/ŭ/ = u (*cup*)	tch (*catch*)
/o͝o/ = oo (*book*)	/h/ = h (*house*)	a (*banana*)	/d/ = d (*dog*)
/o͞o/ = oo (*moon*)	/l/ = l (*leaf*)	/ā/= a-consonant-e	ed (*smelled*)
/âr/ = ar (*star*)	/m/ = m (*mitten*)	(*cake, vacate*)	/j/ = j (*jam*)
/ôr/ = or (*fork*)	/n/ = n (*nest*)	a (*apron*)	g (*gentle, giant,*
	/p/ = p (*pig*)	ay (*tray*)	*biology*)
	/kw/ = qu (*queen*)	/ē/= ee (*feet*)	dge (*edge*)
	/r/ = r (*rabbit*)	e-consonant-e (*athlete*)	ge (*hinge*)
	/w/ = w (*wish*)	e (*equal*)	/k/ = c (*cat, cot, cut,*
	/ks/ = x (*box*)	ee (*three*)	*clam, crab*)
	/y/ = y (*yarn*)	y (*penny*)	k (*keep, kite, sky*)
	/th/ = th (*rather*)	/ī/ = i-consonant-e	ck (*pocket*)
	/th/ = th (*thimble*)	(*five, invite*)	ck (*back*)
	/hw/ = wh (*whistle*)	i (*iris*)	k (*book, milk*)
	/sh/ = sh (*ship*)	y (*fly*)	ke (*make*)
	/zh/ = si (*erosion*)	/ō/ = o-consonant-e	c (*music*)
		(*rope, remote*)	/ng/ = ng (*king*)
		o (*open*)	n (*sink, angle*)
		ow (*snow*)	/s/ = s (*sock*)
		/ū/ = u-consonant-e	c (*grocery, icicle*)
		(*cube, infuse*)	ss (*kiss, discuss*)
		u (*unicorn*)	s (*cactus*)
		ue (*statue*)	ce (*mice*)
		/er/ = er (*fern*)	se (*horse, mouse*)
		or (*world*)	/t/ = t (*table*)
		/au/ = au (*saucer*)	ed (*jumped*)
		aw (*saw*)	/v/ = v (*valentine*)
		a (*ball*)	ve (*have*)
		/oi/ = oi (*boil*)	/z/ = z (*zipper*)
		oy (*boy*)	s (*pansy*)
		/ou/ = ou (*out*)	s (*has*)
		ow (*cow*)	se (*cheese*)

From *Multisensory Teaching of Basic Language Skills, Third Edition* (p. 261).

of spelling choices, students must realize there is a difference between decoding and spelling. When decoding, students look at the printed symbols and translate those graphemes into phonemes. Students have no difficulty reading *gate* because they know that the vowel sound in an *a*-consonant-*e* syllable is pronounced as /ā/.

Table 10.5. Infrequent spellings of vowel sounds

/ă/ = pl<u>ai</u>d, l<u>au</u>gh

/ā/ = r<u>ai</u>n, caf<u>é</u>, st<u>ea</u>k, matin<u>ee</u>, v<u>ei</u>n, <u>eigh</u>t, th<u>ere</u>, th<u>ey</u>, ball<u>et</u>

/au/ = c<u>au</u>ght, br<u>ough</u>t, br<u>oa</u>d

/ĕ/ = h<u>ea</u>d, s<u>ai</u>d, <u>a</u>ny

/ē/ = b<u>ea</u>ch, c<u>ei</u>ling, vall<u>ey</u>, sk<u>i</u>, pr<u>ie</u>st, pet<u>ite</u>

/er/ = doll<u>ar</u>, b<u>ir</u>d, anch<u>or</u>, b<u>ur</u>n, s<u>ear</u>ch, j<u>our</u>nal

/ĭ/ = capt<u>ai</u>n, clim<u>ate</u>, forf<u>ei</u>t, frag<u>ile</u>, g<u>y</u>m

/ī/ = <u>ai</u>sle, k<u>ay</u>ak, h<u>eigh</u>t, t<u>ie</u>, l<u>igh</u>t, n<u>y</u>lon, st<u>yle</u>, d<u>ye</u>, b<u>uy</u>

/ō/ = b<u>eau</u>, b<u>oa</u>t, t<u>oe</u>, d<u>ough</u>

/o͝o/ = p<u>u</u>sh

/o͞o/ = s<u>ou</u>p, d<u>o</u>, sh<u>oe</u>, thr<u>ough</u>, fr<u>ui</u>t

/ou/ = pl<u>ough</u>

/ŭ/ = s<u>o</u>n, bl<u>oo</u>d, t<u>ou</u>ch

/ū/ = b<u>eau</u>ty, <u>Eu</u>rope, n<u>ew</u>

From *Multisensory Teaching of Basic Language Skills, Third Edition* (p. 262).

They can read *bait* because they know that *ai* is pronounced /ā/. Knowing that *eigh* is pronounced /ā/ enables readers to pronounce the word *weight*. All of these words follow frequent, reliable patterns for reading.

Spelling a word starts with sounds, not letter sequences. For spelling, students hear /gāt/, /bāt/, and /wāt/. Except for the initial phonemes, these words sound similar. They all are one-syllable words with medial /ā/ that end in /t/. Students will have little trouble spelling the initial or final sounds, but spelling the medial sounds may be problematic. Without the memory of letter patterns, either because of lack of exposure to print or because of poor orthographic memory, spellers have difficulty knowing whether to use *a*-consonant-*e*, *ai*, or *eigh*. They must be taught that when they hear /ā/ before a final consonant sound, it is most frequently represented with *a*-consonant-*e* (e.g., *cake, insane, equivocate*). With this information, students will be able to spell a high percentage of words with initial or medial /ā/ correctly (Hanna et al., 1966). Not only does their spelling accuracy increase, but also the focus on one spelling establishes that pattern well and actually heightens awareness of other possible spellings of /ā/. If all of the possible spellings of /ā/ are taught at one time, however, then beginning spellers and poor spellers in particular will be overwhelmed with choices. Words such as *bait* and *weight,* which contain less frequent spellings of /ā/, are best learned or memorized as whole words.

Good spellers, who of course are good readers (decoders), begin to weight the frequency of these spellings as they read (Adams, 1990; Foorman, 1994; Lennox & Siegel, 1998; McMurray & McVeigh, 2016; Seidenberg & McClelland, 1989) and are better able to deal with a list that has multiple spellings of one sound. Poor spellers who are poor readers do not receive sufficient exposure to these patterns to weight them. Poor spellers who are good readers do not have adequate sensitivity to letter patterns to determine frequency. The goal of effective spelling instruction is to make the reliability of English orthography obvious to all students by teaching the most frequent, reliable orthographic patterns of English (Post & Carreker, 2002; Post, Carreker, & Holland, 2001).

Morphology

Morphology is the study of morphemes, the smallest units of language that carry meaning (prefixes, suffixes, roots, and combining forms; see Chapters 9 and 14 for more information on morphemes). Morphemic knowledge advances students from the spelling of one-syllable base words to the spelling of one-syllable base words with suffixes and eventually to the spelling of other derivatives (i.e., a base word plus one or more affixes) and multisyllabic words. Knowing suffixes and inflectional morphemes signals to students that /pĭnz/ contains two morphemes or meaningful units: the base word /pĭn/ and the suffix /z/, which makes the word plural; therefore, /z/ is spelled *s* not *z*. Without understanding suffixes and inflectional morphemes, students remain literal in their spellings and write /jŭmpt/ as *jumpt* and /băngd/ as *bangd* because that is what they hear. The understanding that a suffix that begins with a consonant is a consonant suffix and a suffix that begins with a vowel is vowel suffix helps students when they add suffixes to base words to spell derivatives. The final letter of a base word may be doubled or dropped, but this is true only when adding a vowel suffix (e.g., *starring* but not *starrless, hoping* but not *hopful*).

Knowing prefixes and roots facilitates students' spelling of multisyllabic words (Adams, 1990; Brady & Moats, 1997; Henry, 1988). For example, the word *attraction* contains three morphemes. These morphemes serve not only as meaning-filled units but also as spelling units. The word *attraction* can be spelled in chunks instead of sound by sound. Knowing that some consonant prefixes change their spellings for **euphony** (i.e., to ease pronunciation; see Table 10.6), students know to spell a word such as *attraction* with two *t*'s because the *at-* in *attraction* represents a spelling deviation of the prefix *ad-*. The prefix changes the final letter to match the initial letter of the root *tract*. With knowledge of morphology, students can clarify spelling choices and contend with more complex levels of orthography.

Word Origins

Chapter 14 outlines the Anglo-Saxon, Latin, and Greek layers of language in English (see also Henry, 2010). These languages and others have shaped the orthography of English, as evidenced in the spelling of /sh/. Fourteen different spellings

Table 10.6.   Prefixes that change spelling for euphony

Prefix	Prefix changed for euphony
ab-	a-, abs-
ad-	a-, ac-, af-, ag-, al-, an-, ap-, ar-, as-, at-
con-	co-, col-, com-, cor-
en-	em-
ex-	e-, ec-, ef-
in-	il-, im-, ir-
ob-	oc-, of-, op-
sub-	suc-, suf-, sup-, sur-, sus-

From *Multisensory Teaching of Basic Language Skills, Third Edition* (p. 263).

have been noted in English (Bryson, 1990): *sh* as in *ship*; *ch* as in *chef*; *ti* as in *nation*; *si* as in *discussion*; *ci* as in *special*; *xi* as in *anxious*; *sci* as in *conscious*; *sch* as in *schnauzer*; *ce* as in *ocean*; *se* as in *nauseous*; *s* as in *sugar*; *ss* as in *tissue*; *psh* as in *pshaw*; and *chsi* as in *fuchsia*. These spellings represent different layers of language within English: *sh* from Anglo-Saxon; *ch* from French; *ti, ci, si, xi,* and *sci* from Latin; *sch* from German; *ce* from Greek; and *chsi* after German botanist Fuchs. The layers of other languages make English a rich tapestry of words, but they create a confusing orthography, thus compounding the difficulties poor spellers have with spelling. It would seem logical to change orthography to make it less confusing and to make words easier to spell.

There have been attempts to reform English orthography but to no avail. Benjamin Franklin proposed a phonetic alphabet with a better one-to-one letter–sound correspondence, which in the end did not gain much favor. Noah Webster, who advocated educational reform and America's own form of spelling to complement its unique form of government, proposed changes such as *bred* for *bread, laf* for *laugh,* and *crum* for *crumb.* Although these changes were not accepted, Webster was successful in changing the spellings of words such as *honour* to *honor, centre* to *center,* and *publick* to *public.* The American Philological Association, an organization dedicated to spelling reform, made concerted efforts to change the orthography of English in the late 1800s and early 1900s but had little success. In the 1930s, *The Chicago Tribune,* in an effort to increase readership by making words easier to read, used these spellings in their newspaper: *thru, tho,* and *thoro* (Venezky, 1980). Although it seems reasonable to simplify and unify orthography, such attempts have failed. Perhaps this is because changing the orthography of English would mask its rich, interesting history and the interrelatedness of words (e.g., *muscle* is related to *muscular,* which accounts for the silent *c* in *muscle; sign* is related to *signature,* which accounts for the silent *g;* see Henry, 2010).

Rather than bemoan the inconsistencies of English, students can take advantage of information about word origins to refine their spelling knowledge. For example, initially, students are taught that the most frequent, though not the only, spelling of /f/ is *f.* This information serves them well for spelling most words. Knowing that long, scientific terms are usually of Greek origin and that Greek words containing /f/ are spelled with *ph,* students have information that will help them to spell words such as *chlorophyll* and *photosynthesis.* Students will also note that words of Greek origin containing /k/ are often spelled with *ch* and those containing /ĭ/ are often spelled with *y.* Students who know word origins come to understand why some words are spelled in unexpected ways, and, more important, students can determine the appropriate spellings for these words. (See Henry, 1988, 2010, for more on spellings according to word origin.)

REFLECT, CONNECT, and RESPOND
Why is the orthography of English not hopelessly irregular for spelling?

HOW SPELLING ERRORS INFORM INSTRUCTION

Spelling is a skill that must be formally taught (Graham & Santangelo, 2014; McMurray & McVeigh, 2016). Using invented spelling in preschool and kindergarten should be encouraged and supported with phonological awareness training

(Blachman, Ball, Black, & Tangel, 1994, 2000; Castle, Riach, & Nicholson, 1994; Rubin & Eberhardt, 1996). (See Chapter 4 and 6 for activities that can be incorporated into the classroom routine; see also Adams, Foorman, Lundberg, & Beeler, 1998.) By using invented spelling, students learn the essence of spelling—translating sounds to symbols. Good spelling, however, requires more than translating sounds to symbols; it also demands a sensitivity to letter patterns in words. Although invented spelling reinforces sound–symbol correspondences, it does not provide the correct models that students need to build orthographic knowledge. Learning the patterns and rules cannot be left to chance. Correct spelling has a direct impact on students' reading proficiency (Adams, 1990).

Students' spelling errors provide teachers with insights as to the progress of students' understanding of the patterns of the language. Going beyond right and wrong gives teachers an idea of what students know and do not know (Joshi, 1995). As Joshi and Carreker stated,

> The dualist and finite assessment of spelling words as *right* or *wrong* is counter to the nature of spelling development and masks the predictable progression of spelling development. As previously mentioned, spelling proficiency unfolds in a gradual sequence. The progression of the sequence relies on specific underlying phonological and orthographic knowledge that is ultimately consolidated to form conventional spellings. (2009, p. 117)

In addition, scoring spelling words as right or wrong does not give students credit for the spelling patterns they have learned. For example, the spellings of *celebrate* as *selebrate* and *salaprat* are both incorrect and not acceptable as final representations. The student who spells *celebrate* as *selebrate,* however, has greater knowledge of spelling patterns than the student who spells *celebrate* as *salaprat.* Some acknowledgment should be given for what students know about spelling, and the types of spelling errors students make inform instructional decisions.

The IDA (2018) *Knowledge and Practice Standards* suggest that teachers analyze a student's spelling errors to determine if they indicate difficulties with phonological skills versus learning spelling rules versus application of orthographic or morphemic knowledge in spelling. In a study of pre-service and in-service teachers, Carreker, Joshi, and Boulware-Gooden (2010) found that teachers with greater knowledge of language structures were better able to identify the underlying causes of student spelling errors and choose the most appropriate instructional activities. Rubrics can be developed to assist teachers in evaluating a student's spelling knowledge qualitatively. Is this student detecting all the sounds in a word and can he or she accurately discriminate those sounds? Is this student employing conventional patterns and rules? Answering these questions will inform and guide instruction.

Textbox 10.1 presents a sample rubric, with scores from 0 to 5, used to evaluate students' spelling knowledge based on the errors they make. The teacher analyzes students' spelling errors on tests or in daily written work and assigns a score to each error. (A score of 5 is a correct spelling.) The score is an approximation. There is no right or wrong score. The idea is to try to assess what the student knows and needs to know. To do so, the teacher looks at the preponderance of errors, determines the underlying difficulties that are causing students' spelling errors, and decides what instructional activities would best remediate the difficulties.

TEXTBOX 10.1   Sample rubric for qualitative evaluation of spelling errors

0 = Not all sounds are represented (*tk* or *thk* for *thick*).

1 = All sounds are marked, but two or more letters are not reasonable representations of the sounds or extra letters are added (*tig* or *fek* for *thick*; *tickgt* or *thiegk* for *thick*).

2 = All sounds are marked, but one letter is not a reasonable representation of a sound; no extra letters are added (*tik* or *thek* for *thick*).

3 = All sounds are marked with reasonable representations (*thik* or *thic* for *thick*).

4 = The spelling is almost conventional, but a letter is added or doubled (*thicke* or *thickk* for *thick*).

5 = Correct spelling.

———————

From *Multisensory Teaching of Basic Language Skills, Third Edition* (p. 288).

The following sections give examples of errors that would receive a rubric score of 0–4, along with recommendations for how a teacher could instruct a student making these kinds of errors.

Rubric Score of 0

The following are examples of errors assigned a 0 score:

ot for *want*

wt for *want*

wot for *want*

b for *bake*

bk for *bake*

kb for *bake*

By using the rubric presented in Textbox 10.1, a teacher could determine that a student whose errors are consistently scored as 0 would benefit from additional training in phonemic awareness to increase his or her ability to detect all the sounds in a word. The importance of phonemic awareness in learning to read and spell has been well documented (Adams, 1990; Bradley & Bryant, 1983; Goswami & Bryant, 1990; Liberman, Shankweiler, & Liberman, 1989). Spelling begins with the speller's awareness that spoken words are made up of sounds that are represented in print by letters. For the speller to represent those sounds in print accurately, he or she must be able to detect the number of sounds correctly and discriminate them clearly.

Activities that promote phonological awareness, especially phonemic aware-ness, are outlined in Chapter 6 and must be included in beginning reading and spelling instruction. As students prepare to spell words, they need to engage in activities that promote the detection and discrimination of specific sounds in words. The following activities can be used:

- *To heighten sensitivity to the position of a particular sound in a word*: The teacher says a word and asks students to listen for the position of a particular sound in the word. Students repeat the word, listening for the position of the sound. Students indicate the position: initial, medial, or final (see Chapter 5 for activi-ties that explore the concepts initial, medial, and final).

- *To heighten sensitivity to a particular sound in a word*: The teacher says a word and asks the student to listen for a certain sound. The students repeat the word, listening for the sound. If they hear the sound, then they say the sound. If they do not hear the sound, then they say "no."

- *To promote the detection of sounds*: The teacher says a word and asks the students to repeat the word and then say each sound in the word while moving one tile or block for each sound in the word. The students can progress to tiles with letters.

- *To promote spelling by analogy* (Goswami, 1988; Nation & Hulme, 1998): The teacher says a word, and students repeat it. The teacher tells students to change a sound (not a letter name) in the word and to pronounce the new word (e.g., change /s/ in *sat* to /m/ and pronounce the new word, change /t/ in *bat* to /g/ and pronounce the new word).

Rubric Scores of 1 or 2

The following are examples of errors assigned a score of 1 or 2:

uonlt for *want* (1)

wund for *want* (1)

wuant for *want* (1)

canp for *camp* (2)

camb for *camp* (2)

kanp for *camp* (2)

A student with scores of 1 because of the extraneous addition of a letter or letters would benefit from using letter tiles to count the exact number of the sounds in a word. Scores of 1 without additional letters and scores of 2 suggest that although the student perceives the individual speech sounds in words, he or she would benefit from activities that help him or her discriminate similar sounds, such as /ĕ/ and /ĭ/ or /f/ and /th/. Using a mirror can help the students "see" and hear the differences in sounds, such as /ĕ/ and /ĭ/ or /m/ and /n/. To assist students who have difficulties with sounds such as /t/ and /d/ or /s/ and /z/, it is helpful for the student to describe whether the vocal cords vibrate or do not vibrate when a sound is produced. Tables 10.1, 10.2, and 10.3 are resources for describing how sounds look and feel.

Rubric Score of 3

The following are examples of errors assigned a score of 3:

mach for *match*

bak for *back*

brige for *bridge*

fluf for *fluff*

hiting for *hitting*

rakeing for *raking*

A student whose scores are mostly 3s is detecting individual sounds in words accurately and is spelling the words in a reasonable manner. His or her spelling is phonetic. This student would benefit from instruction in a specific spelling pattern, such as final /ch/ after a short vowel in a one-syllable base word is spelled *tch* as in *match* or *itch*, or a specific rule, such as dropping final *e* before adding a vowel suffix as in *raking* or *biked*.

Sounds With Multiple Spelling Patterns

The student who spells *match* as *mach* would receive a score of 3 on the rubric. The student has detected all the sounds in the word and has attached reasonable spellings to each sound but has not spelled the final /ch/ in the conventional way. Because one spelling pattern may not seem overwhelmingly apparent as the best choice, students need to be taught generalizations about the use and frequency of letter patterns in English (Cox, 1977; Post & Carreker, 2002; Post et al., 2001).

When there is more than one spelling pattern for a sound, the best choice of the pattern is based on the frequency of the pattern and the situation of the sound in a word. The situation of the sound (i.e., the particular circumstances of how a sound occurs in a word) may be based on the position of the sound in a word, the placement of accent, the length of the word, the influence of surrounding sounds, or a combination of these factors. Awareness of sounds and syllables in words is important in determining the best choice of spelling patterns. (See Chapters 5 and 9 for activities that promote awareness of accent and Chapter 9 for activities that promote awareness of syllables.) The terms introduced in decoding to express the positions of letters in words—*initial, medial,* and *final*—are also used to describe the positions of sounds in words. *Initial* refers to the first position in a syllable. *Final* refers to the last position in a syllable. *Medial* refers to any position between the first and last positions.

Students need not guess or give up when dealing with the sounds that have more than one frequent spelling pattern. Instead, they consider the situation of the sound that may be represented by more than one spelling. The situation provides clues that will help students in their decision-making process. For example, in considering the spelling of /măch/, students think about possible, frequent spellings of /ch/ (*ch* or *tch*). To decide which spelling is the best choice, students determine the situation of the sound in the word. The sound is in the final position of a one-syllable word, and it comes after a short vowel. On the basis of this situation, students know that *tch* is the best choice for spelling /ch/ in the word *match*. The following examples of spelling patterns show the best choices for spelling sounds according to their situations.

Spelling Choices With Situations Based on Position The sounds /oi/ and /ou/ are examples of sounds whose spelling depends on the sound's position within the word, as described next.

1. When is /oi/ spelled *oi*, and when is it spelled *oy?*

oil	*boy*
ointment	*toy*
boil	*joy*
coin	*enjoy*
joint	*employ*
In initial or medial position, /oi/ is spelled *oi*.	In final position, /oi/ is spelled *oy*. (A less frequent but reliable spelling choice for /oi/ at the end of a syllable is *oy* as in *royal* or *voyage*.)

2. When is /ou/ spelled *ou*, and when is it spelled *ow?*

out	*cow*
ouch	*how*
found	*plow*
shout	*meow*
ground	
In initial or medial position, /ou/ is spelled *ou*.	In final position, /ou/ is spelled *ow*.

(Less frequent but reliable spelling choices that could be introduced later as refinement include the following: /ou/ is spelled *ow* in a one-syllable word before final /l/ or /n/ *owl* or *down*, and /ou/ is spelled *ow* before /er/ as in *shower* or *flower*.)

Spelling Choices With Situations Based on Surrounding Sounds or Letters The sounds /k/ and /j/ are examples of sounds whose spelling in a word depends on the surrounding sounds or letters, as described next.

1. When is /k/ spelled *k*, and when is it spelled *c?*

keep	*cat*
kit	*cost*
sky	*cup*
Before any sound represented by e, i, or y, /k/ is spelled k.	*clasp*
	cramp
	Before everything else, /k/ is spelled *c*.

2. When is /j/ spelled *g*, and when is it spelled *j?*

gem	*jam*
giant	*jot*
biology	*just*
Before any sound represented by *e, i,* or *y,* /j/ is spelled *g*.	Before everything else, /j/ is spelled *j*.

Spelling Choices With Situations Based on Position, Length, and Surrounding Sounds The sounds /ch/, /j/, and /k/, when these occur as a word's final sound, are examples of sounds whose spelling depends on position, word length, and the surrounding sounds, as described next.

1. When is final /ch/ spelled *tch,* and when is it spelled *ch?*

catch	*speech*
sketch	*porch*
pitch	*pouch*
blotch	*belch*
dutch	*sandwich*
Final /ch/ in a one-syllable base word after a short vowel is spelled *tch.*	Final /ch/ after two vowels or a consonant or in a word of more than one syllable is spelled *ch.*

2. When is final /j/ spelled *dge?*

badge
edge
ridge
dodge
fudge
Final /j/ in a one-syllable base word after a short vowel is spelled *dge.*

3. When is final /k/ spelled *ck,* and when is it spelled *c?*

back	*picnic*
peck	*music*
sick	*lilac*
block	
stuck	
Final /k/ after a short vowel in a one-syllable word is spelled *ck.*	Final /k/ in a multisyllabic base word after a short vowel is spelled *c.*

Spelling Choices for Vowels   The sounds /ŏ/, /ŭ/, /ā/, /ē/, / ī/, /ō/, and /ū/ are examples of vowel sounds whose spelling depends on the sound's position within a word, the number of syllables in the word and the stress placed on the syllables, and the surrounding sounds, as described next.

1. What are the best choices for spelling /ŏ/?

odd	*want*
hot	*wash*
top	*wand*
lost	*wasp*
spot	*wall*

The sound /ŏ/ is spelled *o,* except after /w/, when /ŏ/ is spelled *a.*

2. What are the best choices for spelling /ŭ/?

up	*alike*
us	*along*
cup	*parade*
rust	*tuba*
shut	*sofa*

The sound /ŭ/ is spelled *u,* except at the end of an unaccented syllable, when /ŭ/ is spelled *a.*

3. What are the best choices for spelling /ā/?

ate	*day*
ape	*say*
made	*play*
insane	*delay*
evaluate	*repay*
Initial or medial /ā/ before a final consonant sound is spelled *a*-consonant-*e*.	Final /ā/ is spelled *ay*.

table
baby
lady
basic
paper
At the end of a syllable, /ā/ is spelled *a*.

4. What are the best spelling choices for /ē/?

eel	*stampede*
feet	*complete*
green	*extreme*
need	*intervene*
Initial or medial /ē/ in a one-syllable word is spelled *ee*.	Before a final consonant sound in a word of two or more syllables, /ē/ is spelled *e*-consonant-*e*.

meter	*bee*	*tardy*
fever	*see*	*sixty*
even	*free*	*ugly*
evil	*three*	*candy*
At the end of a syllable, /ē/ is spelled *e*.	In the final position of a one-syllable word, /ē/ is spelled *ee*.	In the final position of a word with two or more syllables, /ē/ is spelled *y*.

5. What are the best choices for spelling /ī/?

ice	*fly*
five	*try*
recline	*deny*
excite	*reply*
Initial or medial /ī/ before a final consonant sound is spelled *i*-consonant-*e*.	At the end of a word, /ī/ is spelled *y*.

iris
fiber
tiger
lilac
At the end of a syllable, /ī/ is spelled *i*.

6. What are the best ways to spell /ō/?

rope   *show*
home   *slow*
explode   *window*
trombone   *yellow*
Initial or medial /ō/ before a final   Final /ō/ is spelled *ow*.
consonant sound is spelled
o-consonant-*e*.

open
over
robot
polite
At the end of a syllable, /ō/ is spelled *o*.

7. What is the best way to spell /ū/?

use   *sue*
cube   *cue*
infuse   *rescue*
constitute   *continue*
Initial or medial /ū/ before a final   Final /ū/ is spelled *ue*.
consonant sound is spelled
u-consonant-*e*.

unit
tunic
music
tuna
At the end of a syllable, /ū/ is spelled *u*.

Note: When spelling words with /ū/, it may be necessary to overpronounce or to exaggerate the sound as /yo͞o/.

These spelling patterns offer students a way to manage English orthography for spelling. There will be exceptions to these patterns. It is exciting when students discover the exceptions. To find an exception, students must understand the pattern when it is introduced and remember it. They must compare that pattern with words they hold in memory and realize that there are words that share the same sound but have different spelling patterns. That is active reflection about language. An enthusiastic "Good for you! You found a word that doesn't fit the pattern!" from the teacher affirms that students are thinking about language.

The patterns are not to be memorized. The patterns are established in memory through guided discovery introductions, practice, and opportunities to write through spelling dictation and personal writing. The teacher should direct students' attention to spelling patterns as they occur in the reading. The teacher should refrain from describing the patterns as rules. The term *rule* should be reserved for situations in which a letter in a base word is doubled, dropped, or changed.

Major Spelling Rules   Some words are spelled the way they sound, but certain information needs to be considered before the word is written. For example, the student who spells *cried* as *cryed* would receive a score of 3 on the rubric. The student has detected all the sounds in base word *cry* and has correctly spelled the base word. The student also understands that final /d/ in *cried* represents suffix *-ed*. This error suggests that the student needs instruction in when to change the final *y* in a base word to *i*.

There are five major rules that indicate when a letter should be doubled, dropped, or changed. Two of these rules are used for doubling consonants within a base word. The other three major rules deal with spelling derivatives. They involve a change to the spelling of a base word (i.e., a letter is doubled, dropped, or changed) when adding a suffix. All of the rules are introduced through guided discovery teaching procedures.

The five major rules include the Rule for Doubling the Final Consonant (Floss Rule), the Rule for Doubling a Medial Consonant (Rabbit Rule), the Doubling Rule, the Dropping Rule, and the Changing Rule. Each rule has a set of **checkpoints,** or **markers.** These checkpoints signal students that a letter may be doubled, dropped, or changed. All of the salient checkpoints must be present for a letter to be doubled, dropped, or changed.

The Rule for Doubling the Final Consonant (Floss Rule)   Teachers can use the following discovery words and checkpoints for teaching the Floss Rule.

Discovery words:

tiff

tell

toss

puff

doll

pass

staff

hill

mess

In a one-syllable base word after a short vowel, final /f/, /l/, and /s/ are spelled *ff*, *ll*, and *ss*, respectively. When deciding whether to apply this rule, students must think about these checkpoints: 1) one syllable; 2) short vowel; and 3) final /f/, /l/, or /s/. If all three checkpoints are present, then the final consonant is doubled. If any one of the checkpoints is missing, then the final consonant will not be doubled.

Note: The term *floss* is a mnemonic device that reminds students that *f, l,* or *s* will double in a one-syllable base word after a short vowel.

The Rule for Doubling the Medial Consonant (Rabbit Rule)   Teachers can use the following discovery words and checkpoints for teaching the Rabbit Rule.

Discovery words:

sudden

tennis

mitten

pollen

muffin

In a two-syllable base word with one medial consonant sound after a short vowel, the medial consonant is doubled. The three checkpoints for this rule are 1) two syllables, 2) one medial consonant sound, and 3) a short vowel in the first syllable. If all of the checkpoints are present, then the medial consonant is doubled. If any checkpoint is missing, then the medial consonant will not be doubled. When a reader encounters these words in text, the doubled medial consonants indicate to the reader that the first vowel is short.

Note: The term *rabbit* is a mnemonic device that reminds students that a medial consonant doubles in a two-syllable base word after a short vowel.

The Doubling Rule   Teachers can use the following discovery words and checkpoints for teaching the Doubling Rule.

Discovery words:

hop + ed = hopped

star + ing = starring

red + ish = reddish

begin + er = beginner

When a word ends in one vowel and one consonant and the final syllable is accented (all one-syllable words are accented), and a vowel suffix is being added, the final

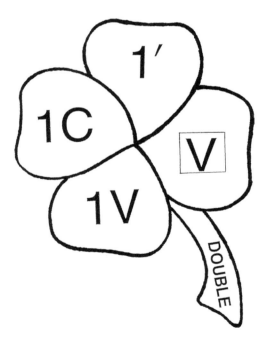

Figure 10.2. Manipulative four-leaf clover indicating checkpoints for the doubling rule: one vowel (1V), one consonant (1C), one accent (1′), and a vowel suffix (a boxed V). When a word has these checkpoints, students add the clover stem, indicating that the final consonant of the base word should be doubled. (From Carreker, S. [2002]. *Scientific spelling* [Rev. ed.; Section 3, p. 7]. Bellaire, TX: Neuhaus Education Center; reprinted by permission.)

consonant is doubled before the suffix is added. There are four checkpoints for consideration: 1) one vowel in the final syllable, 2) one consonant after that vowel, 3) accented final syllable, and 4) a vowel suffix that is being added. If all four checkpoints are present, then the final consonant is doubled. If one checkpoint is missing, then the suffix is just added on. A doubled final consonant before a vowel suffix indicates to the reader that the vowel before the final consonant is short. (For example, in *hopping,* the final consonant is doubled before the vowel suffix and the vowel is short; in *hoping,* the final consonant is not doubled before the vowel suffix and the vowel is long.)

Seven letters in English orthography do not or rarely double. Knowing these seven letters assists students in deciding whether to double a letter. These letters can be taught as a cheer:

h, k

y, j

v, w, x

Never or rarely double in English words.

With this bit of information, students will understand why the *x* in *faxing* or *relaxing* does not double or why the *v* in *river* or *seven* does not double.

The doubling rule is an extremely important rule for students to know for writing, as it is used often in spelling participles and the past tense of verbs. Figure 10.2 (Carreker, 2002) shows a visual aid that students can use to remember the four checkpoints of this rule. The four-leaf clover can be reproduced on green cardstock and cut apart for each student. As students search for the checkpoints in a word, they build the four-leaf clover. If all four leaves of the clover are used, then students are lucky. The stem is added to the clover, and students know they must double the final consonant. If any leaf is missing, then they will not double the final consonant.

The Dropping Rule   Teachers can use the following discovery words and checkpoints for teaching the Dropping Rule.

Discovery words:

bake + er = baker

solve + ed = solved

blue + ish = bluish

house + ing = housing

complete + ed = completed

When a base word ends in *e* and a vowel suffix is being added, the final *e* is dropped before the suffix is added. The two checkpoints are 1) final *e* and 2) a vowel suffix that is being added. If a consonant suffix is being added, then the final *e* is not dropped. As mentioned previously, a single final consonant before a vowel suffix indicates to a reader that the vowel before the final consonant is long.

The Changing Rule   Teachers can use the following discovery words and checkpoints for teaching the Changing Rule.

Discovery words:

try + ed = tried

silly + est = silliest

penny + less = penniless

happy + ness = happiness

When a base word ends in a consonant before a final *y* and a suffix that does not begin with *i* is added, the final *y* changes to *i* before the suffix is added. The checkpoints for this rule are 1) a consonant before a final *y*, 2) final *y*, and 3) a suffix that does not begin with *i*. If the base word has a vowel before the final *y*, then the *y* does not change to *i* (e.g., *boys, enjoying, stayed*). If a suffix that begins with *i* is added, then the *y* does not change to *i* (e.g., *crying, babyish, lobbyist*). The teacher can explain to students that the *y* does not change when adding a suffix that begins with *i* because "two *i*'s are unwise." Of course, when students discover the word *skiing*, the teacher will say, "Good for you!"

Rubric Score of 4

The following are examples of errors assigned a score of 4:

cheeke for *cheek*

golff for *golf*

criyed for *cried*

The student who scores a majority of 4s is aware of spelling patterns, but he or she is overgeneralizing a pattern or rule, such as adding silent *e* when it is not needed or doubling letters that don't need to be doubled. Having the student verbalize a pattern or rule focuses the student's attention on whether a particular pattern or rule is needed. Of course, scores of 5 mean that the student understands and can use knowledge of language structures to spell the words he or she needs: This is the goal of effective spelling instruction.

Irregular Words

Students may make errors when spelling irregular words, as in these examples:

sed for *said*

thot for *thought*

laff for *laugh*

Some words have irregular spellings. The spelling may be unexpected. That is, the orthographic representation does not match its pronunciation (e.g., *should, enough, colonel*). Some irregular spelling words may be **regular words** for reading, but because they contain less frequent representations of sounds, they are classified for spelling as irregular (e.g., *spread, train, teach*). Spelling errors that are related to irregular words suggest that the student does not hold the orthographic images of the words in memory. Each word will need explicit practice to build that orthographic image. Such practice will be described later in this chapter.

SPELLING INSTRUCTION

A meta-analysis by Graham and Santangelo (2014) demonstrated that spelling instruction does improve spelling and, more important, gains in spelling are maintained and generalized over time. This section discusses spelling instruction that targets a specific need, spelling instruction in general classrooms, and spelling instruction for students with dyslexia. In any instruction setting, it is important to remember that spelling is an interactive process that involves phonological and orthographic knowledge (Ehri, 2013, 2014; McMurray & McVeigh, 2016). Spelling instruction enhances this knowledge through synthetic and analytic teaching. Synthetic teaching (i.e., sounds to whole words) systematically builds awareness of sound–letter correspondences and provides a foundation for phonological knowledge and reinforcement of orthographic knowledge. Analytic teaching (i.e., whole words to sounds) builds awareness of letter patterns and provides the foundation for orthographic knowledge and reinforcement of phonological knowledge. Effective lesson planning employs both teaching strategies to provide opportunities for students to develop both phonological and orthographic knowledge.

Small Group Spelling Instruction

The use of a rubric, such as the one presented in Textbox 10.1, can help to identify areas that are consistently interfering with a student's spelling proficiency. Small group instruction targets a need, whether that need is in developing phonological skills, learning a spelling pattern or rule, or applying orthographic or morphemic knowledge to spelling. The idea of small group instruction is informed by student errors. This instruction is focused on students' needs, involves explicit instruction with practice, and is necessary only until the students demonstrate mastery of a skill, a pattern, or a rule and the application of the skill or knowledge.

Whole Group Spelling Instruction

Spelling instruction that requires the copying of words or the memorization of lists is dull and uninspiring. Spelling instruction that engages all students in active, reflective thought about language is exciting. The goal of spelling instruction is to teach the reliable patterns and rules of English for spelling, thereby creating enthusiasm for language. Effective spelling instruction provides students with meaningful lists of words they will use in their academic work.

The following weekly lesson plan for whole group instruction systematically teaches the patterns and rules of English for spelling and provides opportunities for students to generalize and apply this information. The plan allows for modification to meet the needs of students with dyslexia in the general classroom.

Monday (15 minutes). A new spelling pattern (e.g., initial or medial /ou/ is spelled *ou*) or rule is introduced through multisensory guided discovery teaching. Students spell five to seven words with the new pattern or rule. This synthetic teaching ensures that students are systematically learning information about the structure of language for spelling. The words that students practice on Monday become the first words of the weekly spelling list.

Tuesday (15–20 minutes). The rest of the words for the weekly spelling list come from the content area (e.g., words from a map skills unit in social studies). The number of words presented depends on the ages or the needs of the students. Because

Table 10.7. Weekly spelling list with five discovery words from the Monday lesson and 10 words from content areas

Regular	Rule	Irregular
found	mapping	ocean
mouth		country
ouch		east
count		
shout		
north		
south		
west		
globe		
river*		
continent		

*Note that the inclusion of *river* shows an example of how *v* usually is not doubled in English.

From *Multisensory Teaching of Basic Language Skills, Third Edition* (p. 286).

the words are selected from the content area, students will need to know and use them. The need for and use of the words increases the likelihood that students will learn them. Arbitrary lists of words from published spelling series seldom present words commensurate with students' classwork.

Students must analyze the words on the weekly spelling list and decide whether the words are regular words, **rule words,** or irregular words. To be successful with analyzing, students must disengage from what they have learned about decoding. It is true that they will be able to read a word such as *east,* but for spelling purposes, it is considered irregular because *ea* is not the most frequent spelling of /ē/ in initial or medial position of a one-syllable base word. Words such as *eel* or *street* follow the frequent, reliable patterns of the language and would be analyzed as regular words.

The Tuesday lesson provides analytic teaching that ensures that students will look carefully at words to notice how they are spelled. It helps them generalize the patterns and rules students have learned. It engages students in active reflective thought about language. Students cannot decide the category of a word without thinking about all of the aspects of the word.

When students have finished analyzing and sorting the words, they have strategies for learning them. Table 10.7 presents an example of a spelling list that has been analyzed. The regular words are spelled just the way the words sound and can be sounded out. The rule words can be sounded out, but students must remember there is a letter that must be doubled, dropped, or changed before the students write each word. Irregular words have unexpected spellings. The words cannot be sounded out and must be memorized. No more than three or four irregular words should be included in the Tuesday lesson.

The weekly spelling list is easily modified for students with dyslexia in the classroom. Rather than require these students to learn all of the words in the list, the teacher may ask them to be responsible for only the discovery words from the

Monday lesson (e.g., all of the words with medial /ou/ spelled *ou*), or if students are ready, the teacher may ask them to be responsible for all of the regular words in the weekly list.

Wednesday (15 minutes). Students practice the irregular words that were sorted in the Tuesday lesson. Students decide the best way to learn them: using the irregular word procedure, a mnemonic device, or a spelling-based pronunciation. If time permits, students use the dictionary to determine why each word is irregular: 1) the words are from Anglo-Saxon; 2) the words are borrowed from another language; 3) the words are slang or an abbreviated form of a word; 4) the words are borrowed from a proper name; or 5) the words are spelled that way "just because," with no apparent reason listed in the dictionary.

Thursday (15 minutes). The teacher uses the spelling words in various phonological awareness activities segmenting words into sounds, counting syllables, omitting syllables, and changing sounds in words. Students also practice words through word or sentence dictation.

Friday (15 minutes). Throughout the week, students have had the opportunity to analyze, play with, read, and write the spelling words. On Friday, students are tested on the words through word and/or sentence dictation.

Spelling Instruction for Students With Dyslexia

Teaching students with dyslexia to spell is a long, tedious process that requires careful lesson planning. The teacher must plan for success because success builds confidence, and confidence builds independence. Students with dyslexia need spelling instruction that is closely integrated with reading instruction. Because of the exacting demands of spelling on students' complete and accurate recall of letter patterns, students with dyslexia need to spell words with sounds and patterns that have previously been introduced for reading and practiced. Reading words before spelling them heightens students' awareness of orthographic patterns. The number and choices of activities for a spelling lesson will depend on the readiness and needs of the student or students. The teacher will want to plan a rotation of activities that ensures that all areas of spelling are covered regularly. The teacher also will want to discuss the meanings and usages of spelling words to ensure that all of the different layers of language structure are covered in a lesson.

Spelling instruction will most likely need to address phonological processing because it is the primary deficit of students with dyslexia. Without phonemic awareness, students with dyslexia will not be able to develop facility in reading or spelling. Spelling instruction for students with dyslexia should initially build phonemic awareness. Students should engage in activities that require segmenting words into sounds. As students prepare to spell words, they need to engage in activities that heighten the recognition or discrimination of specific sounds, such as listening for a specific sound in a word or listening for the position of a specific sound in a word. After letter–sound correspondences have been introduced for reading, they can be introduced for spelling. These spelling associations are reviewed daily using a sound or spelling deck. Students spell words and derivatives with regular spellings using these sounds. New spelling patterns or rules are introduced as needed. As described in previous sections, multisensory structured guided discovery teaching is used to introduce the new pattern or rule.

When students are ready, the lesson plan is extended. Students begin dictation practice, first with phrases and then with sentences. High-frequency irregular words can be introduced as needed, and students can use the irregular word procedure discussed previously. Analyzing and sorting activities focus students' attention on letter patterns in words, reinforce letter–sound correspondences, and help students generalize patterns and rules. Students can analyze and sort words written on individual index cards by sounds or letter patterns. As they gain greater knowledge of letter patterns, they may analyze and sort words as regular words, rule words, or irregular words. Students can compile a spelling notebook in which they record information about spelling. The notebooks could contain a section for spelling patterns, with one page for each speech sound as illustrated in Figure 10.3. The reliable patterns for each sound are delineated on the pages. Students write words that follow each pattern as well as exceptions to the patterns on each page as the sound and spelling(s) are taught. Students may also have a section for rule words, with one page for each rule, and a section for irregular words, with one page for each letter of the alphabet so that irregular words can be recorded on the pages by first letter. Students may record information in their spelling notebooks once a week during a spelling lesson. On other days, students may simply read information from the notebooks as a means of reviewing spelling information.

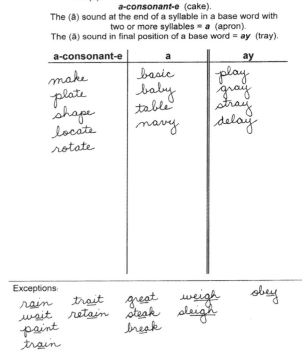

Figure 10.3. Spelling notebook page. This page reviews the most frequent spelling patterns of /ā/. The teacher dictates words that follow these patterns. Students write the words in the correct columns. Words with less frequent patterns that students find as they are reading are written at the bottom of the page. These words are not dictated. (From Carreker, S. [2002]. *Scientific spelling* [Rev. ed.; Student Notebook, p. 2]. Bellaire, TX: Neuhaus Education Center.)

REFLECT, CONNECT, and RESPOND
In what ways do spelling errors inform spelling instruction?

Initial Lesson Plan for Spelling   Teachers can include these activities within an initial lesson plan for spelling: phonological awareness activities, sound dictation, word dictation, and introduction of a new spelling concept.

1. Phonological awareness activities

   The teacher chooses one or two of the following activities:

   - Students repeat words dictated by the teacher and listen for a specific sound.

   - Students repeat words dictated by the teacher and identify the position of a specific sound.

   - Students repeat and segment words dictated by the teacher.

   - Students repeat words dictated by the teacher and change a sound in a word as designated by the teacher to create a new word.

2. Sound dictation

   - The teacher dictates the sounds one at a time.

   - Students echo the sounds, then name and write the letter or letters that spell each sound. (A mirror is available for students who are unable to discriminate the sounds.)

   - The teacher cues students with a key word if they cannot remember the spelling.

   - Each day, the teacher varies the media for the response (e.g., unlined paper, chalkboard, desktop).

3. Word dictation

   - Before students spell words, the teacher reviews the patterns or rules that are germane to the practice session.

   - The teacher dictates the words (as few as 3–4 and no more than 10–12). The words should be homogeneous when students are practicing a new spelling concept and then heterogeneous when students demonstrate mastery of the concept. The teacher should be careful to plan a lesson rotation that includes the spelling of regular words on one day and the spelling of rule words on another day.

   - The teacher provides immediate corrective feedback as needed.

4. Introduction of new spelling concept (synthetic teaching)

   - The teacher introduces a new spelling pattern or rule following a sequential, cumulative order that allows time for concepts to be practiced to mastery.

   - After the new pattern or rule has been introduced, students apply the concept by spelling three to five words with the pattern or rule.

Extended Lesson Plan for Spelling   This extended lesson plan for spelling includes the four activities of the initial lesson plan plus three additional activities. The word dictation activity is expanded to include the dictation of phrases and simple sentences.

1. Phonological awareness activities

2. Sound dictation

3. Word dictation and/or sentence dictation

4. Introduction of a new spelling concept (synthetic teaching)

5. Introduction of a high-frequency irregular word

6. Analyzing or sorting spelling words (analytic teaching)

7. Use of a spelling notebook

Strategies and Techniques for Spelling Instruction

There is not one single method that is best for teaching spelling. Different strategies and techniques such as dialogues, focused practice, and procedures can enhance teaching and learning. Student needs and abilities will dictate which of these teaching strategies or techniques may be most useful.

Procedure for Introducing a Spelling Pattern   The patterns of spelling can be introduced using a guided discovery teaching procedure. The guided discovery teaching procedure uses a Socratic method in which the teacher asks questions to lead students to discover a new spelling pattern. This procedure heightens students' awareness of sounds in words; encourages students to think about how sounds are represented in words; and gives students the opportunity to notice letters in words, thereby heightening their sensitivity to letter patterns.

1. Auditory discovery. The teacher reads five to seven discovery words, which contain the same sound and spelling pattern, one by one. Students repeat each word after the teacher. Students discover the sound that is the same in all of the discovery words and the position(s) of the sound. It is helpful for students to look in small mirrors as they repeat the words. The visual display on the mouth helps students discriminate the sound. Attention to the kinesthetic feel of the mouth also helps students discriminate the sound. **Auditory discovery** heightens students' awareness of a particular sound in words.

2. Prediction. After students have discovered the sound, they predict how the sound might be spelled. The sound students are discovering has been previously introduced for reading. This step encourages students to reflect on their language knowledge.

3. Visual discovery. After students have made their predictions, the teacher writes the discovery words on the board. Students carefully look at all of the words and decide which letter or letters are the same and where the letter or letters are located in the words. They also notice any other common features about the words, such as number of syllables, accent, or surrounding sounds. This step heightens awareness of letter patterns.

4. Verbalization of the pattern. With the discovery of the sound and its spelling, students verbalize the pattern (e.g., final /k/ after a short vowel in a one-syllable word is spelled *ck*) in their own words. Students then apply this information by spelling five to seven new words with the pattern.

Dialogue for Introducing a Spelling Pattern   The following dialogue illustrates how a teacher can introduce a spelling pattern to students.

TEACHER: Listen as I read some words. I want you to repeat each word after me. Listen for the sound that is the same in all of the words. *[The teacher reads the words* pick, sack, luck, clock, *and* peck *one at a time as students repeat.]* What sound (not letter name) do you hear in all of the words?

STUDENTS: /k/

TEACHER: Where do you hear the sound? In what position(s)?

STUDENTS: The sound is in the final position.

TEACHER: Make a prediction about how this sound might be spelled. Think about what you know about the language. How might this sound be spelled? *[Students might predict* c, k, *or* ck.*]* Watch carefully as I write the discovery words on the board. What letter or letters are the same?

STUDENTS: All of the words have the letters *ck*.

TEACHER: In what position(s) do you see the letters?

STUDENTS: The letters *ck* are in final position.

TEACHER: Is there anything else that is similar about these words?

STUDENTS: All of the words have short vowel sounds and have one syllable.

TEACHER: What does the pattern seem to be?

STUDENTS: Final /k/ after a short vowel in a one-syllable word is spelled *ck*.

TEACHER: I want you to apply what you have discovered. I will dictate some words for you to spell.

Focused Practice of Sounds and Patterns   The following activities can be used to provide students with focused practice.

Sound Dictation   Daily review with a sound or spelling deck (**sound dictation**) develops automaticity in translating sounds to spellings (Cox, 1992). Each introduced sound is written on a separate index card. The sounds are represented by letters with appropriate diacritical markings that are enclosed in parentheses or slash marks, such as (ā) or /ā/. The possible spellings of the sound are written on each card. Key words that unlock the spellings of each sound are also written on the cards. While looking at a card that is not shown to the students, the teacher dictates the sound written on the card. Students repeat the sound and name the letter or letters that spell the sound as they write them. If students hesitate about the spelling of a sound, the teacher cues students with the appropriate key word.

When students are spelling sounds with multiple spellings, they repeat the sound and name and write the frequent, reliable spelling choices. For example, if the teacher dictates /ā/, students repeat /ā/ and say, "*a*-consonant-*e, a;* final, *ay.*" In this abbreviated response, the best spelling choices for /ā/ are recognized. Students write this information in shorthand: *a-e, a // ay*. The double slash marks (//) define the spellings according to their positions in words. Everything to the left of the slash marks represents possible spellings of a sound in initial or medial position. Everything to the right represents possible spellings of a sound in final position.

The media that students use to write their responses can be varied daily to provide different kinesthetic reinforcement. Students may write responses on unlined paper, on the chalkboard, on their desktops, on carpet squares, or in salt trays.

Word Dictation　　As each new spelling pattern is introduced, it is practiced to mastery first by using homogenous practice sessions in which every word contains the new pattern. When students demonstrate success in spelling the new pattern, heterogeneous practice sessions that contain the new pattern and previously introduced patterns are used. The words used for these practice sessions are not words that students have memorized or will need to memorize. At first, the words for heterogeneous practice should be one-syllable words that progress from two to three sounds to five to six sounds. When students are ready, they start with the spelling of one-syllable base words with suffixes, then move on to multisyllabic words, and finally, to multisyllabic derivatives. Word dictation practices provide review of sounds and patterns and instill a thinking process for spelling.

A structured procedure can be used for word dictation practice to establish this thinking process for spelling. **S.O.S. (Simultaneous Oral Spelling)** was introduced by Gillingham and Stillman (1960) and adapted by Cox (1992; see Figure 10.4). The steps and rationale are as follows:

1. Look and listen. Students look at the teacher and focus on his or her mouth as he or she dictates the word. By focusing on the teacher's mouth, students use the visual display to clarify the sounds in the dictated word. For example, /f/ will be

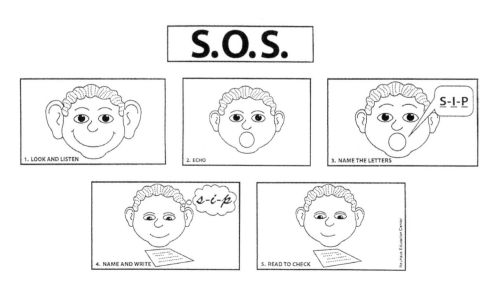

Figure 10.4. Simultaneous Oral Spelling (S.O.S.) procedure. 1) Look and listen, 2) repeat (echo) and segment, 3) name the letters, 4) name and write, and 5) read to check. (From Neuhaus Education Center, Bellaire, TX. *Sources:* Cox, 1992; Gillingham & Stillman, 1960. Reprinted with permission.)

visually displayed with the upper teeth resting on the lower lip, whereas /th/ will be displayed with the tip of the tongue protruding between the teeth.

2. Repeat and segment. Students repeat the word while looking in a small mirror. Using a mirror provides visual cues such as the position of the mouth or the placement of the tongue, teeth, or lips. Repeating the word affirms that students heard the word correctly and gives them additional auditory input and kinesthetic feedback. The kinesthetic feedback clarifies the sounds in the dictated word. For example, with /f/, students feel the upper teeth resting on the lower lip, and with /th/, they feel the tip of the tongue protruding through the teeth.

The segmenting part of this step depends on the kind of word students are spelling and the needs of students. Students initially segment monosyllabic words with two to five sounds. Students segment each word into its constituent sounds. They may use their fingers to mark the sounds. They make a fist, and beginning with the thumb of their nonwriting hand (left palm up for right-handers; right palm down for left-handers) and moving in a left-to-right progression, students extend a finger for each sound that they hear as they segment the word. Instead of using their fingers, students may move counters such as blocks, buttons, or pennies for each sound they hear as they segment the word. Students continue spelling monosyllabic words until they can segment words into constituent sounds with ease.

When students can successfully spell monosyllabic words of five sounds, they are ready to spell derivatives and multisyllabic words. A derivative should be orally separated into morphemic units (e.g., /jŭmpt/ is the base word /jŭmp/ plus the suffix /t/). A multisyllabic word should be segmented into its component syllables. Students may use the fingers of their nonwriting hand, blocks, buttons, or pennies to segment the words into morphemic units or syllables.

3. Name the letters. Before writing the word on paper, students spell the word aloud. This is a rehearsal step for writing. The teacher can guide students to the correct spelling before they write. Naming letters impresses letter sequences in memory (Gillingham & Stillman, 1997). If students have segmented the word using their fingers or counters, then they may want to touch each finger or counter as they spell, thereby reinforcing the sound–letter connection and sequence.

4. Name and write. Students write the word while naming the letters (Cox, 1992; Gillingham & Stillman, 1997). The rationale for this step is that naming letters builds the visual sequence of letters in the word through auditory and kinesthetic input. It is important for students to see the word they have spelled orally. If handwriting is not fluent, then students can use plastic letters or letter cards to spell the words, or the teacher could serve as an **amanuensis** by writing for students on paper or on the board. *Note*: Some students may be more inclined to translate sounds immediately into letters without naming the letters, which is certainly acceptable. The aim is to help students develop a procedure that will be most useful to them.

5. Read to check. After students have written the word, they read the word silently, using their decoding information. Knowing syllable types and syllable-division patterns will aid students' accurate reading of the word and confirmation of the spelling (see Chapter 9). It is permissible, and actually desirable, for a student to write a misspelled word without immediate correction by the teacher. This final step is intended to build independence in determining whether a word is spelled correctly. To monitor a large group in a class environment, the teacher may have students read the word aloud together and then touch and name the letters of this word. The teacher gives appropriate corrective feedback as needed.

The S.O.S. procedure provides a structure for teaching students how to think about the process of spelling a word. Instead of impulsively writing a word on paper, students think about the sounds in the word and how those sounds can be spelled. They also impress the letter sequence in memory by naming the letters, monitor the spelling of the word by naming the letters while writing, and check the spelling by reading the word. In the initial stages of spelling instruction with students with dyslexia, it may be necessary to build an understanding and memory of the five steps gradually by breaking the procedure down into smaller parts. Students may begin with Steps 1 and 2. The teacher says the word, and students repeat the word and segment it into its constituent sounds. Students with recalcitrant spelling deficits may require practice with this abbreviated procedure for several days or weeks.

When students are secure with these two steps, Step 3 may be added, in which students spell the word aloud. When these three steps are secure, students can add Steps 4 and 5, with the teacher serving as the amanuensis. When the teacher writes the word, students can better attend to the letter sequence in the word and do not have to worry about the formation of the letters. Students eventually will complete all five steps of the S.O.S. procedure independently.

Procedure for Teaching Irregular Words   Different procedures can be used to establish irregular words in memory. Various mnemonic strategies help students learn words that contain less frequent patterns. A more structured and multisensory procedure (Cox, 1992; Fernald, 1943; Gillingham & Stillman, 1997) is needed to ensure the learning of some irregular words.

The following procedure uses visual, auditory, and kinesthetic input to assist in the permanent memorization of those words with truly atypical spellings. It is an involved but effective procedure that must be directed by the teacher. The efficacy of the procedure depends on students' naming the letters. This naming of letters as students trace or write is more effective than writing or copying words repeatedly because it focuses students' attention on the letter sequence in the word. The steps and rationale for each step follow:

1. Circle the irregular part. The teacher provides students with a large model of the irregular word on a sheet of paper. Students circle the part of the word that does not conform to the frequent, reliable patterns or rules. Analyzing the irregular part engages students in active reflection of the language. Circling the irregular part draws their attention to the letter patterns in the word. Because many irregular words are from Anglo-Saxon or are borrowed from other languages, a discussion of etymology can provide insight into the unexpected spelling of the word. (See Chapter 14 for a discussion of words from Anglo-Saxon, Latin, and Greek.) Over time, students may begin to recognize patterns in irregular words (e.g., words from Anglo-Saxon are short, common, everyday words with the sound /f/ occasionally spelled as *gh* as in *enough* or *laugh*).

2. Trace a model. Students trace the model word three times, saying the word before they write and naming the letters as they write. Tracing the word while naming the letters provides the consummate multisensory experience. The students reinforce the letter sequence in the word through the visual, auditory, and kinesthetic modalities.

3. Make copies. Students make three copies of the word with the model in view, saying the word and naming the letters of the word as they write. This step extends the multisensory impressing of the letter sequence of the word in memory.

4. *Spell the word with eyes closed.* Students close their eyes and spell the word, imagining the word as they spell. They open their eyes and check the model. They close their eyes and spell the word two more times in this manner.

5. *Write from memory.* Students turn their papers over or fold them so that the model does not show. They write the word three times, saying the word before they write and naming the letters of the word as they write. Because students no longer have a model to rely on, they must call on their memory of the letter sequence of the word that was established through the multisensory input.

Other Procedures for Learning Irregular Words   Some irregular words do not require the intensity of the irregular word procedure just outlined. Instead, using exaggerated or spelling-based pronunciation builds a strong orthographic memory of these irregular words (Cox, 1992; Ehri, Wilce, & Taylor, 1987). Silent consonants often mark that a word will be irregular for spelling. When practicing irregular words, students may pronounce the silent *k* in words such as *knee, knife,* and *knock* or the silent *b* in words such as *comb, limb,* and *crumb* so that they will remember to write the silent *k* or *b* when they spell. Students might exaggerate the pronunciation of *i* as /ī/ in *fragile* so that they will remember to spell the word with an *e* at the end.

Schwa is not uniquely represented in English and therefore is difficult to spell. It is best managed by using the exaggerated or spelling-based pronunciation (e.g., students say /rĭbŏn/ instead of /rĭbŭn/) (Ehri et al., 1987). To remember the spellings of certain irregular words, students could use a mnemonic association: "There is *a rat* in *separate*," "The *capitol* has a *dome*," or "The *principal* is your *pal*" (Moats, 1995). Students could group words in whimsical sentences as a mnemonic device to remember the infrequent spelling patterns that words share: "*Which* *rich* people have so *much* money and *such* big houses?" or "I am *ready* to *spread* the *bread*" (Cox, 1992).

Spelling Homophones

Homophones are words that share the same pronunciation but differ in their orthographic representations (e.g., *plane/plain, to/too/two, red/read*). Published spelling series are notorious for presenting lists of homophones for students to learn. Students often find these words difficult to learn. The problem usually is not the spelling of homophones but rather their usage. Students are not sure when to use which spelling. To alleviate this confusion, homophones should not be introduced in pairs. Often, one word in a pair of homophones is regular for spelling (e.g., *plane*) and the other word is not (e.g., *plain*). Students first should be introduced to the homophone with the regular spelling. When students are secure with the spelling of that word and are clear about its usage, the other homophone can be introduced. If both homophones are irregular for spelling (e.g., *there, their*), then the word with the most frequent usage should be introduced first, followed by the other.

REFLECT, CONNECT, and RESPOND
How is the dualist and finite assessment of spelling words as right or wrong counter to the nature of spelling development?

CLOSING THOUGHTS: TEACHING SPELLING

Spelling serves as a foundation for reading; provides a means of communication; and, even if not rightly or fairly, it is used by society to judge one's level of literacy and intelligence. Spelling is a valuable skill, yet it receives a modicum of attention and respect in schools. It has been reduced to mindless busywork or has been subjugated by the content in writing or has become a vestige of literacy instruction. Perhaps this has happened because of the misconception that English orthography is impossibly irregular and that there is no way to teach it, or because of the perception that spelling is a rote, mechanical skill that does not promote cognition, or because the power of spelling is unknown to too many teachers and administrators.

The time has come to view spelling instruction in a different light. The orthography of English is not hopeless (Kessler & Treiman, 2003). There are frequent, reliable patterns and rules that can be taught, which thus equips students with a system for managing the orthography of English for spelling.

Spelling instruction should be deeply ensconced in a rich study of language structures and take place in a manner that promotes active, reflective thought. Spelling instruction does not distract from the content of writing but rather enhances it by enabling students to choose the words that best express their thoughts instead of those words that are easy to spell. Spelling instruction should be informed by student spelling errors that demonstrate what students know and what they need to know. Effective spelling instruction is engaging, thought provoking, and exciting.

ONLINE COMPANION MATERIALS

The following Chapter 10 resources are available at http://www.brookespublishing
.com/birshcarreker/materials::

- Reflect, Connect, and Respond Questions

- Appendix 10.1: Technology Resources

- Appendix 10.2: Knowledge and Skill Assessment Answer Key

- Appendix 10.3a: Test Your Knowledge and Skill Quiz 1, and 10.3b: Answer Key

- Appendix 10.4a: Test Your Knowledge and Skill Quiz 2, and 10.4b: Answer Key

- Appendix 10.5: Small Group Instruction for Phonological Awareness

KNOWLEDGE AND SKILL ASSESSMENT

1. How many phonemes are in the word *extinct*?

   a. Five

   b. Six

   c. Seven

   d. Eight

2. Which spelling error would receive a 3 using the spelling rubric?

   a. *Spint* for *sprint*

   b. *Tardee* for *tardy*

   c. *Teethe* for *teeth*

   d. *Lenon* for *lemon*

3. A student spells the word *typhoon* as *tifoon*. To promote spelling accuracy, the teacher does what?

   a. Has the student check the spelling in the dictionary

   b. Gives the student the correct spelling of the word

   c. Reminds the student that the word is of Greek origin

   d. Suggests a synonym that the student knows how to spell

4. How many words in this sentence follow the most frequent and reliable spelling patterns for a sound with more than one spelling? *Such clever kids kept the kite in the sky.*

   a. Three

   b. Four

   c. Five

   d. Six

5. How many spelling rules are represented in this sentence? *The silly woman was hitting the flies with a hammer.*

   a. Three

   b. Four

   c. Five

   d. Six

REFERENCES

Adams, M.J. (1990). *Beginning to read: Thinking and learning about print.* Cambridge, MA: The MIT Press.

Adams, M.J., Foorman, B.R., Lundberg, I., & Beeler, T. (1998). *Phonemic awareness in young children: A classroom curriculum.* Baltimore, MD: Paul H. Brookes Publishing Co.

Bear, D.R., Invernizzi, M., Templeton, S., & Johnston, F. (1996). *Words their way: Word study for phonics, vocabulary, and spelling instruction.* Upper Saddle River, NJ: Prentice Hall.

Blachman, B.A., Ball, E.W., Black, R., & Tangel, D.M. (1994). Kindergarten teachers develop phoneme awareness in low-income, inner-city classrooms: Does it make a difference? *Reading and Writing: An Interdisciplinary Journal, 6*(1), 1–18.

Blachman, B.A., Ball, E.W., Black, R., & Tangel, D.M. (2000). *Road to the code: A phonological awareness program for young children.* Baltimore, MD: Paul H. Brookes Publishing Co.

Bradley, L., & Bryant, P.E. (1983). Categorizing sounds and learning to read: A causal connection. *Nature, 303,* 419–421.

Brady, S., & Moats, L.C. (1997). *Informed instruction for reading success: Foundations for teacher preparation.* Baltimore, MD: The International Dyslexia Association.

Bryant, P.E., & Bradley, L. (1980). Why children sometimes write words which they do not read. In U. Frith (Ed.), *Cognitive processes in spelling* (pp. 355–370). London, United Kingdom: Academic Press.

Bryant, P.E., Nunes, T., & Bindman, M. (1997). Children's understanding of the connection between grammar and spelling. In B. Blachman (Ed.), *Foundations of reading acquisition and dyslexia: Implications for early intervention* (pp. 219–240). Mahwah, NJ: Lawrence Erlbaum Associates.

Bryson, B. (1990). *The mother tongue and how it got that way.* New York, NY: Avon Books.

Carreker, S. (2002). *Scientific spelling* (Rev. ed.). Bellaire, TX: Neuhaus Education Center.

Carreker, S., Joshi, R.M., & Boulware-Gooden, R. (2010). Spelling-related teacher knowledge and the impact of professional development on identifying appropriate instructional activities. *Learning Disabilities Quarterly, 33,* 148–158.

Cassar, M., & Treiman, R. (1997). The beginnings of orthographic knowledge: Children's knowledge of double letters in words. *Journal of Educational Psychology, 89*(4), 631–644.

Castle, J.M., Riach, J., & Nicholson, T. (1994). Getting off to a better start in reading and spelling: The effects of phonemic awareness instruction within a whole language program. *Journal of Educational Psychology, 86*(3), 350–359.

Cox, A.R. (1977). *Situation spelling: Formulas and equations for spelling the sounds of spoken English.* Cambridge, MA: Educators Publishing Service.

Cox, A.R. (1992). *Foundations for literacy: Structures and techniques for multisensory teaching of basic written English language skills.* Cambridge, MA: Educators Publishing Service.

Ehri, L.C. (2000). Learning to read and learning to spell: Two sides of a coin. *Topics in Learning Disorders, 20,* 19–49.

Ehri, L.C., & Rosenthal, J. (2007). Spellings of words: A neglected facilitator of vocabulary learning. *Journal of Literacy Research, 39,* 389–409.

Ehri, L.C. (2013). Grapheme-phonemic knowledge is essential for learning to read words in English. In J.L. Metsala & L.C. Ehri (Eds.), *Word recognition in beginning literacy* (pp. 3–40). New York, NY: Routledge, Taylor & Francis Group.

Ehri, L.C. (2014). Orthographic mapping in the acquisition of sight word reading, spelling memory, and vocabulary learning. *Scientific Studies of Reading, 18*(1), 5–21.

Ehri, L.C., Wilce, L.S., & Taylor, B.B. (1987). Children's categorization of short vowels in words and the influence of spelling. *Merrill-Palmer Quarterly, 33,* 393–421.

Fernald, G. (1943). *Remedial techniques in basic school subjects.* New York, NY: McGraw-Hill.

Ferreiro, E., & Teberosky, A. (1982). *Literacy before schooling.* Portsmouth, NH: Heinemann.

Foorman, B.R. (1994). The relevance of a connectionist model for reading for "The Great Debate." *Educational Psychology Review, 6,* 25–47.

Frith, U. (1980). Unexpected spelling problems. In U. Frith (Ed.), *Cognitive processes in spelling* (pp. 495–515). London, United Kingdom: Academic Press.

Frith, U., & Frith, C. (1980). Relationships between reading and spelling. In J.P. Kavanagh & R.L. Venezky (Eds.), *Orthography, reading, and dyslexia* (pp. 287–295). Baltimore, MD: University Park Press.

Fulk, B.M., & Stormont-Spurgin, M. (1995). Spelling interventions for students with disabilities: A review. *Journal of Special Education, 28*(4), 488–513.

Gillingham, A., & Stillman, B.W. (1960). *Remedial training for children with specific disability in reading, spelling, and penmanship* (6th ed.). Cambridge, MA: Educators Publishing Service.

Gillingham, A., & Stillman, B.W. (1997). *The Gillingham manual: Remedial training for children with specific disability in reading, writing, and penmanship* (8th ed.). Cambridge, MA: Educators Publishing Service.

Goswami, U. (1988). Children's use of analogy in learning to spell. *British Journal of Developmental Psychology, 6,* 21–23.

Goswami, U., & Bryant, P. (1990). *Phonological skills and learning to read.* Mahwah, NJ: Lawrence Erlbaum Associates.

Graham, S., & Santangelo, T. (2014). Does spelling instruction make students better spellers, readers, and writers? A meta-analytic review. *Reading and Writing, 23*(9), 1703–1743.

Hanna, P.R., Hanna, J.S., Hodges, R.E., & Rudorf, E.H. (1966). *Phoneme–grapheme correspondences as cues to spelling improvement.* Washington, DC: U.S. Government Printing Office.

Henry, M. (1988). Beyond phonics: Integrating decoding and spelling instruction based on word origin and structure. *Annals of Dyslexia, 38,* 259–277.

Henry, M.K. (2010). *Unlocking literacy: Effective decoding and spelling instruction* (2nd ed.). Baltimore, MD: Paul H. Brookes Publishing Co.

Holmes, V.M., Malone, A.M., & Redenbach, H. (2008). Orthographic processing and visual sequential memory in unexpectedly poor spellers. *Journal of Research in Reading, 31,* 136–156. doi:10.1111/j.1467-9817.2007.00364.x

International Dyslexia Association, The. (2018, March). *Knowledge and practice standards for teachers of reading.* Retrieved from https://dyslexiaida.org/knowledge-and-practices/

Joshi, R.M. (1995). Assessing reading and spelling skills. *School Psychology Review, 24,* 361–375.

Joshi, R.M., & Carreker, S. (2009). Spelling: Development, assessment, and instruction. In G. Reid (Ed.), *Routledge companion to dyslexia* (pp. 113–125). London, United Kingdom: Routledge.

Joshi, R.M., Treiman, R., Carreker, S., & Moats, L.C. (2008/2009). How words cast their spell: Spelling instruction focused on language, not memory, improves reading and writing. *American Educator, 32*(4), 6–16, 42–43.

Kessler, B., & Treiman, R. (2003). Is English spelling chaotic? Misconceptions concerning its irregularity. *Reading Psychology, 24,* 267–289.

Lennox, C., & Siegel, L.S. (1996). The development of phonological rules and visual strategies in average and poor spellers. *Journal of Experimental Child Psychology, 62,* 60–83.

Lennox, C., & Siegel, L.S. (1998). Phonological and orthographic processes in good and poor spellers. In C. Hulme & R.M. Joshi (Eds.), *Reading and spelling development and disorders* (pp. 395–404). Mahwah, NJ: Lawrence Erlbaum Associates.

Liberman, I.Y., Shankweiler, D., & Liberman, A.M. (1989). The alphabetic principle and learning to read. In D. Shankweiler & I.Y. Liberman (Eds.), *Phonology and reading disabilities: Solving the reading puzzle* (pp. 1–33). Ann Arbor: University of Michigan Press.

Lyon, G.R., Shaywitz, S.E., & Shaywitz, B.A. (2003). A definition of dyslexia. *Annals of Dyslexia, 53,* 1–14.

McMurray, S., & McVeigh, C. (2016). The case for frequency sensitivity in orthographic learning. *Journal of Research in Special Educational Needs, 16,* 243–253. doi:10.1111/1471-3802.12079

Moats, L.C. (1994). Assessment of spelling in learning disabilities research. In G.R. Lyon (Ed.), *Frames of reference for the assessment of learning disabilities: New views on measurement issues* (pp. 333–349). Baltimore, MD: Paul H. Brookes Publishing Co.

Moats, L.C. (1995). *Spelling: Development, disabilities, and instruction.* Timonium, MD: York Press.

Moats, L.C. (1996). Phonological spelling errors in the writing of dyslexic adolescents. *Reading and Writing, 8*(1), 105–119.

Moats, L.C. (2005). *Spellography for teachers: How English spelling works (Language essentials for teachers of reading and spelling [LETRS], Module 3).* Longmont, CO: Sopris West Educational Services.

Moats, L.C. (2005/2006). How spelling supports reading: And why it is more regular and predictable than you may think. *American Education, 29*(4), 12–22, 42–43.

Nation, K., & Hulme, C. (1998). The role of analogy in early spelling development. In C. Hulme & R.M. Joshi (Eds.), *Reading and spelling development and disorders* (pp. 433–445). Mahwah, NJ: Lawrence Erlbaum Associates.

Oakland, T., Black, J.L., Stanford, G., Nussbaum, N., & Balise, R.R. (1998). An evaluation of the dyslexia training program: A multisensory method for promoting reading in students with reading disabilities. *Journal of Learning Disabilities, 31*(2), 140–147.

Pollo, T., Kessler, B., & Treiman, R. (2009). Statistical patterns in children's early writing. *Journal of Experimental Child Psychology, 104,* 410–426.

Post, Y.V., & Carreker, S. (2002). Orthographic similarities and phonological transparency in spelling. *Reading and Writing: An Interdisciplinary Journal, 15,* 317–340.

Post, Y.V., Carreker, S., & Holland, G. (2001). The spelling of final letter patterns: A comparison of instruction at the level of the phoneme and the rime. *Annals of Dyslexia, 51,* 121–146.

Read, C. (1971). Pre-school children's knowledge of English phonology. *Harvard Educational Review, 41*(1), 1–34.

Roberts, R., & Mather, N. (1997). Orthographic dyslexia: The neglected subtype. *Learning Disabilities Research and Practice, 12*(4), 236–250.

Rubin, H., & Eberhardt, N.C. (1996). Facilitating invented spelling through language analysis instruction: An integrated model. *Reading and Writing: An Interdisciplinary Journal, 8,* 27–43.

Scarborough, H.S., & Brady, S.A. (2002). Toward a common terminology for talking about speech and reading: A glossary of 'phon' words and some related terms. *Journal of Literacy Research, 34,* 299–336.

Seidenberg, M., & McClelland, J. (1989). A distributed developmental model of word recognition and naming. *Psychological Review, 96,* 523–568.

Share, D.L., & Stanovich, K.E. (1995). Cognitive processes in early reading development: Accommodating individual differences into a model of acquisition. *Issues in Education, 1*(1), 1–57.

Smith, P.T. (1980). Linguistic information in spelling. In U. Frith (Ed.), *Cognitive processes in spelling* (pp. 33–49). London, United Kingdom: Academic Press.

Sterling, C., Farmer, M., Riddick, B., Morgan, S., & Matthews, C. (1998). Adult dyslexic writing. *Dyslexia: An International Journal of Research and Practice, 4*(1), 1–15.

Treiman, R. (1994). Use of consonant letter names in beginning spelling. *Developmental Psychology, 30*(4), 567–580.

Treiman, R. (1997). Spelling in normal children and dyslexia. In B. Blachman (Ed.), *Foundations of reading acquisition and dyslexia: Implications for early intervention* (pp. 191–218). Mahwah, NJ: Lawrence Erlbaum Associates.

Treiman, R. (1998). Beginning to spell in English. In C. Hulme & R.M. Joshi (Eds.), *Reading and spelling development and disorders*. Mahwah, NJ: Lawrence Erlbaum Associates.

Treiman, R., Cassar, M., & Zukowski, A. (1994). What types of linguistic information do children use in spelling? The case of flaps. *Child Development, 65*, 1318–1337.

Treiman, R., Zukowski, A., & Richmond-Welty, D.A. (1995). What happened to the "n" in sink? Children's spelling of final consonant clusters. *Cognition, 55*, 1–38.

Venezky, R.L. (1980). From Webster to rice to Roosevelt. In U. Frith (Ed.), *Cognitive processes in spelling* (pp. 9–30). London, United Kingdom: Academic Press.

West, T.G. (1991). *In the mind's eye*. Buffalo, NY: Prometheus Books.

Technology Resources

Elaine A. Cheesman

PROGRAMS/APPS: SPELLING PHONETICALLY REGULAR WORDS

Effective programs/apps have the following features:

- Letter–sound apps match letters to the most common sound (e.g., short sounds for vowels, /ks/ for *x*, /w/ for *w*).

- Decoding apps present concepts systematically and cumulatively, progressing from easier to more difficult concepts.

- When two or more letters represent a single sound (e.g., *ll, ss, sh, ai, igh, dge*), the grapheme is manipulated in drag-and-drop activities as one unit, not separate letters.

abc PocketPhonics   http://www.appsinmypocket.com

This app combines handwriting practice and spelling of individual graphemes (letters and letter clusters that represent one sound). It uses target spelling–sound correspondence to spell spoken words. It is appropriate for learners ages 7 and older. It uses an educational not a game format.

ABC Spelling Magic series   http://www.preschoolu.com

This series of apps includes both phonemic awareness activities (segmenting oral words presented as photographs) and spelling (spelling words shown as photographs). The mature narration and photographs makes this app series suitable for all ages. In a few two-syllable words, vowels in open syllables are pronounced with the short, not long, sound.

Spelling 1: CVC words

Spelling 2: CCVC and CVCC

Spelling 3: Two-syllable words

Spelling 4: Vowel-consonant-silent-e words

Alpha-read   http://alpha-read.com

This program links letters, key word pictures, and the most common sound. Spelling–sound correspondences are sequenced not in alphabetical order but according to their utility for spelling words (e.g., *a, t, m, s*). The review mode allows teachers or users to select letters to review.

Bob Books—Reading Magic http://bobbooks.com

This program provides decodable, illustrated, interactive stories. The drag-and-drop feature provides practice for the child to spell spoken words in the story. The program orally reads the sentence after all the words are formed. Each story contains four progressively more difficult user tasks.

Lexia Core5 http://www.lexialearning.com

This program addresses phonemic awareness, reading, spelling, and syllable types. It provides engaging, systematic, sequential practice organized by syllable type. It tracks multiple users' progress and provides comprehensive reports.

Montessori Crosswords http://lescapadou.com

This program provides practice spelling one- and two-syllable words in closed syllables (CVC, CCVC, and CVCC), words with consonant digraphs and trigraphs, vowel teams, silent-*e* syllables, and vowel-*r* syllables. Users can choose to focus on one sound or letter cluster or "theme" words (e.g., *city*). The program also gives practice spelling two-syllable words with a schwa vowel (e.g., *tunnel*).

OG Card Deck http://www.mayersonacademy.org

This program presents written graphemes, associated sounds, key words, and articulation video clips. A spelling drill provides sounds for users to spell. It includes multiple spellings for single sounds (e.g., /k/ = *k, c, ck, que*). It is useful for direct instruction by a teacher or independent student review.

Phonics Genius http://www.alligatorapps.com

This app teaches basic and advanced phoneme–grapheme associations using a flashcard format. It pronounces words and highlights vowel spellings. The user may add words.

SoundLiteracy http://soundliteracy.com

For use as a teacher instructional aid, not for independent student use, this digital "tile" has manipulatives for letters and comprehensive collections of graphemes and morphemes.

SpellingCity http://www.spellingcity.com

This program provides practice in spelling, vocabulary, and handwriting, using user-entered or imported word lists from other users or published programs. It is appropriate for Grade 1 through adult.

Starfall ABCs/Starfall Learn to Read http://www.starfall.com

Starfall can be accessed through an identical free (and ad-free) web site and mobile app. It has engaging animations and games for learning letter–sound correspondences. It provides the letter name, not its sound, in the key word for *x* (*x-ray*). A better key word is *box* for /ks/.

PROGRAMS/APPS: SPELLING HIGH-FREQUENCY (SIGHT) WORDS

Effective programs/apps have the following features:

- Derived from the Fry "Instant Word" list of 1,000 most common words (1980) or the Dolch word list of 220 most common words for preschool through third grade.

- Words are presented in small, manageable groups.

- Practice activities develop spelling.

Sight Words by Little Speller   http://www.alligatorapps.com

This app helps the user learn and practice the spelling of 200 Dolch words. It uses a drag-and-drop letters format. Adjustable options are provided to scaffold task difficulty.

Star Speller: Kids Learn Sight Words Games   https://itunes.apple.com/us/developer/teacher-created-materials/id437178006

This app provides practice spelling high-frequency words from the Dolch list. It has nine engaging practice games that involve seeing, hearing, recording, and spelling.

PROGRAMS/APPS: MORPHOLOGY
(PREFIXES, SUFFIXES, LATIN ROOTS, GREEK COMBINING FORMS)

Effective programs/apps have the following features:

- They link the meaning with the spelling of the morpheme.

Roots to Words   http://taptolearn.com

This program has Latin roots and Greek combining forms arranged in meaning categories (e.g., numbers, quantity, shapes). The user selects a meaning category for practice then types the spelling of the morpheme to complete a series of words. It includes several practice activities, which apply the chosen set of morphemes within sentences.

WEB SITES: MATERIALS AND
ACTIVITIES FOR TEACHERS AND LEARNERS

List of English Suffixes   https://www.learnthat.org/pages/view/suffix.html

This is a list of Greek and Latin morphemes, meanings, and sample words and definitions.

Root Words and Prefixes: Quick Reference   https://www.learnthat.org/pages/view/roots.html

This is a list of Greek and Latin morphemes, meanings, and sample words and definitions.

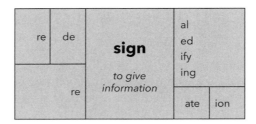

Figure 10.5. Example of output from the Mini Matrix-Maker. (*Source:* Generated with Mini Matrix-Maker. Copyright Neil Ramsden © 2011-2013. All rights reserved. Available at http://www.neilramsden.co.uk/spelling/matrix/. Adapted by permission.)

Word Building and Spelling: Experiments in English Morphology
http://www.neilramsden.co.uk/spelling

This web site has several references and interactive tools for spelling words, including forming plurals and adding suffixes to base words. The Mini Matrix-Maker builds word matrices from a list of word sums provided by the teacher (see Figure 10.5.)

Example word matrix and word sums:

re + de + sign + ed

sign + al

de + sign + ate + ions

Chapter 11

Multi-Modal Handwriting Instruction for Pencil and Technology Tools

Beverly J. Wolf and Virginia Wise Berninger

LEARNING OBJECTIVES

1. To understand the value of explicit instruction and regular practice of handwriting skills

2. To acquire basic skills for teaching handwriting

3. To recognize the values of teaching both manuscript printing and cursive writing

4. To learn why handwriting instruction is important to success in spelling, written language, and learning to read

5. To understand the varied roles of handwriting, computers, and other electronic devices

---

In many textbooks on teaching literacy, handwriting is classified as one of the mechanical skills, along with spelling, punctuation, and grammar. Rarely is handwriting given the importance it deserves in the overall language arts program for typical students or in intervention programs for students with specific learning disabilities (SLDs). Yet, writing disabilities can occur alone or co-occur with reading or oral language disabilities, persist over schooling, and affect a sizable number of students (Katusic, Colligan, Weaver, & Barbaresi, 2009). In this chapter, SLDs refer to specific learning disabilities that can affect the subword level of language (handwriting), the word level of language (word reading and spelling), or the syntax level of language (sentence understanding and construction). That is, handwriting is not a mechanical skill but rather a written language skill at the subword level of language that enables the transcription of sound and morpheme units into spelling written words, which, alone and with other words, enables the translation of ideas into written sentences. Whether teachers are prepared to teach handwriting matters because all students, including those with handwriting disabilities, need to become skilled in accurate, legible, and automatic handwriting to complete writing tasks at school and outside school. The International Dyslexia Association (IDA)'s (2018) *Knowledge and Practice Standards for Teachers of Reading* emphasized

Preparation of this chapter was supported, in part, by grant P50HD071764 from the Eunice Kennedy Shriver National Institute of Child Health and Human Development (NICHD) at the National Institutes of Health (NIH) to the University of Washington Learning Disabilities Research Center.

the importance of understanding component skills, such as handwriting and key-boarding, and related language skills, such as spelling, composing, and translating ideas into written language. Teachers need to know research-based strategies for forming manuscript and cursive letters. This chapter addresses the multisensory techniques recommended for application of the standards and the production strategies for building fluency in letter formation and copying and transcription of written language.

This chapter begins with a history of handwriting instruction, followed by overviews of why handwriting instruction still matters in the computer age and then of how to teach handwriting effectively. These overviews draw on both research and the voice of teaching experience and include practical recommendations. A multileveled language framework for instruction is featured that situates handwriting in the context of the other levels of language in literacy instruction, rather than teaching it as an isolated skill (Berninger & Wolf, 2016; Wolf, Berninger, & Abbott, 2017). Although the multisensory aspects of handwriting instruction have been emphasized—seeing letters, hearing their pronounced names, and feeling the touch sensations of movement—handwriting also has multi-motor aspects: using the hands and fingers to form letters, using the mouth to name letters, and using eye movements to review what is, was, and will be written. Thus, the featured approach in this chapter is multi-modal (multi-motor as well as multisensory) and uses multileveled language for units of increasing size in which handwriting instruction is embedded. The chapter concludes with a vision for the future in which students are prepared to be **hybrid writers** who are skilled in handwriting as well as a variety of technology tools and who are taught to use the various tools for letter production in a variety of literacy tasks within the instructional program at school. Readers are invited to join the mission to translate this vision into reality.

A BRIEF HISTORY OF HANDWRITING INSTRUCTION

The history of teaching handwriting begins in ancient times. Richardson (1995) noted that Plato (428 B.C.E–348 B.C.E.), Seneca (4 B.C.E–65 C.E.), and Quintilian (35 C.E.–100 C.E.) issued instructions to those who taught handwriting. Plato instructed the master to draw lines (letters) for the student to copy. Seneca instructed the teacher to guide the student's hand as the letters were traced. Quintilian recommended using a board with letters cut into it so that the child could keep the pen within the letters to make the letter forms accurately and teaching the sound and shape of a letter simultaneously.

Cursive letters have evolved over time to the more simplified styles of the Palmer, Zaner-Bloser, and D'Nealian methods taught in the United States (Phelps & Stempel, 1987). In a comprehensive review of research on reading, writing, and math disorders for the U.S. Interagency Committee on Learning Disabilities, Johnson (1988) described a shift in the teaching of penmanship. In the late 1800s and early 1900s, penmanship was taught as a separate subject, with copying drills that focused on the form of the letter itself and appropriate posture. After the 1940s, curricular changes led to a broader emphasis on language arts that resulted in less time being devoted to handwriting instruction in schools. This reordering of priorities led to a debate about whether teachers should provide direct instruction in skills and processes or allow children to engage in extensive reading, writing, and speaking experiences without explicit input on component language skills such as handwriting. As personal computers have become more common, school systems have placed even less importance on teaching handwriting. At the same time a growing body of research discussed next supports continued handwriting instruction in the schools.

WHY HANDWRITING INSTRUCTION MATTERS: RESEARCH LESSONS

Research for nearly a half century has supported the importance of teaching handwriting that underlies all levels of written language—letters, written words constructed from letters, and written sentences constructed from multiple words. A few illustrative findings follow.

Students with grade-appropriate handwriting skills are more likely to complete written assignments (McMenamin & Martin, 1980). Handwriting legibility contributes to better spelling skills (Strickling, 1974). Students whose notetaking is slow because of poor handwriting have difficulty with lecture comprehension (Blalock, 1985). Some poor handwriting may be caused by students not having enough training to form letters automatically when rapid writing is needed as a tool to perform assigned writing tasks (Hamstra-Bletz & Blöte, 1990). For most students, however, *graphomotor* skills used in handwriting (planning and sequencing and fine motor control) can be improved with guided practice once correct models are demonstrated, and many models are made available. The part of the brain involved in these graphomotor processes is very near the somatosensory region of the brain that receives sensory input from sequential movement (the kinesthetic sense as well as other senses). Although many do not realize it, the act of writing letters with a writing tool draws not only on motor output but also kinesthetic sensory input, that is, touch sensations related to movement. Thus, a multi-modal approach to handwriting instruction integrates visual input from seeing letter forms, oral motor output from naming letters and producing their corresponding sounds and the associated auditory input from hearing those names and sounds, and kinesthetic input from writing the letters. Moreover, these multi-modal approaches need to be taught for the goals of producing written language to express meaning via words, sentences, and text. Also, students need to be aware that teachers often judge students' abilities and grade them based on the appearance of their written work. To make the case handwriting still matters, we now translate more research findings into evidence-based research lessons for practitioners who teach or assess writing.

The *first research lesson* is that teaching **manuscript handwriting,** sometimes referred to as **printing,** helps children learn to read. Teaching manuscript handwriting led to improved word reading, even though only handwriting was taught, in a randomized, controlled study of low-achieving handwriters in first grade (Berninger et al., 1997). For review of other studies showing that handwriting facilitates reading and written language, see James, Jao, and Berninger (2015). Even in a digital world, most reading material on paper and electronic formats is in manuscript. Learning to produce letters in a format that children encounter when they read will help them read words in the format that they identify more readily because they have learned to form and name (identify) the component letters.

The *second research lesson,* which is related to the first, is that producing letter forms stroke by stroke makes it easier for the brain to perceive the letters in written words during word reading (James et al., 2015; Longcamp, Richards, Velay, & Berninger, 2017). A general principle in cognitive science is that production enhances perception. In addition, these studies have shown that when first learning to identify letters, handwriting them (forming them stroke by stroke) results in greater transfer to improved word reading than does keyboarding (selecting a formed letter on a keyboard). Although these findings do not mean that keyboarding is never appropriate, they do call attention to the contribution of handwriting early in the process of learning to read and write, even in individuals experienced in using thumbs and fingers for pressing to operate phones or laptops.

The *third research lesson* comes from studying both first- and second-graders in learning handwriting, embedded in structured, multileveled language instruction that was also multi-modal, involving multiple sensory and motor systems and grounded in Slingerland methods (Wolf et al., 2017). In first grade, students taught manuscript handwriting embedded in a structured, multi-modal language system were compared to a business-as-usual control group. In second grade, students who received a second year of manuscript instruction were compared to second-grade students who received an initial year of **cursive handwriting** instruction; in both cases, the handwriting instruction was embedded in a structured, multi-modal language system. Results showed the benefit of teaching manuscript in both first grade (to learn to write correctly formed letters that are legible to others) and second grade (to have an additional year of review and practice that helps them learn to write the letters automatically). Introducing cursive instruction without this additional year of manuscript instruction to develop automatic as well as legible handwriting was not as effective. Automaticity allows developing writers to use their limited working memory resources for generating ideas, choosing words, spelling words, and creating sentences, rather than devoting their attention to how to form the letters (Berninger, 1999).

The *fourth research lesson* is less is more. Many teachers, who are currently under intense pressure to ensure their students meet standards on annual tests required by the district and state, do not feel they have the time to devote to handwriting instruction. Yet, research has shown that in the first grade, handwriting lessons of about 15 minutes in duration, with an additional 5 minutes to compose, are effective in learning to form letters and apply letter formation to one's own writing for communication with others (Berninger et al., 1997). A short daily handwriting warm-up, just as athletes warm up with exercises before a game, followed by spelling and composing instructional activities, was effective in developing automatic handwriting in later grades as well (Berninger et al., 2008). Once children have learned to form letters, it is not necessary to drill children in writing the same letters over and over again within a lesson for long stretches of valuable instructional time. Each letter of the alphabet can be practiced in each warm-up but in a different order in each lesson using the following strategy. First, study numbered arrow cues for the order of component strokes in forming each letter, hold the letter form in memory, and then write the letter from memory (Berninger, 2009). Next, move on to spelling and composing activities, which handwriting enables. Also see Wolf and colleagues (2017) for additional ways to guide the handwriting practice and then apply handwriting to other writing activities.

The *fifth research lesson* is that students do benefit from cursive handwriting in Grades 3 and 4. The connecting strokes between letters help link letters into word spelling units and also help increase students' speed in writing words. For those who are introduced to cursive in third grade and review it in fourth grade, cursive alphabet writing skill (the ability to find, access, and produce cursive letters legibly and automatically in alphabetic order) contributed to better spelling and composing in Grades 4–7 than did either manuscript or keyboarding on the same alphabet writing task (finding, accessing, and producing legible, automatic, ordered letters) (Alstad et al., 2015). Cursive handwriting was created to speed up handwriting before the invention of typewriters or computers.

The *sixth research lesson* is that inside the mind, letters are accessed in memory in alphabetic order during reading (Niedo, Lee, Breznitz, & Berninger, 2014) and writing (Berninger, Abbott, Whitaker, Sylvester, & Nolen, 1995). Teaching children to write letters facilitates reading by helping them not only recognize the letters in words but also access them in memory to aid in letter recognition (Niedo et al., 2014). Teaching children to find and write the letter that comes before or after a designated letter in alphabetic order helps them access letters during the composing process (Berninger et al., 1995).

The *seventh research lesson* is that periodic tune-ups in manuscript and/or cursive, in which students practice writing the alphabet from memory, benefit students in Grades 4 and above (e.g., Berninger et al., 2008). Without periodic practice, handwriting, like many other skills, becomes less legible and/or more effortful for many students. Once students learn both manuscript and cursive, they can choose which form of handwriting they prefer—and in fact most students use a mix of formats (Graham, Berninger, & Weintraub, 1998). However, they benefit from brief reviews from time to time of both formats, which they need not only to use in their own writing but also to be able to recognize letters in the writing of others. Students in Grades 4 and above also benefit from exchanging their written composition with peers who then give each other feedback about any illegible letters, which the authors fix so their letters are legible (Berninger et al., 2008). This kind of peer review helps developing writers acquire metalinguistic awareness of the legibility of their own writing, and the students in Berninger and colleagues' (2008) study reported enjoying the process and finding it valuable. Also, school success depends on completing many tasks, which require integrated reading–writing—for example, taking handwritten notes and then using them to generate handwritten summaries or reports at school (Altemeier, Jones, Abbott, & Berninger, 2006). Although laptops may be used for homework assignments, they are not always available in the classroom. Most important, many technology tools currently use handwriting—letter formation by index finger, stylus, or electric pen directly on the screen or pad rather than a keyboard—as is discussed later in this chapter in the section on technology.

REFLECT, CONNECT, and RESPOND
Why should handwriting be considered a language skill?

HOW TO TEACH HANDWRITING: METHODS INFORMED BY TEACHING AND RESEARCH

The following sections describe how to teach handwriting using methods informed by teaching experience and research: specifically, awareness of the stages of handwriting development; use of these stages to inform instruction; the rationale for, and implementation of, a multi-modal, structured language approach; methods for teaching letter formation, including manuscript and cursive; additional instructional strategies not related to letter formation; and finally, handwriting instruction for students with specific learning disabilities (SLDs).

Developmental Stages of Learning Handwriting

Writing development begins before school entry. Infants and toddlers begin to make their own marks on paper, walls, or furniture and then progress to drawing and scribbling. Later preschoolers create strings of letterlike forms and generate invented spellings (Snow, Burns, & Griffin, 1998). During preschool, they have opportunities to trace and copy letters using markers, pencils, and crayons. Models of letters on alphabet strips or letter cards showing upper- and lowercase letters are available for the children to observe. They play with clay to gain finger strength and peg boards to gain fine motor control with fingers. According to Levine (1987), acquiring the skills needed for writing occurs in the following six stages, with variation in the rate of progress, even in typically achieving children.

Stage 1: Imitation—preschool to first grade. Children pretend to write by mimicking letter and number formation but lack precise graphomotor skill. Early warning signs of potential problems may be observed in children who have weaknesses in **fine motor skills** and become frustrated and self-conscious as they notice their peers' proficiency. Hand preference is shown, although it is not fully established in all children.

Stage 2: Graphic presentation awareness—first and second grades. Children learn to form letters. They become aware of the spatial planning of letters that requires thinking about their relative sizes and positions, in relation to lines, spaces, and other letters. Letter reversals are common, sometimes because they overlook **directionality** and **laterality** in letter formation. Fine motor control becomes better developed, and the child relies increasingly on **proprioception** (feedback to the central nervous system from the peripheral nervous system, including muscles and joints in the arms, hands, fingers, and even torso) and **kinesthetic feedback** (sensory feedback from the tactile sense when movement is involved, for example, finger and hand movement in letter formation). Better fine motor control also enables forming of smaller letters, and students progress from needing paper with wide lines within which to place their letters to using paper with narrower lines within which to place the smaller letters. However, lines help them in maintaining proportionality and placing of the letter components in two-dimensional space.

Stage 3: Progressive incorporation—late second to fourth grades. Children produce printed letters with less conscious effort and greater efficiency. They are less preoccupied with the spatial and aesthetic appearance of their writing when they are ready to learn cursive writing, which has the added feature of connecting strokes between the letters. Teachers introduce rules of capitalization, punctuation, syntax, and grammar to incorporate with the handwriting during composing.

Stage 4: Automatization—fourth through seventh grades. Producing legible letters automatically results in improved writing rate and efficiency during composing when children are expected to use correct vocabulary, spelling, grammar, punctuation, and capitalization in their written communication of ideas.

Stage 5: Elaboration—seventh through ninth grades. Writers learn to go beyond the conversational register of everyday speech to communicate in the more complex academic register used in academic subjects at school (Silliman & Scott, 2009).

Stage 6: Personalization-diversification—ninth grade and beyond. Individual style and talent for writing develop. Students who find writing too difficult may never reach this stage.

REFLECT, CONNECT, and RESPOND

What has research shown about effective handwriting instruction?

Providing Instruction Informed by Writing Development

In light of the developmental progression described previously, three principles should inform handwriting instruction: aiming it at a child's developmental level, integrating it with early literacy instruction, and linking it to Common Core State Standards in print.

Aim handwriting instruction at a child's developmental level. Hagin (1983) emphasized that handwriting should be taught at a level appropriate to a child's mastery of visual, motor, kinesthetic, temporal, and spatial skills. Getman (1984) showed that, initially, arm and hand movements that produce the least physiological and cognitive stress came from the shoulder, with the full arm involved in the movements required for forming letters. A student experiencing a problem with the motor act of handwriting often resists writing anything at all because it is tiring, or at best, he or she writes as little as possible (Cicci, 1995).

Integrate handwriting instruction with early literacy instruction. Instruction in writing letters can promote phonemic awareness by teaching letter names and sounds that go with the letters, beginning in kindergarten (Rubin & Eberhardt, 1996). At this point, it is important for children to know the names of the letters and to distinguish between upper- and lowercase letters; that is, alternate forms associated with the same name or letter identity. Snow and colleagues (1998) clearly outlined the handwriting demands for kindergarten and first-grade reading accomplishments; for example, using handwriting to aid in recognizing letters for reading and for written seatwork.

Link handwriting instruction to Common Core State Standards in writing. Within the Common Core State Standards, handwriting standards are provided only for kindergarten and first grade, as described next (National Governors Association Center for Best Practices & Council of Chief State School Officers, 2010; see also The Common Core State Standards Writing Standards for K to 5 and 6 to 12). These include the following:

Kindergarten

- Print many upper- and lowercase letters

- Capitalize the first word in a sentence

- Prints own name (first and last) and the first names of some friends or classmates

- Can write most letters and some words when they are dictated

First grade

- Print all upper- and lowercase letters (letter style is not indicated)

- Demonstrate command of the conventions of standard English capitalization, punctuation and spelling when writing.

- Capitalize dates and names of people.

- Use end punctuation for sentences.

- Use commas in dates and to separate single words in a series.

The standards do not appear to be grounded in research on handwriting or writing development and effective writing instruction (Berninger & Wolf, 2017). Research supports direct, explicit instruction in letter formation and guided practice to become proficient in the task of handwriting across the grades as reviewed earlier in this chapter. Recall that, in Grade 1, children are taught to form the letters so others can recognize them. In Grade 2, they practice until they can form each letter automatically. That is, they do not have to stop and think about each stroke that is needed to form the letter. The process of letter formation is on "automatic pilot," much as when human pilots of a plane rely on a computerized pilot for the routine aspects of flying so they can devote their attention to unexpected conditions that might arise. Once handwriting is on automatic pilot, the writer can devote attention and mental resources to choosing and spelling words, creating sentences, and composing texts to express their ideas and communicate with others.

Multi-Modal, Structured Language Approach to Handwriting

In the field of specific learning disabilities (SLDs), especially for dyslexia, much attention has been given to multisensory methods of literacy instruction, but from the perspective of how the brain plays a role in handwriting, more than sensory input is involved. To begin with, fine motor output also is involved, such as orally naming letters or the sound that goes with one or more letters; sequential writing of a letter by component strokes or a series of letters in a spelled word, with fingers and hand movements. The writer also engages large motor movement (how the arms and even the torso are positioned in space). Moreover, the sensory input involves visual, auditory, and tactile input (from visual feedback from viewed letters, auditory feedback from named letters, and the touch and pressure feedback from the writing tool, respectively). It is also kinesthetic, meaning it involves a tactile sensation for movement, such as when the fingers and hands move through space. In addition, handwriting is not merely a motor act that is integrated with sensory input—language is also involved, in that written words are transformed into orthographic codes that are stored and processed in working memory (Abbott & Berninger, 1993; Berninger, 1998, 2009; Sanders, Berninger, & Abbott, 2018). Although motor skills contribute to handwriting (Graham & Weintraub, 1996), orthographic coding has a more direct relationship to handwriting than do fine motor skills (Abbott & Berninger, 1993).

Instructional Guidelines for Multi-Modal Handwriting Instruction

The Slingerland (1981) handwriting instructional approach emphasizes the Visual-Auditory-Kinesthetic (VAK) associations of sight–sound (grapheme–phoneme) with feel (hand and mouth) of each letter as it is viewed visually, named with auditory feedback, and written with kinesthetic feedback from tactile sensation of movement. Some students learn to write more easily than they learn to read; thus, writing training may take the lead in multisensory language training as these students' strongest pathway to learning (Cox, 1992). In the beginning stages of handwriting, when children are learning to form letters, one activity that can be helpful is forming a large letter shape made in the air with a straight arm (sky or **air writing)** while naming the letter, a key word that begins with that letter, and the letter sound (Slingerland, 1971). Students should be encouraged to verbalize the steps of the movements needed to form a given letter, for example, "*d* begins around like an *a*, tall then a stem is needed." This verbalization helps them to prevent errors as they recall the sequence for forming a letter that might get confused with other similar letters. Also, given research showing attention problems correlate with handwriting problems (Berninger, Abbott, Cook, & Nagy, 2017), forming the letter with gross motor movements and naming the steps of letter formation may help beginning writers pay attention to letter formation and prevent handwriting disabilities. To summarize, multi-modal teaching links listening, speaking, reading, and writing to reinforce the close relationships between letter production and letter perception. See Berninger and Wolf (2016) for currently available instructional materials for displaying upper- and lowercase letters for students, both on classroom walls and at their desk or work space.

When first teaching handwriting, 20–30 minutes per day are necessary to introduce letters, but after all are taught, a daily 5- to 10-minute review of letter forms may be sufficient if students have demonstrated mastery of legible letter formation. The teacher should organize writing instruction with attention to posture, pencil grip, position of the writing surface, and naming the letters before writing them. Children should be instructed to write and then trace over each letter rather than writing the same letter repeatedly because over time students habituate writing without attention to task and letter quality deteriorates (Berninger, 1998, 2009). The Slingerland (1981) format for instruction includes daily practice in moving from one letter to the next smoothly to develop a rhythmic tempo; students form one dictated letter then trace until the next letter or series of letters is named (Slingerland, 1981). If a student is unable to write a letter satisfactorily, then he or she should return to the tracing step at the board or on a large paper pattern. This procedure should be followed meticulously with each letter until all have been learned and written legibly and automatically. In the Slingerland (1981) approach, and in other Orton-Gillingham–based approaches, such as Alphabetic Phonics and Spaulding, which use similar strategies—tracing, copying, and writing from memory—writing practice and review are integrated into the written language lesson to provide success with spelling and written language tasks. Handwriting lessons should consist of teaching new letters, practicing letters already learned, and, if using cursive writing, reviewing and practicing of letter connections. See the *Slingerland Multisensory Approach: A Practical Guide for Teaching Reading, Writing and Spelling* (Slingerland Institute for Literacy, 2008) and corresponding web site for Sample Lesson—Introducing a New Letter and Review.

Uppercase letters are introduced only after students write all lowercase letters automatically and legibly because uppercase letters are used in only about 2% of writing. Some teachers prefer to introduce the capitals needed for student names on an individual basis. See Figures 11.1 and 11.2 for a version of simplified uppercase letters in both manuscript and cursive.

Students will be motivated to improve their handwriting if they take part in deciding which areas need help. The teacher can help students analyze the quality of their writing using generally accepted criteria: correct letter forms, rhythm (fluency), consistent slant, good use of space within and between words and lines, and general appearance (free of excessive strikeovers or erasures). The teacher should set daily goals for the student or group. Although not all individuals have superior handwriting, many can achieve legibility with effort and practice (Texas Scottish Rite Hospital for Children, Child Development Division [TSRHC], 1996) and with setting goals and evaluating if goals are met.

The handwriting lesson also provides an opportunity to teach the correct forms of punctuation marks used while composing. A period should be a dot,

Lowercase Manuscript Letter Forms

All lowercase maunscript letters are made with a
continuous line, except for *f, i, j, k, t,* and *x.*

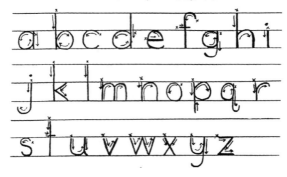

Uppercase Manuscript Letter Forms

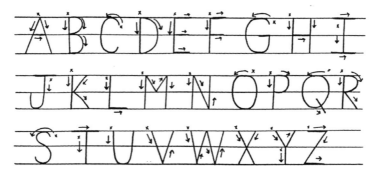

Figure 11.1. Print letters, using a continuous stroke (when possible). (Developed by the Renton School District, Renton, WA; reprinted by permission; versions taught in other school districts may vary slightly.)

with no circling. Commas and apostrophes begin with a dot followed by a slightly curved tail. As each punctuation mark is taught, students should use them in their writing lessons. Students should be taught to attend to margins and spacing, even when practicing individual letters. Daily practice in organizing the writing paper will contribute to the clarity and readability of the finished composing product.

Teaching Letter Formation

Follow these guidelines for teaching letter formation for manuscript and cursive letters.

Manuscript Most public school districts in the United States use manuscript print when introducing handwriting to young children, perhaps because it is typically used in preschools and is the writing style encountered in reading texts in beginning reading instruction. It is not necessary to teach manuscript letter formation in alphabetic order, but the following should be considered:

- Ease of production of the letter
- Continuity of stroke

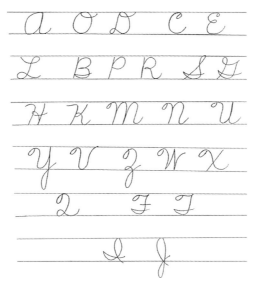

Figure 11.2. Uppercase cursive letters. (From Texas Scottish Rite Hospital for Children, Child Development Division Evaluation and Treatment for Learning Disabilities. [1996]. *Teaching cursive writing* [Brochure]. Dallas, TX: Author; reprinted by permission.)

- Similarity of strokes to those letters previously taught

- Ease of perception and production of the sound associated with the letter

For example, the manuscript letter *l* is the simplest to write, but its sound is more difficult for young children, so it is a poor choice as the first letter to be introduced. It may be taught more easily after a few letters and their sounds have been presented. Students appear to recall the sequence of movements of a given letter better if the instructor verbalizes consistent, precise directions for writing each letter shape. (See Figures 11.3–11.7 for examples of specific verbal directions for forming different letters.) The descriptive phrases should be repeated each time the

a	Around, down.	t	Down, cross.
n	Down, hump.	h	Down, hump.
b	Down, up, around.	u	Down, curve up, down.
o	Around, close.	i	Down, dot.
c	Around, stop.	v	Slant down, up.
p	Down, up, around.	j	Down, hook, dot.
d	Around, up, down.	w	Slant down, up, down, up.
q	Around, down, flag.	k	Down, slant in, out.
e	Across, around, stop.	x	Slant right. Slant left.
r	Down, up, over.	l	Down.
f	Curve, down, cross.	y	Slant right. Slant left.
s	Curve, slant, curve.	m	Down, hump, hump.
g	Around, down, hook.	z	Across, slant, across.

Figure 11.3. Continuous stroke descriptions of print letters. (Used by permission of Neuhaus Education Center, Bellaire, TX.)

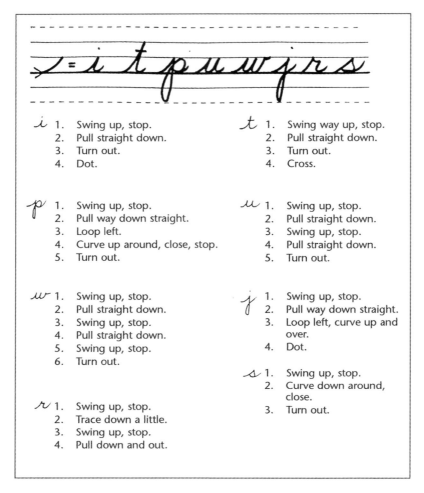

Figure 11.4. Approach stroke: "Swing up, stop." (From Texas Scottish Rite Hospital for Children, Child Development Division Evaluation and Treatment for Learning Disabilities. [1996]. *Teaching cursive writing* [Brochure]. Dallas, TX: Author; reprinted by permission.)

letter is traced or written to reinforce motor memory until the letter shape is automatic (Gillingham & Stillman, 1997; Slingerland, 1971; TSRHC, 1996). Each time students start to write a letter, they should name it as the arm starts to move. To summarize, through multi-modal association of sight, sound, and feel, children integrate each letter name with its visual form and the feel of how the letter is written motorically.

Continuous strokes are relevant to writing some manuscript letters. When a letter such as *h* is taught first, it introduces children to the idea of using a continuous stroke to form a letter because the child starts at the top of the letter, pulls down to the baseline, slides up almost to the midline, curves out and down without lifting the pencil. When a letter such as *t* is taught first, students must lift the pencil to cross the downstroke line; thus, children have more difficulty adjusting to moving their arms without lifting the pencil from the paper when *h* is presented later.

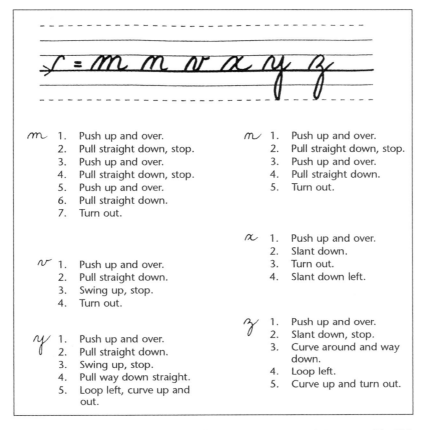

Figure 11.5. Approach stroke: "Push up and over." (From Texas Scottish Rite Hospital for Children, Child Development Division Evaluation and Treatment for Learning Disabilities. [1996]. *Teaching cursive writing* [Brochure]. Dallas, TX: Author; reprinted by permission.)

Letters can also be grouped by similar strokes for teaching. When a letter is learned and practiced, the child will be prepared to use similar arm movements in new letters with similar strokes. For example, it is easier to teach the letter *b* when students have learned to retrace the downward stroke of an *h* and curve up and around. The movements are the same and help students learn new letters more easily. Practical recommendations follow for each of the letter groups.

The h Group   The sound of the letter *h* is easy to hear and reproduce. The print letter form introduces the idea of continuous stroke. Its basic arm movement is also used in letters such as *b, m, n, r,* and *p.* Be prepared to spend considerable time on the letter *b* because of the confusion between *b* and *d.* Slingerland (1971) recommended preparing students for writing the letter *b* with an auditory-motor activity in which students stand and hold their writing arms in front of their bodies. The teacher then separates right- and left-handed students and helps them understand how to move in the direction that handwriting should go.

Right-handed students move their arms away from their bodies, whereas left-handed students move their arms across their bodies. Then, when patterns are introduced at the chalkboard, the teacher verbalizes, "Tall stem down and

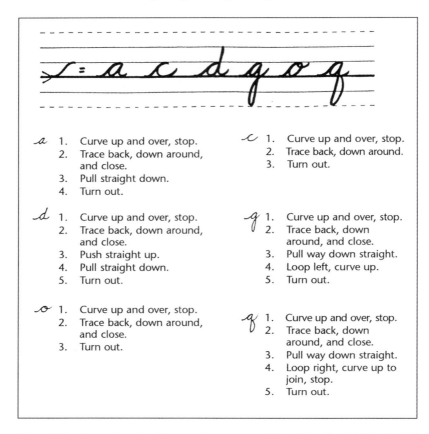

<table>
<tbody>
<tr><td>a</td><td>1.</td><td>Curve up and over, stop.</td></tr>
<tr><td></td><td>2.</td><td>Trace back, down around, and close.</td></tr>
<tr><td></td><td>3.</td><td>Pull straight down.</td></tr>
<tr><td></td><td>4.</td><td>Turn out.</td></tr>
</tbody>
</table>

a
1. Curve up and over, stop.
2. Trace back, down around, and close.
3. Pull straight down.
4. Turn out.

c
1. Curve up and over, stop.
2. Trace back, down around.
3. Turn out.

d
1. Curve up and over, stop.
2. Trace back, down around, and close.
3. Push straight up.
4. Pull straight down.
5. Turn out.

g
1. Curve up and over, stop.
2. Trace back, down around, and close.
3. Pull way down straight.
4. Loop left, curve up.
5. Turn out.

o
1. Curve up and over, stop.
2. Trace back, down around, and close.
3. Turn out.

q
1. Curve up and over, stop.
2. Trace back, down around, and close.
3. Pull way down straight.
4. Loop right, curve up to join, stop.
5. Turn out.

Figure 11.6. Approach stroke: "Curve under, over, stop." (From Texas Scottish Rite Hospital for Children, Child Development Division Evaluation and Treatment for Learning Disabilities. [1996]. *Teaching cursive writing* [Brochure]. Dallas, TX: Author; reprinted by permission.)

away from my body (if right-handed)," and, "Tall stem down and across my body (if left-handed)," to help both right- and left-handed students understand and remember the direction of the letter. The students are expected to subvocalize the stroke patterns, whispering the same language each time they practice the letter *b*.

The a Group　The *a* group consists of letters that start with the same movement as the letter *a* and includes *a, c, d, g, o, q,* and *s*. These letters begin at the 2 o'clock position just below the mid-line. As children begin to form these letters, they should move their pencils at approximately a 45-degree angle toward the midline, curving around toward the baseline. The exaggerated slant typical of beginning writers' letters will become more rounded as the children's writing becomes automatic. The angle of the pencil will eliminate a nearly vertical upward stroke and produce a rounded letter.

Other Groups　The letters *i, j, k, l,* and *t* begin with straight downstrokes, whereas the letters *v, w,* and *x* start with slight slants. If the angle of the first slant is exaggerated, then the resulting letter will be sprawled across the page. The letters *e, u, y,* and *z* do not belong to a particular group.

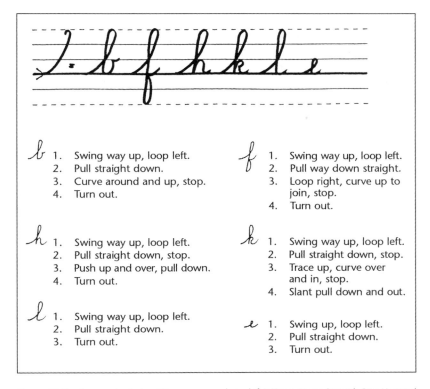

Figure 11.7. Approach stroke: "Curve way up, loop left." (From Texas Scottish Rite Hospital for Children, Child Development Division Evaluation and Treatment for Learning Disabilities. [1996]. *Teaching cursive writing* [Brochure]. Dallas, TX: Author; reprinted by permission.)

Cursive Handwriting Advantages of cursive writing (Cox, 1992; Phelps & Stempel, 1987; TSRHC, 1996) include the following:

- It eliminates a student's need to decide where each letter should begin because all cursive letter shapes begin on the baseline.

- It provides directional movement from left to right.

- It provides unique letter shapes that are not mirror images of other letters.

- It reduces reversals by eliminating the need to raise the pencil while writing a single letter or a series of letters in a word.

Lowercase letters are taught first in cursive handwriting, as in manuscript handwriting. A new letter is introduced each day, and previously learned letters are reviewed and practiced following the introduction of the new one. It is beneficial to follow the order and grouping of cursive letters by the four basic approach strokes (see Figures 11.4–11.7). Students learn the four approach strokes as they learn new letters. Each approach stroke always begins on the baseline and moves from left to right. An arrow is provided to establish a baseline when students practice on the chalkboard or on unlined paper. The drop stroke follows the approach stroke and ties the letter to the baseline. The remaining shape is added to form the letter, which is then finished by a release or connecting stroke. The release stroke is an important part of every letter because it allows for uniform spacing between letters and promotes rhythmic, fluent writing.

After all lowercase letters are learned and can be written legibly, students should practice writing the alphabet in sequence in connected cursive, giving extra attention to the bridge strokes used to connect *b, o, v,* and *w* with the next letter. Extra practice should be provided for frequent combinations such as *br, oa, vi,* and *wh* (see Figure 11.8). Henry (2010) pointed out that third-grade students often need practice in these **linkages** when they are using cursive writing for spelling more complex words. Explicit practice should take place, with students tracing and copying these bridge stroke transitions when difficulties arise.

REFLECT, CONNECT, and RESPOND
What does it mean that handwriting is a language skill best taught in a multileveled language lesson?

Instruction Not Related to Letter Format Formation for Optimizing Handwriting

For optimizing handwriting, it is beneficial to provide instruction not only in letter formation but also in the following areas, discussed next: posture, pencil grasp, writing tool, medium, and paper position.

Figure 11.8. Lowercase cursive bridge strokes between common letter combinations. (From Texas Scottish Rite Hospital for Children, Child Development Division Evaluation and Treatment for Learning Disabilities. [1996]. *Teaching cursive writing* [Brochure]. Dallas, TX: Author; reprinted by permission.)

Good Posture   Poor body position can significantly interfere with coordinating the hand movements in writing (Kurtz, 1994). The student should use a chair with a flat back and a seat that allows the feet to rest flat on the floor, with the hips, knees, and ankles all at 90-degree angles. The desk should be 2 inches higher than the child's bent elbows (Benbow, 1988, as cited in Kurtz, 1994). A desk that is too high will cause the student to elevate the shoulders, which is tiring and restricts freedom of movement, whereas a desk that is too low could cause the student to slouch. The nonwriting hand and arm should be on the desk to hold the paper in place.

Proper Pencil Grasp   The child should use a normal tripod pencil grip (see Figure 11.9). The pencil rests on the first joint of the middle finger with the thumb and index fingers holding the pencil in place and the pencil held at a 45-degree angle to the page. An awkward pencil grip can indicate **finger agnosia.** Using an auxiliary plastic pencil grip or a metal writing frame can aid in changing the fatiguing grip to a normal, less tiring one (Phelps & Stempel, 1985; TSRHC, 1990). Children may need to experiment with pencil grips or a writing frame to determine which one works best for them. Many become frustrated with these implements once the novelty has worn off. The pencil should point toward the shoulder of the writing arm for both left- and right-handed students.

An alert, diligent teacher can help a student change pencil position, but this requires consistency and patience. At any time that the teacher notes incorrect position, he or she can instruct the class as follows.

TEACHER: Stop.

Students place their pencils on the desk with the point toward them.

TEACHER: Pinch.

With the index finger and thumb in a "pinch" position, students lightly grasp their pencils where the paint begins (approximately 1 inch from the point).

TEACHER: Lift.

As the children lift the pencil, it will fall back to correct writing position and rest on the first joint of the middle finger.

After a few practice sessions, students only need to hear, "stop, pinch, lift," to adjust their pencil positions. Teacher perseverance will help students become accustomed to the feel of the new position and use it consistently. After a time, only the one or two children who have continued difficulty will need reminders. The older the child, the more difficulty he or she will have with changing the pencil position.

Writing Tool   While writing, the writer receives kinesthetic feedback from the pressure and touch of moving the writing implement against the paper (Levine, 1987). A No. 2 or softer pencil should be used. Pencils with soft lead require less pressure from the child, thereby reducing fatigue. Children with impaired kinesthetic feedback will benefit from using softer leads, which will not break as the children press firmly in an attempt to receive that feedback when writing (Levine, 1987). Pencils with indentations that help students automatically place fingers in the correct position are now available. Lyra produces a GROOVE pencil, available in two sizes. Stabila sells Move Easy Rollerball Pens and Easy Ergo Pencils. Both manufacturers aim at producing ergonomically designed devices that are comfortable to use and make writing and drawing easier. Lyra pencils may be used

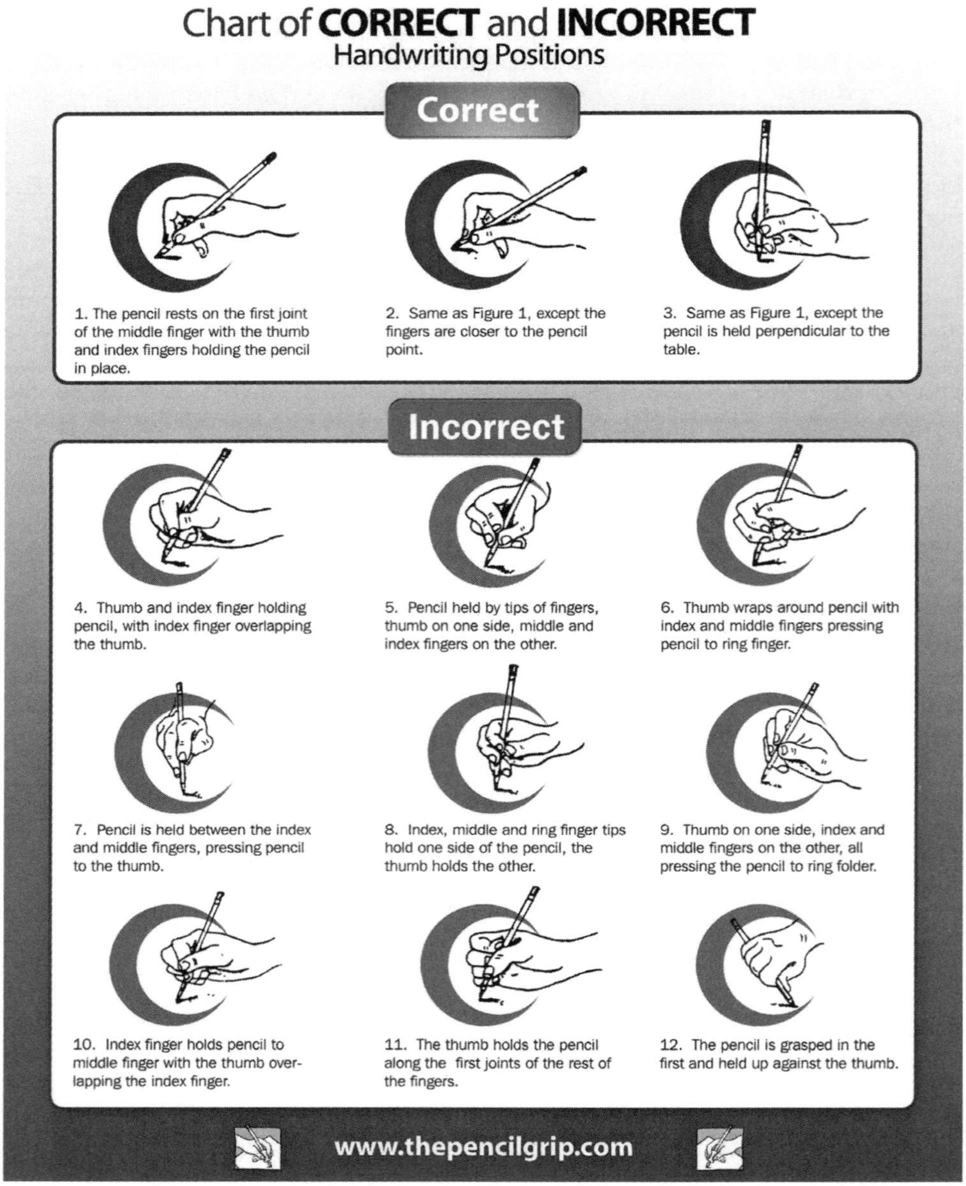

Chart of **CORRECT** and **INCORRECT**
Handwriting Positions

Correct

1. The pencil rests on the first joint of the middle finger with the thumb and index fingers holding the pencil in place.

2. Same as Figure 1, except the fingers are closer to the pencil point.

3. Same as Figure 1, except the pencil is held perpendicular to the table.

Incorrect

4. Thumb and index finger holding pencil, with index finger overlapping the thumb.

5. Pencil held by tips of fingers, thumb on one side, middle and index fingers on the other.

6. Thumb wraps around pencil with index and middle fingers pressing pencil to ring finger.

7. Pencil is held between the index and middle fingers, pressing pencil to the thumb.

8. Index, middle and ring finger tips hold one side of the pencil, the thumb holds the other.

9. Thumb on one side, index and middle fingers on the other, all pressing the pencil to ring folder.

10. Index finger holds pencil to middle finger with the thumb overlapping the index finger.

11. The thumb holds the pencil along the first joints of the rest of the fingers.

12. The pencil is grasped in the first and held up against the thumb.

www.thepencilgrip.com

Figure 11.9. Recognized correct and incorrect writing grips. (From The Pencil Grip. www.thepencilgrip.com; The Pencil Group, P.O. Box 67096, Los Angeles, CA 90067. Reprinted by permission.)

with either hand. Stabilo produces pens and pencils designed for either right- or left-handed writers. Students who have used these devices are enthusiastic about them. Teachers are pleased that there is no need to "fiddle" with adjusting plastic pencil grips. It is preferable to use pencils without erasers; instead of erasing mistakes, the teacher can instruct children to bracket them: *I [wahsed] washed my dog.* This reduces time spent erasing and allows teachers to see the errors children have made and incorporate reteaching into lesson planning.

Medium Letter forms should be introduced using a chalkboard, dry-erase board, or smart board, then unlined paper, then wide-lined paper (1" between rows), next primary-grade lined paper (¾", ½", ⅜"), and finally regular lined notebook paper. The size of the spaces between lines is adjusted downward as the child masters the letter forms. The teacher should watch carefully to see that correct posture, full arm movement, and correct form are maintained. Additional practice utilizing other media, such as carpet squares, salt or rice trays, sand, tabletops, and varying styles of columned paper such as newspaper want ads, will help ensure full arm movement that can vary handwriting practice and make it fun.

Paper Position As early as the ninth century, scribes discovered that a slight slant seemed to be easier to form than a perpendicular stroke (Florey, 2009). To achieve the consistent slant needed in cursive writing, the edge of the paper should be parallel to the writing arm (at about a 45-degree angle to the edge of the desk) and anchored at the top by the nonwriting hand. After the child's writing is small enough to use regular notebook paper, a slant guide (a piece of paper with slanted lines that is positioned beneath the writing paper) can be helpful after the child forms all lowercase letters automatically. Some instructors prefer that a left-handed student write with a backward slant, placing the paper parallel to the left arm; others teach a forward slant to both left- and right-handed students. See Figure 11.10 for examples of both types of slant guides.

It has been suggested that left-handed individuals who write with a hook (the "curled wrist" method) were taught by teachers who insisted all students place their papers in the right-handed position. To avoid smudging the paper and to see what they have written, these left-handed individuals curled their wrists while writing. Athènes and Guiard (1991) showed that the inverted handwriting

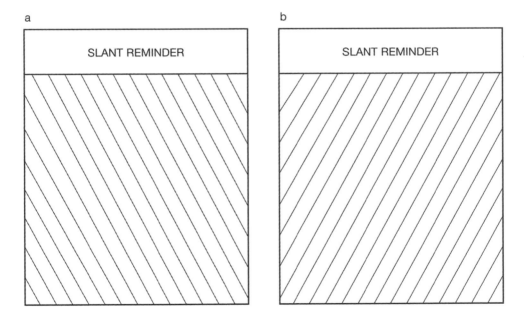

Figure 11.10. Slant reminders for a) left-handers and b) right-handers. (From Texas Scottish Rite Hospital for Children, Child Development Division Evaluation and Treatment for Learning Disabilities. [1996]. *Teaching cursive writing* [Brochure]. Dallas, TX: Author; reprinted by permission.)

posture for left-handers was just as good as that of non-inverters. Bertin and Perl-man (1997) developed a handwriting program for teaching cursive to left-handed individuals that is available commercially. They also have a handwriting program for numerals.

See Figure 11.11 for illustrations of proper posture, pencil grasp, and paper position for both left- and right-handed students. Slingerland and Aho (1985) recommended that when students use cursive, the paper always be slanted with the upper left corner higher for left-handed students and the upper right corner higher for right-handed students. They also suggested that right-handed students keep their papers parallel to the bottom of the desk when using manuscript print. This helps them keep their manuscript letters straight.

Handwriting Instruction for Students With Specific Learning Disabilities

Dysgraphia is unusual difficulty with handwriting, which sometimes affects students' spelling, but not their word reading, decoding, and spelling unless they have co-occurring dyslexia (Berninger, Richards, & Abbott, 2015; Berninger & Wolf,

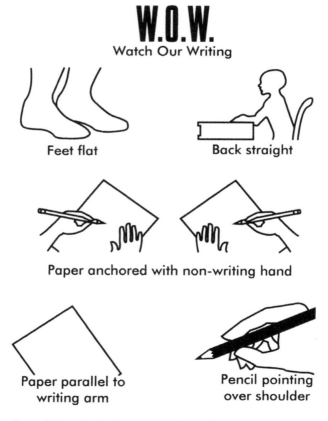

Figure 11.11. Watch Our Writing (W.O.W.) chart. (From Phelps, J., & Stempel, L. [1985]. *CHES's handwriting improvement program* [CHIP]. Dallas, TX: Texas Scottish Rite Hospital for Children; reprinted by permission.)

2016). Children with dysgraphia may express their difficulties with illegible hand-writing and/or slow, nonautomatic letter formation, which has been shown to be related to both finger sequencing and orthographic coding; a finger sequencing difficulty requiring motor planning and control and not just motor production (Richards et al., 2009) and orthographic coding (Abbott & Berninger, 1993; Berninger, Richards, et al., 2015; Sanders et al., 2018).

Dyslexia is a word of Greek origin that means the condition of having impaired word-level reading and spelling skills. In kindergarten, children at risk for dyslexia struggle compared to other children in naming letters, writing letters, and associating sounds with letters. Throughout the early grades, they struggle with oral reading. In some cases, both accuracy and rate of oral reading are impaired, but in other cases, only rate of oral reading is impaired. These students have more difficulty recognizing words on lists without sentence context than in sentences. They tend to have considerable difficulty in orally reading words that are pronounceable in English but have no meaning, like the Jabberwocky words in *Alice in Wonderland*. After the fourth-grade transition to silent reading, they typically exhibit significant problems in silent word reading and written spelling, but oral reading problems may persist, too.

Oral and written language learning disability (OWL LD), also referred to as specific language impairment (SLI) (Berninger, Richards, et al., 2015; Sanders et al., 2018) is unusual difficulty with listening comprehension and reading comprehension and oral and written expression at the syntax level. Students with OWL LD may or may not have co-occurring dysgraphia, but their writing difficulties are not restricted to handwriting problems; they also have difficulty in processing and producing multiple words in syntax in language by ear (listening comprehension), by mouth (oral expression), by eye (reading comprehension), and/or by hand (written expression).

Evidence-based handwriting instruction by human teachers, as described in Berninger (2009) and Berninger and colleagues (1997, 2008), when converted to handwriting instruction by computer teachers, has been shown to be effective in improving the handwriting of students with persisting dysgraphia, dyslexia, and OWL LD in Grades 4–9 (Berninger, Nagy, Tanimoto, Thompson, & Abbott, 2015; Tanimoto, Thompson, Berninger, Nagy, & Abbott, 2015). However, because ADHD co-occurs more often with dysgraphia than dyslexia or OWL LD (Richards, Abbott, & Berninger, 2016), the computerized instruction was designed to help students *pay attention to the sequence of forming component letter strokes* and, in the related spelling and composing instruction, to *pay attention to the sequence of letters in written words, sequence of words in comprehending sentences, and sequence of sentences in composing summaries about read or heard source material.*

Although there has been a longstanding debate about whether individuals with dyslexia produce more reversals and transpositions than those without dyslexia based on Orton (1937), both Vellutino (1979) and Brooks (2003) found that reversals are not related to visual perception. Rather, in a study of 182 children ages 6–18, Brooks, Berninger, Abbott, and Richards (2011) found that some but not all students with or without dyslexia made reversals, but students with dyslexia produced a higher proportion of reversal errors than those without dyslexia in both their letter writing and letter naming. They concluded that reversal errors may be related to inefficiencies or momentary breakdowns in the orthographic loop (letter writing) and/or the phonological loop (letter naming) of working memory.

REFLECT, CONNECT, and RESPOND
What kinds of specialized instruction might students with different kinds of specific learning disabilities (SLDs) need?

EDUCATING HYBRID WRITERS

Twenty-first–century students use both handwriting and keyboarding for producing written language to compose and communicate; this raises the question of how best to educate these hybrid writers. On the one hand, Graham, Berninger, Abbott, Abbott, and Whittaker (1997) found that legible letter writing and automatic letter writing contribute to the amount and quality of written composition in Grades 1–6. Typically developing students in the elementary school grades also wrote more and wrote faster and expressed more ideas when writing by pen than keyboard when they were allowed to hunt and peck (Berninger, 2009). However, when touch typing was taught, handwriting provided an advantage for taking notes when reading source material (Richards, Peverly, et al., 2016b), but touch typing provided an advantage when listening to source material (Thompson et al., 2016). Likewise, King (2005) developed a multisensory approach to touch typing that teaches the position of the keys in alphabetic order. She found that students learn the position of the keys in as little as 30 minutes and then provided practice based on the Orton-Gillingham Approach to instruction (Gillingham & Stillman 1997; King, 2005; Orton, 1966). Computers have other advantages that supplement handwriting rather than eliminate the need for it. Although it is easier to detect errors in printed hard copy than on the monitor, it is easier to make revisions using a word processing program on the computer. The annual tests for assessing whether individual students meet state standards in literacy and other content subjects are increasingly administered by computer. Inadequate computer writing skills by keyboard may contribute to a student not meeting the criterion to pass one or more of the content areas of those exams.

In addition, there are many times and places when only pens or pencils and not computers are available for various writing tasks, or vice versa. For these and other reasons it makes sense to teach students to become hybrid writers who have both handwriting and keyboarding skills (Berninger, 2012, 2013).

At the same time, keyboarding is not the only interface with technology in the computer era. During the preschool years, children learn to press keys on phones and tablets or operate a mouse, which presents its own issues, related to a grip that combines fisting and a pincer grip. They even use fingers or styluses to write on a pad or screen. In a study using computerized instruction, students in Grades 4–9 with or without persisting SLDs despite early intervention were randomly assigned to an order of alternating modes of letter production (finger formation vs. stylus); no significant differences in mode were found on various learning activities showing that one mode was superior to the other (Berninger, Nagy, et al., 2015). However, many students complained that the stylus was not as comfortable as a pencil to grasp and move and that writing letters on a screen resulted in very large letters that looked like "baby handwriting" and made them feel like "babies." Indeed, adding lines to the tablet screen to assist in positioning letters of smaller size on the screen resulted in even greater improvement in handwriting (Tanimoto et al., 2015). It was clear that computers can teach handwriting effectively. This lent additional evidence for the futility of pitting handwriting against computer tools when students in the 21st century benefit from learning how to produce letters by using both handheld pens and pencils and various tools for interfacing with technology to become hybrid writers.

Furthermore, a longitudinal study of manuscript and cursive writing and keyboarding found that printing manuscript letters, writing cursive letters, and finding letters on a keyboard have different early developmental paths (Berninger et al., 2006). Printing letters in manuscript form and finding the manuscript letters on a keyboard had statistically significant correlations in typically developing first-grade students. Printing manuscript letters, writing cursive letters, and finding manuscript letters on a keyboard had statistically significant correlations in typically developing third-grade students. However, different neurodevelopmental processes uniquely predicted automaticity of handwriting or keyboarding—that is, the ability to produce or find letters accurately, quickly, and effortlessly. For printing letters, the unique predictor was orthographic coding, that is, storing letter forms while the letter forms are analyzed in working memory. For writing cursive letters, the unique predictor was inhibition—an executive function in working memory that directs attention to the relevant linguistic information and suppresses the irrelevant linguistic information. Difficulty with inhibition is a working memory marker of dyslexia (Berninger et al., 2006). Training in cursive writing may help individuals with dyslexia because it improves their inhibition. For finding the letters on the keyboard, the unique predictors were orthographic letter-coding skill and rapid automatic naming of letters (phonological loop) in working memory. One implication of these findings is that if an individual student struggles with a particular format of writing by hand or keyboard, individual neuropsychological assessment of the student's profile of strengths and weaknesses in verbal working memory may be warranted.

REFLECT, CONNECT, and RESPOND
What has research shown about teaching computer tools for literacy learning?

TECHNOLOGY

There is a widespread educational practice of using computer tools solely as an accommodation for a handwriting disability. The rationale is that the technology tool will help the student bypass the handwriting disability and work toward the goal of producing written words, sentences, and text without writing them letter by letter with letters formed by producing sequential component strokes (see Thompson et al., 2016).

Research using computerized writing instruction supports an alternative approach—using computers for handwriting instruction, not just accommodation (Thompson et al., 2016). Using computerized instruction employing a variety of tools for writer–computer interface led to improved handwriting, spelling, and composing of students with persisting SLDs despite earlier intervention (Berninger, Nagy, et al., 2015; Tanimoto et al., 2015). See Berninger and Wolf (2016) for practical suggestions for integrating other technology tools in different content areas of the curriculum.

Both inter-individual differences between typically developing writers and those with persisting SLDs and intra-individual differences among the students with SLDs across lessons were found (Niedo, Tanimoto, Thompson, Abbott, & Berninger 2016). This variability among developing writers with and without handwriting struggles serves as a reminder of the importance of tailoring both instruction and accommodations to the learning profile of the individual student. Also, bypass technology, which includes **voice recognition software** and software for dictation, is rapidly evolving and generating new products; it should be selected and implemented with caution and attention to its processing requirements (see Thompson et al., 2016).

Voice Recognition Software

For caveats regarding the ability of voice recognition software to recognize the speech sounds in developing children compared to adults, see the review in Berninger and Amtmann (2003). Voice recognition software may not be effective for children with limited working memory because of the demands of simultaneous tasks. Many children with expressive language difficulties are unable to use voice recognition software effectively because of the complexity of monitoring text and the amount of editing required to transfer their thoughts into language that is grammatical and sensible to others. Very often voice recognition software may be more, rather than less, frustrating for students with SLDs. Voice recognition technology may be a distraction to the other students in the classroom or may be less effective because of background noise. Each student and learning situation must be individually evaluated to monitor the effectiveness of this or any other adaptive tool. The smartpen is a variation that has proven useful for many students, particularly for notetaking. The Pulse Smartpen by Livescribe records and links the audio to what students write so they do not miss words as they struggle to get them on paper.

Educators should consider not only the profile of the learner but also the task requirements for using the technology tool. Effective word processing requires integrating multiple operations, such as selecting, saving, deleting, cutting, pasting, and formulating (Levine, 2003). Spell-checking technology is most effective when children have achieved a fifth-grade spelling level so that their spellings can be recognized by the computer (Berninger, 1998). Students must also have adequate reading ability and a sufficient grasp of vocabulary to discriminate between **homographs** (words that have the same spelling but that sound different and have different meanings) and **homonyms** (words that sound the same and that often have the same spelling but have different meanings). Grammar checks can also be an excellent support for emerging writers.

Word Prediction Software

Word prediction software allows the child to complete a word, phrase, or sentence with only a few keystrokes. The program is based on the letters typed in the word. It generates words beginning in that particular way. As the writer progresses, the program examines syntax and continues to predict the structure of the sentence. As with voice recognition software, the student is expected to keep a number of tasks in working memory. Editing may be helped by programs that read aloud what the child has written. Headphones may be needed in a classroom environment.

Tablet PC and iPAD Apple Software

Computer users can write directly on the computer screen with a stylus or index finger or electric pen. However, observation of children using stylus or index finger in five studies to date in the University of Washington Learning Disabilities Center showed considerable individual differences among students with stylus and finger interfaces (e.g., Niedo et al., 2016). As this and other new bypass technologies are developed and existing ones are refined, continuing research is needed on their effectiveness for individual students, as determined by the students' own individual strengths, weaknesses, and needs.

> **REFLECT, CONNECT, and RESPOND**
> Should handwriting still be taught even though students now have computers? Why or why not?

CLOSING THOUGHTS: TEACHING HANDWRITING

Handwriting is closely linked to other reading skills, writing, oral language, and all content areas of the curriculum. Thus, handwriting instruction should be integrated into curricula designed to help students who have academic difficulties as well as all students. For example, research has shown that students who are unable to take notes and write papers at a grade-appropriate level fall behind not only in notetaking but also in comprehension (Phelps, Stempel, & Browne, 1989). This vital omission can lower overall achievement and affect a child's attitude toward all school learning (Askov & Peck, 1982). Technology should be used not only for accommodations for those with handwriting disabilities but also as part of the instructional program in writing (including handwriting) at school. Choosing the appropriate technology tools to use for instruction (and accommodation if appropriate) should be based on a careful assessment of the student's profile of strengths and weaknesses, the processing requirement of the technology tool, and the writing task(s) at hand. All students, with or without SLDs, should be taught to be hybrid writers skilled in using handwriting and computer tools for letter production and written language composing.

ONLINE COMPANION MATERIALS

The following Chapter 11 resources are available at http://www.brookespublishing .com/birshcarreker/materials:

- Reflect, Connect, and Respond Questions

- Appendix 11.1: Representative Instructional Resources for Educating Hybrid Writers

- Appendix 11.2: Knowledge and Skill Assessment Answer Key

KNOWLEDGE AND SKILL ASSESSMENT

1. How do periodic tune-ups in manuscript and/or cursive, in which students practice writing the alphabet from memory, benefit students?

   a. Without periodic practice, handwriting becomes less legible and/or more effortful.

   b. Practice allows students to recognize letters in the writing of others.

    c.   They assist in integrated reading and writing.

    d.   They assist in use of handwriting on the screen or pad rather than a keyboard.

2.   What are reasons teaching handwriting has value? (Select all that apply.)

    a.   It is a Common Core State Standard.

    b.   Other people can more easily read what a student has written.

    c.   It helps in letter recognition that relates to reading.

    d.   Teachers judge performance more positively.

3.   What are the lessons to be learned from research? (Select all that apply.)

    a.   Handwriting enhances letter recognition and leads to improved word reading.

    b.   Cursive writing links letters into word spelling units.

    c.   Manuscript and keyboarding afford spelling and written language opportunities equal to cursive writing.

    d.   Handwriting as a tool in written language enhances learning.

4.   Which of the following are *not* part of a multi-modal approach to handwriting? (Select all that apply.)

    a.   Visual input from seeing the letter form

    b.   Oral motor output from naming letters and producing their corresponding sounds

    c.   Naming the letters

    d.   Auditory input from hearing letter names and sounds

REFERENCES

Abbott, R., & Berninger, V. (1993). Structural equation modeling of relationships among developmental skills and writing skills in primary and intermediate grade writers. *Journal of Educational Psychology, 85,* 478–508.

Alstad, Z., Sanders, E., Abbott, R., Barnett, A., Hendersen, S., Connelly, V., & Berninger, V. (2015). Modes of alphabet letter production during middle childhood and adolescence: Interrelationships with each other and other writing skills. *Journal of Writing Research, 6*(3), 199–231. http://www.jowr.org/next.html; http://dx.doi.org/10.17239/jowr-2015.06.03.1 #644747: NIHMS644747 [NCBI tracking system #16689920]

Altemeier, L., Jones, J., Abbott, R., & Berninger, V. (2006). Executive factors in becoming writing-readers and reading-writers: Note-taking and report writing in third and fifth graders. *Developmental Neuropsychology, 29,* 161–173.

Askov, E., & Peck, M. (1982). Handwriting. In M.C. Akin (Ed.), *Encyclopedia of educational research* (5th ed., Vol. 2, pp. 764–766). New York, NY: Free Press.

Athènes, S., & Guiard, Y. (1991). The development of handwriting posture: A comparison between left-handers and right-handers. In J. Wann, A.M. Wing, & N. Sovik (Eds.), *Development of graphic skills* (pp. 137–149). London, United Kingdom: Academic Press.

Berninger, V. (1998). *Guides for intervention.* San Antonio, TX: Harcourt Assessment.

Berninger, V. (1999). Coordinating transcription and text generation in working memory during composing: Automatized and constructive processes. *Learning Disability Quarterly, 22,* 99–112.

Berninger, V. (2009). Highlights of programmatic, interdisciplinary research on writing. *Learning Disabilities. Research and Practice, 24,* 68–79.

Berninger, V. (May/June 2012). Strengthening the mind's eye: The case for continued handwriting instruction in the 21st century. *Principal,* 28–31. Retrieved from the National Association of Elementary School Principals' web site: http://www.naesp.org

Berninger, V. (2013, March). *Educating students in the computer age to be multilingual by hand.* Invited commentary on "The Handwriting Debate" NASBE Policy Debate (2012, September) for National Association of State Boards of Education (NASBE), Arlington, VA. Retrieved from http://www.nasbe.org/wp-content/uploads/Commentary-Handwriting-keyboarding-and-brain-development1.pdf

Berninger, V., Abbott, R., Cook, C., & Nagy, W. (2017). Relationships of attention and executive functions to oral language, reading, and writing skills and systems in middle childhood and early adolescence. *Journal of Learning Disabilities, 50,* 434–449. doi:10.1177/0022219415617167 posted online 1/8/16 http://journaloflearningdisabilities.sagepub.com; released to PMC (under embargo)(PMCID:PMC4938801) also PMC5189981

Berninger, V.W., Abbott, R.D., Jones, J., Wolf, B.J., Gould, L., Anderson-Youngstrom, M., & Apel, K. (2006). Early development of language by hand: Composing, reading, listening, and speaking connections; three letter-writing modes; and fast mapping in spelling. *Developmental Neuropsychology, 29*(1), 61–92.

Berninger, V., Abbott, R., Whitaker, D., Sylvester, L., & Nolen, S. (1995). Integrating low-level skills and high-level skills in treatment protocols for writing disabilities. *Learning Disability Quarterly, 18,* 293–309.

Berninger, V., & Amtmann, D. (2003). Preventing written expression disabilities through early and continuing assessment and intervention for handwriting and/or spelling problems: Research into practice. In H.L. Swanson, K.R. Harris, & S. Graham (Eds.), *Handbook of research on learning disabilities* (pp. 345–363). New York, NY: Guilford.

Berninger, V., Nagy, W., Tanimoto, S., Thompson, R., & Abbott, R. (2015). Computer instruction in handwriting, spelling, and composing for students with specific learning disabilities in grades 4 to 9. *Computers and Education, 81,* 154–168. doi:10.1016/j.compedu.2014.10.00NIHMS636683 PubMed Central http://www.ncbi.nlm.nih.gov/pmc/articles/PMC4217090 http://audioslides.elsevier.com/getvideo.aspx? doi=10.1016/j.compedu.2014.10.005

Berninger, V., Richards, T., & Abbott, R. (2015, published online April 21, 2015). Differential diagnosis of dysgraphia, dyslexia, and OWL LD: Behavioral and neuroimaging evidence. *Reading and Writing: An Interdisciplinary Journal, 28,* 1119–1153. doi:10.1007/s11145-015-9565-0 A2 contains supplementary material available to authorized users: NIHMS683238 Publ ID 2615-04-21_0002 PMC ID # forthcoming

Berninger, V., Vaughan, K., Abbott, R., Abbott, S., Brooks, A., Rogan, L., … Graham, S. (1997). Treatment of handwriting problems in beginning writing: Transfer from handwriting to composition. *Journal of Educational Psychology, 89,* 652–666.

Berninger, V., Winn, W., Stock, P., Abbott, R., Eschen, K., Lin, C., … Nagy, W. (2008). Tier 3 specialized writing instruction for students with dyslexia. *Reading and Writing: An Interdisciplinary Journal, 21,* 95–129.

Berninger, V.W., & Wolf, B.J. (2016). *Dyslexia, dysgraphia, OWL LD, and dyscalculia: Lessons from science and teaching* (2nd ed.). Baltimore, MD: Paul H. Brookes Publishing Co.

Bertin, P., & Perlman, E. (1997). *PAF handwriting book for cursive: Right-handed and left-handed models.* White Plains, NY: Monroe Associates.

Blalock, J.W. (1985, November 13). *Oral language problems of learning-disabled adolescents and adults.* Paper presented at the 36th annual conference of The Orton Dyslexia Society, Chicago.

Brooks, A. (2003). Neuropsychological processes related to persisting reversal errors in dyslexia and dysgraphia. *Dissertation Abstracts International, 63*(11A), 3850.

Brooks, A., Berninger, V., Abbott, R., & Richards, T. (2011). Letter naming and letter writing reversals of some children with dyslexia: Symptoms of inefficient phonological and orthographic loops of working memory? *Developmental Neuropsychology, 36,* 847–868.

Cicci, R. (1995). *What's wrong with me? Learning disabilities at home and in school.* Timonium, MD: York Press.

Cox, A.R. (1992). *Foundations for oral literacy: Structures and techniques for multisensory teaching of basic written English language skills.* Cambridge, MA: Educators Publishing Service.

Florey, K. (2009). *Script and scribble*. Brooklyn, NY: Melville House.

Getman, G.N. (1984). About handwriting. *Academic Therapy, 19,* 139–140.

Gillingham, A., & Stillman, B.W. (1997). *The Gillingham manual: Remedial training for children with specific disability in reading, writing, and penmanship* (8th ed.). Cambridge, MA: Educators Publishing Service.

Graham, S., Berninger, V., Abbott, R., Abbott, S., & Whittaker, D. (1997). The role of mechanics in composing of elementary school students: A new methodological approach. *Journal of Educational Psychology, 89,* 223–236.

Graham, S., Berninger, V., & Weintraub, N. (1998). The relationship between handwriting style and speed and legibility. *Journal of Educational Research, 91,* 290–296.

Graham, S., & Weintraub, N. (1996). A review of handwriting research: Progress and prospects from 1980 to 1994. *Educational Psychology Review, 8,* 7–87.

Hagin, R.A. (1983). Write right or left: A practical approach to handwriting. *Journal of Learning Disabilities, 16,* 266–271.

Hamstra-Bletz, L., & Blöte, A. (1990). Development of handwriting in primary school: A longitudinal study. *Perceptual and Motor Skills, 70,* 759–770.

Henry, M.K. (2010). *Unlocking literacy: Effective decoding and spelling instruction* (2nd ed.). Baltimore, MD: Paul H. Brookes Publishing Co.

International Dyslexia Association, The. (2018, March). *Knowledge and practice standards for teachers of reading.* Retrieved from https://dyslexiaida.org/knowledge-and-practices/

James, K., Jao, J.R., & Berninger, V. (2015). The development of multi-leveled writing systems of the brain: Brain lessons for writing instruction. In C. MacArthur, S. Graham, & J. Fitzgerald (Eds.), *Handbook of writing research* (pp. 116–129). New York, NY: Guilford.

Johnson, D.J. (1988). Review of research on specific reading, writing, and mathematics disorders. In J.F. Kavanagh & T.J. Truss (Eds.), *Learning disabilities: Proceedings of the national conference* (pp. 79–163). Timonium, MD: York Press.

Katusic, S.K., Colligan, R.C., Weaver, A.L., & Barbaresi, W.J. (2009). The forgotten learning disability—Epidemiology of written language disorder in a population-based birth cohort (1976–1982), Rochester, Minnesota. *Pediatrics, 123,* 1306–1313.

King, D.H. (2005). *Keyboarding skills* (2nd ed.). Cambridge, MA: Educators Publishing Service.

Kurtz, L. (1994, Fall). Helpful handwriting hints. *Teaching Exceptional Children,* 58–59.

Levine, M. (1987). *Developmental variations and learning disorders.* Cambridge, MA: Educators Publishing Service.

Levine, M. (2003). *The myth of laziness.* New York, NY: Simon & Schuster.

Longcamp, M., Richards, T.L., Velay, J.L., Berninger, V. (2017, Feb. 7). Neuroanatomy of handwriting and related reading and writing skills in adults and children with and without learning disabilities: French-American connections. *Pratiques.* https://pratiques.revues.org/3155 https://www.ncbi.nlm.nih.gov/pmc/articles/PMC5297261

McMenamin, B., & Martin, M. (1980). *Right writing.* Spring Valley, CA: Cursive Writing Associates.

National Governors Association Center for Best Practices & Council of Chief State School Officers. (2010). *Common Core State Standards for English language arts and literacy in history/social studies, science, and technical subjects* (Writing Standards K–5 and 6–12). Washington, DC: Authors.

Niedo, J., Abbott, R., & Berninger, V. (2014, published online April 18, 2014). Predicting levels of reading and writing achievement in typically developing, English-speaking 2nd and 5th graders. *Learning and Individual Differences, 32C,* 54–68. doi:10.1016/j.lindif.2014.03.013 published PubMed Central (PMC) for public access May 1, 2015: http://www.ncbi.nlm.nih.gov/pmc/articles/PMC4058427

Niedo, J., & Berninger, V.W. (2016). Strategies typically developing writers use for translating thought into the next sentence and evolving text: Implications for assessment and instruction. *Open Journal of Modern Linguistics, 6,* 276–292. http://dx.doi.org/10.4236/ojml.2016.64029 Posted on PubMed January 30, 2017 https://www.ncbi.nlm.nih.gov/pmc/articles/PMC526138

Niedo, J., Lee, Y.L., Breznitz, Z., & Berninger, V. (2014*).* Computerized silent reading rate and strategy instruction for fourth graders at risk in silent reading rate. *Learning Disability Quarterly, 37*(2), 100–110. doi:10.1177/0731948713507263 http://www.ncbi.nlm.nih.gov/pmc/articles/PMC4047714

Niedo, J., Tanimoto, S., Thompson, R., Abbott, R., & Berninger, V. (2016). Computerized instruction in translation strategies for students in upper elementary and middle school grades with persisting learning disabilities in written language. *Learning Disabilities: A Multidisciplinary Journal, 21,* 62–78. NIHMS 836952

Orton, J.L. (1966). The Orton-Gillingham approach. In J. Money (Ed.), *The disabled reader: Education of the dyslexic child* (pp. 119–145). Baltimore, MD: The Johns Hopkins University Press.

Orton, S.T. (1937). *Reading, writing, and speech problems in children.* New York, NY: W.W. Norton.

Phelps, J., & Stempel, L. (1985). *CHES's handwriting improvement program* (CHIP). Dallas, TX: Children's Handwriting Evaluation Scale.

Phelps, J., & Stempel, L. (1987). Handwriting: Evolution and evaluation. *Annals of Dyslexia, 37,* 228–239.

Phelps, J., Stempel, L., & Browne, R. (1989). *Children's handwriting and school achievement.* Unpublished manuscript, Texas Scottish Rite Hospital for Children, Dallas.

Richards, T., Abbott, R., & Berninger, V. (2016). Relationships between presence or absence of ADHD and fMRI connectivity writing tasks in children with dysgraphia. *Journal of Nature and Science (JNSCI), 2(12)* e270, 1–5. ISSN 2377-2700 Journal Online: http://www.JNSCI.org NIHMSID 836446 Pub Med: https://www.ncbi.nlm.nih.gov/pmc/articles/PMC5189981

Richards, T., Berninger, V., Stock, P., Altemeier, L., Trivedi, P., & Maravilla, K. (2009). fMRI sequential-finger movement activation differentiating good and poor writers. *Journal of Clinical and Experimental Neuropsychology, 29,* 1–17. To link to this Article: doi:10.1080/13803390902780201 URL: http://dx.doi.org/10.1080/13803390902780201

Richards, T.L, Grabowksi, T., Askren, K., Boord, P., Yagle, K., Mestre, Z., & Berninger, V. (2015). Contrasting brain patterns of writing-related DTI parameters, fMRI connectivity, and DTI-fMRI connectivity correlations in children with and without dysgraphia or dyslexia. *Neuroimage Clinical, 8,* 1–14. http://dx.doi.orgg/10.1016/j.nicl.201503.018 http://www.ncbi.nlm.nih.gov/pmc/articles/PMC4473717

Richards, T., Nagy, W., Abbott, R., & Berninger, V. (2016). Brain connectivity associated with cascading levels of language. *Journal of Systems and Integrative Neuroscience (JSIN), 2,* 219-229. (ISSN: 2059-9781) doi:10.15761/JSIN.1000139 Pub Med Central January 30, 2017 https://www.ncbi.nlm.nih.gov/pmc/articles/PMC5261811

Richards, T., Peverly, S., Wolf, A., Abbott, R., Tanimoto, S., Thompson, R., & Berninger, V. (2016b). Idea units in notes and summaries for read texts by keyboard and pencil in middle childhood students with specific learning disabilities: Cognitive and brain findings. *Trends in Neuroscience and Education, 5,* 146–155. Pub ID TINE73 http://www.journals.elsevier.com/trends-in-neuroscience-and-education.

Richardson, S. (1995). Specific developmental dyslexia: Retrospective and prospective views. In C.W. McIntyre & J.S. Pickering (Eds.), *Clinical studies of multisensory structured language education* (pp. 1–15). Salem, OR: International Multisensory Structured Language Education Council (IMSLEC).

Rubin, H., & Eberhardt, N. (1996). Facilitating invented spelling through language analysis instruction: An integrated model. *Reading and Writing: An Interdisciplinary Journal, 8,* 27–43.

Sanders, E., Berninger, V., & Abbott, R. (2018). Sequential prediction of literacy achievement for specific learning disabilities contrasting in impaired levels of language in grades 4 to 9. *Journal of Learning Disabilities, 51(2),* 137–157. doi:10.1177/0022219417691048

Silliman, E., & Scott, C. (2009). Research-based oral language routes to the academic language of literacy: Finding the right road. In S. Rosenfield & V. Berninger (Eds.), *Implementing evidence-based interventions in school settings* (pp. 107–145). New York, NY: Oxford University Press.

Slingerland, B.H. (1971). *A multisensory approach to language arts: Book I.* Cambridge, MA: Educators Publishing Service.

Slingerland, B. (1981). *A multisensory approach to language arts for specific language disability children: Book 3. A guide for elementary teachers.* Cambridge, MA: Educators Publishing Service.

Slingerland, B., & Aho, M. (1985). *Manual for learning to use cursive handwriting.* Cambridge, MA: Educators Publishing Service.

Slingerland Institute for Literacy. (2008). *The Slingerland multisensory approach: A practical guide for teaching reading, writing and spelling.* Bellevue, WA: Author.

Snow, C.E., Burns, M.S., & Griffin, P. (Eds.). (1998). *Preventing reading difficulties in young children.* Washington, DC: National Academies Press.

Strickling, C.A. (1974). The effect of handwriting and related skills upon the spelling scores of above average and below average readers in the fifth grade. *Dissertation Abstracts International, 34*(07), 3717A.

Tanimoto, S., Thompson, R., Berninger, V., Nagy W., & Abbott, R. (2015). Computerized writing and reading instruction for students in grades 4 to 9 with specific learning disabilities affecting written language. *Journal of Computer Assisted Learning, 31,* 671–689. NIHMS 721216   doi:10.1111/jcal.12110   PMC4743045   https://www.ncbi.nlm.nih.gov/pmc/articles/PMC4743045

Texas Scottish Rite Hospital for Children, Child Development Division (TSRHC). (1990). *Dyslexia training program developed in the Dyslexia Laboratory, Texas Scottish Rite Hospital* [Videotape]. Cambridge, MA: Educators Publishing Service.

Texas Scottish Rite Hospital for Children, Child Development Division (TSRHC). (1996). *Teaching cursive writing* (Brochure). Dallas, TX: Author.

Thompson, R. , Tanimoto, S, Abbott, R., Nielsen, K., Geselowitz, K., Lyman, R., & Berninger, V. (2016). Relationships between language input and letter output modes in writing notes and summaries for students in grades 4 to 9 with persisting writing disabilities. *Assistive Technology Journal.* doi:10.1080/10400435.2016.1199066 Pub Med https://www.ncbi.nlm.nih.gov/pmc/articles/PMC5291827

Vellutino, F. (1979). *Dyslexia: Theory and research.* Cambridge, MA: The MIT Press.

Wolf, B., Berninger, V., & Abbott, R. (2017). Effective beginning handwriting instruction: Multimodal, consistent format for 2 years, and linked to spelling and composing. *Reading and Writing. An Interdisciplinary Journal, 30*(2), 299–317. doi:10.1007/s11145-016-9674-4 2016, July 23 Available as 'Online First' http://link.springer.com/article/10.1007/s11145-016-9674-4 https://www.ncbi.nlm.nih.gov/pmc/articles/PMC5300752

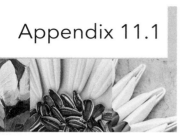

Appendix 11.1

Representative Instructional Resources for Educating Hybrid Writers

HANDWRITING

Benbow, M. (1990). *Loops and groups: A kinesthetic writing system*. San Antonio, TX: Therapy Skill Builders. This program teaches cursive and is for use in third through fourth grade.

Berninger, V. (1998). *PAL Handwriting Program*. New York, NY: Pearson.

Berninger, V., & Abbott, S. (2003). *PAL Research-supported reading and writing lessons. Instructional manual and reproducibles*. San Antonio, TX: Harcourt/PsyCorp. This program is currently distributed by Pearson. See Lesson Sets 3, 7, 9, 10, and 11–15.

Berninger, V.W., & Wolf, B.J. (2016). *Dyslexia, dysgraphia, OWL LD, and dyscalculia: Lessons from science and teaching* (2nd ed.). Baltimore, MD: Paul H. Brookes Publishing Co. This book is also available as an e-book. It covers practical strategies for teaching handwriting.

Bregman, C. (2009). *Move into writing. A lowercase handwriting program*. This book (ISBN: 978-0-692-00235-3) is self-published in consultation with Kristi Komai. It is available by e-mailing cheryl@miwtherapy.com.

Rubel, B. (1995). *Big strokes for little folks*. Tucson, AZ: Therapy Skill Builders. This program is for use in kindergarten through first grade.

Getty-Dubay Productions   http://www.handwritingsuccess.com

This web site offers 10 books, materials, and DVDs, including *Write Now*.

Slingerland Institute for Literacy   http://www.slingerland.org

This web site provides trademark instructional (manuscript and cursive) and assessment materials and teacher training for use in general education or special education classrooms.

Zaner-Bloser Handwriting Program   http://www.zanerbloser.com

This program provides instruction materials by grade, pre-K to Grade 6, for use in general education.

EXPLICIT INSTRUCTION IN KEYBOARDING

Dr. Fry's Computer Keyboarding for Beginners   http://www.teachercreated.com

This self-teaching program is for beginning keyboarders of any age.

Keyboarding Skills   http://eps.schoolspecialty.com

This program by Diana Hanbury King is a supplement to the *Writing Skills* series.

KEYTIME   http://www.keytime.com/

The KEYTIME method is language based and uses color-coded finger patterns.

Ten Thumbs Typing Tutor   http://tenthumbstypingtutor.com

This program teaches the proper way to type without looking at the keys and links to iTunes to let users learn by typing lyrics.

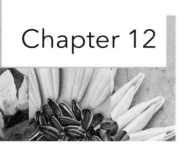

Chapter 12

Fluency in Learning to Read

Conceptions, Misconceptions, Learning Disabilities, and Instructional Moves

Katherine Garnett

LEARNING OBJECTIVES

1. To trace the evolving concept of reading fluency, its importance, and its interconnection with other aspects of learning to read

2. To learn a panoply of instructional methods for developing reading fluency

3. To understand how fluency is more than a particular "stage" of learning to read, being, rather, a pervasive aspect of developing skills, sub-skills, and complex multi-skill performance

4. To identify common misconceptions and pitfalls in approaching students' fluency needs

5. To use insights from this chapter to inform instruction, especially for students with reading/learning disabilities—to prevent reading problems, strengthen early reading, and target intervention for more complex fluency-related skills

This chapter traces the evolving concept of reading fluency, considering it from many angles. What is it? How does it relate to word-reading accuracy? To reading comprehension? What instructional practices develop it? What misconceptions and pitfalls should schools watch out for? What distinct dilemmas developing fluency are experienced by students with reading/learning disabilities?

Investigating these questions draws on cognitive psychology and reading research, along with teaching practices, pointers, cautions, case studies, and two nationwide studies of reading fluency among fourth graders. This rich grounding is meant to inform instruction, especially crucial instruction for students with reading/learning disabilities. The chapter aims to contribute to preventing reading problems, intensifying intervention, and targeting more complex word, phrase, sentence and self-modulated reading skills—for school success and lifelong reading.

WHAT IS FLUENCY?

Fluency is a critical facet of complex skill development. Reading—like playing the piano, driving a car, or juggling—is a complex skill made of myriad sub-skills that require much practice to come naturally. Early stages of piano playing, driving, juggling—and reading—are jerky, slow, uncoordinated, and characterized by great effort and much inaccuracy. With practice, sub-skills smooth out and clusters of sub-skills increasingly operate in synchrony. As practice continues beyond accuracy, performance commences to flow, an indicator that lower level skills no longer consume the mind's narrow bandwidth of conscious attention. So, this freeing up of attention allows the emergent juggler, driver, musician, or reader to deploy attention flexibly. On the early road to becoming fluent, focal attention is literally commandeered by lower level sub-skills, leaving little for coordinating or higher level processing (Topping, 2006).

Fluency is marked by sub-skills sinking below awareness—humming in the background so attention can enliven executive function, such as monitoring and orchestrating. For driving, this means navigating winding roads to reach destinations—safely. For skilled reading, it means making sense while reading along, catching slip-ups, adjusting to winding sentences and other complexities while following where the text is going.

Most of us forget how much time, effort, and repeated experience it took to develop fluent driving (or reading) and what it was like along the way because now it just seems natural. Actually, though, to perform fluently, even at an early level of a complex skill, entails effort and much practice. To gain more advanced performance takes yet more effortful attention to a slew of new sub-skills, often destabilizing overall performance until—with more attentive practice—the newly learned integrates with the well-practiced.

Figure 12.1 captures this process of progressing from basic reading accuracy to fluency, with a rendition of how learners commonly feel. As you review this, pause to consider the toll on students with reading/learning disabilities, whose efforts result in little progress month by month and even year by year.

> ### REFLECT, CONNECT, and RESPOND
> How would you describe the development of complex skills? Can you draw parallels between learning the complex skill of driving a car and the complex skill of learning to read?

Fluency As an Aspect of the Reading Growth Continuum

An important notion here is that fluency is not achieved at one point in time. Rather, it keeps developing—with practice—over a long span. Many educators' first introduction to the notion of fluency was as "a stage of early reading," attained

Effortful accuracy → Reliable accuracy → Word automaticity → Basic reading fluency (decoded and sight words)

Labored focus on accuracy	Some reliable accuracy	Automatic with many words
Word by word	Accurate but labored	Flow
Slow processing	Picking up speed	Increasing rate and flexible
Tiring "work"	Some phrasing	Phrasing and expressiveness
Halting, choppy, tone	Mixed choppiness/prosody	Monitors sense--breakdown → repair
Effortful → little progress	Effortful →progress	Sense of effortlessness
Feeling of incompetence	Feeling of work = growth	Feeling of competence (at basic level)

Figure 12.1. Basic reading fluency: The look, the sound, the feel. (From *Multisensory Teaching of Basic Language Skills, Third Edition* [p. 295].)

when students shift from reading word by word to reading flowingly. This turns out to be an inadequate view; fluency continues to develop along a continuum of increasing linguistic complexity. With practice, both early and later sub-skills continue automatizing—strengthening and integrating, all below conscious attention (Wolf & Katzir-Cohen, 2001). So, fluency is not a "level" but an ongoing process that affects reading across a range of levels. It keeps on affecting reading progress, from early, to competent, to advanced expertise—just as in juggling, driving, and piano playing.

A simple view of this process is as follows: coaching-practice-practice, coaching-practice-practice, coaching-practice-practice-practice-coaching and then—on to Carnegie Hall. Re-conceptualizing fluency as an aspect of reading skill, from early-to-expert, has resounding implications: as reading complexity ratchets up from K to 12, students continue to require explicit foregrounding (teacher coaching) and practice of the critical, and new, sub-skills they encounter, so performance can go from wobbly to accurate to effortless—and well-integrated.

This means that fluency is something of a moving target (Rasinski, 2017; Rasinski & Nageldinger, 2016). A student is fluent at reading text with certain complexities but is not fluent with others. Yes, you get that driver's license at a certain point, but clearly this is only a permit to practice. After several years behind the wheel, surely driving skills are more available, integrated, and swift.

Given this K–12 reconceptualization, it is not so simple to say whether a reader is fluent as that raises the question: *How* fluent, reading *what*? Controlled text with mostly CVC words? *Amelia Bedelia*? The high school earth science text? James Joyce?

Reading and Reading Disability: Building a Reading Brain

As complex skills such as piano playing and reading develop along a fluency continuum, changes in flow, control, and expressiveness are evident—the visible and audible effects of learning plus practice. These same practice effects are evident in brain studies showing activation within and across brain areas and the formation of new neural circuitry. Learning *changes* the brain, both its functioning and its physical structure: Music fluency builds a music brain; reading fluency shapes a reading brain (Fern-Pollak & Masterson, 2014).

Findings show that when students with dyslexia are provided sufficient, phonologically based, structured intervention, not only does reading performance improve, but brain activation patterns and neural connections change as well, coming to resemble those of "normal" skilled readers (Richards & Berninger, 2008; Shaywitz et al., 2004). Students with dyslexia who read without appropriate instruction develop compensatory connections across brain regions that are different from skilled readers' and that are cognitively more demanding (Fern-Pollak & Masterson, 2014). This might explain the fatigue some poor readers experience the longer they read, their lagging progress in fluency, and their frequent fear of being timed.

The mounting evidence that different neural architecture and brain activation patterns distinguish typical readers from those with dyslexia underscores the legitimacy of reading disabilities—they exist (and have existed), despite lingering naysayers. The evidence that appropriate instruction not only improves reading in those with dyslexia but also changes their neural functioning and connectivity, from abnormal to largely normalized, is quite stunning. Such findings about the brain's plasticity have neuroscientists pursuing instructional implications and educational partnerships, both for students with learning disabilities and for the broader normal-range of learners (Butterworth & Kovas, 2013).

So, there is now brain-related confirmation that *what* we teach and *how* absolutely matter. Teaching has consequences on many levels. For reading in particular, methodologies matter. What gets focused on, how systematically, and for how long are all consequential, and instructional features that matter for teaching in general can matter exponentially more for students with reading disabilities. The whats, the hows, and for how long—these not only matter, they can be crucial.

Word Reading in the Grand Complexity of Skilled Reading   Early in learning to read, students cannot modulate tone, tempo, or phrasing; their oral reading is often loud, labored, lurching, and monotone because they are expending attention on lower level skills related to conventions of print, letter recognition, letter patterns, and other sub-skills of word recognition (LaBerge & Samuels, 1974). As word-reading sub-skills become well-practiced, they no longer hijack attention which is set free to shift, as needed, to phrasing, tempo, and self-monitoring.

That is why smooth, expressive reading—a kind of orchestrating—is virtually impossible below a particular threshold of word-recognition skill. In other words, a reader needs sufficient word-level accuracy and ease to move beyond dysfluent reading. It is crucial to not misinterpret as a "comprehension problem" a reader who is coping with many words that are not yet accurate or not easily read. Such inaccuracy and dysfluency signal that there is little bandwidth for distinctions, details, following the thread, or self-monitoring for adjustments—the mind is, literally, all tied up.

Akin to a beam of light, attention illuminates critical features, directing and sustaining cognitive processing to precipitate learning. But, like a light beam, attention does not shine everywhere at once and is easily disrupted. When required at the word level, it is less available for other processing; when recruited for many of the words, the beam of attention cannot dart around to other priorities—oftentimes losing the thread or nuance of meaning. Much like juggling—the novice attends to the balls, first one, up/down—then two, up/over, down/up. Complexity increases—then some joker throws you two more—and the fledgling fluency you were just starting to enjoy collapses. You drop the balls, right? In other words, you are fluent with two balls, but not with more.

In order to attend to successive challenges of increasingly complex text, most of the words must be processed with little conscious attention, recognized under the radar as it were. Reading the words needs to have stabilized from wobbly to accurate—then progressed from more to less effortful—then on to easy and, eventually, virtually effortless.

In addition to swift, effortless, word reading, a host of other sub-skills must go from accurate to effortless, joining the underlying concert. These include morphologic features, syntactic twists and turns, anaphora's pointing finger—all aspects of more complex text, both narrative and expository, that start coming in a barrage as third grade comes to a close (Schwanflugel & Benjamin, 2017; Wolf & Katzir-Cohen, 2001).

REFLECT, CONNECT, and RESPOND

Although not the only skill necessary to fluent reading, *easy word recognition* remains a central aspect. So how should that inform instruction—through the grades? Also, what does it mean that fluency is not, as many people have conceived, simply a stage of early reading development, but is an ongoing process? What are the implications for teaching youngsters of different ages and within different subject areas?

Assessing Fluency: Listening Closely Assessing means discerning what to do—not so easy:

- How easy is effortless?

- How practiced is well-practiced?

- What percentage of words in **continuous text** need to be read with ease?

- How many word trip-ups or slowdowns compromise comprehension?

- What linguistic elements, beyond words, need clarifying and practicing?

- How to trigger students attention to phrasing, navigating grammatical turns, and linguistic pirouettes?

- How, above all, to ensure that readers alert themselves when reading is—and is not—making sense?

The answers to these questions, as in most of life, commence with "It depends." One peek, or score, will not tell the tale. To see requires looking, probing, uncovering what is hidden in plain sight.

Two Peeks: Estimating Accuracy and Rate Word accuracy and rate provide points of departure, though not a full picture. Views differ regarding precise percentages, but a common rule of thumb is

- 93%–100% word accuracy (not more than 3/100 inaccurate) roughly corresponds to an independent level

- 90%–96% word accuracy (4/100–10/100 inaccurate) corresponds to an instructional level

- Below 90% accuracy (more than 10/100) corresponds to a frustration level (Gunther, 2013).

A reading accuracy estimate is commonly calculated with a 100- or 200-word passage, selected because it is anticipated to be within range for the reader.

Reading rate is the other fluency estimate measured during the same passage reading—commonly calculated as words correct per minute (WCPM), with rough norms being 30–70 WCPM for first grade; 50–100 for second; 70–120 for third; 90–140 for fourth; and 100–150 for fifth (Barr, Blachowicz, Bates, Katz, & Kaufman, 2013).

Capturing the Characteristics Accuracy and rate can signal whether reading material is easy, appropriate, or out of bounds for a reader; these also provide a frame for other instruction-related details. So, quantifying accuracy/rate with material expected to benefit a student is an opportune time to capture other characteristics as well: words read with effort, hesitations, self-corrections, noncorrections, awkward phrasing, stumbling over constructions, and barreling through punctuation. Furthermore, post passage probing is important to get a glimpse of the reader's understanding—first by eliciting a retell (prompting with "tell me more about" as needed) and then by posing a few key questions.

Round Two: Exchange and Exploration   After the first read, a stop-and-go interactive re-reading usually offers up many insights. A supported re-read prompts the student to paraphrase "chunks," 1–3 sentence groups (perhaps a paragraph chunk, if deemed appropriate). Paraphrasing text chunks can continue all the way through the passage, if what it uncovers is useful. Like a fine-tooth comb, this chunk-by-chunk paraphrasing unearths confusions—specific word meanings, idioms, and other complexities. And, even beyond that, it can spark reflective strategies—pausing, talking back to text, and checking for understanding. Perhaps most significantly, modulating speed, tone and tempo and routinely recode text into one's own words both secure information in memory and trigger recall.

Of course, teachers do well to untangle confusions before proceeding to the next chunk, clearing the way for more fully following the thread of the passage. During this more exploratory re-read teachers also supply correct renditions of most misread words and briefly convey meanings for unfamiliar terms—the better to see what a student does under scaffolded instruction (a view from the kid's learning edge).

A re-read requires delicate balancing: probing and taking notice, but also giving warm and tangible support throughout. The uncovering process should not feel like testing or quizzing. In fact, from first read to end of session, this "assessing" process can, and should, feel like a supportive joint exploration.

From Early Notions of Reading Fluency to Current Constructs

Although the historical roots of reading fluency, linked to oral reading and reading rate, stretch back from the 1800s to the 1900s (see Rasinski, 2006), its modern debut was sponsored by LaBerge and Samuels' seminal 1974 article, which proposed that young readers' slow, choppy reading represents lack of word automaticity, reflecting the effortful processing of individual words that consumes that narrow beam of conscious attention. This, the researchers pointed out, is in stark contrast to skilled readers, who read words without requiring conscious attention—the words largely reading themselves, releasing attention for other conscious activity. LaBerge and Samuels' instructional linkages were clear and groundbreaking: ensure practice well beyond accuracy; make certain that students reach easy automatic word-recognizing so that attention—that narrow window of consciousness—is freed for other duties.

The term *fluency* migrated from speech-language pathology, where it referred to spoken language—the flow of sounds, syllables, and words which, when impaired, results in slow, blocked, or choppy speech, as in stuttering or cluttering. Because the term *fluency* came to be applied to reading around the same time that *automaticity* was introduced, the two terms were commonly used interchangeably. As it took root in the field of reading, *fluency* asserted itself as the broader concept, referring to flow in reading connected text. *Automaticity* settled in to mean the effect of practicing beyond accuracy—the virtually effortless recognizing of individual words (both in and out of context).

Calculating Fluency and the Untoward Effects of Speeding   A computational estimate of reading fluency has been in wide use for decades (Tindal, Nese, Stevens, & Alonzo, 2016): word accuracy plus reading rate. This fluency estimate commonly has the student read aloud a timed passage and the teacher then calculate WCPM. This simple formula has long been a quick, useful way to assess fluency and to track reading progress:

$$accuracy + rate = reading\ fluency$$

WCPM has recently come under fire for misguiding teachers and students (Rasinski & Nageldinger, 2016). Critics complain that the practice of charting speed has downplayed—even caused neglect of—reading expression and comprehension. They report descriptions of misfocusing on fluency that play out in many schools, with untoward consequences, such as the following:

1. Teachers and students thinking of reading fluency as a matter of speed

2. Timed re-readings as the lens for viewing progress, with the unwitting message that other things—such as trying to make sense, self-questioning, pausing to consider, or changing pace to iron out a stumble or to make a connection—are not "approved" (a version of "damn the torpedoes, full speed ahead")

3. Overestimates about students' understanding of what they are reading because teachers assume the reading is "fluent"

These critiques share commonalities about conveying to struggling readers that reading is an outward exercise, to be speedily dispatched—rather than intent listening to what an author is conveying in the mind's ear.

Speed clearly never was the endgame, and certainly speed can divert both teachers and students from the intense leaning-in to catch meaning. A speed focus, along with other miscuing, can turn students away from their inner monitor, that stealthy sense-sniffer, without whom reading means little (so, who in their right mind would want to do it?). Regular messages promoting speed can diminish students' actively seeking to understand, with teachers unaware of their role in students' passivity and low levels of comprehension. This is a tragic teaching pitfall.

To underscore, speed is not the point, and a speed focus can be harmful; rather, swiftness is one outcome of more fluent reading. Much like driving, pace picks up with proper learning and sufficient practice—not by speeding a lot. Nobody promotes dangerous driving. Why encourage reckless reading, even inadvertently? A reader not paying much mind while reading, not staying alert to sense, is truly in danger.

Professional disaffection seems to have put a damper on fluency building in schools, which is truly alarming. This is not a baby to throw out with the proverbial bathwater; it is too important and necessary an instructional pursuit. Much serious evidence, amassed over decades—and discussed throughout this chapter—demonstrates the power of frequent and intentional building of readers' fluency—in primary grades and beyond (Rasinski & Nageldinger, 2016). Fluency is not a small thing but a major player in skilled proficient reading. Furthermore, fluency-building practices in the classrooms have only recently gained a toehold in schools' practices.

The current speed critique offers legitimate concerns that needed heeding. Currently, fluent reading of connected text is seen as the interplay of expression and comprehension, undergirded with well-oiled skills—an important corrective to the "speed-mostly" prior view. But, make no mistake—major nationwide fluency studies consistency reflect long-term findings that large numbers of fourth-grade readers have significant fluency insufficiencies that seriously impede their learning—alarming evidence that much more work needs doing. This is a clarion call for schooling to get on the stick.

While sensible to heed the news that many classrooms have mis-emphasized speed, it seems equally sensible simply to take corrective measures, like: highlight the misunderstanding, describe its problematic effects, warn new teachers, and encourage all to correct course—teaching kids to modulate and attend to meaning. This is not the first important idea that has produced unforeseen problems; it seems almost the nature of spreading good ideas.

Rasinski and Nageldinger (2016) offer a two-part corrective for the speeding problem:

1. Weed out fluency practices that promote speed per se or steer readers away from monitoring sense. These authors suggest a sensible litmus test for dumping a practice: Notice if it reduces enthusiasm for reading.

2. Keep and refresh practices that have stood the test of fun, those that positively affect motivation to read (e.g., rehearsing for performance; performing plays, poems, reader's theatre, audio- and video-recording of historical speeches).

In their apologia, Rasinski and Nageldinger (2016) offer a trove of examples, laid out in devilish detail for the doing. They also describe missteps in the name of fluency and urge returning to best basics. Their toolkit, available in print and in Kindle format, is a distillation of longtime commitment and well-placed loyalty.

REFLECT, CONNECT, and RESPOND

What has aroused recent concern about schools' fluency-building practices and their negative effects? Offer antidotes—ways to counteract the negative effects, not falling prey to the teaching pitfall. Yet another pitfall is inherent in the image of a youngster juggling two balls and being tossed three more. Explain your own experience of this teaching mis-step, either recalling when it happened to you as a learner or describing your having viewed it firsthand with other learners. Offer examples of what balls might be juggled in terms of teaching basic reading fluency.

Disconnecting Meaning, Even While Reading Flowingly   For some poor readers, surface fluency is not an issue. In fact, it is all too easy for some to sound as if they are reading well, fluently, and expressively while processing only minimally—in other words, while disconnecting. When teachers neglect to notice such disconnects, their students can assume that good reading means sounding good and not a process of wrestling to squeeze out the juice of meaning. And, as such passivity lingers over time, these students are developing a debilitating habit of not interacting with text as they "read."

The mind needs urging to stay in gear during all reading, but the unwelcome fact that meaning can be detached from fluent reading needs to remind us to promote students' monitoring of meaning from the earliest stages of learning to read—and all along the road. Whether a reader's mind grabs onto or lets go of meaning can be affected by what teachers say and neglect to say and how teachers frame practice, point to purposes, and respond to a student's stumbling over confusing text. The look, sound, and feel of students' active *meaning making* are worthy of noticing—and encouraging. For example, when students:

- *Pursue "getting it":* Showing intent facial and body expressions

- *Dig for understanding:* Re-reading, slowing down, and trying different phrasings

- *Notice when the sense derails:* Muttering, "Huh? Say, what? I don't get that"

- *Talk back to the author:* Arguing, "What do you mean by that? What are you saying?"

- *Seek help:* Asking of others, "Somebody, please read this part to me. Can you explain what this means?"

The following are resources for steering clear of speed traps. Figure 12.2 shows strategies for addressing specific "teaching pitfalls" resulting from emphasizing speed over meaning. Figure 12.3 represents how fluency, expression, and comprehension must be actively pursued for meaning.

Teaching potholes *No dangerous driving...*	Watch out! *Avoid reckless reading...*
Mis-emphasis on speed to the detriment of understanding	Change "speed" wording to *modulating* (or modulating tempo), talking about tuning-in to the writer whispering in your ear.
Misconception about the place of speed in fluency instruction	Instead of aiming for speed, aim students towards *getting it clear.* Fluency building is about getting it clearer and clearer. Picking up the pace will happen as an *outcome*—no rush-rush.
Insufficient probing of sense-making in the teacher-student duet as student is reading aloud	If a student does not *ask about* a "confusion"... why not? If he or she cannot retell a page of reading in his or her own words, why not? If he or she can answer some questions but not others, why? *PROBE:* Find the tangle, provide clarity (untangle), note the stumbling block to teach later, perhaps through multiple examples.
Insufficient cuing to self-monitor + adjust for sense	Students need to be *cued* to cock an ear—to listen to the writer who is talking. Students need to alert the inner reader to seek sense, hold onto it, go back when it slips—and adjust to make it clearer. Students need to know that something always goes wrong in reading, *for everyone*—so *good* readers listen and fix. *CUE:* Make it brief, frequent, and more often as coaching to individual kids, then as advice to the group. One of the best cues is the simple self-question: Did that make sense?

Figure 12.2. A warning poster for teachers.

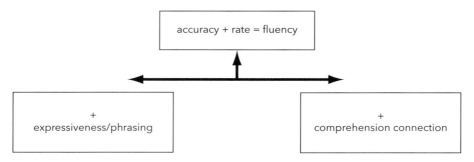

Figure 12.3. More current conceptualization of reading fluency. (From *Multisensory Teaching of Basic Language Skills, Third Edition* [p. 296].)

Depth and Breadth of Definitions of Reading Fluency Current definitions of reading fluency include elements such as word-level accuracy and automaticity, appropriately rapid pace, meaningful phrasing, and connections to comprehension—all in the context of navigating continuous, or connected, text:

- Increases in rate and ease of reading resulting from automaticity of word-level processes (Samuels, 2006)

- Rapidity, smoothness, and effortlessness with little conscious attention to mechanics (Meyer & Felton, 1999)

- The bridge between low-level skills involved in learning to read and high-level skills required for reading to learn (Chall, 1983; Pearson & Johnson, 1978)

- A critical dimension of learning to read, linking word recognition and comprehension, and affecting/intertwining with reading comprehension (Chard, Vaughn, & Tyler, 2002; Kuhn & Stahl, 2000)

- A skill related to accuracy and rate, but not synonymous with them, characterized by phrasing, natural flow of speech, with intonation, stress, and pauses related to author's syntax; meaningful expressiveness (National Assessment of Educational Progress [NAEP], 2002)

- One of the five pillars of reading (along with phonemic awareness, decoding, vocabulary, and comprehension); rapid accurate reading of continuous text with appropriate expression, requiring well-developed word-recognition skills (National Institute of Child Health and Human Development [NICHD], 2000)

- A unique and fundamental component of skilled, proficient reading with close links to comprehension and motivation; ability to read "like you speak," with reasonable accuracy, at a rate appropriate to the task, and with suitable expression (Hasbrouck, 2010)

- Accurate and conversational reading—it flows, is not easily distracted, generalizes across texts, and is maintained over long periods (Torgesen & Hudson, 2006)

- A multidimensional concept related to reading rapidly and modulating the flow of connected text with appropriate prosody—phrasing, stress, juncture, and intonation (Dowhower, 1987; Rasinski & Lenhart, 2007)

TEXTBOX 12.1 Proposed fluency definition

Reading Fluency (in Typical Readers)

Is a fundamental and multidimensional aspect of skilled proficient reading, that

- Requires well-developed word recognition and other language sub-skills at the prelexical, word, phrase, sentence, passage, and discourse levels

- Involves modulating the flow of connected text through phrasing and expression in accord with the author's meanings

- Affects reading from the early years through high school (it is important to, but not restricted to, the early reading years)

- Commonly interacts with comprehension but may disconnect, so pursuing comprehension had best remain a beacon at all levels of reading instruction

- Is marked by ease, flexible adjustments and repairs, increased motivation to read, minimal conscious application of mechanics, and durable performance levels over time (like bike riding)

These definitions increasingly mention comprehension and vocal expression. Less common but noteworthy elements are flexibility, modulation, motivation, and durability over time (attained reading skill stays with you—like riding a bicycle).

This chapter's proposed fluency definition (Textbox 12.1) includes notions from prior definitions, sorted into key requirements, concepts, and observable signs. Details were added to be more explicit and to offer examples discussed later in the chapter. Also, the context *typical readers* has been invoked to point out that fluency is actually separable from understanding, as evident in the atypical reading of those with hyperlexia (Treffert, 2011). Furthermore, the notion of reciprocity was added, following the lead of those (like Rasinski & Nageldinger, 2016) who view fluency as frequently reciprocal with reading comprehension, with each facilitating and being facilitated by the other—the ratio determined by the particulars of the reader and the material.

A further note: It seems important to acknowledge how conceptually close notions of reading fluency and skilled proficient reading are, even while each can be distinguished. This conceptual proximity reflects how fluency increasingly acts in concert with all aspects of reading—quite miraculous, really.

EXPRESSIVENESS, FLUENCY, AND THE COMPREHENSION CONNECTION

Attending to a student reading aloud is hugely informative, directly revealing not only accuracy but also prosody—expressiveness composed of intonation, stress, volume, phrasing, and the like. There has been some controversy over the role of prosody in comprehending (Rasinski, 2004; Torgesen & Hudson, 2006). Expressive reading helps students comprehend when someone reads to them, but it is not yet established whether, how, or how much prosody actually facilitates their understanding when reading on their own.

One view is that prosody simply reflects understanding but does not contribute to it. The other is that, in the main, prosody acts in both directions, facilitating and reflecting understanding. On the likelihood that this reciprocal view is correct at least much of the time and for many students—practices that emphasize expressiveness have been included in this chapter. On the other hand, whether a prosody practice actually affects comprehension is a matter of looking to see. For some students at some ages or stages, it may not help. As always, it is worth testing out.

Whatever the nuanced case about expressiveness, it is amply clear that fluency improves reading comprehension. Why? How does it operate to influence comprehension? First, reading fluency supports verbal working memory. Slow, word-by-word reading strains working memory, making it hard, sometimes impossible, to hold in mind what was just read while also processing the next chunk. Reading words easily and in meaningful chunks (i.e., phrasing) spares working memory—something especially important for those with dyslexia. Second, fluent reading frees attention for a train of thought, a momentary complexity, or for noticing and repairing a breach of sense. These are strategic cognitive moves that develop with use—but they may not develop readily with readers who have been long mired in sluggish lower level processing.

The orchestrated concert of fluent reading reduces the cognitive workload of processing written language. Lessening this load can allow the reader to pause and ponder, question and interact—or simply enjoy. Students with poorly oiled reading sub-skills and insufficient fluency understandably find the reading act laborious, stressful, and truly tiring.

Reading as Listening—A Possible Key

Rasinski and Nageldinger (2016) posit that expressiveness operates both in silent and oral reading and that proficient silent reading, while eventually overtaking oral reading in speed, never fully loses touch with the underlying contours of sounds, phrasing, sentence shapes, and other features of reading aloud. They point to the interior reader, listening—tuning in—when reading both orally and silently. This strong take on reading *as listening* is intriguing and rings true. As an advanced reader, I experience that sort of hearing when I read silently—a sonorousness in my mind's ear. More interesting and even astonishing—I never explicitly shared this when teaching students with reading disabilities, although I have simulated it with the Neurological Impress Method (see the description in the "Methods and Means for Building Fluency" section of this chapter). Actually, sharing this view with students would have helped some of them "get" what it means to tune in.

It seems immensely useful to develop the understanding of reading as listening and practice listening to myself among youngsters who regularly allow confusions to slide by. They may be trying hard but not listening well, which could explain why some comprehend less when reading silently and more when encouraged to read (quietly) aloud (to themselves). Many poor readers likely have little notion, unconscious or otherwise, of readers' active processing, which includes interacting with the writer, following the thread, listening intently, tuning in to a reading voice, and making sense. This active role is important for teachers to convey as part of their ongoing coaching. Other implications include checking in and considering, student by student, whether to engage any of the following:

- Allow oral reading to beyond a student's grade-mates', meaning to delay silent reading

- Cue a student to routinely switch to "out loud" when the reading gets rough

- Help a student listen for phrasing and emphasis, first aloud, then in the mind's ear (maybe we should not use the notion of "silently")

From Listening to *Listening*

This same direct and explicit teaching could, and should, be widely applied to teaching students to listen powerfully to recorded text. Recorded text is an under-appreciated playground for teaching prosody, re-reading, paraphrasing, noticing confusions, and listening more intently—all transferrable skills to reading without recorded accompaniment. Of course, these notions are not new; they circle back to Carol Chomsky's powerful 1976 findings on reading along with taped text. That work needs a major revival, with expansion of the instructional tools and extension into every school system in the country. How can schools *not* be doing this—especially when our adult world is so far into the electronic age that our daily devices can read and write with us.

Why not provide every weak reader, starting at the critical fourth-grade juncture, navigation and comprehension strategies for interacting with recorded text—not only to access content but also to actually improve their reading? Even better, why not arrange instruction in listening to recorded text for all in the fourth- to sixth-grade span, extending support for older students on an as requested basis? To not provide such a powerful, broad-based, educational benefit to all readers seems a huge failing of imagination and will, but perhaps this topic requires its own chapter, book, or movement.

> **REFLECT, CONNECT, and RESPOND**
> What does it mean to "teach" attention to meaning? How would you do that? Perhaps starting with a mini-lesson, initiating an exchange about what we find easy and hard and how we navigate complications. Perhaps by video of a savvy reader interacting with text while reading alone. What could you do to reinforce attention to meaning as your imaginary group of fourth-grade struggling readers sat reading quietly at their seats? What might you do to cue them? How then might you get each of them to cue themselves?

HOW GREAT A PROBLEM IS LACK OF FLUENCY?

Lack of fluency is a widespread problem, impeding progress for many students, just when school heaps a workload uptick atop of their foundation skills (NAEP, 1992, 2002). By fourth grade, students must deploy their mental resources in many directions—sentence-level complexities, new terms, unfamiliar concepts, following a line of argument, interpreting a metaphor, and noticing when the mind goes off the rails of the author's text (Nathan & Stanovich, 1991). Slow and labored reading compromises comprehension, especially as students must expand into denser material, digesting and remembering more unfamiliar information.

Two major initiatives have heightened awareness of fluency as a serious problem for many students nationwide:

1. The National Assessment of Educational Progress (NAEP), also known as the Nation's Report Card, undertook two fourth-grade oral reading substudies (1992, 2002).

2. The National Reading Panel (NRP), convened by Congress to report on the state of reading research and practice, gave prominence to fluency by listing it as one of five major aspects of reading (NICHD, 2000).

National Assessment of Educational Progress

The NAEP (1992) oral reading substudy found that many fourth-grade students across the country had not developed fluent reading on early fourth-grade material. This large-scale study called for fluency instruction in schools as the crucial—and neglected—bridge from the basics to broader and more complex reading. The NAEP's (2002) follow-up 10 years later revealed that the problem had not gone away. Results brought to light that nationwide 30%–40% of fourth-graders do not read an easy fourth-grade passage nearly fluently enough. At this demarcation in schools' reading demands, the famed fourth-grade slump (Chall & Jacobs, 1983, 2003), a significant number of students are ill equipped for the escalation in reading volume and complexity. See Figure 12.4 for this data on oral reading fluency.

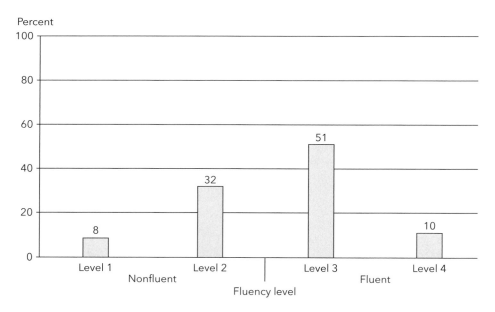

Figure 12.4. Percentage of fourth-grade students by National Assessment of Educational Progress (NAEP) oral reading fluency scale level. (*Note:* These results were not from an unpracticed cold reading; students' oral reading was evaluated only after several prior readings of the same fourth-grade passage.) (From Daane, M.C., Campbell, J.R., Grigg, W.S., Goodman, M.J., & Oranje, A. [2005]. *Fourth-Grade Students Reading Aloud: NAEP 2002 Special Study of Oral Reading* [NCES 2006-469]. U.S. Department of Education. Institute of Education Sciences, National Center for Education Statistics. Washington, DC: Government Printing Office, p. 30. Retrieved from http://nces.ed.gov/nationsreportcard/studies/ors/; reprinted by permission.)

National Reading Panel

The NRP reviewed research and practice, framing its report (NICHD, 2000) in terms of five major components of reading and reading instruction: phonemic awareness, decoding, fluency, vocabulary, and comprehension. The panel gave distinction to fluency as one of these top five facets, which finally precipitated long-needed attention from publishers, researchers, teacher educators, and schools.

The NRP also reviewed fluency intervention studies that included practices such as repeated reading, paired and assisted reading, radio reading, and neurological impress. They concluded that these variations of guided, repeated, oral reading significantly boost fluency, word recognition, and comprehension across a range of elementary grades. These findings were the basis for the panel's recommending fluency-building practices throughout the elementary years—and even for older students whose reading gets stalled in the first- through sixth-grade range.

International Dyslexia Association's Knowledge and Practice Standards

The International Dyslexia Association (2018) issued *Knowledge and Practice Standards for Teachers of Reading*. The fluency instruction section covers many of the bases discussed in this chapter, formulating what teachers and specialists need to understand and be skilled at when working with students with dyslexia and related difficulties.

> **REFLECT, CONNECT, and RESPOND**
> Is fluent reading a common problem in the United States? What is the nationwide evidence? How would you uncover your students' word reading accuracy, connected-text fluency, and active adjusting to make sense as they read?

FLUENCY AND READING/LEARNING DISABILITIES

Children with reading/learning disabilities have difficulty with word-reading accuracy and related sublexical linguistic processes, such as phonological and phonemic skills (Blachman, Tangel, Ball, Black, & McGraw, 1999; O'Connor & Jenkins, 1999). Many of these children also have difficulty accelerating words they read accurately to faster and less effortful levels. This slowness is also reflected on non-reading tasks, including some "naming" tasks, rapid automatic naming, and rapid alternating naming (Denckla & Rudel, 1976; Wolf, 2001) and is viewed as weakness in automatizing rapid oral language processes.

Thus, one or both of the bedrock components of fluency—word accuracy and automaticity—are problem areas for most students with reading/learning disabilities. Regarding accuracy, children with reading/learning disabilities have inordinate difficulty with developing word-reading accuracy, with associating regularities of common spelling patterns (orthography) with their oral counterparts (phonology), and with generalizing those orthographic/phonological correspondences to new words (Torgesen & Hudson, 2006).

Because word recognition, whether of sight or decodable words, is so difficult for these students, interventions tend to teach explicit word reading focused on word analogies and word-part skills (e.g., letter–sound associations, onset–rime, beginning-medial-ending sequencing, sound segmenting and blending, syllable or orthographic patterns). For poor readers—commonly pegged at or below the 25th percentile—intensive word-structure work over a sufficient timespan can establish a foundation. For students at or below the 10th percentile—even more intensive work is required to secure basic word recognition.

But accuracy is not nearly enough. Teaching must systematically build onto and build up reading skills—flexing, extending, weaving together, and practicing in longer and more complex reading contexts. What does it look like to build up reading skills in systematic ways? Three directions are useful, each offering similarities that are not quite the same.

1. Move students' sub-skills along the accurate-to-easy continuum:

   - Sound–symbol associations from accurate-to-easy—*Got it!*

   - Word blending/segmenting from accurate-to-easy—*Hey, look what I can do!*

   - Word recognition to effortless—*Look, Ma, no decoding!*

   - Word combining to easy—*More please!*

2. Move students, as soon as feasible, from single elements to combining: from sounds to words—words to phrases—phrases to sentences to little storybooks (sound-controlled text for extended practice). Too often instruction strands students at a "sound-out" or a "word by word" level, without propelling their skills to phrase reading, sentences and wee book *reading*.

3. Move through a decoding/encoding instructional sequence, new element by new element, adhering to the same systematic integration just laid out. Regular and systematic encoding is as important as decoding, not optional, a frill, or a sometime thing.

The systematic details of reading intervention are not minor, although teachers can unwittingly leave out or under-employ them. Being systematic entails repeated key practices that form daily routines—potent learning routines—the very heart of teachers' skillful means to propel students' reading forward, fluently.

The Good News

Students with a range of reading disabilities who do not establish foundation skills by early in third grade can develop accurate word recognition can increase reading fluency when provided intensive intervention focused on both areas (Torgesen, Rashotte, Alexander, Alexander, & MacPhee, 2003).

The Bad News

Students who are provided effective intervention in later third grade and beyond do not "catch up" in terms of reading fluency. With intervention, their accuracy can reach rough parity with grade peers, but fluency—while it improves over time—remains way behind peers and represents a weakness into adulthood (Pressley, Gaskins, & Fingeret, 2006; Torgesen et al., 2003).

The Interesting News

When early instruction focused on the right stuff with sufficient intensity, even students at lower reading percentiles can reach levels of accuracy and fluency on par with average grade-peers by second or third grade. In reaching that threshold within the second- through third-grade window, students remain up with peers in accuracy, fluency, and comprehension (Torgesen et al., 2003)! In other words, youngsters with serious reading disabilities can stay caught up when given enough of what they need in the primary years. Amazingly, that means that the year-by-year widening gap between students with dyslexia and average readers can be short-circuited—when foundation reading accuracy and fluency develops within the K–3 school years.

These encouraging findings have promoted urgency for early intervention nationwide. Over a series of carefully designed intervention studies, Torgesen and colleagues (2003) delineated the necessary conditions for such effective early reading intervention:

1. Screen early for reading difficulties (phonemic skills, underlying naming speed, and careful attention to early progress).

2. Follow up with intervention that directly focuses on word-level accuracy (phonemic skill and orthographic correspondences), systematic sequencing of instructional elements, and frequent instruction/practice over a sufficient period.

3. Teach through the full cycle: from word accuracy to rapid word recognition and phrased connected text, repeating the cycle with new words, word patterns, word groups, and other linguistic elements.

4. Teach attention to meaning concurrently.

5. Intensify intervention for those below the 25th percentile.

6. Intensify *and* increase the duration of intervention for those below the 10th percentile.

These conditions are doable, but depend on a solid understanding that they are crucial. They will likely need advocates willing to fight for them, especially to protect the time needed for a full set of practices—effective because they are properly focused and systematically carried out (and fun). When schools undertake this full journey—within the early window of opportunity—students reap lifelong benefits.

Sufficient Practice—More Than You Might Think!

Longstanding evidence reveals striking differences between students in the number of practice repetitions needed to reach reliable word reading accuracy (with basic words whose meaning is already familiar). The wide discrepancy is astounding:

- Four to fourteen repetitions for average young readers

- More than 40 repetitions for those with reading difficulties (Reitsma, 1983a, 1983b)

These figures raise alarm that classrooms may vastly underestimate the word practice needs of their weak readers. Some students require far more—and more frequent—word reading practice to reach word-reading accuracy, reliability, and ease! Do we provide that—week in and week out?

Importantly, as youngsters gain tangible skill early on, they feel drawn to reading, so eagerly engage in simple, repetitious reading practice that consolidates the interconnections of their newly forming reading mind. They are motivated to read a lot of easy redundant things—because they can. They love it because they can do it. In contrast, those who cannot, do not.

Those students not reading fluently in the first 3 years of schooling are denied the powerful inner voice of confidence: "I am a reader, smart and capable." An alternate inner narrative commences by second grade, as the poor reader attempts to make sense of why "I can't." As important, such students miss out on all that repetitive imprinting of seemingly simple skills that confident readers practice week by week over 3 years. Torgesen and Hudson (2006) estimated that to catch up in fluency, students with reading disabilities not reaching peer parity by the third grade would have to read massively more (at their own lower reading level) than their peers read over several years!

The Developmental Viewpoint

Wolf and Katzir-Cohen (2001) proposed that fluency is a developmental linguistic process, originating well before learning to read, proceeding through early reading, and extending to sophisticated linguistic complexities in high school and beyond. This comprehensive developmental view was a significant shift, with profound implications for practice from then on:

- Do not wait to work on fluency until students acquire basic reading (generally pegged at standardized scores in the second- through fourth-grade range). Instead, make fluency part and parcel of the earliest reading sub-skills (e.g., letter names, sounds, blending, pattern recognition, word recognition). First, establish each sub-skill to accuracy, then practice more—beyond accuracy to "pretty easy"—then keep on until it comes to mind like magic.

- Fluency building is far from finished just because they are cruising along at second- to fourth-grade reading levels. The next challenge is accuracy with the new elements and new sub-skills related to multisyllable words and other linguistic complexities. These, too, need the attention of instruction and sufficient practice to integrate into fluency at higher levels of reading (Berninger, Abbott, Billingsly, & Nagy, 2001).

Working on Fluency at the Earliest Reading Levels Too often pacing calendars and grade-level thinking result in overloading students who have yet to become fluent at a lower level. Especially for those with weak phonological skill, inefficient linguistic processing, and problems of verbal working memory, the critical early reading sub-skills will require more frequent, fun, and peppy practicing, not only for accuracy, but also for increasingly easy and, eventually, effortless word reading. Instruction often gallops on despite unsteady skills, outpacing learners whose word skills are neither accurate nor even close to effortless.

Working on Fluency With More Advanced Readers Schooling rarely treats advanced linguistic complexities as the skills they are. Rather, these are commonly addressed in the English curriculum as elements to learn *about*, rather than skills to be clarified and practiced from accuracy to fluency. For students with reading/learning disabilities, these advanced skills often pose major blockages to developing further fluency and reading comprehension at higher levels

(Nagy, 2006; Nagy, Berninger, & Abbott, 2006). Important to note, though: these complexities are not necessarily hard to master—when taught. While they may require some instructional attention and practice, they can be learned, sometimes through simply being highlighted, given a memorable name, and practiced with enough multiple examples. This is not to say that casual explaining and a couple of off-the-cuff examples will do it; rather, simple pre-planning examples and a systematic routine for introducing the revisiting can turn into powerful practice routines.

A variety of linguistic complexities crop up in reading material starting at around a fourth-grade level, causing most students to stumble. As the saying goes: where many falter, those with reading disabilities frequently fall. Common stumbling spots include **transition words,** multisyllable words, unfamiliar phrases, idiomatic expressions, confusing sentence contours (especially reversals), within-sentence signal words (or functors), cross-sentence signals (e.g., anaphora), and discourse signals that point the reader toward the author's moves. See Table 12.1 for examples. All teachers (e.g., science, math, social studies, English, special educators) can make critical differences by anticipating unfamiliar linguistic elements that are most common in their fields, ensuring a routine of clarifying, practicing, and revisiting that can be woven into learning routines.

In my long experience, teachers are often perplexed about how to teach these and so resort to unplanned explaining and an example—or two. Such impromptu explaining is never adequate; at the same time, though, it does not take heavy machinery to get these skills in place.

Most of these higher level reading complexities, known as text features, are readily teachable, requiring simply that students understand how the feature works, hear how it sounds, and practice enough examples to navigate it reasonably easily. The planning of examples and the mini-routine can be quite straightforward, repaying with huge dividends:

1. *Read aloud* examples of the feature with helpful expression, then clarify with the students how it is operating in the text.

2. *Name* the feature or, better yet, have students assign a moniker, something to call it, so you can talk about and refer to it. This helps anchor the feature and helps with recall.

3. *Provide* and have students *practice* pre-planned examples. Multiple examples can be enormously potent for learning. Too few examples diminish the power that gets-it-across and can hook it in memory. Students can devise an example of their own making; however, for those with language-based learning disabilities, it is important for teachers to provide multiple punchy examples.

A brief, but regular, routine is a simple and strong means for getting these unfamiliar complexities learned well and in short order.

One might preplan from the text or class reading one to three complexities per lesson (or one per two lessons). Once established, the routine can be also be engaged to spontaneously clarify trip-ups in reading. A practiced brief routine that focused on these at-first-baffling linguistic complexities can sensitize readers to them so that they may pick up more on their own.

Textbox 12.2 offers another 5-minute version of a teaching routine for those text complexities that so often confuse students from fourth grade and above.

Table 12.1.   Examples and notes of linguistic complexities urgently needed by many weak readers in Grades 4–12

Linguistic complexity	Examples	Notes
Sentence forms		
Appositives	The camel, a desert animal, can go for miles without drinking.	Sentence (i.e., thought) complexities are a great human pleasure when one can follow where they lead. For example, "There stood a personage only slightly taller than themselves, but whom they knew at once to be the Great Ta because of a certain unmistakable kingliness about him" (Cameron, 1954, p. 100).
Lists	I won't go unless you clean up your room, get into clean clothes, and find out where little Sue has gone.	
Reversed	I love you, even though you have bad breath. Even though you have bad breath, I love you.	
Cohesive ties		
Backward reference (anaphora)	Dorothy and Toto tip-toed out. *They* worried about every step. *This* made *them* tremble something terrible.	Cohesive ties are certain types of words or clauses that tie together ideas within and between sentences.
Forward reference (cataphora)	Perhaps I shouldn't tell you *this* but it was unzipped all evening.	When the words seem easy but the reader stumbles, consider whether there is an unfamiliar sentence form or cross-sentence tie that needs teaching and practicing (using multiple examples).
Ellipsis (words omitted, assumes the mind fills in)	The cat [that was] hit yesterday by that car has disappeared.	Cohesive ties are an important aspect of teaching English as a second language.
Cohesive ties		
Introductory	Once upon a time; two important ideas animate; it was the best of times	These cohesive ties are also known as *functors, signal words, noncontent words,* and *connectors.* They operate *within* sentences, as well as *across* sentence boundaries and also serve as major markers pointing to where the author is going (discourse signals).
Causals	So, because, thus, as a result of consequently, therefore, furthermore	
Reversals	However, nevertheless, even though, although, in spite of, despite, notwithstanding	Mastering these for reading (as well as writing) is important, especially as they are employed extensively in content-area (information) reading.
Concluding	In conclusion, to summarize, to conclude, in sum	
Sequentials	First, second; at the start, by the end; initially, subsequently; to begin with, in conclusion; primarily, secondarily	*Writing idea:* A cue card with these signal words grouped by type can trigger their use by older students and make the students' essays sophisticated.

Note: "Written language is not just spoken language written down" (Nagy, 2006).
Adapted from *Multisensory Teaching of Basic Language Skills, Third Edition* (p. 304).

TEXTBOX 12.2   **Five-minute multiple example routine**

Introduction (30 Seconds)

Pluck the complexity (word, phrase, sentence, device) out of its context and present it visibly and vividly for all to focus on. Read it aloud—let the students *hear* it. Acknowledge this as a complicated word, phrase, sentence, or discourse signal. (*Caution:* Do not ask questions.)

Clarify (60 Seconds)

Offer a second example of the complexity, one you made up using content closer to the students' frame of reference. Read this one aloud; be sure students take it in. Talk through (or have students join you in talking through) the meaning or purpose—how the complexity works. Then once more, read aloud the initial example from their text so they can *hear* the resonance between the two.

Amplify and Practice (90 Seconds)

Share a third close-to-home example that you created, again by reading it aloud. Help students make connections. Follow with two or three *more* examples, reading each aloud. (If students show readiness, they can read aloud.) Talk together about how the complexity works. Ask two students, one after the other, to read the initial example and then one of the others, for all to hear yet again.

Amplify (30 Seconds)

Suggest or solicit a mascot name for this complexity to make it easier to identify, recall, and talk about (e.g., "butt-ins" for appositives) and use this name going forward. Then, call on students to read the clearest example and to explain in their own words how it works.

Practice (60 Seconds)

Have all students read all sentences (preferably more than once). This can be accomplished in any of several fun ways, such as a muttering free for all for 30 seconds, partners reading the examples to one another, or a student "conductor" calling on groups of three to read three examples in unison.

Extension (30 Seconds)

Seek students' own examples in class, as an exit ticket, or for homework. Be sure to capture all their high-quality examples (with the author's name appended) and add them to the list of examples.

──────────

Note: Timings are only suggested but indicate what to aim for in a "brief" routine.
From *Multisensory Teaching of Basic Language Skills, Third Edition* (p. 305).

> **REFLECT, CONNECT, and RESPOND**
> What are some of the linguistic complexities described in this chapter? Why have they been included in a chapter on developing reading fluency? While the linguistic complexities seem daunting, the brief routines (clarify/ examples/practice) seem simple. Does that fit together for you? What does it mean to "weave" such brief routine into instruction?

METHODS AND MEANS FOR BUILDING FLUENCY

In this section, instructional methods, many mentioned throughout this chapter, are further detailed. Of course, these are simply samples. As skilled teachers become alert to the importance of focusing on sub-skill accuracy and frequent practice for fluency, they can draw on these methods or make up variants of their own. The practices are grouped by whether they focus at the word level, at the phrase, or at the passage level.

Word Work

As Torgesen (as cited in Hasbrouck, 2010) said, "There is no comprehension strategy that compensates for difficulty reading words accurately and fluently." The implication: take instruction beyond accuracy at every step—at the sound-play, letter, word-part, word, and phrase level. Fluency builds over time, picking up momentum from many sources. When securing letter–sound associations, make sure that these connections are accurate, stable, and then so well-practiced that they feel easy. When working on a word set, or word card stack, focus first on accuracy, then practice for greater ease—charting progress as feedback and motivation. This fluency work adds up over days, weeks, and months, fueling increasingly fluent reading at ever-higher levels. Table 12.2 presents in detail the complex cognitive-linguistic skill set that develops from kindergarten through seventh grade.

There are levels of word reading skill from basic to advanced, but in an important sense, word skills are never really complete. Advanced word work (multisyllabic, morphological, etymological) stretches beyond fourth grade, seventh grade, high school, or college. As with musical proficiency, there are gradations, with learners reaching different heights and furthering their skills across genres. For students with reading disabilities, the systematic word work that anchors their basic reading can also benefit them at higher levels.

Hiebert and Fisher (2005) offer a strong case for focusing on morphologically related word sets as a powerful approach to advanced word work. Teaching and practicing words with their morphological siblings creates networks in the reading mind, organized by salient aspects of word structure. (See Chapters 14 and 15 for more on word learning.)

Many students require more interconnection between morphological variants (e.g., *comment* and *commentator, sign* and *signature,* and *kindle, rekindle, kindling*). The mind needs to congregate these related words, rather than have them dispersed to all corners of the mental lexicon. It is important that schooling beyond third grade return to these so that students' repertoires expand while their morphological awareness sharpens. This is not about studying prefixes, suffixes, roots, and word permutations but about seeing and hearing the relatedness among these linguistic siblings, catching hold of the connections and of the different ways they are used, and storing them for easy retrieval from the mental lexicon. In learning to read,

Table 12.2. Reading: A complex cognitive-linguistic skill set

Level	Broad stage	Accuracy to fluency: Skill by skill
Kindergarten to third grade	Foundation building Long runway Lift off Steep initial climb Early aerodynamics Practice reading is required.	Sublexical skills (e.g., letter recognition, sound blending/segmenting, sound–symbol association) Orthographic regularities (spelling patterns) Word recognition: reliable to automatized Simple morphological affixes and derivations Phrasing, expressiveness, breakdown to repair Simple grammar/familiar content Fund of reliably recognized words
Fourth grade: Shift in reading demands	Confident and fluent reader Pilot-in-training permit Handling and flying maneuvers Extended excursions Unfamiliar destinations Reading regularly is required.	Many words recognized at sight Many multisyllabic words read readily Morphological variation (*congress, congressional*) Increased sentence complexity and length Vocabulary (meaning) expansion Increased understanding of idiomatic expressions Passage complexity (cohesive ties) Increasingly unfamiliar content
Seventh grade: Shift in reading demands	Well-developed reader Provisional pilot license A lot of regular reading is required.	Many words recognized at sight Morphological sophistication (*ambulance, ambulatory, perambulator*) Content-area sentence complexities Vocabulary expansion and elaboration Increased conceptual load Complex discourse structures Text that is dense with information

From *Multisensory Teaching of Basic Language Skills, Third Edition* (p. 306).

morphological variants are not to learn *about*; they represent critical word-linking *skills* to master for increasing proficiency. Students with weaknesses in underlying linguistic processes need particular help making these linkages.

How do you teach these? Again, this is straightforward and simple—a matter of multiple examples with which you help the mind catch on to the relatedness of the words. Regularly employ a fun, brief routine introducing morphological word sets (mates, siblings, cousins) and sufficient practice. Word sets can come from a class novel, subject-matter vocabulary, or common sight words in the process of being learned. The following is a sample instructional routine that might take 15–20 minutes to set up the first time but which can then run in 5- to 7-minute "morph-mate" sessions thereafter. Weaving in a routine focus on morphological connections—across the years from 4th to 12th grade—can have profound cumulative effects.

Sample Routine for Morphological Awareness and Skill   This sample routine includes both teaching and practice phases.

Teach It to Fluency

- Provide several sets of easy examples (e.g., *happy, unhappy, happiness, happily; warm, warmer, warmest, warmth*). Read these to the students. With them, come up with a conceptual name for these kinds of related words (e.g., "morph mates"). *Note*: Don't quiz students during this introductory teaching time.

- Provide several more examples appropriate to students' age and stage (e.g., *manage, manager, management; sign, signing, signer, signature, signatory*). Again, read these aloud for all. Do not ask students for illustrative sentences—*provide* those examples. You can also make **semantic maps** with a core word in the center and variants at the ends of the spokes, along with an easy-to-grasp sentence for each morph-mate to show how it is used.

Practice It = Fluency

- Make drill cards, with the core word on Side 1 (e.g., *amble*) and with morphological variants on Side 2 (e.g., *ambling, ambled, ambulate, ambulance*). On separate cards, provide multiple, helpful sentences with each of the morphological variants (one sentence per card), such as "The cowboy and his girl were ambling along the path, acting like they had all the time in the world." "After my car accident, ambulating around the apartment was torturous."

- Create activities (whole class, subgroups, partners) that involve practicing the linking of the core word (Side 1) with the variants (Side 2) and with illustrative sentences with the variants. Be sure students read both the words and the sentences aloud—in a sense, they are training their reading "ear" to increase sensitivity to these word structures. Have students match the variant sentences with the core word (Side 1). *Note*: This morphological work is useful for both early readers (*sit, sitting, sat; wonder, wondering, wonderful*) and for advanced readers with morph mates from fiction and subject areas (*virulent, viral, virus; sign, signer, signature, signifying*).

Phrase Work Leads to Fluency

Once early readers have a store of reliable words, it is valuable to focus on phrasing (Rasinski, 2006). Practice connector words (e.g., *the, and, of, in, at, up, but, over, out*), not on their own but rather in common phrases. Phrase work can propel students who are clinging to accurate but plodding habits to let the words flow as they focus on the phrase. Here are several useful ways to bear down at the phrase level:

- Practice reading phrase cards (e.g., *in a pot, up the hill, into the water, he is coming, she is going, we are waiting*).

- Make large phrase cards; hold them up, one at a time, each for 3 seconds. When they are out of sight, have students read them from short-term memory.

- Find appropriate practice sentences and passages. Have students practice "scooping" by penciling a "scoop line" beneath phrases. They can also scoop phrases using the eraser (fewer marked-up pages). For more on the use of scooping with older students, see Chapter 20.

- Find or create phrased cued text: Thomas Alva Edison/ invented many things/ that are still in use/ today.// He had/ good ideas.// When Edison had ideas,/ he worked on them.// He would try/ many things.//

Re-reading Continuous Text

Re-reading continuous text is a time-honored practice. People re-read deep texts to absorb lifelong nourishment; re-read old favorites for the memories, joy, tears, and laughter; re-read to make better sense of a proposition, a metaphor, or a line of argument. A prominent method for re-reading, developed specifically to increase the fluency of struggling readers, goes under the name of repeated reading.

Repeated Reading   Under the term *repeated reading* is a powerful set of fluency-building procedures first developed by Samuels (1979). Research has confirmed that repeated reading can be effective and has delineated aspects that make it more so.

Meyer and Felton (1999) reviewed repeated reading studies and concluded that the method increases reading speed for a wide variety of readers. From their findings, they recommended these practices:

- Engage students in multiple readings with short, but frequent, fluency practice sessions.

- Use instructional-level text (or decodable text with struggling readers).

- Include measures of progress.

- Provide differentiated teacher support.

Chard and colleagues (2002) highlighted findings from repeated reading studies they considered particularly useful for students with reading/learning disabilities:

- Work on phrasing as part of repeated reading to promote automaticity.

- Include a skilled model to enhance comprehension effects (e.g., live modeling as well as electronic).

- Alert students to stay connected to comprehension, notice when it breaks down, and activate repair strategies.

Note: More procedures from effective repeated reading programs are detailed in the appendices provided in the Online Companion Materials.

Easy or Challenging Material?   Controversy continues over whether passages used for repeated reading should be challenging, moderately challenging, or easy. The "right" answer may depend on the age and other characteristics of the learners and the specific level of reading skill. Differing views also persist about how valuable skilled model reading is as part of repeated reading intervention. Some adult modeling is clearly effective, but how much yields what level of benefit is not yet clear.

Fluency Development Lesson–Rasinski to the Rescue   Rasinski has been a fluency mainstay over years—with good reason. He has written many practical resources, one of the most pivotal being his 2016 defense of doing the right thing in response to recent dampening of schools' fluency efforts. Rasinski not only offers important correctives and methods but also shares outlets for performance-oriented reading materials.

For years, Rasinski's clinic has utilized a Fluency Development Lesson (FDL) with strong empirical results (Rasinski & Nageldinger, 2016) and a simplicity that belies its built-in power. The FDL is an intensification of a common primary grade activity: practicing and performing a poem or other short text, usually undertaken over 4–5 days with one text. Rasinski's FDL tweak uses a short daily session (10–30 minutes) with a new text practiced to fluency each day. Figure 12.5 presents a condensed view of this FDL. The point is to do a short punchy practice,

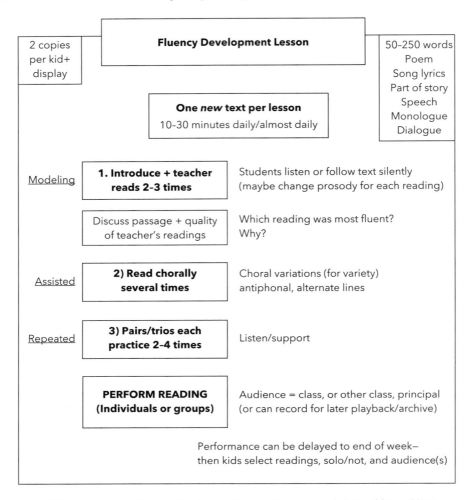

Figure 12.5. Adaptation of Fluency Development Lesson. (*Source:* Rasinski & Nageldinger, 2016.)

do it well, and do it often, and make selections for performance. Within 5 weeks at Rasinski's clinic, students learn to read fluently and with understanding 25–50 poems and other short texts—and perform (i.e., read) them in poetry slams, small-group choral reads, and recorded readings of speeches presented to social studies teachers.

Other Fluency Methods With Continuous Text   Although repeated reading is the most well-known fluency intervention for re-reading continuous text, other methodologies and programs have emerged, using continuous text and incorporating effective and efficient re-reading techniques. Some are "old-time" practices that predate concepts of reading fluency (e.g., choral reading); others grew out of early special education traditions of "precision teaching" (e.g., Great Leaps); and still others have emerged from educators' seeking to motivate struggling readers (e.g., **reader's theatre**).

Reader's Theatre   Reader's theatre has a considerable reputation as a real-world reason to re-read—the imperative to rehearse in preparation for performance. Reader's theatre has interesting aspects that can spur fluency and seriously motivate reading and re-reading. It makes use of performance scripts and a rehearsal process but does not culminate in a full-scale production. Students commonly rehearse sitting on stools with music stands to hold their scripts. They perform in that same format, without costumes, sets, or interactive movement. The teacher/director orchestrates rehearsals (re-readings), urging fluency and expression. Sometimes, readers are taught to scan their line, look up, and then deliver it—a practice that promotes processing in phrases. An interesting twist is reading lines sequentially, rather than assigning character parts to particular students. In this mode, each reader delivers a line, with the next reading the next line, and so forth down the row of readers on their stools. Not being assigned parts requires that everyone perform with the expression of the character, even though characters' lines are spoken by various readers.

Details and variations of repeated reading and reader's theatre can be found on the Internet, where there are also multiple resources and video demonstrations.

Neurological Impress Method (Plus)   The neurological impress method (NIM) was originally developed by Heckelman (1969) and was the focus of two studies with struggling readers in third through sixth grades that found improvement in fluency and comprehension scores (Flood, Lapp, & Fisher, 2005). The researchers added a brief comprehension connection (the "plus") at the end of the original method.

NIM (Plus) is to be used 10 minutes per day, 4 days per week, for 5 or more weeks. General guidelines are as follows:

1. Use instructional-level text (or student-selected).

2. Sit next to and slightly behind the student and read into his or her ear (side of handedness).

3. Slide your finger along text during reading; student rests a finger on top of the teacher's finger.

4. Read the text aloud together, with the teacher setting the pace and modeling skilled expressiveness (phrasing, intonation, pauses). The student's voice trails just behind the teacher's.

5. Gradually release the lead to the student, lowering volume and letting the student's pace overtake the teacher's.

6. Gradually have the student take over the finger-tracking accompanying the reading.

7. *Plus:* After reading, have the student retell the text. Also, talk together about aspects of interest or confusion (prior knowledge connections, high points, humor, unfamiliar vocabulary).

Notes on NIM (Plus) include the following:

- The focus of NIM (Plus) is on fluency and making the voice match the print, so do not correct, teach, or question as you go through the passage.

- The purpose of the extra step is to maintain the comprehension connection, have a brief enjoyable chat, and provide any needed clarification.

- Keep sessions short and fun, no longer than 10 minutes, and acknowledge the student's good work.

Variations on Choral Reading   NIM (Plus) is a variant of choral reading (reading in concert); other variations include whole-class **choral reading**, call and response (**echo reading**), and paired and buddy reading. These variants hold promise for building fluency when done at the appropriate stage of students' reading development. The research to date has been positive (NRP, 2000), so these remain valuable adjuncts to a multidimensional reading program or intervention.

Great Leaps   The Great Leaps reading program (Campbell, 1996) consists of 1-minute timings that make use of three stimuli: phonics, sight phrases, and reading short stories. This is a highly motivating, daily 5- to 10-minute intervention that can be carried out by trained nonteachers. Performance is charted so both students and teachers see and evaluate progress. The program has several levels from elementary to high school, with the K–2 version providing a phonological awareness component (Mercer & Campbell, 1998). Study results show growth in overall reading as well as increased reading rate for middle school students with reading/learning disabilities (Mercer, Campbell, Miller, Mercer, & Lane, 2000).

The Art and Science of Fluency Practice

Fluency work is not a matter of seatwork practicing. It involves teaching (cueing, modeling, explaining, coaching, encouraging, correcting), accompanied by properly framed interactive practice. In the interplay between clear and explicit teaching and interactive, progressive practice, instruction needs also to engage students' understanding of what the fluency work is all about and to gain their informed partnership.

The characteristics of practice text matters; not just any reading material facilitates reading fluency (Hiebert & Fisher, 2005; NICHD, 2000). Elfrieda Hiebert has built a powerful case for the effects of text characteristics in facilitating or hindering learning to read and developing reading fluency (http://textproject .org). Hiebert has amassed evidence that most students who are learning to read require material that is engineered for redundancy. She specifically recommends repeated practice with the 930 most frequent words (see the Zeno list on her text project web site), along with words whose graphophonic patterns are most consistent and most common. The nature of the practice material for developing a reading foundation, most especially the words—their high frequency and their redundancy—can, and does, make a huge difference in whether and how well many children read.

Providing Active Practice (Drill and Thrill)   Drill, another name for active practice, is highly motivating and highly effective, especially when done interactively, with progress charted regularly. Interactive practice enables sub-skills to increase in speed and decrease in focal attention, keys to fluent reading. Classrooms have been known to ignore the basics of effective practice, from drill to distributed practice, intermittent review, and cumulative practice. Drill has been demonized, rather than appreciated for its motivating efficiency at providing needed practice—beyond accuracy. As a result, many students' skills are insufficiently secured—for want of practice. Those with reading/learning disabilities commonly need to be well and explicitly taught—and then to

Practice enough
on the right stuff,
in the right portion size,
with teacher modeling, guidance, and corrections,
with visible feedback from tracking progress,
… and, all the while, helping the mind to remain attuned to sense.

Teaching Self-Monitoring for Sense–The Secret Sauce When targeting speed, prompt the mind to be guided by sense. Share information with students about how all minds get derailed, distracted, or off track and how we all bring our minds back into focus. Self-monitoring is a kind of self-message, triggered by noticing when the mind has slipped up. Developing self-monitoring requires other than pep talks or reminding. Using self-cuing message cards is far more effective for forming self-monitoring habits. By pointing, tapping, or simply winking, teachers can turn students' attention in the direction of the cue card. Messages are frequently formulated as self-questions because these slip into the mind, prompting an inner dialogue. When such an external cue is close up and personal, students start to trigger the habit on their own, shifting their eyes to the card independently and, eventually, shifting their mind's eye. See Figure 12.6 for a sample 3″ × 5″ self-monitoring cue card that can be folded into a tent and placed on the student's desk as a reminder.

REFLECT, CONNECT, and RESPOND

If you had to pick one, which approach to developing reading fluency would you employ regularly? Explain your choice. Which approach could be readily incorporated into a general education elementary classroom?

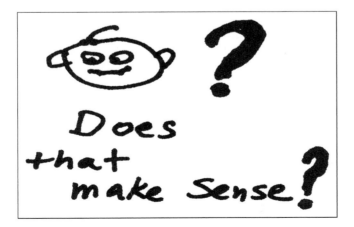

Figure 12.6. A self-monitoring cue card (3″ x 5″ folded tent on student's desk) can nudge the young reader's mind to be guided by sense. (From *Multisensory Teaching of Basic Language Skills, Third Edition* [p. 312].)

CLOSING THOUGHTS: THE ROLE OF FLUENCY IN READING

No one intends for students to be simply fluent readers; the aim is to be active, interacting, sense-seeking readers with accurate, automatic word recognition and other language-navigating skills. Fluency has been largely neglected in classrooms, which has hobbled many readers, even into adulthood. Fluency building needs considerably greater play in the teaching of reading overall and as part of intervention for students with intensive needs. But there is a common and dangerous pitfall—the misconception that fluency work is all about reading faster, which fosters a hurry-up, rush-rush mentality that can throw meaning to the winds. There is much more to developing fluency than acceleration. Keep in mind the instructional takeaways in Textbox 12.3, and consider posting them for continual reference.

Reading is a complex skill with all the richness that entails. Teaching reading is no less complex a skill. There is art, science, and subtlety to teaching reading, especially doing so effectively for students with linguistic weaknesses. Both the teaching and learning are straightforward, while at the same time being mind-bogglingly complex—but with good and sufficient practice, they both are eminently doable.

TEXTBOX 12.3   **Five take-aways for fluency instruction**

The following are five take-aways for fluency instruction. Perhaps post them for reference.

1. Do not assume. Notice signs: frequent pausing, lack of phrasing, little expressiveness, slow or erratic pacing, and tiring effortful effort. Notice at the word level, at the phrase level, and at the increasingly complex sentence level. Explore! Find out! Reading fluency is a set of skills and sub-skills that your instruction can propel to accurate and then to "easy."

2. Do not trade accuracy for speed or sacrifice comprehension—keep the reading mind tuned to sense. Making sense is paramount, and modulating is the key.

3. Do not just teach. Ensure *enough* practice! Kids love that muscular feel of moving from accurate to easy—the thrill of the rep effect! And charting their increases in easy is powerful motivation.

4. Don't short-change practice; distribute it over time. Make full use of short, intense, and frequent teach-it/practice-it sessions (10 minutes, 3-5 times per week, 5 minutes 2 times per day), until easy means *really easy.*

5. *Caution*—students are different. Many respond to timed reading of words or continuous text with alertness and focus; others become anxious. Take care with those distressed by timing pressure; change course and reduce that burden. Remember: Students are different.

ONLINE COMPANION MATERIALS

The following Chapter 12 resources are available at http://www.brookespublishing .com/birshcarreker/materials:

- Reflect, Connect, and Respond Questions

- Appendix 12.1: Knowledge and Skill Assessment Answer Key

- Appendix 12.2: Case Studies

- Appendix 12.3: Assessing Oral Reading Fluency

- Appendix 12.4: Hasbrouck and Tindal's (2006) Oral Reading Fluency Data

- Appendix 12.5: Five Take-Aways for Fluency Instruction

KNOWLEDGE AND SKILL ASSESSMENT

1. Which of the following aspects of reading fluency has grown in emphasis since 2000?

    a. Automaticity

    b. Accuracy and rate

    c. Decoding and encoding

    d. Expressiveness

    e. None of the above

2. Which of the following is *not* accurate?

    a. Reading fluency involves more than acceleration.

    b. Word-by-word reading strains working memory

    c. Improved reading fluency supports improved reading comprehension.

    d. Reading fluency starts early and develops over many years.

    e. None of the above

3. Critics have been increasingly vocal in opposition to particular fluency-building practices, resulting in schools' discontinuing those practices. The criticism focuses on which of the following?

    a. Neurological impress plus (NIM+)

    b. Phrase practice

    c. Repeated reading

    d. Word-level drills

    e. None of the above

4. A 2016 passionate published response to the aforementioned criticism offers well-developed "solutions," highlighting a plan called The Fluency Development Lesson (FDL). Who authored this plan, and what does it focus on?

    a. The National Reading Panel, which delineated the five pillars of reading (one being fluency)

    b. Josef Torgesen, who focused on the Grade 1–3 window for learning to read

    c. LaBerge and Samuels, who focused on automaticity

    d. Rasinski and Nageldinger, who focused on performance-oriented re-reading

    e. None of the above

5. How does increased reading fluency in developing readers support verbal working memory?

    a. By helping students articulate more rapidly.

    b. By encouraging chunking text into meaningful phrases.

    c. By using leveled books.

    d. By emphasizing decoding.

    e. None of the above

REFERENCES

Barr, R., Blachowicz, M., Bates, A., Katz, C., & Kaufman, B. (2013). *Reading diagnosis for teachers: An instructional approach* (6th ed.). Hoboken, NJ: Pearson.

Berninger, V.W., Abbott, R.D., Billingsly, F., & Nagy, W. (2001). Processes underlying timing and fluency of reading: Efficiency, automaticity, coordination, and morphological awareness. In M. Wolf (Ed.), *Time, fluency, and dyslexia*. Timonium, MD: York Press.

Blachman, B.A., Tangel, D.M., Ball, E.W., Black, R.S., & McGraw, C. (1999). Developing phonological awareness and word recognition skills: A two-year intervention with low-income, inner city children. *Reading and Writing: An Interdisciplinary Journal, 11*, 239–273.

Butterworth, B., & Kovas, Y. (2013). Understanding neurocognitive developmental disorders can improve education for all. *Science, 340*(6130), 300–305. doi:10.1126/science.1231022

Cameron, E. (1954). *The wonderful flight to the mushroom planet*. New York, NY: Little, Brown & Co.

Campbell, K. (1996). *Great Leaps reading program*. Gainesville, FL: Diarmuid.

Chall, J. (1983). *Stages of reading development*. New York, NY: McGraw-Hill.

Chall, J.S., & Jacobs, V.A. (1983). Writing and reading in the elementary grades: Developmental trends among low-SES children. *Language Arts, 60*(5), 617–626.

Chall, J.S., & Jacobs, V.A. (2003, Spring). The classic study on poor children's fourth-grade slump. *American Educator*.

Chard, D.J., Vaughn, S., & Tyler, B. (2002). A synthesis of research on effective interventions for building fluency with elementary students with learning disabilities. *Journal of Learning Disabilities, 35*, 386–406.

Chomsky, C. (1976). After decoding: What? *Language Arts, 53*, 288–296.

Daane, M.C., Campbell, J.R., Grigg, W.S., Goodman, M.J., & Oranje, A. (2005). *Fourth-Grade Students Reading Aloud: NAEP 2002 Special Study of Oral Reading* (NCES 2006-469). U.S. Department of Education. Institute of Education Sciences, National Center for Education Statistics. Washington, DC: Government Printing Office. Retrieved from http://nces.ed.gov/nationsreportcard/studies/ors/

Denckla, M.B., & Rudel, R.G. (1976). Rapid automatized naming (R.A.N.): Dyslexia differentiated from other learning disabilities. *Neuropsychology, 14,* 471–479.

Dowhower, S.L. (1987). Effects of repeated reading on second-grade transitional reader's fluency and comprehension. *Reading Research Quarterly, 22,* 389–406.

Fern-Pollak, L., & Masterson, J. (2014). Literacy development. In D. Mareschal, B. Butterworth, & A. Tolmie (Eds.), *Educational neuroscience.* Somerset, United Kingdom: Wiley-Blackwell.

Flood, J., Lapp, D., & Fisher, D. (2005). Neurological impress method plus. *Reading Psychology, 26*(2), 147–160.

Gunther, J. (2013). *Ongoing assessment for reading.* Retrieved from LearnNC: University of North Carolina web site: http://www.learnnc.org/lp/editions/readassess/991

Hasbrouck, J. (2010). *Developing fluent readers white paper.* St. Paul, MN: Read Naturally.

Hasbrouck, J., & Tindal, G.A. (2006). Oral reading fluency norms: A valuable assessment tool for reading teachers. *The Reading Teacher, 59*(7), 636–644.

Heckelman, R.G. (1969). A neurological impress method of remedial reading instruction. *Academic Therapy, 5*(4), 277–282.

Hiebert, E.H., & Fisher, C.W. (2005). A review of the National Reading Panel's studies on fluency: On the role of text. *Elementary School Journal, 105,* 443–460.

International Dyslexia Association, The. (2008, March). *Knowledge and practice standards for teachers of reading.* Retrieved from https://dyslexiaida.org/knowledge-and-practices/

Kuhn, M.R., & Stahl, S.A. (2000). *Fluency: A review of developmental and remedial practices* (CIERA Rep. No. 2-008). Ann Arbor, MI: Center for the Improvement of Early Reading Achievement.

LaBerge, D., & Samuels, J. (1974). Towards a theory of automatic information processing in reading. *Cognitive Psychology, 6,* 293–323.

Mercer, C.D., & Campbell, K.U. (1998). *Great Leaps reading K–2 edition.* Gainesville, FL: Diarmuid.

Mercer, C.D., Campbell, K.U., Miller, M.D., Mercer, K.D., & Lane, H.B. (2000). Effects of a reading fluency intervention for middle schoolers with specific learning disabilities. *Learning Disability Research and Practice, 15*(4), 179–189.

Meyer, M.S., & Felton, R.H. (1999). Repeated reading to enhance fluency: Old approaches and new directions. *Annals of Dyslexia, 49,* 283–306.

Nagy, W. (2006). *Morphological contributions to literacy.* Presentation at the New York Branch of the International Dyslexia Association.

Nagy, W., Berninger, V., & Abbott, R. (2006). Contributions of morphology beyond phonology to literacy outcomes of upper elementary and middle school students. *Journal of Educational Psychology, 98,* 134–147.

Nathan, R.G., & Stanovich, K.E. (1991). The causes and consequences of differences in reading fluency. *Theory Into Practice, 30*(3), 176–184.

National Assessment of Educational Progress (NAEP). (1992). *NAEP oral reading sub study.* Retrieved from http://nces.ed.gov/nationsreportcard/studies/ors/

National Assessment of Educational Progress (NAEP). (2002). *Nation's report card.* Retrieved from http://nces.ed.gov/pubsearch/getpubcats.asp?sid=031#

National Institute of Child Health and Human Development (NICHD). (2000). *Report of the National Reading Panel: Reports of the subgroups. Teaching children to read: An evidence-based assessment of the scientific research literature on reading and its implications for reading instruction* (NIH Publication No. 00-4754). Washington, DC: Government Printing Office.

O'Connor, R.E., & Jenkins, J.R. (1999). The prediction of reading disabilities in kindergarten and first grade. *Scientific Studies of Reading, 3,* 159–197.

Pearson, P.D., & Johnson, D.D. (1978). *Teaching reading comprehension.* Austin, TX: Holt, Rinehart & Winston.

Pressley, M., Gaskins, I.W., & Fingeret, L. (2006). Instruction and development of reading fluency in struggling readers. In S. Samuels & A. Farstrup (Eds.), *What research has to say about fluency instruction* (pp. 47–69). Newark, DE: International Reading Association.

Rasinski, T. (2004). *Assessing reading fluency.* Honolulu, HI: Pacific Resources for Education and Learning.

Rasinski, T. (2006). A brief history of reading fluency. In S. Samuels & A. Farstrup (Eds.), *What research has to say about fluency instruction* (pp. 4–23). Newark, DE: International Reading Association.

Rasinski, T. (2017). Readers who struggle: Why many struggle and a modest proposal for improving their reading. *The Reading Teacher, 70*(5), 519–524.

Rasinski, T., & Lenhart, L. (2007). *Explorations of fluent readers.* Newark, DE: International Reading Association.

Rasinski, T., & Nageldinger, J.K. (2016). *The fluency factor: Authentic instruction and assessment for reading success in the common core classroom* [Kindle ed.] New York, NY: Teachers College Press.

Reitsma, P. (1983a). Printed word learning in beginning readers. *Journal of Experimental Child Psychology, 36,* 321–339.

Reitsma, P. (1983b). Word-specific knowledge in beginning reading. *Journal of Research in Reading, 6,* 41–56.

Richards, T.L., & Berninger, V.W. (2008). Abnormal fMRI connectivity in children with dyslexia during a phoneme task: Before but not after treatment. *Journal of Neurolinguistics, 21,* 294–304.

Samuels, S.J. (1979). The method of repeated readings. *The Reading Teacher, 32,* 403–408.

Samuels, S.J. (2006). Toward a model of reading fluency. In S. Samuels & A. Farstrup (Eds.), *What research has to say about fluency instruction* (pp. 24–46). Newark, DE: International Reading Association.

Schwaneflugel, P.J., & Benjamin, R.G. (2017). Lexical prosody as an aspect of oral reading fluency. *Reading and Writing, 30,* 143–162. doi:10.1007/s11145-016-9667-3.

Shaywitz, B.A., Shaywitz, S.E., Blachman, B.A., Pugh, K.R., Fulbright, R.K., & Skudlarski, P. (2004). Development of left occipitotemporal systems for skilled reading in children after a phonologically-based intervention. *Biological Psychiatry, 55,* 926–933.

Tindal, G., Nese, J., Stevens, J.J., & Alonzo, J. (2016). Growth on oral reading fluency measures as a function of special education and measurement sufficiency. *Remedial and Special Education, 37*(1), 28–40.

Topping, K.J. (2006). Building reading fluency: Cognitive, behavioral and socioemotional factors and the role of peer mediated learning. In S.J. Samuels & A. Farstrup (Eds.), *What research has to say about fluency instruction* (pp. 24–46). Newark, DE: International Reading Association.

Torgesen, J.K., & Hudson, R. (2006). Reading fluency: Critical issues for struggling readers. In S.J. Samuels & A. Farstrup (Eds.), *Reading fluency: The forgotten dimension of reading success* (pp. 130–158). Newark, DE: International Reading Association Monograph of the British Journal of Educational Psychology.

Torgesen, J.K., Rashotte, C.A., Alexander, A., Alexander, J., & MacPhee, K. (2003). Progress towards understanding the instructional conditions necessary for remediating reading difficulties in older children. In B. Foorman (Ed.), *Preventing and remediating reading difficulties: Bringing science to scale* (pp. 275–298). Timonium, MD: York Press.

Treffert, D.A. (2011). Hyperlexia III: Separating "autistic-like" behaviors from autistic disorder; assessing children who read early or speak late. *Wisconsin Medical Journal, 110*(6). Retrieved from https://www.wisconsinmedicalsociety.org/_WMS/publications/wmj/pdf/110/6/281.pdf

U.S. Department of Education, Institute of Education Sciences, National Center for Education Statistics, National Assessment of Educational Progress (NAEP). (2002). *Oral reading study.* Retrieved from http://nces.ed.gov/nationsreportcard/studies/ors/

Wolf, M. (Ed.). (2001). *Time, fluency, and dyslexia.* Timonium, MD: York Press.

Wolf, M., & Katzir-Cohen, T. (2001). Reading fluency and its interventions. *Scientific Studies of Reading, 5,* 211–239.

Chapter 13

Math Learning Disabilities

Katherine Garnett and Colleen Uscianowski

LEARNING OBJECTIVES

1. To stimulate interest in identifying, supporting, and teaching students with math disabilities

2. To lay out instructional paths for education professionals to "see" more clearly, understand more fully, and work more effectively with the foundational math needs of students with dyscalculia—and to share insight that strengthens math instruction with a broader range of students

3. To provide resources that widen the circle of professionals and families who take seriously the needs of students with dyscalculia, encouraging them to band together to school the schools

Eight-year-old Shawn has received special services—speech, occupational therapy, and academic support—since preschool. Shawn's learning disabilities have made reading and writing extraordinarily difficult for him, despite his above-average intelligence and curious mind. In conversation, Shawn often interjects "Whaa…?" prompting others to restate or reword. He commonly has difficulty explaining and easily goes off-track onto related topics. An avid learner, Shawn devours recorded books and video documentaries, viewing them repeatedly. He has talent for three-dimensional creations and can deconstruct—and sometimes reconstruct—anything he gets his hands on.

Shawn's math difficulties have dogged him since kindergarten, but his school paid little attention—especially given the focus on his reading struggles. Now that Shawn is in third grade, the math challenges have acquired new urgency, prompting his mother to reach out to the school team for help with the many math confusions and consequent meltdowns.

Signs of Shawn's math difficulties include

- Immature counting strategies: Counting-all rather than counting-on from the larger number for single-digit combinations that total more than ten, such as $8 + 4$ and $5 + 9$. (He knows facts totaling up to 2–10 but not reliably beyond that.)

- Complete confusion with single-digit multiplication. (He complains, "I just don't get it.")

- Wildly inaccurate answers when hurried or timed.

- Spindly, ill-formed, and poorly spaced written numerals (and handwriting in general).

- Responses to math questions that show some relation to the question but are often way off base.

Examples of off responses are evident in the following sample of exchanges.

Dialogue Exchange 1

Working with tens and ones rods on the desk, Shawn at first responds accurately to sequenced questions.

TEACHER: How many tens? How many ones?

SHAWN: *[Counting tens rods and ones rods]* Three—two.

TEACHER: So, what's the number?

SHAWN: *[Counting by tens and ones]* Ten, twenty, thirty…two. Thirty-two.

TEACHER: *[Following up with a "hiding" game]* I'm holding 42 behind my back. So, how many tens am I holding?

SHAWN: Forty.

TEACHER: Say again? Remember, I took rods from the table. I'm holding them behind my back—they equal 42. So, how many tens does that mean I am holding?

SHAWN: Forty.

TEACHER: You're sure?

SHAWN: Yes, sure.

Dialogue Exchange 2

TEACHER: How many months in a year?

SHAWN: I don't know.

At this, the teacher offers prompting, getting Shawn to accurately recite the names of the months in sequence. Note, as he recites them, he does not tally them on his fingers.

TEACHER: So, how many months in a year?

SHAWN: Twenty-eight.

TEACHER: How did you get that answer?

SHAWN: My mother told me.

TEACHER: Can you keep track of the months you name on your fingers?

SHAWN: I don't understand.

TEACHER: *[Starting to demonstrate tallying on fingers]* January, February, March… like that. Have you ever kept track of things that way?

SHAWN: No.

The teacher makes a mental note that the current month is February, wondering to herself if this relates to Shawn's response.

Dialogue Exchange 3

TEACHER: What is 10 plus 10?

SHAWN: 20.

TEACHER: So, how much is 10 plus 9?

SHAWN: 109.

Shawn insists that 10 and 9 equals 109.

TEACHER: Does that make sense to you—10 and 10 together are 20—but 10 and 9 are 109?

SHAWN: *[Confidently]* Yes—I see it in my mind.

Despite such examples, common over more than 3 years, Shawn's child-study team assures his mother that he does not have a math disability (i.e., **dyscalculia**)—a condition the team admits to never having heard of, nor actually believing in. This stuns his mother, who has lived through many nights of her son's math tantrums and tears. Furthermore, she has been reading about dyscalculia online and is seeking neuropsychological assessment to better assess it. How can these educators see Shawn in class every day and still dismiss his many and obvious confusions with math?

NO ANOMALY—RATHER, A MATTER OF NEGLECT

This scenario is no anomaly. Rather, it traces the contours of a common conundrum facing parents of kids with math learning disabilities—their severe difficulties are rarely recognized. Schools are slow to attend to math underperformance, rarely considering it an area of disability—a case of woeful neglecting of youngsters and families (Butterworth, Varma, & Laurillard, 2011).

The upshot is that schools seldom qualify a student under Specific Learning Disability on the basis of math, even with evidence of severe difficulties and chronic low math scores. Also, when math disability co-occurs with reading and/or writing disabilities, intervention gravitates to reading—leaving even writing problems a distant second, with any significant math needs largely ignored.

Few schools know about special math materials or approaches. Teacher education programs rarely mention dyscalculia or special math methods in the preparation of classroom teachers—or even in preparing educational evaluators, math coaches, or special educators (Butterworth & Kovas, 2013)!

The focus of this chapter is dyscalculia, an underacknowledged disability—underacknowledged both as a singular condition and as one that co-occurs with other learning disabilities, such as dyslexia, dysgraphia, or attention-deficit/hyperactivity disorder (ADHD). Many publications address math teaching and learning; few probe the complexities posed by populations of students with math learning disabilities.

In this chapter, we intend to spur understanding of math disability on behalf of the children, their families, and their schools while anticipating that insights into their special needs will precipitate more skilled math teaching overall—for other youngsters, as well. A circulating truism has it that not all students need Orton-Gillingham reading methodology but that all teachers do. So, perhaps not all children need the full rendition of specially designed math intervention, but certainly their teachers do.

A VIEW FROM WHAT THEY ARE NOT

Math learning disabilities

- Are not rare, although they are unheralded

- Are not a recent phenomenon, although few know much, if anything, about them

- Are not simple but rather pose complexities and challenges in the teaching of math

- Are not inconsequential, precipitating serious schooling, emotional, and life effects

Dyscalculia Is Not Rare

Although underrecognized over the long haul, dyscalculia is not rare, affecting 3.5%–6.5% of the school-age population, a proportion that rivals the numbers of students with dyslexia and also those with specific language impairment. Table 13.1 provides information on the prevalence of dyscalculia and other specific learning disabilities.

Forty to fifty percent of students classified with dyslexia or learning disabilities have some degree of math disabilities (Shalev, 2007). Dyscalculia can also co-occur with ADHD. Disambiguating dyscalculia from ADHD's intrusion on auditory attention or task persistence is complex. See Zentall (2007) for a full view of ADHD/math complexities and targeted instructional guidance.

Table 13.1. Estimated prevalence of five specific learning disabilities (SLD) with National Institutes of Health (NIH) research funding levels 2000-2009

SLD	Estimated prevalence (%)	NIH research funding in U.S $1000s
Dyslexia	4–8	27,283
Dyscalculia	3.5–6.5	1,574
Attention-deficit/hyperactivity disorder	3–6	532,800
Autism spectrum disorder	1	851,270
Specific language impairment	7	28,611

Adapted from Bishop, D.V.M. (2010). Which neurodevelopmental disorders get researched and why? *PloS One, 5*(11), e15112. doi:10.1371/journal.pone.0015112. Originally published in Goswami, U. (2008). *Foresight mental capital and wellbeing project. Learning difficulties: Future challenges.* London, United Kingdom: The Government Office for Science.

Dyscalculia Is Not a Recent Phenomenon

In the late 1800s, an observant medical practitioner wrote about severe problems of math learning in otherwise capable individuals—notably linking dyscalculia, dysgraphia, finger agnosia, and apraxia (Fuson, 1988; Gerstmann, 1940). By the 1920s, pioneers were developing specialized teaching materials and schemes for math learning problems (Gattegno, 1963; Montessori, 1912; Stern, 1949).

By the 1970s, federal special education law mandated "specially-designed instruction" for students with disabilities, including those with Specific Learning Disability (SLD or LD)—one of 13 federally designated educational disability categories (reauthorized as the Individuals with Disabilities Education Improvement Act [IDEA] of 2004, PL 108-446; see the textbox). The LD category encompasses students with average or above-average cognitive capacities who manifest significant problems establishing adequate academic foundations, including learning the foundations of math. Since the federal law was first enacted, math disabilities have continued to be included under LD. Nevertheless, over the intervening half-century math disabilities have been overshadowed by reading disabilities, with which the term *learning disabilities* has become largely synonymous.

Thirteen Categories of Disability in K–12 Federal Education Law

To receive special education services under federal and state law, a student must qualify under 1 of 13 disability classifications. From low-to-high prevalence, these are: Blindness, Visual Impairment, Deafness, Hearing Impairment, Traumatic Brain Injury, Orthopedic Impairment, Other Health Impaired, Multiple Disabilities, Intellectual Disability, Autism, Emotional Disturbance, Speech/Language Disorders, Specific Learning Disability, which include math disabilities (PL 108-446).

Source: IDEA, 2004.

Dyscalculia Is Not Simple

Learning disabilities, including dyscalculia, frequently run in families and persist through the life span, although manifestations vary across time and task (Shalev, 2007). Particular problems can include language inefficiencies (including difficulties of word retrieval), weakness of phonological and/or quantity representation, weakness in linking quantity and symbols, difficulties of finger differentiation, and/or visual neglect.

Considered a neurocognitive developmental disorder, dyscalculia implicates underlying cognitive processes—some math specific and others of a more general nature—which can include linguistic and visuospatial functioning and/or visuomotor coordination, visual and verbal working memory, attention, and language functions. Not yet fully understood, these complex processes reflect ways that neuroscience currently accounts for varying profiles of math learning disabilities (Butterworth et al., 2011).

Dyscalculia Is Not Inconsequential

> The negative repercussions of being engulfed by a (math) learning disability at a young age completely crippled my self-esteem, and by the fifth grade I believed my worth was zero.
>
> —E-mail from a 24-year-old with dyscalculia

Consequences of math disabilities are serious, as shown in the quote from the 24-year-old with dysclaculia. (See Appendix 13.4 for entire e-mail and 4-year follow-up). The erosion of self-confidence can be particularly insidious both in school and life. Negative repercussions span different school subjects and reach into adulthood, interfering with daily life, restricting job prospects, and reducing earning power (Butterworth & Varma, 2013). The misguided notion that being rotten at math is "no big deal" is far from the reality. In fact, there is evidence that dyscalculia can be more debilitating through life than dyslexia (Gross, Hudson, & Price, 2009). Dyscalculia can curtail access to higher education and professional employment, can create financial confusion and vulnerability, and can precipitate day-to-day inadequacies involving money, measuring, time, distance, estimation, and other common worldly skills and understandings.

In sum, math learning disabilities have long been recognized by some, although in general are underappreciated and upstaged by reading disabilities. Reflecting problems of underlying cognitive processing, the condition has seriously adverse effects that can reverberate significantly into adulthood. Despite that, dyscalculia remains undeservedly underidentified and insufficiently addressed; schools hardly have it on their radar at all. Textbox 13.1 places the problem in the broader context of mathematics education in the United States.

Neglecting Dyscalculia Is Not Okay

It is far from okay that math disabilities remain neglected 5 decades after inclusion in federal law; it is not okay that there are scant resources, knowledge, and specialists in this area. Impoverished understanding affects children and teachers in every school as they grapple with real consequences of real disabilities. These inadequacies reflect low societal priority and inadequate funding over a long haul—two serious problems with negative national outcomes (Butterworth &

TEXTBOX 13.1 **The context: Nationwide math teaching/learning**

There is an broader context for the lack of educational attention and know-how about math learning disabilities: the impoverished state of math teaching and learning nationwide. American mathematics is not doing well overall: year upon year, our math performance has lagged behind other countries (Ball & Bass, 2000).

Ginsburg and Pappas (2007) put it baldly: "In one sense, the United States as a whole suffers from underachievement in mathematics" (p. 431).

Kovas, 2013; see also Table 13.1). Math disabilities need far more attention, especially considering the lifelong consequences in today's world, both practical and emotional. (Textbox 13.2 describes the relationships among and between math difficulties, disabilities, and anxiety.)

That which goes unacknowledged remains unaddressed—or worse, can readily be misinterpreted and mistreated. So, in very real ways, the greatest jeopardy may not be having a math disability but rather the attendant misunderstanding and misguided responses. (For examples of misunderstandings and their effects, see

---

TEXTBOX 13.2   **Math difficulties, disabilities, and anxiety**

Not All Math Difficulties Are Math Disabilities

Many factors influence math development—other than learning disabilities. Some math difficulties derive from schooling: inconsistent instruction, insufficient resources, inadequate teacher development and support. Others relate to life circumstances: early experience, poor attendance, effects of poverty. Still others result from broad social attitudes:

- The American myth that math capacities are predominantly inborn.

- The bias that being bad at math is not terrible.

- The distorted notion that girls do not need math.

Such societal wrong-headedness affects U.S. math performance overall, which is consistently miserably low in relation to other countries around the world (Boaler & Zoido, 2016).

Not All Learning Disabilities Include Math Difficulties

There is overlap between reading/writing learning disabilities and math learning disabilities—around 40%–50% (Shalev, 2007). Given such common co-occurrence, it is reasonable to stay alert to students' math needs. On the other hand, this finding also means that approximately half of those with dyslexia do *not* experience math disabilities. Some excel in math from their early years and pursue math-related fields that showcase this prowess and minimize any residual reading or writing weakness.

Math Anxiety

Students with and without math disabilities can be susceptible to math anxiety. Not a disability itself, math anxiety is real and can be serious, with signs such as increased heart rate, sweating, and panic. Children with math anxiety have shown neural responses in brain regions relating to negativity and fear that manifest outwardly as distress or shutdown. Anxiety readily sets off a negative cycle: avoidance, reduced exposure, weaker skills, anxiety, and avoidance. Furthermore, anxiety directly affects working memory, which is crucial to learning day-in and day-out (Chernoff & Stone, 2014; Ramirez, Gunderson, Levine, & Beilock, 2013; Young, Wu, & Menon, 2012).

adults' and parents' commentary in Appendix 13.4: In Their Words.) Butterworth, Varma, and Laurillard (2011) put it starkly from a neurocognitive vantage point: "The typical school environment does not provide the right kind of experiences to enable the dyscalculic brain to develop normally to learn arithmetic" (2011, p. 1050).

MATH FOUNDATIONS–
THREE REALMS FOR TEACHING AND LEARNING

Math disabilities implicate one or all of three broad math learning foundations as shown in Figure 13.1: 1) spatial and numeric concepts, 2) facility with the count system, and 3) language processing. The different kinds of cognitive processing in each realm are cause for much—unseen—confusion. The repertoire of skills and concepts within each realm must be well-developed—and must also match up, or intersect, across the three realms. Teachers, as well as their students, are often unclear about how best to match them up (i.e., ensure the linkages of mental representations, count-system skills, oral language, and written math symbols).

The Realm of Spatial and Numeric Conceptual Underpinnings

Mary's history illustrates the long-term effects of having a weak grasp of spatial and numeric concepts.

The Case of Mary

Mary, a Barnard graduate, experienced many years of math troubles, spending summers from third through sixth grade in tortuous one-to-one math tutoring, making virtually no progress. In adulthood, life events brought on a math-related crisis that pushed her to seek neuropsychological assessment, which, amazingly, revived her sense of herself as a capable person. Mary learned for the first time about the disability she had been wrestling with—dyscalculia. Revved up with the energy of hope, she pressed for special help, passionate to finally "understand" addition and subtraction, and then multiplication and division. The evaluating neuropsychologist took the challenge and, with **Cuisenaire rods**, patiently modeled showing-and-telling, for example, "I can *see and feel* that the light green and red together are as long as the yellow." In time, a number track was added to the work with the rods, showing and strengthening the numeric relationships. Mary repeatedly mirrored actions with the rods while also talking-the-actions to herself. The modeling and words, carefully attended to and mimicked, were like a miraculous revelation to Mary. No one since kindergarten had worked with her at this conceptual level, and even in kindergarten, they did not include such color-coded linear rods, careful and repeated modeling, and the linkages with a corresponding number-track. These carefully delineated verbal and physical activities now, in adulthood, taught her, for the first time, how quantities intersect with the ten-based number system.

Some math disabilities, such as Mary's, are profoundly affected by visuospatial and/or visuomotor processing that undergird the formation of quantity and quantity-relationship concepts. Such math difficulties absolutely require working with well-structured physical representations (not just "visuals)—specifically, linear rods embodying quantities by length and stable color-quantity associations—and

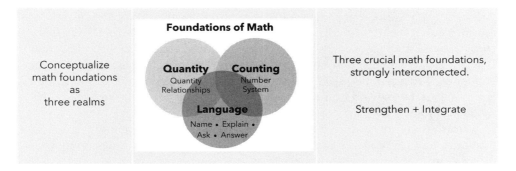

Figure 13.1. Foundations of math.

employing methodical instruction that develops these as mental representations and then language and number system linkages. This is not simply an illustration, but rather repeated variations on the theme so that the mind absorbs the concepts by acting them and talking them. Math dilemmas such as Mary's are foundational—basic basics. Because of schools' proclivity to go on rather than go back, math teaching tends to underdevelop the needed mind-building basics. For a student like Mary, this creates early and persistent confusion about simple addition/subtraction—profound confusion that continues even unto adulthood. Schools are understandably puzzled by their Marys, who read well and exhibit sophisticated language skills, with many superior learning capabilities (remember, she graduated Barnard). In sorting out such a student's strengths and needs, it is worthwhile to probe into the possibility of a broader context known as nonverbal learning disabilities (NLD), which would also implicate handwriting, other organization skills, and understanding of spatial dimensions in social relations and other school areas (e.g., maps, graphic representations). See Rourke (1995) and Tanguay and Rourke (2001) for more on NLD.

The Count System Realm (The Number System, Base-10)

Grant's story illustrates the effects of gaps in number-system knowledge.

The Case of Grant

Grant, a cheeky wisecracking third grader diagnosed with dyscalculia, started having crying fits and refusing to do math in early October. It was as if he had held it together through second grade with the glue of verbal memory and verbalized procedural steps, but now—faced with three-digit confusion and the inexplicability of regrouping—he had lost it. Grant was assessed on a variety of counting skills (see the appendices in the Online Companion Materials), one of which was to count up to 100 and beyond. He whizzed along to the 80s, then the 90s—"97, 98, 99, 100"... *pause* ... "200." Grant's knowledge of the number system clearly dropped off after two digits; his teachers had zero awareness of this limit—or how central it was to all three-digit instruction, causing him complete confusion.

They also had no idea that counting instruction was the key, with well-practiced linkage to number lines. They were blind to his pivotal counting breakdown or how readily he could learn the number system's three-digit logic—probably in two or three 15-minute individualized counting/number line sessions, with some

integrating follow-up. Proceeding with the math curriculum without addressing such count-foundation gaps is like building on sand—with bedrock just a few
steps away. Grant's teachers needed to probe more attentively, checking out not
only basic facts and his understanding of **regrouping** but also his actual number
sequence reading/writing skills and his conceptual math gymnastics on extended
number lines. Not seeing (and directly addressing) what Grant was missing had
made a jumble of the third-grade math in his head.

Worthy of note: Assessing the counting repertoire of high school students
who are weak in math has turned up surprisingly similar lacks in their counting
foundation. (See counting and mental math assessments, Garnett, 2005.)

Some students' math difficulties, like Grant's, stem in large part from lack of a
full repertoire of count-system skills—which go largely unnoticed once grade-level
curriculum moves on. Count-system skills are in the general realm of mental math,
and weakness in this area includes immature strategies, as well as underdeveloped
skills, such as

- Counting the decades—needed to transition from 29 to 30, 39 to 40, and so forth

- Skip counting, first even numbers (to automaticity), then odd (to a lesser level
  of alacrity)

- Counting from any starting number

- Reverse counting—from various starting points

- Counting by 5 from anywhere within the five-sequence—*35, 40, 45, 50* or *60,
  65, 70, 75*

- Counting up and back by 10 from any point, first in the 1–100, then in the
  100–1,000 range

These represent examples of counting "gymnastics" that students need to
become adept at, to perform with ease and agility—and that teachers need to
probe intently when a student displays math trouble. Unfortunately, too little math
instruction peers under the covers for quantity relationship confusions or counting skill breakdowns. Count-system skills can be developed, oftentimes without
great fanfare—but only when the need is noticed. But who, pray tell, is looking for
such weaknesses? Maybe the old critique needs to be turned on its head—instead
of, *you cannot see for looking,* we need to revise it to *you won't see without looking.*

In a literal sense, practicing the mental moves of agile counting actually builds
the rudimentary number line that we mammals are born with (Dehaene, 2011).
Students' counting skill reflects their grasp of the system and, similarly, counting
"workouts" strengthen a weak grasp. Unfortunately, schools' approach to teaching "the system" commonly comes laden with **place-value** verbiage, which largely
mystifies learners because talking about place-value requires linguistic distinctions many youngsters simply do not catch. Also, such talk rarely strengthens the
intuitive pattern-based grasp of the system—while well-practiced counting moves
on a number line to do exactly that. Number lines offer visual-linguistic clarity,
revealing the regular repeating patterns inherent in the base-10 system. Students'
counting prowess on the number line fosters their number sense, mental math,
and self-confidence. See Garnett (2005) and Appendices 13.5–13.7: Garnett's Assessments, as well as Gersten, Clarke, Haymond, and Jordan (2011).

Not Advocating Overextending Counting By Ones Take care not to misconstrue the foregoing discussion as advocating that students' should continually return to counting by ones. Not at all! Of course, early arithmetic is characterized by young children ploddingly practicing one-by-one counting, solidifying their incrementing skills, and synchronizing hand–eye–voice. In time and with practice, counting by ones evolves to increasingly mature strategies (e.g., for 4 and 6, shifting to 6,1,1,1,1 and then to shortcuts such as 6,8,10). Students with math disabilities often stall at the one-at-a-time stage, seeming to resist shifting to more mature mental moves. Why might this be? Perhaps sticking with a methodical mental habit is comforting; perhaps shifting in general feels unsafe; or perhaps there is angst around getting something wrong. In any case, a major aim of math intervention is to help students develop mature and flexible counting/thinking strategies and to wean them off the one-at-a-time early skill. This may require students and teachers agreeing to allow the *time* to think, even if that means slow responding. Both participants need to believe that practicing mature strategies will eventuate in rapid responding!

The Realm of Language Processing

Shawn's story, introduced at the start of this chapter, illustrates how difficulties with language processing can lead to difficulties learning math.

The Case of Shawn

Eight-year-old Shawn shows strength in seeing, feeling, and understanding quantity relationships when he holds them in hand. **Stern blocks** are new to him, but in short order, he has been learning from them with glee. He has stopped prior knee-jerk responding in off ways, instead now tuning-in to the question, envisioning the rods, and then offering a considered response—major progress!

Shawn remains unclear about many terms and explanations, as well as easily confused by math questions, especially when trying to answer rapidly. He also has trouble holding onto the verbal distinctions. Also, he still tends to lose track of his teacher's explanations (rarely tracking with his gaze her pointing, nodding, or accompanying eye-flicks), so he sometimes catches only fragments of the duet conveyed by the word-stream and nonverbal cues. Thus, a focus of his current math instruction is the intersection of verbal and nonverbal indicators he needs to follow.

Some math disabilities, like Shawn's, grow from language difficulties that affect his comprehending teacher talk, using terms, describing coherently without a hands-on understanding. Weak language processing also can negatively affect arithmetic fact fluency, verbal working memory, and recall of sequential procedures. These common language-based math weaknesses can manifest to varying degrees—severe, moderate, or mild. For some students, language confusions accompany math talent (strong conceptual math underpinnings); for others, they come in tandem with weak conceptual grounding. Weak verbal working memory and language confusion can also interfere with the links among concepts, counting, and math talk—connections that are so important to the early years of math learning. For further insight, see Griffin (2005).

REFLECT, CONNECT, and RESPOND
Put Mary, Grant, and Shawn in the headings of three columns and then list descriptive details pertinent to their math needs. Which assessments do

you think might be useful for looking under the covers of each of these students? If there is an assessment need without a corresponding tool, what might your create to fit the bill? (See assessments offered in the appendices as well as others you may know of.)

UNDERSTANDING AND INTERVENTION

Students with math disabilities deserve understanding and intervention. For parents and schools—whose job it is to understand and help—the task is straightforward, although not easy. Drawing on the wisdom of the following directives can keep math intervention on track for those with dyscalculia:

1. Fortify foundation understandings, skills, and language so they are solid and inter-connected.

2. Weave in show-me/tell-me mini routines to refresh the linkages between concepts and language—not simply at one point in time but as an integral part of the advancing math curriculum.

3. Support the emotional dimensions of math learning (courage, persistence, fearless fun).

Principle 1: Fortify Foundations

With special focus, materials, and methods, instruction can strengthen quantity concepts and mapping these onto the number system, as well as connecting math terms and ways of explaining. Ensuring solid foundations may require much playful practice showing concepts with moveable materials, mapping these onto number lines, and associating math terms and ways of explaining. What does it look like? Explicit gamelike practice focusing on the right stuff—with teacher participation to underscore and shift thinking and repeated interactive doing—these are central to intervention. What does it *not* look like? Solo worksheet seatwork, lightly supervised Friday afternoon games, or a sometimes sprinkling of the teacher illustrating with manipulatives.

Take care not to leap to number facts or written computation before establishing enough foundation. Also, attend to the possible dangers of speedy verbal associations and regurgitations. Are such seeming understandings actually unanchored to a student's mental representations?

Principle 2: Weave in Concept/Language Connections

It is hazardous for teachers to simply move on, assuming students' conceptual underpinnings and language connections are firm and fully functional. Thus, as instruction advances, teachers do well to continue cueing students to "show-tell" concept–language connections so these solidify and integrate at deeper levels. Students who routinely practice linkages develop the habit of self-monitoring!

For students like Shawn, concepts, language, and their links may require repeated retrieval over time so that the imprint of concepts and verbal distinctions do not fade or become hard to summon when needed. Reweaving brief retrieval routines can be a powerful teaching habit—sometimes in the intimate whisper of individual feedback and sometimes in thunderclap everyone-show-me "pop-ups."

Principle 3: Remember: Emotions Rule!

Math can evoke confusion, frustration, and defeat in the swirl of word nuances, perplexing explanations, look-don't-touch visuals, and fast-paced teacher questioning. Confusion readily internalizes as negative self-views and debilitating anxieties (e.g., I'm no good at math, My brain doesn't work, Something's wrong with me). The adults on hand often further undermine with remarks about not paying attention, not trying—or offering only mildly reprimanding tones which, over multiple instances, can shut down a child's effort. Fearfulness often sets in, with everyday effects.

A powerful antidote comes in the form of simple acknowledgment of the complexities. Acknowledging a challenge can shrink the fearful monstrousness—and open an emotional space to reveal a shrunken troll.

For more wisdom about changing math misery to joy, see Jo Boaler's resources: https://www.youcubed.org/resource/growth-mindset/. It can be useful to post a teacher cue card such as the one shown in Textbox 13.3 in order to activate your teacher mantras during interactive instruction, noticing, and reconnoitering.

THE DYSCALCULIA KNOWLEDGE BASE

Now, we proceed to explore the evolving knowledge base on dyscalculia in hopes that this provides insight and resources that wend their way into actual practices in schools.

Neuropsychology, Neurobiology, and the Cognitive Sciences

Over recent decades, dyscalculia theory, research, and practical insight have sprouted in a variety of fields. The broader context for this progress follows major new understandings from the 1980s and 1990s regarding children's development of mathematical thinking work which has influenced early childhood programs, the identification of math difficulties, appreciation of critical math foundations, and the honing of instructional principles (Ginsburg, Joon, & Boyd, 2008; Griffin, 2007).

Multiple fields have advanced understanding of dyscalculia, its signs and symptoms, and the characteristics of appropriate instruction. Recent work has even begun to identify brain–mind–performance connections and changes accompanying learning and age, helping to shape instruction for special math needs (Berch & Mazzocco, 1999, 2007; Butterworth, Varma, & Laurillard, 2011; Dehaene, 2011; Geary, 2004). Some cognitive scientists themselves have ventured into creating math-teaching technology (Callaway, 2013; Wilson, Dehaene, Pinel, Revkin, Cohen, & Cohen, 2006).

TEXTBOX 13.3   **Math mantras to teach by**

Fortify Foundations = Solid Understandings

Keep Weaving-in Concepts + Language (Show and Tell)

Remember the Emotional Side

And know that your students' math minds will be grateful for your efforts.

Over time, attempts to classify signs and symptoms of dyscalculia have yielded four groups—deficits of procedural learning, semantic memory, visuospatial functioning, and number knowledge (Stock, Desoete, & Roeyers, 2006). These four groups are further delineated in Figure 13.2, an adaptation of the Dyscalculia Classification chart compiled by the same authors.

This compilation of researchers' views of dyscalculia offers a valuable overview of the terrain, but the four groupings are not definitive—nor are they meant to categorize or diagnose individual students. Rather, they represent a four-way sorting of the manifestations of dyscalculia delineated over time and in varying ways by various investigators.

Pioneers in Specially Designed Math Instruction

The work of math education giants from the 1920s through the 1960s reverberates to this day—particularly contributions from Maria Montessori (1912), Catherine Stern (1949), and Caleb Gattegno (1963, 1987, 2011a). Their influence is more than simply of historical note; it represents basic and enduring understanding, worthy of returning to for sustenance.

Montessori Methods   Maria Montessori, Italy's first female medical doctor and an international educator, began her work at the end of the 19th century and transported it to America in the 1920s, with a resurgence in the 1960s. Montessori's methods grew from her initial teaching of Italian children with developmental delays, expanding to Italian children of poverty and then to children worldwide (Standing, 1998).

She had a gift for child watching and saw this as key to effective teaching, so she trained educators to observe carefully in order to "follow the child." She also discerned critical mental developments in early arithmetic learning and the ways by which young minds constructed these, first outwardly with quantities of things and then in mind. From this, she concluded that math learning is grounded in strong tangible concepts that develop out of the child's interactions with structured—visible-graspable-movable—materials that correspond to quantities in relationship to other quantities (the 5ness-of-5 in relation, say, to the 3ness-of-3). *Note:* The term *quantity,* used here, is referred to elsewhere as *amount, magnitude, number, number-in-a-set,* or *numerosity.*

Montessori math materials, many of which she and her colleagues created, remain in use today. Her early childhood math work has made lasting cultural imprints, even while comprehensive use of her methods remains somewhat sequestered within the Montessori schools community.

I endeavored to put the number system into such concrete form that the child would see and grasp its *structure*. Thus he can discover in a short time the system of numbers which the human mind took centuries to develop.

—Stern (1949, p. xxiii)

Stern Structural Arithmetic   Catherine Stern's groundbreaking work is as relevant today as when Albert Einstein praised it. Stern was a contemporary of both Einstein and Montessori. After receiving her doctorate in physics, she turned to her passion for education, working at first in a Montessori kindergarten. Subsequently emigrating to the United States, she assisted the famed gestalt psychologist Max Wertheimer, and imbibed through him the prevailing psychological constructs of the age. Stern's experiences set the context for her own ideas about concept-grounded math materials and hand–eye–mind, movable and tangible pedagogy.

PROCEDURAL DEFICITS
Operational dyscalculia (Geary, 2004)
Procedural (Kosc, 1974)

Difficulties with
Procedures in (written) calculation
Sequencing multiple steps in complex procedures
Planning or execution of complex operations
Mental calculations
Routines

As well as
Immature strategies
Many mistakes with complex procedures
Time-lag in arithmetic procedures
Poor understanding of concepts in procedures

SEMANTIC MEMORY DEFICITS
R-S profile (Rourke & Conway, 1997)
Semantic memory deficits (Geary, 2004)

Difficulties with
Acquisition of number facts
Retrieval of numerical facts
Semantic-acoustic aspect of linguistic domain
Conceptual knowledge terms
Language comprehension
Passive vocabulary
Orally presented terms

As well as
Low accuracy in mental calculation
Slow speed of mental and written calculation
Irregular reaction times
High error rate
Wrong associations in retrieval
Low enumerating speed for figures, symbols, numbers, and quantities

VISUOSPATIAL DEFICITS
Practognostic dyscalculia (Kosc, 1974)
Nonverbal learning disorder (Rourke & Conway, 1997)
Visualspatial subtype (Geary, 2004)

Difficulties with
Placing numbers on a number line
Understanding geometry
Abstraction
Temporal order or planning
Novel and complex tasks
Symbol recognition
Insight in and notions of space

Disturbance in
Setting out objects in order according to magnitude
Visuospatial memory
Visual imaginative faculty
Enumerating groups of objects
Estimating and comparing quantities

Difficulties with
Inversions and reversals in numbers
Misinterpretation of spatially represented information
Visual neglect

As well as
Misalignment and misplacements of digits
Nonverbal impairments
Eventually dyspraxia

NUMBER KNOWLEDGE DEFICITS
Verbal-Lexical-Graphical-Ideognostic dyscalculia (Kosc, 1974)
Arabic dyscalculia, Pervasive dyscalculia (von Aster, 2000)

Difficulties with
Understanding Arabic notation, math ideas, and relations
Abstract number comprehension
Transcoding between the different modalities
In size comparison
Number ordering
Enumeration
Number dictation

Disturbance in
Number knowledge
Basic sense of numerosity
Encoding the semantics of numbers
Number reading
Number writing
Number production

Figure 13.2.   Specific deficits associated with dyscalculia (procedural, semantic memory, visuospatial, number knowledge). (*Source:* Dyscalculia Classification chart, Stock, Desoete, & Roeyers, 2006.)

Stern laid out systematic methods for developing the mind's grasp of quantities and their relationships with one another, using color-coded blocks of increasing lengths from 1 to 10 (see Figure 13.3). She structured teaching activities with the number blocks that students arranged within wooden number-frames (also color-coded) and number-tracks (see Figure 13.4). These materials revealed clearly and vividly the various quantity *concepts* in action, such as comparing, increasing/decreasing, and combining/separating—and the related quantity *relationships*, such as same/different, more/less, short/long, shorter/taller, short/shorter/shortest, long/longer/longest, near/far, and close/distant. Guided play with the comparative-length materials aimed at forming representations in the mind; the language interchanges served to reflect and anchor the work with the materials. Such a potent combination, all wrapped in gamelike activities, gave students confidence in their powers of reasoning—and was a world apart from the memorizing and mechanical educational methods of the day.

The Stern program makes tangible the number-system foundation. The number line is in the form of a physical numbered track, into which students slide Stern blocks as they play out quantity relationships. Repeated game playing reinforces the correspondences between quantities and the count system. The blocks in the track exemplify, through action, the ways that quantities map directly onto the base-10 number system, a powerful embodiment.

Materials matter, but teacher–student exchange is crucial as well, involving reciprocal showing, asking, doing, and telling—linking up the concrete visual, actions, and language. In other words, they fortify connections among visuospatial, kinesthetic, numeric, and linguistic dimensions. Such highly interactive multisensory practices establish and strengthen the bonds among quantity concepts, the count system, and language by requiring translations from one to another—in reciprocal directions.

Stern's work has carried on in clinical settings nationwide—a school district here, a teacher preparation program there, and it is shared among many

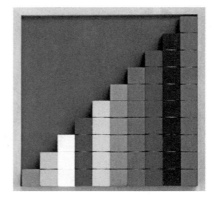

Figure 13.3. Stern blocks in ten-frame. (From Stern, M.B. & Gould, T.S. [1998]. *Structural Arithmetic I, II, III: Teachers Guide and Workbooks.* Cambridge, MA: Educators Publishing Service. Reprinted by permission.)

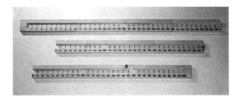

Figure 13.4. Number track for Stern blocks. (From Stern, M.B. & Gould, T.S. [1998]. *Structural Arithmetic I, II, III: Teachers Guide and Workbooks.* Cambridge, MA: Educators Publishing Service. Reprinted by permission.)

in-the-know learning specialists. It remains a beacon for special educators who work with perplexingly slow and math-confused youngsters. Wonderful materials, games, and guides are found at http://www.sternmath.com (Stern & Gould, 1998; Stern, Stern, & Gould, 1966). Currently available only on the second-hand market, the seminal volume *Children Discover Arithmetic* (Stern & Stern, 1971) needs reissuing; it is a trove of wisdom and practicality.

Gattegno's Visible Tangible Mathematics Caleb Gattegno, arguably the 20th century's most influential math educator, stumbled into a chance encounter with Georges Cuisenaire, which eventuated in spreading the Belgian teacher's diminutive math rods worldwide. Color-coded and of graduated lengths from 1–10, these are now called Cuisenaire rods, although Gattegno originally dubbed them Algebricks because they behave the way numbers do—in the same way that the Stern blocks do. (Cuisenaire rods are depicted in Figure 13.5.) The linear numeric character, with color-specific redundancy, is why both sets of materials are considered by many to be the best tools building math foundations. Shaping instruction with either Stern blocks or Cuisenaire rods can result in robust mental models and strong underlying number sense because their lengths make obvious

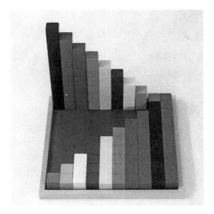

Figure 13.5. Cuisenaire rods 1–10 in a double-staircase number frame. (From http://sternmath.com/teaching-with/10-box.html. Used by permission.)

their relationships (with color underscoring the distinctions) and also obviously correspond to distance on a related number line, or track (e.g., it is immediately visible that 56 + 10 = 66, 66 + 10 = 76, or 403 + 10 = 413 when planting the 10-rod at each of the starting numerals).

Gattegno created guides for using the rods and also authored math textbooks grounded in visible, tangible concepts. The influence of his contributions to mathematics education has been profound, as has his prolific work in other areas: *The Silent Way* (foreign language); *Words in Color* (2011b; beginning reading); and explorations of teaching-learning, learning-effort, and awareness as the root of learning. Gattegno's works—essays, textbook series, manuals, and videos of his teaching, remain accessible through a company he originally founded, now at http://www.educationalsolutions.com.

Current Trailblazers in Specially Designed Math Instruction

In addition to the powerful work of pioneers, current trailblazers have spawned resources for developing math foundations in students with dyscalculia. These include books, articles, research, toolkits, as well as trainings and web sites rich in guidance and insight. Over recent decades, this instructional work has borne reciprocal effects—both fueling current dyscalculia pursuits in other fields and also drawing on research findings (Bird, 2017; Butterworth & Yeo, 2004; Chinn & Ashcroft, 2017; Griffin, 2007; Griffin, Case, & Siegler, 1994).

Ronit Bird is prominent among current instructionally oriented specialists. Over many years, she has taught students with dyscalculia and created powerful resources for 6- to 14-year-olds (Bird, 2017; see also http://www.ronitbird.com). Materials matter—so, as a connoisseur of math materials for dyscalculia, Bird is well worth emulating; she knows the value of Cuisenaire's color-distinct, graspable/movable, length model, and she eschews other materials and practices that are largely decorative or fluff, rather than vivid and demonstrative embodiments of math concepts. The following are staples in Bird's math pantry:

- Multiple sets of Cuisenaire 1–10 rods (at least two sets per student) with the accompanying structured number tracks and frames

- Many additional stashes of 10s and 1s rods

- Dice, dominoes, and cards—dot patterns all

- A slew of highly targeted gamelike activities that sharpen the math focus and ensure serious practice for each individual

Bird offers a panoply of videos, books, free downloads, and intensive games, all of which reflect her expertise with learners and her effectiveness with their teachers. The particularity of Bird's methods extends their usefulness to a broad range of students stumbling on the math path. As is the case with dyslexia intervention, principles and practices crucial for students with dyscalculia, like Shawn, are beneficial as well for many of his classmates who are simply stumbling.

Sharon Griffin, an influential researcher and clinician, worked for many years with students failing to thrive in mathematics and with their teachers (Harvard Education Letter, 2007). In her collaboration with Robbie Case, Griffin focused on the critical groundwork children need to connect with schools' first math teaching (Griffin & Case, 1997). Her work eventuated in a powerful program, Number Worlds—much sought after but long available only through her informal Worcester,

MA, workshop. Number Worlds has now been commercially published, along with a solid empirical history of its effectiveness (Griffin, 2015).

Griffin also provides a clarion call about what it takes to reach youngsters with serious math learning difficulties. Methods, yes. Materials, of course. Understanding and skill, without question. But, at the very core, Griffin places the *fun* of math learning! It is that fearless fun that keeps kids going, even in the face of challenge—words to the wise about *all* intervention (Griffin, 2007).

Cognitively Guided Instruction (CGI; Carpenter, Fennema, Franke, Levi, & Empson, 1999) is a problem-based approach not specifically pitched toward math disabilities. CGI is a valuable supplement, even at an early math level. The program employs scenarios, or story problem solving that systematically scaffolds students' talking about their math moves. CGI's strength is its well-structured modeling and explicit guidance; youngsters are not left to make math discoveries with little support, nor are they inundated with multiple methods. Rather, the program provides systematic examples and coaching as students talk-listen in increasingly comprehensible ways. Teachers incorporating CGI into their intervention mix report that their students with learning disabilities respond with renewed enthusiasm and effort and with increased participation during math time.

REFLECT, CONNECT, and RESPOND

Explore what you can find on the web about Stern Arithmetic and Number Worlds. Comb the possibilities, seeking a stronger feel for these resources. Find related videos or readings. Describe what you learned that is different from, or goes beyond, the information in this chapter.

Notes on Using Foundation Math Interventions

The foundation interventions described here are well developed and sharply focused, each offering potent means for fostering students' sense of their own math powers to figure things out. The interventions can be used with learners of different ages as follows:

- The Stern or Bird systems, or a combination, are appropriate for intensive tutoring and small groups at various ages. (If combined, the teacher needs to choose between using Cuisenaire rods and Stern blocks because the size and color systems are not the same.)

- Cuisenaire rods and accessories can be particularly appropriate for teen and adult foundation work. Guidance and games from Bird and Stern can apply.

- Griffin's Number Worlds is a good fit for preventative intervention in early-grade classrooms but can also be appropriate for tutoring and small groups.

- CGI, a worthy tool for every teacher's kit, scaffolds students' math language—naming, asking, answering, and explaining—and clarifies the easily confusable language of math teaching. It is best considered as an addition to a fuller foundation program.

- The work of Maria Montessori and Caleb Gattegno continues to inspire schools and programs. Their legacies also remain valuable at a clinical level—for insight into particular dilemmas and for thinking more deeply about teaching and its effects. Their manuals, materials, seminal books, and current-day practitioners offer untarnished wisdom and treasure.

In sum, interest in dyscalculia, first documented at the turn of the 19th century, has waxed and waned since, always on the periphery of schooling concerns. It has clearly not garnered the attention lavished on dyslexia. In recent decades, interest from diverse fields has sown many seedlings. There is finally a respectable base of dyscalculia research, theory, and instructional practice—all in dire need of funding and fanfare. A priority need is nationwide dissemination of math learning disabilities information and support for families and schools who are, in large measure, clueless. A few extremely well-crafted foundation interventions are available; unfortunately, these are rarely on display in schools.

For example, Shawn's mother pleaded for help with her son's math difficulties and was met with denial that the problem exists. When Shawn's co-teachers offered to look into special resources, school administrators insisted they stick to the curriculum, with one accommodation—they could reduce the number of practice problems required of him.

> How can it be that Shawn's math disability is summarily dismissed, despite the evidence and despite his qualifying since preschool for special services under Learning Disability?

In Shawn's school life, he has clearly been ill served and, accordingly, his mother has chosen to remove him from the school.

But what if Shawn's co-teachers had been encouraged to pursue special intervention, to be responsive and appropriate to his obvious math foundation-building needs? What if they had been allowed to make instruction appropriate, with materials and methods suitable to his needs? Most likely, even with permission, they would have felt stranded with many sensible, important, and unanswered questions, such as the following:

- What does responsive and appropriate mean for this student?

- We should "meet him where he is," but where is that?

- What is a proper starting focus, and how do we determine that?

- What is the toolset for this work—the powerful materials and guidance, the means for specially designed foundation math intervention?

- What are key teaching routines we need to refine in order to be effective?

Avoid Assuming–Look to See–Conceptualize

Next we discuss a three-pronged mini-guide to addressing these teachers' rightful question. It might be useful to post this as a mantra, or cue card, for planning, teaching, and assessing.

Avoid Assuming, Steering Clear of Assumptive Teaching Examples of knee-jerk assumptions are as follows:

- We already used manipulatives; we did that.

- He needs basics, so work on basic facts.

- Stick to teaching him the steps.

- Don't have him explain. He talks in confused ways.

Such *a priori* notions are likely to be hazardous as instructional guides because they cover up, rather than reveal and address underlying learning, math, and math learning needs.

Look to See What's With the Foundation–Attend, Notice, Probe   Can the student:

- Show and tell quantities 1–10 and their relationships using number rods along with rudimentary explaining

- Subitize (recognize at a glance) 1–3 items in random display and 2–5 items in arrays (e.g., dominos, dice, ten-frames)

- Use simple counting skills with ease—counting forward to 10, then 20; counting-on from varying points within 2–10, then 2–20; touch-counting using one-to-one correspondence; tally-counting on fingers

- Write and read the numerals 1–10, then the numerals 20–30, and show physical representations of these (number rods, number line, fingers)

- Use more advanced counting skills with ease—counting forward to 50, then to 100 from varying starting points, counting back, skip counting, counting through the decades, counting forward or back by 10s from varying points, counting forward or back by 25s, counting higher and higher into the hundreds-plus

- Demonstrate counting with number rods and boxes and a number track

- Write, read, and demonstrate with rods math symbols and equations in different number notation formats

- Understand and use math terms

- Understand the language of math instruction and generate explanations and reasoning

- Understand and make up number stories

In other words, look under the covers—actually see what is in place or missing, clear or confused, strong or unreliable, easy or unsteady. The profile you uncover will guide how you review, revisit, or build from the ground up. Of equal importance, this probing will point to what to weave in, even as you advance in the math curriculum.

Conceptualize Clearly–Crucial, Critical, Core? Or Fuzzy Fluff   The term *foundational* means "sufficient to build upon, to support subsequent layers." A useful conception of foundational math learning spans three kinds of mental structures that support the layers of elementary arithmetic and subsequent mathematical concepts and skills: 1) hand-to-mind quantity and quantity relationship representations; 2) varied, strong, and flexible counting skills, including the reading and writing of numerals; and 3) corresponding language distinctions—along with the interconnecting of these foundation realms, or three ways of thinking. (See quantity, counting, and language in Figure 13.6.)

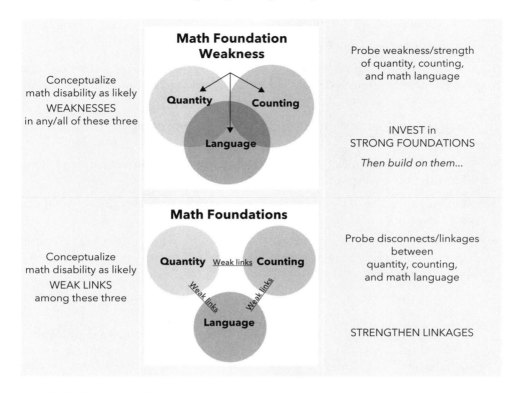

Figure 13.6. Weaknesses + Weak Links.

A number of foundation interventions bear down on these realms and their interconnections, especially the Bird (2017) materials, Stern Arithmetic materials and games (Stern & Stern, 1971; http://www.sternmath.com), and the Number Worlds curriculum (Griffin, 2015). Other well-targeted, but less comprehensive, materials include Garnett (2005) and Carpenter, Fennema, Franke, Levi, and Empson (1999).

Assessing in Three Realms—Quantity, Counting, and Language

Now alert to the dangers of assumptive teaching, you have in mind a potent math foundation conceptualization and in hand powerful tools. So, it is time to simply get started teaching, with an inquiring mind and the guidance of Bird, Stern, Griffin, and Garnett, whose work is foundational, focused, and fun. Exploratory teaching will now reveal particulars about Shawn's needs, where to bear down, and how to nuance the teaching moves.

Other ways of looking under the covers (i.e., assessing), including prior reports, homemade math probes, published instruments, and in-depth conversations with parents and teachers, can, of course, be undertaken before instruction, but these can just as well fit into early-stage instruction. Starting with teaching can actually yield more by noticing-without-knowing first and following up with more systematic uncovering—interviews, targeted assessments, and made-up probes. (See Appendices 13.5–13.7 for counting and other assessments.)

Starting with teaching may sound heretical, but it is not actually so. Exploratory instruction can reveal much (that is otherwise assumed). The key is to stay alert and notice and note what energizes, what activates, what needs to be broken down, and what is known that can be a starting place. Such ongoing "tuning" will be critical to the progress of a student with serious math confusions.

Working from a powerful conception of what math foundations are—like that provided by the three realms of quantity, counting, and language and their linkages—can profoundly influence how one sees, what gets noticed (i.e., result of assessing). Understanding key areas directs the gaze, pointing at what to look for and to take note of. Remember, even with the best tools, only you can see for looking. Even a stellar intervention program will not go far without the teacher's noticing the clues and cues for slowing, shifting, backtracking, or bearing down—in other words, noticing what is in front of you and, as Montessori put it, following the child.

The interplay of teaching–noticing–adjusting reveals what Shawn (or Mary or Grant) *gets,* what each can do easily—not only where and how each falters, stumbles, or falls into confusion. Probing the edges of both adeptness and trip-ups opens the teaching view to see more—and more clearly. Figure 13.7 offers sample questions for probing. Probes and prompts make visible what to add, subtract, emphasize, weave in, and practice as parts of ensuing instruction.

Shawn, Mary, and Grant

These three learners vividly demonstrate that exploring math's quantity, counting, and language foundation is important—crucial, in fact. How, otherwise, can you glean what needs doing?

The time and care spent strengthening the foundations and their connectivity can pay back in lifetime skills. Schools unfortunately often hold different views, opting to press on in full gear with grade-level math or to back up to basic facts and procedural how-tos, as if these were the target needs. Although particular aspects of grade-focused math can remain in the mix for these students, those aspects (and expectations) need careful culled, adapted, and undergirded by foundation work. Pursued on its own, grade-level math for Shawn, Mary, or Grant will stall progress and compound confusion.

Not developing the foundations and their connectivity will result in fragments piling onto a weak base, immature skills, or completely confused language processing—without teachers even seeing these underlying stumbling stones.

The common alternative, pivoting to basic facts and procedures, results in negatively narrowing the math path, while continuing to neglect the actual fundamentals—yet another prescription for stalled progress. Basic facts and procedures will not scaffold thinking to reach more mature counting strategies or firm-up math's spatial, nonverbal grounding; they do not forge linkages and do not untangle the web of confusing terms. Ungrounded fragments do not stick, integrate, or form the base on which to build more math learning (see Figure 13.8). Furthermore, increasing fragmented learning without developing the web of understandings reinforces the student's experience that math is not fun, not comprehensible, and "not for me."

What About Number Facts in Basic Operations?

Becoming nimble with basic number facts and well-practiced with procedures (algorithms) is important—as are the foundations they are built on. The underlying substrate is more commonly neglected, too often wrongly assumed to be intact.

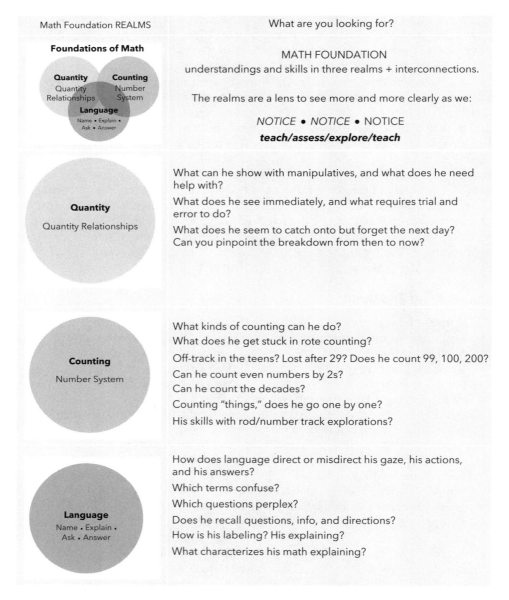

Figure 13.7. Exploring math foundations in three realms.

So, checking out and strengthening quantity, language, and the gamut of counting skills is important first.

The solid ground required before working on typing down basic facts is being sure that the student is very clear about the relevant operation (+, –, ×, /)—that he or she can readily demonstrate with materials, rods, drawings, and number lines and explanations. The details of this clarity include

1. Writing, reading, and demonstrating the operation in its various algorithmic formats

2. Recognizing whether an answer will be an increase or decrease, "in the ballpark" or "out-to-lunch"

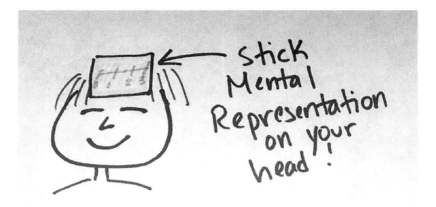

Figure 13.8. Mental representation.

3. Knowing and showing that

   a. Adding congregates quantities.

   b. Subtracting separates constituent quantities.

   c. Both addition and subtraction compare quantities.

   d. Addition can undo subtraction and vice-versa.

   e. The parts of addition can be in any order (are swappable); not so for subtraction.

   f. Multiplication is repeated addition of the same quantities (and can be represented by the area of squares and rectangles).

   g. Division partitions or distributes quantities.

   h. Addition and multiplication are commutative (swappable).

   i. Subtraction and division do not commute.

Robust basic fact understandings also include Shawn and Grant being easily able to bring a representation to mind. They need explicit cuing to shift from showing/telling with rods to envisioning-in-mind. Their working with number rods made math principles such as commutativity ($7 + 8 = 8 + 7$) and friendly facts ($3 + 6 = 9, 6 + 3 = 9, 9 - 3 = 6, 9 - 6 = 3$) self-evident, but—for both boys—summoning this to mind as needed took much practice, teacher cuing, and a self-triggering cue card to "think of making it with your rods" (or tens-frame, etc.).

Furthermore, Shawn needed extended work with math terms, writing/reading numerals, and the different-looking written algorithms and ensuring these remained bonded with his quantity understandings. Shawn's teachers find it hard to always realize how math terms, numerals, and written algorithms are symbolic pointers, not concepts themselves. What they point to must be well secured in mind, accessible, and well tethered to a slew of different-looking symbolic variations, both oral or written.

Next, both Shawn's and Grant's teachers pinpoint which facts were already solid so they can link those with less-solid facts (e.g., $5 + 5$ linked to $5 + 6$ or 5×5 linked to 5×6). Research on number-fact linking interventions shows mixed outcomes (Garnett, 1992, 2012; Ansari, 2015). For Grant, the thinking-linking strategies form a foundation and backup system that, with practice, shifts to his retrieving them directly from memory; for Shawn, the shift to direct retrieval does not occur. Instead, he continues with thinking-linking strategies that, with much use, eventually gain in ease of retrieval. For both boys increases in reliability and alacrity came from practice thinking, not from trying to speed up. Practicing thinking-linking short cuts (with as few mental steps as possible) in manageable-sized groupings and with the mind in gear resulted in their abandoning the torturously long counting-by-one strategies they had previously used.

Nuance is important—with Grant, bearing down on the thinking steps and practicing in small-enough groupings; with Shawn, extending distributed practice; for both boys, a critical nuance was helping them stay focused on the right things (the thinking link), rather than half-attending in semi-distracted verbal recitation.

Using Number Fact Charts and Calculators   When working on procedural steps or engaged in problem solving, students deserve to freely use a number fact chart—a stylish, pocket-sized reference that makes visible the entire network of basic facts, with each answer to be found consistently at the same crossroad coordinates—and supports memory. These values are not present with a calculator for basic facts, so calculator look-up is not useful for this purpose. On the other hand, calculators are helpful for checking end-of-process answers or substep calculations in complex problems.

Weaving Foundation Strands Into Ongoing Instruction   As previously emphasized, concepts, counting skills, and math-language need initially to be well-developed—and then threaded through instruction, rather than abandoned or relegated to a review heap. These foundations actually need further integrating—to strengthen connections, ensure easy mental access, and link up with new learning. As ongoing math concepts and skills are taught, this sort of brief but regular weaving-in of earlier basics also helps learners make connections and see this new "math topic" as actually just a variation on what they know. The following is a particular way such weaving could play out: a possible template for Do it–Show me–Tell me routines.

Such reweaving is effective as a habitual aspect of instruction—a second-nature part of math interactions—not a once-in-a-while add-on. When establishing math foundations, create a Do–Show–Tell routine, ensuring it is well-practiced and easily triggered. As instruction advances, building on the foundations, the teacher routinely weaves in Do–Show–Tell as a common part of teacher–student exchanges—frequently when overseeing individual target students (as 1-minute micro-routines) and daily, or at least three times per week with groups (3-minute mini-routines). The purpose is to get students to press pause, a self-monitoring habit to routinely step back from close-up work to consider and connect with the bigger picture. Prodding students to do, then pause, show and tell promotes shifting from procedures to reasoning, from answering to pausing on whether an answer makes sense. Important caveat: The intent of the directions "show me" and "tell me" is not to list the procedural steps—but rather to "show" how you DO IT with materials (paperclips, linear rods, number lines), what it looks like—and then to "tell" WHAT YOU DID with the things, to talk your walk.

Shawn's Pause That Refreshes   Just this kind of pause routine has changed Shawn's answering 109 when posed 10 + 9. He has even begun to initiate a focused pause on his own. As he is about to answer a teacher question or written problem, he says it aloud, shifts his mind to the mental representation (his inner image, or memory of the ten-frame, rods, or number line)—and, *only then,* answers. When asked to "show me/tell me," he can readily tell what he envisioned and show it with rods and/or a number line. In this pause, Shawn intercepts the mindless rush-rush that disconnects him from math sense. Given how potent this pause is, Shawn's teachers have him practice these mental moves, routinely requesting show/tells in 30-second pop-ups. This is creating easy thinking for Shawn, a mindful habit that thoroughly thrills him.

Jo Boaler asserts that strong math learners commonly are not fast; they pause and consider (Boaler & Zoido, 2016). Boaler warns that American schools often sacrifice math learning in pursuit of speed; she advocates doing away with timing because it can hinder as many students as it may motivate. An alternate take on this would be to assert the value of kids' differences, arranging timing for those who delight in it and no timing for those who, like Shawn, hate it. Boaler's point, more generally, is about strong math performance not being about speed, but about easily and clearly conceiving of the math you are doing, making sense of it, and taking the time to envision, connect, or think with it. Doing all of those regularly gets you faster and firmer at meaning-filled math. Shawn's pause procedure is starting to show just those effects.

REFLECT, CONNECT, and RESPOND

Discuss your response to the idea that assessing can be profitably undertaken during teaching. How might you use the three-realm conceptualization to guide your ongoing noticing, probing, and checking further into a student's needs? Here's a big one: How might you become more skilled at noticing?

CLOSING THOUGHTS: DYSCALCULIA AND INTERVENTION

Many students with serious math difficulties will need specialized foundation work to make headway. Some will require special instruction at advanced levels as well, but others will proceed to middle school needing little further help, especially as language-laden arithmetic gives way to the increased spatial basis of higher branches of mathematics. For students with visuospatial strengths, the dilemmas they experienced in elementary school that overtaxed verbal memory (for facts and procedures) can recede and the students can emerge to shine at higher math.

The pace of students' progress with foundation intervention clearly varies with the nature and severity of their difficulties. Some show early intervention effects, as though a light had switched on in a dim room. Others show slow initial progress requiring painstaking instructional moves to develop quantity relations, mental math, and/or math language. Although foundation intervention programs provide crucial roadmaps and guides, they will always need adjusting because students with dyscalculia come with differing strengths, diverse difficulties, and various versions of mental "trick-knees." When teachers attentively notice and bear down on needs as these come into view, they are providing responsive clinical teaching. When teachers do that routinely and also follow-up by weaving micro-practices into ongoing instruction—*that* is highly skilled specially designed instruction.

Progress is possible—on an appropriate path, with timely adjustments and enough mindful practice—along with acknowledgment of the difficulties and the progress. As Shawn makes efforts that show visible effects, no matter how small the steps, he is now noticing and feeling that progress acutely. As he experiences understanding and knows what he is doing, Shawn recalibrates his mind view, increasingly sensing—maybe even believing—that his math brain really does work after all.

For Shawn and compatriots who attend every school in the nation, the needle on dyscalculia has barely budged in half a century, despite expectations of free appropriate public education with specially designed instruction addressing the individual needs of students with disabilities, which include math disabilities that too few have heard of or believe exist.

Much needs to change. An urgent task—too long delayed—is to reach families and schools with information and the wherewithal to disseminate current kid-insight and teaching expertise to all the critical school participants, which includes parents. Math learning disabilities are legitimate and approachable, with potential benefits to a wide range of math learners. Dyscalculia poses a formidable challenge, for which resources have been insufficient at all levels—the level of research; program creation; and dissemination across schools, classroom, clinics, and families.

How can we concoct creative algorithms for approaching this multistep, complex, societal math problem? One proposal is for participants from all aspects of this work to congregate much more. Parents, teachers, coaches, math educators, neuropsychologists, and researchers need to gather together. As a launching pad, check out the many resources offered in tandem with this chapter. (See Appendices 13.1 and 13.3 for resources available online and in print.) See also Figure 13.9, and share it with colleagues.

REFLECT, CONNECT, and RESPOND

Before you read this chapter, what were your ideas and/or experiences related to students with significant math difficulties? What two to three notions from the chapter were the most mind-shifting for you? What barriers to doing right by students with math learning disabilities did you glean from this chapter? Have you had your own experiences with such barriers? If yes, describe. A challenge: Sketch out a three-pronged plan you might set in motion to surmount the obstacles.

ONLINE COMPANION MATERIALS

The following Chapter 13 resources are available at http://www.brookespublishing.com/birshcarreker/materials:

- Reflect, Connect, and Respond Questions
- Appendix 13.1: Technology Resources (see also the web links listed in Appendix 13.3: Math Resources)
- Appendix 13.2: Knowledge and Skill Assessment Answer Key
- Appendix 13.3: Math Resources
- Appendix 13.4: In Their Words
- Appendix 13.5: Counting Assessment
- Appendix 13.6: Computation Assessment

A cue card for teachers

Specially Designed Intervention for Dyscalculia

involves sharpening teaching focus and intensity on:

1. CONCEPTS—robust mental models of quantity + quantity relationships with language links

2. COUNT SYSTEM—the starting steps of mental math.

   It's about developing nimble oral counting, both with physical number lines and on one's mental number line. Count-system skills are a set of flexible mental moves, a kind of cognitive acrobatics: counting on, up and up, the decades, up-one/down-one, by even twos, by odd twos, by ten from any number, back by ten from any number, and so forth.

   Pitfall: Careful not to encourage relentless one-by-one counting. Rather, facilitate mature strategic counting.

   This includes READING and WRITING numerals 1–10, then 1–20, then 1–50, then 1–100+

   - In conjunction with nimble counting on the number line

   - With connection to quantities and the number line (the count/number "system"!)

3. LANGUAGE—both understanding and using.

   Name, ask, answer, describe, and explain—also, understanding teacher mathtalk plus, interconnecting these three:

   - Link physical and mental representations, the number system (number line), and language.

   - Keep connections from fading—probing individuals in brief Do–Show–Tell routines.

Teaching skills for effective intervention and for building higher math on this foundation:

TIME + PATIENCE—for developing robust mental representations + strong language links, before proceeding far into written problems or procedures.

DIRECT INSTRUCTION—Modeling, scaffolding, feedback, and multiple examples for

- Physical and mental representations (concepts)

- Language links (naming, describing, asking, answering, explaining)

- Basic facts and linking facts

- Continuing to stitch math fragments together with frequent show and tell

TASK ANALYSIS looking and probing

… at the curriculum hinge points for what confuses and what has not stuck.

CONFUSION and GLITCHES

- Use student confusions/glitches as guides for tailoring next-step planning.

- Teach thinking/deciding—tie in meaning-minders, check-ins, and tie-backs.

ENOUGH PRACTICE—more than you would think.

- It's crucial for practice to be interactive, supervised, and sharply focused.

- Practice thinking, practice linking, practice telling, practice asking, practice connections, and do most of it through games and gamelike activities—FUN!

- DO NOT practice ad nauseam or without the mind in gear.

Figure 13.9. Cue card for teachers: Specially designed intervention

KNOWLEDGE AND SKILL ASSESSMENT

1. This chapter offers a conceptualization of the broad foundations of the elementary arithmetic curriculum grouped into which of the following?

    a. Basic number facts and computations steps

    b. Quantity concepts, the count system, and math language

    c. Commutativity, counting-on, and one-to-one correspondence

    d. The mental number line and subitizing

    e. None of the above

2. Which intervention programs target foundation-level math learning?

    a. Catherine Stern's *Stern Arithmetic*

    b. Ronit Bird's *Toolkit* and online resources

    c. Sharon Griffin's *Number Worlds*

    d. All of the above

    e. None of the above

3. Which of the following is true, based on current evidence?

    a. Math learning disabilities commonly precipitate referrals to special education.

    b. Few students with reading disabilities also have math disabilities.

    c. Dyscalculia usually has less debilitating life effects than dyslexia.

    d. Math teachers commonly know little to nothing about math disabilities.

    e. All of the above

4. Which of the following is inaccurate?

    a. Activities with Cuisenaire rods and Stern blocks target difference aspects of math.

    b. Students' ready recall of basic number facts is important.

    c. Games are a major feature of Ronit Bird's program.

    d. Gymnastic sorts of counting on the number line are part of foundation-level math.

    e. None of the above

REFERENCES

Ansari, D. (2015). *Understanding developmental dyscalculia: A math learning disability* [Webinar and Transcript]. Retrieved from https://www.ldatschool.ca/math/understanding-developmental-dyscalculia-a-math-learning-disability/

Ball, D., & Bass, H. (2000). Interweaving content and pedagogy in teaching and learning to teach: Knowing and using mathematics. In J. Boaler (Ed.), *Multiple perspectives in mathematics teaching and learning* (pp. 83–104). Westport, CT: Ablex Publishing.

Berch, D.B., & Mazzocco, M.M.M. (1999) (2007). *Why is math so hard for some children? The nature and origins of mathematical learning difficulties and disabilities.* Baltimore, MD: Paul H Brookes Publishing Co.

Bird, R. (2017). *The dyscalculia toolkit: Supporting learning difficulties in maths* (3rd ed.). London, United Kingdom: SAGE Publications.

Bishop, D.V.M. (2010). Which neurodevelopmental disorders get researched and why? *PloS One, 5*(11), e15112. doi:10.1371/journal.pone.0015112

Boaler, J., & Zoido, P. (2016, Nov. 1). Why math education in the U.S. doesn't add up. *Scientific American Mind.*

Butterworth, B. (1999). *What counts: How every brain is hardwired for math.* New York, NY: Free Press.

Butterworth, B., & Kovas, Y. (2013). Understanding neurocognitive developmental disorders can improve education for all. *Science, 340*(6130), 300–305. doi:10.1126/science.1231022

Butterworth, B., & Varma, S. (2013). Mathematical development. In D. Mareschal, B. Butterworth, & A. Tolmie (Eds.), *Educational neuroscience* (pp. 201–236). Chichester, United Kingdom: Wiley.

Butterworth, B., Varma, S., & Laurillard, D. (2011). Dyscalculia: From brain to education. *Science, 332*(6033), 1049–1053. doi:10.1126/science.1201536

Butterworth, B., & Yeo, D. (2004). *Dyscalculia guidance: Helping pupils with specific learning difficulties in maths.* Abingdon, Oxford: Nelson Publishers.

Callaway, E. (2013). Number games. *Nature, 493*(7431), 150.

Carpenter, T.P., Fennema, E., Franke, M.L., Levi, L., & Empson, S.B. (1999). *Children's mathematics: Cognitively guided instruction.* Portsmouth, NH: Heinemann.

Chernoff, E.J., & Stone, M. (2014, June). An examination of math anxiety. *Ontario Mathematics Gazette, 52*(4), 29.

Chinn, S., & Ashcroft, R.E. (2017). *Mathematics for dyslexics and dyscalculics: A teaching handbook* (4th ed.). Oxford, United Kingdom: John Wiley & Sons.

Dehaene, S. (2011). *The number sense: How the mind creates mathematics* (Revised and updated.). New York, NY: Oxford University Press.

Fuson, K.C. (1988). *Children's counting and concepts of number.* New York, NY: Springer-Verlag.

Garnett, K. (1992). Developing fluency with basic number facts: Intervention with students with learning disabilities. *Learning Disabilities Research & Practice, 7*(4), 210–216.

Garnett, K. (2005). *Fact fluency foundations guide: Laying the foundation for math fact fluency.* [Print resource within *FASTT Math*.] New York, NY: Tom Snyder Productions/Scholastic Publications. Retrieved from http://www.ldonline.org/article/5896

Garnett, K. (2012). *Math and learning disabilities.* Retrieved from http://www.Smart KidswithLD.org

Gattegno, C. (1963). *For the teaching of mathematics.* New York, NY: Educational Solutions.

Gattegno, C. (1987). *The science of education part 1: Theoretical considerations.* New York, NY: Educational Solutions.

Gattegno, C. (2011a reissue). *Gattegno mathematics textbooks 1–4.* New York, NY: Educational Solutions.

Gattegno, C. (2011b reissue). *Words in color.* New York, NY: Educational Solutions.

Geary, D.C. (2004). Mathematics and learning disabilities. *Journal of Learning Disabilities, 37*(1), 4–15. doi:10.1177/00222194040370010201

Gersten, R., Clarke, B., Haymond, K., & Jordan, N. (2011). *Screening for mathematics difficulties in K–3 students.* Portsmouth, NH: RMC Research Corporation, Center on Instruction. Retrieved from http://www.centeroninstruction.org

Gerstmann, J. (1940). Syndrome of finger agnosia, disorientation for right and left, agraphia and acalculia local diagnostic value. *Archives of Neurology & Psychiatry, 44*(2), 398–408. doi:10.1001/archneurpsyc.1940.02280080158009

Ginsburg, H.P., Joon, S.L., & Boyd, J.S. (2008). Mathematics education for young children: What it is and how to promote it. *Social Policy Report: Giving Child and Youth Development Knowledge Away, XXII*(1).

Ginsburg, H.P., & Pappas, S. (2007). Commentary on Part III, Section VI: Instructional interventions and quantitative literacy. In D.B. Berch, M.M.M. Mazzocco, & H.P. Ginsburg (Eds.), *Why is math so hard for some children? The nature and origins of mathematical learning difficulties and disabilities* (pp. 431–440). Baltimore, MD: Paul H. Brookes Publishing Co.

Goswami, U. (2008). *Foresight mental capital and wellbeing project. Learning difficulties: Future challenges.* London, United Kingdom: The Government Office for Science.

Griffin, S. (2005). Fostering the development of whole-number sense: Teaching mathematics in the primary grades. In National Research Council, *How students learn: History, mathematics, and science in the classroom* (pp. 257–308). Washington, DC: The National Academies Press. Retrieved from https://www.nap.edu/read/10126/chapter/6

Griffin, S. (2007). Early intervention for children at risk of developing mathematical learning difficulties. In D. Berch & M.M.M. Mazzocco (Eds.), *Why is math so hard for some children? The nature and origin of mathematical learning difficulties and disabilities.* Baltimore, MD: Paul H. Brookes Publishing Co.

Griffin, S. (2015). *Number worlds: A prevention/intervention math program applying games and manipulatives in math intervention curriculum to foster enhanced conceptual understanding of numbers.* New York, NY: McGraw-Hill.

Griffin, S., & Case, R. (1997). Re-thinking the primary school math curriculum: An approach based on cognitive science. *Issues in Education, 3*(1), 1–49.

Griffin, S., Case, R., & Siegler, R. (1994). Rightstart: Providing the central conceptual prerequisites for first formal learning of arithmetic to students at-risk for school failure. In K. McGilly (Ed.), *Classroom lessons: Integrating cognitive theory and classroom practice* (pp. 24–49). Cambridge, MA: Bradford Books MIT Press.

Gross, J., Hudson, C., & Price, D. (2009). *The long term costs of numeracy difficulties.* London, United Kingdom: Every Child a Chance Trust, KPMG.

Harvard Education Letter. (2007). An interview with Sharon Griffin. Doing the critical things first: An aligned approach to preK and early elementary math. *Harvard Education Letter, 23*(2), 1–4.

Individuals with Disabilities Education Improvement Act (IDEA) of 2004, PL 108-446, 20 U.S.C. §§ 1400 *et seq.*

Kosc, L. (1974). Developmental dyscalculia. *Journal of Learning Disabilities, 7,* 164–77.

Montessori, M. (1912). *The Montessori method.* New York, NY: Schocken Books.

Ramirez, G., Gunderson, E., Levine, S., & Beilock, S. (2013). Math anxiety, working memory and math achievement in early elementary school. *Journal of Cognition and Development, 14*(2), 187–202.

Rourke, B.P. (Ed.). (1995). *Syndrome of nonverbal learning disabilities: Neurodevelopmental manifestations.* New York, NY: Guilford.

Rourke, B., & Conway, J.A. (1997). Disabilities of arithmetic and mathematical reasoning: Perspectives from neurology and neuropsychology. *Journal of Learning Disabilities, 30*(1), 34–46.

Shalev, R.S. (2007). Prevalence of developmental dyscalculia. In D.B. Berch, & M.M.M. Mazzocco (Eds.), *Why is math so hard for some children? The nature and origins of mathematical learning difficulties and disabilities.* Baltimore, MD: Paul H. Brookes Publishing Co.

Standing, E.M. (1998). *Maria Montessori: Her life and work.* New York, NY: Penguin.

Stern, C. (1949). *Children discover arithmetic: An introduction to structural arithmetic.* New York, NY: Harper & Row.

Stern, C., & Stern, M.B. (1971). *Children discover arithmetic: An introduction to structural arithmetic* (Revised and enlarged). New York, NY: Harper & Row.

Stern, C., Stern, M., & Gould, T.S. (1966). *Experimenting with numbers.* New York, NY: Houghton Mifflin.

Stern, M.B., & Gould, T.S. (1998). *Structural arithmetic I, II, III: Teachers guide and workbooks.* Cambridge, MA: Educators Publishing Service.

Stock, P., Desoete, A., & Roeyers, H. (2006). Focusing on mathematical disabilities: A search for definition, classification and assessment. In S.V. Randall (Ed.) *Learning disabilities: New research* (pp. 29–62). Hauppage, NY: Nova Science.

Tanguay, P.B., & Rourke, B.P. (2001). *Nonverbal learning disabilities at home: A parent's guide.* London, United Kingdom: Jessica Kingsley.

von Aster, M. (2000). Developmental cognitive neuropsychology of number processing and calculation: Varieties of developmental dyscalculia. *European Child & Adolescent Psychiatry, 9*(Suppl 2), S41. doi:10.1007/s007870070008

Wilson, A.J., Dehaene, S., Pinel, P., Revkin, S.K., Cohen, L., & Cohen, D. (2006). Principles underlying the design of "The Number Race," an adaptive computer game for remediation of dyscalculia. *Behavioral and Brain Functions, 2*(19).

Young, C.B., Wu, S.S., & Menon, V. (2012). The neurodevelopmental basis of math anxiety. *Psychological Science OnlineFirst.* doi:10.1177/0956797611429134

Zentall, S.S. (2007). Math performance of students with ADHD: Cognitive and behavioral contributors and interventions. In D.B. Berch & M.M.M. Mazzocco (Eds.), *Why is math so hard for some children? The nature and origins of mathematical learning difficulties and disabilities* (pp. 219–243). Baltimore, MD: Paul H. Brookes Publishing Co.

Technology Resources

Katherine Garnett and Elaine A. Cheesman

MATH LEARNING DISABILITIES: SELECTED INTERVENTIONS

Chapter 13 discussed four current trailblazers in specially designed math instruction; online resources are available for each of the four approaches.

Ronit Bird, *The Dyscalculia Toolkit* and other resources   http://www.ronitbird.com

Ronit Bird created a collection of games, videos, and teaching resources to assist students with dyscalculia. Her physical books include *Overcoming Difficulties with Number* (2009), *The Dyscalculia Resource Book* (2011), and *The Dyscalculia Toolkit* (2017). Her rich resources for teachers and parents include free downloads, videos, and clear guides. Available downloads include

- Maths Games: Card Games for Addition & Subtraction
- Number Games to Improve Maths
- Maths Games: Dice & Domino Games
- Number Games to Improve Maths
- Exploring Numbers Through Dot Patterns (Dyscalculia & Dyslexia Friendly Game Activities)
- Understanding Times Tables
- Exploring Numbers Through Cuisenaire Rods (Dyscalculia & Dyslexia Friendly Game Activities)

Sharon Griffin, *Number Worlds* https://www.mheducation.com/prek-12/program/microsites/MKTSP-TIG05M0.html

Number Worlds (McGraw Hill Education) spans pre-kindergarten through Grade 8. It focuses on conceptual understanding of the number system. Warm-up activities address computational fluency; lessons explore quantities using hands-on manipulatives. Children's number understandings are grounded in these physical materials before they are asked to compute and use symbolic numbers. *Number Worlds* also places an emphasis on oral language, with students learning to describe their number manipulations.

Catherine Stern, *Stern Math*   http://sternmath.com

Stern Math spans pre-kindergarten through Grade 5. It uses color-coded 1–10 blocks in well-structured frames and tracks to teach the foundation of number sense and operations. Students learn the relationship among numbers and the foundation of our number system as they are guided through a developmentally appropriate set of activities and games.

Cognitively Guided Instruction (CGI)

CGI is a worthy tool for every teacher's kit. See the following CGI resources online:

The Impact of Cognitively Guided Instruction [Video] Heinemann (https://blog .heinemann.com/impact-cognitively-guided-instruction-video/)

Starting Out With Cognitively Guided Instruction [Video] Heinemann (http://www .heinemann.com/blog/starting-cognitively-guided-instruction/)

CGI Video Resources Teachers Development Group (http://www.tdgnetwork.org/)

Cognitively Guided Instruction Video information Monterey Bay Area Math Project (http://mbamp.ucsc.edu/information-on-cgi-videos/)

Teachers can also learn more about CGI through the following text: Carpenter, T.P., Fennema, E., Franke, M.L., Levi, L., & Empson, S.B. (1999). *Children's mathematics: Cognitively guided instruction.* Portsmouth, NH: Heinemann.

PROGRAMS/APPS FOR MATH FOUNDATION (WRITING, QUANTITY, COUNTING, AND LANGUAGE)

Effective programs/apps have the following features:

- They do not require extensive reading or reading skills.

- They provide clear illustrations of concepts.

Dexteria Dots—Get in Touch with Math   http://www.dexteria.net

This app reinforces the concept of comparing quantity. The user makes equal dots or compares dots by separating or combining dots to produce a value. For beginners, larger dots represent greater values, and smaller dots represent smaller values.

DysCalculator   https://itunes.apple.com/us/app/dyscalculator/id508012847?mt=8; https://play.google.com/store/apps/details?id=com.shapehq.dyscalculator&hl=en

This app calculator shows the relationship between numbers and numerals in four ways (the digit, e.g., 4; the spelled-out number, e.g., four, audio, and a bargraph). It reads numbers, thus linking quantity with language. One can use the app to solve equations with extended operations. It also rounds numbers.

Jungle Fractions   http://jungleeducation.com

This app provides visual assistance with quantity, comparisons, and counting in fractions. It orally reads both text and numerals, thus assisting with the language of mathematical concepts. Both learn and game modes use engaging formats and provide immediate feedback with animated animals.

Jungle Geometry　http://jungleeducation.com

This app provides visual assistance with quantity and comparisons in line measurement, names of shapes, names of angles, and other geometric concepts. It orally reads both text and numbers, thus assisting with the language of mathematical concepts. Both learn and game modes use engaging formats and provide immediate feedback with animated animals.

Letter School/Cursive Letter School　http://www.letterschool.com

These two apps provide engaging practice in naming and writing numerals from 1 to 10. With a choice of fonts, they provide starting and mid-point clues. The practice is engaging, with increasing difficulty, independent writing, and progress monitoring reports.

Math Vocabulary　http://www.mathlearningcenter.org

This app and web-based program is available in English and Spanish. It links math terms, examples, and definitions for an extensive collection of content.

Native Numbers　https://itunes.apple.com/us/app/native-numbers/id570231808?mt=8

Native Numbers is a number sense app for the iPad (available in free and paid versions). Appropriate for ages 4–7, it includes number representation, number relations, ordering, and counting. It is considered particularly well done and systematic. It is being researched by Daniel Ansar at Western Ontario University (daniel.ansari@uwo.ca).

Number Frames　http://www.mathlearningcenter.org

This app and web-based program is a virtual manipulative to help students see, compare, and compute quantities up to 100.

Number Line　http://www.mathlearningcenter.org

This app and web-based program develops counting skills with a virtual number line. It helps students visualize number sequences and skip-counting. It also illustrates strategies for counting, comparing, and all four operations, plus fractions, decimals, and negative numbers.

Number Pieces　http://www.mathlearningcenter.org

This app and web-based program is a set of virtual Cuisenaire rods.

The Number Race by Anna Wilson & Stanislas Dehaene, 2005
http://www.thenumberrace.com/nr/home.php?lang=en

This adaptive game software was designed and programmed by the author of this site. It is free and is designed to improve number sense in dyscalculia. So far research suggests that it is most useful for children age 4–7. It is currently available in English (U.S.), French, Dutch, German, and Spanish.

Number Rack　http://www.mathlearningcenter.org

This app and web-based program shows rows of moveable colored beads to develop skills of quantity and counting.

Numbers and Counting http://eggrollgames.com

This intuitive app links subitizing with matching numerals.

Oh No! Fractions http://learningworksforkids.com/apps/oh-no-fractions/

This app develops the concept of quantity in fractions. The interactive manipulatives help the user compare, add, subtract, multiply, and divide fractions. The app presents a pair of fractions and challenges the user to find a common denominator, add, or decide which is larger. Bar graphs show the answers in "show me" or "prove it" modes.

Subitize Tree http://www.doodlesmithink.com

Subitizing is instantly seeing how many are represented, like the dots on dice or dominoes. This engaging game provides independent practice and reinforces the concept of quantity using a variety of representations (e.g., dominoes, dice, fingers on hands, playing cards). Players can choose a specific representation to practice, change the amount of time the images are displayed, and select the range of numbers used.

Ten Frame Fill http://www.classroomfocusedsoftware.com

This app reinforces quantity relationships. It shows a ten frame with virtual tokens. The player is shown an addition problem and a complementary subtraction problem and asked, "How many more are needed to make 10?" The players can drag tokens of another color or touch the number for the correct response.

PROGRAMS/APPS FOR OPERATIONS PRACTICE (MATH FACTS)

Bedtime Math http://bedtimemath.org

This app presents short authentic scenarios with daily math problems presented in three different levels of difficulty.

Decimal Squares http://www.decimalsquares.com/

This site provides virtual manipulatives on decimal understanding.

Flash Card Match for Add and Subtract or Multiply and Divide
http://eggrollgames.com

In these flash-card apps, the numbers and equations are spoken, thus developing math language skills. The user can select the number range and time limits for practice.

Five-0 DLX http://www.codevandal.com

This strategy game is "Scrabble with Numerals." Each sequence must add up to a multiple of 5.

iDevBooks http://idevbooks.com

This is a collection of 26 math operations (add, subtract, multiply, divide, and fractions) apps that the user can purchase in sets or individually; some are free. The app illustrates how to solve problems, from simple to complex, including regrouping numbers and long division.

MathBase by Richard Glemburg   http://www.mathbase.co.uk

This U.K. software was designed by a special education teacher and focuses on basic number concepts. More advanced modules are also available as pupils progress.

MathTopia   http://www.TopShelfLearning.com

This is an engaging game that involves solving the four operations in separate games as it builds math fluency.

National Library of Virtual Manipulatives   http://nlvm.usu.edu/en/nav/category_g_4_t_2.html

This site is great for teaching algebra, with some very visual examples of abstract concepts. See also the home page: http://nlvm.usu.edu/en/nav/vlibrary.html

Sums Stacker   http://www.MathDoodles.com

This strategy game challenges the user to produce different sums in three different stacks. It presents values in numerals, dice, Roman numerals, and designs.

Thinking Blocks—K–6   http://www.thinkingblocks.com/

This site has virtual manipulatives ("blocks") students use to understand problems.

BROAD-RANGING PROGRAMS/APPS FOR MATH FOUNDATIONS AND MATH OPERATIONS

Cool Math   http://www.coolmath.com/algebra/index.html

This site keeps students strongly engaged with math and logic games. It also provides practice problems with worked-out answers.

Gamequarium   http://www.gamequarium.com/algebra.htm

This site provides algebra games, videos, and other free resources.

Geogebra   http://www.geogebra.org

This site provides free materials and interactive software for geometry, algebra, statistics, and calculus.

Math Learning Center   http://catalog.mathlearningcenter.org/apps

This site provides free apps for early geometry, number sense, and place value.

Motion Math   http://motionmathgames.com

This program provides instructional math games for the iPad, with many different games at different levels. A research study supports Motion Math's effectiveness:

Ricoscente, M.M. (2013). Results from a controlled study of the iPad fractions game Motion Math. *Sage Journals, 8,* 4.

Advanced Reading/Literacy Skills

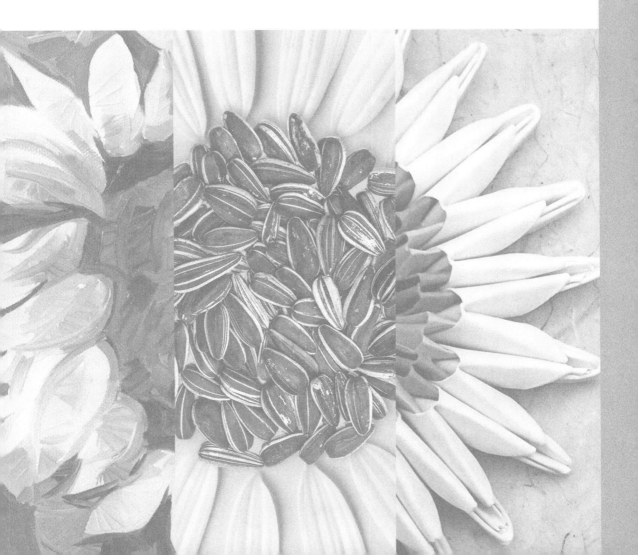

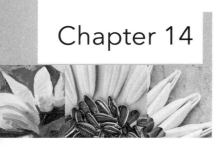

Chapter 14

The History and Structure of Written English

Marcia K. Henry

LEARNING OBJECTIVES

1. To understand the structure and origins of English words
2. To consider a framework for studying, reading, and spelling English words
3. To acquire strategies for teaching decoding and spelling

This chapter presents a short history of written English and introduces the structure of English orthography—the English spelling system. English is a dynamic language, and numerous historical forces shaped the development of written English. The historical perspective is of primary importance to studying word formation in English. As Nist (1966) and Venezky (1970) asserted, English orthography begins to make sense when understood from an historical perspective.

An understanding of the historical forces that influenced written English, along with a grasp of the structure of the English spelling system, provides teachers and their students with a logical basis for the study of English. Students who recognize letter–sound correspondences, syllable patterns, and morpheme patterns—the meaningful word parts such as bases (often called roots), prefixes, and suffixes—in words of Anglo-Saxon, Latin, and Greek origin have the strategies necessary to read and spell unfamiliar words.

The *Knowledge and Practice Standards for Teachers of Reading*, developed by the International Dyslexia Association's (IDA) Professional Standards and Practices Committee in 2010, include the Knowledge of the Structure of Language. Content knowledge categories include Phonology (the speech system), Orthography (the spelling system), and Morphology. The standards recognize the importance of understanding the etymology of words and the "broad outline of historical influences on English spelling patterns, especially Anglo-Saxon, Latin (Romance, including French) and Greek" (IDA, 2010, p. 6). The Orthography section also emphasizes the need to recognize orthographic rules and patterns in English and identify the basic syllable types in English spelling. In the Morphology section, the standards recognize the necessity to "identify and categorize common morphemes in English, including Anglo-Saxon compounds, inflectional suffixes, and derivational suffixes; Latin-based prefixes, roots, and derivational suffixes; and Greek-based combining forms" (IDA, 2010, p. 6).

The English spelling system is said to be opaque (or deep or nontransparent) in contrast to transparent (or shallow) orthographies, such as Finnish and Italian. In transparent orthographies, letters and their pronunciations have almost one-to-one correspondence. In English, however, many words do not carry this relationship. Yet, many psycholinguists believe that English is more transparent than tradition-ally thought. In their studies of the consistency in English graphemic represen-tation of speech sounds, Hanna, Hodges, and Hanna concluded that the results "indicated that our written code is not so inconsistent that analysis of phoneme–grapheme correspondences cannot provide the basis for teaching spelling" (1971, p. 76). They found that roughly 80% of the phonemes contained in the traditional spelling vocabulary of elementary school children used the alphabetic principle in their letter representations. Pinker noted, "Indeed, for about eighty-four percent of English words, spelling is completely predictable from regular rules" (1994, p. 190).

Most teachers who subscribe to teaching the structure of English begin teach-ing letter–sound correspondences, often called phonics, and move on to teaching syllable and morpheme patterns. Morphemes include Anglo-Saxon compound words and affixes (the prefixes and suffixes added to base words); Latin bases (or roots), prefixes, and suffixes; and Greek bases, often called roots or combining forms. The importance of teaching more than basic phonics cannot be stressed enough. Venezky (1970) proposed that morphemes as well as phonemes play lead-ing roles in the English orthography. He referred to morphophonemic relation-ships in which certain morphemes kept their written spelling while changing their phonemic forms. Balmuth noted that

> It can be helpful to readers when the same spelling is kept for the same morpheme, despite variations in pronunciation. Such spellings supply clues to the meanings of words, clues that would be lost if the words were spelled phonemically, as, for example, if *know* and *knowledge* were spelled *noe* and *nollij* in a hypothetical phonemic system. (2009, p. 207)

Seidenburg (2017) emphasized that in order to maintain continuity, related words are spelled the same despite differences in pronunciation. He provided an interesting discussion of the spelling of *sign* and how it won out over *sine, segn*, and *syne*, pointing out: "Preserving information about morphological structure won out over spelling-sound consistency" (2017, p. 133). He went on to say, "The spellings of many words are a compromise between the conflicting demands of the alphabetic and morphological principles" (2017, p. 133). Cooke (2016) posited the example of the different pronuncia-tions of the Latinate base *cred* in *credit, credential, credence* and *incredulous*.

Brown (1947) found that 80% of English words borrowed from other lan-guages came from Latin and Greek. Therefore, teaching relatively few Latin and Greek roots provides students with the key to unlocking hundreds of thousands of words. In fact, new research concluded that even young children benefit from being exposed to morphology and etymology in first and second grades. Ebbers (2008) found that second graders encounter inflections, compounds, and deriva-tions in both narrative and informative text. Apel and Henbest gained support in their study of first through third graders "for how students might use morphologi-cal problem solving to read unknown multimorphemic words successfully" (2016, p. 148). Bowers and Kirby (2010) and Bowers and Cooke (2012) emphasized the importance of including morphology in literacy instruction, especially for less able and younger students. Their work was inspired by the Latin and Greek scholar Michel Rameau (2000). Devonshire, Morris, and Fluck (2012) concluded that using explicit instruction of morphology and etymology should be taught in addition to traditional phonics beginning as early as kindergarten and first grade.

▌ REFLECT, CONNECT, and RESPOND
▌ What are the three major strategies available to decode unfamiliar words?

HISTORY AND ENGLISH ORTHOGRAPHY

Knowing the historic origins of words, the etymology, provides clarification for the spelling of many words. The web site https://www.etymonline.com is an excellent source for the etymology of most words.

Historically, English is one of the youngest among the important languages of the world. The original inhabitants of the British Isles, the Celts, spoke a different language in the **Indo-European** family. They were conquered by Julius Caesar in 54 C.E. (Common Era).

The Britons continued to speak Celtic, whereas the Romans spoke Latin. The Romans departed and returned almost a century later and stayed for nearly 400 years. During the fifth century C.E., Germanic groups—the Jutes, Saxons, and Angles—began to settle in different parts of England. They did not speak the Celtic language and did not practice the Celtic religion (Balmuth, 2009). Rather, Anglo-Saxon became the dominant language and the vocabulary revolved around the people, objects, and events of daily life. The Roman alphabet, which the Romans had adapted from Greek via Etruscan, was reintroduced to the British Island by Christian missionaries at this time.

Five major factors shaped the English language during the period of Old English between 450 and 1150 C.E.: Teutonic invasion and settlement; the Christianizing of Britain; the creation of a national English culture; Danish–English warfare, political adjustment, and cultural assimilation; and the decline of Old English as a result of the Norman Conquest (Nist, 1966). During this time, Germanic, Celtic, Latin, Greek, Anglo-Saxon, Scandinavian, and French words entered Old English. Nist explained that, at the end of the period, "language was no longer the basically Teutonic and highly inflected Old English but the hybrid-becoming, Romance-importing, and inflection-dropping Middle English" (1966, p. 107).

The period of Middle English (1150–1500) heralded great changes in the native tongue of Britain. Early Middle English (1150–1307) sounded much like present-day German. Claiborne estimated that after the Norman Conquest "more than ten thousand French words passed into the English vocabulary, of which 75 percent are still in use" (1983, p. 112). Anglo-French compounds (e.g., *gentlewomen, gentlemen; faithful, faithfulness*) appeared during this period. Spelling based on French such as the *our* in *journey, ch* pronounced as /sh/, and the *que* as /k/ in *antique* also occurred during this time.

A renewed Latin influence penetrated the language during the period of Mature Middle English (1307–1422) in the 14th and 15th centuries. Chaucer wrote *The Canterbury Tales* in the late 1300s. This was the time of the Renaissance, which brought a wave of cultural advancement. Hanna and colleagues observed,

> The Latin vocabulary was felt to be more stable and polished and more capable of conveying both abstract and humanistic ideas than was a fledgling language such as English. Further, Latin was something of a lingua franca that leaped across geographical and political boundaries. (1971, p. 47)

Many of the words used in English today are borrowed from the Latin of this period, including *index, library, medicine,* and *instant.* During the time of Mature Middle English, Latin affixes entered the language in great numbers. Prefixes (e.g., *ad-, pro-*) and suffixes (e.g., *-ent, -ion, -al*) were added to word roots to form words such as *adjacent, prosecution,* and *rational* (Claiborne, 1983).

The written word grew in importance during the period of Late Middle English (1422–1600). English pressman William Caxton introduced the printing press to England and printed books using the English spoken in London by the well-to-do. Many spelling conventions were set into place at this time. Also, words from Greek and Romance languages enriched English enormously during the English Renaissance. The Romance languages include Latin-based languages (e.g., Portuguese, Spanish, French, Italian, and Romanian). French contributions at this time included final *que* pronounced as /k/ as in *masque, pique,* and *opaque.*

During the periods of Late Middle English and Early Modern English, the sound patterns of the language, especially the vowel sounds, underwent changes. Nist commented that

> The changes in the pronunciation from the Mature Middle English of Chaucer to the Early Modern English of Shakespeare, insofar as these tense vowels were concerned, were so dramatic that Jespersen [1971] has named their phonemic displacement the Great Vowel Shift. (1966, p. 221)

The vowel shift resulted in certain vowel sounds being articulated in new positions and ensured a sharp separation between phonology and spelling. For example, in Chaucer's time, the vowel sound in *bide* was pronounced like /ē/ in *bee,* but in Shakespeare's time, it shifted to /ā/ as in *bay.* This shift caused problems for spellers; Hanna and colleagues explained that "stabilized spellings now came to represent different sounds" (1971, p. 49).

Changes continued through the periods of Authoritarian English (1650–1800) and Mature Modern English (1800–1920) to reach the pronunciation of today. The period from 1920 to the present has been called World Power American English as English becomes the global language for much of the Internet and international trade. New words continue to form. In the early 2000s, words related to the real estate and financial crises brought us the new words *subprime* and *bailout.* In addition, new immigrants to the United States bring greater linguistic diversity. More recently, in the second decade of the 2000s, new terms based on advancing technology include *app, hashtag, tweet,* and *google.*

English, then, is a **polyglot,** and the Anglo-Saxon, Latin (Romance), and Greek languages all played a role in establishing the words as they are spoken and written today (Balmuth, 2009; Hanna et al., 1971; Nist, 1966). Claiborne noted,

> The truth is that if borrowing foreign words could destroy a language, English would be dead (borrowed from Old Norse), deceased (from French), defunct (from Latin) and kaput (from German). When it comes to borrowing, English excels (from Latin), surpasses (from French) and eclipses (from Greek) any other tongue, past or present. (1983, p. 4)

REFLECT, CONNECT, and RESPOND

Claiborne (1983) called English a *polyglot.* What does this mean, and how is it important in teaching about the structure of English words?

FRAMEWORK FOR CURRICULUM AND INSTRUCTION

One framework for teaching a decoding and spelling curriculum is based on word origin and word structure (Henry 1988a, 1988b, 2010a, 2010b). The three origin languages most influential to English are Anglo-Saxon (a term that includes early Germanic, Scandinavian, and other contributing languages), Latin, and Greek. Teachers who understand the historical origins of words enhance their presentation of reading instruction. The major structural categories are letter–sound correspondences, syllables, and morphemes. By teaching all of the components of this framework, teachers can ensure that their students will learn the primary patterns found in English words. Teachers are encouraged to use a multisensory approach for teaching each component so that students will simultaneously link the visual symbol with its corresponding sound and form the pattern accurately (see Chapter 9).

Teaching phonics offers a strategy for decoding and spelling that works when the letter–sound correspondence system carries all of the demands of word analysis. When students do not recognize syllabic and morphological patterns, however, they are constrained from using clues to identify long, unfamiliar words. In our experience, most decoding instruction largely neglects the instruction of syllable and morpheme patterns, perhaps because these techniques are thought to be useful only for the longer words found in literature and subject-matter text beyond second or third grade, at which point decoding instruction becomes virtually nonexistent in most schools.

Figure 14.1 represents the categories in the word origin and word structure framework. Each entry in the matrix corresponds to words of Anglo-Saxon, Latin, or Greek origin that are related to letter–sound correspondences, syllables, or morphemes. In the following sections, pre-reading instruction and the major components of the framework are discussed.

Phonological Awareness

Liberman and her colleagues (Liberman, 1973; Liberman & Liberman, 1990; Liberman & Shankweiler, 1985, 1991; Liberman, Shankweiler, Fischer, & Carter, 1974) noted that children's phonological awareness, or understanding of the role that sounds play in the English language, is extremely important in learning to read. Phonemic awareness, which is only one component of phonological awareness, is the awareness that speech is made up of discrete sounds and the ability to manipulate sounds into words. Before learning letter–sound correspondences, often called *phonics*, children benefit from training in phonological awareness. Phonological awareness is an awareness of all levels of the speech sound system, including rhymes, stress patterns, syllables, and phonemes. Students practice rhyming, segmentation, and blending (see Chapter 6) before learning letter names and letter formation (see Chapter 5).

Phonics

Balmuth (2009), as well as Adams (1990), Chall (1983), Chall and Popp (1996), Ehri (2005), and Richardson (1989), provided insights on the importance of phonics in education since the 19th century. When learning phonics, students must link the graphemes and phonemes of English. Linguists note there are 40–44 phonemes in English but many more ways to spell the sounds heard in words. Letter–sound

	Letter–sound correspondences	Syllable patterns	Morpheme patterns
Anglo-Saxon	Consonants Single Blend Digraph _bid_ _step_ _that_ Vowels Short/long -r/-l Digraph m_a_d/m_a_de b_ar_n b_oat_	Closed: _mad_ Open: _go_ VCe: _lame_ Vowel team: _boat_ Consonant -le: _tumble_ r-controlled: _barn_	Compound _shipyard, hardware_ Affix _read, reread, rereading get bid, forbid, forbidden_
Latin	Same as Anglo-Saxon but few vowel digraphs Schwa prevalent (ə): _direction_ _spatial_ _excellent_	Closed: _struct, flect_ VCe: _scribe, vene_ r-controlled: _port, form_	Affix _construction erupting conductor_
Greek	_ph_ for /f/–_phonograph_ _ch_ for /k/–_chorus, scholar_ _y_ as /ĭ/–_symphony_ Also–_ps, rh, pn, mn, pt_	Closed: _graph, gram_ Open: _photo, micro_ Unstable digraph: _poet_	Compound _microscope hemisphere physiology_

Figure 14.1. Word origin and word structure matrix. (_Source:_ M. Henry, 1988b. Matrix adapted from Henry, M.K. [2010], _Unlocking literacy: Effective decoding and spelling instruction._ Baltimore, MD: Paul H. Brookes Publishing Co. Adapted with permission.)

correspondences are the relationships between the consonant and vowel letters (graphemes) and their corresponding sounds (phonemes).

Teachers generally use dictionary markings (phonic symbols) as guides to pronunciation. Linguists and specialists in speech-language disorders tend to use symbols from the International Phonetic Alphabet. (See Moats, 1995, 2010, as well as Chapters 3 and 10, for further information on phonetics, identifying and describing speech sounds, and articulating specific sounds.)

Syllable Patterns

Syllables are units of spoken language consisting of a vowel sound or a vowel–consonant combination. Groff (1971) emphasized that syllables are not units of writing, grammar, or structure. He noted that the boundaries of syllables rather than the number of syllables in a word cause difficulty in their analysis. He made the distinction between how linguists divide words based on morphemic boundaries and how dictionaries divide syllables based on sounds. For example, linguists usually divide the word _disruptive_ as _dis|rupt|ive_ (prefix, root, and suffix), whereas dictionaries usually divide the word as _dis|rup|tive_, based on pronunciation. Groff wondered whether teaching syllable division is an important part of teaching reading. Although this argument continues, it is useful for teachers to know the six major syllable types and the predominant syllable division patterns because children will read multisyllabic words in the primary grades and will find syllable division useful in pronouncing and hyphenating words.

Morpheme Patterns

A morpheme is the smallest meaningful linguistic unit. Prefixes (beginnings), suffixes (endings), and bases or roots are the morphemes that are helpful for students learning to read and write because they appear in literally hundreds of thousands of words (Brown, 1947; Henry, 1993). Students learn that free morphemes can stand alone whereas bound morphemes cannot. Affixes are always bound, but bases can be either free (e.g., *spell* in *respelling*) or bound (e.g., *spect* in *respecting*). By knowing the common morphemes, students enhance not only their decoding and spelling skills but also their vocabulary skills. Related to morphology is the study of etymology, the origin and history of a word.

> ### REFLECT, CONNECT, and RESPOND
> What is a morpheme? Why is an understanding of morphemes important for reading teachers to have and impart to students?

THE ANGLO-SAXON LAYER OF LANGUAGE

Words of Anglo-Saxon origin are characterized as the common, everyday, down-to-earth words that are used frequently in ordinary situations. These words come mostly from Germanic, Anglo-Saxon, and Scandinavian words. Nist provided a clever example of Anglo-Saxon words:

> No matter whether a man is American, British, Canadian, Australian, New Zealander, or South African, he still *loves his mother, father, brother, sister, wife, son and daughter; lifts his hand to his head, his cup to his mouth, his eye to heaven and his heart to God; hates his foes, likes his friends, kisses his kin and buries his dead; draws his breath, eats his bread, drinks his water, stands his watch, wipes his sweat, feels his sorrow, weeps his tears and sheds his blood; and all these things he thinks about and calls both good and bad.* (1966, p. 9)

As the Nist passage shows, most words of Old English origin consist of one syllable and represent everyday objects, activities, and events. Although consonant letters are fairly regular (i.e., each letter corresponds to one sound), vowels are more problematic. Words that are learned early on in school are often considered "irregular" because the spellings are not the usual vowel spellings. It should be mentioned that no words are actually "irregular;" their spellings are based on their history. Some students often need to memorize the spellings of these "outlaw" words, such as *rough, does, only, eye, laugh, blood,* and *said,* because the vowels do not carry the normal short (lax) or long (tense) sound associated with these spellings. When students understand the etymology of these words, they are no longer "irregular."

Letter-Sound Correspondences

Anglo-Saxon letter–sound correspondences are the first symbol–sound relationships taught to children learning to read and spell. Consonant letters (e.g., *b, c, d, f, m, p, t*) represent the speech sounds produced by a partial or complete obstruction of the air stream. The consonant pairs *gn, kn,* and *wr* are Anglo-Saxon forms. Vowel letters (i.e., *a, e, i, o, u,* and sometimes *y* and *w*) represent the sounds that are created by the relatively free passage of breath through the larynx and oral cavity.

Graphemes are organized either in consonant or vowel patterns. Single-letter consonant spellings seldom vary; each letter stands for a specific sound. The letters *c* and *g*, however, have more than one possible pronunciation: a hard and soft sound. The letter *c* usually has the sound of /k/ as in *carrot* but becomes soft before *e, i,* and *y,* as in *cell, city,* and *cypress*. Likewise, the *g* in *go* or *gas* is hard, whereas *g* before *e, i,* and *y* is soft as in *gem, ginger,* and *Gypsy*. The letter *s* is usually pronounced as /s/ as in *snake* but sometimes has the /z/ sound as in *dogs*. The letter *x* at the end of a word makes the sound of /ks/ as in *box* but makes the sound of /z/ at the beginning of some words. These words, such as *xylophone* and *xenophobe,* are usually of Greek origin.

Consonant blends (sometimes called *consonant clusters*), which are made up of two or three adjacent consonants that retain their individual sounds in a syllable, are common (e.g., *bl* and *mp* in *blimp; spl* and *nt* in *splint*). In contrast to blends, consonant digraphs, which evolved in Middle English times, are two or more adjacent letters that form only one speech sound. Often, one of the letters of a consonant digraph is *h* (e.g., *sh* in *ship, ch* in *chump, th* in *this, wh* in *when*).

Vowel graphemes tend to be more difficult to learn than consonant graphemes because they can represent more than one sound and are often difficult to discriminate. Single vowels are generally either short or long. Words often contain clues, referred to as markers, that indicate whether the short or long sound should be used. A vowel with a consonant after it in the same syllable carries the short sound (e.g., *cat, let, fit, fox, fun*). In contrast, a vowel at the end of a syllable becomes long or "says its own name" (e.g., *go, baby, pilot*). A silent *e* at the end of a word, as in *shape* and *vote,* also signals that the word has a long vowel sound. A doubled consonant, as in *pinning* and *cutter,* marks that the preceding vowel has a short sound. The doubled consonant cancels the long-vowel signal that would otherwise be given by the *i* in *ing* and the *e* in *er*.

Students will also read words with a vowel plus *r* or *l*. The vowel sounds are often neither short nor long. These patterns are best taught as combinations, such as *ar* in *star, or* in *corn, er* in *fern, ir* in *bird, ur* in *church,* and *al* in *falter*.

Vowel digraphs consist of two adjacent vowel letters that represent one sound (e.g., *oa, ee, oi, ou, au*); these often occur in words of Anglo-Saxon origin. A vowel digraph usually occurs in the middle of a word. Vowel digraphs are often difficult for students to acquire because of their variability and because of interference from previously learned associations. They can be divided into two sets—those that are fairly consistently linked to a single sound (e.g., *ee, oa, oi, oy*) and those that may have either of two pronunciations (e.g., *ea* in *bead* or *bread, ow* in *show* or *cow*). (It should be noted that linguists differentiate between the terms *vowel digraph* and *diphthong*. Both contain two adjacent vowels letters in the same syllable. Diphthongs contain two vowels with a slide or a shift in the middle; they include *au/aw, oi/oy,* and *ou/ow*.) Balmuth provided the historical origins of vowel digraphs and diphthongs and noted that during Middle English times, diphthongs were "especially varied in spelling because of the confusions that resulted from the separation of the written *i* and *y* and the introduction of the *w* and other French spelling conventions" (2009, p. 102).

By the end of the second grade, children should have mastered all of the common letter–sound correspondences and related spelling patterns (see Chapter 10). For example, children need to learn when to use *c* rather than *k* at the end of a one-syllable word or *tch* rather than *ch*. The appendices in the Online Companion Materials provide examples of instruction on reading and writing words containing new target patterns.

Syllable Patterns

Words of Anglo-Saxon origin have a variety of syllable patterns. Students first learn that each syllable must contain a vowel. Children generally have less difficulty with hearing syllables in words than with identifying the syllables in written words (Balmuth, 2009; Groff, 1971). Therefore, teachers often begin by having children say their own names and count the number of syllables. Students also begin to listen for accent or stress in words of more than one syllable. Teachers can help students discover that words of Old English origin (e.g., *sleep, like, time*) tend to retain the accent when affixes are added (e.g., *asleep, likely, timeless*).

The major types of syllables are 1) closed, 2) vowel-consonant-*e,* 3) open, 4) vowel pair (or vowel team), 5) consonant-*le,* and 6) *r*-controlled (see Moats, 1995, 2010; Steere, Peck, & Kahn, 1971). Teachers generally introduce closed syllables first. In these syllables, the single vowel has a consonant after it and makes a short vowel sound (e.g., *map, sit, cub, stop, bed*). The final *e* in a vowel-consonant-*e* syllable makes the vowel long (e.g., *made, time, cute, vote, Pete*). An open syllable contains a vowel at the end of the syllable, and the vowel usually has a long sound (e.g., *me,* /mē/, and *hobo,* /hōbō/). Stanback (1992) found that closed syllables alone make up 43% of syllables in English words. Open syllables and closed syllables together account for almost 75% of English syllables. A vowel pair (or vowel team) syllable contains two adjacent vowel letters as in *rain, green, coil,* and *pause.* Children learn the long, short, or diphthong sound of each pattern. A syllable ending in *-le* is usually preceded by a consonant that is part of that syllable. For example, *bugle* has a long *u* because the *gle* stays together and makes *bu* an open syllable. *Tumble,* in contrast, contains *tum* and *ble;* with *tum* being a closed syllable. *Little* requires two *t*s to keep the *i* in *lit* short. As discussed previously, vowel sounds in *r*-controlled syllables often lose their identity as long or short and are coarticulated with the /r/ (as in *star, corn, fern, church,* and *firm*).

Students also need to learn some common rules for syllable division so that multisyllabic words are easier to read and spell. By understanding and practicing identification of the various syllable types in one-syllable words first, readers will recognize these common syllable types as they learn to divide words into syllables. Understanding how to spell the vowel sounds in syllables gives readers an advantage and a more productive grasp of syllable-division rules. Readers may recognize syllable-division patterns such as vowel-consonant-consonant-vowel (VC|CV) and others (V|CV as in *hobo* and VC|CCV as in *hundred*). These are useful separations to know when analyzing unfamiliar words (see Chapter 10).

Morpheme Patterns

Anglo-Saxon morphemes are found in both compound (e.g., *football, blackboard*) and affixed words (e.g., *lovely, timeless*). These words tend to be simple because they contain regular orthographic features. Compound words generally comprise two short words joined together to form new, meaning-based words (e.g., *blackboard* suggests a *black board, football* refers to a *ball* for kicking with one's *foot*). Computer technology has been the impetus for many new compound words, such as *software* and *shareware.*

Words can also be expanded by affixing prefixes and suffixes to the base. These bases, or free morphemes, can stand alone as words, such as *like* or *hope.* Morpheme affixes have two forms. Inflectional morphemes indicate grammatical features such as number, person, tense, or comparison (e.g., *dog, dogs; wait, waits; walk, walked; small, smaller*). Derivational morphemes, in contrast, change one part of speech to another, chiefly by adding affixes to root words (e.g., *hope, hopeless, hopelessly* (see Chapters 9 and 10).

Students begin learning morpheme patterns by adding suffixes to words requiring no change in the base form (e.g., *help, helpless; time, untimely*). Soon after that, they must learn suffix addition rules that affect some base words, such as the rule about when to drop a final *e* or double a final consonant or change *y* to *i* (*skate, skating; baby, babies*; see Chapter 10).

THE LATIN LAYER OF LANGUAGE

The Latin layer of the English language consists of words used in more formal settings. Latinate words are often found in the literature, social studies, and science texts in upper elementary school and later grades.

Letter–Sound Correspondences

Many students expect Latin-based words to be more complex because they are longer than Anglo-Saxon–based words. Yet, in most cases, the words follow simple grapheme–phoneme correspondences. Single consonants are identical to those found in Anglo-Saxon bases, but words of Latin origin contain fewer vowel digraphs. Most Latin bases contain short vowels as in *dict, rupt, script, struct, tract, tens, pend,* and *duct*. The consonant combination *ct* is a signpost for words of Latin origin, as in *contradict, construct,* and *viaduct*.

Latin-based digraphs generally appear in suffixes such as *-ion, -ian, -ient,* and *-ial*. When these vowel digraphs come after the letters *c, s,* and *t,* they combine with those letters as the /sh/ sound as in *nation, politician, partial, social,* and *admission* (*-sion* is also pronounced as /zhən/ in words such as *erosion* and *invasion*.) The schwa (/ə/), or neutral vowel sound in an unstressed syllable, is often found in words of Latin origin.

Syllable Patterns

Latin bases tend to be closed (e.g., *rupt, struct, script*), vowel-consonant-*e* (e.g., *scribe, vene*), and *r*-controlled (e.g., *port, form*). The accent usually falls on the base, but stress patterns can be fairly complex when adding derivational suffixes. Wade-Wooley and Heggie (2015) discussed the importance of stress assignment. The schwa (/ə/) is common in longer words of Latin origin such as *excellent* and *direction*. When one pronounces *excellent,* for example, stress occurs on the first syllable, so the initial *e* receives the regular short sound. The following two *es,* appearing in unstressed syllables, have the schwa sound (/ə/). Listening for the unstressed vowels in open and closed syllables is an advanced skill that students with reading difficulties need to learn. Students who can discover the stem (e.g., *excel*) often will be able to spell the longer word.

Morpheme Patterns

Although Old English–based words can make up compound words (e.g., *houseboat*) and can become affixed (e.g., *hopelessly*), Latin roots usually are affixed but can be compounded (e.g., *aqueduct, manuscript, artifact*). Nist provided another key example: "So great, in fact, was the penetra*tion* of Latin *af*fixing during the *Re*nais-*sance* that it quite *un*did the Anglo-Saxon habit of *com*pounding as the leading means of word form*ation* in English" (1966, p. 11).

Words of Latin origin become affixed by adding a prefix and/or a suffix to the base, which rarely stands alone (e.g., *rupt, interrupt*; *mit, transmitting*; *struct, reconstructing*). For example, the prefix *in-* can be added to the bound morpheme *spect* to get *inspect*, and the suffix *-ion* can be added to get *inspection*. (*Note:* Some sources, such as Barnhart, 1988; Gillingham & Stillman, 1957; and *Webster's New Universal Unabridged Dictionary*, 1983, explain *-tion* and *-cian* as noun suffixes. Actually, *-ion* and *-ian* are the suffixes added to bases such as *invent* and *music*, respectively; Cox, 1980; Henry, 2010a. Teachers and students need to know that *-ion* and *-ian* are the suffixes but that these are often preceded by *t, s,* or *c*.)

The final consonant of a Latin prefix often changes based on the beginning letter of the base. For example, the prefix *in-* changes to *il-* before roots beginning with *l* (e.g., *illegal, illicit*); to *ir-* before roots beginning with *r* (e.g., *irregular*); and to *im-* before roots beginning with *m, b,* and *p* (e.g., *immobile, imbalance, important*). These alliterative prefixes, called "chameleon prefixes" by Gillingham and Stillman (1956), are found in several forms (see Henry, 2010a, 2010b; Henry & Redding, 1996).

Latin bases form the basis of hundreds of thousands of words (Brown, 1947; Henry, 1993, 2010a). These bases are useful not only for decoding and spelling words but also for enhancing vocabulary. Students can readily observe the prefixes, roots, and suffixes in such words as *prediction, incredible, extracting,* and *reconstructionist.* Although most words of Latin origin follow regular letter–sound correspondences, some do not. Morphophonemic relations are the conditions in which certain morphemes keep their written spelling when affixes are added, although their phonemic forms change. This concept provides students with a logical reason for many English spellings. Cooke (2016) cited the example of the different pronunciations of *cred* in *credit, credential, credence,* and *incredulous.*

REFLECT, CONNECT, and RESPOND
Describe the characteristics of words with Latin origins.

THE GREEK LAYER OF LANGUAGE

Greek-based words also entered English by the thousands during the Renaissance to meet the needs of scholars and scientists. In addition, Bodmer noted that "the terminology of modern science, especially in aeronautics, biochemistry, chemotherapy, and genetics" (1944, p. 246) is formed from Greek. Greek bases are often called *combining forms* and generally compound to form words. Words of Greek origin appear largely in science textbooks (e.g., *microscope, hemisphere, physiology*). The following passage from a middle school science text shows not only how short words of Anglo-Saxon origin mix with longer Romance words but also how the scientific terminology is couched in words of Greek origin.

> Suppose you could examine a green part of a plant under the *microscope.* What would you see? Here are some cells from the green part of a plant. The cells have small green bodies shaped like footballs. They give the plant its green color. They are called *chloroplasts.* A single green plant cell looks like this. *Chloroplasts* are very important to a plant. As you know, plants make their own food. This food-making process is called *photosynthesis.* It is in these *chloroplasts* that *photosynthesis*

takes place. (Cooper, Blackwood, Boeschen, Giddings, & Carin, 1985, p. 20; italics added for emphasis)

Letter-Sound Correspondences

Greek grapheme–phoneme correspondences are similar to those of Old English, but words of Greek origin often use the sounds of /k/, /f/, and /ĭ/ represented by *ch*, *ph*, and *y*, respectively, such as in *chlorophyll*. These unique consonant combinations were introduced by Latin scribes and make words of Greek origin easily recognizable (Bodmer, 1944). Less common Greek letter–sound correspondences, found in only a handful of words, include *mn* in *mnemonic*, *rh* in *rhododendron*, *pt* in *pterodactyl*, *pn* in *pneumonia*, and the better known *ps* in *psychology* and *psychiatry*.

Syllable Patterns

Syllable types most prevalent in Greek-based words are closed (CVC, as in *graph*) and open (CV, as in *photo*). In addition, a unique type of syllable can be found, that of adjacent vowels in separate syllables (CV|VC), as in *theater, create,* and *theory*. These vowels appear in distinct syllables and therefore have distinct sounds. Syllable division in words of Greek origin generally follows the rules given for Old English words, especially the rules for open syllables (e.g., *phono, photo, meter, polis*). For example, the letter *y* sounds like short *i* in closed syllables (e.g., *symphony, gymnasium*), and these syllables are divided after the consonant. The letter *y* sounds like long *i* in open syllables (e.g., *cyclone, gyroscope, hyperbole*), and these syllables are divided immediately after the *y*. Combining forms such as *semi, hemi,* and *micro* do not follow traditional V|CV or VC|CV division. CVVC words such as *create* and *theory* are divided between the vowels (*cre|ate, the|or|y*). Students rarely need to depend on strategies for syllable division because they learn the patterns as wholes.

Morpheme Patterns

If students recognize relatively few Greek bases (or combining forms), then they can read and spell many words. As students learn the common Greek forms that hold specific meaning, such as *micr(o), scope, bi(o), graph, heli(o), meter, phon(o), phot(o), aut(o),* and *tele*, they begin to read, spell, and understand the meaning of words such as *microscope, telescope, phonoreception, telephoto, telescopic, photoheliograph, heliometer, biography,* and *autobiography*. (*Note*: Suffixes can be added, as in the last two examples.) Many Greek bases are often called prefixes because they appear at the beginning of words (e.g., *auto* in *autograph, hyper* in *hyperbole,* and *hemi* in *hemisphere*). Numeral prefixes such as *mono* (1), *di* (2), *tri* (3), *tetra* (4), *penta* (5), *hexa* (6), *hepta* (7), *octa* (8), *nona* (9), *deca* (10), *centi* (100), and *kilo* (1,000) become useful in the study of mathematics and geometry.

Ehrlich (1972); Fifer and Flowers (1989); Fry, Polk, and Fountoukidis (1996); Henry (2010a, 2010b); and Henry and Redding (1996) provided numerous resources for words containing both Latin- and Greek-based words. Specific instructional activities can be found in the latter three sources.

REFLECT, CONNECT, and RESPOND

How is understanding the structure and origin of English words important for teaching decoding and spelling?

CLOSING THOUGHTS: TEACHING THE ORIGIN AND STRUCTURE OF ENGLISH

Perfetti asserted that "only a reader with skilled decoding processes can be expected to have skilled comprehension processes" (1984, p. 43). Children's understanding will be enhanced when they are able to grasp words important to the gist of a story or to the meaning of text.

Teachers who comprehend the origins of the English language along with the primary structural patterns within words can improve their assessment skills, enhance their understanding of reading and spelling curricula, communicate clearly about language issues, and effectively teach useful language strategies to their students. Influences on English orthography stem from the introduction of letters and words from diverse origins. When teachers and their students understand the historical basis and structure of written English, they can better understand the regularities as well as the very few irregularities in English words.

Young students will use these language strategies to decode and spell short, regular words as well as Old English compound words and words using common prefixes and suffixes. Older students and adult learners receiving instruction in more advanced language structure will focus on Latin and Greek roots and affixes.

Finally, students of all ages often enjoy learning about the structure and origins of English words. Students who are learning English as a second language find that English is quite regular after all and is not a language of exceptions. Children with or without specific language disabilities benefit as they learn effective and efficient strategies to read and spell numerous words.

ONLINE COMPANION MATERIALS

The following Chapter 14 resources are available at http://www.brookespublishing .com/birshcarreker/materials:

*   Reflect, Connect, and Respond Questions

*   Appendix 14.1: Technology Resources

*   Appendix 14.2: Knowledge and Skill Assessment Answer Key

*   Appendix 14.3: Sample Lesson for Anglo-Saxon Letter–Sound Correspondences: *ar* and *or*

*   Appendix 14.4: Sample Lesson for Latin Bases

*   Appendix 14.5: Sample Lesson for Greek Bases (or Roots or Combining Forms)

*   Appendix 14.6: Resources

KNOWLEDGE AND SKILL ASSESSMENT

1.   Which is not one of the major influences of English?

     a.   Latin

     b.   Greek

     c.   Anglo-Saxon

     d.   Russian

2. Words from Old English tend to be what?

   a. Short, common words

   b. Polysyllabic words containing a base and affixes

   c. Technical words found in math and science content words

   d. All of the above

3. Latinate and Greek-based words entered the English language in large numbers during what time period?

   a. Renaissance

   b. Norman Conquest

   c. Reign of Julius Caesar

   d. Settlement in the New World

4. *Illiterate, rejection, survival,* and *intervention* are words from which language?

   a. Anglo-Saxon

   b. French

   c. Latin

   d. Greek

5. Letter–sound correspondences unique to Greek include which of the following?

   a. *ea, ou,* and *aw*

   b. *ph* as /f/, *ch* as /k/, and *y* as /ĭ/

   c. *que* and *ch* as /sh/

   d. None of the above

6. *Spect, duct,* and *rupt* are examples of what?

   a. Bound bases

   b. Suffixes

   c. Prefixes

   d. Free bases

REFERENCES

Adams, M.J. (1990). *Beginning to read: Thinking and learning about print.* Cambridge, MA: The MIT Press.

Apel, K., & Henbest, V.S. (2016). Affix meaning knowledge in first through third grade students. *Language, Speech, and Hearing Services in Schools, 47,* 148–156.

Balmuth, M. (2009). *The roots of phonics: A historical introduction* (Rev. ed.). Baltimore, MD: Paul H. Brookes Publishing Co.

Barnhart, R.K. (1988). *The Barnhart dictionary of etymology.* New York, NY: H.W. Wilson.

Bodmer, F. (1944). *The loom of language.* New York, NY: W.W. Norton.

Bowers, P.N., & Cooke, G. (2012). Morphology and the common core: Building students' understanding of the written word. *Perspectives on Language and Literacy, 38*(1), 31–35.

Bowers, P.N., & Kirby, J.R. (2010). Effects of morphological instruction on vocabulary acquisition. *Reading and Writing, 23*(5), 515–597.

Brown, J.I. (1947). Reading and vocabulary: 14 master words. In M.J. Herzberg (Ed.), *Word study* (pp. 1–4). Springfield, MA: Merriam-Webster.

Chall, J.S. (1983). *Learning to read: The great debate revisited.* New York, NY: McGraw-Hill.

Chall, J.S., & Popp, H.M. (1996). *Teaching and assessing phonics.* Cambridge, MA: Educators Publishing Service.

Claiborne, R. (1983). *Our marvelous native tongue.* New York, NY: Times Books.

Cooke, G. (2016, Oct. 16). *English morphology: How meaning takes shape* [Online Webinar].

Cooper, E.K., Blackwood, P.E., Boeschen, J.A., Giddings, M.G., & Carin, A.A. (1985). *HBJ science* (Purple ed.). Orlando, FL: Harcourt Brace.

Cox, A.R. (1980). *Structure and techniques: Multisensory teaching of basic language skills.* Cambridge, MA: Educators Publishing Service.

Devonshire, V., Morris, P., & Fluck, M. (2012). Spelling and reading development: The effect of teaching children multiple levels of representation in their orthography. *Learning and Instruction, 25,* 85–94.

Ebbers, S. (2008). Morphological word families in narrative and informational text. In Y. Kim, V.J. Risko, D.L. Compton, D.K. Dickinson, M.K. Hundley, R.T. Jimez, & D. Well Rowe. (Eds.), *57th yearbook of the National Reading Conference* (pp. 203–218). Oak Creek, WI: NRC.

Ehri, L.C. (2005). Learning to read words: Theory, findings, and issues. *Scientific Studies of Reading, 9*(2), 167–188.

Ehrlich, I. (1972). *Instant vocabulary.* New York, NY: Pocket Books.

Fifer, N., & Flowers, N. (1989). *Vocabulary from classical roots.* Cambridge, MA: Educators Publishing Service.

Fry, E.B., Polk, J.D., & Fountoukidis, D.L. (1996). *The reading teacher's new book of lists* (3rd ed.). Upper Saddle River, NJ: Prentice Hall.

Gillingham, A., & Stillman, B.W. (1956). *Remedial training for children with specific disability in reading, spelling and penmanship* (8th ed.). Cambridge, MA: Educators Publishing Service.

Groff, P. (1971). *The syllable: Its nature and pedagogical usefulness.* Portland, OR: Northwest Regional Educational Laboratory.

Hanna, P.R., Hodges, R.E., & Hanna, J.S. (1971). *Spelling: Structure and strategies.* Boston, MA: Houghton Mifflin.

Henry, M.K. (1988a). Beyond phonics: Integrated decoding and spelling instruction based on word origin and structure. *Annals of Dyslexia, 38*(1), 259–275.

Henry, M.K. (1988b). Understanding English orthography: Assessment and instruction for decoding and spelling (Doctoral dissertation, Stanford University, 1988). *Dissertation Abstracts International, 48,* 2841-A.

Henry, M.K. (1993). Morphological structure: Latin and Greek roots and affixes as upper grade code strategies. *Reading and Writing, 5*(2), 227–241.

Henry, M.K. (2010a). *Unlocking literacy: Effective decoding and spelling instruction* (2nd ed.). Baltimore, MD: Paul H. Brookes Publishing Co.

Henry, M.K. (2010b). *WORDS: Integrated decoding and spelling instruction based on word origin and word structure.* Austin, TX: PRO-ED.

Henry, M.K., & Redding, N.C. (1996). *Patterns for success in reading and spelling.* Austin, TX: PRO-ED.

International Dyslexia Association, The. (2010). *Knowledge and practice standards for teachers of reading.* Baltimore, MD: Author.

Jespersen, O. (1971). *Growth and structure of the English language.* New York, NY: The Free Press.

Liberman, I.Y. (1973). Segmentation of the spoken word and reading acquisition. *Bulletin of the Orton Society, 23,* 65–77.

Liberman, I.Y., & Liberman, A.M. (1990). Whole language vs. code emphasis: Underlying assumptions and their implications for reading instruction. *Annals of Dyslexia, 40*(1), 51–78.

Liberman, I.Y., & Shankweiler, D. (1985). Phonology and the problems of learning to read and write. *Remedial and Special Education, 7,* 8–17.

Liberman, I.Y., & Shankweiler, D. (1991). Phonology and beginning reading: A tutorial. In L. Rieben & C.A. Perfetti (Eds.), *Learning to read: Basic research and its implications* (pp. 3–17). Mahwah, NJ: Lawrence Erlbaum Associates.

Liberman, I.Y., Shankweiler, D., Fischer, F.W., & Carter, B. (1974). Explicit syllable and phoneme segmentation in the young child. *Journal of Experimental Child Psychology, 18*(2), 201–212.

Moats, L.C. (1995). *Spelling: Development, disability, and instruction.* Timonium, MD: York Press.

Moats, L.C. (2010). *Speech to print: Language essentials for teachers* (2nd ed.). Baltimore, MD: Paul H. Brookes Publishing Co.

Nist, J. (1966). *A structural history of English.* New York, NY: St. Martin's Press.

Perfetti, C. (1984). Reading acquisition and beyond: Decoding includes cognition. *American Journal of Education, 93*(1), 40–60.

Pinker, S. (1994). *The language instinct: How the mind creates language.* New York, NY: William Morrow.

Rameau, M. (2000). *Real spelling.* http://www.Realspelling.fr

Richardson, S.O. (1989). Specific developmental dyslexia: Retrospective and prospective views. *Annals of Dyslexia, 39,* 3–23.

Seidenberg, M. (2017). *Language at the speed of sight.* New York, NY: Basic Books.

Stanback, M.L. (1992). Syllable and rime patterns for teaching reading: Analysis of a frequency based vocabulary of 17,602 words. *Annals of Dyslexia, 42,* 196–221.

Steere, A., Peck, C.Z., & Kahn, L. (1971). *Solving language difficulties.* Cambridge, MA: Educators Publishing Service.

Venezky, R.L. (1970). *The structure of English orthography.* The Hague, The Netherlands: Mouton.

Wade-Wooley, L., & Heggie, L. (2015). Implicit knowledge of word stress and derivational morphology guides skilled readers' decoding of multisyllabic words. *Scientific Studies of Reading, 19*(1), 21–30.

Webster's new universal unabridged dictionary (2nd ed.). (1983). New York, NY: Simon & Schuster.

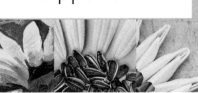

Appendix 14.1

Technology Resources

Elaine A. Cheesman

PROGRAMS/APPS

Effective programs/apps have the following features:

• They provide information on word origins (etymology).

Lexia Core5   http://www.lexialearning.com

This program provides engaging, systematic, sequential practice in Latin roots and Greek combining forms. It includes vocabulary and comprehension activities as well. It tracks multiple users' progress and is appropriate for kindergarten through adult.

Voyage of Ulysses   http://elasticoapp.com

This app provides highlighted prose narration of stories from Ulysses's voyage, such as The Cyclops and the Trojan Horse. It provides background about word origins. It shows each tale's location on a map; animation deepens text comprehension.

Word Hippo   http://www.wordhippo.com

This web site provides the meaning of a word and also synonyms, antonyms, words that rhyme with it, sentences containing it, the derivatives, and etymology. It includes U.K. and U.S. spellings.

WEB SITES: MATERIALS AND ACTIVITIES FOR TEACHERS AND LEARNERS

Dictionary.com   http://www.dictionary.com

This site provides user-friendly definitions, synonyms, antonyms, sample sentences, and illustrated language of origin.

List of English Suffixes   https://www.learnthat.org/pages/view/suffix.html

This is a list of Greek and Latin morphemes, meanings, and sample words and definitions.

Online Etymology Dictionary   http://etymonline.com/

This web site is a comprehensive collection of the history of thousands of English words, including slang. Each entry contains the dates of the earliest year for which there is a written record of that word and the word histories. The site also contains an extensive glossary of abbreviations for language terms.

Root Words and Prefixes: Quick Reference https://www.learnthat.org/pages/view/roots.html

This is a list of Greek and Latin morphemes, meanings, and sample words and definitions.

Vocabulary.com http://www.vocabulary.com

This web site is designed for older students and adults. It offers semantically connected words and examples from sources written for adults (e.g., *The New Yorker*).

Wordnik http://www.wordnik.com

This site allows the user to enter any word or phrase to reveal definitions, etymologies, and examples in sentences from various sources. It is more appropriate for adults and older students.

Your Dictionary http://www.yourdictionary.com

This site includes simple definitions with examples, synonyms, quotes, word origins, and related forms.

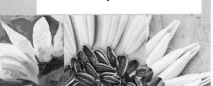

Chapter 15

Working With Word Meaning

Vocabulary Instruction

Nancy E. Hennessy

> We are verbivores, a species that lives on words, and the meaning and use of language are bound to be among the major things we ponder, share and dispute.
>
> —Pinker (2007, p. 24)

LEARNING OBJECTIVES

1. To understand the contributions of vocabulary to reading proficiency
2. To understand the nature of vocabulary acquisition
3. To acquire a knowledge of a comprehensive approach to vocabulary instruction
4. To acquire a knowledge of evidence-informed strategies and activities aligned with a comprehensive approach

---

Words are uniquely human. Individuals are literally surrounded by them from birth onward, and their understanding of word meaning allows them to communicate thought. But what do you know about the word *vocabulary* and its influence on who you are, not only individually but also as an educator?

Dictionary.com defines *vocabulary* as "the words of a language." Others view it as one's knowledge of words and word meanings or an individual's lexicon or mental dictionary of words that can be used receptively (i.e., listening, reading) and expressively (i.e., speaking and writing). Kamil and Hiebert described vocabulary as the "kind of words that students must know to read increasingly demanding text with comprehension" (2005, p. 4). Perfetti and Stafura identified one's lexicon as "a central connection point between the word identification system and the comprehension system" (2013, p. 24). We also could define it as a critical focus for reading instruction.

Despite a long-standing consensus on the pivotal role of vocabulary and its well-supported contributions to literacy development and academic performance, recognition of the importance of vocabulary instruction has taken time. The National Reading Panel (NRP; National Institute of Child Health and Human Development [NICHD, 2000]) identified vocabulary as an essential component of reading instruction and acknowledged its critical role in reading achievement. The Common Core State Standards (CCSS; National Governor's Association, Center for Best Practices, & Council of Chief State School Officers, 2010), in the areas of

English Language Arts (ELA) and Language, reference its importance for multiple purposes (speaking, reading, writing), specifying related standards at each grade level. Prompted by these and state standards, coupled with an increased focus on core curriculum resources, there is a growing awareness of the need to consider multiple aspects of word meaning and effective vocabulary instruction.

Understanding all dimensions of word meaning and their relationship to instruction requires a deep knowledge base for translation to practice. Knowing the research and possessing disciplinary knowledge related to this topic are necessary for making informed decisions. What then, should a teacher of reading know about vocabulary? The International Dyslexia Association's (2018) *Knowledge and Practice Standards for Teachers of Reading* provided guidance for both the preparation and continuing professional development of educators. The contents of this chapter align with these standards and are intended to ultimately provide the knowledge necessary to support the design and delivery of effective instruction for all students.

Take a moment now to consider what you know about vocabulary or need to learn more about prior to reading this chapter (see Figure 15.1). Questions at the end of each section prompt reflection on learning and connection to your practices.

VOCABULARY AND READING PROFICIENCY: A REVIEW OF THEORETICAL MODELS

Proficient reading demands the development, coordination, and interaction of multiple skills that develop over time. Reading is too complex to be explained by one theory, but a brief review of related models can inform your understanding of the complexity of reading and provide insight into contributing skills, such as vocabulary, as well as interrelationships critical to the reading process.

Question Do you know and/or understand	Yes	No	Maybe
1. The role of vocabulary (semantics) in developing proficient reading?			
2. The relationship of vocabulary to word recognition and comprehension and other major contributors to reading and writing?			
3. The sources of wide differences in student vocabularies?			
4. The role of vocabulary in comprehension?			
5. The nature of vocabulary acquisition?			
6. The multidimensional nature of word meaning, including associations, antonyms, synonyms, multiple meanings, parts of speech, semantic overlap, and semantic features?			
7. The role and characteristics of direct and indirect instruction?			
8. Effective strategies and activities for before, during and after reading?			
9. The critical components of lesson planning, including goals, word choice, instructional routines and activities, as well as materials necessary for effective instruction?			

Figure 15.1. Self-assessment. (*Source:* The International Dyslexia Association's [2010] *Knowledge and Practice Standards for Teachers of Reading.*)

The **Simple View of Reading** (Gough & Tunmer, 1986), a model that is well represented in the literature, has served as the basis of a number of studies. It defines reading comprehension as the product of decoding or word recognition and linguistic or listening comprehension (R = D x C). The Simple View holds that there can be no reading comprehension when either factor equals zero. But is the Simple View of Reading all that simple? What are the components of the language or listening comprehension factor, and what role does vocabulary play?

A brief discussion of the **Four-Part Processing Model for Word Recognition** (Rayner, Foorman, Perfetti, Pesetsky, & Seidenberg, 2001; Seidenberg & McClelland, 1989) and Scarborough's (2001) Reading Rope Model serves to clarify and elaborate on the components of the Simple View of Reading, including the contribution of vocabulary.

Four-Part Processing Model for Word Recognition

This model provides a framework for understanding the neural systems involved in reading words and insight into the underlying processes. Four unique, complex, yet interrelated systems contribute to word recognition: the **phonological, orthographic, meaning,** and **context processors.** These provide an explanation of how the reader maps sound onto print and the role of word meaning. Delving into the function of, and interactions between, each processing system provides clarity about the contributions to word recognition when and if each does its job well. Consider an example of how each contributes to reading the word *catch:*

- Phonological processor: identification of sounds (phonemes) (e.g., /k/ - /ă/ - /ch/)

- Orthographic processor: recognition of letter and letter patterns (graphemes) (e.g., *c, a, tch*)

- Meaning processor: access to semantic network and varied meanings (e.g., If you *catch* an item moving through the air, then you seize it with your hands; if you *catch* an animal or person, you capture them)

- Context processor: use of language experiences and context to confirm word recognition and meaning (e.g., We will *catch* the 6:00 a.m. train into the city)

Although each processor is primarily responsible for its own task, they simultaneously coordinate and support each other; hence, they are interdependent. Each also has to perform accurately as well as automatically. Although this model is a rather simplistic explanation for a complex task, it provides a basic understanding of how different processing systems, including meaning, contribute to and work together for automatic word recognition. The model also provides insight into potential sources of student difficulty and classroom practices.

Reading Rope Model of Reading Development

Scarborough's (2001) Rope, shown in Figure 15.2, provides an analogy for understanding how skilled reading—the fluent execution and coordination of word recognition and text comprehension—develops.

The skills represented in the word recognition strands of the rope represent the primary focus of instruction in the early grades and the major contributor, at that point, to reading comprehension. Language comprehension abilities

LANGUAGE COMPREHENSION

BACKGROUND KNOWLEDGE
(facts, concepts, etc.)

VOCABULARY
(breadth, precision, links, etc.)

LANGUAGE STRUCTURES
(syntax, semantics, etc.)

VERBAL REASONING
(inference, metaphor, etc.)

LITERACY KNOWLEDGE
(print concepts, genres, etc.)

WORD RECOGNITION

PHONOLOGICAL AWARENESS
(syllables, phonemes, etc.)

DECODING (alphabetic principle,
spelling-sound correspondences)

SIGHT RECOGNITION
(of familiar words)

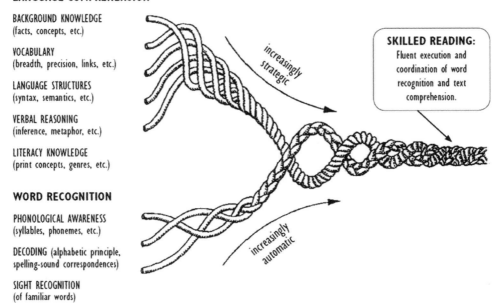

SKILLED READING:
Fluent execution and
coordination of word
recognition and text
comprehension.

increasingly strategic

increasingly automatic

Figure 15.2. The reading rope. (From Scarborough, H. [2003]. Connecting early language and literacy to later reading [dis]abilities: Evidence, theory and practice. In S.B. Neuman & D.K. Dickinson [Eds.], *Handbook of early literacy research* (pp. 97–110). New York, NY: Guilford Press; reprinted by permission.)

become more influential as students gain competency in word-reading skills and are capable of reading texts independently. Vellutino, Tunmer, Jaccard, and Chen concluded that "language comprehension becomes the dominant processing in reading comprehension when the reader has acquired enough facility in word identification to comprehend in written language text what would be normally comprehended in spoken language" (2007, p. 26). Catts, Hogan, Adolf, and Barth (2013) also showed that the combination of word recognition and listening comprehension account for significant variability in reading comprehension, but the unique contributions change over time, with listening comprehension becoming increasingly more important.

The strands that represent language comprehension include a focus on vocabulary. This model is particularly informative regarding the specific or independent role of word meaning in proficient reading while also reminding that all of the processes and skills represented work together and develop over time. For example, consider the connections between word meaning, background knowledge, and language structures (syntax). Words do not exist in isolation but rather as part of a connected network of meaning reflecting **schema.** Word meanings do not live apart from their syntactic function; it is a dimension of their meaning. The rope model prompts thinking about vocabulary and how it works in concert with other skills to construct meaning. These models not only provide insight into the development of skilled reading but also call attention to individual component processes and skills, such as vocabulary, along with their respective roles and contributions to word recognition and reading comprehension.

Vocabulary serves as the bridge between word level processes of phonics and the cognitive processes of comprehension.

—Kamil and Hiebert (2005, p. 4)

THE VOCABULARY CONNECTION: WORD RECOGNITION AND COMPREHENSION

The Word Recognition Connection

Although the relationship between vocabulary and comprehension is self-evident, the role of vocabulary in developing phonological awareness and word recognition may not be as apparent. Phonological awareness is, in part, a product of vocabulary development, with both being precursors to reading proficiency (NICHD Early Child Care Research Network [ECCRN], 2005). It is theorized that words are stored holistically in the young child's lexicon and gradually become more segmented during the preschool and early school years. As a child's vocabulary grows, he or she becomes more aware of phonological similarities and discovers that it is more efficient to remember and recognize words in terms of their constituent parts rather than as whole entities (Lonigan, 2007). This change in representations of words to representations of segmental units is described in the lexical restructuring model (Walley, Metsala, & Garlock, 2003). Phonological restructuring of words depends on vocabulary growth and is thought necessary for developing explicit phoneme awareness. A review of early literacy studies indicates concurrent and longitudinal correlations between phonological awareness and oral language skills in preschool and beyond (Lonigan, 2007), and a more recent study also confirms strong correlations between receptive and expressive language and phoneme awareness (Cassano & Schickedanz, 2015).

The Comprehension Connection

Although vocabulary facilitates phonological awareness and word recognition in students, its power lies in its relationship to reading comprehension. Scarborough indicated that "reading comprehension deficits are essentially oral language limitations" (2001, p. 98). Vocabulary has predictive value for later reading comprehension. The strength of its contribution to skilled reading has been documented over time, and the relationship between early word knowledge and elementary, middle, and secondary grade-level performance has been well established. Both causal and correlational links between vocabulary and comprehension reflect the importance and complexity of their relationship. In addition, there is evidence for a reciprocal relationship between vocabulary and comprehension, with reading comprehension influencing the growth of vocabulary knowledge during the school years (Nagy, 2005; Stanovich, 1986). Vocabulary is not an isolated component of reading instruction but rather a complex capability that influences both word recognition and comprehension. Insight into the role of vocabulary in reading proficiency should inform practice.

VOCABULARY ACQUISITION: INFANCY TO PRESCHOOL AGE

Language is an essential characteristic of being human. Acquisition is complex and complicated, beginning in infancy and continuing across a lifetime. Infants come into the world capable of perceiving and producing sounds. Infants initially use gestures (e.g., waving or lifting up their arms) to communicate. The speech stream of those around them (e.g., parents, caregivers, siblings) is perceived holistically rather than consisting of meaningful units (e.g., sounds, syllables, words). As children grow physically, however, so does their ability to analyze and discern phonemes, syllables, and words. Infants eventually parse out the sounds of their native language and combine them to repeat and produce words. Words must have some relevance to prompt acquisition (i.e., an understanding that words reference objects, events, and actions). Thus, infants' first words usually relate to things in their environment or to actions related to their needs (e.g., *ba-ba/bottle*). Young children typically learn words receptively (through listening) before using them expressively (speaking). Their understanding of words is greater than their ability to produce them, as evidenced by how they use general terms to identify different objects with similar features (e.g., all animals with four legs are "doggies").

Between 18 and 24 months, children acquire words at an amazing rate. McLaughlin (1998) estimated the average number of expressive vocabulary words acquired by age 24 months to be 200–300. This "spurt," or "vocabulary burst," period is marked by the ability to make inferences about relationships between words and referents, even after as little as one exposure. This phenomenon is described as **"fast mapping"** (Carey & Bartlett, 1978) and is sufficient to promote partial knowledge of word meaning. Building a deeper representation of a word, slow mapping, requires multiple exposures in different contexts. As children's labels for objects, people, and actions grow, so does their syntactical awareness. In other words, they no longer just imitate or memorize language; they also analyze, extract, and even experiment with rules of speech that govern stringing words together for asking and telling. Chomsky (1965) suggested that children are equipped with an innate "universal grammar."

Early Informed Oral Language Environments

Rich and responsive language experiences from infancy to preschool age directly influence oral language acquisition that, in turn, is highly predictive of later reading abilities. Children learn language by participating in the linguistic environment around them, with gaps in oral language emerging very early. The critical role of parents, caregivers, and preschool educators in creating and nurturing informed

> Without fluent and structured oral language, children will find it very difficult to think.
>
> —Bruner (1983, p. 24)

oral language environments is undisputable. Both the home environment and preschool setting can be incredibly influential on children's achievement (NICHD, ECRN, 2005). Adults in these environments have countless informal and formal opportunities to teach vocabulary intentionally and incidentally but are often unaware of when and how they can create these productive experiences for children. Combined findings from multiple studies show that young children benefit from both implicit and explicit approaches to language development (Neuman & Wright, 2013). Consider these two general approaches to vocabulary acquisition: productive and purposeful oral language interactions, and purposeful and productive book reading.

Productive and Purposeful Oral Language Interactions

Adult talk that is responsive to beginning and later language attempts influences a young child's language development. Productive parent–child and preschool provider–child interactions depend on the nature of language input (e.g., word expansion) and the use of different contexts (e.g., book reading), as well as the content of speech (Landry & Smith, 2007). Most parents, educators, or caregivers would assert that they regularly talk with the children in their care. Although the number of words children hear is important, the differences in quality and the nature of conversation most affect language development. Teacher–child language interactions that include cognitively challenging conversations have been identified as a critical mark of quality instruction. The importance of planning for both informal and formal instruction cannot be overlooked in preschool settings. It takes a vocabulary-attuned adult to purposefully incorporate activities that focus on developing word meaning.

Studies (Rowe, 2012; Weizman & Snow, 2001) also suggest that parents can support their children's vocabulary acquisition at different points in development by exposure to varied types of talk, including the use of more sophisticated vocabulary and decontextualized language such as explanation or story telling (narrative). Moats and Paulson (2009) recommended that parents and caregivers purposefully use language-stimulation techniques that include taking the time to describe what the child is doing, talking about what the adult is doing, and/or expanding on a child's expressive language. Preschool providers can also support parents by sharing suggestions and resources such as those found in *Talking on the Go* (Dougherty & Paul, 2007). This book is chock-full of activities, based on everyday experiences and normal routines, that can serve as a basis for conversation. The authors provide multiple ways parents can engage children, beginning at birth through preschool, in productive oral language experiences. Consider the possibilities while strolling through the aisles of the supermarket with a 3- to 4-year-old:

- Identify and discuss the attributes of hard, soft, rough, and smooth by having the child feel a hard carrot, soft bread, smooth apples, and/or a rough pineapple.

- Name cleaning items in the store, and talk about how they are used (e.g., broom, cleansers, soaps, brush, cloth, dish soap).

- Ask questions about cleaning items that are placed in the cart, such as "What do we use to sweep the floor?" and "What do we wash clothes with?"

Similar informal opportunities abound throughout the day or during planned activities at home or in the preschool environment. A walk outside can generate conversation about multiple topics, such as identifying items that can be collected (e.g., leaves) and compared by describing shapes, textures, colors, and sizes (focus on attributes)—or a ride in the car can be the basis for discussing all that one sees. Have you ever played "I Spy" while taking a trip, making use of color, size, and category as clues?

Preschoolers need food, shelter, love; they also need the nourishment of books.

—Whitehurst (2013, p. 8)

Purposeful and Productive Book Reading

Purposeful and productive book reading provides unique opportunities for children to acquire both oral language and early print concepts. Multiple studies affirm the contribution of early book reading to language and literacy development.

Often, the vocabulary found in children's books is far richer than that of every-day conversation. Book reading can also serve as a powerful knowledge-building activity, particularly when books chosen reflect varied topics and content area. The availability of books for preschoolers, both in the home and at school, is also a criti-cal contributor to future academic success (Neuman & Dickinson, 2001).

A consistent finding regarding shared book reading is the importance of including interactive reading activities. The structure and nature of the verbal interactions directly influences language development and ultimately literacy skills. Trivette and Dunst (2007) conducted a secondary analysis of *The What Works Clearinghouse* original research syntheses (updated 2015) on the effectiveness of three different reading interventions often used in preschool settings: shared book reading, shared interactive book reading, and **dialogic reading.** These approaches all involve an adult reading a book to an individual or a small group of children. However, the level of interaction is more extensive with interactive or dialogic reading. Their findings indicate that the more involved and engaged children are during reading, the more positive the results. Marulis and Neumann (2010) also conducted two meta-analytic reviews of varied preschool vocabulary interven-tions and programs. In most of the studies reviewed, word meanings were intro-duced within the context of authentic texts and discussed before, during, and after story book reading. While effect sizes varied for different subject groups, including at-risk students, the authors reported overall "impressive gains," particularly when instruction was explicit and intentional. They also identified that the most effective interventions included child-friendly definitions as well as multiple opportunities for student response and interaction. In addition, in a related meta-analysis, Neu-man and Wright (2013) reported that student gains were most obvious when the interventions were delivered by individuals with the most knowledge of how lan-guage is acquired.

The foundation for literacy development begins early and is rooted in oral language development. Informed language environments provide multiple oppor-tunities for vocabulary acquisition. Purposeful oral language interactions and pro-ductive **shared reading** provided by preschool providers, parents, and caregivers play critical roles.

REFLECT, CONNECT, and RESPOND
What is the potential role of the parent, caregiver, or preschool provider in early vocabulary acquisition? Why is this information relevant to you?

VOCABULARY ACQUISITION: SCHOOL AGE TO ADULTHOOD

Young children, who are naturally inquisitive about words, appear spongelike in their receptivity to learning new words; however, vocabulary learning extends over a lifetime. Children's innate curiosity about words and their need to com-municate continue to fuel their desire to acquire and deepen word knowledge. However, as students move through school, increasing academic demands often become a strong motivating factor. Some researchers report that kindergarteners come to school recognizing 4,000–5,000 base words, and the average high school graduate has a lexicon of 40,000–50,000 words (Biemiller, 2012). Most agree that students learn approximately 3,000 words per year, or about 7 words per day (Beck, McKeown, & Kucan, 2002). Acquisition of word meaning is a complex and com-plicated process that is incremental, interrelated, and multidimensional in nature

(Nagy & Scott, 2000). Other avenues of acquisition, in addition to oral language environments, become necessary contributors. Informed practitioners also recognize that effective instruction requires more than writing a lesson plan or even choosing a program. An understanding of the following topics is necessary to inform the design and delivery of effective instruction:

- Levels of understanding of word meaning

- Dimensions of word learning

- Goals of instruction

- Instructional framework

- Comprehensive instructional approaches

Levels of Understanding of Word Meaning

A student's ability to use words receptively (listening, reading) and expressively (talking, writing) is dependent on his or her levels of understanding. So, what are these levels, and how do they differ?

- *Breadth of vocabulary* usually refers to the size of an individual's mental lexicon. It denotes how many words a learner recognizes or knows at a certain level (Nation, 2001). Breadth does not specifically address how well each of these words is known.

- *Depth* refers to the richness of word knowledge that the individual possesses about known words; thus, it is the measure of how well an individual knows a word. Depth is not an all-or-none concept. As depth of word knowledge increases, words can be used more flexibly, and their meaning can be readily appreciated and accessed within multiple contexts (Anderson & Freebody, 1981; Beck, McKeown, & Kucan, 2002; Stahl, 1998).

- *Fluency* refers to the rate at which the individual accesses the meaning of a word. As word meanings deepen as a result of experience, the time it takes to gain access to specific meaning decreases, thus influencing reading proficiency (Wolf, Miller, & Donnelly, 2000).

A student's breadth, depth, and access to word meaning facilitate participation, development of ideas and concepts, comprehension of text, and expression of thoughts in different ways. For example, in a study of third graders, Tannenbaum, Torgesen, and Wagner (2006) indicated the importance of breadth for performance on reading outcome assessments as well as the relationship between depth and performance on classroom-based academic tasks. Other studies (Li & Kirby, 2014) confirmed the different contributions of each, such as comprehension measures (breadth) and writing tasks (depth). As the student moves from a basic understanding of the word to fully understanding all of its dimensions, the influence of this understanding on academic literacy tasks becomes more significant. Calfee and Drum described this deep understanding as involving and facilitating "precision of meaning; facile access; the ability to articulate one's understanding; flexibility in application of knowledge of a word; the appreciation of word play; the ability to recognize; to define; to use expressively" (1986, pp. 825–826). Knowing the differences between these levels and their connections to academic demands can and should directly influence the practitioner's thinking about instructional focus and approaches.

Dimensions of Word Learning

We have addressed levels of understanding: so, how does that relate to varied dimensions of word knowledge? Acquisition of word meanings is incremental and involves interrelated skills. This understanding changes over time depending on multiple factors, including instruction and experience. Think about a child's understanding of a simple word such as *dog* and how that might change or grow incrementally as the child encounters or interacts with different dogs and as he or she notices different characteristics (e.g., size, looks), behaviors (e.g., docile, aggressive), and even varied roles of dogs (e.g., service, rescue). Based on experiences and perhaps instruction, the student's understanding of the word *dog* may

> Words are not isolated units of language but fit into many interlocking systems and levels. Because of this, there are many particular things to know about words and many degrees of knowing.
> —Nation (2001, p. 33)

consist of interrelated information that is phonological, orthographic, semantic, syntactic, and pragmatic in nature. This network or word schema for *dog* may eventually include literal and figurative meanings (e.g., *dog* days of summer), use as a noun or verb (e.g., *dogged* by worries), synonyms (e.g., *mutt*), and subcategories such as dog heroes (e.g., *Bolt*). Thus, Nation (2001) suggested that facets of word knowledge can include the components shown in Figure 15.3.

When these representations of word meaning are rich and have many associated concepts, the precise meaning is more readily available and allows for more rapid access to word meaning (Perfetti, 2007). Understanding that knowledge of word meaning is complex should influence the practitioner's thinking about goals and instructional practices that develop targeted levels of understanding.

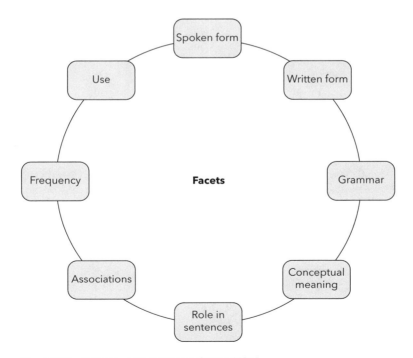

Figure 15.3. Critical questions. (*Source:* Graves, 2006.)

Goals of Instruction

Although some might argue that the primary goal of vocabulary instruction should be its influence on comprehension, a broader perspective includes the development of and access to an academic lexicon that allows students to not only listen and read with comprehension but also to express understanding and thinking orally and in writing.

Instructional goals are usually reflective of varied levels of understanding demanded by particular academic tasks and are often related to expectations set by individual state standards or CCSS. The CCSS's focus on the increased use of informational text and the student's ability to work with the academic language and respond and express understanding in varied formats has highlighted the need to attend to vocabulary instruction. For example, a review of the College and Career Readiness Standards for Reading and Language, as well as grade specific expectations, provided guidance for goal setting:

Anchor Standards for Reading

Craft and Structure

- Interpret words and phrases as they are used in a text, including determining technical, connotative, and figurative meanings, and analyze how specific word choices shape meaning or tone (Common Core State Standards Initiative, 2018, p. 10).

Standards for Language

Vocabulary Acquisition and Use

- Determine or clarify the meaning of unknown and multiple-meaning words and phrases by using context clues, analyzing meaningful word parts, and consulting general and specialized reference materials, as appropriate.
- Demonstrate understanding of figurative language, word relationships, and nuances in word meanings.
- Acquire and use accurately a range of general academic and domain-specific words and phrases sufficient for reading, writing, speaking, and listening at the college and career readiness level; demonstrate independence in gathering vocabulary knowledge when encountering an unknown term important to comprehension or expression. (Common Core State Standards Initiative, 2018, p. 25)

Additional considerations include school/district curriculum goals as well as the individual student's level of performance. The individualized education program (IEP), designed for students found eligible for special education, calls for the identification of goals related to specific needs that have surfaced through team analysis of multiple sources of data. These, in concert with teacher knowledge of classroom demand, provide direction for educators as they set learning objectives for their students.

Instructional Framework

Given the sheer number of words in the English language, the critical role word knowledge plays in reading proficiency, and the multidimensional nature of word learning, it is not surprising that effective instruction requires a multi-faceted approach. In fact, a review of the literature revealed varied pathways to vocabulary acquisition for the school-age student. At first glance, there appear to be many differences, but a closer look yields support for a four-part instructional framework. Graves provided the following guidelines, which also reflects the literature on this topic (2006, pp. 4–8):

- Provide rich and varied language experiences

- Teach individual words

- Teach word-learning strategies

- Foster word consciousness

Other recommendations, found in the National Reading Panel Report's (NICHD, 2000) meta-analysis of effective practices, include direct teaching of vocabulary and acquisition through incidental learning, along with the use of computer technology. Ebbers and Denton (2008) also provided guidance specific to students with language-based learning disabilities:

- Use explicit instruction.

- Apply cognitive and metacognitive strategies.

- Incorporate questioning approaches.

- Use collaborative engagement involving verbal interactions.

- Provide many opportunities for practice with teacher feedback.

Informed instruction requires an understanding of multiple aspects of vocabulary acquisition, including the nature of word learning, degrees and dimensions of meaning, and goals for instruction. Each of these plays a critical role as educators consider implementing a four-pronged instructional framework that develops the lexicon necessary for students to meet the academic demands of the educational setting.

REFLECT, CONNECT, and RESPOND
Why is it important to know the difference between breadth, depth, and access to word meaning? How might an understanding of the facets or dimensions of word knowledge influence instruction? Which of these aspects of word learning are most relevant to you?

Comprehensive Instructional Approaches

A comprehensive approach to the design and delivery of instruction includes a recognition of these varied aspects of word learning as well as inclusion of evidence-based practices. The following discussion of an instructional framework and aspects of each approach provides direction for practical application (see Figure 15.4).

Intentional on purpose instruction	Incidental on purpose instruction	Independent word learning strategies

Word choice
Principles of vocabulary
   instruction
Instructional routines
Processing and practice activities
	Rich oral language classroom
	   environments
	Structured shared reading
	Structured independent reading
		Dictionary
		Context clues
		Morphemic analysis

	Word consciousness	

Figure 15.4. Instructional framework.

Intentional on Purpose Instruction   A meaningful approach to vocabulary instruction requires the direct teaching of individual words. This involves teaching word meaning intentionally and intensively, knowing that students need both depth of and access to meaning. The design and delivery of such instruction requires careful consideration of word choice, principles of vocabulary instruction, and instructional routines as well as activities that provide adequate practice and processing necessary to develop deeper understanding of word meaning.

Word Choice   Educators are faced with critical choices as they consider the number of words in the English language and the dilemma posed by the richness of vocabulary used in academic texts and settings. Dictionaries have close to 300,000 words, with new words added yearly. A review of 5 million words sampled from third- through ninth-grade school texts resulted in an estimate of 88,500 word families in printed school English (Nagy & Anderson, 1984). Why so many? The English language is "promiscuous!" Although English is primarily based in the Anglo-Saxon, Romance, and Greek layers of language, it also borrows from other languages as it grows. A review of grade-level narrative and informational texts also confirms how many academic and technical words are critical to meaning. There are just too many words to teach directly and intentionally. In fact, the majority of word meanings are learned incidentally. So, how many words can a teacher target for explicit instruction and for what purpose? Most in the field agree that optimally 10–15 words per week can be taught directly and in depth (Beck et al., 2002; Biemiller, 2012). This equates to approximately 300–400 words per year, which is a fraction of the thousands of words acquired each year. How then, do educators decide which words to target? An understanding of the types of words typically encountered in text—academic, domain-specific, and high-frequency words—can inform decision making. See Table 15.1 for an explanation of these three categories.

The nature of words themselves, some more common than others, some more reflective of academic texts, others domain specific, and some crossing content boundaries, influences criteria for word choice. A review of the literature reveals commonality as well as some differences regarding word choice. The most common words, those used in everyday interactions, are usually not the target for

Table 15.1.   Types of words encountered in text

Academic	Domain specific	High frequency
Essential to understanding and communicating ideas within and across disciplines Usually morphologically and semantically complex Abstract and often have more than one definition Usually derived from the Latin layer of the English language (consisting of prefixes, roots, suffixes)	Common to a specific subject area or discipline More technical in nature Relate directly to the topic May have just one meaning Usually derived from the Latin and Greek layers of the English language (consisting of prefixes, roots, suffixes and compounding forms)	Do most of the work in text Encountered over and over Words of everyday conversations Necessary foundation for working with academic and technical vocabulary Usually derived from the Anglo-Saxon layer of the English language
Examples *approach* *concept* *distribution* *interpretation* *process*	Examples *alkaloid* *equilateral* *molecule* *symbiosis* *tangent*	Examples *family* *enough* *old* *someone* *think*

direct instruction, given that they are typically acquired independently. Rather, those words that students are less likely to learn on their own and that are necessary for participation in academic tasks drive word choice for teaching younger and older students. Most researchers agree that students must learn academic vocabulary words that are multifunctional (cutting across domains) and that are critical to understanding text. Stahl (2004) described academic vocabulary as synonymous with the vocabulary of school. Given the focus on informational text, there is also increased attention on technical or discipline-specific vocabulary.

Although educators traditionally rely on their teacher editions or curriculum guides as a source for word choice, they also need an informed eye as they select texts for multiple purposes and strategically identify words for targeted instruction. A discussion of some well-known approaches, such as Beck and colleagues' (2002) teacher-friendly criteria, provides additional guidance. Beck and her colleagues suggested that educators choose words based on these criteria:

- *Importance and utility*: Words that are characteristic of mature language users and appear frequently across a variety of domains.

- *Instructional potential*: Words that can be worked in a variety of ways so that students can build deep knowledge of them and of their connections to other words and concepts.

- *Conceptual understanding*: Words for which students understand the general concept but that will help students provide precision and specificity in describing the concept.

They also classify words by three tiers, suggesting the primary focus be on Tier 2:

- *Tier 1 words* are common, basic words that are used in everyday conversations and that most children know; they are not usually the target of instruction (e.g., *family, someone, think*).

- *Tier 2 words* are more sophisticated and are often used by mature language users in speech and writing; they are found across a variety of texts and domains; they are often the target of instruction. (e.g., *approach, concept, process*).

- *Tier 3 words* have more narrow and specific roles in language; these words are not necessarily familiar to mature language users. They are more specific to a domain or content; they are technical and more likely to be taught through explanation in context; they may not be the focus of intentional instruction (e.g., *equilateral, molecule, homeostasis*).

The lines between the tiers are not crystal clear, and teacher judgment will always be a critical variable. Knowing what their students know, their individual needs as well as the academic demand, is key to selecting words for instruction. For example, informed practitioners recognize that Tier 1 words may be the starting point for some students and instruction of Tier 2 words for English language learners should include relationships to cognates. Beck and colleagues (2002) have not developed lists for each tier because they do not want teachers to believe there is "one set of must-know words," although they do acknowledge that some of the more well-known word lists do reflect the properties of their tiers (McKeown, Beck, & Sandora, 2012).

Biemiller's sequential approach, described in *Words Worth Teaching* (2010), provides another alternative for word choice. Although he acknowledged the importance of recognizing those words that most students know, Biemiller focused on word meanings that those students with larger vocabularies know and used this as a basis for identifying words for instruction. The result was a list of high-priority "root" words (11,000) for Grades K–6. He also provided an instructional framework identifying targets for pre-kindergarten (concrete and relational), primary (concrete, relational, symbolic), and upper-middle grades (academic, relational, symbolic). Coxhead (2000) also constructed a list of 570 useful root words and derivatives based on words that appear frequently in a wide range of academic texts. These are most relevant for students in middle school and beyond.

Finally, Graves (2006) proposed posing four critical questions to facilitate choice of words (see Figure 15.5). Practitioners might consider these guiding questions as they preview and prepare text(s), an essential first step for instruction. If one's responses are "yes," then the word is a potential candidate for intentional instruction of individual word meaning or for application of independent word learning strategies (e.g., use of context, morphology).

Although we are focused on word choice for intentional teaching, educators also need to consider those words that they will "incidentally on purpose teach" as well as those that provide opportunity for the teaching and application of "independent word learning strategies." Identification of words for these different purposes can be accomplished at the same time, using relevant guiding questions such as those suggested next.

- *Incidental on purpose instruction:* Are there words that led themselves to "point of contact teaching"? Can I briefly provide a substitution, synonym, or brief explanation within the text?

- *Independent word learning strategies:* Are there words that can be used to teach, then practice independent word learning strategies (use of context or morphemes)?

Consider the example shown in Table 15.2 for students in second through third grade, who are learning about civil rights and segregation and reading narratives such as *The Story of Ruby Bridges* by Robert Coles and expository text from online sources such as Newslea (http://www.newslea.com) (e.g., Civil Rights Activists: Ruby Bridges).

Within a school setting, collaborating on, developing, and implementing a common approach, including agreed-on criteria within and across grade levels

Question	Yes	No
Is understanding the word important to understanding the selection in which it appears?		
Are students able to use context, structural word analysis, or dictionary skills to discover the word's meanings?		
Can working with this word be useful in furthering the student's context, structural analysis, or dictionary skills?		
How useful is this word outside of the reading selection currently being read?		

Figure 15.5. Facets of word knowledge. (*Source:* Nation, 2001.)

Table 15.2. Words for instruction

Intentional–words	Incidental–point of contact	Independent word learning strategies
civil rights	*cabin*	Context:
event	*crop*	*angry*
segregation	*marshals*	*confident*
courageous	*janitor*	Morphology:
anxious	*credit*	*desegregation*
		inequality

for identifying vocabulary, is very effective. Having chosen words for instruction, educators need to focus on the nature of instruction for each of the approaches (intentional, incidental, and word learning strategies).

Principles of Vocabulary Instruction   Intentional instruction is synonymous with explicit teaching. It is structured, systematic, and characterized by clear explanations and/or demonstrations of targeted skills or concepts, and it includes opportunities for practice with feedback and independent application (Archer & Hughes, 2011). There is strong evidence supporting the direct teaching of the meanings of targeted words and the use of related instructional principles (NICHD, 2000). According to Coyne and colleagues (2007), direct instruction is more effective when it reflects validated principles of curricular design, such as conspicuous teaching, which calls for clear, consistent, carefully designed teacher actions regarding explanations, modeling, and opportunities for practice and review.

> Decades of research clearly demonstrate that for novices (comprising virtually all students), direct, explicit instruction is more effective and more efficient than partial guidance.
>
> —Clark, Kirschner, and Sweller (2012, p. 7)

Explicit intentional instruction is facilitated by an instructional routine, but this must be aligned with evidence-based instructional principles, focus on developing varied dimensions of word knowledge, and opportunities to use targeted words receptively and expressively. Stahl and Fairbanks (1986) and others have identified foundational principles for instruction. Stahl (2005) elaborated on and further explained these:

1. Using definitional and contextual information

   - Definitional information may include synonyms, antonyms, examples, nonexamples, and differences in related words.

   - Contextual information is provided by discussing meaning in different sentences from context, scenarios, creation of sentences, and silly questions.

2. Providing multiple exposures to targeted words by using words orally and in written expression in different contexts individually and collaboratively

3. Engaging in deep processing of word-generating information that ties the word to known information and build connections; activities may include extended discussions, categorization, and semantic mapping

Instructional Routines   A vocabulary routine, aligned with these evidence-based instructional principles, scaffolds and supports intentional instruction of individual words. Sample routines can be found in the literature. For example,

Paynter, Bodrova, and Doty (2005) suggested six concrete steps for learning words that represent a combined effort of teacher and student:

1. The teacher identifies the new word and elicits students' background knowledge.

2. The teacher explains the meaning of the new word and clears up confusion.

3. Students generate their own examples.

4. Students create a visual representation of the new word.

5. Students engage in experiences that depend on their understanding of the new word.

6. Students engage in vocabulary games and activities to help them remember the word and word meaning.

Moats (2009) recommended a similar routine based on both principles of instruction and dimensions of word meaning, including attention to linguistic structure.

The following simple routine and a more complex routine (briefly described later in this section) build on these examples, reflect what we know about effective vocabulary instruction, and provide organizational guidance for before, during, and after reading. Although they are designed for explicit intentional instruction, components of these routines are also applicable to incidental on purpose instruction and the teaching of word learning strategies. The simple routine shown in Table 15.3 also purposefully acknowledges the role of phonological, orthographic, and syntactical as well as definitional and contextual information.

The relationship between high-quality representation of words and access to meaning was established previously. These representations consist of not only semantic but also phonological and orthographic information. Students need opportunities to consider sounds, syllables, morphemes, and spellings within words—hence, the attention in this routine to linguistic as well as definitional and contextual information.

The routine demands practitioner preparation beyond word choice. The development of a student-friendly definition is also important. These definitions explain word meanings in everyday language and in complete sentences. Dictionary definitions are based on an Aristotelian view of meaning that sorts words by category and by how the word differs from other members of the category or genus (Stahl, 2005). Although it is important for students to understand the relationship of a word to others and to category, and its distinguishing or

Table 15.3.   Simple vocabulary routine

Teacher behavior	Student behavior	Critical connections
Pronounces targeted word and discusses structure and/or asks questions about linguistic structure.	Listens to teacher pronounce targeted word. Responds to questions.	Phonology Morphology Syntax
Asks student to repeat.	Echoes targeted word.	Phonology
Explains the meaning in everyday language.	Listens to explanation of meaning.	Semantics Definitional
Provides examples from context and other situations. Asks students for example.	Provides examples reflecting own experience.	Contextual

different features, the explanation needs to be expressed in language that students can understand and use. Individuals do not speak in "dictionary-ese." A word-meaning map serves both teacher and student by providing a format for the development of definitions while allowing for user-friendly language. Consider the example shown in Figure 15.6 that uses one of the identified words, *segregation*, related to civil rights. Similar maps can be used for other parts of speech (e.g. verbs, adjectives).

Context is also integral to understanding meaning. The text can and should be considered as the primary source, even if the teacher has to adapt the language based on student need. At the same time, practitioners need to create or elaborate on meaning by providing additional scenarios or other contexts for word use. Questioning and prompts can facilitate thinking about word meaning and possible connections with other words. Remember, students will require many opportunities to process and practice words in varied contexts if they are to use them receptively and expressively.

What might the routine look like and sound like if the targeted word is *segregation*?" See the following sample teacher dialogue.

TEACHER: We are going to learn about the word "segregation" today.

Listen as I say the word and get ready to echo. [*Teacher says the word.*]

How many syllables did you hear in "segregation?" [*Students respond.*]

I wonder if you know what part of speech this word is? Here's a hint. Does it answer the question who or what? [*Students respond.*] Yes, it is a noun.

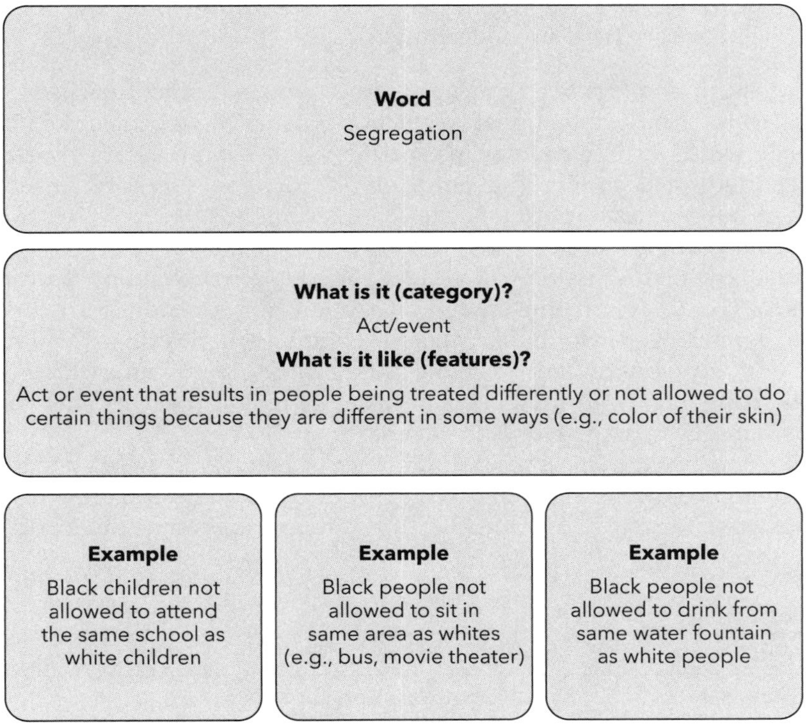

Word
Segregation

What is it (category)?
Act/event

What is it like (features)?
Act or event that results in people being treated differently or not allowed to do certain things because they are different in some ways (e.g., color of their skin)

Example
Black children not allowed to attend the same school as white children

Example
Black people not allowed to sit in same area as whites (e.g., bus, movie theater)

Example
Black people not allowed to drink from same water fountain as white people

Figure 15.6.   Sample noun word meaning map.

TEACHER: This word is about someone purposefully treating you differently. Think about someone separating you from others or not allowing you to do certain things because you are different in some way. This happened in our country to black people (African Americans) because of the color of their skin. Black children could not go to school with white children. They went to separate schools. Black people had to drink from separate water fountains and sit in separate places on a bus. These are examples of "segregation." *[Teacher pauses as students take in the explanation and examples.]*

TEACHER: In our story, black and white children went to separate schools until the 1960s. Even though there was a civil rights law that did not allow this, it still was happening. In 1960, a judge ordered four black girls to go to two white elementary schools. Segregation was against the law. Six-year-old Ruby Bridges went to first grade at the William Frantz Elementary School in New Orleans. She was the first black child to integrate this school. *[Teacher pauses.]* Have you ever been separated or not allowed to do something because you are different? *[Teacher allows time for a few students to respond.]*

TEACHER: Listen and watch as I write this word on the board. The word is "segregation." Listen again as I spell it by syllable: "seg – re – ga – tion." Repeat it yourself, and spell it quietly as you write. *[Teacher allows time for students to repeat the word to themselves and write it.]*

A more complex routine elaborates on the components of the simple routine, including additional adaptations such as the use of visuals, gestures, and possibly connections to cognates, while also identifying opportunities for the practice and processing necessary for deep understanding.

Processing and Practice Activities   Processing and practice activities are an essential component of intentional instruction but may also be integrated into incidental and word learning strategy instruction. A range of necessary exposures has been reported for deep learning. For example, McKeown and Colleagues (1985) and others have indicated that it may take as many as 12–20 meaningful exposures for students to know a word.

The following discussion will surface varied expressive and receptive opportunities for 1) identifying connections and relationships between words, 2) using or applying knowledge of words, and 3) representing word meanings (see Table 15.4).

1. Identifying connections and relationships between words can include teaching semantic relationships (through semantic mapping and other means) and using concept maps. Each of these is described next.

Teaching semantic relationships. Words are not remembered in isolation but rather in networks of connected meaning. Strategies and activities based on semantic relationships are effective for all students. One example is semantic mapping, which

Table 15.4.   Processing and practice activities

Connections	Use	Representations
Semantic maps	Questions, examples…	Pictures
Semantic feature analysis	Conversation prompts	Gestures and movement
Concept maps	Writing stems	Word walls

focuses on varied features of words, such as categories, subcategories, synonyms, antonyms, or multiple meanings. Useful procedures for developing a semantic map, based on category, might include the following (Stahl & Kapinus, 2001):

- Identifying the targeted topic/word.

- Brainstorming and discussing words that go with the targeted topic/word.

- Generating categories for the brainstormed words.

- Reading the selection and adding additional terms and categories from the text when appropriate.

Consider this example that reflects a third-grade unit/reading selection about weather and requires an understanding of words related to storms. A brainstorming session might initially surface words such as *northeaster, hurricane, blizzard, wind, heavy rain, snow, flooding, loss of electricity,* and *downed trees* (see the semantic map shown in Figure 15.7). Note that after reading, students might add tornadoes, ice storms, thunderstorms, and additional consequences and characteristics.

Students, particularly those with language learning disabilities or English language learners, may need additional scaffolding when creating semantic maps. Teachers can support these students by providing sets of related words (reflecting subcategories) that engage students in partner or group discussion prior to mapping.

Other activities that foster understanding of relationships include semantic feature analysis and semantic gradients or scaling for synonyms and antonyms. For instance, the more semantic features individual words share, the more synonymous they are, with the reverse being true for antonyms. Using semantic gradients or scaling, teachers can foster an understanding of shades of difference in meaning. This is important as authors choose precise words for text. Consider the differences between *sad* and *despondent* and those words that are similar (*pained, down, gloomy, dejected, miserable, depressed*). Each word is just a bit different from the others, even though they are close in connotation. What other words might your students generate? Consider an activity that asks them to place and explain their words on a continuum reflecting a little sad to very sad?

Using concept maps. Concept maps are similar to semantic maps. For example, the original Frayer Model or Four Square (Frayer, Frederick, & Klausmeier, 1969) generally calls for a definition, characteristics of a word, and examples and

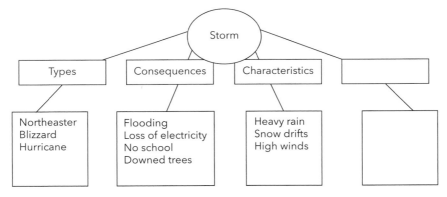

Figure 15.7. Semantic map. (From *Multisensory Teaching of Basic Language Skills, Third Edition* [p. 475].)

nonexamples. Variations on this model might include substituting personal connections, a picture, or synonyms/antonyms for examples/nonexamples. Consider the variation shown in Figure 15.8, in which students craft their definition of an identified word (e.g., *segregation*) and provide examples/facts, a visual, and words that could be confused with the targeted word.

2. Using or applying knowledge of words can include using words in conversation and discussion, including extension activities that incorporate questions, examples, and personal connections, as well as using words in writing. Each of these is described next.

Questions, examples, and connections. Engaging students in conversations and discussions related to critical concepts and targeted words provides the opportunity to express understanding and make connections beyond ideas presented within the text. Beck and colleagues (2002) developed several extension activities that probe individual word meanings and relationships. These incorporate using questions, examples, and personal connections so that students have the opportunity to work with definitional and contextual information and engage in deep processing of word meaning. Figure 15.9 provides sample activities based on words related to civil rights and segregation. Providing opportunities for using vocabulary in productive conversations is important throughout the school day.

Writing response. Writing about a text enhances understanding and is a tool for developing reading skills as well, particularly for older students (Graham & Perin, 2007). As a National Commission on Writing (2003) report succinctly stated:

> If students are to make knowledge their own, they must struggle with the details, wrestle with the facts, and rework raw information and dimly understood concepts into language they can communicate to someone else. In short, if students are to learn, they must write. (2003)

When teachers ask students to use their vocabulary words in written response, they provide opportunity for translating ideas into precise language. Teachers can scaffold writing tasks by beginning at the sentence level, creating sentence stems related to current learning and providing vocabulary **word banks.** As the students' writing skills progress, assignments can include varied types of purposeful paragraphs, focused on big ideas or themes that require the use of targeted vocabulary.

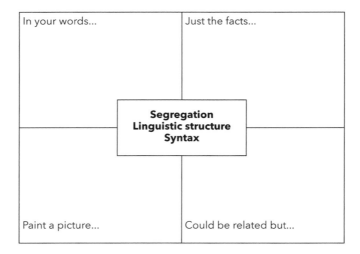

Figure 15.8. Variation on a four square.

If I say something that would be considered coura- geous, then say "courageous." *To do something that no one else has done before that is scary.*	Questions, reasons… *Why would someone be anxious? What does it mean to treat someone equally?*
Applause, applause! Clap how much you would like to be described as *courageous cowardly*	Describe a time when *You were courageous You were anxious*

Figure 15.9. Questions, examples, and connection activities. (*Source:* Beck, McKeown, & Kucan, 2002.)

3. Representing word meanings can include representing them through visuals and physical responses. Each of these is described next.

Visuals. The use of visual representations is effective with young and older students as well as those with individual needs. Although graphic organizers can represent semantic relationships visually, there are many other options. Pictures can be accessed electronically (clip art), drawn by hand, or created digitally to represent meaning. A key to effective use is the student's ability to explain how the visual illustrates word meaning. Following explicit teaching of word meaning, students are often prompted to write their own definitions of words, create pictures, and generate examples. These are typically recorded on index cards, in notebooks, in logs, or in journals. Consider the pictures from a middle school student's notebook, shown in Figure 15.10, that depict the meanings of these words (moving from left to right): *analysis, bewilderment, muted,* and *ascend.*

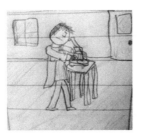
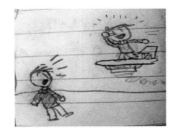
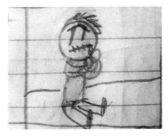
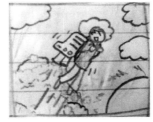

Figure 15.10. Seventh-grade student's vocabulary notebook. (Used with permission of Will Wagner.)

Teachers can also create visual displays such as vocabulary word walls arranged by category, alphabetical order, or even initial sound. Applications abound!

Physical response. A limited number of studies have examined the use of movement in learning word meaning. Beck, Perfetti, and McKeown (1982) designed an activity that grouped specific words from a reading passage by the semantic category "How We Move Our Legs." Students were taught a specific set of movements for each word (e.g., *stalk, trudge*). As words were encountered during oral reading of the passage, students acted them out. Students were enthusiastic about this activity, and researchers reported success with putting motions to words. Paynter and colleagues (2005) described a sixth-grade activity involving words associated with parts of a tree, such as *crown, trunk, xylem, sapwood, phloem,* and *bark.* After instruction and creating word cards with a definition and picture, students thought about the position their word would occupy in a drawing of a tree. Then, instead of drawing it, students became the tree by placing themselves on the floor to represent each of their words. The use of gesture, particularly for English language learners, is supported in the literature (Kelly, McDevitt, & Esch, 2009). The teacher's introduction and rehearsal of word meanings, coupled with linguistic features, visuals, and gesture, engages multiple senses. The combination of modalities holds promise for the learning and retention of targeted words for all students.

A consideration of frameworks and then, a comprehensive approach provides a road map for effective instruction. Vocabulary-attuned teachers understand the importance of incorporating multiple methods into the design and delivery of instruction. Intentional or explicit instruction of individual words demands a working knowledge of foundational principles, word-choice criteria, and routines that address dimensions of word meaning and essential processing and practice activities.

REFLECT, CONNECT, and RESPOND

What have you learned about the role of direct (intentional on purpose) instruction? What would you consider most significant in terms of your own practice?

Good vocabulary teaching involves a lot of talk and practice using language.

—Nonie LeSaux (2014, p. 11)

Incidental on Purpose Instruction   As noted previously, a comprehensive approach (see Figure 15.5) is necessary to ensure vocabulary acquisition for students to participate successfully in academic environments. Given the breadth of vocabulary that is essential for students to demonstrate understanding, it is obvious that intentional instruction alone, while necessary, is not sufficient. Thus, it is time to consider the role of incidental on purpose instruction.

Vocabulary-attuned teachers know that when language environments are purposefully rich, students are immersed in words through listening, reading, speaking, and writing activities. They recognize the need to create multiple on purpose opportunities for students to hear, see, and use other words informally, to provide incidental on purpose instruction. Although this approach will differ somewhat from intentional instruction, there will be overlap, and there are opportunities to use some of what has been discussed.

Rich Oral Language Classroom Environments   The nature of the student's word environment, coupled with developing a positive disposition toward word learning, has the potential of being a powerful instructional resource throughout life. Opportunities are plentiful once practitioners are aware of the importance of word-rich surroundings. An intentional focus on elevating teacher talk and creating opportunities for student talk is essential. Consider that not all language environments are equal or sufficiently robust to create a lexicon adequate to meet academic demand. Most adult conversation is simple and usually consists of the same 5,000–10,000 words. The vocabulary-attuned teacher takes responsibility for being more reflective and selective about his or her own oral language. This requires a conscious effort because everyday spoken language is less formal than academic vocabulary, which often carries with it many important concepts that students need to know. In a study of a reading intervention for middle school students, LeSaux (2014) found that increased literacy growth was more reflective of the quality of teacher talk than the intervention itself.

What are the possibilities within the school environment? Morning Meeting, a staple in early grades, provides innumerable opportunities for incidental on purpose learning. Consider the scaffolded word wall (see Figure 15.11) that a second-grade teacher uses to prompt daily informal conversations about feeling words. Note the display of the prompt (How are you feeling?), the related visuals, and the synonyms introduced to date that represent a range of feelings from annoyed to elated.

Everyday chatter about classroom activities and procedures also provides opportunities to use more sophisticated "ten- to twenty-dollar" words that students may not know or typically use. Think about the varied ways a teacher might ask students to "walk" to lunch. Substitutions for *walk*, coupled with a physical demonstration, could include semantic relatives such as *amble, strut, march, saunter,* or *meander.* A questioning student could be complimented for being *inquisitive* or *curious*; successfully completing a class project could be labeled as *fulfilling* or *exhilarating.* Teachers can purposefully point out when their students use valuable words. In turn, students can be asked to *look out* or *listen* for such words themselves. Just such an activity resulted in a third grader constructing a chart of words she had read or heard that interested her (see Table 15.5). She also decided on her own

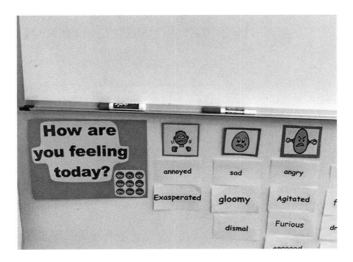

Figure 15.11.   Morning meeting word wall. (Used with permission of Becky Smith, AIM Academy.)

Table 15.5.   Sampling of valued words

Value	Words*
$5	habitat
	courage
	forecast
$10	prejudice
	metaphor
	hostility

*Some spellings have been corrected; words were spelled phonetically.

values! Think about the conversation a teacher might have with this student about her choice of value alone!

Both the texts and topics of the classroom provide opportunity for content-specific discussions and the weaving of vocabulary throughout conversations. A structured approach, such as the use of language frames or prompts, scaffolds student talk and can deepen understanding. Younger students can be prompted to identify and categorize related words, describe attributes, and use words to retell readings. Simple expressions, such as *are you saying, say more,* and *can you say it again in a different way,* are effective and support students in restating, revising, and elaborating their understanding of words and their conceptual connections. Rich discussions depend not only on word meaning but also content knowledge. Approaches for older students, such as Academic Conversations (Zwiers & Crawford, 2011) or Socratic Circles (Zwiers, 2014), provide opportunity to use both and should be guided by the identification of core discussion skills such as the following:

- Elaborate and clarify
- Support ideas with examples
- Build on and challenge a partner's ideas
- Paraphrase
- Synthesize conversation points (Zwiers & Crawford, 2011, p. 31)

Structured Shared Reading   Reading aloud or shared book reading, particularly in preschool and the early grades, is a common practice and acknowledged as an important source of language development. Less attention has been given to the value of reading aloud for older students; yet, there is evidence that even after children learn to read independently, they benefit from listening to text read aloud. Carlisle and Katz (2005) reported that studies show that kindergarteners and sixth-graders learn words by listening to books read aloud and that this activity can facilitate the understanding of complex texts. In addition, their benefit has been documented for special populations, including children with limited vocabulary and language delays (Crain, Thoreson, Dale, & Phillips, 1999; Hargrave & Senechal, 2000). Students who struggle with word recognition, such as those with dyslexia, benefit from hearing text at their listening comprehension level.

If the focus for shared reading is word meaning, the text selected should contain challenging words that are not typically found in the student's lexicon. Although much of the research has focused on the use of narrative texts, there is an increasing awareness of the importance of using informational text across the grades. Selecting text, whether for intentional and/or incidental instruction, is critical because students across grade levels need to build word meaning and schema related to the academic concepts of content. At the same time, it may be necessary to differentiate for students who do not know the basic words of oral language and to identify appropriate resources (e.g., Vadasy & Nelson, 2008).

Shared reading is also most productive when preplanned and structured. For example, practitioners need to prepare the text by identifying those words that provide opportunity for "point of contact" teaching (Stahl, 2005). Simply put, words can be quickly explained as they are encountered by providing synonyms, using the context or visuals. Questions related to word meaning should be developed and when possible, opportunities identified for use of words. Older student can also be taught to tune into and note interesting words for discussion following reading (Paynter, Bodrova, & Doty, 2005). Remember, students will not reap the potential benefits if the text is simply read and no response is required.

Structured Independent Reading   Once students acquire automatic word-reading skills, wide reading emerges as the major source of vocabulary development. Cunningham and Stanovich (1991) found that out-of-school reading is a powerful predictor of vocabulary and knowledge. Book reading has also been correlated with vocabulary growth and subsequent academic achievement. Even independent reading can be structured and purposeful. Students can be instructed to search for and surface intriguing words and/or to respond to generic questions that become the focus for impromptu sharing with peers.

The work of Anderson, Wilson, and Fielding (1988) has been informative in understanding student differences in wide reading while undoubtedly creating some discomfort given what is known about the diminishing reading habits of many children. They studied fifth-grade students' reading habits over several months. Based on daily diary recordings, Anderson and colleagues estimated and extrapolated how many words per year students read based on the percentage of time spent reading independently. Their data are somewhat alarming given the importance of wide reading as a primary source of word learning. For example, they estimated that a child at the 80th percentile (based on amount of independent reading time) read more than 20 times as much as the child at the 20th percentile.

Other factors also influence word learning during independent reading. Besides structure and amount, Carlisle and Katz (2005) identified the number of times a word is repeated in text, nature of clues to word meaning (context), and the difficulty of the text itself as important. Book choice and activities are a critical consideration for all of these reasons. The NRP (NICHD, 2000) recognized that children need to read for varied purposes and read texts at varied levels of difficulty, with some being read for enjoyment and others for more specific purposes. Although there has been debate about which books will most effectively promote vocabulary acquisition, there is some consensus. Decodable and leveled texts build critical foundational skills and are generally not sufficient to build a more sophisticated vocabulary. More challenging texts that provide opportunity for students to see and work with vocabulary in content-rich contexts are better suited to this purpose (Kamil & Hiebert, 2005; LeSaux & Harris, 2015). Until students can read these, teachers should guide their students in choosing books at the upper end of their independent level and support them in reading those at their instructional level.

Of course, availability and access to text are necessary conditions. Teachers need collections that allow for choice but also books that contain the rich language and repetition necessary to grow word and world knowledge. Book baskets or library collections should contain varied genres linked to developing specific grade-level themes or academic content as well as books that can be taken home and read for enjoyment.

Struggling readers tend to read fewer and easier books. Providing access to age- and grade-appropriate texts through **assistive technology,** while simultaneously providing intervention and/or intensive instruction for word recognition difficulties, is imperative. Otherwise, these students often become victims of the Matthew effect (Cunningham & Stanovich, 1998), falling further and further behind their peers in exposure and experience with the contents of rich text. New technologies, as well as some familiar ones (e.g., Learning Ally, Kurzweil 3000, Kindle, Intel Reader), allow them to read with their ears.

Purposefully creating language-rich experiences and environments is critical to vocabulary acquisition. Vocabulary-attuned teachers plan for incidental on purpose opportunities, including structured conversations, and shared and independent reading that support the learning of word meanings.

REFLECT, CONNECT, and RESPOND

What have you learned about the role of indirect or incidental on purpose instruction (intentional on purpose instruction)? What would you consider most significant in terms of your own practice?

Independent Word Learning Strategies A comprehensive approach (as was shown in Figure 15.3) acknowledges that acquiring word meaning independently requires the use of word learning strategies. Learning how and when to use these tools, including the use of the dictionary, context clues, and morphology, maximizes the potential of word learning.

Dictionaries The dictionary can be a valuable resource and reference tool if students understand how and when to use it. Dictionaries are a source of information on linguistic structure, etymology, syntax, and meaning. However, they often present some obstacles to understanding, such as truncated definitions and a lack of contextual information.

A number of prerequisite skills are needed for independent dictionary use, not the least of which are reading and spelling skills that may be problematic for struggling readers. In addition, dictionaries usually work best when the student has some sense of the targeted word's meaning. Explicit instruction in sub-skills such as alphabetical order, use of guide words, symbols, abbreviations, and overall format is necessary. Knowing that definitions typically include category or synonym as well as features or characteristics that differentiate the word from other similar words can be useful.

Not all dictionaries are created equal; some are more student friendly, such as the *Longman Dictionary of American English, Fourth Edition* (2007), which includes contextual information. Other resources include online dictionaries (e.g., http://www.merriam-webster.com), online thesauruses (e.g., http://www.visualthesaurus.com), and *The Visual Dictionary* (http://visualdictionaryonline.com), which provides more than 6,000 visual images on 15 different themes (e.g., the animal kingdom, the human body, energy).

Context Clues The context in which a word is used may be a rich source of information related to word meaning. However, educators should not assume that it will always be helpful. Some contexts do not yield clues, and some even confound understanding. Beck and colleagues (2002) studied contexts and identi-fied a continuum of usefulness related to context. She and her colleagues identified four categories of clues: mis-directive (directs the student to incorrect meaning), nondirective (provides no direction), general (provides general direction), and directive (provides specific direction for the correct meaning). Using the context effectively is dependent on understanding the nature of context clues coupled with the student's linguistic knowledge and experiences.

Context clues are broadly interpreted as including any meaning cues that sur-round the unfamiliar word within the context, including linguistic information (e.g., words, phrases, sentences) and nonlinguistic information (e.g., illustrations, typographic features). They potentially can be used to infer the word's meaning (Edwards, Font, Baumann, & Boland, 2012). Analyzing the context for linguistic clues typically involves searching the surrounding text for syntactic cues (based on word order) or semantic cues (meaning information) to determine the meaning of a targeted word. A student's use of context is also dependent on the following (Blachowicz & Fisher, 2010):

- Knowing why and when to use context.

- Having a general idea about clues that may be provided by context.

- Knowing how to look for and use these clues.

Most important, students need explicit instruction and opportunity for prac-tice and feedback using this independent word learning strategy. More intensive instruction, specific to cues and increased amounts of guided practice, may be neces-sary for students with language-based learning disabilities or for English language learners. A basic approach for upper elementary students (Lubliner, 2005, p. 58) prompts students to use the following clues while reading:

- Consider the context (read the sentence, paragraph, or passage for clues).

- Look for comma clues (meanings sometimes hide within commas [e.g., definition]).

- Look for explanation clues (sometimes provided in adjacent sentences).

- Look for feeling clues (other words that represent a feeling or emotion).

- Look for opposition clues (words such as adversative or conditional conjunc-tions, e.g., *but, even though, however*).

Baumann, Edwards, and colleagues (2003) have explored the effectiveness of teaching middle school students to use word part clues and context clues sepa-rately and in conjunction with each other. Their results indicated that students who were taught specific types of context cues could and did use this knowledge to infer meanings of unfamiliar words. They recommended teaching five common types of clues found in text; these are listed with examples in Table 15.6.

Morphemic Analysis   Morphology plays an essential role in literacy develop-ment. Strong correlations have been identified between morphological awareness and school-age literacy success in reading, writing, and spelling (Wolter, Wood, & D'zatko, 2009). Morphological awareness is the student's ability to understand, ana-lyze, and manipulate morphemes with an explicit awareness of their meaning. It accounts for unique variance in vocabulary knowledge beginning in kindergarten

Table 15.6.   Context clues

Clues	The author...
Definition	Explains the meaning of the word in the sentence or selection.
Synonyms	Uses a word similar in meaning.
Antonyms	Uses a word nearly opposite in meaning.
Example	Provides one or more examples of words or ideas.
General	Provides several words or statements that give clues to the word's meanings.

Source: Baumann, Edwards, Boland, & Font (2012, p. 147).

and increases over time (Carlisle, 2000). Not surprising, students who are better readers tend to be more aware of morphemes and their meanings than students who struggle with reading (Carlisle & Rice, 2002).

Morphemes are defined as the basic units of language learning that carry meaning; morphemes include base words, roots, prefixes, suffixes, and Greek combining forms. Morphemic analysis allows students to independently parse words into parts to infer meaning of unknown words. Not unlike context clues, the ability to use this independent word learning strategy depends on the content of the text and the student's knowledge. For example, an understanding of the meaning of Latin roots, Greek forms, prefixes, and suffixes is critical. Informed instruction includes explicit instruction of morphemes and their meanings, based on a logical sequence of the most common Latin roots and Greek forms, words, prefixes and suffixes in our language.

Baumann, Edwards, and colleagues (2003), in the study previously cited, suggested the following strategy for using morphemic analysis to determine word meaning:

- Look for the root word—a single word that cannot be broken into smaller words or word parts. See if you know what it means.

- Look for a prefix—a word part added to the beginning of a word that changes its meaning. See if you know what the prefix means.

- Look for a suffix—a word part added to the end of a word that changes its meaning. See if you know what the suffix means.

- Put the meanings of the root word, prefix, and suffix together. See if you can build the meaning of the word.

A fourth consideration, specific to English language learners, is the teaching of cognates when applicable. Cognates are words in two languages that share a similar meaning, spelling, and pronunciation, such as in *activities* in English and *actividades* in Spanish (see Table 15.7). Up to 40% of all words in English have a

Table 15.7.   Examples of English cognates

English	Spanish
accident	accidente
brilliant	brillante
cause	causa
center	centro

Adapted from *Multisensory Teaching of Basic Language Skills, Third Edition* (p. 331).

related word in Spanish. Identifying the English word and its cognate provides a clue or anchor for word meaning. The Colorín Colorado site (http://www.colorincolorado.org) offers multiple ideas and resources on how to use cognates, including a comprehensive cognate reference list.

A comprehensive approach to word learning also includes a focus on developing independent word learning strategies. The vocabulary-attuned teacher recognizes that students need tools to learn words on their own as they read independently. This includes the use of dictionaries, context clues, and morphemic analysis.

REFLECT, CONNECT, and RESPOND

What have you learned about the role of independent word learning strategies? How might you apply this information to your practice?

Word Consciousness   The vocabulary-attuned teacher (see Figure 15.5) also has to attend to word consciousness, which in many ways pervades the other components of comprehensive instruction. It has been conceptualized as "a cluster of diverse types of knowledge and skills that lead to an awareness of words and a flexible engagement with their use" (Stahl & Nagy, 2006). It has also been defined as an interest in and awareness of words (Graves & Watts, 2002). Those who are word conscious might be described as being "word omnivores." They are attracted to interesting words read or heard, recognize their communicative powers, and are meta-linguistically responsive to all aspects of a word, including linguistic structure and semantic connections.

> Successful language users develop word consciousness, or "an awareness of and interest in words and their meanings."
> —Graves (2006, p.7)

Although this component of instruction has not yet been fully researched, it is considered promising and one that educators should consider. Based on findings from an intervention project designed to increase word consciousness instruction, Scott, Miller, and Flinspach (2012) hypothesized that informal instruction affects vocabulary acquisition by increasing meta-cognitive and meta-linguistic awareness and knowledge as well as the appreciation and enjoyment of words. Word consciousness can be nurtured in several ways in the educational setting by a thoughtful teacher. Johnson, Johnson, and Schlicting (2012) identified seven word play categories, shown in Table 15.8, as potential sources of student activities.

Table 15.8.   Word play categories

Category	Examples	
Figurative language	Idiom	*Button your lip.*
Word associations	Homophones	*Bow (incline) or bow (knot)*
Word formations	Acronyms	*IT, NEA, LOL*
Word manipulations	Palindromes	*Noon, mom, level*
Word games	Tongue twisters	*Who sells seashells by the seashore?*
Ambiguity	Ambiguous words and phrases	*Break, light*
Onomastics	Origin of names	*Adam's apple*

Multiple resources for both incidental and intentional instruction exist. For example, Dr. Seuss, Shel Silverstein, and Richard Lederer's works contain multiple examples of the subtleties of language. *Super Silly Sayings That Are Over Your Head: A Children's Illustrated Book of Idioms* (Snodgrass, 2004) is specifically designed for children who have difficulty with expressions that say one thing and mean another. The author uses illustrations to depict the differences between the literal and abstract meanings of expressions. Homophones are explored in *How Much Can a Bare Bear Bear* (Cleary, 2007). *The King Who Rained* (Gwynne, 1970) targets multiple meanings, and *The Phantom Tollbooth* (Juster, 2001) takes students on a journey to the fantasy world of *Dictionopolis,* where they encounter fascinating words from music, mathematics, science, and other fields.

The final component of a comprehensive approach to vocabulary instruction, word consciousness, calls for the vocabulary-attuned teacher to develop word-attuned students by engaging them in varied activities such those described as word play.

REFLECT, CONNECT, and RESPOND
What role does word consciousness play in your practice?

Assessment

Understanding assessment types, their purpose, and the use of data to inform effective vocabulary practices is a fundamental competency for all educators. Screening, progress monitoring, outcome, and diagnostic assessment are all terms that educators should not only recognize but in some cases own, particularly in environments that utilize multi-tiered system of supports or response to intervention frameworks. Assessment of vocabulary is critical, challenging, and problematic for practitioners. It is critical because assessment serves multiple purposes, including

Table 15.9. Assessment tools

Assessment types	What is the purpose?	What do we have?
Screening	To identify students at risk for reading failure efficiently and effectively; predictive factors include vocabulary knowledge	Predictive Assessment of Reading-PAR (Red-e Set Grow, 2014) *Peabody Picture Vocabulary Test-Fourth Edition (PPVT-4; Dunn & Dunn, 2007)
Progress monitoring	To evaluate student progress in identified risk areas and determine effectiveness of intervention provided	Predictive Assessment of Reading-PAR (Red-e Set Grow, 2014) *Formative assessments
Diagnostic	To identify specific strengths and weaknesses in specific areas compared to age and grade level peers; to diagnose specific learning disability and/or determine eligibility for special education services	Peabody Picture Vocabulary Test-Fourth Edition (PPVT-4; Dunn & Dunn, 2007) Test of Language Development-Fourth Edition (TOLD-4; Newcomer & Hammill, 2008) Comprehensive Assessment of Spoken Language-Fourth Edition (CELF-4; Semel, Wiig, & Secord, 2003)
Outcome	To determine overall effectiveness of curriculum and instruction within a school, district; vocabulary assessment is usually one dimensional	High stakes state assessments

*Recommended alternatives

informing instruction; it is challenging and problematic because, with the exception of diagnostic tests, there is a general lack of measures that target vocabulary. However, those tools that are available should be used to inform instruction for all students (see Table 15.9).

It has been suggested that educators rely more on formative or classroom-based assessment as a possible solution to the lack of measures for monitoring progress. Coyne and colleagues examined the effectiveness of ongoing curriculum-based mastery measures (based on their vocabulary intervention) and found that "formative assessment that measured whether students were learning target vocabulary was a good indicator of whether students were responding to intervention" (2015, p. 56). Pearson, Hiebert, and Kamil (2012) also recommended the development of school/classroom assessments of vocabulary knowledge to progress monitor and provided direction, suggesting the following item content and format:

- *Definition*: write a definition.

- *Context:* identify meaning within context.

- *Semantic network*: express knowledge of related words.

Others (Scott, Flinspach, & Vevea, 2010) informally assess word knowledge by asking students to respond to questions related to whether they had seen the word, their level of confidence regarding meaning, and their identification of general category and probable meaning. This seems reminiscent of informal word knowledge surveys often used before and after vocabulary instruction. Although diagnostic assessment measures are plentiful, it is obvious there is more work to be done regarding screening and progress monitoring tools. Classroom educators also need guidance on the construction of informal measures and how to use the data as well as additional standardized tools.

Assessment data from multiple sources is necessary for effective vocabulary instruction for all students. Although availability of varied assessment tools is somewhat challenging, educators do have sufficient resources to make informed decisions.

 REFLECT, CONNECT, and RESPOND
How do you assess vocabulary instruction?

CLOSING THOUGHTS: WORKING WITH WORD MEANING

Proficient reading requires the development, coordination, and interaction of multiple language processes and skills. Among these, vocabulary emerges as one of the most critical, contributing not only to word recognition but also to directly influencing comprehension. Many consider vocabulary to be the bridge between these two factors that are necessary for skilled reading. In the school setting, vocabulary plays an essential role in constructing and expressing meaning across disciplines and is a necessary component of reading instruction. Students arrive at school with wide differences in vocabulary knowledge (Biemiller & Slonin, 2001). These are often evident in children from low socioeconomic status backgrounds, English language learners, and those with language-based learning disabilities. An understanding of the potential reasons for vocabulary acquisition and deficits is necessary for educators and specialists as they collaborate on the design of differentiated instruction for all students.

> **REFLECT, CONNECT, and RESPOND**
> How does vocabulary contribute to reading proficiency? How do children acquire word meaning before they enter school? Explain this statement: Acquisition of word meaning is a complex and complicated process that is incremental, interrelated, and multidimensional in nature. How would you describe a comprehensive approach to vocabulary instruction? What insights have you gained about vocabulary instruction?

ONLINE COMPANION MATERIALS

The following Chapter 15 resources are available at http://www.brookespublishing .com/birshcarreker/materials:

- Reflect, Connect, and Respond Questions

- Appendix 15.1: Technology Resources

- Appendix 15.2: Knowledge and Skill Assessment Answer Key

- Appendix 15.3: Additional Online Resources

KNOWLEDGE AND SKILL ASSESSMENT

1. What does vocabulary knowledge contribute to?

    a. Phonological awareness

    b. Word recognition

    c. Comprehension

    d. All of the above

2. How would you describe the acquisition of word learning?

    a. Incremental

    b. Interrelated

    c. Multidimensional

    d. All of the above

3. The number of word meanings a student recognizes refers to what?

    a. Breadth of vocabulary

    b. Depth of vocabulary

    c. Sight word vocabulary

    d. All of the above

4. A comprehensive approach to vocabulary instruction for the school-age child includes what?

    a. Direct instruction

    b. Indirect instruction

    c. Word learning strategies and word consciousness

    d. All of the above

5. Which of the following is a principle of effective vocabulary instruction?

    a. Use of multisensory instruction

    b. Provision of definitional and contextual information

    c. Use of concept mapping

    d. None of the above

6. Why are strategies and activities based on semantic relationships important?

    a. Words are learned in isolation

    b. Words are learned in networks of meaning

    c. Words are learned indirectly

    d. Words are learned in context

7. Teaching students to use context to determine word meaning is an example of what?

    a. Indirect approach to word learning

    b. Word consciousness approach

    c. Direct approach to word learning

    d. Independent word learning strategy

8. Which of the following is an example of an effective indirect instructional approach?

    a. Using an instructional routine

    b. Using strategies to determine word meaning

    c. Immersing students in rich language environments

    d. Using word play activities

REFERENCES

Anderson, R.C., & Freebody, P. (1981). Vocabulary knowledge. In J. Guthrie (Ed.), *Comprehension and teaching: Research reviews* (pp. 77–117). Newark, DE: International Reading Association.

Anderson, R.C., Wilson, P.T., & Fielding, L.G. (1988). Growth in reading and how children spend their time outside of school. *Reading Research Quarterly, 23*, 285–303.

Archer, A.L., & Hughes, C.A. (2011). *Explicit instruction: Effective and efficient teaching (What Works for Special-Needs Learners)*. New York, NY: Guilford.

Baumann, J.F., Edwards, E.C., Boland, E., & Font, G. (2012). Teaching word learning strategies. In J.F. Baumann & E.J. Kame'enui (Eds.) *Vocabulary instruction: Research to practice* (2nd ed., pp. 117–139). New York, NY: Guilford.

Baumann, J.F., Edwards, E.C., Boland, E., Olejnik, S., & Kame'enui, E.J. (2003). Vocabulary tricks: Effects of instruction on morphology and context on fifth grade students' ability to derive and infer word meaning. *American Educational Research Journal, 40*, 447–494.

Beck, I.L., McKeown, M.G., & Kucan, L. (2002). *Bringing words to life: Robust vocabulary instruction.* New York, NY: Guilford.

Beck, I.L., McKeown, M.G., & Kucan, L. (2008). *Creating robust vocabulary: Frequently asked questions and extended examples.* New York, NY: Guilford.

Beck, I.L., Perfetti, C., & McKeown, M.G. (1982). Effects of long-term vocabulary instruction on lexical access and reading comprehension. *Journal of Educational Psychology, 74*(4), 506–521.

Biemiller, A. (2010). *Words worth teaching: Closing the vocabulary gap.* Columbus, OH: SRA/ McGraw-Hill.

Biemiller, A. (2012). Teaching vocabulary in the primary grades: Vocabulary instruction needed. In J.F. Baumann & E.J. Kame'enui (Eds.), *Vocabulary instruction: Research in practice* (2nd ed., pp. 28–40). New York, NY: Guilford.

Biemiller, A., & Slonin, N. (2001). Estimating root word vocabulary growth in normative and advantaged populations. *Journal of Educational Psychology, 93,* 498–510.

Blachowicz, C., & Fisher, P.J. (2010). *Teaching vocabulary in all classrooms.* Boston, MA: Allyn & Bacon.

Bruner, J. (1983). *Child's talk: Learning to use language.* New York, NY: W.W. Norton.

Calfee, R.C., & Drum, P.A. (1986). Research on teaching reading. In M.C. Wittrock (Ed.), *Handbook of research on teaching* (3rd ed., pp. 804–849). Mahwah, NJ: Lawrence Erlbaum Associates.

Carey, S., & Bartlett, E. (1978). Acquiring a single word. *Papers and Reports on Child Language Acquisition, 15,* 17–29.

Carlisle, J.F. (2000). Awareness of the structure and meaning of morphologically complex words: Impact on reading. *Reading and Writing: An Interdisciplinary Journal, 12*(3), 169–190.

Carlisle, J.F., & Katz, L.A. (2005). Word learning and vocabulary instruction. In J.R. Birsh (Ed.), *Multisensory teaching of basic language skills* (2nd ed., pp. 345–376). Baltimore, MD: Paul H. Brookes Publishing Co.

Carlisle, J.F., & Rice, M.S. (2002). *Improving reading comprehension.* Timonium, MD: York Press.

Cassano, C.M., & Schickedanz, J.A. (2015). An examination of the relations between oral vocabulary and phonological awareness in early childhood. *Literacy Research: Theory, Method, and Practice, 64,* 227–248.

Catts, H.W., Hogan, T.P, Adlof, S.M., & Barth, A.E. (2013). *The simple view of reading. Changes over time.* Boulder, CO: Poster Presentation Scientific Studies of Reading.

Chomsky, N. (1965). *Aspects of a theory of syntax.* Cambridge: MA: The MIT Press.

Clark, R.E., Kirscher, P.A., & Sweller, J. (2012). Putting students on the path to learning: The case for fully guided instruction. *The American Educator, 36*(10), 6–11.

Cleary, B. (2007). *How much can a bare bear bear?* Minneapolis, MN: Millbrook.

Coles R. (1995). *The story of Ruby Bridges.* New York, NY: Scholastic.

Common Core State Standards Initiative. (2018). *College and career readiness anchor standards for language.* Retrieved from http://www.corestandards.org/ELA-Literacy/CCRA/L/

Coxhead, A. (2000). A new academic word list. *TESOL Quarterly, 34,* 213–238.

Coyne, M.D., Cappozzoli-Oldham, A., Cuticelli, M., & Ware, S.M. (2015). Using assessment data to make a difference in vocabulary outcomes. *Perspectives on Language and Literacy, 41*(3), 52–56.

Coyne, M.D., McCoach, B., & Kapp, S. (2007). Vocabulary intervention for kindergarten students: Comparing extended instruction to embedded instruction and incidental exposure. *Learning Disability Quarterly, 30*(2), 74–88.

Crain W., Thoreson, C., Dale, P.S., & Phillips S. (1999). Enhancing linguistic performance: Parents and teachers as book reading partners for children with language delays. *Topics in Early Childhood Special Education, 19*(1), 28–39.

Cunningham, A.E., & Stanovich, K.E. (1991). Tracking the unique effects of print exposure in children: Associations with vocabulary, general knowledge, and spelling. *Journal of Educational Psychology, 83,* 264–274.

Cunningham, A.E., & Stanovich, K.E. (1998). What reading does for the mind. *American Educator, 22,* 8–15.

Dougherty, D.P., & Paul, D.R. (2007). *Talking on the go: Everyday activities to enhance speech and language development.* Rockville, MD: American Speech-Language-Hearing Association.

Dunn, L.M., & Dunn, D.M. (2007). *Peabody Picture Vocabulary Test–Fourth Edition* (*PPVT-4*). New York, NY: Pearson Clinical.

Ebbers, S.M., & Denton, C.A. (2008). A root awakening: Vocabulary instruction for older students with reading difficulties. *Learning Disabilities Research & Practice, 23*(2) 80–90.

Edwards, E.C., Font, G., Baumann, J.F., & Boland, E. (2012). Teaching word-learning strategies word meanings. In J.F. Baumann & E.J. Kame'enui (Eds.), *Vocabulary instruction: Research to practice* (2nd ed., pp. 139–159). New York, NY: Guilford.

Frayer, D., Frederick, W.C., & Klausmeier, H.J. (1969). *A schema for testing the level of cognitive mastery.* Madison: Wisconsin Center for Education Research.

Gough, P.B., & Tunmer, W.E. (1986). Decoding, reading and reading disability. *Remedial and Special Education, 7,* 6–10.

Graham, S., & Perin, D. (2007). *A report to Carnegie foundation: Writing next.* New York, NY: Alliance for Excellent Education.

Graves, M.F. (2006). *The vocabulary book: Learning and instruction.* New York, NY: Teachers College Press.

Graves, M.F., & Watts, S.M. (2002). The place of word consciousness in a research-based vocabulary program. In J. Samuels & A.E. Farstrup (Eds.), *What research has to say about reading instruction* (3rd ed., pp. 140–165). Newark, DE: International Reading Association.

Gwynne, F. (1970). *The king who rained.* New York, NY: Simon & Schuster.

Hargrave, A.C., & Sénéchal, M. (2000). Book reading interventions with language-delayed preschool children: The benefits of regular reading and dialogic reading. *Early Childhood Research Quarterly, 15,* 75–90.

International Dyslexia Association, The. (2010). *Knowledge and practice standards for teachers of reading.* Baltimore, MD: Author.

International Dyslexia Association, The. (2018, March). *Knowledge and practice standards for teachers of reading.* Retrieved from https://dyslexiaida.org/knowledge-and-practices/

Johnson, D.D., Johnson, B.V.H., & Schlicting, K. (2012). Language play: Essential for Literacy. In Baumann, J. F. & Kame'enui, E. (Eds.), *Vocabulary instruction: Research to practice* (pp. 190–210). New York, NY: Guilford.

Juster, N. (2001). *The phantom tollbooth.* New York, NY: Random House.

Kamil, M.L., & Hiebert, E.H. (2005). The teaching and learning of vocabulary. In E.H. Hiebert & M.L. Kamil (Eds.), *Teaching and learning vocabulary: Bringing research to practice* (pp. 1–26). Hillsdale, NJ: Lawrence Erlbaum Associates.

Kelly, S.D., McDevitt, T., & Esch, M. (2009). Brief training with co-speech gesture lends a hand to word learning in a foreign language. *Language and Cognitive Processes, 24,* 313–334.

Landry, S.H., & Smith, K.E. (2007). Parents support of children's language provides support for later reading competence. In R.K. Wagner, A.E. Muse, & K.R. Tannenbaum (Eds.), *Vocabulary acquisition: Implications for reading comprehension* (pp. 32–51). New York, NY: Guilford.

LeSaux, N. (2014). Focus on deeply words that matter. *Best practices.* Retrieved from http://www.ngreach.com

LeSaux, N.K., & Harris, J.R. (2015). *Cultivating knowledge, building language.* Portsmouth, NH: Heinemann.

Li, M., & Kirby, J.M. (2014). The effects of vocabulary breadth and depth on English reading. *Applied Linguistics, 36*(5), 611–634.

Longman dictionary of American English (4th ed.). (2007). Essex, United Kingdom: Pearson.

Lonigan, C.J. (2007). Vocabulary development and the development of phonological awareness skills in preschool children. In R.K. Wagner, A.E. Muse, & K.R. Tannenbaum (Eds.), *Vocabulary acquisition: Implications for reading comprehension* (pp. 15–31). New York, NY: Guilford.

Lubliner, S. (2005). *Getting into words: Vocabulary instruction that strengthens comprehension.* Baltimore, MD: Paul H. Brookes Publishing Co.

Marulis, L.M., & Neumann, S.B. (2010). The effects of vocabulary training on word learning: A meta-analysis. *Review of Educational Research, 80*(3), 300–335.

McKeown, M., Beck, I., Omanson, R., & Pople, M. (1985). Some effects of the nature and frequency of vocabulary instruction on the knowledge and use of words. *Reading Research Quarterly, 20*(5), 522–535.

McKeown, M., Beck, I.L., & Sandora, C. (2012). Direct and rich vocabulary instruction needs to start early. In J.F. Baumann & E.J. Kame'enui (Eds.), *Vocabulary instruction: Research to practice* (2nd ed., pp. 17–33). New York, NY: Guilford.

McLaughlin, S. (1998). *Introduction to language development.* San Diego, CA: Singular.

Moats, L.C. (2009). *The mighty word: Building vocabulary and oral language* (2nd ed.). Longmont, CO: Sopris West Educational Services.

Moats, L.C., & Paulson, L.H. (2009). *Early childhood LETRS.* Longmont, CO: Sopris West Educational Services.

Nagy, W. (2005). Why vocabulary instruction needs to be long-term and comprehensive. In E.H. Hiebert & M.L. Kamil (Eds.), *Teaching and learning vocabulary: Bringing research to practice* (pp. 27–44). Mahwah, NJ: Lawrence Erlbaum Associates.

Nagy, W.E., & Anderson, R.C. (1984). How many words are there in printed school English? *Reading Research Quarterly, 19,* 304–330.

Nagy, W.E., & Scott, J.A. (2000). Vocabulary processes. In M.L. Kamil, P.B. Mosenthal, P.D. Parson, & R. Barr (Eds.), *Handbook of reading research* (Vol. III, pp. 269–284). Mahwah, NJ: Lawrence Erlbaum Associates.

Nation, I.S.P. (2001). *Learning vocabulary in another language.* Cambridge, United Kingdom: Cambridge University Press.

National Commission on Writing. (2003). *The neglected R: The need for a writing revolution.* Retrieved from https://www.nwp.org/cs/public/print/resource/2523

National Governor's Association, Center for Best Practices, & Council of Chief State School Officers. (2010). *Common core state standards.* Washington DC: Author.

National Institute of Child Health and Human Development. (2000). *Report of the National Reading Panel: Reports of the subgroups. Teaching children to read: An evidence-based assessment of the scientific research literature on reading and its implications for reading instruction* (NIH Publication No. 00- 4754). Washington, DC: Government Printing Office.

National Institute of Child Health and Human Development, Early Child Care Research Network (NICHD-ECCRN). (2005). Pathways to reading: The role of oral language in the transition to reading. *Developmental Psychology, 41,* 428–442.

Neuman, S.B., & Dickinson, D.K. (Eds.). (2001). *Handbook of early literacy research.* New York, NY: Guilford.

Neuman, S.B., & Wright, T.S. (2013). *All about words: Increasing vocabulary in the common core classroom PreK–2.* New York, NY: Teachers College Press.

Newcomer, P.L., & Hammill, D.D. (2008). *Test of Language Development, Fourth Edition (TOLD-4).* Austin, TX: PRO-ED.

Paynter, D.E., Bodrova, E., & Doty, J.K. (2005). *For the love of words: Vocabulary instruction that works in grades K–6.* San Francisco, CA: Jossey-Bass.

Pearson, D.P., Hiebert, E.H., & Kamil, M. (Eds.) (2012). Vocabulary assessment: Making do with what we have. In J.F. Baumann & E.J. Kame'enui, *Vocabulary instruction: Research to practice* (2nd ed., pp. 231–256). New York, NY: Guilford.

Perfetti, C. (2007). Reading ability: Lexical quality to comprehension. *Scientific Studies of Reading, 11*(4), 357–383.

Perfetti, C., & Stafura, J. (2014). Word knowledge in a theory of reading comprehension, *Scientific Studies of Reading, 18*(1), 22–37.

Pinker, S. (2007). *The stuff of thought: Language as a window into human nature.* New York, NY: Viking/ Penguin Group.

Rayner, K., Foorman, B.F., Perfetti, C.A., Pesetsky, D., & Seidenberg, M.S. (2001). How psychological science informs the teaching of reading. *Psychological Science in the Public Interest, 2*(2), 31–74.

Red-e Set Grow. (2014). *Predictive Assessment of Reading (PAR).* Clemmons, NC: Author.

Rowe, M.L. (2012). A longitudinal investigation of the role of quantity and quality of child-directed speech in vocabulary development. *Child Development, 83*(5), 1762–1774.

Scarborough, H. (2001). Connecting early language and literacy to later reading (dis)abilities: Evidence, theory and practice. In S.B. Neuman & D.K. Dickinson (Eds.), *Handbook of early literacy research* (pp. 97–110). New York, NY: Guilford.

Scott, J., Miller, T., & Flinspach, S.L. (2012). Developing word consciousness: Lessons from a highly diverse fourth grade classrooms. In J.F. Baumann & E.J. Kame'enui (Eds.), *Vocabulary instruction: Research to practice* (2nd ed., pp. 169–188). New York, NY: Guilford.

Scott, J.A., Vevea, J.L., & Flinspach, S.L. (2010, Dec.). *Vocabulary growth in fourth grade classrooms: A quantitative analysis of Year 3 in the VINE project.* Paper presented at the annual meeting of the Literacy Research Association.

Seidenberg, M.S., & McClelland, J.L. (1989). A distributed, developmental model of word recognition and naming. *Psychological Review, 96,* 523–568.

Semel, E., Wiig, E.H., & Secord, W.A. (2003). *Clinical Evaluation of Language Fundamentals–Fourth Edition (CELF-4).* New York, NY: Pearson.

Snodgrass, C.S. (2004). *Super silly sayings that are over your head: A children's illustrated book of idioms.* Higanum, CT: Starfish Specialty Press.

Stahl, S.A. (1998). *Vocabulary development: From reading research to practice.* Brookline, MA: Brookline Books.

Stahl, S.A. (2004). Scaly? Audacious? Debris? Salubrious? Vocabulary learning and the child with learning disabilities. *Perspectives, 30,* 5–13.

Stahl, S.A. (2005). Four problems with teaching word meanings (and what to do to make vocabulary an integral part of instruction). In E.H. Hiebert & M.L. Kamil (Eds.), *Teaching and learning vocabulary: Bringing research to practice* (pp. 95–114). Mahwah, NJ: Lawrence Erlbaum Associates.

Stahl, S.A., & Fairbanks, M.M. (1986). The effects of vocabulary instruction: A model-based meta-analysis in. *Review of Educational Research, 56*(1), 72–110.

Stahl, S.A., & Kapinus, B.A. (2001). *Word power: What every educator needs to know about teaching vocabulary.* Washington, DC: National Education Association.

Stahl, S.A., & Nagy, W.E. (2006). *Teaching word meanings.* Mahwah, NJ: Lawrence Erlbaum Associates.

Stanovich, K.E. (1986). Matthew effects in reading: Some consequences of individual differences in the acquisition of literacy. *Reading Research Quarterly, 21,* 360–406.

Tannenbaum, K.R., Torgesen, J.T., & Wagner, R.K. (2006). Relationship between word knowledge and reading comprehension in 3rd grade children. *Scientific Studies of Reading, 10,* 381–398.

Trivette, C.M., & Dunst, C. (2007). Relative effectiveness of dialogic, interactive, and shared reading interventions. *CELL Review, 1*(2) 1–6.

Vadasy, P., & Nelson, J.R. (2008). *Early vocabulary connections: Important words to know and spell.* Longmont, CO: Sopris West Educational Services.

Vellutino, F.R., Tunmer, W.E., Jaccard, J.J., & Chen, R. (2007). Components of reading ability: Multivariate evidence for a convergent skills model of reading development. *Scientific Studies of Reading, 11*(1), 3–32.

Walley, A.C., Metsala, J.L., & Garlock, V.M. (2003). Spoken vocabulary growth: Its role in the development of phoneme awareness and early reading ability. *Reading and Writing: An Interdisciplinary Journal, 16,* 5–20.

Weizman, Z., & Snow, C.E. (2001). Lexical input as related to children's vocabulary acquisition: Effects of sophisticated exposure and support for meaning. *Developmental Psychology, 37,* 265–279.

What Works Clearinghouse. (2015). *IES intervention report: Shared book reading.* Retrieved from http://www.ies.ed.gov

Whitehurst, G. (2013). The dialogic reading method. In M. Bjerregaard, C. Judd, & J. Judd, *Chatter batter: Four stories for speech development.* Bloomington, IN: AuthorHouse.

Wolf, M., Miller, L., & Donnelly, K. (2000). Retrieval, automaticity, vocabulary elaboration, orthography (RAVE-O): A comprehensive, fluency-based reading intervention Program. *Journal of Learning Disabilities, 33,* 375–386.

Wolter, J.A., Wood, A., & D'zatko, K. (2009). The influence of morphological awareness on first-grade children's literacy development. *Language, Speech, and Hearing Services in the Schools, 40*(3), 1–13.

Zwiers, J., & Crawford, M. (2011). *Academic conversations: Classroom talk that fosters critical thinking and content understanding.* Portland, ME: Stenhouse.

Zwiers, J. (2014). *Building academic language: Meeting common core standards across disciplines, grades 5–12* (2nd ed.). San Francisco, CA: Jossey-Bass.

Technology Resources

Elaine A. Cheesman

PROGRAMS/APPS: VOCABULARY

Effective programs/apps have the following features:

- They avoid presenting unrelated words.
- They organize vocabulary words/phrases by shared relationships, topic, or content (e.g., beach words: *sand, shell, kelp*; words with Latin root "rupt": *disrupt, rupture*).
- They provide repetition and multiple exposures within small groups of target words.

Comparative Adjectives   http://www.alligatorapps.com

This app allows students to select the picture that matches the oral comparative adjective (e.g., *taller*) or superlative adjective (e.g., *tallest*). It is appropriate for younger students.

Homophones   http://www.alligatorapps.com

This app provides practice using the correct homophone in sentences and opportunities for reading and using the correct homophones. It presents some homophones in seven engaging games. The optional text-to-speech feature reads sentences.

Irregular Verbs   http://www.alligatorapps.com

This app gives practice reading and using correct verb forms. It presents some homophones in seven engaging games. The optional text-to-speech feature reads sentences. This app is appropriate for younger students and English language learners.

Lars and Friends https://www.amazon.com/Carla-Susanto-Lars-and-Friends /dp/B00M8BDAOM

This app teaches collective nouns (e.g., a tower of giraffes, a mob of kangaroos) through an animated, narrated story. It is appropriate for younger children.

Phrasal Verb Machine and Phrasalstein http://thephrasalverbsmachine.org

This site addresses idiomatic verb phrases (*lock up, turn off*). Using it requires good reading skills or a reading assistant. (No text-to-speech feature is available.) The Phrasal Verbs view allows the user to view animation of a given phrase (learn mode). The Exercise view allows the user to choose the phrase to match the phrasal verb. The site has Spanish and Italian options available. It is appropriate for older students.

The Right Word by Connor Duggan https://itunes.apple.com/us/app/the-right-word/id761529361?mt=8

This app shows frequently misused words within the context of a sentence. Using it requires reading skills. The app includes four games to practice and test skills. It is appropriate for older students and adults.

Word Hippo http://www.wordhippo.com

This web site provides the meaning of a word and also provides synonyms, antonyms, words that rhyme with it, sentences containing it, the derivatives, and etymology. It includes U.K. and U.S. spellings.

Wordflex Touch Dictionary http://wordflex.com

This site provides the oral pronunciation of a main word in U.S. or British accents. It shows word relationships as networks of semantic word associations. Word webs are organized by the parts of speech (e.g., noun, verb), phrases, and derivatives. Words listed include phrasal verbs (*walk away, pull out*). Dynamic word trees can be moved and rearranged. The site is appropriate for older students and teachers.

PROGRAMS/APPS: MORPHOLOGY (PREFIXES, SUFFIXES, LATIN ROOTS, GREEK COMBINING FORMS)

Effective programs/apps have the following features:

- They link the meaning with the spelling of the morpheme.

Lexia Core5 http://www.lexialearning.com

This site provides engaging, systematic, sequential practice in Latin roots and Greek combining forms. It includes vocabulary and comprehension activities as well. It can track multiple users' progress. It is appropriate for kindergarten through adult.

Roots to Words http://www.taptolearn.com

This site presents morphemes organized by category—Numbers, Quantity, Shapes, Directions, Comparison, Time and Distance, See 'N Speak, Not or

Against, Body and Life, Movement, People, Feelings, Life Cycle, Anatomy I, and Anatomy II. It provides several activities to link spelling, meaning, and related words. Using this site requires reading skills. Four activities are provided to reinforce skills.

SpellingCity   http://www.spellingcity.com

This site provides practice spelling, vocabulary, and handwriting using user-entered or imported word lists. In the paid version, users can access and share lists with published textbooks. The site is appropriate for Grade 1 through adult.

WEB SITES: MATERIALS AND ACTIVITIES FOR TEACHERS AND LEARNERS

Dictionary.com   http://www.dictionary.com

This web site provides user-friendly definitions, synonyms, antonyms, sample sentences, and illustrated language of origin.

Florida Center for Reading Research   http://www.fcrr.org

This web site has thousands of downloadable "Center" activities in all five components of reading: phonemic awareness, phonics, fluency, vocabulary, and comprehension. It also has research and resources for teachers.

List of English Suffixes   https://www.learnthat.org/pages/view/suffix.html

This is a list of Greek and Latin morphemes, meanings, and sample words and definitions.

Longman Dictionary and Thesaurus   http://global.longmandictionaries.com

This site provides clear definitions using only 2,000 common words. It has special features for education (e.g., flashcards, teacher resources, printable worksheets, search on idiomatic phrases, synonyms and word histories.)

Root Words and Prefixes: Quick Reference   https://www.learnthat.org/pages/view/roots.html

This is a list of Greek and Latin morphemes, meanings, and sample words and definitions.

Vocabulary.com   http://www.vocabulary.com

This web site is designed for older students and adults. It offers semantically connected words and examples from adult sources (e.g., *The New Yorker*).

Word Building and Spelling: Experiments in English Morphology
http://www.neilramsden.co.uk

The Mini Matrix-Maker builds word matrices from a list of word sums the user provides (see Figure 15.12).

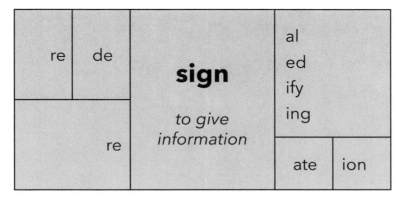

Figure 15.12. Example of output from the Mini Matrix-Maker. (*Source:* Generated with Mini Matrix-Maker. Copyright Neil Ramsden © 2011–2013. All rights reserved. Available at http://www.neilramsden.co.uk/spelling/matrix/. Adapted by permission.)

Example word matrix and word sums:

re + de + sign + ed

sign + al

de + sign + ate + ions

Wordnik   http://www.wordnik.com

This site allows the user to enter any word or phrase to reveal definitions, etymologies, and examples in sentences from various sources. This site is more appropriate for adults and older students.

Your Dictionary   http://www.yourdictionary.com

This dictionary includes simple definitions with examples, synonyms, quotes, word origins, and related forms.

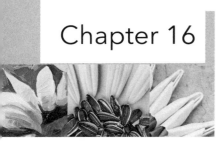

Chapter 16

Strategies to Improve Reading Comprehension in the Multisensory Classroom

Eileen S. Marzola

LEARNING OBJECTIVES

1. To identify major shifts in the focus of reading comprehension resulting from the Common Core State Standards, research-validated target areas of comprehension instruction, and new 21st-century literacies and to explain their implications for reading teachers

2. To describe the historical role of comprehension in reading instruction and literacy research from the 1960s through the present

3. To identify general strategies good readers use and articulate overarching principles for developing students' comprehension (e.g., assessing understanding, building listening comprehension, working with sentences and with longer texts)

4. To understand and describe common sources of students' difficulties with reading comprehension (e.g., dyslexia, narrow focus on fluency, limited background knowledge)

5. To identify specific research-validated strategies for comprehension instruction and steps for implementing these, including use of reciprocal teaching to enhance students' use of multiple strategies

Since the last edition of this text was published, an important shift of focus has occurred in the national goals for reading comprehension instruction in the schools. The Common Core State Standards (CCSS) for English Language Arts and Literacy in History/Social Studies, Science, and Technical Subjects (Council of Chief State School Officers [CCSSO] & National Governors Association Center for Best Practices [NGA Center], 2010) have brought comprehension instruction into a new era with their call to focus more on complex expository text with integrated academic vocabulary to prepare students for college, career, and life. Although the standards for English Language Arts have been set, decisions about exactly what to teach and how to teach it have been deferred to states, districts, schools, and teachers. Although that sounds promising, schools unfortunately are not excelling in teaching students to be proficient readers.

The latest report from the National Assessment of Educational Progress (NAEP; National Assessment Governing Board, 2015) showed that, compared to 2013 scores in reading, 2015 scores are not different at Grade 4 and are lower at

Grade 8. To complicate matters, as recently as 2011, Kucan, Hapgood, and Palincsar noted that 85% of teachers lack a theoretical framework to guide how they teach comprehension. In the past, teachers frequently had students practice specific skills independently, such as finding the main idea. Yet, research by Taylor, Pearson, Peterson, and Rodriguez (2003) has confirmed that these routine, isolated practice-oriented approaches result in much lower growth rates for students' reading comprehension than more strategic approaches. So what supports do teachers need to meet these evolving standards for reading instruction?

MAJOR SHIFTS IN READING COMPREHENSION INSTRUCTION

The CCSS web site (http://www.corestandards.org) cited several key shifts in the standards for English Language Arts.

1. Regular practice with complex texts and their academic language. This shift calls for a progressive development of reading comprehension, with attention paid to informational text gradually increasing as students move through the grades. In the first Appendix of the CCSS (http://www.corestandards.org/assets/Appendix_A .pdf), a rationale for this progression is presented:

> In brief, while reading demands in college, workforce training programs, and life in general have held steady or increased over the last half century, K–12 texts have actually declined in sophistication, and relatively little attention has been paid to students' ability to read complex texts independently. These conditions have left a serious gap between many high school seniors' reading ability and the reading requirements they will face after graduation. (p. 2)

The CCSS evaluate text complexity through attention to three areas (Core Standards Appendix, pp. 4, 5, 7):

- Qualitative dimensions of text complexity (particularly "levels of meaning, structure, language conventionality and clarity, and knowledge demands")

- Quantitative dimensions of text complexity (including "readability measures and other scores of text complexity") (*Note:* A broader discussion of text complexity can be found in Hiebert and Pearson [2014].)

- Reader and task considerations (attention to "reader variables such as motivation, knowledge and experiences and task variables, such as purpose and the complexity generated by the task assigned and questions posed").

Within this recommendation is an additional focus on increasing student mastery of academic vocabulary that can appear in a variety of content areas (National Assessment Governing Board, 2015). Baumann and Graves (2010) noted two general categories of academic vocabulary that are commonly used. They defined "domain-specific academic vocabulary" as words used in disciplines such as biology, geometry, civics, and geography (e.g., *photosynthesis, isosceles*). The second category, "general academic vocabulary," includes broader terms that appear across content areas (e.g., *ignite, form, process*). The broad impact a robust knowledge of academic vocabulary can have on comprehension has been confirmed many times (see Miller, 2002; Marzano, 2012; Nagy & Townsend, 2012).

2. Reading, writing, and speaking grounded in evidence from texts, both literary and informational. This recommendation marks a shift away from answering questions that can be answered primarily from students' background knowledge and experience and a move toward questions that require a close reading of the text. Text-dependent questions should require inferences drawn from students' reading.

Fisher and Frey (2012) presented useful guidelines for teachers to explore the qualities and uses of text-dependent questions as well as examples thereof. Text-dependent questions require that students go back to the text to locate evidence supporting their responses. Recall should not be the focus of those questions, the authors caution: "The emphasis should be on using explicit and implicit information from the text to support reasoning" (2012, p. 70). Fisher and Frey explored a progression of six categories of text-dependent questions, increasing in text complexity from general understandings and key details, through vocabulary and text structure, author's purpose, inferences, and finally opinions, arguments, and intertextual connections. McKenna (2002) suggested "clustering questions," beginning with clusters of literal questions and following that with an inference question. The use of literal questions helps the reader to elicit information from the text that will assist him or her to draw an appropriate inference.

Examples of text-dependent questions across these categories with links to specific texts can be found in Fisher and Frey's article (2012, pp. 71–73). Examples are also available on many web sites, including Achieve the Core (see http://achievethecore.org/category/1158/ela-literacy-text-dependent-questions).

3. Building knowledge through content-rich nonfiction. The importance of students being immersed in information about the world around them so that they can gain general knowledge and vocabulary is stressed here. For 4th grade, the recommended percentage of passages is split equally between literary and informational passages, but by 12th grade, literary passages are expected to comprise 30% of students' reading, with the suggestion that informational passages comprise 70%. Coupled with this is a recommendation that assessments echo this distribution. Targeted categories of question types are also shifting. For example, fourth-grade percentage targets for questions addressing different cognitive skills range from 30% for locating/recalling information to 50% for integrating/interpreting information and 20% for critiquing and evaluating information. Those percentage targets shift to 20%, 50%, and 30% by 12th grade (National Assessment Governing Board, 2008).

As of this writing, 42 states, four territories, and the District of Columbia have adopted the CCSS. (See http://www.corestandards.org/standards-in-your-state/ for most current information.) Twenty-one states are revising the standards, but most of those are not making significant changes. The vast majority of changes involve clarifying wording and not content in order to make the standards more accessible to educators and the public (Sparks, 2017).

Setting these standards is one thing, but providing support for teachers to meet them is an entirely different issue. The results of a recent *Education Week* survey of teachers from elementary, middle, and high schools in states that have adopted the standards yielded very mixed reviews about their experiences with professional development, resources, and other aspects of the standards. Although teachers' confidence about their general ability to teach the standards in their classes is growing, few teachers polled expressed confidence in their skills to teach students who are learning English, students who have disabilities, academically at-risk students, and low-income students (Zubrzycki, 2017). Yet, the standards expect all students to be successful in reaching these new goals. Also troubling is the fact that more teachers indicate that they know the CCSS, but they are less positive about adequate materials available to them and professional development to assist their implementation of the standards. The information presented in this chapter will hopefully support teachers' understanding of "what works" for teaching a wide range of students how to comprehend increasingly complex text in both narrative and expository formats.

> ### REFLECT, CONNECT, and RESPOND
> What instructional goals for reading comprehension are emphasized within the CCSS? How have these goals influenced the ways schools and teachers approach reading instruction?

RESEARCH-VALIDATED TARGETED AREAS FOR INSTRUCTION IN READING

The five Pillars of Reading introduced by the National Reading Panel in 2000 essentially remain with new studies reaffirming their validity (Butler, Urrutia, Buenger, & Hunt, 2010). Research support for instruction in phonics, phonemic awareness, fluency, reading comprehension, and vocabulary to ensure skilled reading continues. However, the introduction of the CCSS for Kindergarten through 12th grade in English Language Arts has provoked a shift of emphasis. These standards have established the key goal of supporting students' ability to comprehend increasingly challenging literary and informational texts in any printed or electronic form in order to prepare them for college and careers. Decisions about what and how to teach are reserved for the states, but the standards clearly emphasize a more profound focus on expository texts, beginning as early as kindergarten. As a result, more attention needs to be paid to determining effective strategies to meet this goal and evaluate progress toward achieving it. It has also led to growth of Internet-based and technology resources that can give these students some of the support they need to meet their literacy goals. These resources are discussed later in the chapter.

The primary factors affecting a skilled reader's comprehension of text have not changed. They include the following (Carlisle & Rice, 2002):

- Accurate, fluent word reading

- A broad base of vocabulary knowledge

- Access to robust background knowledge

- An awareness of sentence, paragraph, and text structure

- Ongoing monitoring of comprehension

- Application of strategies where appropriate

In addition to these basics, some new areas of concern have arisen relatively recently. For example, with the growth of response to intervention (RTI) as a framework for evaluating the effectiveness of strategies used with struggling students, educators have been compelled to determine best practices to monitor progress in comprehension (see Chapter 7 on assessment for more about progress monitoring). Comprehension challenges facing English language learners (ELLs) have taken a more visible place in the field (see Chapter 19 for information about language and literacy development among ELLs). Finally, the growing call to apply comprehension skills judiciously to Internet content has invigorated discussion among researchers and practitioners.

This chapter explores some of the more pressing challenges educators face related to reading comprehension. How can they best tackle obstacles their students face when they are asked to comprehend a wide range of texts? After a brief history of how comprehension instruction has changed since the 1960s, this chapter presents a developmental framework for comprehension, followed by a review of research-supported strategies as well as other promising methods designed to improve this essential reading skill within a multisensory learning environment.

A HISTORICAL PERSPECTIVE ON COMPREHENSION

Although Durkin (1993) described reading comprehension as the "essence of reading" and Adams, Treiman, and Pressley (1998) described it as the "ultimate goal of reading education," much of the reading research before 2000 focused on understanding the development of word reading as well as improving instruction for children who struggle with reading at the word level. During the more limited occasions when instructional strategies for comprehension were proposed, they were rarely validated by controlled studies to see whether their adoption improved student performance (for reviews, see Adams et al., 1998).

Comprehension instruction was largely absent from classrooms throughout the 1960s and 1970s (Durkin, 1979; Williams, 1987). Durkin's observational studies of reading instruction in fourth-grade classrooms revealed that during more than 4,000 minutes of reading, only 20 minutes of comprehension instruction were observed. Instead of the focus being on teaching comprehension, the spotlight was on testing it. Research conducted in the late 1990s showed that attention to comprehension in instruction was still woefully underrepresented in classrooms (Pressley, 2000; Taylor, Pearson, Clark, & Walpole, 1999). More recent research unfortunately has not indicated any appreciable improvement in instructional time devoted to comprehension instruction (Dewitz, Leahy, Jones, & Sullivan, 2010). In addition, there is no indication that instruction is getting better as students progress through the grades. In 2009, a study was published indicating that in secondary content area classrooms, only 3% of instructional time was devoted to teaching effective comprehension strategies (Ness, 2009).

For many years, students were required to answer questions included at the end of packaged reading selections as a way of testing comprehension and sometimes stimulating discussion and/or reflection. This was done even though little thought had been given to the steps readers go through to process and understand what they read. Most often, teachers spent no time instructing students about the strategies required to answer those questions (Maria, 1990). At best, if difficulties were noted in responding to questions after reading a text, a quick dip into a specific skill exercise (e.g., finding the main idea, drawing inferences, determining sequence) was a common recommended prescription (and frequently the only one). There was little, if any, transfer to real text reading. Allington (2001) labeled this approach "assign and assess" because no instruction was provided with the materials used. This method rarely met students' needs. Activities were usually completed silently, with no direct instruction. Students were expected to acquire useful comprehension strategies through self-discovery, but many students were not able to discover effective reading strategies without teacher modeling.

Through the 2000s, a great deal of reading comprehension instruction was constructivist in nature, although this has shifted slightly in response to the CCSS's emphasis on textual evidence, as discussed in the next section. A constructivist approach focuses on the distinctive knowledge base each reader brings to the text and results in a unique interpretation of the text for each reader (Williams, 2002). The role of the teacher in this model is one of facilitator. Instruction is organized around discussion, with each student contributing his or her own interpretation that can be expanded and refined as discussion evolves.

CLOSE READING

As noted by Serafini, the concept of close reading "permeates the CCSS and suggests a particular way of reading and responding to texts" (2013/2014, p. 299). The "Anchor Standards" for College and Career Readiness for Reading, highlighted in the English Language Arts Standards within the CCSS, require students to read closely to "determine what the text says explicitly and to make logical inferences from it and cite specific textual evidence when writing or speaking to support conclusions drawn from the text" (CCSSO & NGA Center, 2010). Serafini went on to say how this focus on the specific content of the text demands that readers pay increased attention to "the language and structure of texts; various elements of literature, such as plot, character, and setting; figures of speech, for example, metaphors and symbols, and the use of symbols, motifs, and literary archetypes" (2013/2014, p. 300). Focusing on the explicit text marks a shift away from teachers' encouragement of readers making personal connections to what they are reading and recording those responses in literature response journals (Keene & Zimmerman, 1997; Miller, 2002). Not all researchers in reading agree with this shift, however. Serafini, for example, cautions:

> Readers make sense of the texts they encounter not by staying within the four corners of a text, but by using their background knowledge of the world; their previous experiences with text; their understandings of language; the context of the text's production, dissemination, and reception; *and* the text itself to construct meaning. (2013/2014, p. 301)

> ### REFLECT, CONNECT, and RESPOND
> How does current reading instruction strike a balance between close reading and constructivist approaches? How does this differ from the approaches reading teachers typically used during the latter decades of the 20th century?

STRATEGIES USED BY GOOD READERS

Much of the research conducted in the past about reading comprehension focused on strategies used by good readers. Table 16.1 outlines the differences between behaviors of good and poor readers before, during, and after reading. Good readers have many strengths that prevent them from encountering the pitfalls experienced by less skilled readers. For example, good readers understand the complexities of the reading process. They can identify key ideas from the text they are reading, and they are aware of text structures that can assist their comprehension (e.g., headings, subheadings). Good readers rarely allow themselves to get too lost in the text they are reading. They monitor their comprehension and know how to

Table 16.1.   Behaviors of good and poor readers before, during, and after reading

Good readers	Poor readers
Before reading	
Activate prior knowledge	Begin to read without preparation
Understand what they need to do and set a purpose for reading	Are unaware of their purpose for reading
Are self-motivated to read	Tend to read only because they have to
Make positive self-statements about their progress	Make negative self-statements about their progress
Choose strategies that are appropriate for the task	Begin to read without any specific plan or strategy in mind
During reading	
Are focused	Are distracted easily
Monitor their understanding as it is occurring	Are often unaware of their lack of understanding
Anticipate and predict what is likely to happen next	Read just to get it over with
Are able to use fix-up strategies if their comprehension gets off track	Do not know what to do to help themselves if they begin to lose understanding
Can use context to understand the meaning	Do not recognize which new vocabulary is important
Recognize and use text structure to support their comprehension	Do not recognize any organization within the text
Organize and integrate new information	Tend to add on rather than integrate new information with what they already know
After reading	
Think about what was read	Stop both reading and thinking
Summarize main ideas in some manner	
Seek more information from other sources	
Affirm that their success is a result of their effort	Believe that any success they experience is a result of luck

From Deshler, D.D., Ellis, E.S., & Lenz, B.K. (1996). *Teaching adolescents with learning disabilities: Strategies and methods* (2nd ed., p. 68). Denver, CO: Love Publishing. Originally adapted by Deshler et al. (1996) from Grover, H., Cook, D., Benson, J., & Chandler, A. (1991). *Strategic learning in the content areas.* Madison: Wisconsin Department of Public Instruction.

employ fix-up strategies (often re-reading) to get back on track before they have gone too far astray. Good readers tend to have a stronger background knowledge and vocabulary foundation than poor readers. They have knowledge of a variety of reading strategies and use them effectively. They are flexible in adjusting their understanding of the topic to fit in new information.

In contrast to the powerful behaviors of good readers, poor readers have a weak understanding of the variables that are part of the reading process. They struggle to separate important from unimportant information in text. They are often unaware of text structures that could aid their understanding. Even if they do not understand what they are reading, they still continue reading until the end. Completing the task, rather than understanding the text, becomes the primary goal. Finally, poor readers do not make adjustments in their background knowledge to accommodate the new information they are acquiring. Instead, they make adjustments in the information they are absorbing so that it fits with their previous understanding (Deshler, Ellis, & Lenz, 1996).

> **REFLECT, CONNECT, and RESPOND**
> Review the strategies listed in this section, and list three key differences between what good readers do and what weaker readers do when they read a text. Have you ever observed these or other behavioral differences in the classroom? Jot down notes about what differences in reading behavior look like among students with whom you work.

SOURCES OF COMPREHENSION DIFFICULTIES

Individuals who are strong comprehenders bring much to the complexities of the reading task. They carry with them rich experience with literacy and an understanding of text structure; strong oral language ability; breadth of background knowledge (including understanding of both high-utility and content-specific vocabulary); accurate, fluent decoding skills; and efficient, active comprehension strategies, including monitoring their understanding of their interactions with text (Gambrell, Block, & Pressley, 2002; Shaywitz, 2003). Individuals who struggle to comprehend may have deficits in any one of these areas. In addition, the source of difficulty may change as students age (Aaron, Joshi, & Williams, 1999). For example, Aaron and colleagues (1999) reported that weak word-reading skill was the major contributor to poor reading comprehension for third graders, but by fifth and sixth grades, word reading and listening comprehension played equal roles in comprehension performance, with word-reading fluency also playing a crucial role.

Most teachers would agree that two essential tools required for good reading comprehension are strong general language comprehension skills and accurate, fluent word-reading skills (Gough, 1996; Torgesen, 1998). Comprehension cannot occur without them. Discussions of these factors have dominated the literature. For many years, educators believed that when individuals had at least average intelligence and could decode accurately and fluently, good reading comprehension would naturally follow (Allington, 2001; McNeil, 1987). Few would deny the critical importance of accurate, fluent decoding as a requirement for strong comprehension (Adams, 1990; Ehri, 1998; see Chapters 9 and 12 for more on this topic). However, there has been a growing awareness of other factors that promote successful development of skilled comprehension of text. For example, a robust as well as active prior knowledge base, a rich vocabulary foundation (see Chapter 15), and employment of metacognitive strategies are also fundamental components of the reading process.

Dyslexia and Comprehension Difficulties

Individuals with dyslexia, although certainly not the only group who may struggle with comprehension issues, have the most profound difficulty with reading text in general. Dyslexia is a language-based disorder, and some individuals with dyslexia may have more pronounced deficits in language beyond difficulty with written language comprehension. Individual deficits in oral language, syntax, morphology, semantics, pragmatics, and understanding narrative structure will negatively affect reading comprehension for those individuals with more global language impairments. (See Chapter 3 for more about the relationship between oral language and reading.)

Many times, however, an individual with dyslexia's difficulty with language is much more apparent at the word-reading level. Students with dyslexia as well as other individuals with poor reading performance may appear to be poor comprehenders when, in reality, their difficulties lie in decoding accuracy and reading fluency. If an individual has strong listening comprehension skills but stumbles when asked to demonstrate understanding of something read independently, it is often because higher order thinking and reasoning skills cannot be accessed until the words on the page can be read accurately and fluently. Individuals who have dyslexia, as well as those with general decoding weaknesses, must allocate their efforts to sound out words strategically at the expense of using that same effort to monitor comprehension strategically (Rose & Dalton, 2002). Pressley stated it succinctly: "If the word-level processes are not mastered (i.e., recognition of most words is not automatic), it will be impossible to carry out the higher order processes that are summarized as reading comprehension strategies" (2000, p. 551).

Balancing Fluency and Comprehension

Another group of individuals is not able to maintain the balance between reading fluency and reading comprehension. They focus too much on the word level and fail to derive meaning from what has been read. When asked what is the most important part of reading, getting all of the words right or understanding what has been read, they answer without hesitation, "Getting all of the words right." They miss the point of reading; they are not always aware of when they become lost in the text; and, if they are aware, they lack the active comprehension strategies needed to get themselves back on track. One of the most important benefits of the latest focus on strategy use is that it encourages readers to recognize that the goal of reading is to gain meaning and to monitor their progress toward that goal on a continuous basis (Willingham, 2006/2007).

REFLECT, CONNECT, and RESPOND
Struggling readers with or without disabilities may focus heavily on decoding words and reading words fluently. How does this affect their comprehension of the text?

The Role of Background Knowledge in Reading Comprehension

Gaps in background knowledge and weak vocabulary development can have a significant effect on comprehending text (Hirsch, 2003, 2006; McKeown & Beck, 1990; Stahl, 1991; Willingham, 2007). Most widely used basal reading programs unfortunately do not offer the strong background knowledge that students need to develop more sophisticated reading skills (Dewitz et al., 2010; Walsh, 2003). Broadening readers' exposure to nonfiction texts is one important path students can take to deepen their background knowledge and enrich their vocabularies. Yet, Moss (2008) noted a significant gap between the NAEP's recommendation for inclusion of nonfiction texts and what was actually found in two widely used basal reading programs in California. In addition, poor readers often struggle to understand how and when to use their background knowledge to generate missing details or bolster weak connections in text (Cain & Oakhill, 1999).

Hirsch, who founded the Core Knowledge Foundation in 1986, has probably done more to draw attention to the role of background knowledge in facilitating comprehension than anyone. Hirsch draws on the work of Hart and Risley (1995), who documented the extreme gap in vocabulary development in children from different socioeconomic backgrounds, comparing low-income households receiving public assistance to working-class and professional households. Hirsch proposed that the dramatic drop in scores on national reading tests experienced by students in the fourth grade who come from low-income families arises because of a large language gap between advantaged and disadvantaged students. He also observed that reading tests in earlier grades are heavily focused on testing more basic reading skills such as decoding, and it is not until fourth grade that the differences in vocabulary and background knowledge show their effect (Hirsch, 2003).

Lack of adequate background knowledge can have a particularly negative effect on higher level comprehension skills such as inferencing (Willingham, 2006). Authors frequently use a verbal shorthand to communicate ideas. For example, a story about a character "meeting his Waterloo" is an abbreviated way of communicating his defeat. If the reader has no background knowledge of Bonaparte's defeat at Waterloo, however, then he or she will be hard pressed to make sense of the reference. Students who have a rich fund of background knowledge process new information more deeply, make more significant connections between what is new and what is known, and, in general, will learn more (Willingham, 2006).

Probably the most widely used approach to building background knowledge through the grades has been through teacher read-alouds addressing rich content materials coupled with audiovisual supports and engaging discussion. For a more systematic approach to incorporating specific content into instruction, Hirsch's (2009) Core Knowledge Sequence for students in kindergarten through Grade 8 has been adopted by many schools, and in 2004, the American Federation of Teachers recommended this program to fill the background knowledge gap for children in these grades. Today, there is also a wide assortment of audio-supported books available. Learning Ally (http://www.learningally.org) provides human-narrated audio textbooks and literature that allow students with documented print disabilities to maintain connections to the current curriculum, even if they lack the reading skills to tackle these texts independently. Text-to-speech software available on most computers is an assistive technology tool that allows anyone to see any text on the screen and hear it read aloud at the same time. Sometimes a computer-generated voice is used, but Apple computers, for example, allow the selection of a variety of human voices with varying speeds of presentation. Also see Appendix 16.4: Supplementary Materials for more ideas and helpful resources.

REFLECT, CONNECT, and RESPOND
How can differences in students' socioeconomic circumstances contribute to gaps in reading comprehension? What can reading teachers do to close these gaps?

CONTINUUM OF COMPREHENSION DEVELOPMENT WITHIN A MULTISENSORY TEACHING ENVIRONMENT

The continuum of comprehension development begins at the word level and progresses through increasingly complex units of text. The more students are actively involved in their learning, the more the retention and application of strategies are apparent. Students with dyslexia as well as others with poor reading skills benefit from multisensory learning that captures their attention. Involving at least two or more modalities in teaching simultaneously helps students to solidify their grasp of the strategies they are being taught (see Chapter 2).

When Adams and her colleagues (1998) reviewed research on reading comprehension instruction, they concluded that silent reading and independent seat work were not nearly as effective as active verbal modeling by the teacher coupled with active, vocal student practice of basic comprehension techniques, including summarizing, questioning, and predicting. This model of active involvement by both student and teacher may begin at the earliest levels of instruction.

Aural activities coupled with opportunities for students to articulate the strategies they are using to comprehend text are good ways to begin comprehension instruction. Creating and using visual representations of the text's organization as well as its content through graphic organizers adds yet another modality. As students gain in skill, they can demonstrate their understanding through drawing or writing. Examples of specific strategies to involve students actively as they create meaning from text are woven throughout the rest of this chapter.

Beginning Comprehension Instruction

Planning for instruction must begin with a good assessment (see Chapter 7). Is a student having difficulty reading the words with accuracy and fluency? How extensive (and accurate) is the student's prior knowledge? Vocabulary? Does the size of the text affect the student's comprehension?

Can the student make sense of what he or she reads when only a sentence or a short paragraph is presented? What happens when the individual is asked to retell what he or she has read? Is the student able to make connections between what is known and what is new? Can the individual answer questions when answers are explicitly stated in the text? Is there evidence of higher level thinking, or is the student bound to the concrete level of understanding? Is there evidence of self-monitoring of comprehension, or is the student merely "word-calling?" Is there any evidence of active repair strategies if something read obviously does not make sense? Is there a difference between the student's silent and oral reading comprehension? What about listening comprehension? All of these are important questions that need to be explored to determine which strategies will be most effective for which students.

Developing Listening Comprehension Skills

Students who have dyslexia and others who have not yet mastered decoding skills need not wait until they become fluent readers to begin addressing comprehension. Instruction can be started early by bypassing reading altogether and focusing instead on an aural level (Williams, 2002). Reading high-quality narratives and rich informational texts can also play an important role in building and expanding important background knowledge and vocabulary.

Kindergarten and even preschool-age children can improve their comprehension performance through experiences that support both oral language and reading skills. If students have adequate listening skills, then stories can be read to them and oral discussion can be the mode of instruction. Students can be encouraged to "read" picture books to hone their comprehension skills. Describing the characters and actions in pictures begins the process of comprehension. It also sets the tone for helping students to focus on what factors come into play in comprehending text. Students can listen to stories read by older students, parents, teachers, and other adults. At this age, students can participate in analytic conversations in which they practice connecting events in stories with their own experiences. They can learn about predictable story structure and use graphic organizers, such as story maps, to aid their recall and retelling of stories. They can be engaged in drawing inferences, making predictions, analyzing characters, and following sequences of events. They can be exposed to rich vocabulary and background knowledge within meaningful contexts. Teachers can begin modeling their own thinking at this early level.

Visual presentations (e.g., short films or stories on CD-ROMs coupled with conventional text stories) may entice young children's attention and draw them more deeply into stories they hear. A word of caution is necessary here, however. If the ultimate goal is reading comprehension, then nontext presentation should not be overemphasized. That would reduce the amount of textual language the children hear, and familiarity with the linguistic features of written language fosters the acquisition of reading comprehension (Williams, 2002).

Developing Reading Comprehension at the Sentence Level

There are times when decoding and fluency are in place, yet an individual still struggles to gain meaning from the page. Once students have adequate decoding skills to begin to read independently, the unit size of the presentation must be considered. Some students may need to begin at the word level as they develop their understanding of the meanings of single words (see Chapter 14), whereas the sentence level may be the most appropriate starting point for other students. A wide range of studies has shown that there is a strong association between a robust grasp of sentence grammar and reading performance (Fowler, 1988; Siegel & Ryan, 1988; Weaver, 1979). Children with good grammatical awareness may be able to monitor their oral reading accuracy better (Cain, 2007; Carlisle & Rice, 2002).

Carnine, Silbert, and Kame'enui (1990) described a sequence of sentence comprehension activities designed to teach students how to identify what has happened in a sentence, who was involved, when the event occurred, where the event took place, and why the event happened. Using this strategy can serve as a foundation for comprehension activities using larger chunks of text later.

The question words *who, what, when, where, why,* and *how* are used during this exercise. A prerequisite skill for engaging in this activity is the ability to repeat five- to seven-word statements (e.g., *The girl skipped up the street. The boy jumped over the fence*). If individuals cannot retain the information in a sentence long enough to repeat it, then they are unlikely to be able to recall the information needed from those sentences to answer simple questions. Although not presented by the authors of this strategy, a possible option for students who have difficulty recalling information presented orally may be to have them *see* the complete sentence and parse it that way.

Instruction begins with the introduction of *who* and *what* questions and is followed by extensive practice until the students can answer questions independently. A model for instruction utilizing this strategy may be found in Appendix 16.5 in the Online Companion Materials.

It is not enough, however, to require students to identify syntactical elements and explain their function. Carlisle and Rice (2002) promoted having students dig deeper into the internal structure of sentences by creating, combining, and expanding sentences. Although they admitted that these strategies have not been evaluated with children with reading or learning disabilities in controlled research studies, they reported that clinical experience of several reading experts including Maria (1990) and McNeil (1987) have suggested that they are helpful for struggling readers. Eisenberg (2006) also highlighted the positive effects of sentence combining on reading comprehension for school-age children with language impairments.

Helping students to become more familiar with the role of conjunctions in compound and complex sentences may be particularly useful for building sentence comprehension. Carlisle and Rice (2002) advised teaching conjunctions in related groups, including teaching those that express "adversative" roles (e.g., *but, however, even though*) with those that play causal roles (e.g., *so, because, as a result*). Among the activities they recommended are highlighting conjunctions in text to draw students' attention to them, rewording sentences using different but similar conjunctions such as *but* and *even though,* and combining sentences using specific conjunctions.

A student's lack of understanding of pronoun referents or cohesive ties is another common obstacle to sentence comprehension (Carlisle & Rice, 2002). Helping students match cohesive ties with their antecedents is helpful in this regard. For example, suppose students read the following sentences:

Sally ran down the stairs to the parlor on Christmas morning to open her gifts. Her sister, Mary, got there before her.

The teacher might ask: Whose sister is Mary? Where did Mary go?

Carlisle and Rice suggested other activities, including deleting pronouns from a passage and then having students fill in the blanks, having students substitute pronouns for unnecessarily repeated names, and identifying strategies that they might use when pronoun referents are ambiguous (e.g., reading on in the text for further clues).

A useful series by Carlisle (1999) also addressed the "anatomy" of the sentence, emphasizing the relationships between sentence parts, including cause and effect, chronology, and comparisons. Once students demonstrate understanding of the application of these important concepts at the simple sentence level, they may be asked to respond to multiple sentences, paragraphs, and eventually longer texts.

REFLECT, CONNECT, and RESPOND

Why is it important for teachers to build students' listening comprehension and comprehension of written sentences in addition to working with longer texts?

GOOD READER STRATEGIES FOR COMPREHENDING LONGER TEXTS

A major goal for teachers of reading is to teach poor readers to use strategies that good readers use spontaneously. Can this be done? The explicit teaching of reading comprehension strategies has fortunately been highly effective (Deshler, Ellis, & Lenz, 1996; National Institute of Child Health and Human Development [NICHD], 2000; Sweet & Snow, 2002). It is one thing, however, to be able to demonstrate that a student has mastered the steps to a reading comprehension strategy but quite another to have evidence that using the strategy has been generalized to daily reading experiences. Students need to know not only how to operationalize the strategies but also why they are learning them and under what conditions they should apply them. Mason and Au (1986) outlined six steps to ensure that comprehension strategies will not only be learned but also applied:

1. Set the stage by discussing how reading activity changes depending on the purpose for reading and the nature of the text.

2. Explain and model the steps in the strategy. Begin with clear, simple examples.

3. Present more than one situation or one kind of text in which the strategy would be useful.

4. Provide many opportunities for practice, starting with easy examples.

5. Encourage students to think out loud when they use the strategy so that they can correct misunderstandings or mistakes.

6. Have students suggest times and conditions when they would use the strategy on their own. When these occasions arise, remind students to use the strategy.

Research-Validated Strategies for Comprehension Instruction

With the Reading First program, a component of the No Child Left Behind Act of 2001 (PL 107-110), major financial awards were made available to states that demonstrated that they were using scientifically based reading programs in their schools. The result was a flood of interest in scientifically validated strategies to improve instruction. A foundation of research has been building that shows which cognitive processes are involved in text comprehension and which comprehension strategies are most effective for improving the skills of students who struggle to understand what they read.

Once researchers have a good picture of what is working and what is ineffective when a student reads, the next question is how to choose which strategies to teach. How do researchers know which strategies are truly effective? In 1997, an important step was taken in gathering and disseminating information about the effectiveness of different approaches used to teach children to read. At that time, Congress approached the Director of NICHD at the National Institutes of Health, in consultation with the Secretary of Education, to form a national panel to review research-based knowledge on reading instruction. The result of this collaboration was the *Report of the National Reading Panel* (NRP; NICHD, 2000). Evaluating reading comprehension was one of the research areas the panel chose to evaluate.

After identifying almost 500 studies on comprehension published since 1970, the NRP (NICHD, 2000) applied a strict selection process, choosing only those studies that were relevant to instruction of reading or comprehension among typical readers; were published in a scientific journal; had an experiment involving at least one treatment and an appropriate control group; and, if possible, had random assignment of subjects to treatment and control groups. Application of these criteria whittled the number of studies down to about 200. Before conclusions could be drawn about the effectiveness of the strategies selected, the next step for the panel was to select only those studies that had an experimental effect that was "reliable, robust, replicable, and general" (p. 4-42).

The NRP (NICHD, 2000) identified 16 categories of comprehension instruction, 7 of which appear to have a strong scientific basis for concluding that they improve comprehension in typical readers:

1. Comprehension monitoring, in which readers learn how to be aware of their level of understanding as they read

2. Cooperative learning, in which students work together in pairs or small groups as they learn reading strategies

3. **Graphic** and **semantic organizers** (including **story maps**) that help students make graphic representations of the material they are reading in order to bolster comprehension

4. Question answering, in which teachers ask questions and students receive immediate feedback about their responses

5. Question generation, in which students ask themselves questions to clarify understanding

6. **Story structure,** in which students learn how to use the structure of the text to help them recall content to answer questions about what they have read

7. Summarization, to encapsulate and remember important ideas from the text

Many of these strategies have also been included in an eighth category, multiple strategies. In general, the research suggested that teaching a combination of techniques to bolster comprehension works the best (NICHD, 2000). When these seven strategies are used appropriately, they improve recall, question answering, question generation, summarization of text, and ultimately result in improved performance on standardized comprehension tests.

Although not identified as one of the "super seven" strategy categories, the other eight categories (integrating strategies into the normal curriculum, listening actively, mental imagery, **mnemonics** [including pictorial aids and key words], building prior knowledge, **psycholinguistic strategies** relating to learning relevant knowledge about language, teacher preparation to learn effective transactional strategies, and the vocabulary–comprehension relationship) should not be dismissed. Many were eliminated because there were simply too few studies in a category to determine the scientific merit of the treatment. Two categories in particular, building prior knowledge (discussed earlier in this chapter) and the vocabulary–comprehension relationship (see Chapter 15), have risen to prominence in the recent literature. The strong research base for the "super seven" strategy categories cannot be denied, however.

Comprehension Monitoring   Pressley, Brown, El-Dinary, and Afflerbach wrote that comprehension monitoring may be defined as "the active awareness of whether one is understanding or remembering text being processed" (1995, p. 218). Comprehension monitoring can also be seen as one of the two components of self-regulation as they apply to reading: 1) monitoring and evaluating comprehension and 2) implementing strategies when comprehension breaks down (Klingner, Vaughn, Dimino, Schumm, & Bryant, 2001). The second component may also be looked at as "strategic effort" (RAND Reading Study Group [RRSG], 2002). The temptation to go on automatic pilot and just read on is common for nonstrategic, weak readers. They are much less likely to be tuned in to the need for comprehension monitoring than strong readers (Oakhill & Yuill, 1996).

The goals of comprehension monitoring are to help readers to become aware of whether they are understanding a text as they read and, equally important, to help them identify where their understanding has been blocked. Children as young as first graders can be taught to ask themselves questions as they read and monitor their understanding:

- Does this make sense?

- Do I understand what I am reading?

- What does this have to do with what I already know?

- What will happen next?

Steps readers can take when their comprehension monitoring reveals a roadblock to their understanding include

- Identifying the difficulty

- Using **think-aloud** procedures that highlight where and when the difficulty began

- Restating what was read

- Looking back through the text (re-reading)

- Looking forward in the text to find information that might help (reading ahead)

When comprehension-monitoring strategies were taught to students in second through sixth grade in the studies reviewed by the NRP (NICHD, 2000), improved detection of text inconsistencies and memory of the text were noted as compared with the performance of control groups. In addition, students also made gains on standardized reading comprehension tests. Transfer and generalization of this strategy were critical outcomes of instruction.

Cooperative Learning   Diversity in classrooms has been increasing dramatically since the 1990s. In addition to rising numbers of children who come from homes where English is not the first language (Hodgkinson, 1991), more children are coming from families below the poverty level (Pallas, Natriello, & McDill, 1989). Also, growing populations of children with disabilities are appearing in general education classrooms. The typical range of academic performance in urban classrooms is 5.4 years (Jenkins, Jewell, Leicester, & Troutner, 1990). Classroom teachers' instructional skills are being challenged as never before as they try to meet the wide range of students' needs. Cooperative or **collaborative learning** is a promising alternative for teaching students with mixed abilities in the same class.

Students are engaged in cooperative learning when involved in clearly defined activities in which they work together to achieve their individual goals. A related approach, collaborative learning, is described by Harris and Hodges as "learning by working together in small groups, so as to understand new information or to create a common product" (1995, p. 35). Research has demonstrated growth in elementary school–age children in reading competence when they work collaboratively on structured activities (Greenwood, Delquadri, & Hall, 1989; Rosenshine & Meister, 1994). The benefits of cooperative learning are clear. The creators of the Collaborative Strategic Reading (CSR) program noted that

> Cooperative learning fosters the development of higher-level reasoning and problem solving skills. Cooperative learning is effective in diverse classrooms that include a wide range of achievement levels, and has been recommended by experts in the fields of multicultural education, English as a second language (ESL), special education and general education. (Klingner et al., 2001, p. 6)

In addition, the NRP's summary evaluation of cooperative learning stated, "Having peers instruct or interact over the use of reading strategies leads to an increase in the learning of the strategies, promotes intellectual discussion and increases reading comprehension" (NICHD, 2000, p. 4-45). The panel also cited the social benefits of this approach in addition to students' increased control over their own learning.

Collaborative Strategic Reading   The From Clunk to Click Collaborative Strategic Reading program is drawn from original research conducted by Klingner, Vaughn, Hughes, Schumm, and Elbaum (1998). It was designed primarily for students in third through eighth grade who are in mixed-level classrooms and are reading expository or content-area text drawn from textbooks. Although the program was designed with middle school students in mind, adaptations for high school students are also included in the instructional materials (Klingner & Vaughn, 2000; Klingner, Vaughn, Boardman, & Swanson, 2012).

Students work together to reach five main goals as they read these content-area selections:

1.   Discuss the material.

2.   Help each other understand it.

3.   Encourage each other to do their best.

4.   Learn collaborative skills while mastering content.

5.   Learn comprehension strategies that are likely to improve reading comprehension.

Each student must participate with a partner or as part of a small group in a cooperative or collaborative learning environment. Students assume specific, meaningful roles within the group as they work on clearly outlined tasks. In some programs, students may exchange roles as part of their activity. All students contribute to the overall success of the group. In this CSR program, at least three roles are essential: leader, "clunk" expert, and "gist" expert. Other roles are included in the program, but they may be shared because they require fewer discrete skills: encourager, announcer, and timekeeper. Roles and responsibilities of each member of the group, as described next, are clearly outlined on cue cards or sheets that can be referred to as needed.

- *Leader:* Helps the group stay on track and guides members in using the four strategies: Preview, Click and chunk, Get the gist, and Wrap up.

- *Announcer:* Makes sure that each member of the group participates by sharing his or her good ideas.

- *Clunk expert:* Helps the group members figure out words they do not understand and clarify any misunderstandings they may have.

- *Gist expert:* Works with the group to decide on the best gist (main idea to write in their learning logs for each section of the reading assignment).

- *Encourager:* Watches the group and lets group members know when they are doing something well.

- *Timekeeper:* Helps the group complete the reading assignment in a timely manner.

Each member of the group has a cue sheet. These sheets have scripted dialogue to help students know what to say as they assume their roles. Descriptions of extensive practice activities, including question stems, question types, time allotment sheets, learning logs, and graphic organizers, are included in the manual for the program. (For more information on question types, see the description of the Question-Answer Relationships section.)

This CSR program's plan for strategic reading includes three phases of activity: before reading, during reading, and after reading. Before reading, students preview by brainstorming what they already know about the topic and predicting what they will learn about the topic when they read the passage.

During reading, students identify and repair "clunks," the parts of text that were hard to understand, including challenging vocabulary. See Textbox 16.1 for

---

TEXTBOX 16.1   Clunk expert's cue sheet

1. What is your clunk?

2. Does anyone know the meaning of the clunk?

    YES
    - Announcer, please call on someone with their hand raised.
    - Ask them to explain how they figured out the clunk.
    - Everyone, write the meaning in your Learning Log.

    NO
    - If NO, follow these steps until you know the meaning of the clunk and are ready to write it in your Learning Log.

        STEP 1:   Read the sentence with the clunk and look for key ideas to help you figure out the word. Think about what makes sense.

        Raise your hand if you can explain the meaning of the clunk.
        (If NO, go to STEP 2)

        STEP 2:   Reread the sentence with the clunk and the sentences before and after the clunk looking for clues.

        Raise your hand if you can explain the meaning of the clunk.
        (If NO, go to STEP 3)

        STEP 3:   Look for a prefix or suffix in the word that might help.

        Raise your hand if you can explain the meaning of the clunk.
        (If NO, go to STEP 4)

        STEP 4:   Break the word apart and look for smaller words that you know.

        Raise your hand if you can explain the meaning of the clunk.
        (If NO, go to STEP 5.)

        STEP 5:   Ask the teacher for help.

    From Klingner, J.K., Vaughn, S., Dimino, J., Schumm, J.S., & Bryant, D. (2002). *Collaborative Strategic Reading: Strategies for Improving Comprehension.* Longmont, CO: Sopris West, p. 91; reprinted by permission of Sopris West Educational Services.

a sample cue sheet for the clunk expert that includes examples of fix-up strategies. Students also work at getting the gist of the text during reading. They identify the most important person, place, or thing in the section they are reading and then identify the most important idea about that person, place, or thing.

After reading, students wrap up. They identify which questions will check their understanding of the most important information in the passage and then determine whether they can answer those questions. Finally, they review what they have learned.

Research evaluating the effectiveness of CSR, most of which was conducted after the NRP (NICHD, 2000) review, has been promising. For example, when middle school students in fourth and sixth grade engaged in CSR activities were compared with others in a control group, CSR students outperformed the controls on standardized comprehension tests. Even more encouraging was that students who were low achievers showed the greatest gains (Klingner et al., 2001). Another study showed gains in vocabulary knowledge based on text read by ELLs engaged in CSR (Klingner & Vaughn, 2000). A study reported in 2016 showed that students with learning disabilities who received CSR in general education classrooms made significantly greater gains in reading comprehension than students in comparison classrooms (Boardman et al., 2016).

Peer-Assisted Learning Strategies **Peer-Assisted Learning Strategies (PALS)** is another popular cooperative learning strategy with a strong research base. Although it was originally designed to work in second- through sixth-grade classrooms, kindergarten and high school versions of the strategy have been added. A Spanish manual is also available for Grades 2–6 (Fuchs, Mathes, & Fuchs, 2001).

In the original model, teachers implement three 35-minute PALS sessions each week. Students are paired by the teacher so that a higher and a lower performing student work together. The teacher splits the class in half and pairs the highest performer in the top half of the class with the highest performer in the bottom of the class and so forth. PALS sessions are quite structured and include frequent verbal interaction and feedback between tutor and tutee.

An exchange of roles within the pairs is built in so that each student has the opportunity to assume the role of both tutor and tutee during each session. It is important to note, however, that the higher performing student in each pair reads first for each activity, serving as a model for the lower performing reader. Material chosen for reading is literature that is appropriate for the lower performing reader. Each 35-minute session is divided into three 10-minute segments for partner reading, paragraph shrinking, and prediction relay, plus an additional 2 minutes are used for a retelling activity that follows partner reading. The remaining time is used for setting up and putting away materials during transitions.

The goal of partner reading is to improve reading accuracy and fluency (Simmons, Fuchs, Fuchs, Hodge, & Mathes, 1994). In paragraph shrinking, students develop comprehension through summarizing and identifying the main idea (Doctorow, Wittrock, & Marks, 1978; Palincsar & Brown, 1984). In prediction relay, students practice formulating expectations about what is likely to follow in their reading. Students who practice making predictions have been shown to improve in reading comprehension (Palincsar & Brown, 1984).

Within PALS, pairs of students are assigned to one of two teams. They earn points from the teacher for being engaged in their reading activities and helping their partners in a constructive and collaborative manner. Each student acting as the tutor also awards points as activities are completed successfully. Point cards represent joint effort, progress, and achievement. At the end of each week, the points are tallied for each team, and the winning team is announced and cheered for. Students are assigned to new pairs and new teams every 4 weeks.

Careful training is required to make PALS work in classrooms. Teachers are expected to model key procedures and allow students to role-play them. It usually takes about seven 45-minute sessions for teachers to train their students. The first session is a general orientation in which students learn how set up materials, be a helpful partner, use a scorecard, and report points. After this first orientation session, each of the three reading activities takes about two 45-minute sessions to teach. Teachers are encouraged to teach one PALS activity at a time, taking at least a week to practice an activity before introducing a new one.

PALS has been approved by the U.S. Department of Education's Program Effectiveness Panel for inclusion in the National Diffusion Network of effective educational practices. Research conducted in second- through sixth-grade classes where PALS has been implemented has shown an enhancement of reading development in low and typically achieving students as well as students with learning disabilities (Fuchs, Fuchs, Mathes, & Simmons, 1997; Simmons et al., 1994).

Cue cards that may be used by reading partners are found in Figure 16.1. The content of PALS reading activities may be found in Appendix 16.8 in the Online Companion Materials.

Graphic and Semantic Organizers A graphic or semantic organizer is a visual representation of knowledge. It is essentially a diagram or picture that structures information to demonstrate relationships. Research has shown its

---

Prompt Card 1: Retell

1. What did you learn first?
2. What did you learn next?

Prompt Card 2: Paragraph Shrinking

1. Name the who or what.
2. Tell the most important thing about the who or what.
3. Say the main idea in 10 words or less.

Prompt Card 3: Prediction Relay

Predict _____ What do you predict will happen next?

Read _____ Read half a page.

Check _____ Did the prediction come true?

Figure 16.1. Partner reading question cards from Peer-Assisted Learning Strategy (PALS). (From Fuchs, D., Fuchs, L.S., Simmons, D.C., & Mathes, P.G. [2008]. Partner reading question cards from Peer Assisted Learning Strategy [PALS]. In *Peer assisted learning strategies: Reading methods for grades 2-6, revised edition.* Nashville, TN: Vanderbilt University. © The Fuchs Research Group; reprinted by permission.)

effectiveness for a wide range of purposes (Kim, Vaughn, Wanzek, & Wei, 2004), including the following:

- Generating lists of character traits with supporting evidence within narrative text (See Figure 16.2 for an example of a character map.)

- Deepening understanding of unfamiliar vocabulary (See Figure 16.3 for an example and also Chapter 15 for more on vocabulary word study.)

- Depicting relationships in expository texts in social studies or science (See Figure 16.4 for an example of an animal map.)

- Activating background knowledge and setting a purpose for reading (see Figure 16.5)

- Helping students to see the text structure of stories, which can enhance students' ability to retell stories they have heard or read themselves (see Textbox 16.2)

The NRP, in its review of research on graphic or semantic organizers, cited three important uses for these visual cues: "(1) help students focus on text structure while reading, (2) provide tools to examine and visually represent textual relationships, and (3) assist in writing well-organized summaries" (NICHD, 2000, p. 4–73).

The most robust finding of the studies reviewed by the NRP (NICHD, 2000) was that using graphic organizers can facilitate memory of the content of what has been read for many students. This may be the result of having a means to retrieve information in a more organized manner because clear relationships between

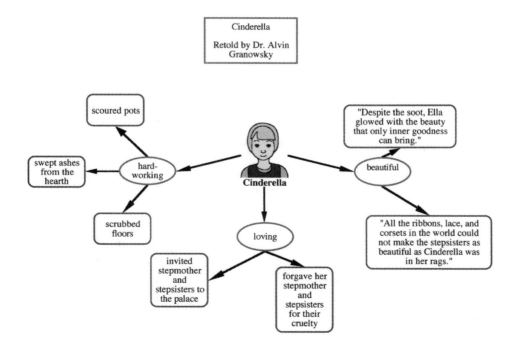

Figure 16.2.   Character map. (Diagram created in Kidspiration® by Inspiration® Software, Inc.) (Text of story from *That Awful Cinderella*, © 1993, Steck-Vaughn. All Rights Reserved. Used with permission of Harcourt Achieve.)

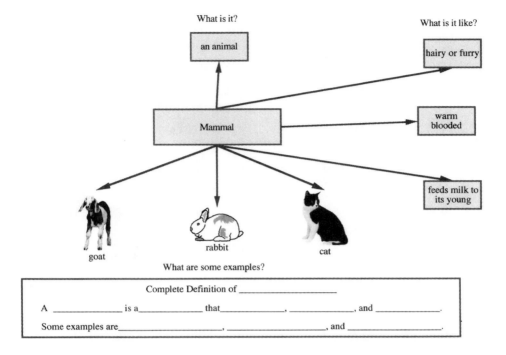

What is it?

an animal

What is it like?

hairy or furry

Mammal

warm blooded

feeds milk to its young

goat

rabbit

cat

What are some examples?

Complete Definition of _____

A _____ is a _____ that_____, _____, and _____.

Some examples are_____, _____, and _____.

Figure 16.3. Word structure map. (Diagram created in Kidspiration® by Inspiration® Software, Inc.)

concepts or events are displayed visually. This may also generalize to better comprehension and achievement, particularly in content-area instruction.

Pearson and Johnson talked about comprehension as the process of "building bridges between the new and the known" (1978, p. 24). If a reader has some accurate and appropriate knowledge of the topic, then that building can be accomplished more easily. K-W-L is one comprehension strategy that uses a structured graphic organizer and has facilitated that process for many struggling readers.

K-W-L (Ogle, 1986) and K-W-L Plus (Carr & Ogle, 1987) are procedures that have been used to help both elementary and secondary students to become more active readers of expository text. The two strategies are essentially the same except that in K-W-L Plus, semantic mapping and written summaries have been added to the three basic K-W-L steps.

K-W-L stands for three basic cognitive steps that are often particularly challenging to students with learning disabilities but that are essential to reading comprehension:

K Accessing what I already **K**now about the topic (activating prior knowledge)

W Deciding what I **W**ant to learn (setting a purpose for reading, including deciding what categories of information or ideas are likely to be discovered)

L Recalling what I **L**earned as a result of my reading (including integrating that new information with what I already know)

The teacher plays a critical role in students' mastering this strategy by acting as both a guide and model for the think-aloud strategies that are essential for

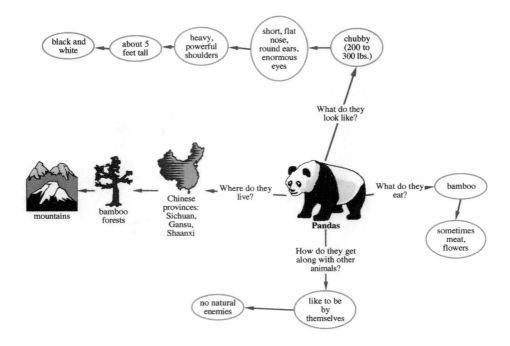

Figure 16.4. Brainstorming map. (Diagram created in Kidspiration® by Inspiration® Software, Inc.)

K-W-L's implementation. Steps for the K-W-L Strategy may be found in Appendix 16.6 in the Online Companion Materials.

The "categories of information we expect to use" section of the K-W-L strategy sheet (Ogle, 1986; see Figure 16.5) is particularly useful for creating written summaries or expanded writing about the topic at hand. For example, when reading a text about an animal, some of the expected categories might be appearance, habitat, food, and behavior. If the topic is a person, then categories might include information about birth, childhood, family influences, education, pivotal life events, important contributions, and death. Each category of information can represent a new paragraph.

Generating these categories early in the K-W-L procedure helps students select and organize information for their writing. Ogle (1986) suggested discussing with students how the results of their brainstorming could help them to generate categories. For example, in the brainstorming graphic organizer about pandas shown in Figure 16.4, student attention could be brought to the fact that many of the terms relate to the way pandas look. The name of a category they can expect to use, therefore, might be appearance. That category would then be written on the bottom of the K-W-L strategy sheet (Ogle, 1986; see Figure 16.5).

The results of research on K-W-L and K-W-L Plus conducted by Carr and Dewitz (1988) indicated that these strategies are effective in helping students learn new social studies content, develop both literal and inferential comprehension, and improve their summary-writing skills. Vaughn and colleagues (2006) noted significant effects for comprehension improvements using K-W-L among other strategies with first-grade ELLs at risk for reading problems. The K-W-L reading strategy is very widely used today in classrooms where students are actively exploring expository text.

KWL Strategy Sheet

1. K—What we know	W—What we want to find out	L—What we learned and still need to learn

2. Categories of information we expect to use

    A.   E.

    B.   F.

    C.   G.

    D.

Figure 16.5. K-W-L strategy sheet. (From Ogle, D.M. [1986, February]. K-W-L: A teaching model that develops active reading of expository text. *The Reading Teacher, 39,* 565; copyright © 1986 by International Reading Association; reprinted by permission.)

The NRPs summary evaluation of graphic and semantic organizer instruction noted students' improvements in remembering what they read after they used this strategy. The panel also suggested that "this may transfer, in general, to better comprehension and achievement in Social Studies and Science content areas" (NICHD, 2000, p. 4-45).

Question Answering Good readers ask themselves questions before, during, and after reading. Yet, many students do not self-question spontaneously. They need to have good models of questioning during all three periods of the reading process to have an effect on their comprehension. Results of the

---

TEXTBOX 16.2 **Story-retelling strategy**

Setting:	Who, What, When, Where
Trouble:	What is the trouble/problem to be solved?
Order of Action:	What happened to solve the problem? (correct/logical order)
Resolution:	What was the outcome (resolution) for each action?
End:	What happened in the end?

From Bos, C.S. (1987). *Promoting story comprehension using a story retelling strategy.* Paper presented at the Teachers Applying Whole Language Conference, Tucson, AZ.

NRP's (NICHD, 2000) review of research on questioning confirmed that teaching question-answering strategies can improve student performance in this area. Teaching these strategies before, during, and after reading can have a positive effect on students' comprehension of text.

Before Reading   Teacher questions before reading can help teachers to evaluate (and if necessary supplement and/or modify) students' prior knowledge about a topic. The *K* segment of the K-W-L strategy outlined previously, for example, functions well in this role. Activating prior knowledge and then organizing it into schema can integrate learning more readily into an existing framework. Asking predictive questions before reading also helps to set readers' purposes for reading and can improve motivation to read. Forming hypotheses about what will happen next has been shown to aid comprehension (Hammond, 1983).

During Reading   Teachers asking questions during reading can help their students to direct their attention to important sections of the text, monitor their comprehension, and serve as a catalyst to get them to activate fix-up strategies when comprehension is blocked.

After Reading   Questions asked after reading can encourage students to reprocess what they have read, thereby creating new associations as they review information. If students are to learn to be good self-questioners, then they need to see their teachers as strong models. Although teachers may ask a question or two before reading to motivate students' interest, questioning by the teacher often functions primarily as an evaluative activity following reading (Durkin, 1979). Questions can have a more far-reaching effect, however, if they are used to teach more than to test. Quality of questions asked, feedback given to student responses, and instruction in how to answer challenging questions are critical to the success of this process.

Attention must obviously be paid to the quality of questions teachers ask. Yet, when researchers have looked at this area, the findings have been dismal. For example, Guszak (1967) observed that about 70% of the questions teachers asked were literal and required only recognition (locating information in the text) or recall (answering from memory) of factual information. Worse yet, the majority of the questions asked neglected literal understanding of essential information presented in stories (e.g., characters, plot, sequence of critical events) in favor of "trivial factual makeup of stories" (1967, p. 233).

Although the need to ask students text-related questions that tap both literal and inferential comprehension is important, questions that extend the discussion beyond the text should also be posed. However, many struggling readers are unsure of what to do if answers to questions are not immediately obvious. Raphael (1982) found that students did not employ effective strategies when reading and answering questions. Instead of applying specific strategies to meet the demands of different kinds of questions, she found that many readers' approaches to answering questions fell into two broad categories: 1) They overrelied on the content of the text and neglected their own background knowledge, or 2) they ignored the text and answered questions only from their prior experiences. It is obvious that applying either of these approaches exclusively negatively affects question-answering skill.

Questioning the Author: The Teacher as Facilitator in Talking About Texts   Questioning the author is one of the more popular approaches for engaging children in literature discussion groups (Beck & McKeown, 2006; Beck, McKeown, Hamilton, & Kucan, 1997). In this "content" approach, the teacher engages students in open, meaning-based discussion of the text as he or she initiates "queries" rather than questions after a segment of text has been read. Beck and colleagues described the role of questions as tools to assess student comprehension, in contrast to "queries" that "are designed to assist students in grappling with text ideas as they construct meaning" (1997, p. 23). Questions, in Beck and colleagues' view, focus on encouraging students to recall what they have read. Queries support students as they are in the process of building an understanding of what they are reading.

Three types of "initiating queries" begin the process. After a segment of text has been read and summarized the teacher may ask

1. What is the author trying to say here?

2. What do you think the author wants us to know?

3. What is the author talking about?

After the entire selection is read, "follow-up queries" commence, with the goal of clarifying and elaborating on students' thinking:

1. What does the author mean here?

2. That's what the author said, but what did the author mean?

3. Does that fit in with what the author has told us before?

4. How does this fit in with what the author has told us?

5. But does the author tell us why?

6. Why do you think the author tells us this now?

In addition to these queries, special queries are designed for narrative text, including

1. How do things look for this character now?

2. How does the author let you know that something has changed?

3. How has the author worked that out for us?

4. Given what the author has already told us about the character, what do you think he or she is up to?

5. How is the author making you feel right now about these characters?

6. What is the author telling us with this conversation?

If readers do encounter blocks to their understanding, then they need to be aware of what cognitive processes are involved in their own reading as they employ fix-up strategies to correct their comprehension difficulties. Teacher modeling of the process readers go through when they struggle to understand words, phrases, clauses, sentences, or longer chunks of text is critical to learning this strategy. Students need to know that even good readers encounter obstacles to their understanding as they read; that it is perfectly acceptable to stop when that occurs;

and, most important, that there are effective strategies students can use to bypass those blocks. (See more about monitoring understanding later in this chapter.)

Although this constructivist model has been noted to be effective for many students (Allington, Guice, Michelson, Baker, & Li, 1996), Williams argued, "This constructivist approach would not fully meet the needs of students with learning disabilities, who have been shown to respond well to structured, direct instruction" (2002, p. 129). Weak readers can be taught to improve their thinking and reasoning skills and can be taught interactive reading strategies to bolster their comprehension of text (Simmons, Fuchs, Fuchs, Mathes, & Hodge, 1995). Many of these effective strategies are discussed next.

Categorizing Questions to Aid Comprehension   Learning how to categorize questions into those that can be answered by referring back to the text and those that require higher level thinking based on personal knowledge can be an effective strategy to improve question-answering performance. Pearson and Johnson (1978) created a model to describe three different types of questions that teachers can ask to help their students to develop both text-related comprehension skills (literal and inferential comprehension) and those that go beyond text (critical analysis, interpretation, generalization, and extension of ideas from the text):

1. *Text explicit:* The answer to this type of question can be cleanly lifted verbatim from the text.

2. *Text implicit:* Rather than being explicitly stated, the answers to these questions are suggested in the text. It may be necessary to gather information from several sentences or integrate information from larger sections of text in order to answer this type of question.

3. *Script implicit:* Connecting the reader's background knowledge with information from the text is required to answer this kind of question.

There is a relationship between children's recall of passages they have read and the types of questions they have been asked. If they are asked text-explicit questions, then they recall parts of the text verbatim. If they are asked text-implicit questions, then they tend to draw more inferences from text. If they are asked script-implicit questions, then they make more interpretive and evaluative connections between their own prior knowledge and new information from their readings (Wixson, 1983). For children to be able to respond to a variety of question levels, then they must be given opportunities to observe good models and practice extensively.

Question–Answer Relationships   Raphael (1982, 1984, 1986) and Raphael and Au (2005) designed an instructional program called Question–Answer Relationships (QAR), which is based on Pearson and Johnson's (1978) taxonomy. The program was designed to help students label the type of questions being asked and then, as they considered both the text and their prior knowledge before they answered a question, use this information to assist them in formulating answers. The strategy can also be used to generate questions. More information about the QAR Strategy may be found in Appendix 16.7 in the Online Companion Materials.

At the beginning, the teacher needs to provide a lot of modeling and immediate feedback as students begin to assume responsibility for labeling the relationships. Students progress from shorter to longer texts and build independence by moving from group to independent activities. After the two broad QAR categories have been mastered, the teacher repeats the teaching sequence with the two subcategories under each: Right There and Think and Search for In the Book questions, and Author and You and On My Own for In My Head questions. (See Figure 16.6 for an illustration of the cue card used to explain the QAR strategy to students.)

The most important things about the QAR strategy are that students not only learn to identify different categories of questions, but they also use this information as a signal to try different strategies to answer those questions. Students become active learners who come to value both their own prior knowledge about a topic and the information the author of the text has presented to them.

After reviewing 17 studies on question-answering instruction, the NRP (NICHD, 2000) noted student improvement both in answering questions after reading passages and in strategies of finding answers.

Question Generation   The NRP's review of the research found "the strongest scientific evidence for the effectiveness of asking readers to generate questions during reading" (NICHD, 2000, p. 4-45). It has the strongest evidence for a single reading comprehension strategy among the seven listed. An eighth, which combines several strategies, including self-questioning, is also promising for struggling readers. Self-questioning has been demonstrated to distinguish effective readers and learners from those who have more difficulty with reading (Bransford et al., 1982; Cote & Goldman, 1999).

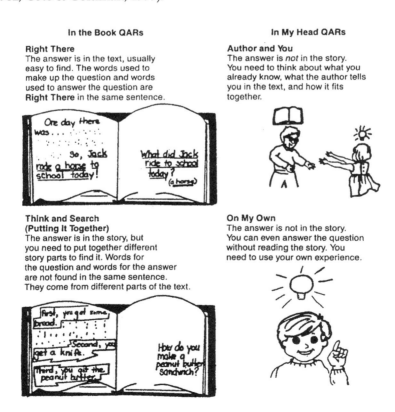

In the Book QARs

Right There
The answer is in the text, usually easy to find. The words used to make up the question and words used to answer the question are **Right There** in the same sentence.

**Think and Search
(Putting It Together)**
The answer is in the story, but you need to put together different story parts to find it. Words for the question and words for the answer are not found in the same sentence. They come from different parts of the text.

In My Head QARs

Author and You
The answer is *not* in the story. You need to think about what you already know, what the author tells you in the text, and how it fits together.

On My Own
The answer is not in the story. You can even answer the question without reading the story. You need to use your own experience.

Figure 16.6.   Illustrations to explain Question-Answer Relationships (QARs) to students. (From Raphael, T.E. [1986]. Teaching question answer relationships, revisited. *The Reading Teacher, 39*[6], 519; copyright © 1986 by International Reading Association; reprinted by permission.)

Strickland, Ganske, and Monroe stated, "Readers who don't think while they read do not generate questions. The most direct and effective way for teachers to help students do this is by demonstrating self-questioning through think-alouds" (2002, p. 162). Opening a window for students onto the kind of self-questioning good readers do as they read can in fact be a powerful strategy. The Questioning the Author strategy discussed previously in this chapter is one promising approach to increasing students' awareness about how good readers process (and sometimes struggle with) what they read. There are also other more systematic, explicit methods (e.g., the ReQuest strategy) that can be used to promote students to begin to "interrogate" the text.

ReQuest   As early as 1969, Manzo demonstrated that students could be taught to create their own questions. His technique, ReQuest, was designed to "improve the student's reading comprehension by providing an active learning situation for the development of questioning behaviors" (1969, p. 123). ReQuest can be used with either narrative or expository text and is effective in starting students on the road to active comprehension. It emphasizes modeling, an important feature of cognitive behavior modification. ReQuest has been shown to be particularly effective in helping students focus their attention on the text and pay attention to detail. ReQuest follows a simple sequence:

1. *Silent reading:* The students and the teacher silently read a common segment of text (from one to two sentences, to one to two paragraphs).

2. *Student questioning:* The teacher closes the book, and students ask him or her as many questions as possible. The teacher models appropriate answers and also provides substantial feedback to students about the questions they generate. Students are asked to "try to ask the kinds of questions a teacher might ask in the way a teacher might ask them" (Manzo, 1969, p. 124).

3. *Teacher questioning:* The students close their books, and the teacher asks the questions. The teacher helps students sharpen their questions by modeling good questioning behavior that includes a range of question types (see the previous discussion of QAR for ideas).

4. *Repetition of sequence:* When questions are exhausted, the students and the teacher read the next segment of text and repeat the procedure. New sections of the text should be integrated with old sections. Questions may relate to new and old sections.

5. *Predictions:* When enough text has been processed for the students to make predictions about the remainder of the text, the exchange of questions stops. The teacher asks predictive questions ("What do you think the rest of the story will be about? Why do you think so?")

6. *Reading:* The teacher and the students read to the end of the passage, verifying and discussing predictions made.

ReQuest was first tested under clinical conditions with students receiving one-to-one remedial instruction, but both Manzo (1969; Manzo & Manzo, 1993) and others (Mason & Au, 1986) have supported its effectiveness when it is used with larger groups. In order to encourage students to generalize questioning to other situations, Bos and Vaughn (1998) advised cuing students to remember to stop while reading and ask themselves questions as they did during ReQuest.

In its summary evaluation of question generation, the NRP (NICHD, 2000) cited significant scientific evidence that instruction on question generation during reading improves reading comprehension in terms of memory and answering questions based on text as well as integrating and identifying main ideas through summarizing. The panel recommended this strategy as part of a multiple-strategy instruction program. (Using multiple strategies is discussed later in this chapter.)

Story Structure   The bulk of texts used in elementary school reading are stories. Story structure pertains to how stories and their plots are organized into a predictable format that includes characters, setting, problem, goal, action, and outcome (or resolution of the problem). When students are taught about story structure, they have an easier time retelling stories within a logical framework. They also show improvements in asking and answering *who, what, when, where, why,* and *how* questions about the story (NICHD, 2000).

Idol (1987) developed a simple story map with a visual representation of story components and their relationship to one another (see Figure 16.7). She offered one straightforward approach for presenting story mapping in a classroom:

1. *Model:* After introducing the purpose of the strategy, the teacher presents the story elements that are on the story map. The teacher reads a story out loud and stops periodically when story elements are presented in the text. If certain story elements are not presented explicitly, then the teacher needs to model the thinking required to generate the inferences. Students label the parts and write them in the appropriate places on the story map.

2. *Lead:* Students read the story and complete their story maps independently. The teacher gives students feedback about their maps and encourages them to add details they may have omitted.

3. *Test:* Students read a story, generate a story map, and then answer questions that relate to the story elements on the map (e.g., Who are the characters in the story? Where did the story take place? What was the main problem in the story?).

Four optional supports to the story mapping strategy may be helpful for some students. These additions to classic story structure instruction may facilitate recall of story elements for students and spur more active reading of text.

In the first modification, students who have difficulty remembering story elements may use a "five finger retelling" (Stahl, 2004). In this strategy, each finger is used as a reminder or prompt for an element in story structure: characters, setting, problem, plot, and resolution/solution. A chart may serve as an additional reminder of these elements.

For a second modification using the elements from the story map, Bos (1987) proposed a mnemonic, STORE, to help students to retell the story. See Textbox 16.2 for a cue card for this story retelling strategy.

For a third option, the Project Read Language Circle (http://www.projectread.com) created a set of Primary Story Boards with story elements on sticky notes. Students can use the sticky notes to flag the elements of the story as they read. A fourth option is Story Stickies (http://www.storystickies.com). This tool produces both blank and story-specific sticky notes that allow students to take notes under specific categories (e.g., characters, settings, main ideas, predictions, vocabulary).

According to the NRP (NICHD, 2000) report, instruction in story structure improves students' ability to understand stories, answer questions about them,

Simple Story Map

Name _____   Date _____

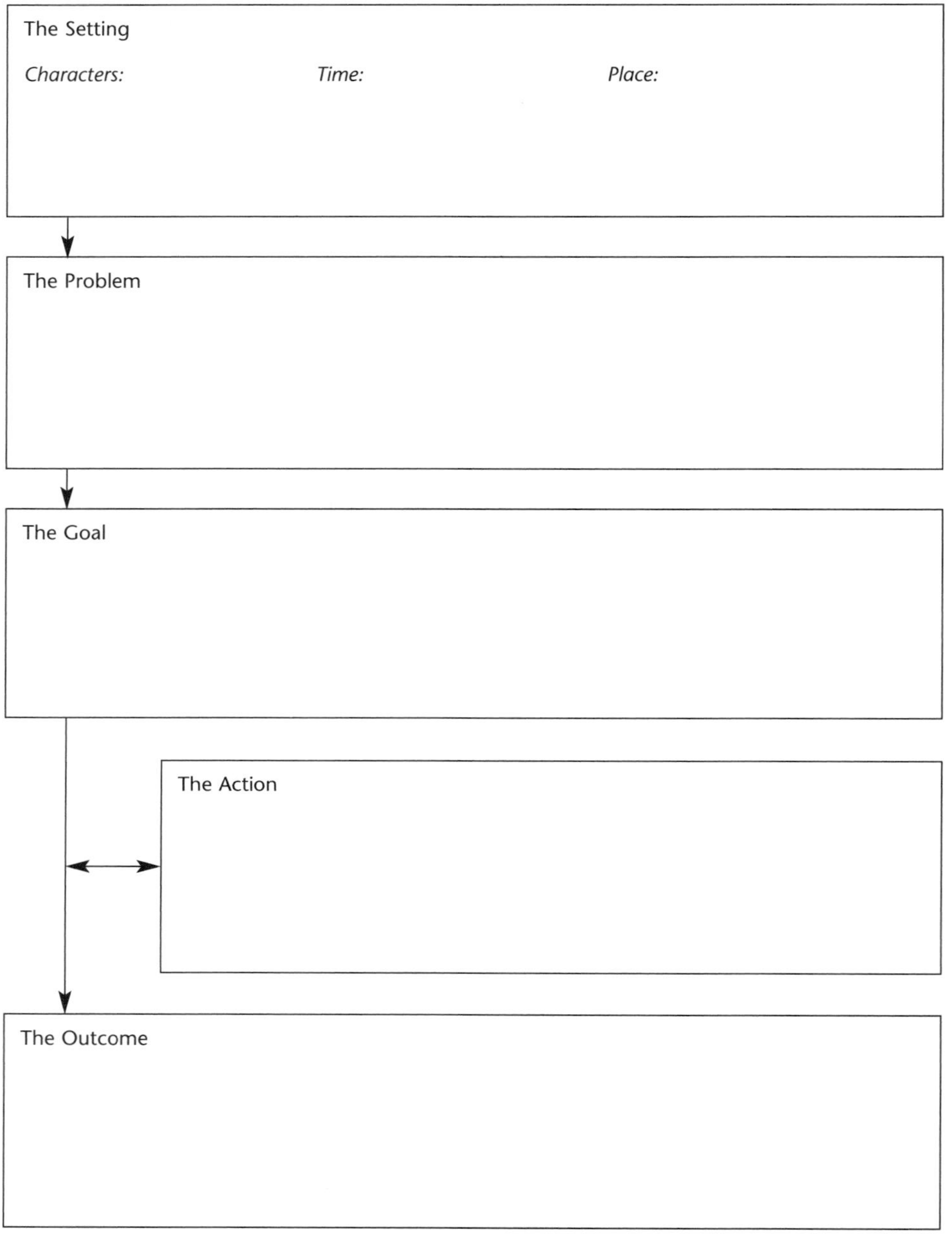

The Setting

Characters: *Time:*   *Place:*

The Problem

The Goal

The Action

The Outcome

Figure 16.7   Simple story map. (From Idol, L. [1987]. Group story mapping: A comprehension strategy for both skilled and unskilled readers. *Journal of Learning Disabilities, 20,* 199; reprinted by permission.)

and remember what was read. The weakest readers benefit the most from this strategy, although even strong readers improve their performance after instruction.

Summarization and the RAP Paraphrasing Strategy In order to summarize, students must orchestrate three important tasks (NICHD, 2000, p. 4-92):

1. Decide what are "the most central and important ideas in the text"

2. "Generalize from examples or from things that are repeated"

3. "Ignore irrelevant details"

Researchers who have studied the behaviors of students with learning difficulties have long been aware that these tasks are particularly challenging for these students (Brown & Palincsar, 1982; Graves, 1986; McCormick, 1992; Wong, 1979).

The University of Kansas Center for Research on Learning (Schumaker, Denton, & Deshler, 1984) developed the RAP Paraphrasing Strategy, which helps students bypass these difficulties and improve their ability to recall the main ideas and important facts from expository text they have read. Each step in RAP involves a variety of strategic questions and prompts that are described in step-by-step detail in written materials. These materials can be obtained only as part of guided professional development experiences that are offered throughout the nation and are designed to ensure high-quality implementation with students. This program is one of several research-based programs designed for teachers to use as they teach learning strategies to students. Visit the University of Kansas Center for Research on Learning web site at http://www.kucrl.org for more information.

The RAP Paraphrasing Strategy has three specific steps:

1. Read a paragraph.

2. Ask yourself, "What were the main idea and details in this paragraph?"

3. Put the main idea and details into your own words.

Prior to implementing these steps, the teacher begins by describing the rationale for learning RAP. If students learn to put information into their own words, they will more likely think about what they have read and understand and remember it. Next, the general conditions under which the strategy may be used are noted. Students will be able to use the strategy any time they are reading something in paragraph form that they want to understand and remember. Finally, the teacher shares the positive results that students can expect after learning and applying the strategy.

Next, the teacher describes the three steps of the strategy. As students do Step 1, the teacher reminds them to think about the meaning of the words they are reading. As students do Step 2, they are guided to look back over the paragraph quickly to find the main idea and details. The teacher reminds them that the first or last sentence, key vocabulary, and repetitions of the same word or words in the whole paragraph often give hints about the main idea. Important details are related to that main idea. As students prepare for Step 3, the teacher then describes how to locate the main idea. Throughout the description of the strategy, students are reminded of certain requirements of each paraphrased statement (Schumaker et al., 1984):

• It must contain a complete thought, with a subject and a verb.

• It must be totally accurate.

- It must have new information and must not be a repetition of something that was already said.

- It must make sense.

- It must contain useful information.

- It must be in the students' own words.

- Only one general statement per paragraph is permitted.

As students continue to learn the strategy, modeling by the teacher (and by students); verbal practice; controlled practice with short, simple passages; advanced practice; and generalization become integral parts of the instruction.

The NRP's (NICHD, 2000) final evaluation of summarization as a targeted strategy was quite positive. The panel noted that this is a sound method for connecting ideas and making generalizations from text. Other benefits were also listed for summarization, including improving memory of what is read, both for free recall and for answering questions. This strategy has been incorporated successfully into other multiple strategy interventions, most notably Reciprocal Teaching (discussed next). In addition, PALS and CSR include a summarization step in their approaches.

Multiple Strategies and the Reciprocal Teaching Method   Although research on individual reading strategies has yielded many positive results, these strategies may even be more powerful when they are combined into a multiple strategy instructional program. As the NRP noted, "This method finds considerable scientific support for its effectiveness, and it is the most promising for use in classroom instruction where teachers and readers interact over texts" (NICHD, 2000, p. 4-46).

Reciprocal teaching (Palincsar & Brown, 1984) is probably the most well-known method for teaching multiple comprehension strategies. It has even been replicated in an Internet-focused format (Coiro, Knoebel, Lankshear, & Leu, 2008; Leu et al., 2008; McVerry, Zawilinski, & O'Byrne, 2009).

This approach combines several of the most effective comprehension strategies reviewed by the NRP (NICHD, 2000): prediction, questioning, seeking clarification when comprehension monitoring reveals confusion, and summarization.

As a reciprocal teaching lesson begins, the teacher explains the purpose of the work the students and teacher will do together and describes the four strategies they will be using in the lesson. The teacher models the activity, and the students try to emulate the process. Throughout the lesson, the teacher provides corrective feedback so that students have ample opportunity to be supported in their steps to independence. Students read passages silently that are appropriate to their age and ability. Young children (or very weak readers) may have passages read aloud to them. After a passage has been read, children are asked to state the topic and summarize the important information they have read.

The teacher always models the reciprocal teaching procedure first, but eventually a student is chosen to act as the teacher and asks an important question about the passage that was just read. Next, he or she will summarize, making a prediction and, if necessary, asking for clarification of confusing terms or concepts. The teacher provides support during this process by prompting students to guide them in the right direction, instructing (reminding them about the important steps to the procedure if they have forgotten), modifying the activity for students who appear to be stuck, or asking for other students to step in and help.

Carlisle and Rice (2002) cautioned practitioners to make sure that sufficient time is devoted to the instructional process in reciprocal teaching, that they allow adequate chances for students to practice the strategies, and that they provide continued guidance and support for students to reach independent application of the embedded strategies. Rosenshine and Meister's (1994) review of the research on reciprocal teaching concluded that more time should be spent teaching the individual strategies directly before beginning the more interactive segment of the technique.

The Miami-Dade County Public Schools developed a project to provide Reciprocal Teaching support materials (http://pers.dadeschools.net/prodev/reciprocal_teaching.htm). Lesson plans and instructional materials, including student cue cards and bookmarks, may be found on the site.

Reciprocal teaching is similar to CSR, discussed earlier. Klingner et al. (2001) acknowledged that CSR is an outgrowth of reciprocal teaching and, in fact, used reciprocal teaching in their earlier work (Klingner & Vaughn, 1996). After adopting many changes to reciprocal teaching over time, they felt that they had created a substantially different approach that deserved its own name (Klingner et al., 2001). An outline of the differences the authors cited between CSR and reciprocal teaching may be found in Table 16.2.

> **REFLECT, CONNECT, and RESPOND**
> Review the strategies within this section, Research-Validated Strategies for Comprehension Instruction. Identify one strategy that is less familiar to you or that you have not used very frequently. How could you incorporate this strategy within a current unit of instruction or use it to help a particular student who struggles with comprehension? Jot down notes about how you might implement the strategy in a lesson or intervention plan.

Comprehension Challenges for Twenty-First–Century Students: New Literacies

More and more students use the Internet to locate, understand, and use information online. Current research points to the need for students to develop new comprehension strategies and skills to read and gain meaning from this resource (Biancarosa & Snow, 2004; Coiro, 2003, 2005; Lacina & Mathews, 2012; Mangen, Walgermo, & Bronnick, 2013; Sutherland-Smith, 2002). As the RAND Reading Study Group (RRSG) noted, "Accessing the Internet makes large demands on individuals' literacy skills; in some cases, this new technology requires readers to have novel literacy skills, and little is known how to analyze or teach those skills" (2002, p. 4). In addition to understanding how search engines work and how information is organized on web sites, students need to develop higher levels of inferential reasoning as well as comprehension monitoring strategies to effectively use these new literacies (Coiro, 2005).

Members of the New Literacies Research Team at the University of Connecticut have accepted the challenge of identifying the key literacy skills that need to be developed to enable students to use Internet resources effectively during content

Table 16.2.   How reciprocal teaching and Collaborative Strategic Reading (CSR) differ

Reciprocal teaching	Collaborative Strategic Reading
Designed primarily for use with narrative text	Designed primarily for use with expository text
No *brainstorming* before reading	Students *brainstorm* to activate prior knowledge as part of preview (before reading).
Students predict what they think will happen next before reading each paragraph or segment of text.	Students only *predict* as part of the Preview strategy (before reading), making informed guesses about what they think they will learn.
Students *clarify* words or chunks of text they don't understand by rereading the sentences before and after the sentence they don't understand and/or asking a peer for assistance.	Students use fix-up strategies to clarify *clunks* (words they don't understand). • Reread the sentence. • Reread the sentences before and after. • Break apart the word and look for smaller words they know. • Look for a prefix or suffix they know. • Look at the picture for clues. • Ask for help.
Students *summarize* the paragraph or segment of text they have just read.	Students *get the gist* of the paragraph or segment of text they have just read, identifying "the most important who or what" and the most important thing about the who or what. They then say the gist in ten words or less.
Students *generate questions* after each paragraph or segment of text they have just read.	Students only *generate questions* as part of a *wrap up* after they have read the entire day's selection. Students answer each other's questions.
No *review* after reading	Students *review* what they have learned after reading the day's selection.
8–12 students in the group; the teacher in the group	An entire class is divided into *cooperative groups* of 2–5; the teacher circulates rather than staying with a group.
No learning logs	Students record their previews, clunks, questions, and what they've learned in individual *CSR Learning Logs*.
The leader (a student) facilitates the discussion about a paragraph or section of text; this role rotates after each paragraph.	Every student in the group has a meaningful role; one of these roles is to be the leader. Roles are assigned for an entire lesson (only rotating biweekly in some classes).
No cue cards	Students use *Cue Cards* to help them implement their roles and the comprehension strategies.

From Klingner, J.K., Vaughn, S., Dimino, J., Schumm, J.S., & Bryant, D. (2002). *Collaborative Strategic Reading: Strategies for Improving Comprehension*. Longmont, CO: Sopris West, p. 7; reprinted by permission of Sopris West Educational Services.

area lessons. Leu, Kinzer, Coir, and Cammack (2004) have identified five New Literacies for Online Reading Comprehension:

1.   Identifying important questions

2.   Locating information

3.   Critically evaluating that information

4.   Synthesizing information

5.   Communicating the answers to others

To identify important questions, the first new literacy, students need to learn how to formulate a question or define a problem. Sub-skills within this topic include understanding the question; narrowing, expanding, and/or refining the question as needed; and knowing when there is a need to shift the question because of new information accessed or lack of information available. To locate information on the Internet, the second new literacy, students need to know how to use a search engine or other methods to locate an information resource. They must then be able to evaluate information they have found, identify any biases, and know how to verify it through alternative or primary sources—all skills that fall under the third new literacy, critically evaluating online information. To develop the fourth new literacy, synthesizing what they have accessed, they need to be able to integrate information from multiple resources including those that are text based, multimedia based, or a combination thereof. Finally, students need to be able to organize and communicate their findings.

The New Literacies community is asking more questions than providing definitive answers to those questions. Researchers in this community acknowledge that reading comprehension is likely to be the primary focus of investigation because the Internet and other information and communication technologies are focused primarily on information and learning from text (Leu et al., 2004).

> **REFLECT, CONNECT, and RESPOND**
> What is one skill you can teach students to help them use Internet resources effectively? Describe how and why you would make this skill an instructional focus for the age group with whom you work (or plan to work).

ONLINE RESOURCES FOR COMPREHENSION INSTRUCTION

Although there has been an increase in the number of online resources available to teachers, students, and parents, there has been little guidance or instruction in how to use these resources well. In general, practice precedes research and preparation for teachers to make the best use of online supports. Increased attention to meeting the needs of the nation's nearly 5 million ELLs and those who do not have mastery of basic decoding skills needed for accessibility to more sophisticated text has also been evident. This has led to provision of a growth of Internet-based and technology resources that can give these students some of the support they need to meet their literacy goals. A selection of these resources teachers may find useful may be found in the Online Companion Materials.

CLOSING THOUGHTS: NEXT STEPS
FOR COMPREHENSION INSTRUCTION

Students should not have to struggle to gain meaning from text, whether that text is found in a book, a magazine, or on the Internet. As Stanovich noted, "Students who do not read well read less and when they read less, they learn less" (1986). As a result, students' comprehension difficulties complicate their learning in all academic areas (Chall, 1996). Although Pressley's observations conflict with common philosophy and practice in many schools today, they must be acknowledged:

> Despite the improvements in fluency and knowledge permitted by extensive reading, the "read, read, read" approach does not lead to as active meaning construction during reading as occurs when students are taught explicitly to use and articulate comprehension strategies when they read. (2000, p. 554)

There are many powerful, research-supported strategies that hold promise for struggling readers who may be able to decode but who still strive to understand what they read. Although a good amount is known about effective (and ineffective) reading comprehension strategies, many questions remain unanswered. Many issues continue to be troubling: concerns about understanding the multiple sources of variance in the reading comprehension process and outcomes, continuing national demand for high literacy skills that coexists with stagnant reading test performance, weak teacher preparation, minimal or ineffective reading comprehension instruction in the schools, and a persistent achievement gap between children of different demographic groups.

In 2000, the RRSG was formed when the U.S. Department of Education's now-defunct Office of Educational Research and Improvement (OERI) asked RAND to look at how OERI could improve the quality and relevance of research that the agency funded (RRSG, 2002). When the final report was released in 2002, the authors recommended that teachers "must teach comprehension explicitly, beginning in the primary grades and continuing through high school" (p. xii). The authors strongly advised that while maintaining methodological rigor, potential research must be "usable" and directed toward improving classroom practices, enhancing curricula, enriching teacher preparation, and producing better and more informative assessments of reading comprehension. As part of this initiative, the RRSG recommended that these questions be addressed:

- What instructional conditions should accompany strategy instruction to encourage students to generalize strategic approaches to learning across texts, tasks, contexts, and different age levels?

- How should teachers of poor comprehenders who are in general education classes prioritize time and instructional emphasis among the many competing calls for their attention to everything from building fluency to teaching vocabulary, using computer technology, and improving reading skills?

- What variations in instructional time and practice optimize opportunities for students who are ELLs to improve their comprehension skills?

The RRSG's research agenda for reading comprehension promised to "build new knowledge that will be helpful to all concerned with reading education—practitioners, teacher educators, policymakers, and parents" (Sweet & Snow, 2002, p. 47). Teachers now have a much better understanding about what works (and what does not work) to improve children's comprehension of increasingly complex text. They are being given an opportunity to have a huge effect on the lives of children now and on their futures. Nothing can replace the power of a well-trained teacher providing direct instruction using research-validated strategies to enhance reading comprehension development. The time is ripe to seize the opportunity and build on what they already know to prepare students to be productive, literate adults in the 21st century.

ONLINE COMPANION MATERIALS

The following Chapter 16 resources are available at http://www.brookespublishing .com/birshcarreker/materials:

- Reflect, Connect, and Respond Questions

- Appendix 16.1: Technology Resources

- Appendix 16.2: Knowledge and Skill Assessment Answer Key

- Appendix 16.3a: Test Your Knowledge and Skill—Bonus Quiz Questions and 16.3b: Answer Key

- Appendix 16.4: Supplemental Resources (additional online and print resources for teaching comprehension)

- Appendix 16.5: A Model for Instruction to Develop Reading Comprehension at the Sentence Level

- Appendix 16.6: K-W-L Strategy

- Appendix 16.7: QAR Strategy

- Appendix 16.8: Peer-Assisted Learning Strategies (PALS)

KNOWLEDGE AND SKILL ASSESSMENT

1. What has been the most significant change in recommendations for reading comprehension instruction because of the CCSS for English Language Arts?

   a. Mandated comprehension strategies to be used in all classrooms

   b. Increased focus on using expository texts in all grades

   c. A list of recommended programs to be used for instruction

   d. The use of mandated tests for every state

   e. Increased focus on using narrative texts in all grades

2. The National Assessment Governing Board recommendations for the percentages of literary versus informational texts increases the most through the grades for teaching which skill?

   a. Locating/recalling information

   b. Critiquing and evaluating information

   c. Integrating/interpreting information

   d. Identifying sources of information

   e. Connecting prior knowledge to reading content

3. The National Reading Panel indicated that which single comprehension strategy had the strongest scientific evidence for effectiveness?

   a. Use of graphic organizers

   b. Asking readers to generate questions during reading

   c. Summarization

   d. Ample practice answering questions after reading text silently

   e. Oral reading of text before answering questions

4. Which of the following is the major contribution to weak comprehension for young children?

    a. Inadequate vocabulary knowledge

    b. Poor listening comprehension

    c. Limited background knowledge

    d. Weak word reading skill

    e. Poor motivation

5. Teachers should begin comprehension instruction by doing what?

    a. Providing multiple opportunities for children to write the answers to questions related to texts they have read

    b. Reading aloud multiple engaging books

    c. Completing a good assessment

    d. Devoting more time to students reading silently

    e. Previewing pertinent vocabulary

REFERENCES

Aaron, P.G., Joshi, M., & Williams, K.A. (1999). Not all reading disabilities are alike. *Journal of Learning Disabilities, 32,* 120–137.

Adams, M.J. (1990). *Beginning to read: Thinking and learning about print.* Cambridge, MA: The MIT Press.

Adams, M.J., Treiman, R., & Pressley, M. (1998). Reading, writing and literacy. In W. Damon (Series Ed.) & I.E. Sigel & K.A. Renninger (Vol. Eds.), *Handbook of child psychology: Child psychology in practice* (Vol. 4, pp. 275–355). New York, NY: Wiley.

Allington, R.L. (2001). *What really matters for struggling readers: Designing research-based programs.* New York, NY: Longman.

Allington, R., Guice, S., Michelson, N., Baker, R., & Li, S. (1996). Literature-based curricula in high poverty schools. In M.F. Graves, P. van den Broek, & B.M. Taylor (Eds.), *The first R: Every child's right to read* (pp. 73–96). New York, NY: Teachers College Press.

Baumann, J.F., & Graves, M.F. (2010). What is academic vocabulary? *Journal of Adolescent & Adult Literacy, 54,* (1), 4–12.

Beck, I.L., & McKeown, M.G. (2006). *Improving comprehension with questioning the author: A fresh and expanded view of a powerful approach.* New York, NY: Scholastic.

Beck, I.L., McKeown, M.G., Hamilton, R.L., & Kucan, L. (1997). *Questioning the author: An approach for enhancing student engagement with text.* Newark, DE: International Reading Association.

Biancarosa, G., & Snow, C.E. (2004). *Reading next: A vision for action and research in middle and high school literacy.* A report to Carnegie Corporation of New York. Washington, DC: Alliance for Excellent Education.

Boardman, A.G., Vaughn, S., Buckley, P., Reutebuch, C., Roberts, G., & Klingner, J. (2016). Collaborative strategic reading for students with learning disabilities in upper elementary classrooms. *Exceptional Children, 82*(4), 409–427.

Bos, C.S. (1987). *Promoting story comprehension using a story retelling strategy.* Paper presented at the Teachers Applying Whole Language Conference, Tucson, AZ.

Bos, C.S., & Vaughn, S. (1998). *Strategies for teaching students with learning and behavior problems* (4th ed.). Boston, MA: Allyn & Bacon.

Bransford, J.D., Stein, B.S., Vye, N.J., Franks, J.J., Auble, P.M., Mezynski, K.J., & Perfetto, G.A. (1982). Differences in approaches to learning: An overview. *Journal of Experimental Psychology, 111,* 390–398.

Brown, A.L., & Palincsar, A.S. (1982). Including strategic learning from texts by means of informed, self-control training. *Topics in Learning and Learning Disabilities, 2*(1), 1–17.

Butler, S., Urrutia, K., Buenger, A., & Hunt, M. (2010). *A review of the current research on comprehension instruction.* Portsmouth, NH: National Reading Technical Assistance Center.

Cain, K. (2007). Syntactic awareness and reading ability: Is there any evidence for a special relationship? *Applied Psycholinguistics, 28,* 679–694.

Cain, K., & Oakhill, J.V. (1999). Inference making ability and its relation to comprehension failure in young children. *Reading and Writing, 11,* 489–503.

Carlisle, J.F. (1999). *Beginning reasoning and reading.* Cambridge, MA: Educators Publishing Service.

Carlisle, J.F., & Rice, M.S. (2002). *Improving reading comprehension.* Timonium, MD: York Press.

Carnine, D., Silbert, J., & Kame'enui, E.J. (1990). *Direct instruction reading* (2nd ed.). Columbus, OH: Charles E. Merrill.

Carr, E., & Dewitz, P. (1988). *Teaching comprehension as a student-directed process.* Paper presented at the meeting of the International Reading Association, Toronto, Canada.

Carr, E., & Ogle, D. (1987). K-W-L Plus: A strategy for comprehension and summarization. *Journal of Reading, 30,* 626–631.

Chall, J. (1996). *Stages of reading development* (2nd ed.). Orlando, FL: Harcourt.

Coiro, J. (2003). Reading comprehension on the Internet: Expanding our understanding of reading comprehension to encompass new literacies. *The Reading Teacher, 56*(5), 458–464.

Coiro, J. (2005). Making sense of online text. *Educational Leadership, 63*(2), 30–35.

Coiro, J., Knoebel, M., Lankshear, C., & Leu, D.J. (2008). *Handbook of research on new literacies.* Mahwah, NJ: Lawrence Erlbaum Associates.

Cote, N., & Goldman, S. (1999). Building representations of informational text: Evidence from children's think-aloud protocols. In H. Van Oostendorp & S. Goldman (Eds.), *The construction of mental representations during reading* (pp. 169–193). Mahwah, NJ: Lawrence Erlbaum Associates.

Council of Chief State School Officers (CCSSO) & National Governors Association Center for Best Practices (NGA Center). (2010). *Common Core State Standards.* Retrieved from http://www.corestandards.org

Deshler, D.D., Ellis, E.S., & Lenz, B.K. (1996). *Teaching adolescents with learning disabilities: Strategies and methods* (2nd ed.). Denver, CO: Love Publishing.

Dewitz, P., Leahy, S.B., Jones, J., & Sullivan, P.M. (2010). *The essential guide to selecting and using core reading programs.* Newark, DE: The International Reading Association.

Doctorow, M., Wittrock, M., & Marks, C. (1978). Generative processes in reading comprehension. *Journal of Educational Psychology, 70,* 109–118.

Durkin, D. (1979). What classroom observations reveal about reading comprehension. *Reading Research Quarterly, 14,* 518–544.

Durkin, D. (1993). *Teaching them to read* (6th ed.). Boston, MA: Allyn & Bacon.

Ehri, L. (1998). Word reading by sight and by analogy in beginning readers. In C. Hulme & R.M. Joshi (Eds.), *Reading and spelling development and disorders* (pp. 87–111). Mahwah, NJ: Lawrence Erlbaum Associates.

Eisenberg, S. (2006). Grammar: How can I say it better? In T. Ukrainetz (Ed.), *Contextualized language intervention* (145–194). Eau Claire, WI: Thinking Publications.

Fisher, D., & Frey, N. (2012). Text-dependent questions. *Principal Leadership, 13*(1), 70–73.

Fowler, A.E. (1988). Grammaticality judgments and reading skill in grade 2. *Annals of Dyslexia, 38,* 73–74.

Fuchs, D., Fuchs, L.S., Mathes, P.G., & Simmons, D.C. (1997). Peer assisted learning strategies: Making classrooms more responsive to diversity. *American Educational Research Journal, 34,* 174–206.

Fuchs, D., Fuchs, L.S., Thompson, A., Svenson, E., Yen, L., Al Otaiba, S., … Saenz, L. (2001). Peer-assisted learning strategies in reading: Extensions for kindergarten, first grade, and high school. *Remedial and Special Education, 22,* 15–21.

Fuchs, D., Mathes, P.G., & Fuchs, L.S. (2001). *Peer-assisted learning strategies: Reading methods for grades 2–6* [Teacher manual]. Nashville, TN: Vanderbilt University.

Gambrell, L.B., Block, C.C., & Pressley, M. (2002). Introduction: Improving comprehension instruction: An urgent priority. In C.C. Block, L.B. Gambrell, & M. Pressley (Eds.), *Improving comprehension instruction* (pp. 3–16). San Francisco, CA: Jossey-Bass.

Gough, P.B. (1996). How children learn to read and why they fail. *Annals of Dyslexia, 46,* 3–20.

Granowsky, A. (1973). *That awful Cinderella*. Lexington, MA: D.C. Heath.

Graves, A.W. (1986). Effects of direct instruction and metacomprehension training on finding main ideas. *Learning Disabilities Research, 1*(2), 90–100.

Greenwood, C.R., Delquadri, J.C., & Hall, R.V. (1989). Longitudinal effects of classwide peer tutoring. *Journal of Educational Psychology, 81,* 371–383.

Grover, H., Cook, D., Benson, J., & Chandler, A. (1991). *Strategic learning in the content areas.* Madison: Wisconsin Department of Public Instruction.

Guszak, F.J. (1967). Teacher questioning and reading. *The Reading Teacher, 21,* 227–234.

Hammond, D. (1983). How your students can predict their way to reading comprehension. *Learning, 12,* 62–64.

Harris, T.L., & Hodges, R.E. (Eds.). (1995). *The literacy dictionary: The vocabulary of reading and writing.* Newark, DE: International Reading Association.

Hart, B., & Risley, T.R. (1995). *Meaningful differences in the everyday experience of young American children.* Baltimore, MD: Paul H. Brookes Publishing Co.

Hiebert, E.H., & Pearson, P.D. (2014). Understanding text complexity: Introduction to the special issue. *Elementary School Journal, 115,* 153–160.

Hirsch, E.D., Jr. (2003, Spring). Reading comprehension requires knowledge—of words and the world: Scientific insights into the fourth-grade slump and the nation's stagnant comprehension scores. *American Educator, 27,* 10–22, 28–44.

Hirsch, E.D., Jr. (2006). *The case for bringing content into the language arts block and for a knowledge-rich curriculum core for all children.* Retrieved from https://www.aft.org/periodical/american-educator/spring-2006/building-knowledge

Hirsch, E.D., Jr. (2009). *Core Knowledge Sequence: Content and skill guidelines for grades K–8.* Charlottesville, VA: Core Knowledge Foundation.

Hodgkinson, H. (1991). Reform versus reality. *Phi Delta Kappan, 73,* 9–16.

Idol, L. (1987). Group story mapping: A comprehension strategy for both skilled and unskilled readers. *Journal of Learning Disabilities, 20*(4), 196–205.

Jenkins, J.R., Jewell, M., Leicester, N., & Troutner, N.M. (1990). *Development of a school building model for educating handicapped and at-risk students in general education classrooms.* Paper presented at the annual meeting of the American Educational Research Association, Boston, MA.

Keene, E.O., & Zimmerman, S. (1997). *Mosaic of thought: Teaching comprehension in a reader's workshop.* Portsmouth, NH: Heinemann

Kim, A.H., Vaughn, S., Wanzek, J., & Wei, S. (2004). Graphic organizers and their effects on the reading comprehension of students with LD: A synthesis of research. *Journal of Learning Disabilities, 37*(2), 105–118.

Klingner, J.K., & Vaughn, S. (1996). Reciprocal teaching of reading comprehension strategies for students with learning disabilities who use English as a second language. *Elementary School Journal, 96,* 275–293.

Klingner, J.K., & Vaughn, S. (2000). The helping behaviors of fifth-graders while using collaborative strategic reading (CSR) during ESL content classes. *TESOL Quarterly, 34,* 69–98.

Klingner, J.K., Vaughn, S., Boardman, A., & Swanson, E. (2012). *Now we get it! Boosting comprehension with collaborative strategic reading.* San Francisco, CA: Jossey-Bass.

Klingner, J.K., Vaughn, S., Dimino, J., Schumm, J.S., & Bryant, D. (2001). *From clunk to click: Collaborative strategic reading.* Longmont, CO: Sopris West Educational Services.

Klingner, J.K., Vaughn, S., Hughes, M.T., Schumm, J.S., & Elbaum, B. (1998). Academic outcomes for students with and without learning disabilities in inclusive classrooms. *Learning Disabilities Research and Practice, 13,* 153–160.

Kucan, L., Hapgood, S., & Palincsar, A.S. (2011). Teachers' specialized knowledge for supporting student comprehension in text-based discussions. *Elementary School Journal, 112*(1), 61–82.

Lacina, J., & Mathews, S. (2012). Using online storybooks to build comprehension. *Childhood Education, 88*(3), 155–161.

Leu, D.J., Coiro, J., Castek, J., Hartman, D.K., Henry, L.A., & Reinking, D. (2008). Research on instruction and assessment in online reading comprehension. In *Comprehension instruction: Research-based best practices.* New York NY: Guilford. Retrieved from https://newliteracies.uconn.edu/wp-content/uploads/sites/448/2014/07/Leu_et_al_Final_Chaptersinglespaced.pdf

Leu, D.J., Kinzer, C.I.K., Coiro, J.L., & Cammack, D.W. (2004). Toward a theory of new literacies emerging from the Internet and other information and communication technologies. In R.B. Ruddell & N. Unrau (Eds.), *Theoretical models and processes of reading* (5th ed., pp. 1568–1611). Newark, DE: International Reading Association.

Mangen, A., Walgermo, B.R., & Bronnick, K. (2013). Reading linear texts on paper versus computer screen: Effects on reading comprehension. *International Journal of Educational Research, 58,* 61–68.

Manzo, A. (1969). The ReQuest procedure. *Journal of Reading, 13,* 123–126.

Manzo, A.V., & Manzo, U.C. (1993). *Literacy disorders: Holistic diagnosis and remediation.* Orlando, FL: Harcourt.

Maria, K. (1990). *Reading comprehension instruction: Issues and strategies.* Timonium, MD: York Press.

Marzano, R.J. (2012). A Comprehensive approach to vocabulary instruction. *Voices from the Middle, 20*(1), 31–25.

Mason, J.M., & Au, K.H. (1986). *Reading instruction for today.* Glenview, IL: Scott Foresman.

McCormick, S. (1992). Disabled readers' erroneous responses to inferential comprehension questions: Description and analysis. *Reading Research Quarterly, 27,* 54–77.

McKenna, M.C. (2002). *Help for struggling readers: Strategies for grades 3–8.* New York, NY: Guilford.

McKeown, M.G., & Beck, I.L. (1990). The assessment and characterization of young learners' knowledge of a topic in history. *American Educational Research Journal, 27,* 688–726.

McNeil, J.D. (1987). *Reading comprehension.* Glenview, IL: Scott Foresman.

McVerry, J.G., Zawilinski, L., & O'Byrne, W.I. (2009). Navigating the Cs of change. *Educational Leadership, 67*(1). Retrieved from http://www.ascd.org/publications/educational-leadership/sept09/vol67/num01/Navigating-the-Cs-of-Change.aspx

Miller, D. (2002). *Reading with meaning: Teaching comprehension in the primary grades.* Portland, ME: Stenhouse.

Moss, B. (2008). The information text gap: The mismatch between non-narrative text types in basal readers and 2009 NAEP recommended guidelines. *Journal of Literacy Research, 40,* 201–219.

Nagy, W., & Townsend, D. (2012). Words as tools: Learning academic vocabulary as language acquisition. *Reading Research Quarterly, 47,* 91–108.

National Assessment Governing Board, U.S. Department of Education. (2008). *Reading framework for the 2009 National Assessment of Educational Progress.* Washington, DC: U.S. Government Printing Office.

National Assessment Governing Board, U.S. Department of Education. (2015). *Reading framework for the 2015 National Assessment of Educational Progress.* Washington, DC: U.S. Government Printing Office.

National Institute of Child Health and Human Development (NICHD). (2000). *Report of the National Reading Panel: Reports of the subgroups. Teaching children to read: An evidence-based assessment of the scientific research literature on reading and its implications for reading instruction* (NIH Publication No. 00-4754). Washington, DC: Government Printing Office.

Ness, M.K. (2009). Reading comprehension strategies in secondary content area classrooms: Teacher use of and attitudes toward reading comprehension instruction. *Reading Horizons, 49*(2). Retrieved from http://scholarworks.wmich.edu/cgi/viewcontent.cgi?article=1052&context=reading_horizons

No Child Left Behind Act of 2001, PL 107-110, 115 Stat. 1425, 20 U.S.C. §§ 6301 *et seq.*

Oakhill, J., & Yuill, N. (1996). Higher order factors in comprehension disability: Processes and remediation. In C. Cornoldi & J. Oakhill (Eds.), *Reading comprehension difficulties: Processes and intervention* (pp. 69–92). Mahwah, NJ: Lawrence Erlbaum Associates.

Ogle, D.M. (1986). K-W-L: A teaching model that develops active reading of expository text. *The Reading Teacher, 39,* 564–570.

Palincsar, A.S., & Brown, A. (1984). Reciprocal teaching of comprehension-fostering and comprehension-monitoring activities. *Cognition and Instruction, 1,* 117–175.

Pallas, A.M., Natriello, G., & McDill, L. (1989). The changing nature of the disadvantaged population: Current dimensions and future trends. *Educational Researcher, 18,* 16–22.

Pearson, P.D., & Johnson, D.D. (1978). *Teaching reading comprehension.* Austin, TX: Holt, Rinehart & Winston.

Pressley, M. (2000). What should comprehension instruction be the instruction of? In M. Kamil, P. Mosenthal, P.D. Pearson, & R. Barr (Eds.), *Handbook of reading research* (Vol. III, pp. 545–562). Mahwah, NJ: Lawrence Erlbaum Associates.

Pressley, M., Brown, R., El-Dinary, P., & Afflerbach, P. (1995). The comprehension instruction that students need: Instruction fostering constructively responsive reading. *Learning Disabilities Research and Practice, 10,* 215–224.

RAND Reading Study Group (RRSG). (2002). *Reading for understanding: Toward an R & D program in reading comprehension.* Retrieved from http://www.rand.org/publications/MR/MR1465/MR1465.pdf

Raphael, T.E. (1982). Teaching children question-answering strategies. *The Reading Teacher, 36,* 186–191.

Raphael, T.E. (1984). Teaching learners about sources of information for answering comprehension questions. *Journal of Reading, 28,* 303–311.

Raphael, T.E. (1986). Teaching question-answer relationships, revisited. *The Reading Teacher, 39,* 516–522.

Raphael, T.E., & Au, K.H. (2005). QAR: Enhancing comprehension and test taking across grade and content levels. *The Reading Teacher, 59*(3), 206–221.

Rose, D., & Dalton, B. (2002). Using technology to individualize reading instruction. In C.C. Block, L.B. Gambrell, & M. Pressley (Eds.), *Improving comprehension instruction* (pp. 257–274). San Francisco, CA: Jossey-Bass.

Rosenshine, B., & Meister, C. (1994). Reciprocal teaching: A review of the research. *Review of Educational Research, 64*(4), 479–530.

Schumaker, J.B., Denton, P.H., & Deshler, D.D. (1984). *The paraphrasing strategy (learning strategies curriculum).* Lawrence: University of Kansas.

Serafini, F. (2013/2014). Close readings and children's literature. *The Reading Teacher, 67*(4) 299–301.

Shaywitz, S. (2003). *Overcoming dyslexia: A new and complete science-based program for reading problems at any level.* New York, NY: Alfred A. Knopf.

Siegel, L.S., & Ryan, E.B. (1988). Development of grammatical-sensitivity, phonological, and short-term memory skills in normally achieving and learning disabled children. *Developmental Psychology, 24,* 28–37.

Simmons, D.C., Fuchs, D., Fuchs, L.S., Hodge, J.P., & Mathes, P.G. (1994). Importance of instructional complexity and role reciprocity to class-wide peer tutoring. *Learning Disabilities Research and Practice, 9*(4), 203–212.

Simmons, D.C., Fuchs, L.S., Fuchs, D., Mathes, P.G., & Hodge, J.P. (1995). Effects of explicit teaching and peer tutoring on the reading achievement of learning-disabled and low-performing students in regular classrooms. *Elementary School Journal, 95,* 387–408.

Sparks, S.D. (2017). Common Core revisions: What are states really changing? *Education Week's blogs: Curriculum matters.* Retrieved from http://blogs.edweek.org/edweek/curriculum/2017/01/common_core_revisions_what_are.html

Stahl, K.A.D. (2004). Proof, practice, and promise: Comprehension strategy instruction in the primary grades. *The Reading Teacher, 57*(1), 598–609.

Stahl, S.A. (1991). Beyond the instrumentalist hypothesis: Some relationships between word meanings and comprehension. In P. Schwanenflugel (Ed.), *The psychology of word meanings* (pp. 157–178). Mahwah, NJ: Lawrence Erlbaum Associates.

Stanovich, K.E. (1986). Matthew effects in reading: Some consequences of individual differences in the acquisition of literacy. *Reading Research Quarterly, 21,* 360–406.

Strickland, D.S., Ganske, K., & Monroe, J.K. (2002). *Supporting struggling readers and writers.* Portland, ME: Stenhouse Publishers.

Sutherland-Smith, W. (2002). Weaving the literacy web: Changes in reading from page to screen. *The Reading Teacher, 55,* 662–669.

Sweet, A.P., & Snow, C. (2002). Reconceptualizing reading comprehension. In C.C. Block, L.B. Gambrell, & M. Pressley (Eds.), *Improving comprehension instruction* (pp. 17–53). San Francisco, CA: Jossey-Bass.

Taylor, B.M., Pearson, P.D., Clark, K.F., & Walpole, S. (1999). Effective schools/accomplished teachers. *The Reading Teacher, 53*(2), 156–159.

Taylor, B., Pearson, P., Peterson, D., & Rodriguez, M. (2003, September 1). Reading growth in high poverty classrooms: The influence of teacher practices that encourage cognitive engagement in literacy learning. *Elementary School Journal, 104*(1), 3–28.

Torgesen, J.K. (1998, Spring/Summer). Catch them before they fail. *American Educator,* 1–8.

Vaughn, S., Mathes, P., Linan-Thompson, S., Cirino, P., Carlson, C., Pollard-Durodola, S., … Francis, D. (2006). Effectiveness of an English intervention for first-grade English language learners at risk for reading problems. *Elementary School Journal, 107*(2), 153–180.

Walsh, K. (2003, Spring). Basal readers: The lost opportunity to build the knowledge that propels comprehension. *The American Educator, 27*, 24–27.

Weaver, P. (1979). Improving reading comprehension: Effects of sentence organization instruction. *Reading Research Quarterly, 15*, 127–146.

Williams, J. (1987). Educational treatments for dyslexia at the elementary and secondary levels. In R. Bowler (Ed.), *Intimacy with language: A forgotten basic in teacher education* (pp. 24–32). Baltimore, MD: The International Dyslexia Association.

Williams, J. (2002). Using the theme scheme. In C.C. Block & M. Pressley (Eds.), *Comprehension instruction: Research-based best practices* (pp. 126–139). New York, NY: Guilford.

Willingham, D. (2006, Spring). How knowledge helps. *American Educator, 30*, 30–37.

Willingham, D. (2006/2007, Winter). The usefulness of brief instruction in reading comprehension strategies. *American Educator, 30*, 39–45, 50.

Willingham, D. (2007, Summer). Can critical thinking be taught? *American Educator, 30*, 8–19.

Wixson, K. (1983). Questions about a text: What you ask about is what children learn. *The Reading Teacher, 37*, 287–293.

Wong, B.Y.L. (1979). Increasing retention of main ideas through questioning strategies. *Learning Disability Quarterly, 2*(2), 42–47.

Zubrzycki, J. (2017). Common-Core materials hard to find, poll says. *Education Week, 36*(17), 1, 7, 9.

Technology Resources

Elaine A. Cheesman

Effective programs/apps have the following features:

- They have text-to-speech option when appropriate.

- They have simultaneous text highlighting and narration.

- In connected text, article *a* is pronounced /u/ as in *up*, not /ā/ as in *ape*.

- They focus on components that affect a reader's comprehension of text—background knowledge, language structures (phrase, clause, sentence, paragraph), verbal reasoning (e.g., inference, figurative language), and genre. The associated component(s) are identified in parentheses next to the web site of the program/app.

Inspiration/Kidspiration   http://www.inspiration.com; language structures

This graphic organizer app provides multiple templates for different text structures/genre. For comprehension, students should complete the appropriate graphic organizer. The app has speech-to-text ability.

Interactive Book Apps   http://loudcrow.com or http://www.oceanhousemedia .com; genre, background knowledge

These apps provide simultaneous highlighting of narrated text. The user may tap to access the pronunciation of individual words.

Intro to Geography: United States; Intro to Geography: World   http://www. montessorium.com; background knowledge

This program allows the user to match map shapes to states (United States) and countries. It is fully narrated; no reading skills are needed. Organized by geographic area, the program presents small bits of information and provides systematic and cumulative instruction and review. It is appropriate for older students.

Kindle Books   http://www.Amazon.com; vocabulary, text structures, genre

The user may purchase or download free books from http://www.Amazon.com or http://www.gutenberg.org. Within the text, the user may tap a word to access its definition, pronunciation, and translation into numerous languages. Many orally narrated titles are available. The teacher can attach the device to an overhead projector.

Mind the Gap http://mindthegapapp.com; vocabulary, language structures, verbal reasoning, genre

This program allows the user to type missing words within paragraphs. Its 500 texts span multiple genres and 15 subject areas. The program can limit options to function words. Different levels are available (not for beginners). Arcade mode is available for idioms, proverbs, and so forth. The program is appropriate for older students and English language learners.

Rainbow Sentences http://mobile-educationstore.com; language structures

This program allows students to construct grammatically correct sentences with given words, using the drag-and-drop feature with individual words or with phrases. It has a color-coding option and manuscript and cursive options. It is appropriate for young children.

Sentence Reading Magic 1 and 2 http://www.preschoolu.com; language structures

This program allows the user to arrange words into complete sentences. It contains 324 two-, three-, four-, and five-word sentences, using decodable text with short vowels and consonant blends or high-frequency words. Manuscript or cursive fonts may be used. The program is appropriate for younger students.

Voyage of Ulysses http://elasticoapp.com; genre, background knowledge

This app provides an abridged, prose version of Homer's epic (tales include The Cyclops and The Trojan Horse). Text is narrated in British English or Italian. The app shows each tale's location on a map. Interactive animation deepens comprehension. Sometimes the user must activate animation to progress to the next story.

Chapter 17

Composition

Evidence-Based Instruction

Judith C. Hochman and Betsy MacDermott-Duffy

LEARNING OBJECTIVES

1. To consider the impact of explicit writing instruction on students of any proficiency level in all grades and content areas

2. To acquire strategies for teaching sentence-, paragraph-, and composition-level writing

3. To understand that sentences are the building blocks of all writing

4. To contemplate how to immediately integrate explicit writing instruction in all subjects

---

Many believe that writing is the most difficult of the language arts both to teach and to learn because of the simultaneous and complex cognitive, social, and linguistic demands required to complete a writing task. Yet, almost 50% of teachers report that they received minimal to no preparation for teaching writing in their teacher certification programs (Graham, 2008), and as a result, many teachers do not feel adequately prepared to teach writing. Lack of teacher preparation and knowledge can translate into ineffective instruction.

According to the latest National Assessment of Educational Progress in Writing (NAEP), (National Center for Education Statistics [NCES], 2012), approximately 75% of students tested in the United States in Grades 4–12 have only partial mastery of the prerequisite knowledge and skills required for writing competency. In order to address this deficit, the Common Core State Standards (CCSS; National Governors Association Center for Best Practices, 2010), were developed with a set of benchmarks to ensure college and career readiness. Their objective is to define a set of anchor standards and rigorous expectations for each grade level in language arts and literacy, including writing. Although the CCSS established student learning goals, teachers need direction and training about how to provide writing instruction in order to reach the objectives.

Research supports providing an early foundation in writing, often beginning as oral language activities in the primary grades. Not only is this seen as developmentally appropriate (National Association for the Education of Young Children

---

[NAEYC], 1998), but there is also considerable evidence that writing about content greatly enhances learning (Bangert-Drowns, Hurley, & Wilkinson, 2004; Graham & Hebert, 2010; Hebert, Gillespie, & Graham, 2013). To achieve the best outcomes, writing instruction should be integrated into every content area and at all grade levels from elementary through high school. Writing and thinking are inextricably linked. In order to enhance their knowledge of content, students should write about it. When students write about what they are learning, they gain more knowledge than if they are taught writing as a separate activity and assigned topics unrelated to the content in their classes.

Many individuals with excellent reading and speaking skills experience problems with writing. However, those with learning and language difficulties face especially formidable obstacles. These students have difficulties with decoding, spelling, word retrieval, and syntax that are often exacerbated by a limited vocabulary. Therefore, writing with clarity and accuracy is often significantly compromised. In addition, weak organizational skills often accompany learning and language problems. The inability to distinguish essential from nonessential information and to set forth facts or ideas in logical order can impede students as they try to generate well-organized paragraphs and compositions. Writing problems remain a persistent learning disability personally, academically, and vocationally for many adults who were not taught specific strategies as students (Scott, 2005). There is little, if any, explicit instruction in written language (Scott, 2005). This is especially true in the higher-level skills: revision, organization, and modifications for a particular audience. Often, it is assumed that mastery of the conventions of written language will naturally follow fluent decoding and good reading comprehension, but novice and poor writers need extensive practice with component writing skills in order to become proficient writers.

According to the *Knowledge and Practice Standards for Teachers of Reading* published by the International Dyslexia Association (IDA; 2018), between 15% and 20% of young students exhibit significant weaknesses with language processes. Beyond the skills outlined in the IDA *Knowledge and Practice Standards,* teachers need training in research-based strategies that will improve student writing at all levels in order to meet the written language expectations of the 21st century.

A growing body of research regarding the connection of writing to critical thinking, oral language, and comprehension has catapulted writing to the forefront of national attention. The development of writing in three distinct modes—narrative, expository, and argumentative—should be the primary aim of written language instruction. However, writing activities which center on self-expression rather than on communication with a reader, are frequently the major focus in elementary schools and even in some middle schools. Imaginative stories, personal narratives, poems, journal writing, and descriptions involving personal perceptions are assigned in many classes, often with little or no guidance from the teacher. Although the CCSS does not exclude creative assignments, the standards place a strong emphasis on students' ability to reason critically and write sound arguments on substantive topics and issues. Because many students tend to write the way they speak, a great deal of practice is necessary for unified, coherent written expression. Given the limited time teachers have to provide instruction in writing, their goal should be to help students develop a solid underpinning in those writing skills that are required most often academically and in the workplace: writing that explains or informs.

Working memory and executive function play critical roles in the develop-ment of writing proficiency. Executive function (see Chapter 8) affects all aspects of memory, attention, and language. Writers require them when they

- Strategize (select a topic)

- Initiate actions for a writing task (choose sources, gather information)

- Plan approaches (outline)

- Organize information (sequence and order details and evidence)

- Inhibit diversions

- Sustain tasks and motivation

- Assess outcomes against plans

- Institute needed changes (revise and edit).

The demands on working memory when writing are enormous. Working memory requires simultaneous processing of a multitude of tasks at higher cog-nitive levels than are required in other areas of skills acquisition. They have to plan ahead, as well as sequence and organize information. Both working memory and executive function require selective attention, as well as sustained and divided attention, span of attention, and the ability to shift attention (Singer & Bashir, 2004). Teachers of young children should keep these demands in mind when giving them writing assignments since letter formation, spelling, capitalization, punctuation and usage may not be at the levels of automaticity that would allow the students to focus on the higher level cognitive tasks, such as meaning, purpose, audience, syntax and semantics.

This chapter describes strategies and activities for writing sentences, para-graphs, and compositions, as well as for revising. Although they are presented in a linear structure, many should take place concurrently. Every strategy provides opportunities for differentiation for both developing and proficient writers.

SENTENCES

The importance of allocating a great deal of time crafting sentences cannot be over-stated. They are the foundation of all writing. If a student is not proficient in craft-ing sentences, the student's ability to construct coherent, unified paragraphs and compositions will be significantly compromised. Sentence activities are the bed-rock for revising and editing skills and play a major role in reading comprehension.

Sentence activities have two primary purposes. The first goal is to enable stu-dents to write complex sentences in addition to simple, active, declarative ones. Specific strategies to create varied and more linguistically interesting sentences can result in better writing, improved oral language, and better reading comprehension (Graham & Perin, 2007; Hillocks, 1984; Maria, 1990; Neville & Searls, 1991; Scott, 2005; Shanahan, 2004). When students can produce complex sentences in writing, they will process them better while reading text that is densely loaded with facts and **embedded clauses,** such as **relative clauses**. The second goal is to improve revision and editing skills, which enhance both the flow of composing as well as the writer's analytical thinking. Students' knowledge of grammar and the functions of the parts of speech is enhanced by emphasizing sentence structure and sentence activities (Scott, 2002).

Sentence strategies should be practiced both orally and in writing and can be adapted to be more or less challenging, depending on the age and ability of the students.

Sentences and Fragments

The IDA's *Knowledge and Practice Standards* identify grammatical sentence structure and sentence processing as important component abilities. For kindergarten literacy, the CCSS calls for teachers to design instruction that will encourage students to produce complete sentences in shared oral language activities, and by Grade 4, students should be able to independently write complete sentences and recognize and correct inappropriate fragments and **run-on sentences.** Learning the varied sentence structures needs to be reinforced throughout the grades (declarative, interrogative, imperative, and exclamatory; simple, compound, complex, and compound-complex). Through oral activities and then to written activities embedded in content, students can effectively learn to identify **fragments** and sentences while demonstrating comprehension of important information.

To teach these skills, first the teacher guides the students to identify and correct fragments. Then, the students distinguish between sentences and fragments in lists. They correct the fragments and provide capitalization and punctuation to the sentences. After that, the students have to find and correct fragments in texts. The final step is to find and correct fragments in their own writing.

The following sentence and fragment activities can reinforce vocabulary knowledge and spelling, as well as demonstrate the difference between fragments and sentences.

Example for Developing Writers Use an activity such as the following to teach developing writers to distinguish between sentences and fragments and change fragments into complete sentences.

TEACHER: A sentence tells us who or what did what. Tell me whether groups of words you hear (or read) are sentences or not: *need water to grow.* Does that tell us what needs water to grow?

STUDENT: No, that's not a sentence.

TEACHER: Correct. It's a fragment, which is only part of a sentence. Change the fragment into a complete sentence by adding what needs water to grow.

STUDENT: Plants need water to grow.

TEACHER: That's right. That's a complete sentence.

Identify & Convert Fragments

1. _F_ a political map
   A political map features cities, capitals and borders.

2. _F_ where people live
   A map illustrates where people live.

3. _S_ a legend explains what the symbols mean
   A legend explains what the symbols mean.

4. _F_ on a physical map
   Mountains and rivers can be found on a physical map.

Figure 17.1. Example of student work practicing identifying fragments and sentences and then correcting them. Copyright © 2017 The Writing Revolution. All rights reserved. Published with Permission.

Example for Proficient Writers Use an activity such as the following to reinforce proficient writers' understanding of sentences and fragments by having them supply a missing subject or predicate.

TEACHER: On a physical map

STUDENTS: Mountains, rivers and deserts can be found on a physical map.

Students often speak in fragments (incomplete sentences), and many of them do the same when they write. Students should be able to identify and correct fragments in a list or a paragraph before attempting to find and correct them in their own work.

When students understand the concept of a complete sentence they can look for and correct fragments in text. Unlike the examples in Figure 17.1, the fragments in Figure 17.2 are capitalized and punctuated, making them more difficult to find. This activity requires the student to read closely to find and to demonstrate knowledge by correcting errors.

Scrambled Sentences

According to the early grade-level goals from the CCSS, students are expected to produce complete sentences with correct punctuation and capitalization, and in

Identify & Convert Fragments

Jupiter and "the Mighty Ones" are not so mighty. Jupiter fears being discovered as weak. To keep humans poor and ignorant. He fears humans gaining fire from Prometheus. If they gain knowledge and health. As a result, Jupiter resorts to tricks to keep humans from gaining power. Clearly, Jupiter and the gods wants to maintain their power over humans.

He wants to keep humans poor and ignorant.
If they gain knowledge and health, Jupiter will no longer have power.

Figure 17.2. Example of fragments embedded in text. Copyright © 2017 The Writing Revolution. All rights reserved. Published with Permission.

the IDA *Knowledge and Practice Standards* teachers are charged with having knowledge of sentence structure.

Rearranging words that are out of sequence into sentences and adding the correct punctuation and capitalization reinforces the concept of sentence boundaries and the grammatical roles of words in a sentence. Scrambled sentences should not be too complex or have too many words. Younger students may need to be given the first word of the sentence with the first letter capitalized. The following examples of scrambled sentences could be given to developing and proficient writers.

Examples for Developing Writers

yellow **the** flew bird away

The _____

ants spiders **A**rmy and kill catch

_____

Examples for Proficient Writers

in the means name Esperanza "hope" English

_____

ended without the War of 1812 a victory

_____

Sentence Types: Statements, Questions, Exclamations, and Commands

The ability to vary the sentence types is an important tool for writing topic and concluding sentences as well as varying the sentence structures within text. The following examples show practice activities to help developing and proficient writers learn to vary sentence types.

Example for Developing Writers

Change statements into questions (and vice versa).

The yellow bird flew away.

Did the yellow bird fly away?

Examples for Proficient Writers

Write sentences about the following topic.

Topic: Fractions

Statement: A fraction is a part of something.

Question: Can you give me the definition of a fraction?

Command: Divide a circle into two equal parts.

Exclamation: I want half of that candy bar!

Topic: Van Gogh

*Declarative:** *The Starry Night* depicts a village in southern France.

*Interrogatory:** Did the impressionist movement influence Vincent van Gogh?

*Imperative:** Study Van Gogh's work.

*Exclamatory:** Van Gogh was brilliant!

*Some teachers of older students prefer to use these synonymous terms for the sentence types.

It is just as important to have students generate questions as it is to have them respond to the questions. For example, the teacher can show primary-grade students a picture and ask them what question(s) the picture suggests. Older students should be asked to anticipate essay questions on upcoming tests or produce questions after assigned reading and reading comprehension exercises. Research indicates that this exercise enhances reading comprehension (Graham & Hebert, 2010).

Conjunctions

Conjunctions (also called connectives or linking words) join words, phrases, and clauses. Their purpose is to link or relate parts of a sentence. For a list of conjunctions with their definitions, see Textbox 17.1. Teachers may use this as a reference and insert it in students' notebooks to aid them in independent writing.

Conjunctions help student write extended responses, which provide the reader with more information and encourage analytical thinking. In addition, conjunctions foster close reading as the student looks for textual evidence. Conjunction activities also serve as checks for comprehension. Students who learn to write using conjunctions are better able to connect relationships between ideas, a skill necessary to compose effective compositions and argumentative essays.

The conjunction *because* tells why, the conjunction *but* indicates a change of direction, and the conjunction *so* explains cause and effect.

TEXTBOX 17.1 **Conjunctions most frequently used in texts and student writing**

CONJUNCTIONS

Conjunctions join words, phrases, and clauses to each other. They help make writing clear and linguistically rich.

There are four kinds of conjunctions:

1. *Coordinating conjunctions:* A coordinating conjunction joins two or more independent clauses (*and, but, or, yet, not, for, so*).

2. *Correlative conjunctions:* A correlative conjunction is a pair of words that joins independent clauses.

Both . . .and	*either . . .or*	*neither . . .nor*
just as . . .so	*not only . . .but also*	*whether . . .or*

3. *Subordinating conjunctions:* A subordinating conjunction introduces an adverb clause and signals the relationship between that clause and the main idea.

   Common subordinating conjunctions:

after	*if*	*than*	*when*
although	*in order*	*that*	*where*
as	*once*	*that*	*while*
as if	*regardless*	*though*	
because	*since*	*unless*	
before	*so that*	*until*	

4. *Conjunctive adverbs:* A conjunctive adverb connects independent clauses and can be considered both a conjunction and an adverb. Independent clauses connected by a conjunctive adverb must be separated by a semicolon, not just a comma. Conjunctive adverbs often begin sentences.

   Common conjunctive adverbs:

also	*however*	*moreover*	*similarly*
anyway	*incidentally*	*namely*	*still*
besides	*indeed*	*nevertheless*	*then*
certainly	*instead*	*next*	*therefore*
finally	*likewise*	*now*	*thus*
furthermore	*meanwhile*	*otherwise*	*undoubtedly*

Asking students "Why did the colonists settle near rivers?" will not yield as much information or require as much thinking as asking them to complete the following sentence stems:

- The colonists settled near rivers because . . .

- The colonists settled near rivers, but . . .

- The colonists settled near rivers, so . . .

The following examples show sentence-completion activities for developing and proficient writers that help them learn to use conjunctions to connect ideas.

Examples for Developing Writers

The American flag is an important symbol because *it represents the fifty states and thirteen colonies.*

The American flag is an important symbol, but *it is not always respected.*

The American flag is an important symbol, so *most United States citizens are grateful for what it represents.*

Examples for Proficient Writers

The British invaded the colonies because *they were threatened by repeated acts of rebellion.*

The British invaded the colonies, but *they faced fierce resistance.*

The British invaded the colonies, so *they could maintain control.*

Students should learn to write sentences beginning with subordinating conjunctions. Linguistically complex sentences reflect frequently used written language structures, often with one or more dependent clauses beginning a sentence. The following examples show activities that teach developing and proficient writers to complete sentences beginning with dependent clauses.

Examples for Developing Writers

After the bird flew south, *Rocket practiced writing the alphabet.*

If Charlotte didn't write words on her web, *Wilbur would have been killed.*

Even though seeds need water, *be careful not to give them too much.*

> **Examples for Proficient Writers**
>
> Although both plant and animal cells have many of the same organelles, *they are not exactly alike.*
>
> While plant cells need chloroplasts to create food, *animal cells don't need them because animals eat to get food.*
>
> Since cells are the building blocks of life, *all living things have cells.*

Appositives

Choosing words and phrases to convey ideas precisely and provide support for ideas in writing have been identified in new standards as areas that will necessitate continued attention throughout the grades as these structures are applied to progressively more sophisticated writing and speaking. Appositives exemplify one of these structures and although they are frequently seen in writing, they rarely used when speaking.

An appositive is often referred to as a phrase that renames the subject of a sentence or another noun. It can be a brief or lengthy combination of words. Along with sentence types and subordinating conjunctions, appositives also provide a strategy for writing topic and concluding sentences. They provide the reader with more information and vary sentence structure.

Students need to know that an appositive is a noun or noun phrase that provides the reader with more information about the noun next to it. They need to see examples and then provide their own. The following activity illustrates how a teacher might explain the concept of appositives.

TEACHER: How would you describe Washington, D.C.?

STUDENT: The capital of the United States

TEACHER: We call a phrase that gives us another name for the subject or noun an appositive. Now say a sentence using the appositive.

STUDENT: Washington, D.C., the capital of the United States, is a beautiful city.

Students should be able to distinguish between various types of clauses and appositives. The following activity illustrates how a teacher might show students how to do so.

TEACHER: Does this sentence have an appositive in it? John is very strong and lifts weights.

STUDENT: No.

TEACHER: Can you rephrase it and add an appositive?

STUDENT: John, a strong person, lifts weights.

TEACHER: Tell me a topic sentence about Gandhi using an appositive.

STUDENT: Gandhi, a pacifist, led India's independence movement.

The following additional examples illustrate how developing and proficient writers might use appositives in their writing.

Examples for Developing Writers

Giraffes, *the world's tallest mammals*, are endangered.

Bullying, *mistreating another person*, is unacceptable behavior.

Examples for Proficient Writers

Emperor Qin Shi Huang initially conceived the Great Wall of China, *a symbol of the country's strength*, in the third century B.C. as a means of preventing invasions by barbarians.

The Nobel Peace Prize, *one of five Nobel awards,* is given to individuals who have promoted peace between nations.

Sentence Combining

Sentence combining is a technique for combining simple sentences into longer, more complex ones and is one of the most effective ways to teach grammar and usage. Traditional grammar instruction, typically taught in isolation, has produced slight negative effects on student writing (Graham & Perin, 2007; Saddler, 2012). Gaining knowledge about basic grammar within content is most effective. Students need plenty of practice combining short, declarative sentences using pronouns, commas, and conjunctions as needed. More capable writers may also be taught to use colons and semicolons. Activities like the following can be used to practice this skill.

TEACHER: *[Asks students to combine short, active, declarative sentences using conjunctions and explains that repetition can be avoided by using pronouns.]*

Combine these sentences using a conjunction: John was at the bus stop. John's car was being repaired.

STUDENT: John was at the bus stop because his car was being repaired.

The following additional examples illustrate how developing and proficient writers might practice combining sentences.

Examples for Developing Writers

TEACHER: Combine the following sentences using a conjunction and a pronoun.

Mulan wanted to fight.

Mulan was a girl.

STUDENT: Mulan wanted to fight, but she was a girl.

Examples for Proficient Writers

TEACHER: Combine the following sentences using a subordinating conjunction
and an appositive.

The periodic table is a chart of chemical elements.

The chart displays the elements in horizontal rows.

The elements are displayed horizontally in order of increasing atomic number.

*The elements are displayed vertically in order of the structured similarity of
their atoms.*

STUDENT: The periodic table, a chart of chemical elements, displays them horizontally in order of increasing atomic number and vertically in order
of the structural similarity of their atoms.

Sentence Expansion

This strategy requires students to anticipate what a reader needs to know and to
provide that information. It also teaches notetaking skills and promotes written
language structures. In addition, sentence expansion helps students to summarize
and serves as a comprehension check.

To teach sentence expansion, the teacher should display the question words
who, what, when, where, why, and *how* and then give students a kernel sentence, a
simple sentence without modifiers, such as *Jane ran* or *The candidates debated.* Next,
the teacher should ask the class to expand the **sentence kernel** by using one, two,
three, or more of the question words. The teacher, not the students, should select
the question words. When the students are writing independently, they can decide
which question words to use in order to provide a reader with more information

When introducing this strategy, it is best to begin with *when, where,* or *why.*
If *who* or *what* are used, they must refer to a pronoun in the kernel (e.g., He *fought
the British. Bill dropped* it.)

Responses to the question words should be written in key words and phrases
on the dotted lines placed after the question words. Older students should use
abbreviations and notetaking symbols when appropriate. (see Figure 17.3) In
elementary school, learning to use symbols should begin with equal signs (=),
"and" (+, &) symbols, and the sideways arrow indicating leads to or results in (→).
Symbols are important for sentence expansion, annotating, note taking and creating the outlines discussed later in this chapter. Research indicates that taking notes
by hand, rather than on a laptop is more efficient and effective in helping students
differentiate between essential and nonessential information. In addition, it boosts
comprehension, and enables retention. Note taking is a critical feature in helping
students outline paragraphs and compositions before drafting them (Mueller &
Oppenheimer, 2014; Willingham, 2017).

Kernel sentences should not be commands because the students may be confused about *what* or *who* when the subject is inferred. The response to *when* should
always come first in the expanded sentence because that structure reflects one frequently noted in written language: *On April 9, 1865, the Civil War ended.*

Give students practice converting sentences into key words and phrases. As
they become more proficient, they can add symbols and abbreviations.

SYMBOLS

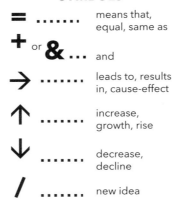

Figure 17.4 illustrates how a teacher might provide practice for proficient writers to convert sentences into key words, phrases, symbols, and abbreviations. Students can reverse this process and turn key words, phrases, symbols, and abbreviations into sentences.

Example for Developing Writers Figure 17.5 shows an example of sentence expansion by a developing writer. Note that it contains only key words and no symbols or abbreviations.

Example for Proficient Writers Figure 17.6 shows an example of sentence expansion of a proficient writer. Note key words, symbols, and abbreviations.

Grammar and Usage

The parts of speech and their usage should be taught within the writing program. Teaching grammar within sentence activities helps students gain an

Convert sentence into key words, phrases, abbreviations, & symbols

1. Artifacts are man-made objects.

   artifacts = man-made objects

2. Weapons, pottery, bowls, and tools are examples of artifacts.

   Weapons + pottery + bowls + tools = artifacts

3. Artifacts can give clues about ancient civilizations.

   artifacts → clues / ancient civs

Figure 17.4. Example of sentence expansion by a developing writer. Note that there are only key words and no symbols or abbreviations. Copyright © 2017 The Writing Revolution. All rights reserved. Published with Permission.

Sentence Expansion

Pyramids were built.

When: ancient times

Where: Egypt

Why: protect body of deceased pharaoh

Expanded sentence:

In ancient times, pyramids were built in Egypt
to protect the body of the deceased pharaoh.

Figure 17.5. Example of sentence expansion of a proficient writer. Note key words, symbols, and abbreviations. Copyright © 2017 The Writing Revolution. All rights reserved. Published with Permission.

understanding of how parts of speech are used in context, which proves especially useful when students are expected to revise and edit their own work or assigned passages. An activity such as the following one can be used to reinforce students' understanding of the parts of speech.

TEACHER: *[Asks students to change nouns to pronouns.]* The tarantula hid.

STUDENT: It hid.

TEACHER: *[Asks students to change tenses from present to past (or from present to future or vice versa).]* The tarantula sheds its exoskeleton.

STUDENT: The tarantula shed its exoskeleton. The tarantula will shed its exoskeleton.

TEACHER: *[Asks students to insert an adjective, an adverb, and a prepositional phrase.]* The tarantula attacked.

STUDENT: The gigantic tarantula attacked swiftly.

Sentence Expansion

He called a meeting.

Who: Old Major

When: 3 days b/4 he died

Where: Manor Farm

Why: encourage animals to revolt

Expanded sentence:

Three days before he died, Old Major called a
meeting at Manor Farm to encourage the
animals to revolt.

Figure 17.6. Practice for proficient writers to convert sentences into key words, phrases, symbols, and abbreviations. Students can reverse this process and turn key words, phrases, symbols, and abbreviations into sentences. Copyright © 2017 The Writing Revolution. All rights reserved. Published with Permission.

TEACHER: *[Asks students to use an appositive after a proper noun (As noted earlier, an* **appositive** *is a second noun, placed beside the first noun to explain it more fully; it usually has modifiers).]* George Washington was a brilliant general.

STUDENT: George Washington, our first president, was a brilliant general.

Topic Sentences

The topic sentence of a paragraph should clearly state the writer's objective. The teacher should show students how to generate topic sentences for given topics. He or she explains to the students that the topic sentence is the leading sentence of the paragraph (Morgan, 2001).

Students must be able to distinguish between topic sentences and supporting details. Selecting the topic sentence from a group of sentences is a beneficial activity. For example, students might be asked to select the topic sentence among the following:

- Try to see a Broadway show.

- The Metropolitan Museum of Art is a fantastic place to visit.

- New York City is a great place to visit.

- The New York Botanical Garden is beautiful.

Students can learn to write more interesting topic and concluding sentences in the early grades by using the sentence types. Then, as they become more proficient, they can learn to use subordinating conjunctions and appositives to write better topic and concluding sentences. An activity such as the following can be used to provide practice.

TEACHER: Create three different topic sentences using the strategies that we learned. Use New Orleans as the topic.

STUDENTS: Visit New Orleans. *[sentence type: a command]*

New Orleans, a beautiful city, is popular with tourists. *[includes appositive]*

After visiting New Orleans, it's easy to see why it's a popular tourist destination. *[includes subordinating conjunction]*

REFLECT, CONNECT, and RESPOND
Use the two primary goals for sentence strategies to develop an explanation of the importance for practice in sentence activities.

PARAGRAPHS AND COMPOSITIONS

The CCSS emphasize the importance of nonfiction reading and expository writing from the earliest grades through high school. The standards place a strong emphasis on writing as a means of demonstrating knowledge. It is suggested that writing be taught in the context of expository text related to science, social studies, literature and current events.

Five Writing Modes

Students should practice writing five types of paragraphs in preparation for writing compositions and to enhance their reading comprehension: narrative, expository, descriptive, compare and contrast (a type of expository writing), persuasive and argumentative.

Narrative writing relates events in chronological order, and sentences can be sequenced using transition words, such as *first, next, then,* and *finally.* Narratives are often assigned to younger and less skilled writers (Alley & Deshler, 1979). Written in the first person (narrator as a participant) or third person (narrator as an observer), this type of composition is helpful when it is based on a process or a class experience. Older students are often assigned narratives to describe historical events or a scientific process. Textbox 17.2 provides a list of frequently used transition words and phrases.

Expository writing explains or informs. Students typically are asked to define, discuss, criticize, list, compare, contrast, explain, justify, and summarize. The topic sentence of a paragraph or thesis statement of a composition should clearly express the writer's purpose or claim. Because this type of assignment is the kind of writing most frequently required in school, in the workplace, and in life, it deserves the most instructional time.

The **compare-and-contrast composition,** a type of expository writing, highlights the similarities (comparisons) and differences (contrasts) among two or more people, places, things, ideas, or experiences. A conclusion is sometimes developed from the facts presented.

Descriptive writing taps the five senses in order to effectively transmit experiences about people, places, things, and thoughts. Varied and vivid vocabulary is especially important when developing a descriptive passage. Brainstorming and generating lists of adjectives, adverbs and more precise nouns and verbs are appropriate activities to use in conjunction with descriptive writing lessons. It is often beneficial to employ spatial and visual terms in descriptive writing, such as *beyond, underneath, below, above, to the left,* and so forth.

In **persuasive** or **pro/con** or **argumentative writing,** the writer tries to convince a reader to adopt a certain point of view. Persuasive writing, the least challenging of the three, requires no evidence and is usually assigned to elementary students. It is based on the writer's personal experience. Pro and con paragraphs require the writer to present both sides of an issue in a neutral tone. Argumentative essays, on the other hand, call for students to defend a thesis using reason and logic and to marshal evidence in support of claims (Hochman & Wexler, 2017).

To prepare students to write argumentative essays, teachers should have them first practice arguing both sides of a question, in separate paragraphs, and provide evidence to support each side. A student might plan or write a pro paragraph arguing that Andrew Carnegie was a captain of industry and a con paragraph taking the position that he was a "robber baron."

As difficult as it is to learn to write an argumentative essay, it is a skill that will serve students well. This kind of writing is frequently assigned in college, and students will be at a serious disadvantage if they encounter it there for the first time. It is also a skill students will generally find useful in later life both in the workplace and personally. Of all the writing genres, it is the most effective at sharpening analytical faculties. Learning to construct and defend an argument will force students to think logically and critically.

TEXTBOX 17.2   Transition Words and Phrases

1A: Time and Sequence	1B: Time and Sequence	2: Conclusion
first	initially	in conclusion
second	previously	in closing
in addition	soon	in summary
after	later on	as a result*
last	at last	consequently*
then	additionally	finally
next	currently	therefore*
also	earlier	so*
before	meanwhile	thus*
finally	ultimately	in the end
	during	

3: Illustration	4: Change of Direction	5: Emphasis
for example	however	especially
for instance	even though	in particular
specifically	in contrast	obviously
particularly	otherwise	above all
as an illustration	on the other hand	most
namely	although	importantly
such as	but	primarily
expressly	yet	certainly
like	instead	particularly
including	on the contrary	moreover
in particular		notably
		keep in mind

*In addition to conclusion signals, these words or phrases can be used to indicate cause and effect.

The ability to write a reasoned, evidence-based argument is critical for college and career readiness. The foundation for writing analytical argumentative essays can be laid in the primary grades. For example, learning to demonstrate change of direction with *but*, then using transitions such as *on the other hand, although,* and *however,* are important in presenting claims or counterclaims. The transitions that illustrate a point, *specifically* and *for example,* are helpful when introducing evidence. Younger students can begin to use these strategies, even at the sentence level, without being required to write a fully developed argumentative paper, as in the following examples:

- Presenting a counterclaim, then a claim: *Plants need water to grow. However, too much water will kill them.*

- Presenting evidence: *Global warming is endangering some species. Specifically, the population of Adélie penguins along the West Antarctic Peninsula is declining.*

It is important that students know how to develop a good paragraph before moving on to compositions. Many students are encouraged prematurely to write at length about a topic, thus confusing quantity with quality. The chances are that if students write too much too soon, they will not stick to the topic, they will repeat themselves, and they will not proofread or learn how to revise their writing effectively.

The Writing Process

The following four steps should be required for most writing assignments:

- Planning and outlining

- Drafting

- Revising

- Editing

Planning and outlining, revising, and editing are the most important. Therefore, they should be given the most instructional time.

Planning and Outlining Planning is the point at which students begin to organize information and ideas systematically and sequentially. Teachers should model the planning and outlining process as a whole-class activity. Class discussions that establish the topic, purpose, and audience of the paragraph or composition are essential. Practice is needed to distinguish between relevant, less essential, and nonessential details. Main ideas and important supporting details can then be categorized and sequenced on the outline.

A plan for a paragraph or composition should be presented. Linear outlines help writers see the overall structure of a paragraph or composition (see Figures 17.7–17.10). They support analytical thinking through explicit instruction of organizational strategies for varied text structures. Outlines enhance the ability to link related ideas, and they help avoid repetitive or tangential information (Hochman & MacDermott-Duffy, 2015). In addition, the format reminds the writer to provide sufficient support for the topic sentence or **thesis statement.** All of these activities should initially be done as a class with plenty of teacher demonstrations and guidance.

Multiple outlines can be generated without moving on to drafts since the importance of a plan cannot be overestimated. As students become proficient, they can be expected to develop outlines independently whenever a paragraph or composition is assigned.

Three useful outline forms are as follows:

- **The Single Paragraph Outline (SPO)** is used for developing a single paragraph and is intended to help students discern the basic structure of a paragraph: topic sentence, supporting details, and concluding sentence (see Figures 17.7 and 17.8).

Single Paragraph Outline

T.S. Winter, the coldest season of the year, takes place from December until March.

weather　1. cold + snow / short days

dangers　2. icy roads + sidewalks/frostbite

activities　3. sledding/ice skating/snowmen

clothes　4. scarves, mittens, hats, heavy coats

C.S. Even though there can be problems, many people love winter!

Figure 17.7. Example of developing writer using a Single Paragraph Outline. Copyright © 2017 The Writing Revolution. All rights reserved. Published with Permission.

- **The Transition Outline** is effective when younger students are beginning to write compositions of two or three paragraphs (see Figure 17.9).

- **The Multiple Paragraph Outline (MPO)** is for developing compositions of three or more paragraphs as students are preparing to write more advanced compositions and argumentative essays (Hochman & Wexler, 2017; see Figure 17.10).

After students have mastered a particular outlining format, they should proceed to writing drafts.

Single Paragraph Outline　Students must master several preliminary skills before they can develop an SPO independently (see Figures 17.7 and 17.8). First, they should be able to distinguish topic sentences from supporting detail sentences. Then, they need to learn to produce a topic sentence for a given topic. Students eventually should be able to use the three strategies for writing topic sentences: a sentence type, a subordinating conjunction, and an appositive.

The only complete sentences on the SPO are the topic and concluding sentences. Therefore, another prerequisite skill is learning how to write details on the

Single Paragraph Outline

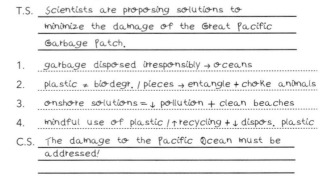

T.S. Scientists are proposing solutions to minimize the damage of the Great Pacific Garbage Patch.

1. garbage disposed irresponsibly → oceans

2. plastic ≠ biodegr. / pieces → entangle + choke animals

3. onshore solutions = ↓ pollution + clean beaches

4. mindful use of plastic / ↑ recycling + ↓ dispos. plastic

C.S. The damage to the Pacific Ocean must be addressed!

Figure 17.8. Example of proficient writer using a Single Paragraph Outline. Copyright © 2017 The Writing Revolution. All rights reserved. Published with Permission.

Transition Outline (3 Paragraphs)

Name: _____ Date: _____

Topic: _Thanksgiving_

1st ¶ – T.S. A long time ago Pilgrims started a holiday called Thanksgiving, which we still celebrate today.

History

1. hardships in England
2. Mayflower → new world → escape persecution
3. Native Americans helped / feast "Thanksgiving"

2nd ¶ – T.S. Today, Thanksgiving is a time when families get together.

Tradition

1. hours spent / preparing traditional feast
2. everyone gathers / Macy's parade / football
3. feast / turkey + trimmings + delicious desserts

3rd ¶ – T.S. Also, Thanksgiving is a reminder to appreciate all we have.

Thankful

1. thankful for good health
2. free country → vote / travel
3. grateful for relationships / friends + family

C.S. Thanksgiving is a truly meaningful holiday!

Figure 17.9. Transition Outline example. Copyright © 2017 The Writing Revolution. All rights reserved. Published with Permission.

dotted lines using key words, phrases, and later, when students are more proficient, symbols and abbreviations (e.g., Sugar + Stamp = Townshend Acts = taxation w/o representation --> Revolutionary War). This is a precursor to effective notetaking, a skill vital for extracting the main points from texts or oral presentations, for annotating and for better recall.

The last prerequisite skill for developing outlines is writing a concluding sentence, which is often a rephrasing of the topic sentence or, in an opinion piece, a call to action. The three options for writing topic sentences can be used for concluding sentences, as seen on the topic of climate change:

1. Appositive: *Climate change, a dangerous threat to the planet, needs to be addressed by all nations.*

2. Subordinating conjunction: *Unless the threat of climate change is addressed, the planet will be in danger.*

3. Sentence type (exclamation): *Climate change is a threat to the future of the planet!*

Many activities can focus on one feature of the SPO—specifically, sequencing details in chronological order; eliminating details from a list or a paragraph that does not relate to the topic sentence; selecting appropriate details from a list that

Multiple-Paragraph Outline

Topic: Mosquito-born Diseases

Thesis Statement: Even though Dengue fever has become pandemic, it is not safe to unleash genetically-altered mosquitos into the environment.

Main Idea	Details
Introduction ¶1	G S T (above)
¶2 risks (claim) X T.S.	• insecticides → resistance / toxic • Dengue / ↑ 100 countries / 14 B ppl. • no vaccines / must find solutions
¶3 benefits (counterclaim) X T.S.	• vital to protect health • less damaging than pesticides / need res. • initial results positive / Brazil
¶4 risks (claim) X T.S.	• unknown consequences • alter ecosystems / agri. havoc • modifying DNA → accident → superbug
Conclusion ¶5	rephrase T S G

Figure 17.10. Multiple Paragraph Outline example. Copyright © 2017 The Writing Revolution. All rights reserved. Published with Permission.

support the topic sentence; and practicing outlining topics with varied text structures (problem–solution, cause–effect, pro–con, compare–contrast, narrative).

The following sequence is suggested to develop an SPO with developing writers:

- Introduce a topic and provide background information (e.g., Thanksgiving).

- Identify the audience (e.g., people who do not know about the holiday).

- Identify the purpose (e.g., explain history and traditions).

- Provide a topic sentence for the students or generate several as a class.

- Elicit supporting details about the topic and categorize them for the dotted lines on the outline (e.g., history, traditions, food, thankful). Write the details as key words, phrases, abbreviations, and symbols.

- Distribute a blank SPO to each student.

- If more than one topic sentence is generated, ask the students to write their preferred one on their outline. Then, either as a class, in small groups, or individually select the most relevant details. The students write the related details on the dotted lines using key words and phrases, symbols and abbreviations.

- Generate a concluding sentence.

Transition Outline   The Transition Outline (see Figure 17.9) can be introduced after the students have had experience writing single paragraphs and are ready to move to longer compositions. Some students will be able to go directly to MPOs, described in the next section, but others may need an intermediate step. The Transition Outline provides an overview of the whole composition, including topic sentences and details for every paragraph. A concluding sentence is not necessary for any paragraph other than the last one; however, students may have to learn how to use transitional sentences between paragraphs. The first topic sentence has to be broad enough to cover all the paragraphs, as does the concluding sentence.

Multiple Paragraph Outline   The MPO (see Figure 17.10) is designed for students who are ready to develop unified, coherent compositions of three or more paragraphs with formal introductions and conclusions. This type of essay poses a number of challenges for students with learning disabilities. Students must initially be guided to select topics that are neither too broad nor too narrow. Sufficient background knowledge, appropriate sources, and a specific purpose for writing as well as the audience must be established. The thesis statement should present a claim or summarize the main point of the essay.

Unlike the SPO, the main idea of each paragraph in an MPO is not written as a topic sentence but as a category on the left side of the MPO outline (e.g., pro, con; cause, effect; similarities, differences; first reason, second reason). As with the other outlines, the supporting details should be written on the dotted lines as notes, such as phrases or key words, symbols, and abbreviations. The MPO helps students learn to write an introduction, body paragraphs, and a conclusion. This outline enables students to adhere to their theme, state their purpose, and present their points or evidence by providing a clear visual diagram of the entire work.

The teacher does not need to move in sequence from three-, to four-, to five-paragraph compositions because the number of paragraphs usually depends on the topic and the number of categories needed to write fully about the subject. For example, a book report may require three paragraphs, with categories such as introduction, plot summary, and opinion. A topic such as pollution might have four categories: introduction, causes, effects, and a conclusion that might present possible solutions. A presidential biography may require five categories: introduction, early life, career, presidency, and conclusion.

Depending on the topic, most MPOs require a thesis statement, which drives the entire essay. The body paragraphs support the thesis with details that present relevant evidence. Students need to understand that the points the writer wishes to emphasize should be at the end of the composition because that is where they will have the most impact on a reader. The last sentences of an essay are as important as the first ones.

To develop a complete MPO, the following sequence is suggested:

- Select the topic.

- Identify the purpose and audience.

- Develop the thesis statement.

- Write the main idea for each paragraph in the left-hand column. Each paragraph must relate to the thesis statement.

- After determining the main idea for each paragraph, write the supporting details in the right-hand column. Each supporting detail should relate directly to the main idea of the paragraph.

Writing introductions is often difficult for students. They might add details that belong in the body paragraphs or fail to convey to the reader the composition's purpose and plan of development. An introduction should consist of at least three sentences, and the last sentence should be the thesis statement. The first sentence should be a general statement, and the second sentence should be a specific statement (Lunsford & Connors, 1995). The following introduction follows that structure.

General statement: Thomas Jefferson is remembered for significant accomplishments during his presidency.

Specific statement: The acquisition of the Louisiana Territory from France is considered by many historians to be his most outstanding achievement.

Thesis statement: As a result of the Louisiana Purchase, Jefferson significantly increased the size of the United States, opened up new trade routes, and marked the beginning of the nation as a world power.

The prerequisites for writing effective introductions include the ability to do each of the following:

- Distinguish between general, specific, and thesis statements.

- Write general statements when given specific and thesis statements.

- Write general and specific statements when given a thesis statement.

Conclusions begin with a rephrase thesis statement, followed by a specific and then a general statement, as in the following example.

Thesis statement rephrased: With the Louisiana Purchase, Jefferson opened trading opportunities and almost doubled the size of the United States.

Specific statement: The acquisition of 828 square miles began the westward expansion.

General statement: Jefferson's decision to purchase the Louisiana territory led to the nation's role as a world leader.

Drafting   Drafting begins with writing paragraphs or compositions based on SPOs, Transition Outlines, or MPOs. Developing writers should limit their writing to one paragraph of five or six sentences because longer papers tend to discourage attempts to revise and edit. An activity can end with an outline or with a revision if the objectives of the lesson have been met. However, a draft should not be left uncorrected or unimproved. Revisions and edits should always be expected. A teacher may decide to end an activity with a corrected draft instead of moving on to a final copy.

Revising and Editing   The sentence and outlining strategies provide the foundation for developing the skills to improve written work. Revision refers to the clarification or alteration of the meaning or structure of a draft. This is in contrast to editing, which involves proofreading and correcting errors in grammar, punctuation, syntax, and spelling. Editing usually receives more instructional time, although revision is just as important, if not more so.

Throughout the revision process, the teacher should stress that even proficient writers rework their drafts at least two or three times and that the better the writer, the more often the draft will be rewritten. Students will require a great deal of direct instruction, demonstrations, and group participation as they correct and improve their work. They need to understand that their goals should be compositions that flow smoothly, are properly organized, and maintain the reader's interest. Teachers' comments and feedback should be explicit and plentiful during drafting and during revising. "Add more details" is too vague for helpful feedback. Directions to the students should, to the extent possible, reflect the sentence activities with which students are familiar: "Use an appositive in your topic sentence," or "Start with *when*." (If revision is the instructional goal, producing a final copy may not be necessary.)

A simple paragraph with no spelling, capitalization, or punctuation errors is a useful tool for teaching revising and will be referred to here as an unelaborated paragraph (Hochman, 2009; Hochman & Wexler, 2017). In these paragraphs, the students focus only on revision because editing is not an issue. An unelaborated paragraph, together with the specific instructions students are given for improving it, are important tools for preparing them to improve their own writing. Teachers need to provide ample whole-class demonstrations for revising prior to allowing students to work in pairs, in small groups, or independently. Teachers should follow these steps when students are revising:

- Revise the unelaborated paragraph with the whole class.

- Put the unelaborated paragraph on the board and have students suggest improvements.

- Have students work in pairs and small groups to improve the unelaborated paragraph with specific instructions.

- Have students work together or independently to improve the unelaborated paragraph without instructions.

- Have students improve their own work, given teacher feedback.

- Have students improve their own work independently.

Figure 17.11 shows an example of a revise-and-edit activity for a developing writer, and Figure 17.12 shows an example of a revise-and-edit activity for a proficient writer.

Revising an unelaborated paragraph

The Titanic was a big ship. It sank. Many passengers died. There are new regulations.

- Expand the T.S. (telling when and where).
- Use an appositive in the T.S.
- Combine (first two) sentences.
- Answer "why" in the third sentence.
- Use examples after the fourth sentence starting with an illustration transition.
- Write a C.S. beginning with a conclusion transition.

On April 14, 1912, the Titanic, a huge ocean liner, sank in the North Atlantic. 1500 passengers died when the ship hit an iceberg. After the tragedy, many new safety regulations had to be followed by passenger ships. For example, more life boats, safety drills and intensive training of the crew were required. In the end, the sinking of the Titanic led to new improvements in maritime safety for future generations of travelers.

Figure 17.11. Example of a revise-and-edit activity for a developing writer. Copyright © 2017 The Writing Revolution. All rights reserved. Published with Permission.

In our experience, students are all too frequently given credit for the quantity of their written work rather than for the quality. They should be reminded regularly that clarity and accuracy, not length, are their goals.

Transitions are taught as students learn to revise. Transitions are often called signal words because they signal, or indicate, a relationship between ideas. Although they are usually not grammatically connected to a sentence, they make text smoother and help minimize the confusion that fragmented statements can cause. Teaches should point out to students that commas set off most, but not all, transitions. Transitions may begin sentences, link thoughts within sentences, or help unify sentences

Revising an Unelaborated Paragraph

Wetlands are in danger. Wetlands are habitats. Wetlands provide many things. Humans are affecting the wetlands. They should be protected.

- improve TS and CS
- expand sentences
- add a transition
- combine sentences
- add an example
- vary sentence starters
- use an appositive
- vary vocabulary

Wetlands, areas like swamps and marches, are being destroyed. This is a major problem because these areas are habitats for many species and provide food, timber, improved water quality, and recreation. Humans are filling in wetlands for residential, commercial, and industrial development. As a result, the continental United States has lost half of its original 221 million acres of wetlands. Since wetlands are important for ecosystems, humans need to protect what is left of them.

Figure 17.12. Example of a revise-and-edit activity for a proficient writer. Copyright © 2017 The Writing Revolution. All rights reserved. Published with Permission.

and paragraphs. Because they help writers avoid short, choppy sentences, correctly used transitions are vital to coherent paragraphs and compositions.

Students tend to overuse transitions, so teachers should assign activities that present blanks where specific transitions should be used, along with a list of transition choices. They should show students examples of writing with and without transitions so they can see how these signal words create fluent, more coherent writing. They can display charts of transitions as an easy reference and as a reminder to use them.

Teachers should introduce transitions in the order in which they appear on Textbox 17.2. (Please note that these transitions are the ones often used in student writing, and this is not an exhaustive list.) Time and sequence transitions should be taught first, followed by conclusions and illustration transitions. The remaining two groups can be taught in any order. (See Textbox 17.2 for examples of transitions.)

1. *Time and sequence.* Time and sequence transitions are used to order events in a composition that relates a series or a process. They help demonstrate the logical order of a narrative and divide time order into the tenses (past, present, and future).

2. *Conclusion.* Conclusion transitions appear at the beginning of the last sentence in a paragraph or in the last paragraph of a composition. In shorter works, writers can use a conclusion that focuses on a solution or on their point of view. There is a difference between stating a conclusion and summing up an idea, although sometimes the two overlap. More able students can practice deciding when it would be better to use a summation rather than a conclusion. The conclusion transitions indicated by an asterisk signal cause and effect. Students should use them at the end of cause-and-effect paragraphs and compositions.

3. *Illustration.* Illustration transitions are used to give examples, to support a detail, and/or to explain or elaborate on a statement. They must communicate a clear representation of the idea or event.

4. *Change of direction.* Use change-of-direction transitions with contrasting thoughts.

5. *Emphasis.* Emphasis transitions prove a point or statement or reaffirm something the writer has already stated. They are often used in persuasive essays, letters of complaint, and formal requests. They provide emphasis in writing that is issue oriented. Often, emphasis transitions can be used interchangeably with conclusion transitions. In addition to conclusion signals, these words or phrases can be used to indicate cause and effect.

Assignments should be kept brief. When longer compositions are expected, they should be assigned in segments, which makes revision and editing a less daunting task. The teacher should provide students with checklists for revising and editing. Typical items include the following, with variations for age and ability:

- Does your draft follow your outline?

- Is your topic sentence or thesis statement clearly stated?

- Are your supporting details clear and in order?

- Do the details support the topic sentence?

- Did you use different types of sentences?

- Do your sentences vary in length?

- Are there sentences that should be combined or expanded?

- Did you use transition words or phrases?

- Did you provide support or evidence using example and illustration sentences?

- Are your word choices repetitive? Vivid? Precise?

- Have you checked for run-on sentences? Fragments? Spelling, punctuation, or capitalization errors?

- Have you checked tense and number agreement?

At first, only a few items should be selected from the checklist to provide a focus for the students as they improve and correct their work. As they become more adept, more checklist items can be added. Teachers should remind students to revise style first and then edit the mechanics.

In addition to listing specific items on the checklist, it is often helpful for teachers to give developing writers explicit instructions that will add flair to their compositions, such as "Add an appositive," "Insert a transition word," or "Add when and why." At first, teachers will have to show students exactly where to place the words and phrases. In time, students will be able to see where to insert them independently. Much attention should also be given to the selection of strong and varied nouns and verbs as well as modifiers. Teachers should encourage students to use transitions even at the beginning stages of paragraph development. Moreover, sentences should vary in length and style. Although short, simple, active, declarative sentences are useful for emphasis, too often they are the only forms used by less skillful writers. Using appositives, conjunctions, transitions, and beginning sentences with *when* will raise the level of linguistic complexity, reflect written structures, and enhance the quality of the students' writing.

Finally, students should routinely read their work aloud. This can take place during sentence activities and the drafting or revising and editing stages. Students can read to a partner, to a small group, or to the entire class. One purpose of oral reading is to sharpen proofreading capabilities. Many students are able to correct their errors more accurately and effectively when they read their written work aloud. Another goal is to enhance critical listening skills of the audience. The writer's classmates can contribute suggestions based on the checklist for revision and editing.

Writing a Final Copy   It is not advisable to spend precious instructional time recopying or retyping written work for final copies. Therefore, teachers must be selective about which writing assignments should be developed to this stage. If final copies are produced, every effort should be made to display them. Students should be given opportunities to see their written work on bulletin boards or published in a class journal, school or local newspaper, or parent bulletin. Writing letters that will accomplish a purpose or elicit a reply can also be rewarding.

REFLECT, CONNECT, and RESPOND

How do each of the four steps for writing assignments support analytical thinking and organization for a writer?

CLOSING THOUGHTS: TEACHING WRITING

National assessments and standards now oblige schools to adopt methods with research-based strategies that help teachers effectively teach writing, but explicit instruction of narrative and expository writing skills is given too little time in most schools and too often is treated as a separate subject. Too often, students are given writing assignments and expected to complete them with minimum guidance. Teachers of all subjects and grades should be able to learn about best practices for writing instruction as part of all teacher certification programs. In order to acquire both skills and knowledge most effectively, writing assignments must be embedded in content. Writing is a powerful learning tool and will enhance the teaching of content, not slow it down.

The key to helping all students, especially those with learning and language disabilities, to become proficient writers is to provide them with a model that has clear goals and scaffolded activities for achieving them. Writing provides multiple opportunities for students to gain important word and world knowledge, be better able to reflect, develop social cognition, and enhance their reading comprehension in order to deeply learn, analyze content, and enhance their ability to succeed.

REFLECT, CONNECT, and RESPOND

Why is writing about content key for student learning?

ONLINE COMPANION MATERIALS

The following Chapter 17 resources are available at http://www.brookespublishing.com/birshcarreker/materials:

- Reflect, Connect, and Respond Questions

- Appendix 17.1: Technology Resources

- Appendix 17.2: Knowledge and Skill Assessment Answer Key

KNOWLEDGE AND SKILL ASSESSMENT

1. Which of the following statements is true?

   a. Fluent decoding and reading comprehension lead directly to mastery of the conventions of written language.

   b. Writing activities should focus on student self-expression in elementary school.

   c. The focus of writing instruction should be on skills required most often academically and in the work place.

   d. Sentence, paragraph, and composition writing activities should follow a linear structure.

2. If students are taught to use conjunctions in their writing, they can do what?

    a. Create more extended responses

    b. Correct run-ons

    c. Better understand sentence boundaries

    d. Vary sentence types (declarative, interrogative, imperative, exclamatory)

3. Which type of writing would involve the most use of time and sequence transition words?

    a. Narrative

    b. Expository

    c. Persuasive

    d. Descriptive

4. Which *two* prerequisite skills create an effective introduction?

    a. Taking notes using key words, phrases, abbreviations, and symbols

    b. Using different strategies to combine sentences

    c. Distinguishing between general, specific, and thesis statements

    d. Developing a general statement from a topic

5. How would you describe the revision process?

    a. It is used to correct errors in punctuation, grammar, syntax, and spelling.

    b. It is used to clarify or alter meaning or structure of a draft.

    c. It is most effective when completed independently by students.

    d. It is most effective when teachers provide students with needed changes.

REFERENCES

Alley, G.R., & Deshler, D.D. (1979). *Teaching the learning disabled adolescent strategies and methods.* Boulder, CO: Love Publishing Co.

Bangert-Drowns, R.L., Hurley, M.M., & Wilkinson, B. (2004). The effects of school-based writing-to-learn interventions on academic achievement: A meta-analysis. *Review of Educational Research, 74*(1), 29–58.

Graham, S. (2008). *Effective writing instruction for all students.* Retrieved from http://doc.renlearn.com/KMNet/R004250923GJCF33.pdf

Graham, S., & Hebert, M.A. (2010). *Writing to read: Evidence for how writing can improve reading.* Washington, DC: Carnegie Corporation of New York.

Graham, S., & Perin, D. (2007). *Writing next: Effective strategies to improve writing of adolescents in middle and high schools.* Washington, DC: Alliance for Excellent Education.

Hebert, M., Gillespie, A., & Graham, S. (2013). Comparing effects of different writing activities on reading comprehension: A meta-analysis. *Reading and Writing, 26,* 111–138.

Hillocks, G., Jr. (1984). What works in teaching composition: A meta-analysis of experimental treatment studies. *American Journal of Education, 93,* 133–170.

Hochman, J. (2009). *Teaching basic writing skills: Strategies for effective expository writing instruction.* Longmont, CO: Sopris West.

Hochman, J., & MacDermott-Duffy, B. (2015). Effective writing instruction: Time for a revolution. *Perspectives on Language and Literacy, 65(1),* 31–37.

Hochman, J., & Wexler, N. (2017). *The writing revolution: A guide to advancing thinking through writing in all subjects and grades.* San Francisco, CA: Jossey Bass.

International Dyslexia Association, The. (2010, March). *Knowledge and practice standards for teachers of reading.*

Lunsford, A., & Connors, R. (1995). *St. Martin's handbook* (3rd ed.). New York, NY: St. Martin's Press.

Maria, K. (1990). *Reading comprehension instruction: Issues and strategies.* Parkton, MD: York Press.

Morgan, C.G. (2001). *When they can't write.* Timonium, MD: York Press.

Mueller, P.A., & Oppenheimer, D.M. (2014, April). The pen is mightier than the keyboard. *Psychological Science, 23.*

National Association for the Education of Young Children. (NAEYC). (1998). *Learning to read and write: Developmentally appropriate practices for young children.* Washington, DC: Author.

National Center for Education Statistics (NCES). (2012). *The Nation's Report Card: Writing 2011* (NCES 2012–470). Washington, DC: U.S. Department of Education, Institute of Education Sciences.

National Governors Association Center for Best Practices, Council of Chief State School Officers. (2010). *Common Core State Standards.* Washington, DC: Author.

Neville, D.D., & Searls, E.F. (1991). A meta-analytic review of the effect of sentence-combining on reading comprehension. *Reading Research and Instruction, 31,* 63–76.

Saddler, B. (2012). *Teacher's guide to effective sentence writing.* New York, NY: Guilford.

Scott, C.M. (2002). Sentence comprehension instruction. In J.F. Carlisle & M.S. Rice (Eds.), *Improving reading comprehension: Research-based principles and practices* (pp. 115–127). Timonium, MD: York Press.

Scott, C.M. (2005). Learning to write. In A.G. Kamhi & H.W. Catts (Eds.), *Language and reading disabilities* (pp. 233–273). Boston, MA: Allyn & Bacon.

Shanahan, T. (2004). Overcoming the dominance of communication: Writing to think and learn. In T.L. Jetton & J.A. Dole (Eds.), *Adolescent literacy research and practice* (pp. 59–74). New York, NY: Guilford.

Singer, B.D., & Bashir, A.S. (2004). Developmental variations in written composition skills. In C.A. Stone, E.R. Silliman, B.J. Ehrren, & K. Apel (Eds.), *Handbook of language and literacy: Development and disorders* (pp. 559–582). New York, NY: Guilford.

Willingham, D.T. (2017, April 2). *New studies show the cost of student laptop use in lecture classes* [Blog]. Retrieved from http://www.danielwillingham.com/daniel-willingham-science-and-education-blog/new-studies-show-the-cost-of-student-laptop-use-in-college-lectures

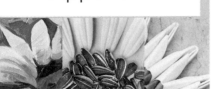

Appendix 17.1

Technology Resources

Elaine A. Cheesman

Effective programs/apps have the following features:

- They provide intensive, focused practice on specific skills of written expression.
- They provide proofreading assistance that also explains the nature of the errors.

Ginger Software   http://www.gingersoftware.com

Originally created for English language learners, this program (for desktop and mobile devices) helps users improve written expression by checking grammar, punctuation, and contextual spelling (e.g., *there/they're/their*). When it detects an awkwardly worded sentence, it offers suggestions to rephrase sentences. The thesaurus suggests more interesting words without prompting. It includes a free translator that translates passages between 50 languages, including those with different orthographies such as Chinese and Arabic. It has human voice text-to-speech capabilities.

Grammarly   http://www.grammarly.com

This program helps the writer improve writing by checking grammar, punctuation, and spelling. Errors are not corrected automatically; the writer must correct each error manually. Brief explanations of the errors help the user learn about his or her mistakes. The free version of Grammarly supports word documents, e-mail, and social and media posts. It corrects contextual spelling (e.g., *there/they're/their*), punctuation, subject–verb disagreement, and grammar. The premium version detects more sophisticated errors, reports statistics on each type of error, and analyzes for plagiarism. For those writing academic papers, the premium version has settings for specific writing styles (e.g., APA, MLA). School site licenses are available. (*Note:* At this time, there is no version for iPads or other mobile devices.)

Inspiration/Kidspiration   http://www.inspiration.com

This is a graphic organizer computer program and a complementary app for organizing paragraphs and longer text. It contains multiple templates for different text structures and genres. With a tap, one can alternate views from visual "mind map" to a traditional outline. To help comprehend text, the user or teacher can select and complete a graphic organizer. To help the writer brainstorm and organize paragraphs and longer works, the user can select an appropriate template or create a new one starting from scratch. Once complete, the user can e-mail, print, or export the outline and/or mind map to a Word or text document. This program and app are good for adults, older students, and English language learners.

Irregular Verbs   http://www.alligatorapps.com

This app provides practice reading and using correct verb forms. It presents homophones in seven engaging games. The optional text-to-speech feature reads sentences.

No Red Ink   http://www.NoRedInk.com

This web site helps students improve grammar and writing skills with an engaging, interactive platform. With the free version, users can create pretests, assign content lessons, provide extensive practice, and assess learning. The site asks the user to identify a few interests and friends and then places these names within the exercises. The self-paced practice lessons provide immediate feedback, increasing levels of help, and explanations when users do not understand. Teachers can track individual student progress with color-coded charts.

PrepositionBuilder   http://www.Mobile-educationstore.com

This mobile app presents an image and a narrated sentence with three preposition options. The user drags one preposition to complete the sentence. If the user selects the wrong preposition, the picture changes to show the correct meaning of the chosen preposition with oral feedback. Statistics track individual progress; reports can be e-mailed to parents and teachers. The app supports multiple users; it covers the 28 most common prepositions, with 300 images. It was named the Best Teaching App for 2012 (Teachhub.com).

Rainbow Sentences   http://mobile-educationstore.com

This program provides practice constructing grammatically correct sentences with given words. The user forms sentences using the drag-and-drop feature with individual words or by phrase. There are several layers of scaffold supports, including a color-coding option for words, phrases, or placeholders. It features both manuscript and cursive options. There is a version for older students.

Sentence Reading Magic 1 and 2   http://www.preschoolu.com

To practice forming sentences of varying lengths, the user arranges words into complete sentences. An adult voice reads it to the user. Each app contains 324 two-, three-, four-, and five-word sentences. Both apps feature decodable text for sentences and two sight-word activities. Sentence Reading Magic 1 has CVC words with short vowels; Sentence Magic 2 has words with short vowels and consonant blends. Users can work in manuscript or cursive fonts and select a male or female voice.

Vocabulary.com   http://www.vocabulary.com

Teachers can use existing lists, upload text from books, or create original lists of up to 10 words. Students can then practice the spelling and review the meaning of these words online using a multiple-choice format that includes extra information about each word. The existing "featured" lists contain text from literature, nonfiction, historical documents, morphology, speeches, and current events reported in newspapers. It also has downloadable PDFs of confusable words (e.g., *affect* and *effect*) under "Choose Your Words." The free version allows users to create classes of up to 50 students, invite students, and assign words. Students can view their progress online. The web site has two versions for desktop and tablet platforms.

Word Hippo　http://www.wordhippo.com

For those who want to find better words, this web site is a user-friendly thesaurus suitable for young and old. It provides the meaning of a word plus synonyms, antonyms, words that rhyme with it, sentences containing it, derivatives, and etymology. It includes U.K. and U.S. spellings.

Wordflex Touch Dictionary　http://wordflex.com

This app is a "movable thesaurus." It shows word relationships as networks of semantic word associations. The word web is organized by the parts of speech (e.g., noun, verb), phrases, and derivatives. It also includes phrasal verbs (*walk away, pull out*). These dynamic word trees can be moved and rearranged. The resulting word web can be printed on a poster!

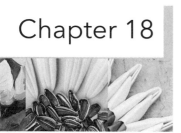

Chapter 18

Designing the Learning Environment and Planning Multisensory Structured Literacy Lessons

Judith R. Birsh, Jean Schedler, and Robin Anderson Singer

LEARNING OBJECTIVES

1. To create an effective classroom context that enhances the physical space and emotional climate to maximize time spent on instruction

2. To implement the principles of research-based support of systematic instruction for teaching the Structured Literacy process

3. To become familiar with the history and evolution of the Orton-Gillingham Approach (OGA)

4. To write and deliver Multisensory Structured Literacy (MSL) lessons that include evidence-based instructional components

5. To understand the benefits for teachers and students of planned Multisensory Structured Literacy lessons engaging all of the language systems in the content of learning to read

High-quality professional learning around multisensory teaching of basic language skills occurs in a **context** (learning environment) through a **process** (the **Orton-Gillingham Approach,** or **OGA**) with specific **content** (elements of Structured Literacy). This chapter provides a roadmap that you, as a teacher, can use to structure for success these three critical variables—context, process, and content (see Figure 18.1)—to provide instruction that integrates the teaching of reading, spelling, handwriting, and written expression using a comprehensive approach. The information in this chapter is directly aligned with the International Dyslexia Association (IDA)'s (2018) *Knowledge and Practice Standards for Teachers of Reading.* When teachers have the opportunity to learn about these reading-related concepts and then engage in explicit reading instruction carefully specified in the Knowledge and Practice Standards, students score higher on reading achievement tests than those with less well-prepared teachers (Al Otaiba, Lake, Scarborough, Allor, & Carreker, 2016). With the guidance of this chapter, teachers can learn to deliver their pedagogical content knowledge, using evidence-based, systematic, explicit,

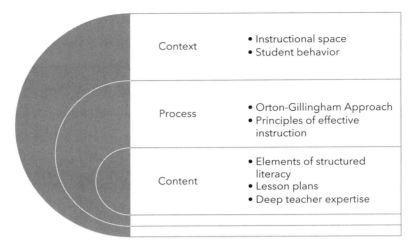

Figure 18.1.   Context, process, content.

multisensory instruction, along with the help of practicums and mentorships in well-organized classrooms.

The first section of this chapter examines the context (learning environment) or setting for teacher instruction and student learning. This section describes the essentials of creating an organized classroom environment—ways to utilize the physical space and organize and maintain materials effectively, and in so doing, to facilitate student behaviors that are most conducive to learning. Thus, the learning environment consists of both external factors (physical space and materials) and internal factors (the emotional climate and expectations in a classroom and the ways these influence students). Effective classroom procedures need to be in place to maximize time spent on instruction.

The second section of this chapter discusses the process or the implementation of **diagnostic and prescriptive instruction,** through teachers' deep knowledge and continuous study of the essential features of evidence-based Structured Literacy (Chapter 2). This enables teachers to create sensitive and responsive instruction, providing differentiated, active learning opportunities for students to build and master all components of language. The core principles of OGA are outlined, followed by the essential elements of systematic instruction and principles of designing and delivering effective lessons.

The third section of this chapter connects the content of Structured Literacy with the process of the OGA and explains how to develop lesson plans. It describes how to plan and organize lessons that contain all of the elements for building literacy, coupled with ongoing monitoring of progress and sensitivity to differentiating instruction to meet individual students' needs. Sample lesson plans are provided in the last part of this section to demonstrate how all of the levels of language content can be combined into an integrated whole for introducing new concepts, providing opportunities for guided practice, and reviewing while intensely focusing on students' most essential needs to accelerate their learning. Underpinning these lessons is the positive belief that these students will be successful due to their teachers' relentless dedication and informed instruction. Here is where research on what to teach, practical experience on how to teach, and intensive teacher preparation and mentoring come together.

The need to teach literacy explicitly is firmly supported by research. In addition, the Individuals with Disabilities Education Improvement Act (IDEA) of 2004 (PL 108-446) makes clear the critical role of instruction for preventing and identifying learning disabilities with the incorporation of response to intervention (RTI). The previous chapters have provided ample evidence of the need to teach literacy explicitly and detailed information about the literacy content to be taught. The essential content of literacy instruction (cognitive and linguistic) is well established based on converging scientific evidence since the 1980s (National Institute of Child Health and Human Development [NICHD], 2000).

CONTEXT

Context is the setting for the teacher instruction and student learning—the internal and external learning environment.

The Learning Environment

Student instruction takes place within the context of a classroom or learning environment. Taking time to organize the teaching space allows teachers to remove potential obstacles that could prevent students from becoming expert learners. Without an organized classroom and appropriate student behavior, it is difficult, if not impossible, for teacher instruction and student learning to be successful. School schedules are set up according to instructional time blocks that allocate a specific amount of time to instruction in specific subjects. The focus of this section is to ensure that classroom time is used for effective and meaningful instruction; achieving this goal also requires using instructional space effectively, organizing classroom materials, planning transitions, and fostering productive student behavior (see Table 18.1).

Designing Instructional Space

The classroom is defined here as the space that you have been assigned to instruct your students. This space might be a room with four walls and a door, a space marked off by bookcases, an alcove in a hallway, or a space no bigger than a broom closet. However big or small or permanent or temporary, it is the space in which you are assigned to teach.

The organization of the instructional space begins even before the students enter the room. First, you must consider the arrangement of the furniture and lay it out, and second, you must organize instructional and student materials used during the lesson.

Table 18.1. Elements of the learning environment that promote student success

Components of the classroom culture	Instructional space	Student behavior	Teacher instruction and student learning
Components that use time	Layout of furniture: chairs, desks, and so forth Organization: teaching materials before, during, after instruction	Classroom procedures Executive function	Delivery of lesson and student engagement in learning

Organization of Furniture in the Instructional Space Your plan for organizing that space must be carefully thought out. There is no one right plan or organization to any given space. Rather, the space must work for you as the teacher and for the specific students assigned to it. Often, this means doing the best you can with few resources in terms of physical space, desks, whiteboards, and chalkboards.

The main teaching space is the first space to plan. Begin by standing in the space and mentally listing available classroom furniture (e.g., desks, file cabinets, tables, whiteboards, Smart boards, easels, bulletin boards, shelves, cubbies). Ask yourself these questions:

- Where will you stand during the major portion of classroom instruction (or sit if it is a small-group tutorial setting)?

- Where are the boards located in relation to your position? Sometimes boards can be moved or added if necessary.

- Where will the other teaching equipment (e.g., easels, projectors) used during daily instruction be placed?

- How best can the student desks be arranged so that all students can see you during instruction? What works best for you and them—desks in rows, touching, or in a four-square pattern?

Are the desks the correct size for your students? Students should be able to sit comfortably with their feet flat on the floor and knees not hitting the bottom of the desk. Take the time at the beginning of the year to adjust the desks to fit each student's size and body. You may need to trade desks with other teachers or add wooden boxes for your shorter students to rest their feet. Where will students keep their books and supplies? What works best for you and your students should be the deciding factor. Do you want them to keep their materials in their desks? If lockers are available, what will be kept in them? Even if the desks have space for supplies, you may still want to have students keep supplies and books in an assigned tote located elsewhere in the classroom so that during instruction they have only the needed materials at their desks. It may take several attempts to get the board(s), easels, projector, digital equipment, and student desks to fit and work in the teaching space.

The next decision is where to locate your teacher's desk(s). Decide where to place and how to situate the teacher desk(s), filing cabinets, and bookcases that are to be used exclusively by you and/or classroom assistants. It is often a good idea to locate the teacher desk(s) and confidential materials away from the student traffic pattern. If you plan to have students sit with you at your desk for individualized instruction, plan how that area will work as well. Planning the teacher's space may require slight changes to the instructional space. Organizing the teacher's space is discussed more in the next section.

The small-group instructional area or study center is the third important space to plan. This could be a reading corner and/or a learning center based on a topic of study.

Once different classroom areas of use have been identified and the furniture is placed in its respective area, check the traffic pattern that results from the current placement of furniture. Ask the following questions:

- Are the students able to enter and exit the classroom without bumping into desks, bookcases, and tables stacked with papers?

- Is the teacher's desk still situated so that it will be undisturbed by students?

- Is there still a place to easily store and gain access to confidential information, such as tests and progress reports, away from students?

- Where will students place papers they are handing in for grading?

- Where will sets of workbooks, teacher's manuals, card decks, reading lists, dictation materials, and alphabet letters and other manipulatives be stored?

- Where are the pencil sharpener, other classroom supplies, and trash can located?

- Is there a space or desk set off as a quiet corner if needed?

- How will the bulletin boards and countertops (if any) be used?

- How will computer time be assigned for practice and **review** activities?

Every need and movement of students, from the time they enter the classroom until they exit, must be arranged for what will be most efficient. The classroom setup may not be perfect; however, it needs to be well thought through to determine what works best for your teaching style, the students assigned to your class, and the furniture and space available. After your classroom has been set up, take a critical look around the room with an eye toward limiting classroom distractions.

Finding what works best for you may take several attempts, extending over several years, but you will be fine-tuning the physical surroundings of the instructional environment with a heightened awareness of your needs as the teacher and your students' needs for logical, systematic order in the classroom's physical environment.

Organization of Teaching Materials   Organization of materials encompasses organizing 1) the space used exclusively by you as the teacher, 2) physical teaching materials, such as notebooks, and 3) teacher transitions. You must be efficient in having available the materials necessary for a lesson to be successful in keeping students actively and productively engaged in learning.

Teacher's Personal Space   Organizing a teacher's personal space is often overlooked; yet, it is so critical for effective, efficient instruction. Begin by thinking of all of the requests made of you as a teacher by students, administrators, colleagues, student teachers, and parents. As a teacher, you need to have easy access to documentation that may be requested by school personnel and supervisors. Students request materials such as paper, tape, scissors, passes, and forms. If you store these items on your desk, then consider how to make them readily accessible without students accidentally having access to confidential materials. Take time to set up folders or files (on a computer if possible) for confidential student information, information for parents, routine memos from the administration, and committee information. Complete this organization prior to students' arrival. Your plan for organizing your desk, drawer space, and desktop supplies, as well as setting up any filing cabinets, bookcases, and storage closets, needs to be well thought out for accessibility and keeping daily clutter to a minimum. Make your personal space efficient so that you do not dread sitting down to a disheveled desk at the end of a productive day. Having everything organized ensures the items are readily accessible and do not become distractions or disruptions to implementing the lesson.

Teaching Materials   Teaching materials include the physical materials used by the teacher and students. At the start of a school year, teaching materials are usually neatly stacked and ready for use. As the school year progresses, however, the stacks become untidy, materials are lost or damaged, and needed supplies get depleted. At the beginning of the year, set up labeled shelves or containers to accommodate materials critical to the success of your lessons. Each group or individual student should have the core daily lesson materials in a clearly marked bin, which could also contain card decks for review and teaching new concepts, current reading lists, workbooks, manipulatives, extra pencils, and index cards. Student notebooks should be nearby. For older students, it is helpful to number electronic devices and assign each student a specific one. Provide a labeled storage box that can hold the entire set of electronic devices at the end of the lesson, and store them in the same place on the shelf for the entire year. Setting up computers and scheduling time for your students to practice and review becomes part of the learning process. This thoughtful attention to detail will enable the lessons to move efficiently and smoothly, thereby preventing the loss of precious time needed for learning and positive teacher–student interactions.

Planned Transitions   The third aspect of organization that needs to be planned for is transitions. Teachers, as well as their students, have transitions in their academic day—from subject to subject or from instructional group to instructional group, including from one discrete instructional component to the next within a lesson. Although teachers are usually thoughtful about making sure they have all materials needed for implementing a lesson, they also must spend time planning what to do with teacher and student materials at the end of a specific lesson or component so that the next subject or instructional group can be initiated efficiently. Furthermore, keeping track of teaching and student materials during each lesson component leads to better planning and **scaffolding** of instruction for the next day. For example, enclosed plastic folders with multiple sections are ideal for students for holding letter tiles, writing boards, and composition books.

An effective teacher organizes and maintains the classroom learning environment to maximize the time spent engaged in productive activities and minimize the time lost during transitions or disruptions due to disciplinary action (Mather & Goldstein, 2008). Taking the time to get your personal space organized; set up a system for storage of instructional materials; and find a way to efficiently access teaching materials before, during, and after instruction contributes to a productive classroom environment.

Student Behavior

Within society, certain prosocial behaviors are expected for different contexts. Humans develop schemas regarding what comprises appropriate and inappropriate behavior for a given context. For example, individuals learn what behavior is appropriate in public swimming pools, elegant restaurants, rock concerts, and schools. Teachers expect positive student behavior in their classroom. Teachers need positive guidance strategies to teach these skills and reinforce positive and appropriate student behavior.

Teachers may focus too narrowly on the curriculum without allocating enough time to developing positive student behavior. Kilpatrick (2015) cited Morgan and colleagues' (2008) study that showed that some of the behavior problems in schools demonstrate a reciprocal relationship between poor reading and behavior problems in classrooms. However, both behavior and attitudes are key elements of the classroom climate. Berninger and Wolf stated,

> Emotional climate is defined by teacher attitudes toward students and student attitudes toward one another. Teachers provide the emotional safety that encourages students to take risks and allows student to make mistakes. Freedom to make mistakes is necessary for learning. (2016, p. 183)

Positive student interactions are important for creating a healthy emotional climate. One way to visualize the importance of positive student interactions is to think of each student as an individual drinking glass whose size varies according to the amount of attention that each student requires. A student will strive to keep his or her glass full of attention. To some students, it does not matter whether the attention is positive or negative, rather that attention is given. Your objective is to keep each glass filled to the brim with positive attention. False praise does not work. If students know the expectations for a classroom in terms of behavior, participation, or routine, many opportunities for giving praise will occur naturally. Use these opportunities to compliment students who require a lot of attention. It will take concerted and conscientious efforts on your part not to criticize an attention-seeking student for what he or she is doing wrong. Rather, you should keep an eagle eye out for ways to sincerely and appropriately compliment such a student for specific actions that merit praise. Beware of false praise, however, which is often more general and less tangible. For example, praising a student for better behavior after he or she has repeatedly been disruptive is false praise. Sincere praise is to compliment the student for the specific appropriate behavior—for example, "You really worked through those steps carefully of dividing that word into syllables before you read the word." The goal is to drain the negative attention from the glass and fill the glass to the brim with positive attention.

Classroom Procedures How do you instill positive classroom behavior in your students? Building a positive environment begins with thinking through expected student behavior and classroom procedures from the moment students enter the classroom. These expectations need to be explained to the students, clearly understood by them, and reinforced by you in a positive manner. The next key piece is to maintain consistent rules and expectations from one day to the next. It is important to take the time to reinforce the established rules and expectations (even if it reduces the amount of instruction)—and it is better to do so at the beginning of the year than to have instruction repeatedly disrupted throughout the year. When reinforcing classroom expectations, explain these in a patient, nonjudgmental tone. Firmly repeat what the students may already know but have yet to internalize. Once classroom rules and expectations have been established, the key is to be consistent and follow through on upholding them. Students are more successful in environments in which they know what to expect. They need to be held accountable for classroom rules and expectations on the days when everything is going well, as well as on the days when nothing is going right. For example, one middle school special education teacher successfully used only one rule in her classroom: "You are responsible" (E.F. Bitler, personal communication, 2004). Her focus was to keep the rule simple and applicable to the real world. Whatever the difficulty (lost homework, broken pencil, inappropriate behavior), the student is held responsible for the action as well as determining an appropriate solution. Teachers may need to model how to determine or problem-solve an appropriate solution.

Teachers need to ensure that the classroom is a safe environment for students to take academic risks, explore friendships, learn to negotiate a classroom setting, and learn appropriate expectations and behaviors that are transferable to the outside world. Students must know it is a safe place where unexpected negative things will not happen. It is okay to be incorrect; it is not okay to not try. There will be time and opportunity to develop social skills. Students will learn how to be students. They will be explicitly guided toward learning appropriate expectations and behaviors. A well-managed classroom is task oriented and predictable. This kind of environment has

- A high level of student involvement with work
- Clear student expectations
- Relatively little wasted time, confusion, or disruption
- A relaxed and pleasant climate

It is important to bond and connect with all students but especially with students who have experienced limited academic success. A key behavior is to establish eye contact during teaching and while conversing with a student. When you first meet, shake hands and look the student in the eye. It may feel corny, but this is a powerful first tool for establishing a unique, caring connection. Using students' names is critical, especially with adolescents. Both of these practices are powerful constructive tools in providing positive attention.

Once students begin to feel that you are approachable, it is critical that you practice active listening. Active listening involves maintaining attention to the students by simultaneously looking at the students while they are talking and keeping focused on what is being said. It is important not to interrupt the student. Acknowledge that you have listened by neutrally responding to what the student has said, even though you might disagree. This will often require momentarily setting aside your agenda for a student so that you can hear and understand what information or request the student wishes to convey. Additional information at the SkillsYouNeed web site supports the effectiveness of active listening: https://www.skillsyouneed.com/ips/active-listening.html.

Current brain research has shown that fear and anxiety are detrimental to learning. A positive approach is required to structure a classroom environment for success (National Science Council on the Developing Child, 2010). Dr. Becky Bailey (*Conscious Discipline,* 2000) offers a relationship-based community model of classroom management in which seven basic skills are practiced through which teachers and students are empowered to control themselves and to relate to others. The seven basic skills are composure, encouragement, assertiveness, choices, positive intent, empathy, and consequences. Another approach around which to frame classroom behavior expectations is positive guidance. Positive guidance is based on the belief that child guidance should focus on a child's self-control rather than focusing exclusively on behavioral outcomes. Teachers are able to guide student behavior by establishing predictable routines, setting clear rules, and modeling kindness and respect (Dumro, Jablon, & Stetson, 2011).

Assuring students that you will not ask them to do what you have not taught them nor what they have not yet learned is another important way to gain their confidence. This helps to eliminate guessing and encourages them instead to practice the strategies you are instructing them to use to master the intricacies of the language. Being successful on a daily basis builds trust and confidence so much that students are quick to recognize your inadvertent use of something in a lesson they have not yet learned.

Using less teacher talk is another key strategy to improve student–teacher interactions. By using active listening and structuring lessons to engage learners by using **Socratic questioning,** a skillful teacher is able to use what students already know to further their understanding and to help them integrate their knowledge of the components of reading.

Effective teachers know that it is important to acknowledge each student, engage in meaningful feedback dialogues during teachable moments, and recognize individual student successes. Other ways to engage students positively are to establish classroom traditions to celebrate successes and to disclose something meaningful about yourself. During student–teacher interactions, it is important to genuinely convey an attitude of respect, make yourself available for individual questions, and care enough to make a difference by doing what is needed to assist the student.

Appendix 18.3: Building Block Checklist for Effective Classroom Management (Schedler & Bitler, 2004), is available in the Online Companion Materials. You can use this checklist to review your current practices and to evaluate any further actions you need to enhance your classroom environment.

REFLECT, CONNECT, and RESPOND
Context examines both classroom organization and student behavior. Choose one and discuss how a teacher might structure that element for success.

Executive Function Behaviors and Universal Design for Learning   Executive function is a term used to describe a set of mental processes that helps people connect past experiences with present action. Individuals use executive function when performing such activities as planning, organizing, strategizing, and paying attention to and remembering details (National Center for Learning Disabilities [NCLD], 2008). According to Kaufman (2010), executive function is an issue for everyone, not just children and adults with particular diagnostic labels. There are two core strands of executive functioning: the metacognitive strand and the social-emotional regulation strand. Both strands are critical in terms of students not only meeting academic requirements but also managing themselves in the classroom.

To promote executive functioning, establish positive student behavior that facilitates productive learning by having clear expectations that students understand, along with familiar routines and classroom schedules. This creates secure learning environments where students are comfortable to take risks, practice, and construct knowledge, with scaffolding, support, and specific feedback from the teacher. With explicit instruction and sufficient practice, students learn to regulate their behavior to ensure productive learning. As Monica Gordon-Pershey explains in her discussion of executive function in Chapter 8, students learn to minimize distractions, limit multitasking, set task goals, and promote internal motivation, and "executive function allows learners to flexibly adjust their thinking and behaviors." In addition, "Executive functions allow school-age and adolescent learners to persevere so that they can learn and accomplish a multitude of academic learning tasks and social behaviors."

Universal design for learning (UDL) is a framework for instruction organized around three principles based on the learning sciences. These principles guide the design and development of a curriculum that is effective and inclusive for all learners (Rose & Gravel, 2010). UDL guidelines are organized around three principles: 1) provide multiple means of representation; 2) provide multiple means of action and expression; and 3) provide multiple means of engagement (Rose & Gravel, 2010). Visit the National Center on Universal Design for Learning (http://www.udlcenter.org/aboutudl/udlguidelines) for the complete research, examples, and resources supporting the guidelines. As of late, UDL has been incorporated in the definition of comprehensive literacy in the Every Student Succeeds Act (ESSA) of 2015 (PL 114-95; (Baglieri & Shapiro, 2017).

The Center for Applied Special Technology (CAST) suggested that UDL is an evidence-based response to adapting curricula because current technologies have provided clear and diverse images of brain activity among and within learners. Therefore, flexible ways of instructing students are essential, and Rose and Meyer asserted that this flexible nature of teaching "activates specific brain networks associated with learning" (2000). To promote learning they proposed preventing three central barriers: the ways in which materials and instruction are represented, the ways in which learners express what they have learned, and the ways in which learners engage in learning.

According to Baglieri and Shapiro,

> Instruction derived through UDL is equivalent to conceptualizing teaching as a way to offer a spectrum of possibility. Planning with the assumption that learners are individuals who will benefit from a variety of materials, interactions, experiences, and opportunities better attends to the tenets of the most noted learning theories. (2007, p. 180)

In review, a classroom environment has three components: 1) instructional space, 2) student behavior, and 3) student instruction and student learning (see Table 18.1, for a review of these elements). When you take the needed time to structure for success both the instructional space and student behavior, then time within the content block is available to focus on your lesson plan and interaction with the student. The next section looks at how to plan for student learning, adjusting instruction as needed.

REFLECT, CONNECT, and RESPOND
How do the components of executive function support or complement positive student classroom behavior?

PROCESS

Process is the action or steps taken. Process is the vehicle that moves the learning forward with carefully planned lessons. So, which approach should be implemented within the context of learning to read?

In July 2014, the IDA Board of Directors chose a name—Structured Literacy—that would encompass all approaches to reading instruction that conform to IDA's (2018) *Knowledge and Practice Standards*. The board noted, "The term 'structured literacy' is not designed to replace Orton Gillingham, multisensory or other terms in common use. It is an umbrella term designed to describe all of the programs that teach reading in essentially the same way" (Malchow, 2014). In addition, IDA found

> A great body of research shows that the approach to reading instruction developed for children with dyslexia works best for all beginning readers…. Structured Literacy…is a highly structured, recursive, cumulative, phonics-based approach that combines the written word with other senses to enhance memory and learning of written language. (IDA, 2018)

IDA said, "Structured Literacy prepares students to decode words in an explicit and systematic manner. This approach not only helps students with dyslexia, but there is substantial evidence that it is more effective for all readers" (2015). The context for Structured Literacy arises from the imperative to provide evidence-based reading instruction for all students.

This section on process begins with a brief history of the work of Anna Gillingham and Bessie Stillman in the 1930s and 1940s, followed by a listing of instructional principles that guide how Structured Literacy elements are taught. Next, the research that supports systematic instruction is considered as it applies to carrying out that type of instruction. Following that, how both teachers and students benefit from precisely planned lessons, ending with a discussion of effective and sustainable professional learning.

The Orton-Gillingham Approach (OGA): History and Evolution

The lesson plan, evolved from the original OGA, provides a solid background for expert teachers (Gillingham & Stillman, 1956, 1997). The OGA to remedial instruction began in the 1930s when Anna Gillingham and Bessie Stillman collaborated to develop remedial techniques based on Dr. Samuel T. Orton's neurological explanation for language learning disabilities (Orton, 1937). Dr. Orton's approach was derived from his neuropsychiatric background and his case studies of children whose individual learning differences and instructional needs did not mesh with the sight word method reading curriculum then being used in the traditional classroom (Henry & Brickley, 1999).

In 1932, Dr. Orton appointed Anna Gillingham, an experienced psychologist at the Ethical Culture School in New York, as a research fellow in language disabilities at the Language Research Project of the New York Neurological Institute. Gillingham had recognized and worked with bright children with academic problems for many years.

She and Bessie Stillman, a gifted teacher, researched ways to organize remedial techniques to meet the unique needs of students who were struggling to read and spell. Gillingham and Stillman explained that their efforts were fueled because "such children present a challenge which customary teacher training does not enable the teacher to meet" (1956, p. 1). What emerged from their meticulous work was a system of teaching language-related skills incorporating letter sounds, syllables, words, sentences, and writing contained within a daily lesson plan which detailed all aspects of the alphabetic phonetic approach to reading and spelling.

The instruction was to be direct, explicit, sequenced, systematic, cumulative, and intensive. In contrast to the sight word method prevalent at the time, their technique was based on the close association of visual, auditory, and kinesthetic elements to teach the phonetic units step by step. Teaching was responsive and intensive, with many opportunities for corrective feedback as each element was taught and practiced.

These basic multisensory teaching techniques to remediate reading problems are still used today, with some adaptations (Gillingham & Stillman, 1997;

International Dyslexia Association, 2018). See Chapter 2 for a full description of the principles of Structured Literacy and how these strategies of direct, explicit instruction are implemented and supported by research.

What has evolved over time is the essence of lesson planning, which is now consistent with the effort to implement evidence-based instructional approaches to teach all readers. Many programs rely on these important instructional design principles of lesson planning to meet the needs of diverse learners. Some examples of programs developed from the original OGA are Gillingham and Stillman (1956), Slingerland (1994), Spalding (2003), Alphabetic Phonics (Cox, 1984), Multisensory Teaching Approach (Smith, 1987), Sonday System (Sonday, 1997), Wilson Reading System (Wilson, 2002), and Project Read (Greene, 2017) (see Chapter 2 for the origins of Multisensory Structured Literacy).

The principles of instruction are the processes or delivery style for instruction in literacy to be effective. Teachers need to learn and practice the "how" of instruction, in addition to the "what" or elements of Structured Literacy (see Table 18.2).

Research That Supports Systematic Instruction

Until the 2000s, there was neither research that offered evidence on how to teach the most deeply struggling readers, nor research on lesson planning for intensive reading intervention incorporating all of the language components in a single lesson. The same common hallmarks of skillful teaching of literacy subskills established by the OGA are now supported by research. Instruction for struggling readers must be direct, explicit, sequenced, systematic, cumulative, and intensive (Youman & Mathers, 2013).

Direct, Explicit, Sequenced It is important to understand what is meant by the terms *direct, explicit,* and *sequenced* when applied to effective teaching, especially for students who continue to struggle with reading at any level. To be *direct* means to say or define what students are going to learn and why. It may also involve demonstrating or modeling, which can then be copied by students. *Explicit* teaching is marked by stating concepts clearly and leaving no room for confusion or doubt, as well as teaching the precise steps to learn a particular skill. Teaching *sequentially* means that students learn language concepts in a logical order, from the simplest to the more complex, and then take each concept from reading to spelling and then into comprehension and writing. According to Moats,

> The teacher-directed, systematic, sequential, explicit approaches that work best (Archer & Hughes, 2011; Clark, Kirschner, & Sweller, 2012; Rosenshine, 2012) are receiving much less discussion than they deserve. The risk, of course, is that even larger numbers of students will fail to become independent readers and writers. (2012, p. 20)

Clark, Kirshner, and Swelling (2012) noted that

> Decades of research clearly demonstrate that *for novices* (comprising virtually all students), direct, explicit instruction is more effective and more efficient than partial guidance. So, when teaching new content and skills to novices, teachers are more effective when they provide explicit guidance accompanied by practice and feedback. (2012, p. 26)

Systematic, Cumulative, Intensive Systematic lessons adhere to a fixed plan or method and are easily depended on by the student. The outcome of this kind of instruction is that students gain knowledge of the language and how it works

Table 18.2. Principles of code-based* instruction

Direct-explicit (not implicit)	*Direct*—Direct teaching of all concepts involves continuous student-teacher interaction. Inferential learning of any concept cannot be taken for granted. *Explicit*—Instruction is clearly and succinctly stated, not implied through examples.
Systematic, sequential, and cumulative (not incidental)	*Systematic*—A systematic approach to the content means that any explicitly taught concept about language or orthography is situated within a system that has a defined and overarching conceptual structure. The teacher can place each element of the system in relation to language organization as a whole (Moats, in press). *Sequential*—Print-speech concepts and correspondences range from simple to complex, from transparent to elusive, and from highly reliable to highly variable (Moats, in press). *Cumulative*—Each concept must be based on those already learned. Taught concepts must be systematically reviewed.
Synthetic and analytic	*Synthetic (deductive)*—Synthetic means that students learn the sound-symbol correspondences individually and then blend them as they read syllables and whole words (Moats, 2017). *Analytic (inductive)*—Inductive instruction presents the whole and teaches how this can be broken down into its component parts.
Comprehensive and inclusive	*Comprehensive and Inclusive*—All levels of language are addressed, often in parallel.
Diagnostic-prescriptive	*Diagnostic*—The teaching plan is based on careful and continuous assessment of the individual's needs. *Prescriptive*—Deep knowledge is required to interpret potential underlying variables to deliver prescriptive instruction.
Progress from skills to functional use	Instruction during every lesson moves from teaching skills, to functional use and application of skills.
Consistent use of Structured Literacy vocabulary	Consistent use of explicit vocabulary during instruction and discussion of language concepts builds the necessary vocabulary for both beginning and later learning.
Use of multisensory instructional strategies	The goal of simultaneous multisensory instruction is to foster automatic integration of auditory, visual, and kinesthetic-motor modalities regardless of which modality carries the initial stimulus.

Code-based means that reading instruction is organized around a defined progression of speech-to-print associations and concepts (Moats, 2017).

cumulatively. Each new piece of information is carefully and successively added over time and reinforced by practice and review. Intensive instruction often occurs daily for an extended period and focuses on specific components of reading proficiency for students who need extra time to develop them, often on a one-to-one basis, including extensive practice and high-quality feedback (Rosenshine, 2012). What is a priority depends on what students need to know based on a good assessment and ongoing progress monitoring (see Chapter 7 for more information about assessment).

There is a validated reason for everything included in each lesson. Researchers have pinpointed components essential for reading instruction—phonemic awareness, alphabetic code, fluency, vocabulary, and comprehension (NICHD, 2000)—and others include spelling and writing as well (Moats, 2012; Youman & Mathers, 2013). Lessons should contain a few targeted reading skills, and the instructional pace needs to reflect a focus on short introductions, with various ways to review and practice. In addition, both Moats and Youman and Mathers recommended extended time for one-on-one instruction, with active learning on the part of the student and high-quality teacher feedback. These students require a lot of support and carefully scaffolded instruction based on progress monitoring—going from easy to difficult while also ensuring that the students master the skill or strategy before moving on (Rosenshine, 2012).

The 17 Principles of Effective Instruction are listed next to emphasize that the art of teaching includes expertise in both content knowledge and the process or delivery principles. Rosenshine called these principles the "research-based strategies all teachers should know" (2012, p. 12). Structured lesson planning supports and deliberately integrates these components, thus giving the teacher a scaffold on which to build the sequence of the individualized curriculum for the students. Furthermore, a thorough review of reading remediation studies and programs for deeply struggling readers reveals that programs that were explicit provided guided practice, distributed practice over time, targeted feedback and support, and assessment are most beneficial (Youman & Mathers, 2013). Teachers and students both benefit from the explicit systematic approach, but for different reasons, discussed in the following sections. (See Chapter 2 for the comprehensive elements of structured language lessons.)

---

17 Principles of Effective Instruction (Rosenshine, 2012)

Begin a lesson with a short review of previous learning.

Present new material in small steps with student practice after each step.

Limit the amount of material students receive at one time.

Give clear and detailed instructions and explanations.

Ask a large number of questions, and check for understanding.

Provide a high level of active practice for all students.

Guide students as they begin to practice.

Think aloud, and model steps.

Provide models of worked-out problems.

Ask students to explain what they have learned.

Check the responses of all students.

Provide systematic feedback and corrections.

Use more time to provide explanations.

Provide many examples.

Reteach material when necessary.

Prepare students for independent practice. Monitor students when they begin independent practice.

Adapted from Rosenshine, B. (2010). Principles of instruction: Research-based strategies that all teachers should know. *Educational Practices Series, 21*, p. 7. Brussels, Belgium: International Academy of Education (IAE); Geneva, Switzerland: International Bureau of Education (IBE).

REFLECT, CONNECT, and RESPOND

Process speaks to actions. Eight actions (or pairs) are listed for the OGA (see Table 18.2). Select one pair, and explain why it is effective.

Benefits of Planning Multisensory Structured Literacy Lessons

Multisensory Structured Literacy lessons benefit both teachers and students.

Benefits for Teachers Berninger explained that structured lesson planning ensures that teachers include

> All levels of language in the same instructional session: the subword level (phonological awareness, letter formation and orthographic awareness); the word level (multiple strategies for connecting spoken and written words while spelling); and [the] text level (constructing sentences and discourse). (1999, p. 20)

A typical lesson follows this pattern:

- Review of sounds and letters previously taught

- Phonemic awareness activities incorporated at appropriate levels

- Systematic review of words for oral reading

- Words incorporated into separately read sentences and short paragraphs of connected text based on what has been taught

- Spelling words from dictation that reflect the same letter patterns

- New concepts carefully introduced and linked to students' prior knowledge through guided **discovery learning**

- Handwriting integrated deliberately to help reinforce the memory for letter sounds and forms and to stress automaticity and legibility of writing

- Oral reading of narrative and expository texts using appropriate materials with an emphasis on accuracy and fluency

- Activities for comprehension strategies and composition

- Direct instruction of vocabulary development

Expert teacher preparation and supportive mentoring ensure that teachers create lesson plans that are cumulative and build the concepts for reading and spelling one step at a time. In summary, this carefully crafted lesson plan ensures a comprehensive presentation in which all components of language are practiced and reviewed systematically in tightly focused, deliberately paced, intensive lessons. Program fidelity can be addressed in this cyclical teaching format. See Table 18.3 for a summary of lesson planning benefits for both teachers and students.

REFLECT, CONNECT, and RESPOND

Discuss the benefits for teachers of creating a Structured Literacy lesson plan.

Benefits for Students The strong emphasis on language instruction brings the students face to face with exactly what they are having the most trouble figuring

Table 18.3. Benefits of lesson planning

For teachers	For students
All levels of language are incorporated in the same instructional period.	There is structure and consistency to each lesson.
Multisensory learning provides many student responses and teacher feedback opportunities.	Active participation within a daily prescribed order helps keep focus on building skills.
Diagnostic and prescriptive approach allows adaptation and differentiation for student learning.	Instruction includes charts for visual reminders and manipulatives to prompt strategies using all sensory systems.
Lessons make use of well-defined scope and sequence of language concepts.	Lessons allow for integration of skills learned and connection of new learning to acquired skills.
Lesson plans help organize skills, materials, and presentation.	Consistency and structure promote student organization.
Lessons have appropriate pacing with short intervals of intensive instruction.	Students have time to review and practice what they are learning.

out for themselves. The lively interaction between teacher and students encourages reflection on the language forms they are learning that underlie reading, spelling, and writing.

How Planning Provides Structure   Structured lesson planning is essential for successfully teaching students with language learning disabilities and attention issues for many important reasons. From the students' point of view, the lessons fit their need for structure, limits, and an anxiety-free atmosphere in which to learn. Students do not like surprises or last-minute changes that can confuse them and affect their performance. They like to know what is coming next to prepare for it (Frank, 2002). The lessons adhere to a daily structure to ensure that students feel secure, knowing that the lesson is stable, predictable, and designed for their success. The lesson agenda is often displayed on a chart using words and symbols for the activities listed. The students and teacher refer to this agenda as the lesson progresses. Often, students use a paper clip to mark each step on the chart as they work through each task in order. They are frequently surprised at the fast pace and amount accomplished at the end of the session.

How Planning Promotes Active Participation   Presenting activities in the same order removes students' anxiety over time. Students know what to expect and when. Because the activities rotate rapidly, none lasting more than 10 minutes, student attention is better focused. In addition, students' active participation increases through verbalizing, generalizing, and comparing and contrasting language elements while students build the structure of the language for themselves.

How Planning Uses Visual Reminders   Most systems have a structured lesson chart that is a visual reminder of the order of the lesson and, incidentally, how students are slowly mastering the components of written language (Smith, 1989). Spelling, handwriting, and composition lessons have procedure charts that prompt the students to use the strategies they are learning. These familiar structured procedures promote readiness for learning (see Chapters 8, 9, 10, 11, and 16).

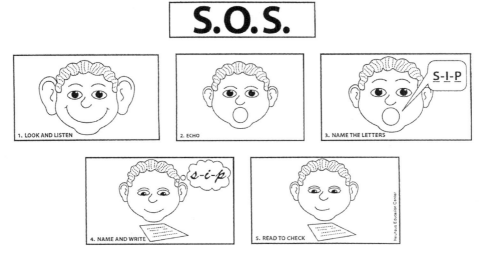

Figure 18.2. Simultaneous Oral Spelling (SOS) procedure. 1) Look and listen, 2) Repeat (echo) and segment, 3) Name the letters, 4) Name and write, 5) Read to check. (From Neuhaus Education Center, Bellaire, TX. *Sources:* Cox, 1992; Gillingham & Stillman, 1960. Reprinted with permission.)

Figure 18.2 illustrates the multisensory procedure for spelling practice, Simultaneous Oral Spelling (SOS).

How Planning Facilitates Guided Discovery Learning **Guided discovery learning** happens when new material or concepts are carefully prepared and presented to students that relate logically to what they already know. By using this process, students can deduce what is new. They will remember more readily what they have been allowed to discover. The lesson planning approach described here does not support the theory that learning something new should be unguided or partially guided but supports the theory that novice learners and "nearly everyone else thrives when provided with full, explicit instructional guidance (and should not be asked to discover any essential content or skills)" (Clark et al., 2012, p. 6). Clark and colleagues also affirmed, "Evidence from controlled, experimental (a.k.a. 'gold standard') studies almost uniformly supports full and explicit instructional guidance rather than partial or minimal guidance for novice to intermediate learners" (2012, p. 11).

For example, when teaching the digraph *ck,* the first part of the new learning is auditory discovery that the teacher uses while having the students repeat words with that ending and listening for and identifying the final sound in each word. They already know the sounds of *c* and *k* as /k /in their recall memory. Then, when the teacher writes the same words on the board, they discover visually that the final /k/ sound is now made by the two letters together after a short vowel. Students are introduced to digraph *ck* through guided discovery. They see the digraph and say "digraph ck"; next, they discover the key word *truck*. Then, they skywrite, naming the letters, sounds, and key words before they trace and write digraph *ck* several times on paper. This exemplifies both guided discovery and direct explicit instruction in conjunction with the use of multisensory modalities: saying, listening, seeing, skywriting, and writing on paper.

Discovery learning has the following advantages:

- It makes students partners in learning.

- Students understand and connect the new learning to prior knowledge, supporting students and increasing memory.

- Students discover the information through multisensory guided discovery.

- Teachers report that once they start using discovery learning instruction in their Structured Literacy instruction classes, it changes the way they teach everything.

How Planning Helps You Use Language About Language   Another consideration when planning and executing Multisensory Structured Literacy lessons is to use a consistent vocabulary together with students. It is not any vocabulary, but one that is a logical, consistent way of referring to the language elements you are working on. You will be setting up a vocabulary for later learning as well. By using language about language, both students and teachers need to think metalinguistically. Martin referred to **metalinguistics** as "an awareness of language as an entity that can be contemplated; crucial to early reading ability, to understanding discourse patterns in the classroom, and to analyzing the language being used to teach the language that must be learned" (2011, p. 710).

Some examples of important metalinguistic terms are as follows:

- *Initial, medial* and *final:* These refer to the position of letters and letter groupings in words for reading and spelling.

- *Before* and *after:* These are used to describe the positions of letters in the alphabet and letters and sounds in words.

- *Voiced* and *unvoiced:* These describe how speech sounds are articulated.

- *Blocked* and *unblocked:* These pertain to speech sounds that are sustained or not sustained in their production (e.g., /p/ and /g/ are blocked; /e/ and /o/ are unblocked).

- *Vowels* and *consonants:* Vowels are open speech sounds, and consonants are constricted or obstructed by the teeth, tongue, or lips.

- *Syllable:* This refers to a spoken or written unit that is organized around a vowel.

- *Accented* and *unaccented:* These terms refer to accent, what Martin described as the "stress or emphasis on one syllable in a word or on one or more words in a phrase in a sentence" (2011, p. 699).

- *Prefix* and *suffix:* These are affixes attached to the beginning or end of a word that can change its meaning or grammatical class. (See Chapter 14 for more about affixes.)

- *Digraphs:* These consist of two vowels or two consonants in the same syllable representing one speech sound (e.g., *ck, ee*).

- *Diphthong:* A combination of two adjacent vowel sounds within the same syllable, also known as a gliding vowel.

- *Schwa sound* (/ə/): This is a nondistinct, unaccented vowel sound that sometimes sounds like short /u/ (e.g., *cotton*).

Using the same linguistic terms from lesson to lesson helps build up a common vocabulary about concepts that need to be taught directly. In addition, such use of these and other terms gives students and teachers a common way to describe, discuss, and discover new concepts; review what they have learned; and make corrections themselves (Birsh, 2006).

How Planning Integrates All Language Systems   Careful planning guarantees that many layers of structured language processing are practiced, integrated, and applied systematically based on an organized curriculum. Students experience short, intensive, interactive activities that integrate reading, writing, and spelling. What they read, they write; what they write, they read; what they read, they spell. Students are taught to use all pathways to learn in every lesson as they work on letter sounds, reading words, spelling, handwriting, vocabulary, comprehension, and composition. This seamless presentation ensures that the basic skills needed for students to become skilled readers are not presented in a disjointed and disconnected way. Grasping written language concepts presents difficulties for students, especially when attention is a problem. Therefore, activities are short and focused, with small steps taken in sequence, from easy to more complex. The teacher keeps the lesson interesting with the rapid changing of learning modalities (visual, auditory, and tactile–kinesthetic) and media. Students learn to accept and even anticipate variety within the structure (Tucker, 2003). Necessary repetition builds toward mastery while all taught concepts are maintained in the lessons (Wilson, 1988, 2002). New learning and practice with prior learning are well balanced. Review is necessary for purposes of fluency and automaticity of each level of the essential components of reading and writing.

REFLECT, CONNECT, and RESPOND
Discuss the benefits for students of participating in a Structured Literacy lesson.

Role of the Professional Learning Community

How do you integrate knowledge and skill in the delivery of an effective lesson? What is the process for becoming an effective literacy teacher and diagnostician? We cannot leave this section on process without referencing the importance of professional learning for the teacher.

Given the fast pace of new information surrounding learning and the brain, it is difficult to stay current. School-based experts are busy with the day-to-day needs of the students and the school. Professional learning partners or external partners are experts in the field who assist in-school subject matter experts and others by providing high-quality learning experiences in both subject matter and effective professional learning practices. Through every point of the teaching continuum, beginning with high-quality mentoring and coaching, teachers engage in the active, sociocultural construction of their professional knowledge in the form of professional learning communities and collegial and collaborative forums, which fuel their capacities to promote effective learning as well as provide resources for the school community—teachers and parents. Educators are guided by the larger professional community by attending conferences and workshops from local and national educational organizations, by participating in webinars, or by keeping abreast of current articles and research found in professional journals.

Pasi Sahlberg, Finnish educator and school improvement activist, stated, "I think the greatest misconception around professional learning is that teaching is a mechanistic construction of separate parts that can be absorbed and that anybody can do. In other words, that teaching is easy" (2017, p. 3).

The contents of this book have been constructed with separate parts; each chapter a complete field of study. This chapter provides a road map for how to weave all the chapters into a complete lesson for the benefit of teachers and students. It takes more than these printed words for you to become a knowledgeable, skilled, and sensitive literacy teacher. It takes learning, experience, and practice within the context of a professional learning community. It will take both a coach, who is a short-term, task-based professional, and a mentor for a long-term, two-way relationship to become a highly effective teacher. The quality (not quantity) of literacy instruction is critical.

REFLECT, CONNECT, and RESPOND
Describe what is involved in participating in a professional learning community and how this contributes to teachers' deep understanding of creating and implementing Structured Literacy lessons.

CONTENT

Content is the "what" of instruction. The content of Structured Literacy, discussed in the previous chapters is phonology, phonics, morphology, syntax, text-reading fluency, vocabulary, and semantics-comprehension, handwriting and composition. This section describes how to develop lesson plans that include all the linguistic components of literacy and how to build a lesson plan from simple to complex, and known to unknown. Samples of both daily and weekly lesson plans are provided. In addition, the similarities and differences of lesson plans for Tier 1, Tier 2, and Tier 3 will be discussed. Here is where research on what to teach, practical experience, and intensive teacher preparation come together.

Multisensory Structured Literacy Lesson Plan

Other chapters in this book describe the linguistic components of literacy, such as alphabet and letter knowledge (Chapter 5), phonology and phonological awareness, including phonemic awareness (Chapter 6), the role of decoding in reading (Chapter 9), spelling (Chapter 10), handwriting (Chapter 11), fluency (Chapter 12), vocabulary (Chapter 15), comprehension (Chapter 16), composition (Chapter 17), and assessment (Chapter 7). Structured lesson planning supports and integrates these components, giving the teacher the framework to deliver the systematic sequence of concepts and skills in the individualized curriculum the students need to master. Spalding described how lesson planning brings together "the content to be taught, the most effective way to teach it and the principles of learning and instruction" (2003, p. 193).

This section highlights common features of various curricula, research-based principles of learning and instruction, and lesson plan formats implementing planning through a variety of organizing strategies.

The sample lesson plans provide examples of how a plan varies based on the Structured Literacy levels students need. Beginning teachers may find them particularly useful.

Common Features and Language Concepts
for Classroom Reading Teachers and Literacy Specialists

Discrete components of language are included in the daily lesson plan to build the associations necessary for successful reading, spelling, and writing. The language components are modified for each student or group and for different levels of instruction. Not all components appear every day; they are rotated through the weekly lesson plans to help students establish mastery across the linguistic concepts. The list that follows is an amalgam of Structured Literacy lesson components derived from research and accredited teacher education programs:

- The alphabet sequence and letter recognition and naming

- Phonemic awareness activities

- Reviewing sound–symbol associations learned in previous lessons, using letter decks, and reviewing letter clusters, using cards and key words to aid memory

- Spelling these same sounds to integrate reading and spelling

- Introducing new sounds and language concepts and/or reviewing previously introduced concepts for reading and spelling

- Reading phonetically regular words in lists and sentences with letter patterns already taught and developing automatic recognition of high-frequency sight words to build automaticity

- Vocabulary study

- Reading connected, controlled, and/or decodable text to develop fluency

- Spelling and writing words and sentences from dictation, using words from reading practice

- Handwriting practice, with explicit instruction in letter formation

- Comprehension and listening strategies for use with connected text

- Oral language practice and written composition

It is necessary for these discrete components of language to be incorporated into lesson planning (see Chapter 1, Figure 1.3).

Research-Based Principles of Learning and Instruction

During 10 years of research on 1,000 students with dyslexia, the Texas Scottish Rite Hospital in Dallas developed a way to integrate these elements in a lesson plan to facilitate learning. From the research, certain elements were shown to be essential to successfully teaching students (Cox, 1984). One element is a daily lesson plan that follows a set format. Cox suggested four types of structure that are essential in the remediation of language-related skills:

1. Ordered daily presentation of activities and materials
2. Precise steps in procedures
3. Rapid rotation of activities
4. Periodic measurement of progress (Cox, 1984, p. 35)

The lesson activities are short and focused, with small steps taken in sequence, at first easy and then more difficult. The principles of instruction include multisensory presentation of each component of the lesson using visual, auditory, and tactile–kinesthetic cues. The simultaneous presentation through these modalities within the daily structure of the lesson plan ensures learning.

Lesson Plan Formats

A lesson plan is a working document for the success of both the teacher and the student. Examples of different formats are a daily lesson plan, a weekly lesson plan, and a summary worksheet or scope and sequence, which denotes student progress. Begin with formats provided by a certified trainer or coach. However, once experienced in implementing the steps in the curriculum from basic to complex, you may begin to fine-tune lessons to match your style of instruction.

How to Begin   Begin by identifying the individual components of the reading lesson in the suggested daily lesson plan along with the sequence of these components. When you begin planning for a group of students or an individual, you can assume nothing about the students' previous mastery of material.

If prior progress monitoring, educational evaluations, or report cards are available, then refer to them to identify the highest level of mastery attained for each component (see Chapter 7). If a student is new to a reading tutorial approach, administer a quick probe of all skills, beginning with letter names and sounds. Each student must be evaluated to determine what material has been mastered and what knowledge is yet to be learned or needs to be reviewed. Once lessons have begun, succeeding steps will be driven by assessment data obtained from records of informal curriculum-based probes and later formal testing. It is important for students to know what they know and for you to be aware of the gaps in students' skills. For students struggling with reading, it is a well-accepted axiom that remediation starts at the beginning and goes as slowly as necessary and as quickly as possible.

Creating a Daily Lesson Plan   A lesson plan can be thought of as a concrete way to analyze the needs of each student.

A detailed daily lesson plan is needed to plan and organize skills, materials, and presentations. When you sit down to plan lessons, keep long-term goals in mind according to the curriculum scope and sequence that delineates the discrete components of language and subskills to be mastered. When teachers are new to this kind of instruction, it often takes 2 or even 3 hours while using assessment materials to plan and organize the materials for a 1-hour tutorial. You will find the planning process becomes easier after teaching through all of the elements of the curriculum with several different groups of students. For this kind of expert, dedicated instruction to be successful, it is important to have the ongoing support of administrators and instructional team members, along with parent input, to carry it out.

The first daily lesson plan is generally an assessment or review of the student's known skills that are to be mastered in each lesson component. Every program has a beginning series of skills to be mastered. For example, check new students for knowledge of the following: the alphabet, sequence, letter names, phonemic awareness of beginning sounds of words, writing upper- and lowercase print letters, some consonant sounds and short vowel sounds on cards, spelling individual sounds, and blending sounds into words (Sonday, 1997).

A variety of daily and weekly lesson plan formats are provided here for review. Their Structured Literacy components (listed earlier in the chapter), are derived from research and accredited teacher education programs. Figure 18.3 is an example of a beginning-level daily lesson plan after several consonants and two short vowels have been introduced. Figure 18.4 is an example of a more advanced daily lesson plan after the students have progressed to two-syllable words for reading and spelling. The students have worked with the dropping rule and spelling derivatives. The students have also been introduced to four syllable types: closed, vowel pair, vowel-*r*, and vowel-consonant-*e*. The daily lesson plan shown in Figure 18.4 introduces the open syllable.

For a description of the precise steps in a multisensory introduction of letter sounds and concepts, see Chapters 5, 6, 9, and 10 for teaching elementary students and Chapter 20 for older students. The times given for each lesson component are approximate. Teachers may or may not have the opportunity to include every component each day; by using the weekly lesson plan, however, all activities will be incorporated consistently over time. Figures 18.3 and 18.4 list chapters from this book that contain information and guidance on what can be included in each step of the daily lesson plan for beginners and those at an intermediate level, respectively.

REFLECT, CONNECT, and RESPOND

Choose a daily lesson plan, either beginning level (see Figure 18.3) or intermediate level (see Figure 18.4). Given that lesson plans are built on the known, identify for each section what the student already knows.

Creating a Weekly Lesson Plan   In addition to a daily lesson plan, a weekly lesson plan is also needed. This can be in a separate plan book or more often in the same plan book if there is enough space. Some teachers use a lesson planner. If the planner contains a block for each class, use each block for one lesson component instead. Sometimes a 9″ × 12″ sketch pad is used to accommodate daily and weekly plans on the same page. When you first begin to organize lesson plans, each daily plan may require a full sheet of paper. As you become more experienced with planning and implementing the lessons, five daily lessons can be recorded on a single sheet of paper or in a teacher's plan book.

The weekly plan enables you to always be looking ahead to focus the direction of the instruction. In that way, you can ensure that the same components are practiced using different multisensory pathways and media. It is easy to fill a lesson with instructional activities; the real expertise is to continue moving the lessons and the instruction forward. Pacing is the most difficult skill for inexperienced teachers to acquire because it only comes with experience. If you are a novice teacher, working with both a daily and a weekly lesson plan format (under the guidance of a coach and/or instructional team) enables you to begin to see when instruction is moving too quickly or too slowly. As mentioned previously, the idea is to move as quickly as possible but as slowly as necessary. By sketching out five lessons and then adjusting the plan on a daily basis, you can begin to recognize and pace instruction based on students' performance. Figures 18.5 and 18.6 provide a model for a weekly lesson plan that shows the interplay of new information,

Instructional components (A typical lesson follows this pattern.)	Approximate time	Refer to...	Teacher's notes
ALPHABET KNOWLEDGE AND PHONEMIC AWARENESS *Alphabet Knowledge* Students touch and name the letters of the alphabet in sequence as warm-up. Students match plastic uppercase letters to grid of alphabet letters on a mat. *Phonemic Awareness* Ask students if these words rhyme: *pill/hill, tip/lip, yes/my, run/sun, mice/nice, now/nap.*	5 minutes	Chapters 5 and 6	
READING PREVIOUSLY TAUGHT LETTERS AND SOUNDS Show letter cards for students to name for quick drill. Give key words and sounds: i, t, p, n, s, a, l, d, f, h, g, o. Use irregular word deck: *said, the, of, one.*	3 minutes	Chapter 9	
SPELLING SOUNDS Using a spelling deck (cards bearing letters and sounds introduced for reading), dictate sounds to students, who repeat the sounds, say the letter names, and write them on chalkboard: /ĭ/, /t/, /p/, /n/, /s/, /ă/, /l/, /d/, /f/, /h/, /g/, /ŏ/.	3 minutes	Chapter 10	
HANDWRITING Students practice writing *d* on folded newsprint paper. Students trace the letter three times while listening to guided stroke description: "Curve under, over, stop, back around, up, down, release." Students make three copies, saying the letter name each time.	3 minutes	Chapter 11	
MULTISENSORY DISCOVERY OF LETTER OR CONCEPT Provide multisensory introduction of digraph *ng* using guided discovery of sound, letters, key words, and mouth position. Discovery words: *sing, sang, sting, ding* Reinforce with sky writing, handwriting, reading the sound, and spelling the sound.	5 minutes	Chapters 2, 9, 10, and 11	
ORAL READING REVIEW FOR ACCURACY AND FLUENCY Students prepare and read orally closed-syllable words: *hint, stand, tint, slap, split, spat, spin, snap, nips, plant. Dad lifts the sand in a tin pan.*	5–10 minutes	Chapters 9 and 12	
SPELLING REVIEW OF PREVIOUSLY TAUGHT PATTERNS Give warm-up, with review of sounds to be spelled: /ĭ/, /t/, /s/, /a/, /l/, /f/, /h/. Review Floss Rule and spell these words: *sniff, tiff, staff, till, hill, spill.*	5–10 minutes	Chapter 10	

(continued)

Figure 18.3. Beginning-level daily lesson plan.

Instructional components (A typical lesson follows this pattern.)	Approximate time	Refer to. . .	Teacher's notes
ORAL LISTENING STRATEGIES AND COMPREHENSION Read "The Tortoise and the Hare" to students. Have students retell the fable with a graphic organizer for stories (simple story map).	10 minutes	Chapter 16	
ORAL LANGUAGE PRACTICE AND VOCABULARY Introduce vocabulary: *boasted, plodding, patient.* Have students find and discuss meanings for the descriptive words from the story, use words in sentences, and enter words in the vocabulary section of their language notebooks.	10 minutes	Chapters 3, 15, and 16	

review of concepts, and practice in controlled lists and texts for reinforcement and the variety of multisensory interactions between teacher and students. As the week unfolds, you will adjust the lesson plan to suit students' needs.

The explicit and systematic instruction used in these lessons plays an important role in efforts to improve reading instruction and link instruction to how children are identified with learning disabilities. Using the RTI criteria to assess and identify struggling readers calls for a three-tiered system of intervention (see Chapter 7). In this data-based decision-making model, teachers target and plan their lessons according to their students' identified weaknesses.

Tier 1 involves screening students for reading difficulties in preschool, kindergarten, and first grade and placing them in research-based literacy programs emphasizing the five critical components of early reading (phoneme awareness, phonics, fluency, vocabulary, and comprehension; NICHD, 2000) in the general education classroom. Tier 2 is the provision of small-group intervention and progress monitoring to support students with similar needs for effective instruction in reading along with the general education program. For children who do not progress in reading at a reasonable rate, Tier 3 would include special education services using scientifically based programs with progress regularly monitored (Fletcher, Coulter, Reschly, & Vaughn, 2004).

The lesson plan is the very backbone of RTI. The National Center on Response to Intervention explained that through the lesson plan, reading teachers are able to "adjust the intensity and nature of…intervention depending on a student's responsiveness" (2010). Regarding the three-tier system of intervention programs in U.S. public schools for students struggling with reading, Dickman, Hennessy, Moats, Rooney, and Tomey (2002) noted that Structured Literacy lessons should fit into the third tier of intervention in special education for the poorest readers. Merely using direct instruction and strategy instruction, however, is not sufficient. Students engaging in second- and third-tier intervention must have "structured teaching of language systems" (Dickman et al., 2002, p. 24).

Structured language interventions must be intensive to be effective. As students reach the third grade, up to 2 hours daily are necessary to remediate severe reading disabilities. Remediation programs with demonstrated effectiveness, staffed by teachers with appropriate training in language and explicit instruction, should be available to older poor readers in lieu of other academic requirements.

Instructional component	Approximate time	Refer to...	Teacher's notes
ALPHABET AND DICTIONARY, PHONOLOGICAL AWARENESS, AND MORPHOLOGY STUDY Students review the definition of accent ("When we accent something, our mouths open wider, and our voices are louder and higher.") Instructor shows an example sequence when the third letter is accented: ab**C**′, de**F**′, gh**I**′. Using the alphabet strip, students recite the alphabet, accenting the third letter.	5 minutes	Chapters 5, 6, 9, and 14	
REVIEW OF LETTERS, SOUNDS AND WORD PARTS PREVIOUSLY TAUGHT Students say the sounds represented by symbols in the letter card deck. Students also use a deck of word parts: suffixes, prefixes, and roots.	3 minutes	Chapters 9 and 20	
MULTISENSORY DISCOVERY OF LETTER OR CONCEPT Students learn vowels in open syllables through auditory/visual discovery. Discovery words: *able, ogle, idle, bugle* Explain to students, "All words end in final stable syllables; the first syllable is open and accented. A vowel in an open, accented syllable is long. Long vowels say their names." **sta′**|ble **ri′**|fle **no′**|ble	10 minutes	Chapters 2, 9, 10, and 20	
ORAL READING PRACTICE FOR ACCURACY AND FLUENCY Read words with vowels in open syllables: *table, cradle, trifle, stable, ruble, sable, title, maple, staple.* Read sentences: *The wooden cradle was carved from pinewood.* Read a review list of words and a short story in a controlled reader.	10 minutes	Chapters 9, 12, and 20	
SPELLING OF PREVIOUSLY TAUGHT PATTERNS Students spell on paper from *dictation: maple, stifle, table, noble, bugle, staple, stable.* Students categorize list of words for spelling as regular, irregular, or rule words: *tank, tail, swimming.* Students write sentences from dictation: *The fish nibbles on the worm on the hook.*	10 minutes	Chapters 10 and 20	
HANDWRITING (*does not occur every lesson*) Students practice writing capital letters *T, S,* and *I* in cursive.	5 minutes	Chapter 11	
EXTENDED READING AND WRITING Goal is accuracy, fluency, and comprehension. Students read from connected decodable text with controlled vocabulary that is geared to the students' levels. Students write sentences using vocabulary they are reading and spelling.	10 minutes	Chapters 9, 16, 17, and 20	

(continued)

Figure 18.4. Intermediate-level daily lesson plan.

Instructional component	Approximate time	Refer to. . .	Teacher's notes
COMPREHENSION AND LISTENING STRATEGIES Read students' stories or expository texts that match their ages and interests. Include comprehension strategies (see Chapter 14).	5 minutes	Chapters 16 and 8	
ORAL LANGUAGE PRACTICE AND COMPOSITION Begin expanding written sentences using *where* and *when*. Practice orally, starting with basic simple sentences: *The baseball player left his mitt (where?). Molly called her best friend Sara (when?).*	5 minutes	Chapters 3, 15, and 17	

As Dickman and colleagues pointed out, "Accommodations and modifications are never a substitute for intensive remediation" (2002, p. 25).

Lesson Plans Across the Tiers

Explicit and systematic instruction used in structured language lessons is critical to improving reading instruction for all children. Reading instruction across the tiers requires both different contexts or settings and differences in process (intensity and duration) for each tier. Tier 1 is quality reading instruction for all children. Tier 2 is focused reading instruction for a few children. Tier 3 is very focused reading instruction for very few children. Table 18.4 provides an overview of the instructional tiers and how different aspects of instruction differ across tiers. Although the content of instruction (IDA *Knowledge and Practice Standards*) does not change across the tiers, the setting, number of students, and intensity of instruction do change.

First, the instructional setting is different for each tier of instruction. Instructional tiers differ in intensity and duration. Intensity is reflected both in the smaller group size and the increased individual student response opportunities. Duration can be reflected in the number of sessions and/or the time spent in the session. Literacy instruction across the tiers will differ in setting, intensity, duration, materials, and depth of teacher knowledge.

To capture the difference in Tier 1, Tier 2, and Tier 3 instruction, you need to examine additional components of the respective lesson plans: materials, teacher language, anticipated student responses and next steps, and notes on student performance.

- *Materials* — With each tier of instruction, the materials used must be compatible. For example, the materials to teach blends to a classroom may include examples of all two-letter blends. Materials to teach blends to Tier 2 may be limited to the set of *s*-blends (*st, sm, sk, sw, sp, sc, sl, sn*). Materials used to teach blends to Tier 3 students may start with a picture sort of five *s*-blends because the student(s) struggle to differentiate among the second sounds in a blend.

- *Teacher language of instruction* — The lesson plans for the different tiers of instruction differ in the teacher language of instruction. Often, the teacher is able to give an example of a language concept but struggles to provide a clear

Instructional component	Day 2	Day 3
ALPHABET KNOWLEDGE AND PHONEMIC AWARENESS	*Alphabet knowledge* Students touch and name the alphabet on strip. Students practice accent and rhythm, naming the letters in pairs. Students accent the first letter of pairs (**A**'B, **C**'D, **E**'F). *Phonemic awareness* Students add a sound to a word: add /p/ to the beginning of these words: *each, in, age, ill, itch.*	*Alphabet knowledge* Students touch and name the alphabet on strip. With model available, students put plastic letters in alphabetical order. *Phonemic awareness* Students identify the sound at the beginning of each word: *beach, ball, bark, boil, bus.* (Students use mirrors to check lips.)
READING: REVIEW OF LETTERS AND SOUNDS PREVIOUSLY TAUGHT	Show letter cards for students to name and give key words and sounds for quick drill: *i, t, p, n, s, a, l, d, f, h, g, o, a,* and (new card) *ng.* Use irregular word deck: *said, the, of, one.*	Repeat Day 2 activity.
SPELLING SOUNDS	Dictate sounds to students, who repeat the sounds, say the letter names, and write them on rice tray: /ĭ/, /t/, /p/, /n/, /s/, /l/, /d/, /f/, /h/, /g/, /ŏ/, /ă/, /k/, and (new sound) /ng/.	Repeat Day 2 activity, using table top instead of rice tray.
MULTISENSORY DISCOVERY OR REVIEW OF LETTER CONCEPT	*Review of Day 1's new concept* Review /ng/ sound, letters, key word (king), and mouth position. Review digraph *ng* final: *sing, hang, long.* Discover /ng/ medial *(link, sank, honk)* where /ng/ is represented by letter *n* (key word: *sink*). Students draw *g*-curve on *n* to mark new sound: ŋ.	*Review of Day 1's new concept* Review /ng/ sound, letters, key words, and mouth position. Reinforce with sky writing, handwriting, reading sound, spelling sound (sometimes *n* = /ng/). Students put /ng/ in student notebook, with spelling examples of digraph ng and n with key words.
ORAL READING PRACTICE FOR ACURACY AND FLUENCY	Students prepare and read orally words with *ng* and other short *a* words: *pat, tang, lap, sat, pang, sap, sang, dad, fang.* Read sentences with *ng* words.	Students prepare and read orally words with short *i*: *sit, hit, tip, dip, tin, pin, lid, did, pig, sis.* Read controlled sentences for fluency.
SPELLING OF PREVIOUSLY TAUGHT SOUNDS AND RULES	Give warm-up, with review of sounds to be spelled: /ĭ/, /p/, /n/, /s/, /ŏ/, /t/, /d/, /g/, /l/. Review suffix -*s* rule (/z/ and /s/ = s): *pins, pots, tops, digs, dogs, logs, nips.* Students write sentences from dictation: Dan sits on the logs.	Give warm-up, with review of sounds to be spelled: /h/, /ĭ/, /l/, /s/, /f/, /p/, /ŏ/. Review Floss Rules and suffix -*s* rule, and have students spell words from dictation: *hills, pills, fills, dolls, sills.* (Also discuss word meanings.)
HANDWRITING	Review guided stroke description for letters *d, p,* and *a.* At the chalkboard, students practice *a, p,* and *d,* connecting them in random order: *adp, pda, dpa.*	Review guided stroke description, and have students begin practice connecting bridge letter *o.* Students trace *op, od,* and *og* on folded newsprint. Students write copies after tracing.

(continued)

Figure 18.5. Days 2 and 3 of a 5-day weekly lesson plan, beginning level. (From *Multisensory Teaching of Basic Language Skills, Third Edition* [p. 475].)

Instructional component	Day 2	Day 3
ORAL LISTENING STRATEGIES AND COMPREHENSION	Reread fable ("The Tortoise and the Hare") to students. Using a simple story map as a prompt, have students describe the actions of the hare.	Using a simple story map, have students describe the cations of the tortoise.
ORAL LANGUAGE PRACTICE AND VOCABULARY	*Vocabulary* List adjectives used in the fable to describe the hare.	*Vocabulary* List adjectives used in the fable to describe the tortoise.

explanation. For example, an example of a consonant blend would be *sl* as in *slip*. An explanation would be "Two letters that come together to form two sounds."

- *Anticipated student response*—The different tiers of instruction are structured to provide individual responses from individual students. Teacher language is precise and targeted to elicit precise and targeted student responses. This individualization provides the teacher with sharp insight into individual student strengths and errors. The teacher language of instruction is structured to elicit a response that will reflect the student's understanding of the targeted language concept.

- *Next steps if student response is different than anticipated*—When a student answer is different than anticipated or incorrect, the teacher will need to know which questions to ask next to support the student in his or her learning. Each instructional tier requires an increase in teacher expertise. The teacher language of instruction becomes more precise to puzzle out the barriers to student learning. An ever-increasing teacher knowledge and expertise is required to diagnose and then implement, in the moment, the effective instruction.

- *Notes on student performance*—The student performance notes are written as quick reminders to the teacher after completion of the lesson. Tier 1 notes might be a quick reminder of how the lesson went and might identify which students need additional support in terms of more practice and/or a Tier 2 support. Teacher notes taken during a Tier 2 lesson (4–5 students) document where individual students continue to struggle in order to review or reteach in the next lesson. Teacher notes also record progress and mastery to determine when students are ready to participate exclusively in Tier 1 and no longer need the second dose of instruction provided in Tier 2. Tier 3 notes are focused exclusively on the specific students and their strengths and weaknesses such as what worked, the amount of review needed, and the specific concepts needing review and practice.

Lesson Plans for Structured Literacy Instruction   Instruction using Multisensory Structured Literacy techniques, OGA, and/or Structured Literacy was originally delivered in a small group and/or pull-out setting. It is only recently that Structured Literacy is being taught to an entire class; thus, the education field is in the midst of the challenges of making the transition from small-group to

Instructional component	Day 4	Day 5
ALPHABET KNOWLEDGE AND PHONEMIC AWARENESS	*Alphabet knowledge* Students touch and name the alphabet on strip. Point to a letter on the alphabet strip. Students name what comes after and before the letter. *Phonemic awareness* Using the letter tiles *p* and *b*, students point to the first sound in dictated words: *pill, bat, pet.*	*Alphabet knowledge* Students touch and name the alphabet on strip. Students play Alphabet Bingo. *Phonemic awareness* Students add /d/ to the beginning of each syllable: *ear, esk, ock, og, ust, oll, ive, ime, itch.*
READING: REVIEW OF LETTERS AND SOUNDS PREVIOUSLY TAUGHT	Repeat Day 2 activity.	Repeat Day 2 activity.
SPELLING SOUNDS	Repeat Day 2 activity on chalkboard.	Repeat Day 2 activity on lined paper.
MULTISENSORY DISCOVERY OR REVIEW OF LETTER CONCEPT	*Introduction of new concept* New letter *c* = /k/ before *a, o,* and *u* Visual discovery: *can, cop, cup.* Students form linkages with key word *cup* and letter *c* pronounced as /k/. Reinforce with sky writing, handwriting, reading sound, and spelling sound. Students add *c* to the /k/ page in their notebooks.	*Review of digraph <u>ng</u> and <u>n</u> before /k/* Present mixed review of *ng* and *nk* words presented during the week: *sing, sang, song, sing, dong, gong, tank, pink, honk, stink.* Students read sentences and underline *ng*: He sa<u>ng</u> a so<u>ng</u>.The bell went di<u>ng</u>-do<u>ng</u>.
ORAL READING PRACTICE FOR ACCURACY AND FLUENCY	Students prepare and read orally nonsense words with *c* read as /k/ before *a* and *o*: *cass, coll, caff, scad, scop, scap.* Read sentences with review of new sight words *said, of, the,* and one: *One of the cops said "Stop!"* *Pat spills one of the cans of pop.* Students draw boxes around words containing the suffix *-s*, which says /s/ or /z/.	Prepare mixed review of words read this week, through use of a deck of word cards or words listed on the board or on chart paper: *tank, gang, tong, sing, king, sting, pink, honk, dank, sink, lank, stink, cast, cod, can, cop, cap.* Students read sentences listed on chart paper or on strips.
SPELLING OF PREVIOUSLY TAUGHT SOUNDS AND RULES	Students review suffix *-s* rule, referring to their notebooks. Students write sentences rom dictation: *Sis fills the gas can.* *Tad pats the cats.* *One of the kids hits the logs.*	Have students explain the Floss Rule and the suffix *-s* rule. Have students give two examples for each. Students write sentence from dictation: *The dog sniffs the pan and spills the fat.*
HANDWRITING	Students write five previously learned letters three times each (to stress size proportion). Each student places a star by one of each letter than he or she feels is best.	Students write five tall letters (*k, h, t, l, d*) three times each (to stress size proportion). Each student places a star by one of each letter than he or she feels is best.

(continued)

Figure 18.6.   Days 4 and 5 of a 5-day weekly lesson plan, beginning level. (From *Multisensory Teaching of Basic Language Skills, Third Edition* [p. 476].)

Instructional component	Day 4	Day 5
ORAL LISTENING STRATEGIES AND COMPREHENSION	With aid of graphic organizer, students identify and explain the turning point of the fable "The Tortoise and the Hare."	Students identify which character they feel they are most like or give a situation when they were most like each character.
ORAL LANGUAGE PRACTICE AND VOCABULARY	*Vocabulary* Students list adjectives used to describe the turning point of the fable.	Students lay graphic organizers on the table and generate one or two clear, concise sentences for each map.

whole-class instruction. All teachers need to know and understand the elements of Structured Literacy. Each element has a unique developmental scope and sequence, in addition to when and how it is woven into Scarborough's rope of skilled reading. (Hollis Scarborough's reading rope of skilled reading is shown in Figure 15.2 in Chapter 15.) The sequence of a lesson plan begins with the smallest elements and gradually builds on the simple to the complex aspects of written language. See Table 18.5 for a sample lesson sequence that progresses in this way.

Many of these learning activities were previously done separately during the school day and were not necessarily related. The weekly spelling list had its own scope and sequence, independent of the phonics lesson, independent of the story being read in reading group. Structured Literacy instruction requires all components of learning to read support and complement each other. The other requirement is that integrated instruction take place within a holistic time slot. Whatever the student reads is immediately followed by spelling. There is a structured procedure for spelling, in which error correction happens immediately after the misspelling occurs. Specific teacher error correction language guides and supports the student to identify and correct his or her own spelling error.

OGA manipulative materials sufficient for whole-class instruction continue to be developed. Print materials and manipulatives are giving way to web-based

Table 18.4. Overview of instructional tiers

	Tier 1	Tier II	Tier III
Setting	Entire classroom	Learning center in classroom	Pull-out
Average time spent on teacher-led instruction	30–50 minutes	30–50 minutes	20–50 minutes
Number of students	Approximately 25+	Small group; approximately 5	Very small group; 1–3
If a teacher were to call on 5 students every minute	Each student would get called on about 10 times per class period	Each student would get called on about 50 times per class period	Each student would get called on 90 times or more per class period
Location of teacher during instruction	Standing in front of the classroom	Usually sitting at a table with all the students	Sitting to directly face the student(s)
Student oral response to instruction	Choral responses and some individual responses	Choral responses with round-robin responses	Individual responses with a few choral or round robin responses

Table 18.5. Sequence of a lesson plan from simple to complex

Component	Skill
Phonemic awareness (review of previously learned material)	Awareness of the sounds of our language; ability to manipulate sound (no print)
Letter names (review of previously learned material)	Ability to say the alphabet; ability to recognize letters
Phonics	Mapping sounds onto print
Read sounds (review)	
Spell sounds (review)	Whatever one reads, one then spells
Read words (review)	Build sounds and letters into words
Spell words (review)	Whatever one reads, one then spells
Introduce new concept	
Read connected text–sentences, phrases, and short stories	

applications and the use of individual student devices. Scripted teacher guides are being written to support teachers as they learn new material and new techniques.

The Tier 1 Lesson Plan   A Tier 1 lesson plan provides the sequence of instruction similar to that shown in Table 18.5. The materials for each component, which may be print materials or the web-based application, may be listed. Sometimes the lesson plan will include the scripted teacher language, with the expected correct student response. The focus of a Tier 1 lesson plan is the teacher—providing the teacher with the scope, sequence, materials, and teacher language to deliver Structured Literacy instruction to a whole class. Tier 1 is quality reading instruction for all children. At Tier 1, it may be possible to write a draft of a week's worth of lessons.

The Tier 2 Lesson Plan   A Tier 2 lesson is focused instruction for a few children. The Tier 2 lesson plan is focused on previously taught skills for a few children who need more—more time, more instruction, or more practice. The lesson plan format remains the same as shown previously, moving from simple to complex, known to unknown; and what the student reads, he or she then immediately spells. At Tier 2, the lesson plan may resemble a template, providing spaces for the teacher to carefully select which concepts need to be focused on and which letters, sounds, words, or sentences to use during instruction. There is an additional column to record notes regarding student performance. The focus of Tier 2 instruction in a smaller setting is for the teacher to have the opportunity to unpack the student learning, diagnose where the difficulty is occurring, and deliver a **prescriptive** approach to support student success. A Tier 2 lesson plan can usually be written at the conclusion of each lesson, with room for minor adjustments during the delivery of the lesson.

The Tier 3 Lesson Plan   A Tier 3 lesson is very focused instruction for very few children. Tier 3 instruction occurs in a small quiet space, separate from the classroom, using different materials from those used for whole-class instruction, with only one or two children in the group, with a highly qualified teacher of Structured Literacy knowledge and experience. The lesson plan is highly individualized and unique to the student(s), and it evolves during instruction. The highly qualified teacher is constantly diagnosing and then prescribing; he or she is constantly tweaking the lesson based on the student performance. For example, listening to student sound production may result in a lesson focused on voiced and unvoiced consonant pairs, cleaning up "vowelization" of specific consonants, or focused repeated practice of weak but accurate sounds.

Based on how a student does with sounds that are read, the teacher determines which sounds the student will be asked to spell. This then determines the sounds that will be the focus in words to be read and then words to be spelled. All the while the highly experienced professional who possesses deep learning is carefully guiding the student toward success with precise teacher language of instruction. Tier 3 instruction is highly technical and precise to the needs of the student. A Tier 3 lesson plan is completed as the lesson unfolds, based on student performance, or it is well thought out and deliberate, providing constant assessment because it is constructed concurrently with the student as he or she goes through the lesson sequence.

The lesson plan is a vehicle that moves the lesson forward, a record of the student learning process, and a teacher roadmap of the instructional journey. A highly effective teacher with deep knowledge is able to avoid inadvertent potholes through insightful scaffolding of the content and skills from the solid known that gradually makes the transition into the unknown. The amount of detail in the lesson itself and the lesson plan is dependent on the needs of the student.

> ### REFLECT, CONNECT, and RESPOND
> Explain each component in the organization of Chapter 18: context, process, and content.

CLOSING THOUGHTS: PLANNING THE LEARNING ENVIRONMENT AND LESSONS

Be exhilarated by making needed changes to your classroom—your space, your interactions with your students, and your lesson planning. This chapter has aimed to provide you with fresh ideas and a new perspective for teaching reading to all children. Use Appendix 18.3: Building Block Checklist for Effective Classroom Management to reflect on what you are currently doing and what you want to do differently.

> Change done to you is debilitating; change done by you is exhilarating.
>
> —Anonymous

A lesson plan for Multisensory Structured Literacy instruction is the framework for interaction between the teacher and the student. It is designed to support teachers in their efforts to teach the linguistic content to be mastered, using the most effective ways to teach according to informed principles of learning and instruction. These kinds of lessons highlight the progression of time-intensive activities, which include reviews of previously taught information, practice in all levels of language, and introducing new concepts based on a systematic curriculum. Careful planning builds the foundation for discovery learning and enables both the teacher and the students to work within a framework designed for explicit instruction. Time spent ensuring that each part of the lesson includes multisensory components provides students with multiple opportunities to be active participants in the learning process.

This chapter is about change: change in classroom organization (context); change in how you deliver instruction (process), and change in elements of reading instruction (content). In previous editions of this book, this chapter emphasized focused instruction for a few children (Tier 2) and very focused instruction for very few children (Tier 3). Now, teachers are looking at how to deliver quality reading instruction for all children in a classroom setting (Tier 1), based on new information coming from research on the brain and learning. Teachers are taking responsibility for their own professional learning, identifying their areas of strengths and needs in their own professional journey.

We have set out to assist teachers on this journey: to assist them in structuring the learning environment for success (context) and implementing proven and effective delivery techniques (process) while using deep knowledge of all the elements involved in learning to read (content). The journey will last a lifetime, for you will never stop learning. Along the way, you will be enriched by both children and colleagues.

ONLINE COMPANION MATERIALS

The following Chapter 18 resources are available at http://www.brookespublishing.com/birshcarreker/materials:

- Reflect, Connect, and Respond Questions
- Appendix 18.1: Structured Literacy Lesson With Apps
- Appendix 18.2: Knowledge and Skill Assessment Answer Key
- Appendix 18.3: Building Block Checklist for Effective Classroom Management
- Appendix 18.4: Sample One-Day Lesson Plan
- Appendix 18.5: Lesson Plan Template

KNOWLEDGE AND SKILL ASSESSMENT

1. Which of these objectives is not a key element to ensure that classroom time is used for effective and meaningful instruction?

   a. Using instructive space effectively

   b. Organizing classroom materials

   c. Criticizing an attention-seeking student for what he or she is doing wrong

   d. Planning transitions

   e. Reinforcing positive productive student behavior

2. In order to gain student confidence, which is *not* helpful?

   a. Allowing them to guess when asked about a new concept

   b. Helping them to be successful on a daily basis

   c. Using Socratic questioning to elicit new information

d. Engaging in meaningful feedback dialogues

e. Reviewing recently learned concepts

3. Which reading activities are essential components of research-based Structured Literacy?

a. Review of sounds and letters previously taught

b. Phonemic awareness activities at appropriate levels

c. Systematic review of words for oral reading

d. Spelling words from dictation that reflect the same letter patterns

e. All of the above

4. Which of the following is a principle of code-based reading instruction?

a. Students experience inferential learning of the alphabet code.

b. Language concepts are taught in order from transparent to elusive.

c. Levels of language are taught in isolation to ensure mastery.

d. Highly variable print-speech concepts are taught early in the sequence.

e. All of the above

5. The weekly lesson plan does which of the following?

a. Contains each individual element taught to date

b. Ensures that a new concept is taught daily

c. Ensures that the instruction keeps pace with the prescribed curriculum

d. Enables the instructor to always be looking ahead to focus the direction of the instruction

e. All of the above

REFERENCES

Al Otaiba, S., Lake, V.E., Scarborough, K., Allor, J., & Carreker, S. (2016). Preparing beginning reading teachers for K–3: Teacher preparation in higher education. *Perspectives on Language and Literacy, 42*(4).

Archer, A.L., & Hughes, C.A. (2011). *Explicit instruction: Effective and efficient teaching.* New York, NY: Guilford.

Baglieri, S., & Shapiro, A. (2017). *Disability studies and the inclusive classroom: Critical practices for embracing diversity in education.* New York, NY: Routledge.

Bailey, B.A. (2000). *Conscious discipline: 7 basic skills for brain smart classroom management.* Ovieto, FL: Loving Guidance.

Berninger, V.W. (1999). The "write stuff" for preventing and treating writing disabilities. *Perspectives, 25*(2), 20–22.

Berninger, V.W., & Wolf, B.J. (2016). *Dyslexia, dysgraphia, OWL LD, and dyscalculia: Lessons from science and teaching* (2nd ed.). Baltimore, MD: Paul H. Brookes Publishing Co.

Birsh, J.R. (2006). What is multisensory structured language? *Perspectives, 32*(4).

Clark, R.E., Kirschner, P.A., & Sweller, J. (2012, Spring). Putting students on the path to learning. *American Educator, 36*(1), 6–11.

Cox, A.R. (1984). *Structures and techniques: Multisensory teaching of basic language skills.* Cambridge, MA: Educators Publishing Service.

Cox, A.R. (1992). *Foundations for literacy: Structures and techniques for multisensory teaching of basic written language skills.* Cambridge, MA: Educators Publishing Service.

Dickman, G.E., Hennessy, N.L., Moats, L.C., Rooney, K.J., & Tomey, H.A., III. (2002). *Response to OSEP Summit on Learning Disabilities.* Baltimore, MD: The International Dyslexia Association.

Dumbro, L., Jablon, J., & Stetson, C. (2011). *Powerful interactions: How to connect with children to extend learning.* Washington, DC: NAEYC Online Store.

Every Student Succeeds Act (ESSA) of 2015, PL 114-95, 129 Stat. 1802, 20 U.S.C. §§ 6301 *et seq.*

Fletcher, J.M., Coulter, W.A., Reschly, D.J., & Vaughn, S. (2004). Alternative approaches to the definition and identification of learning disabilities: Some questions and answers. *Annals of Dyslexia, 54*(2), 304–331.

Frank, R. (with Livingston, K.E.). (2002). *The secret life of the dyslexic child: How she thinks, how he feels, how they can succeed.* Emmaus, PA: Rodale Press.

Gillingham, A., & Stillman, B.W. (1956). *Remedial training for children with specific disability in reading, spelling and penmanship* (5th ed.). Cambridge, MA: Educators Publishing Service.

Gillingham, A., & Stillman, B.W. (1960). *Remedial training for children with specific disability in reading, spelling, and penmanship* (6th ed.). Cambridge, MA: Educators Publishing Service.

Gillingham, A., & Stillman, B.W. (1997). *The Gillingham manual: Remedial training for children with specific disability in reading, spelling, and penmanship* (8th ed.). Cambridge, MA: Educators Publishing Service.

Greene, V.E. (2017). *Project Read.* Bloomington, MN: Language Circle enterprises.

Henry, M.K., & Brickley, S.G. (1999). *Dyslexia: Samuel T. Orton and his legacy.* Baltimore, MD: The International Dyslexia Association.

Individuals with Disabilities Education Improvement Act (IDEA) of 2004, PL 108-446, 20 U.S.C.§§ 1400 *et seq.*

International Dyslexia Association, The. (2015). *Effective reading instruction for students with dyslexia. In just the facts.* Retrieved from https://dyslexiaida.org/effective-reading-instruction/

International Dyslexia Association, The. (2018, March). *Knowledge and practice standards for teachers of reading.* Retrieved from https://dyslexiaida.org/knowledge-and-practices/

Kaufman, C. (2010). *Executive function in the classroom: Practical strategies for improving performance and enhancing skills for all students.* Baltimore, MD: Paul H. Brookes Publishing Co.

Kilpatrick, D.A. (2015). *Essentials of assessing, preventing, and overcoming reading difficulties.* Hoboken, NJ: John Wiley & Sons.

Malchow, H. (2014, July). Structured literacy: A new term to unify us and sell what we do. *The Examiner.* Retrieved from https://dyslexiaida.org/ida-approach/

Martin, M. (2011). *Multisensory teaching of basic language skills* (3rd ed.). Baltimore, MD: Paul H. Brookes Publishing Co.

Mather, N., & Goldstein, S. (2008). *Learning disabilities and challenging behaviors: A guide to intervention and classroom management* (2nd ed.). Baltimore, MD: Paul H. Brookes Publishing Co.

Moats, L. (2012, Fall). Reconciling the Common Core Standards with reading research. *Perspectives on Language.*

Moats, L. (2017, Summer). Can prevailing approaches to reading instruction accomplish the goals of RTI? *Perspectives on Language and Literacy.* Baltimore, MD: The International Dyslexia Association.

Moats, L. (in press). Phonics and spelling: Learning the structure of language at the word level. In D. Kilpatrick, M. Joshi, & R. Wagner (Eds.), *Reading problems at school.* New York, NY: Springer.

Morgan, P.L., Farkas, G., Tufts, P.A., & Sperling, R.A. (2008). Are reading and behavior problems risk factors for each other? *Journal of Learning Disabilities, 41*(5), 417–436.

National Center for Learning Disabilities (NCLD). (2008). Executive function fact sheet. In *LD Online. The educator's guide to learning disabilities and ADHD.* Retrieved from http://www.ldonline.org/article/24880

National Center on Response to Intervention. (2010, April). *Essential components of RTI—A closer look at response to intervention.* Retrieved from http://www.rti4success.org/sites/default/files/rtiessentialcomponents_042710.pdf

National Institute of Child Health and Human Development (NICHD). (2000). *Report of the National Reading Panel: Reports of the subgroups. Teaching children to read: An evidence-based assessment of the scientific research literature on reading and its implications for reading instruction* (NIH Publication No. 00-4754). Washington, DC: Government Printing Office.

National Science Council on the Developing Child. (2010). *Persistent fear and anxiety can affect young children's learning and development: Working paper no. 9.* Retrieved from http://www.developingchild.net

Orton, S.T. (1937). *Reading, writing and speech problems in children.* New York, NY: W.W. Norton.

Rose, D.H., & Gravel, J.W. (2010). Universal design for learning. In P. Peterson, E. Baker, & B. McGraw (Eds.), *International encyclopedia of education* (pp. 119–124) Oxford, United Kingdom: Elsevier.

Rose, D.H., & Meyer, A. (2000). Universal design for learning. *Journal of Special Education Technology, 15*(1), 67–70.

Rosenshine, B. (2012, Spring). Principles of instruction: Research-based strategies that all teachers should know. *American Educator, 36*(1), 12–19, 39.

Sahlberg, P. (2017, April). *The Learning Professional, 38*(2), 3.

Schedler, J., & Bitler, E.F. (2004). *A classroom management secret: Keep the glasses full.* Workshop presented at the annual conference of the New York Branch of the International Dyslexia Association, New York.

Slingerland, B.H. (1994). *A multi-sensory approach to language arts for specific language disability children.* Cambridge, MA: Educators Publishing Service.

Smith, M. (1987). *Multisensory teaching approach.* Cambridge, MA: Educators Publishing Service.

Smith, M.T. (1989). *MTA classroom charts.* Cambridge, MA: Educators Publishing Service.

Sonday, A. (1997). *The Sonday System: Learning to read.* Bloomington, MN: Winsor Corporation.

Spalding, R.B. (2003). *The writing road to reading: The Spalding method for teaching speech, spelling, writing, and reading* (6th rev. ed.). New York, NY: HarperCollins.

Tucker, V. (2003). *Planning multisensory structured language lessons.* Manuscript in preparation.

Wilson, B.A. (1988). *Wilson Reading System: Teacher's guide and student material.* Oxford, MA: Wilson Language Training. Available from http://www.wilsonlanguage.com

Wilson, B.A. (2002). *Wilson Reading System instructor manual* (3rd ed.). Millbury, MA: Wilson Language Training.

Youman, M., & Mathers, N. (2013). Dyslexia laws in the USA. *Annals of Dyslexia, 63,* 133–153.

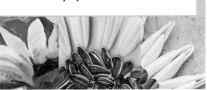

Appendix 18.1

Structured Literacy Lesson With Apps

Elaine A. Cheesman

For full descriptions, see the Online Companion Materials for each chapter.

Instructional component	Programs/apps for independent practice/homework
Alphabet knowledge	Alphabet Dots Game
	DotToDot
	Letter Case
	Letter Quiz
	SpellingCity (alphabetizing)
Reading and spelling decks	Alpha-read
	OG Card Deck
Multisensory introduction or review of letter or concept	SoundLiteracy (Teacher-led instruction)
Reading practice	abc PocketPhonics
	ABC Reading Magic 1–5
	Blending SE
	English Words: Everybody Learns
	Fry Words
	Fry Words Ninja
	Interactive Books
	Lexia Core5
	Phonics Genius
	PocketPhonics Stories
	Reading Ninja (Word Automaticity)
	Sentence Reading Magic
	Sight Words
	Sight Wordy (Photo Touch)
	Starfall ABCs and Learn to Read
Spelling	A+ Spelling Test
	ABC Spelling Magic 1–3
	Bob Books–Reading Magic
	Homophones Sight Words (Little Speller)
	Irregular Verbs
	SpellingCity
	Star Speller: Kids Learn Sight Words Games
	Starfall Learn to Read

(continued)

Instructional component	Programs/apps for independent practice/homework
Handwriting	Cursive Writing Wizard
	Cursive LetterSchool
	Handwriting Without Tears: Wet Dry Try
	Star Dot Handwriting
Comprehension and composition	Ginger Software
	Grammarly
	Inspiration/Kidspiration Maps
	Interactive Books
	Intro to Geography (World and United States)
	Lars and Friends
	Kindle Books; Project Gutenberg
	Mind the Gap (for older students and adults)
	No Red Ink
	Preposition Builder
	Rainbow Sentences
	The Right Word
	Vocabulary.com
Oral language and vocabulary	Comparative Adjectives
	The Right Word
	Roots to Words
	Word Analogy
	Word Flex

The following general resources are also helpful for teaching reading/language arts:

Learning disAbilities (1997) http://www.vineyardvideo.org

> A six-part DVD series that clearly demonstrates, in actual teaching situations, the strategies, content, and techniques of Structured Literacy covered in the chapters of *Multisensory Teaching of Basic Language Skills, Fourth Edition.* (Consulting Editor: Judith R. Birsh, Ed.D. Produced by Robert and Marjory Potts, Vineyard Video Productions.)

UCNLEARN (you see and learn) https://www.ucnlearn.com

> UCNLEARN provides products for dyslexia therapists as well as ESL/ELL and general-education classroom teachers to help make their students successful in learning to read and spell. With color and high-quality graphics, the materials bring spelling rules, reading concepts, and vocabulary root words to life.

Instructional Strategies for Specific Populations and Skill Areas

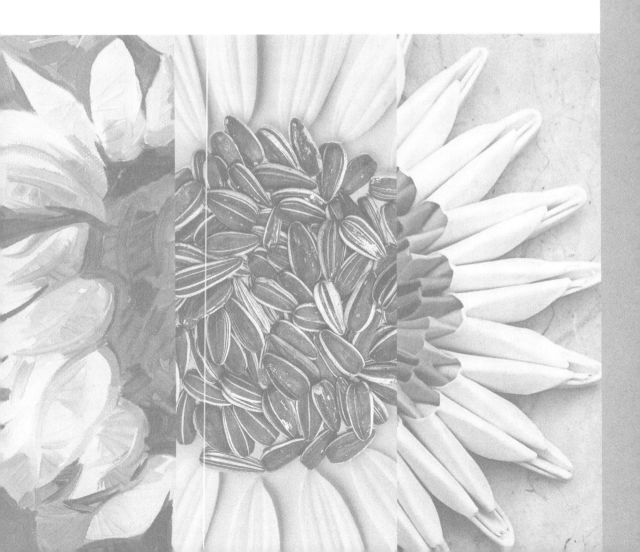

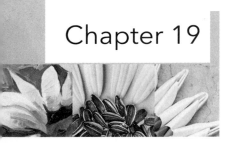

Chapter 19

Language and Literacy Development Among English Language Learners

Elsa Cárdenas-Hagan

LEARNING OBJECTIVES

1. To understand first and second language acquisition stages

2. To understand evidence-based strategies for teaching reading to English language learners

3. To understand how to build a framework for literacy instruction that addresses the commonalities between the native language and the second language

4. To understand how to build second language vocabulary knowledge

5. To understand the necessary components for implementing response to intervention/ multi-tiered systems of support among English language learners

The number of English language learners (ELLs) in the United States has increased. By the year 2030, 40% of the school-age population is predicted to speak a language other than English (Camarota, 2012). Due to the increasing number of ELLs in public schools, there has been much research to determine effective practices for this student population. However, much more is needed because these students come from diverse backgrounds, their language proficiency is varied, and the school settings and programs available to them are also varied. Finally, the teachers who serve them may or may not have the credentials for working with ELLs. It is necessary for instructors to understand how to best develop ELLs' academic language and literacy skills. It is also well known that the majority of ELLs in the United States speak Spanish in the home (Snyder, de Brey, & Dillow, 2018). Therefore, understanding the components of Spanish and how they relate to English can be beneficial for literacy instruction amongst this student population.

The first section of this chapter reviews the changing demographics in the United States and the need for understanding how to best instruct a diverse population. In addition, the response to intervention (RTI), multi-tiered systems of support (MTSS) model, and its implications for ELLs are discussed in the second section. The third section discusses the connections between language components and literacy in the context of learning a second language; for the purpose of extending most teachers' knowledge base, this section briefly reviews the structure of the Spanish language, its phonology, morphology, orthography, and syntax. The fourth section discusses multisensory techniques for literacy development in Spanish, the most commonly spoken language of ELLs. The fifth section describes the transfer of language and literacy skills from the native language to the second language using a well-designed, evidence-based instructional approach. The final section describes how to serve adolescent ELLs.

DEMOGRAPHICS

An estimated 10.9 million school-age children speak a language other than English at home, and 4.6 million of these students are identified as ELLs (McFarland et al., 2017). In addition, approximately 80% of these students speak Spanish in the home. It is also projected that 1 out of every 5 students will be an ELL by the year 2050 (Fry & Gonzalez, 2008). The dropout rate for Hispanic youth is 10%; Hispanic youth in the United States are more likely to drop out of school than other youth (McFarland et al., 2017). Literacy outcomes among this population have been unsatisfactory, as 79% read at a basic or below basic level (McFarland et al., 2017). This booming population primarily speaks Spanish and must achieve academic English language skills in order to obtain higher levels of English literacy skills. Therefore, educational achievement of Hispanic youth must a priority.

Schools today face the challenge of teaching English to students whose primary language is Spanish. Many of these students live in poverty. Approximately 30% of Hispanic children live below the poverty level, defined as a family of four with earnings of less than $24,036 (Jiang, Granja, & Koball, 2017). Children in poverty experience fewer opportunities for rich language interactions (Fernald, Marchman, & Weisleder, 2013; Hart & Risley, 2003). These children may enter school with limited world knowledge and limited exposure to reading and literature in their first language in addition to the English language. There is no doubt that it is necessary to concentrate on increasing the educational achievement of these language-minority students.

ELLs' academic achievements have historically been below those of their monolingual English-speaking peers. Results from the National Assessment of Educational Progress (NAEP), conducted in 2015, described 64% of all children reading at a basic or below basic level—in contrast to the 79% of Hispanics who scored at basic or below basic level in reading when compared with non-Hispanic Caucasians. How can an ELL acquire a second language and become literate in that language when his or her first language and literacy skills are not fully established? Educators must understand the oral language proficiency levels and the literacy skills of ELLs and thus prescribe effective instructional techniques to meet their individual needs.

Several federal laws describe how schools should serve ELLs in public institutions. For example, the Every Student Succeeds Act (ESSA) of 2015 (PL 114-95) and the No Child Left Behind (NCLB) Act of 2001 (PL 107-110) have held schools accountable for serving all students, including those who speak English as a second language. The Individuals with Disabilities Education Improvement Act (IDEA) of 2004 (PL 108-446) also recommends RTI or MTSS models for identifying and serving students with learning difficulties. These laws protect all students in public schools but especially those who are ELLs.

THE RESPONSE TO INTERVENTION/
MULTI-TIERED SYSTEMS OF SUPPORT MODEL

The RTI/MTSS model is a commitment to address individual students' needs. Implementing this framework increases the likelihood of identification and treatment of students who struggle with learning to read. The needs of ELLs are more closely considered, and the overrepresentation of language minority youth in special education programs is reduced because the RTI/MTSS model requires universal screening and high-quality instruction for all students in the general education classroom. This is considered the first tier of instruction. Two elements are implemented—an analysis of classroom instruction and necessary modifications—before certain students receive more intensive instruction (the second and third tiers of this model). Progress monitoring tools are also necessary and help educators to make data-driven decisions regarding differentiated instruction. Supplemental instruction is provided to struggling readers in a small-group setting with no more than five students in the group, which is the second tier of instruction. Thus, if students make adequate progress, then they receive classroom instruction only (Tier 1). If they need more assistance, then a minimum of 30 minutes of intervention per day is provided in a small-group setting (Tier 2). If necessary, instructors provide even more intense instruction (Tier 3) before referring the student to special education services (Vaughn & Fuchs, 2003).

This framework holds potential for linguistically diverse students as a mechanism for making data-informed instructional decisions, identifying and meeting the specific needs of ELLs, and reliably identifying ELLs who may be at risk for reading disabilities. The following features are necessary for implementation of an RTI/MTSS model for ELLs: 1) appropriate, research-based reading instruction and interventions specifically designed for ELLs; 2) culturally responsive teaching strategies and principles; 3) professional development and strategic coaching for teachers regarding English as a second language and second language literacy considerations; and 4) appropriate assessments, screening tools, and progress monitoring tools that consider an ELL population in their development and implementation (Project ELITE, Project ESTRELLA, Project REME, 2015).

Regarding the first feature listed (i.e., appropriate instruction and interventions) numerous studies related to effective interventions for ELLs and their implications for practice are described in the *Institute for Education Sciences Practice Guide* (Gersten et al., 2007). These features of instruction are described in this chapter in more detail. To incorporate the second feature (i.e., culturally responsive teaching strategies), teachers can attempt to engage ELLs with information relevant to their culture. It is also necessary to expand their knowledge and experience of other cultures. However, instructors must first understand the features of ELLs' primary language and their culture. This knowledge can be incorporated into instruction and can be a link for learning. This chapter discusses features of the Spanish language as a link to learning English language and literacy.

Other challenges to implementing RTI/MTSS include the fact that many assessments and progress monitoring tools are not designed for ELLs. Therefore, it is necessary to determine the exact population of students on which the tests have been validated. In addition, instructors must understand first- and second-language literacy development so they can consider the language proficiency levels for identification and intervention purposes. For example, if the ELL is at the initial stages of second language acquisition, his or her reading comprehension skills in

English will not likely be at an average performance level when compared to a monolingual English-speaking student's skills. Interventions will more than likely need to incorporate English language support and oral language opportunities within the literacy development lessons.

Numerous studies have described the positive outcomes of ELLs in intervention groups (Linan-Thompson, Vaughn, Prater, & Cirino, 2006; Richards-Tutor, Baker, Gersten, Baker, & Smith, 2016; Vaughn, Cirino, et al., 2006; Vaughn, Mathes, et al., 2006). These studies focus on developing the language and literacy skills necessary for successful reading. Each of these intervention studies includes explicit opportunities to develop oral language while also developing reading skills. Therefore, a thorough understanding of language and literacy development within and across languages is necessary to provide effective language and literacy instruction.

> ## REFLECT, CONNECT, and RESPOND
> How can educators ensure that the necessary components of an RTI/MTSS model are incorporated at the school and classroom level?

LANGUAGE COMPONENTS AND LEARNING A SECOND LANGUAGE

Humans have the capacity to learn to converse and read in multiple languages. However, many variables can affect one's ability to achieve high levels of language and literacy skills in two or more languages. These include having opportunities early in life to be exposed to language- and literacy-rich environments in more than one language (Lesaux & Siegel, 2003). Another important factor is participation in classrooms with highly trained instructors who can facilitate language and literacy growth in a systematic and cumulative manner in more than one language. Cross-language relations to build oral language proficiency can also have positive student outcomes (Prevoo, Malda, Mesman, & Ijzendoorn, 2016). Many countries require students to graduate with mastery of literacy in more than one language. It is an achievable goal when evidence-based language and literacy instruction is incorporated in a systematic, explicit, and cumulative manner.

It is also well known that cognitive skills transfer and there is a cognitive advantage to **biliteracy** (Shakkour, 2014). A foundation in the first language can benefit second language development. Moreover, exploring the common "ties" of languages is extremely beneficial for biliteracy, especially for the Spanish language, which has many similarities to the English language. Both languages are based on the alphabetic principle, share common sounds, and share common words and word parts derived from Latin. Thus, some linguistic elements can transfer from one language to the other. Focusing on the similarities of Spanish and English can promote biliteracy. ELLs' understanding of concepts in the second language can be facilitated by explicit instruction in the commonalities between the two languages.

Spanish is considered a Romance language. Like English, it is based on an alphabetic system. Both languages have distinct systems: phonology, semantics, morphology, syntax, and pragmatics. Orthography is the written system of a language (spelling) and relies on phonology and morphology. Phonology includes the study of the sounds of a language and incorporates the rules that determine how sounds can be combined. Morphology includes the study of word meanings and the structure of the language. This means understanding morphemes, the smallest units of meaning in a language. Morphemes include word parts such as roots, prefixes, and suffixes. Semantics encompasses word, phrase, and sentence meanings. Syntax, another language system, includes the rules for word usage and word order. One might describe pragmatics as the social rules of a language necessary for language usage (Bloom & Lahey, 1978). Pragmatics includes rules for conversation, such as turn-taking and initiating a topic appropriately. Bloom and Lahey defined language as the integration of content (semantics and morphology), form (syntax and phonology), and use (pragmatics). This model can be applied to all languages. A strong foundation in language is necessary for literacy development. In fact, at the written level of language is the system of orthography, which incorporates the rules for how sounds can be represented in print. Knowing sound–symbol relationships assists students with spelling development. In addition, some spelling and morphological patterns in Spanish transfer to English and can facilitate mastery of English orthography.

Language and Literacy Connections

Language is a natural system. Humans have the ability to understand and communicate. Reading is also a language-based process. However, reading is not a natural process: it is a skill that must be taught. Thus, the ability to read one's language system should be developed through instruction. Language skills are necessary to develop reading skills successfully. For example, phonology is necessary for phonological awareness, phonics, and orthography development. Morphology is necessary for understanding the structure of text, which contributes to comprehension. Semantics is necessary for understanding the meaning of the words that are read. In fact, young dual language learners demonstrate the ability to expand semantics across languages (Durán, Hartzheim, Lund, Simonsmeier, & Kohlmeier, 2016). In addition, exposure to content-related read alouds can have a positive impact on language development for ELLs (Pollard-Durodola et al., 2016). Pragmatics is necessary for composing and creating written language that is comprehensible and appropriate for one's audience. ELLs may not be familiar with the pragmatics of the language and may need support to learn colloquial expressions, social nuances, and nonverbal aspects of communication (Cárdenas-Hagan, 2016). Biliteracy, therefore, requires knowing phonology, morphology, syntax, and pragmatics in both Spanish and English. Working with students in small groups is helpful for engaging students in using their pragmatic language skills. These skills can be facilitated through role playing and through giving a topic and determining how students maintain the topic and take turns. Often, there are differences across cultures and in the social and academic use of language. Instructors must understand the pragmatic features of multiple languages and cultures.

Spanish and English can serve mutually as resources for second language acquisition. Understanding the structure of one language facilitates the acquisition of the second. Children who are provided with explicit instruction in all components of language and literacy are more likely to achieve biliteracy.

According to Bialystok (2002), when children learn literacy skills in their weaker language at the same time as they learn to read in their strong language, the transfer of skills from the dominant language facilitates literacy attainment in the weaker language. Individual differences in reading ability account for the variance in performance. Bialystok also reported that intact language proficiency skills increase the probability for literacy acquisition. Chiappe, Siegel, and Wade-Woolley (2002) determined that children with different backgrounds and cultures

acquired basic literacy skills in a similar manner. Alphabet knowledge and phonological processing, including phonological and phonemic awareness, were important contributors to children's early literacy performance. Phonological awareness
is the ability to process, segment, and manipulate the sounds and syllables of a
language; it includes skills such as rhyming, identifying sounds and syllables, and
adding or deleting sounds and syllables within words. Phonemic awareness is
the ability to process and manipulate phonemes, the smallest units of sound. In
Spanish, phonemic awareness tended to be more highly related to literacy than
rhyme identification and syllable identification (Francis & Carlson, 2003). Therefore, it is important for ELLs to have early language and literacy opportunities in
the native and second language. A strong foundation in the native language can
lead to strong second language and literacy development. In addition, preventing
reading disabilities is possible when individuals have the opportunity to learn
in an explicit, systematic manner (National Institute of Child Health and Human
Development [NICHD], 2000).

REFLECT, CONNECT, and RESPOND

How does knowledge of the structure of the native language inform English
literacy instruction? How does knowledge of second language acquisition
stages inform literacy instruction?

Spanish Phonology and Orthography

Phonology is the system of rules that determine how sounds exist and can be combined in a language. Processing and understanding sounds of a language can be
considered as foundational skills for reading English. Proficient Spanish readers
also transfer phonological awareness skills to their reading (Quiroga, Lemons-
Britton, Mostafapour, Abbott, & Berninger, 2000). Although Spanish is a syllabic
language, in that it has reliable syllable patterns, knowing sounds (phonemes) at
the beginning of reading instruction can assist with predicting future reading ability (Francis & Carlson, 2003). The Spanish language has 23 phonemes (Barrutia &
Schwegler, 1994): 5 vowel sounds and 18 consonant sounds. In addition, variations
in Castilian Spanish include /th/ and /zh/.

   The structure of the Spanish language consists of common syllable patterns.
Some of the most common syllable patterns also exist in English. The Spanish consonant–vowel (CV) pattern, as in *ma, pa, la,* and *sa,* is a basic syllable pattern and
can be combined to form a CV-CV pattern, as in the words *mala, pala, sala, masa,*
and *pasa.* Thousands of words can be formed from this common syllable pattern,
which is regular in Spanish. The CV-CV pattern is divided after the first vowel.
The vowel–consonant–vowel (VCV) syllable pattern is also common in the Spanish
language. It can be divided after the first vowel. Spanish words such as *uno, oso,*
and *ala* represent this syllable pattern. (The VCV syllable type does not constitute
the entire word in English as previously demonstrated in the Spanish words: *uno,
oso, ala.*) Another common syllable pattern is the VC/CV pattern, as in the Spanish
words *lista, isla, esta, hasta,* and *norte.* This syllable pattern is also common in the
English language. In Spanish and English, the VC/CV pattern is divided between
the two consonants. Reading teachers will utilize these common syllable patterns
to practice reading multisyllabic words. In Spanish, the CVC syllable pattern is
present, but fewer words in Spanish than in English utilize this pattern. Words in
Spanish with this pattern include *mes, dos, las, gis,* and *luz.* Words in English using

this pattern include *pat, met, his, cot,* and *cut*. (See Chapter 9 for more on English syllable patterns and decoding.)

There are syllable types in English that will need to be explicitly taught. Those include the open, closed, vowel-pair, vowel-*r*, vowel-consonant-*e*, and final stable syllables. Some of these letter combinations or syllable patterns exist in the Spanish language. For example, open and closed syllables are present but are not taught in this manner because the vowel sounds in Spanish do not change. Spanish-speaking ELLs will have difficulty with the vowel-consonant-*e* pattern because they will tend to produce the final *e*. In Spanish, the pattern of a vowel and the letter *r* exists but is not taught in this manner because vowel sounds are regular and do not change.

ELLs will need to understand when vowel sounds are pronounced as short or long sounds in the English language. They will need to learn vowel-*r* syllables and unfamiliar vowel pairs, such as *ea, ei,* and *ou*. Vowel pairs such as *oi, ai,* and *eu* exist across the two languages; however, the pronunciation is not the same. Letter patterns that look similar to those in English, such as final stable syllable patterns, exist in Spanish. For example, the words *palacial* and *edición* are similar to the English final stable syllables *-cial* and *-tion*. Patterns in English with final *-le* will need to be explicitly taught because Spanish speakers tend to produce the final silent letter *e*. Knowing English syllable types and the similarities and differences among the two languages will assist students with learning to read. Table 19.1 compares the syllable types across the English and Spanish languages.

Table 19.2 categorizes vowel sounds by three mouth positions. The vowel sounds produced in the back of the mouth are /o͞o/ and /ō/. When /o͞o/ and /ō/ are uttered as in *uno* and *hola*, they produce high and middle tones, respectively. The vowel /ä/ is produced in the central position of the mouth and has a low tone as in the Spanish word *amigo*. The long and short vowels /ē/ and /ĕ/ are produced toward the front of the mouth and have high and middle tones as in the Spanish words *iguana* and *elefante*.

Spanish consonant sounds can be characterized by the placement of the tongue and the **manner** of production. (See Table 19.3 for comparison; Table 19.4 shows the placement and manner of production for English consonants.) The sounds /b/ and /p/ are made with the two lips and are considered **bilabial** sounds (e.g., *bate, beso, piano, peso*). The manner in which they are produced is considered a stop because the air is abruptly stopped by the lips when the sound is produced.

Table 19.1.   English and Spanish syllable types

English syllable type	Spanish syllable type
Closed syllable *tĕn*	Closed syllable–Vowel sounds do not change *tĕn*
Open syllable *no*	Open syllable–Vowel sounds do not change *no*
Vowel-consonant-*e* *base*	Vowel-consonant-*e* (*e* is pronounced) in Spanish *base*
Vowel-*r* syllable *arc*	Vowel-*r* syllable *arco*
Vowel pair syllable *automobile*	Vowel pair syllable *automóvil*
Final stable syllable *emotion*	Final stable syllable *emoción*

From Multisensory Teaching of Basic Language Skills, Third Edition (p. 610).

Table 19.2. Spanish vowel sounds, by tone and mouth position

	Anterior position of mouth	Central position	Posterior position of mouth
Low	/ē/		/u/
Middle		/ĕ/	/o/
High		/ä/*	

*This is the obscure /äw/ as in the Spanish word *mañana*.
From *Multisensory Teaching of Basic Language Skills, Third Edition* (p. 610).

The consonant sound /f/, a labiodental sound, is produced with the upper teeth placed on the lower lip. It is a fricative sound because it is produced by the friction of the teeth on the lower lip. The Spanish word *fiesta* begins with this sound. Speakers of Castilian Spanish produce the fricative sound /th/, which is produced like the English /th/ sound as in *bath*. This sound may also be produced as a dialectal variant for the /s/ sound in Spanish. The ridge behind the front teeth is known as the **alveolar ridge.** Sounds such as /n/ and /s/, which are produced with the tongue touching this ridge, are categorized as **alveolar** sounds. The Spanish words *sol* and *noche* begin with alveolar sounds. **Palatal** sounds are produced by the tongue touching the palate in the medial position. The Spanish words *yoyo* and *llanta* begin with the palatal sound /y/. Speakers of Castilian Spanish produce this sound as /zh/.

Sounds such as /k/ and /g/ are produced close to the structure in the back of the mouth known as the **velum.** These two particular **velar** sounds are categorized as stops because the air is stopped abruptly by the tongue (e.g., *kilo, gusano*).

By comparing the placement of the tongue and the manner of production of Spanish consonant sounds in Table 19.3 with those of English consonant sounds in Table 19.4, the well-informed teacher can understand the commonalities and possible sources of difficulty in learning the sounds in a second language. For example, the /ng/ sound can be difficult to produce for ELLs; however, it does exist in Spanish, as represented by the letter *n* before the /k/ sound as in *nunca*. In English,

Table 19.3. Spanish consonant sounds

Manner	Placement					
	Bilabial	Labiodental	Alveolar	Palatal	Velar	Glottal
Stops	/b/, /p/[a]				/k/, /g/	
Nasal	/m/		/n/	/ñ/[b]		
Fricative		/f/, /v/[a]	/s/	/ks/	/h/[c], /w/	x[d]
Affricate				/ch/		
Liquids			/r/, /l/, /rr/	/y/		

[a]Some dialects of Spanish do not use the /v/ sound and use the bilabial /b/ sound in its place. English language learners would benefit from learning these two sounds because they correlate with English sounds and thus facilitate the transfer to English.

[b]The /ñ/ sound in Spanish can be an alveolar-palatal nasal sound.

[c]The /h/ sound exists in Spanish and is spelled with the letter *j* or the letter *g* before *e* or *i*.

[d]The /x/ sound is a glottal fricative as in the words *Xavier* and *Oaxaca*.

From *Multisensory Teaching of Basic Language Skills, Third Edition* (p. 611).

Table 19.4. English consonant sounds

Manner	Bilabial	Labiodental	Interdental	Alveolar	Palatal	Velar	Glottal
			Placement				
Stops	/b/, /p/			/t/, /d/		/k/, /g/	
Nasals	/m/			/n/			
Fricatives		/f/, /v/	/th/, voiced /th/, unvoiced	/s/, /z/	/sh/, /zh/	/h/	
Affricates					/ch/, /j/		
Liquids				/l/, /r/			
Glides	/hw/, /w/				/y/		

From *Multisensory Teaching of Basic Language Skills, Third Edition* (p. 611).

the letter *n* before the /k/ sound is produced as /ng/, as in the word *sink*. The Spanish sound represented by the letter *ñ* is not represented in English. Although the letter *r* transfers from Spanish to English, the sound is mostly trilled in Spanish and is not as trilled in English. It is also important to understand the medial *r* in Spanish when placed between two vowels is soft and not trilled; rather, it is pronounced as a **flap** sound. (A flap sound is produced when the tongue strikes against another articulator, such as the palate, and then returns to its rest position.) The flapping of medial Spanish *r* is similar to the flap sounds of medial *d* and *t* in English as in the words *battle* and *ladder. Cara* and *pera* are examples of Spanish words with a medial flap. Therefore, medial *r* between two vowels transfers to medial *t* and *d* in English.

English has a total of 44 phonemes represented by 26 alphabetic symbols. Many sounds in Spanish and English directly transfer from one language to the other. The place, manner, and production are directly related in English and Spanish. As noted previously, this facilitates the acquisition of phonology in the two languages. Table 19.5 illustrates the common consonant sounds between the two languages.

Table 19.5. Common sounds of Spanish and English

Manner	Bilabial	Labiodental	Interdental	Alveolar	Palatal	Velar	Glottal
			Placement				
Stops	/b/, /p/			[a]		/k/, /g/	
Nasals	/m/			/n/			
Fricatives		/f/, /v/	/th/[b]	/s/		/h/	
Affricates					/ch/, /zh/[b]		
Liquids				/l/ /r/[c]			
Glides	/w/				/y/		

[a]The /t/ and /d/ sounds in Spanish are dental as they are produced in a slightly more forward position of the mouth than the English /t/ and /d/ sounds.

[b]The unvoiced /th/ sound and the /zh/ sound exist in Castilian Spanish and in English.

[c]The symbol represents the flap sound, which occurs as a medial in the American English pronunciation of the words ladder and bottle and in Spanish words *cara* and *pera*.

From *Multisensory Teaching of Basic Language Skills, Third Edition* (p. 612).

Although Spanish and English have some sounds in common, the orthographic representations of some of these sounds may differ. For example, /h/ is spelled with the letter *h* in English but with the letters *j* or *g* (before *e* or *i*) in Spanish. The /w/ sound exists in Spanish. In English, this sound is spelled with the letter *w*. In Spanish, it can be heard in words such as *guante,* pronounced /gwahn-teh/, or *cuando,* pronounced as /cwahn-do/ in English. This sound is produced in Spanish when the letter *g* or *c* is followed by *u*.

Spanish consists of a transparent orthographic system in that the correlations between the sounds and the symbols are regular and reliable. The English orthographic system is more complex because the English language contains more rules and irregularities. It appears that the development of spelling is similar in English and Spanish, however; students begin by understanding the sounds of a language and the representation of these sounds by symbols. Next, they learn the patterns and morphological influences on spelling. Arteagoitia, Howard, Louguit, Malabonga, and Kenyon (2005) noted that Spanish spelling knowledge can transfer to English spelling abilities. Cárdenas-Hagan and Carlson (2009) suggested Spanish spelling can influence English spelling, and errors can result from overgeneralization of Spanish to English. One example would be using the Spanish letter *i* for the English long *e* sound. Errors may also be a result of Spanish sound approximations for English phonemes not present in Spanish. One example would be digraph *ch* for the English letter *j*. The difference between these two sounds is voicing, and these students can benefit from working with voiced and voiceless pairs of sounds, including /s/ and /z/, /f/ and /v/, and /sh/ and /zh/. Table 19.6 depicts the voiced and voiceless pairs of sounds and their relationship across Spanish and English.

Finally, as students transfer to the English language, they may overgeneralize English spelling for English words, as do monolingual English speakers. Knowing the Spanish orthographic system does not negatively influence English spelling; instead, it is a more natural progression for developing spelling among bilingual students (Arteagoitia et al., 2005). Therefore, it is important for teachers to understand that spelling patterns transfer from one language to another. For example, in Spanish as well as English, the letter *c* before *a, o, u,* or consonants is produced as /k/. The sound of the letter *c* before *e* or *i* changes to the /s/ sound as in the English words *mice* and *cinema* and the Spanish words *centavo* and *cinco*. The spelling of the letter *g* before *a, o, u,* and consonants is produced as /g/ in English and Spanish. When the letter *g* is immediately before *e* or *i,* however, the sound changes to /j/ in English (e.g., *gem, gin*) and /h/ in Spanish (e.g., *gente, gigante*). Instructors must understand the language and spelling development levels of their bilingual students in order to better design spelling instruction.

Table 19.6. Voiced and voiceless sounds

Language	Voiced	Voiceless
Spanish/English	/b/	/p/
Spanish/English	/d/	/t/
Spanish/English	/v/	/f/ produced as labiodental sounds
Spanish/English	/g/	/k/
English	/j/	/ch/
English	/zh/	/sh/
English	/th/	/th/

Spanish Morphology

Morphology, the study of morphemes, assists second language learners in decoding by improving the accuracy and rate of reading words (Ramirez, Chen, Geva, & Luo, 2011; Verhoeven & Perfetti, 2011). Understanding morphemes also provides a foundation for vocabulary development and spelling in both Spanish and English (see Chapter 9 on decoding and Chapter 14 on English morphology and etymology). For example, the Spanish word *xilófono* has the morpheme *fono*, which means *sound*. Another example is the word *incompleto*, which contains the morpheme *in-*, meaning *not*. The Spanish word *adorable* includes the morpheme *-able*, which means *able to do*. Teachers can take advantage of the fact that Spanish has morphemes whose meanings are similar in English. These morphemes can take the form of base words, roots, prefixes, and suffixes that carry meaning (see Chapters 9 and 14). Studying morphemes can assist children in developing reading as well as increase vocabulary skills. Instruction on word parts can increase morphological awareness among ELLs, which is further described as positively improving reading (Marinova-Todd, Siegel, & Mazabel, 2013).

Approximately 60% of English is derived from Latin (Lindzey, 2003). Spanish **cognates**, which are words that are similar in meaning and spelling with words in English and other languages, are extremely useful for ELLs. One study showed that Spanish cognates and word knowledge facilitated English vocabulary and reading comprehension (Durgunoglu, Nagy, & Hancin-Bhatt, 1993) and another described how morphological awareness contributes to reading comprehension in a second language (Kieffer & Lesaux, 2012). Studying word families as groups of words helps readers infer meaning, especially when encountering words in context (Anderson & Nagy, 1992). Studies show that learners can transfer morphological awareness skills from their first language to facilitate language and literacy development in a second or third language (Ramirez, 2017). Hancin-Bhatt and Nagy (1994) reported that Spanish-speaking elementary students are not likely to recognize cognates spontaneously. They will need explicit attention to the cognates in a systematic manner. Morphology is helpful for learning words and word meanings in a first and second language.

Spanish Syntax

The Spanish language has its unique grammatical rules. In Spanish, as well as English, children learn the concept of nouns, which name a person, animal, place, thing, or idea. Verbs are considered action words. Adjectives and adverbs have a primary job, to describe. Adjectives describe nouns and adverbs describe verbs. Although these parts of speech are the same across the two languages, placing them in a sentence in the grammatically correct order is what often causes the most difficulty when learning a language. In Spanish, for example, the adjective typically follows the noun. To describe pretty hair, one would say *pelo bonito*, with the noun placed before the adjective.

To learn the grammatical rules, an ELL may learn the rules in his or her native language and then apply or compare them with the rules of English syntax. For example, nouns in Spanish have either a masculine or feminine gender. Thus, if a teacher is male, then he is referred to as *maestro* in Spanish. Nouns denoting males or animals that are males end in the letter *o*. Nouns denoting females or animals that are generally feminine must end with the letter *a*. A female teacher therefore is referred to as *maestra*. Spanish speakers must not only learn nouns but must also learn how to apply the rules of gender. Therefore, ELLs should be able to understand the concept of nouns; they have learned how to use both nouns and the rules of gender for nouns, and they do not have to learn the latter for English.

The Spanish language has three regular classes of verbs, with infinitives ending in *-ar, -er,* and *-ir.* The regular tenses of verbs are formed by dropping the *-ar, -er,* and *-ir* and adding the endings shown in Table 19.7.

Spanish adjectives ending in *o* change the *o* to *a* in the feminine gender. Adjectives ending in a vowel other than *o* have the same form for masculine or feminine. Adverbs related to manner are often formed in Spanish by adding the suffix *–mente* to the feminine form of the adjective, as seen in Table 19.8.

Common Ties Between Spanish and English

Instructors can facilitate English language literacy development by providing instruction that builds on native language and literacy knowledge.

Alphabets   There are 30 letters and digraphs that are regarded as individual letters in the Spanish alphabet, and 26 letters in the English alphabet.

Spanish: a b c ch d e f g h i j k l ll m n ñ o p q r rr s t u v w x y z

English: a b c d e f g h i j k l m n o p q r s t u v w x y z

Although some in academia may recommend that the letters *ch, ll, ñ,* and *rr* be removed from the Spanish alphabet, students at risk for reading difficulties benefit from the one-to-one letter and sound correspondence that is regular and stable.

Spanish and English have five letters to represent the vowels. Spanish vowels have consistent sounds and consistent spellings. They can also be combined to form diphthongs—two adjacent vowels in a syllable that blend together to make a new sound. English vowels have less consistent sounds and spellings. They can be short or long, form digraphs and diphthongs, or have unaccented sounds. English vowel sounds can have more than one frequent spelling.

The sequential order of the English and Spanish alphabet is similar. In some cases, it is useful for teachers to remove the digraphs from the Spanish alphabet; however, doing so can cause a decrease in the one-to-one letter–sound correspondence within the Spanish alphabet during early reading instruction. Struggling readers require regularity of the language and literacy system.

Table 19.7.   Regular Spanish verb endings

Person	Verb ending		
	-ar	-er	-ir
yo	-o	-o	-o
tú	-as	-es	-es
el, ella, usted	-a	-e	-e
nosotros	-amos	-emos	-imos
vosotros	-amaís	-eis	-is
ellos, ellas, ustedes	-an	-en	-en

From *Multisensory Teaching of Basic Language Skills, Third Edition* (p. 613).

Table 19.8. Adjectives and adverbs

	Adjectives		Adverbs
	Masculine	Feminine	
	rápido	rápida	rápidamente
	lento	lenta	lentamente
	correcto	correcta	correctamente
	triste	triste	tristemente
	alegre	alegre	alegremente

From *Multisensory Teaching of Basic Language Skills, Third Edition* (p. 614).

As noted previously, many sounds and symbols transfer from the Spanish language to English. There are 23 phonemes in Spanish compared with English, which contains 44 sounds. Consonant phonemes that directly transfer from English to Spanish include: /b/, /ch/, /d/, /f/, /g/, /k/, /l/, /m/, /n/, /p/, /s/, /t/, /v/, /w/, and /y/ (see Figure 19.1). English and Spanish sound systems can be described by their articulatory manner of production. These concepts are useful for literacy in the two languages.

Diphthongs   Table 19.9 depicts the Spanish–English consonant and diphthong correlations, respectively. Notice that the Spanish vowels can combine to form diphthongs. Diphthong spellings such as *oy* and *au* directly transfer to the English language. If a Spanish vowel pair is accented, then the two vowels are produced separately and are not combined (e.g., *oído, tía*).

INSTRUCTION OF SPANISH LANGUAGE COMPONENTS

Reading in two languages is possible when students' strengths and knowledge base are considered. The National Reading Panel (NRP; NICHD, 2000) reported important findings regarding the development of English reading skills. The results acknowledged the importance of direct, systematic instruction in phonological

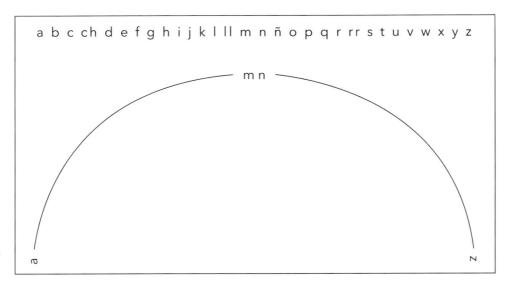

Figure 19.1. Alphabet sequence mat for the Spanish Alphabet. (From *Multisensory Teaching of Basic Language Skills, Third Edition* [p. 615].)

Table 19.9. Spanish-to-English diphthong correlations

Spanish	English
ai (*bailarina*)	i (*light, like*)
au (*autobús*)	ou (*out*)
ey (*rey*)	ey (*they*)
ei (*peine*)	a (*pay*)
oi, oy (*oigan, voy*)	oi, oy (*oil, joy*)
ia (*media*)	ya (*yarn*)
ua (*cuando*)	wa (*wand*)
ie (*hielo*)	ye (*yet*)
ue (*cuete*)	we (*went*)
io (*radio*)	yo (*yoke*)
uo (*cuota*)	uo (*quote*)
iu (*ciudad*)	yu (*yule*)
ui (*cuidar*)	we (*week*)

From *Multisensory Teaching of Basic Language Skills, Third Edition* (p. 615).

awareness, letter knowledge, phonics, vocabulary, reading fluency, and reading comprehension as skills important for successful reading development. Considering the challenge of biliteracy, learning to read in two languages can be facilitated by transferring these same skills from one language to the other. The following exercises, which are similar to those used in English reading instruction, were developed to facilitate teaching reading in Spanish. The first groups of activities presented address several levels of phonological awareness in a developmental progression of difficulty.

Phonological Awareness

Phonological awareness skills can transfer across languages when students have opportunities to build these skills in their native language and English. This can occur in program models such as transitional bilingual education (Branum-Martin, Ta, Garnaat, Burta, & Francis, 2006). The first activities under the category of phonological awareness involve rhyming in the native language and English. Making connections with words that are similar in sound patterns can be helpful. The following sections also describe alliteration and syllable-level activities and, finally, phoneme blending and segmenting activities.

Rhyme Identification   When children rhyme, they are manipulating an initial sound or cluster of sounds. This is sound manipulation and is a necessary step toward achieving a higher level of phonological awareness, such as phoneme manipulation. Students and the teacher can utilize mirrors and observe that only the initial sound is substituted when rhyming words, as illustrated in the activity below.

Teacher	*Students*	*Teacher*	*Students*	*Teacher*
(Digan = Say)		(¿Riman? = Do they rhyme?)		(Cambiamos ... por ... = We change ... for ...)
Digan *mía tía*.	mía tía	¿Riman?	Sí	Cambiamos /m/ por /t/.
Digan *sol gol*.	sol gol	¿Riman?	Sí	Cambiamos /s/ por /g/.

Digan *las mas.*	las mas	¿Riman?	Sí	Cambiamos /l/ por /m/.
Digan *sí no.*	sí no	¿Riman?	No	Cambiamos todos los sonidos. (We change all of the sounds.)
Digan *luna cuna.*	luna cuna	¿Riman?	Sí	Cambiamos /l/ por /k/.

Next is an English activity with sounds that transfer across Spanish and English.

Teacher	*Students*	*Teacher*	*Students*	*Teacher*
Say *mess, less.*	mess, less	Do they rhyme?	Yes	We changed /m/ to /l/.
Say *den, ten*	den, ten	Do they rhyme?	Yes	We changed /d/ to /t/
Say *boo, soy*	boo, soy	Do they rhyme?	No	We changed all the sounds.

Rhyme Generation   Rhyme generation is the ability to produce rhyming words. The teacher can scaffold this skill by using flashcards of Spanish letters. The ultimate goal is for students to perform this skill by listening. Therefore, the teacher dictates words that end in the same VC or VCV pattern and asks the students to change the initial sound. One example is the ending *-asa*. Children can change the initial sound and generate rhyming words: *asa, casa, masa, pasa, taza.* Other endings include *-eso, -ano, -ala, -elo,* and *-una.* The same activity can be implemented in English, and instructors may begin by using the common sounds across languages whenever possible.

Activities such as the following can be used to help students generate rhymes.

TEACHER: Digan *mis.* (Say *mis.*)

STUDENTS: Mis

TEACHER: Digan una palabra que rime con *mis.* (Say a word that rhymes with *mis.*)

STUDENTS: Gis

The teacher continues the activity with the following Spanish words: *sol, las, mes, gato, casa, luna, pino, nido, mal, pala,* and *usa.*

The same activity can be implemented in the English language using consonant and vowel sounds that transfer from Spanish to English.

TEACHER: Say *bee.*

STUDENTS: Bee

TEACHER: Say a word that rhymes with *bee.*

STUDENTS: Me.

The teacher can continue with words such as *ten, no,* and *too* because these sounds transfer from Spanish to English.

Alliteration Repetition and Identification   Alliterations are called *trabalenguas* in Spanish. It is important to initially have students repeat the alliteration and identify the common initial sound. Later, students can sing and generate Spanish alliterations. Here are a few examples to use with students:

1. Mí mamá me mima.

2. ¿Cómo Como? Como, como, como.

3. Tres tristes tigres tragan tres tragos.

4. Pepe Pecas pica papas con un pico pica papas Pepe Pecas.

The same activity can be implemented in English, but students will need to understand the vocabulary and grammatical features of the alliteration. It can be helpful to use some of the words that look and sound similar across languages such as Spanish and English.

1. Manuel makes mangos.

2. Lisa likes lemons.

3. Sam sees Susie.

Alliteration Generation   The teacher can scaffold the ability to produce alliterations by providing the first two words of the alliteration and asking the students to extend the alliteration with words that begin with the same initial sounds. As students progress, they can generate their own alliterations. This activity can be implemented in Spanish and English, as in the following example.

Teacher	Students
Manuel mira ____ _____.	mangos, melones, mapas
Consuelo come __ _____.	carne, coco, cacahuates
Tania toca _____ _____.	tomates, tamales, timbres
Daniel da _____ _____.	dinero, donas, dulces

Teacher	Students
Manuel makes __ _____.	mangos, melons, maps
Consuelo cooks __ _____.	cookies, cocoa, cranberries
Tania touches __ _____.	tomatoes, tamales, tacos
Daniel dumps __ _____.	dirt, doughnuts, dishes

Syllable Blending   Children are asked to listen, repeat, and blend syllables to form words. They can use counters or their fingers to blend syllables and form words. This activity can be implemented in Spanish and English, as in the following examples.

Teacher	Students	Teacher	Students
(Digan = Say)		(La palabra es = The word is)	
Digan /mä/ /sä/.	/mä/ /sä/	La palabra es	masa
Digan /lo͞o/ /nä/.	/lo͞o/ /nä/	La palabra es	luna
Digan /säl/ /gō/.	/säl/ /gō/	La palabra es	salgo
Digan /bä/ /tĕ/.	/bä/ /tĕ/	La palabra es	bate
Digan /mĕ/ /sä/.	/mĕ/ /sä/	La palabra es	mesa

Teacher	Students	Teacher	Students
Say /mä/ /mä/.	/mä/ /mä/	The word is	mama
Say /tu/ /nä/.	/tu/ /nä/	The word is	tuna

Say /t/ä /co/.	/t/ /ä /co/	The word is	taco
Say /sun/ /ny/.	/sun/ /ny/	The word is	sunny
Say /yo/ /yo/.	/yo/ /yo/	The word is	yoyo

Syllable Omission Students can clap their hands, use counters, or use their fingers to practice syllable omission activities. They can also use their bodies and move from left to right as they repeat the syllables and then omit the movement when they delete a syllable. Total physical body response is a technique that will assist ELLs. Deleting an initial or a final syllable is easier than deleting a medial syllable, so the teacher should first ask students to delete initial and final syllables before moving on to deleting medial syllables. See the following activities in Spanish and English.

Teacher	Students	Teacher	Students
(Digan = Say)		(Ahora digan … sin … = Now say …)	
Digan *mango*.	mango	Ahora digan *mango* sin *man*.	go
Digan *batería*.	batería	Ahora digan *batería* sin *a*.	baterí
Digan *yogur*.	yogur	Ahora digan *yogur* sin *gur*.	yo
Digan *rápido*.	rápido	Ahora digan *rápido* sin *rá*.	pido
Digan *piano*.	piano	Ahora digan *piano* sin *pi*.	ano

Teacher	Students	Teacher	Students
Say *mango*.	mango	Now say *mango* without *man*.	go
Say *battery*.	battery	Now say *battery* without *y*.	batter
Say *yogurt*.	yogurt	Now say *yogurt* without *gurt*.	yo
Say *rapidly*.	rapidly	Now say *rapidly* without *ly*.	rapid
Say *piano*.	piano	Now say *piano* without *pi*.	ano

Phoneme Blending Students can listen, repeat, and blend sounds to form words. They can use counters or their fingers to illustrate the concept of blending phonemes. This activity can be implemented in Spanish and English, as in these examples.

Teacher	Students	Teacher	Students
(Digan = Say)		(La palabra es = The word is)	
Digan /s/ /ä/ /l/.	/s/ / ä / /l/	La palabra es	sal
Digan /m/ /ĕ/ /s/.	/m/ /ĕ/ /s/	La palabra es	mes
Digan /g/ /ō/ /l/.	/g/ /ō/ /l/	La palabra es	gol
Digan /g/ /ä/ /s/.	/g/ /ä/ /s/	La palabra es	gas
Digan /b/ /ä/ /t/ /ĕ/.	/b/ /ä/ /t/ /ĕ/	La palabra es	bate

Teacher	Students	Teacher	Students
Say /s/ /ä/ /l/ /t/.	/s/ / ä/ /l/ /t/	The word is	salt
Say /m/ /ĕ/ /s/.	/m/ /ĕ/ /s/	The word is	mess
Say /g/ /ō/ /l/.	/g/ /ō/ /l/	The word is	goal

| Say /g/ /ă/ /s/. | /g/ / ă/ /s/ | The word is | gas |
| Say /b/ /ă/ /t/. | /b/ / ă / /t/ | The word is | bat |

Phoneme Substitution   Students can use their mirrors to view the position of the mouth as they substitute the initial sounds. Phoneme substitution activities can be implemented in Spanish and English, as in these examples.

Teacher	Students	Teacher	Students
(Digan = Say)		(Cambia … por … = Substitute/change … for …)	
Digan *mesa*.	mesa	Cambia /m/ por /p/.	pesa
Digan *luna*.	luna	Cambia /l/ por /t/.	tuna
Digan *sal*.	sal	Cambia /s/ por /m/.	mal
Digan *gato*.	gato	Cambia /g/ por /p/.	pato
Digan *cena*.	cena	Cambia /s/ por /p/.	pena

Teacher	Students	Teacher	Students
Say *port*.	port	Change /p/ to /f/.	fort
Say moon.	moon	Change /m/ to /n/.	noon
Say *salt*.	salt	Change /s/ to /m/.	malt
Say *got*.	got	Change /g/ to /p/.	pot
Say *cent*.	cent	Change /s/ to /d/.	dent

Alphabet Knowledge

Alphabet knowledge can be taught using manipulatives. Activities such as singing the alphabet, placing letters in order, and identifying missing letters can be performed in Spanish as well as English. The alphabet activities described in Chapter 5 can be incorporated into reading instruction in Spanish. One example is sequencing and manipulating plastic letters into an arc and teaching the sequential order of the alphabet (see Figure 19.1). The same procedures incorporated for acquiring alphabet knowledge in English can be utilized in Spanish. In addition, games that focus on a missing letter or a game of alphabet bingo can be used (see Chapter 5). As students begin to master phonological awareness and letter knowledge, they are prepared to learn letter–sound correspondences.

Letter-Sound Correspondences

Children learn new sounds by listening to words with common initial sounds, looking at the letter that represents the sound, and feeling their mouth and throat as they produce the sounds. They discover the letter, a key word, and a sound to facilitate the letter and sound correlation. Using flashcards depicting each letter, key word, and sound is helpful as students learn the letter–sound correspondences. Activities such as the following can be used to develop understanding of letter–sound correspondences.

TEACHER: Digan *pala, pesa, punto.* (Say *pala, pesa, punto.*)

STUDENTS: *Pala, pesa, punto*

TEACHER: ¿Cuál sonido oyeron? (What sound did you hear in the beginning of the words?)

STUDENTS: /p/

TEACHER: Miren su boca. ¿Está abierta o cerrada? (Look at your mouth. Is it open or closed?)

STUDENTS: Cerrado por los labios. (Closed by the lips.)

TEACHER: ¿Es vocal o consonante? (Is it a vowel or consonant?)

STUDENTS: Es consonante. (It is a consonant.)

TEACHER: La palabra clave es *piano*. (The key word is *piano*.)

STUDENTS: *Piano*.

TEACHER: Letra *p*, piano, /p/. (Letter *p*, piano, /p/.)

STUDENTS: Letra *p*, piano, /p/. (Letter *p*, piano, /p/.)

The same procedure can be implemented in English, and often similar key words and sounds can be incorporated across languages to facilitate mastery of letter and sound correspondences in two languages.

TEACHER: Say *pet, point, pup*.

STUDENTS: *Pet, point, pup*

TEACHER: What sound did you hear in the beginning of each word?

STUDENTS: /p/

TEACHER: Look at your mouth. Is it open or closed?

STUDENTS: Closed by the lips.

TEACHER: Is it a vowel or consonant?

STUDENTS: It is a consonant.

TEACHER: The key word is *piano*.

STUDENTS: *Piano*.

TEACHER: Letter *p*, piano, /p/.

STUDENTS: Letter *p*, piano, /p/.

It is important for Spanish speakers to learn letter–sound correspondences in order to learn to decode. In one program, Spanish speakers are exposed to sounds, symbols, and words that directly transfer to the English language (Cárdenas-Hagan, 1998). For example, when learning the short *e* vowel sound, students learn the key word *elefante* (elephant). This letter, sound, and word can directly transfer to English, thereby facilitating the knowledge of letter–sound correlations from one language to the next. Letters, sounds, and key words in Spanish and English are illustrated in Table 19.10. Figure 19.2 shows key word pictures and letters.

> **REFLECT, CONNECT, and RESPOND**
> How can knowledge of the sound structure of the native and second language affect spelling instruction?

Table 19.10.   Letters, sounds, and key words

Letter	Sound(s)	Spanish key word	English key word
b	/b/	bate	bat
c	/k/	cámara	camera
d	/d/	doctor	doctor
e	/e/	elefante	elephant
f	/f/	fuego	fire
g	/g/	ganso	goose
i	/i/	iguana	iguana
k	/k/	kilo	kilo
l	/l/	limón	lemon
m	/m/	mama	mother
n	/n/	nido	nest
p	/p/	piano	piano
r	/r/	rosa	rose
s	/s/	sol	sun
t	/t/	tomate	tomato
y	/y/	yoyo	yoyo
x	/ks/	saxofón	saxophone

From Cárdenas-Hagan, E. (2000). *Esperanza training manual* (p. 18). Brownsville, TX: Valley Speech, Language, and Learning Center; reprinted by permission.

Word Study

ELLs can benefit from learning Latin and Greek word parts. This is especially true for Spanish-speaking students because many English words are based on Latin roots. Students can learn the meanings of words parts, which can extend their word knowledge. Teachers can incorporate key words within the following activities to

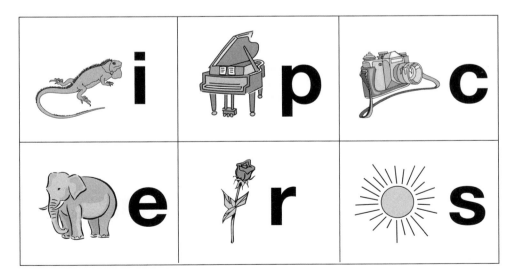

Figure 19.2.   Key word pictures and letters. (From Cárdenas-Hagan, E. [1998]. *Esperanza; A multisensory Spanish language program* [Reading deck cards]. Brownsville, TX: Valley Speech, Language, and Learning Center. Adapted by permission)

teach beginning word study through a process of auditory, visual, and tactile/kinesthetic discovery, as in the following examples.

Auditory Discovery   Use an activity like this one for auditory discovery.

TEACHER: Estudiantes saquen sus espejos y miren su boca mientras que repiten estas palabras que tienen la misma raíz: *teléfono, micrófono xilófono.* (Students, take out your mirrors and look at your mouth as you repeat these words that have the same root: *telephone, microphone, xylophone.*)

STUDENTS: *Teléfono, micrófono, xilófono*

Visual Discovery   Use an activity such as this one for visual discovery.

TEACHER: Miren el pizarrón mientras que yo escribo las palabras *teléfono, micrófono, xilófono.* Cada palabra tiene la misma raíz. La raíz es ____. (Look at the board as I write the words *telephone, microphone,* and *xylophone.* Every word has the same root. The root is _____.)

STUDENTS: Fono (phone)

Tactile-Kinesthetic Discovery   Use an activity such as this one for tactile–kinesthetic discovery.

TEACHER: Miren y toquen mi teléfono. Yo uso el teléfono para oír los sonidos de la voz de otra persona. Miren y toquen mi xilófono. Ustedes pueden escuchar el sonido de este instrumento. Miren el micrófono. Ustedes pueden escuchar los sonidos de mi voz muy recio. Entonces el significado es _____. (Look at and touch my telephone. I use the telephone to listen to the sounds of another person's voice. Look and touch my xylophone. You can listen to the sounds of this instrument. Look at the microphone. You can hear the sounds of my voice. It is loud. Therefore, the meaning of *phone* is _____.)

STUDENTS: Sonidos (sounds)

TEACHER: Miren la tarjeta de la raíz *fono.* La palabra clave es *micrófono.* Conocen otras palabras con la raíz *fono?* (Look at this card with the root *phone.* The key word is *microphone.* Do you know other words with this root?)

STUDENTS: Audífonos, fonología, megáfono (audiophones, phonology, megaphone)

TEACHER: Muy bien. Ahora pueden usar estas palabras con la raíz *fono.* (Very good. Now you can use these words with the root *phone.*)

Ahora pueden crea oraciones con las palabras *audífonos, fonología, y megáfono.* (Now you can create sentences with the words *audiophones, phonology,* and *megaphone.*)

Tables 19.11–19.14 are helpful to teachers working with ELLs. Tables 19.11–19.13 display the correlations between Spanish and English prefixes, suffixes, and roots, respectively, and their meanings in both languages. Reaching beyond phonics and basic orthographic patterns, these comparisons can lead to a wider understanding of the similarities and differences in the meaning units of Spanish and English.

Table 19.11. Spanish prefixes and their English correlations

Spanish		English	
prefix	Meaning	prefix	Meaning
ante-	antes	ante-	before
anti-	contra	anti-	against
con-	unión	con-	with
contra-	contra	contra	against
des-	negación	dis-	not
dis-	oposición	dis-	not
ex-	afuera de	ex-	outside of
extra-	más	extra-	above
in-	no	in-	not
inter-	entre	inter-	between
intro-	dentro	intro-	within
multi-	mucho	multi-	many
pre-	antes	pre-	before
pro-	por	pro-	for
re-	repetir	re-	again
sin-	con	syn-	with
sub-	debajo	sub-	under
super-	sobre	super-	above
trans-	al otro lado	trans-	across
tri-	tres	tri-	three
uni-	uno	uni-	one

From Cárdenas-Hagan, E. (2015). *Esperanza training manual* (p. 88). Brownsville, TX: Valley Speech, Language, and Learning Center; reprinted by permission.

This study of word parts can increase vocabulary knowledge among ELLs (Graves, August, & Mancilla-Martinez, 2013). Students can write the affixes and roots on index cards with their meanings and examples on the back to form a deck for review and practice during reading lessons. Teachers may use the graphic organizer shown in Table 19.14 as a tool for multisensory introduction of base words and affixes. It is also useful to highlight the morphemes and words that exist across the first and second language. Understanding the similarities and differences can deepen students' understanding of the words across languages.

In addition, some words are cognates between languages. Some are similar in orthography and meaning (true cognates). Other cognates have different orthography and meanings (false cognates). For example, the word *largo* in Spanish means *long*. The English word *large* looks similar, but the meaning is different. Teachers will need to be aware of true and false cognates. (See examples of each in Table 19.15.)

Syntax

The Spanish language has the same parts of speech with the same functions as English: nouns, verbs, articles, adjectives, adverbs, conjunctions, and prepositions. Knowing the rules of one language and their similarities and differences with the second language's rules is helpful for learning to read and write. Students can be taught these similarities between Spanish and English:

Table 19.12. Spanish suffixes and their English correlations

Spanish		English	
suffix	Meaning	suffix	Meaning
-able	capaz de	-able	able to
-ancia	forma de ser	-ance	state of being
-ano	nativo	-an	native of
-ante	alguien que	-ant	one who
-cial	en relación con	-cial	related to
-ción	estado de	-tion	state of being
-encia	estado de	-ence	state of being
-idad	calidad	-ity	quality of
-ido	en relación con	-id	related to
-ista	alguien que	-ist	one who
-itis	inflamación	-itis	inflammation
-ito	diminutivo	-ite	related to
-ivo	causa de	-ive	causing
-lento	en relación con	-lent	relating to
-osis	enfermedad	-osis	disease
-oso	lleno de	-ous	full of
-sión	estado de	-sion	state of being
-tad	forma de ser	-ty	state of being
-undo	en relación con	-und	related to
-ura	estado de	-ness	state of being

From Cárdenas-Hagan, E. (2015). *Esperanza training manual* (p. 89). Brownsville, TX: Valley Speech, Language, and Learning Center; reprinted by permission.

- Nouns name a person, place, thing, or idea.
- Verbs are used for depicting action.
- Articles come before a noun.
- Adverbs describe verbs.
- Adjectives describe nouns.
- Conjunctions connect thoughts.
- Prepositions are words that relate to other words.

As noted previously, although the parts of speech are the same, learning the rules for how to order words in a sentence correctly (syntax) often poses a challenge for ELLs. Activities such as the following can be used to help students develop understanding of Spanish syntax.

TEACHER: Miren, yo hablo español. Miren, ahora yo camino. Miren, ahora yo brinco. (Look, I speak Spanish. Look, I walk. Look, I jump.)

Digan *hablo, camino, brinco.* (Say *hablo, camino, brinco.*)

Estas palabras son verbos. Cada palabra termina en la letra *o.* El verbo es *hablar.* En el presente indicativo pongo la letra *o* al final de cada palabra. Ahora pueden usar el verbo *apagar.* (These words

Table 19.13. Spanish roots and their English correlations

Spanish		English	
root	Meaning	root	Meaning
audi	oír	audi	to hear
auto	solo	auto	by itself
cent	cien	cent	one hundred
ducto	guiar	duct	to lead
fam	fama	fam	famous
fin	final	fin	final
fono	sonido	phono	sound
graf	escribir	graph	written
gram	peso	gram	weight
kilo	mil	kilo	one thousand
liber	libre	liber	free
lingua	lengua	lingua	tongue
logía	estudio de	ology	study of
luna	lunar	luna	moon
metro	medida	meter	measure
novel	nuevo	novel	new
port	cargar	port	carry
semi	mitad	semi	half
tract	estirar	tract	to pull
trans	cruzar	trans	across
vis	ver	vis	to see
voc	voz	voc	voice

From Cárdenas-Hagan, E. (2015). *Esperanza training manual* (p. 90). Brownsville, TX: Valley Speech, Language, and Learning Center; reprinted by permission.

are verbs. Each word ends in the letter *o*. The verb is *hablar*. In the present indicative I place the letter *o* at the end of each word. Now you can use the verb *apagar*.)

STUDENTS: Yo apago.

TEACHER: Muy bien usaron la leta *o* al final del verbo *apagar*. (Very good. You used the letter *o* at the end of the verb.)

Sigue con los verbos: *hallar, lavar llamar, llevar, recomedar, sacar, tirar, trabajar, pintar, visitar*. (Continue with the following verbs: *hallar, lavar llamar, llevar, recomedar, sacar, tirar, trabajar, pintar, visitar*.)

Comprehension for English Language Learners

Reading comprehension is the ultimate goal of reading. That is, one reads to understand and extract meaning from text. For excellent reading comprehension to occur, ELLs must be able to decode words, sentences, and paragraphs with accuracy and fluency, in addition to excellent memory, vocabulary, background knowledge, and language comprehension (Quirk & Beem, 2012). All of these skills must be in place for excellent reading comprehension, and ELLs typically lag behind

Table 19.14.　Enseñanza de prefijos, sufijos o raíces (in Spanish and English)

Descubrimiento auditivo	*Nombra tres palabras con el prefijo, sufijo o raíz.* Los estudiantes repitan la palabra. Los estudiantes nombren el prefijo, sufijo o raíz que oyeron.
Visual	La maestra escribe tres palabras en el pizarrón. Los estudiantes pueden ver el prefijo, sufijo o raíz.
Significado kinestético	La maestra usa cada palabra en una oración.
	La maestra puede demostrar el significado de la palabra.
	La maestra usa las tarjetas de prefijos, sufijos o raíces.
	Los estudiantes escriben una oración para cada palabra.
	Los estudiantes usan y escriben las palabras en sus cuadernos de vocabulario.
Auditory discovery	*Name three words with a prefix, suffix, or root.* The students repeat the words. The students name the prefix, suffix, or root that they heard.
Visual discovery	The teacher writes three words on the board. The students can see the prefix, suffix, or root.
Kinesthetic discovery	The teacher uses each word in a sentence.
	The teacher can demonstrate the meaning of the word.
	The teacher uses prefix, suffix, or root cards.
	The students write a sentence for each word.
	The students use the words and write them in their vocabulary notebook for further reference.

From *Multisensory Teaching of Basic Language Skills, Third Edition* (p. 626).

their English-speaking peers in their reading comprehension levels (McFarland et al., 2017). This is not surprising because ELLs are expected to develop their oral language, reading and comprehension skills in a second language with ease and efficiency in a simultaneous manner. This is not required of monolingual English speakers, who have extended periods of time to develop listening and speaking skills before they achieve high levels of reading and writing. Therefore, ELLs will need many opportunities to develop their oral language, listening, and vocabulary skills. Young ELLs in preschool develop vocabulary skills that can enhance future listening comprehension and literacy skills (Mancilla-Martinez, Gámez, Vagh, & Lesaux, 2016). In addition, ELLs can benefit from interactive shared book reading (Giroir, Grimaldo, Vaughn, & Roberts, 2015). For ELLs whose native language is

Table 19.15.　True versus false cognates

True cognates		False cognates	
English	Spanish	English	Spanish
animal	animal	pie	pie
doctor	doctor	large	largo
kilo	kilo	embarrassed	embarazada
capital	capital	ten	ten
natural	natural	red	red
jaguar	jaguar	sin	sin
cereal	cereal	son	son
zebra	zebra	fin	fin

From *Multisensory Teaching of Basic Language Skills, Third Edition* (p. 622).

Spanish, many words that are cognates can help students increase their English vocabulary (August, McCardle, & Shanahan, 2014).

ELLs will also need to expand their background knowledge because this will help to improve their comprehension. To build ELLs' background knowledge, teachers should explore and use a central theme or topic. The theme can be discussed in order to introduce new vocabulary and concepts that are unfamiliar to ELLs. Teachers can also select books centered around the theme that are related to the content areas, such as math, science, social studies, and language arts. When bilingual books are available, using them can also enhance ELLs' comprehension. Teachers can target language development while increasing students' general knowledge. It is important to teach relevant vocabulary and fill in the gaps of ELLs' background knowledge. Teachers should use multiple examples of language targets so students can subsequently use the same targets. Teachers can explore and expand knowledge through questioning and prior knowledge. They can anticipate students' reactions and ask reaction questions: "Do you agree with this? Yes or no?" Teachers can also model effective questioning techniques.

In addition, teachers should remember to set a purpose for reading and use text structure to build a mental model. Teaching ELLs to be cognizant of text structure aids their reading comprehension (Geva & Ramirez, 2015). Teachers can make text more comprehensible by connecting words and phrases. Students can practice linking pronouns with their referents. Sentence combining and sentence construction can also help ELLs' comprehension.

The use of passive voice is challenging for ELLs. Teachers should, therefore, use text that incorporates active voice before text that uses passive voice. They should teach comprehension strategies and apply the strategies across multiple texts. Teachers should prepare questions whose answers can be found in the text. Students can engage with a partner for think and search questions, which require ELLs to make inferences and put two thoughts together. Teachers should also explore questions that are considered "between the author and me" and require the student to make inferences that go beyond the text. Comprehension monitoring helps ELLs to stay engaged with the text and make sure they understand what they are reading. ELLs can also engage in think-alouds. They can make predictions about what they are about to read. They can also visualize in their minds the context of what they have read, which assists with reading comprehension.

According to the NRP (NICHD, 2000), the use of multiple strategies for reading comprehension can be beneficial. The acronym **3PV 3RQ** incorporates the evidence-based strategies for reading comprehension with adaptations for ELLs: determining purpose, preparing a connection, predicting, working with vocabulary, reading, reviewing, and answering questions:

- *Purpose*—ELLs need to know the purpose of the text that is to be read. The teacher should explain the purpose in simple terms.

- *Prepare a connection*—ELLs need to have prior knowledge that is related to the content of the text. The teacher should begin with text that is culturally and linguistically relevant and then move to text that may not be as familiar.

- *Predict*—The teacher should provide ELLs with the opportunity to predict the content of the text from the title or any visuals that can be helpful for creating a prediction. This provides the teacher with a better understanding of the students' thought processes and their potential understanding.

- *Vocabulary*—The teacher should select vocabulary words that are necessary to understand the text and that can be used across the content areas. The teacher should remember to provide multiple exposures and opportunities to use the words. Also, the teacher should remember to make cross-language connections when possible.

- *Read*—Students can be provided the opportunity to read the text for accuracy. ELLs can benefit from reading the text once to build reading fluency and then reading it again for reading comprehension and paying particular attention to the text structure, which can enhance comprehension.

- *Review*—ELLs can benefit from a review of the content. The use of graphic organizers and visuals can enhance comprehension.

- *Question*—Students can answer questions before, during, and after reading. ELLs can focus on whether they understand what they are reading. Students should also generate questions because this can further enhance comprehension.

REFLECT, CONNECT, and RESPOND
What are some strategies for increasing vocabulary among ELLs, and why are these methods recommended?

Writing Among English Language Learners

Writing is a complex process. ELLs' writing is dependent on their oral language proficiency, their linguistic and cultural backgrounds, their world knowledge, and extensive instructional opportunities (Baker et al., 2014). Instructors must understand each of these variables to provide comprehensive written language instruction. Multiple opportunities for writing can occur when reading and writing instruction are integrated across the curriculum.

When teaching ELLs, one must take into consideration their oral language skills, which lay the foundation for written language skills. Therefore, instructors must consider ELLs' first and second language development. By understanding the levels of native language and second language oral proficiency, teachers can better understand how these levels may relate to writing proficiency. It is also important to incorporate the similarities that exist across languages. For instruction, teachers should capitalize on the similarities. The next step for instruction will include systematic and explicit writing instruction including new concepts that do not transfer across languages.

Students must be able to read and write. In classrooms, teachers may find it challenging to teach writing to ELLs. ELLs can develop academic written language skills. However, instructors must be prepared to provide ELLs with the foundational skills for writing. That is, ELLs may need to learn how to construct sentences and paragraphs through explicit instruction (Bowman-Perrot, Herrera, & Murry, 2010). These students may need a review of the grammatical structures of the second language and knowledge on how to expand sentences. In addition, learning text types can enhance writing instruction. Common text types might include narrative, expository, descriptive, and persuasive texts, to name a few. The use of graphic organizers to present these text types can be helpful to ELLs. The use of graphic organizers can be considered a scaffold for ELLs' instruction and thus can provide support for improving their written language skills.

Handwriting is a foundational skill for written language. The majority of ELLs in the United States speak Spanish as their native language (McFarland et al., 2017), and most of the letters of the Spanish alphabet exist in English. Therefore, if a student can write all of the letters of the alphabet in Spanish, he or she can write them in English. If students cannot write the letters with great legibility, then they can benefit from handwriting instruction. The same techniques for handwriting with monolingual English speakers can be incorporated and utilized with ELLs. The goal is for the student to write the letters with automaticity, accuracy, and legibility. Some ELLs may have been provided formal instruction in handwriting and others may not have had direct instruction in handwriting. Those ELLs who are foreign born may have received instruction in cursive handwriting prior to print handwriting. Therefore, instruction must be designed to meet the individual's needs.

Another foundational skill for written language is grammar. Students must be able to understand the grammatical features of the language, including the parts of speech, and the grammatical structures through which these parts of speech can be put together to form phrases and sentences. They must know the function of nouns, verbs, adjectives, adverbs, and prepositions, to name a few of the grammatical elements of the language. The good news is that other languages consist of these same grammatical features. Instruction can begin with defining the role of articles, nouns, and verbs in the English language and the use of grammatical structures to form simple and complex sentences. Some of the similarities and differences between the Spanish and English language capitalization, punctuation, and grammatical rules are shown in Table 19.16.

ELLs will need to build their syntax knowledge in the second language in order to be effective writers. Teachers can obtain a written language sample and determine the grammatical structures that are intact in the first and second language. For example, teachers can observe whether the students use complete sentences or

Table 19.16. Similarities and differences between the Spanish and English language capitalization, punctuation, and grammatical rules

English	Spanish
Nouns name a person, place, or thing.	Nouns name a person, place, or thing.
Nouns have gender when something is male or female (*woman, man, tiger, tigress*).	Nouns are either masculine or feminine (*perro/perra, gato/gata*).
When a word ends in *s, sh, ch, v, x,* or *z,* add *-es.*	When a word ends in a vowel add *-s.* When a word ends in a consonant add *-es.*
Proper nouns are capitalized.	Proper nouns are capitalized except common nouns, such as days of the week.
Verbs are words used to describe action. Verbs have tenses such as present and past.	Verbs are words used to describe action. Verbs have tenses such as present and past.
Adverbs are words that modify verbs.	Adverbs are words that modify verbs.
Adjectives are words that modify a noun. Adjectives appear before the noun.	Adjectives are words that modify a noun. Adjectives appear after the noun.
Exclamation point is used at the end of the sentence to alert the reader that something exciting has been stated.	Exclamation point is used at the beginning and at the end of the sentence to alert the reader that something exciting has been stated.
Question mark is used at the end of the question.	Question mark is used at the beginning and at the end of the question.

simple sentences and whether their sentences are complex or primarily simple sentences. In this way, the students' level of vocabulary, syntax, and orthography can be analyzed and instruction can be differentiated to meet their individual needs. Students can also be provided with rubrics to check for specific features that are necessary to improve their written language skills.

Once again, it is important to make sure ELLs use the correct capitalization and understand the similarities and differences between the native language and second language. For example, in Spanish, the days of the week or the months of the year are not capitalized as in English. ELLs will need direct instruction regarding capitalization skills in the second language. Punctuation marks also vary across languages. For example, the question mark and the exclamation point in Spanish are marked at the beginning of the sentence, unlike in the English language.

ELLs will also need to understand how stress and accent can change the meaning of a sentence in English, as in this example:

He is walking home.

He *is* walking home.

He is *walking* home.

He is walking *home.*

In addition, ELLs will need to learn how to expand or elaborate sentences for their writing. Teachers can ask questions to help ELLs generate more detailed sentences, as in these examples.

To expand a sentence.	The boy jumped.
How did the boy jump?	The boy jumped very high.
What kind of boy?	The tall boy jumped very high.
When did the boy jump?	The tall boy jumped very high today.
Where did the boy jump?	The tall boy jumped very high today in the basketball gym.
Why did the boy jump?	The tall boy jumped very high today in the basketball gym to score 2 points.

Teachers should use culturally and linguistically appropriate and relevant topics for ELLs to make connections and expand sentences, as in the following example.

What do you eat?	I eat tortillas.
What kind of tortillas?	I eat corn tortillas.
When do you eat tortillas?	I eat corn tortillas for lunch and dinner.
Where do you eat tortillas?	I eat corn tortillas for lunch and dinner at my house.
Why do you eat tortillas?	I eat corn tortillas for lunch and dinner at my house because they are tasty.

ELLs need to refer to charts with examples of grammar and punctuation. In addition, they need pictures that are relevant to them, such as anchor charts with pictures. Teachers should simplify existing rubrics so ELLs can understand the rubric. Teachers can add pictures or symbols if needed. Teachers should make sure to have culturally and linguistically appropriate text and topics so that ELLs can make connections.

Teachers should provide model texts for ELLs. They should try to make the model texts culturally relevant and linguistically appropriate for the ELLs' level of second language learning. They should teach the writing process, as described in Chapter 17, across genres, and use simplified anchor charts.

Writing should be integrated across the curriculum. Students write to communicate, but they also write to learn. Not only do ELLs need expert models of writing; they also need authentic opportunities to write that are meaningful and linguistically appropriate. ELLs can benefit from writing to learn. During reading math, science, or social studies lessons, writing can be incorporated with the goal of increasing students' writing opportunities and helping them learn content in more depth. Students can begin with prewriting activities. Instructors can then encourage ELLs to create reports, essays, or poems in relation to topics and the core content area. ELLs will thus have increased opportunities to write and to learn across the content areas.

REFLECT, CONNECT, and RESPOND
How can writing instruction among ELLs be differentiated?

ADOLESCENT ENGLISH LANGUAGE LEARNERS

Only 21% of **Hispanic** eighth-grade students achieve a proficient or above proficient level in reading (Snyder et al., 2018). In addition, the percentage of Hispanic students in the United States continues to increase. Many of these students speak Spanish in the home and need to further develop the English language. By the time an ELL is in secondary education, this student is required to have mastered academic language skills and advanced literacy skills in order to participate in and master challenging content area instruction.

The Adolescent English Language Learner Literacy Advisory Panel (Short & Fitzsimmons, 2007) suggested that, compared with their monolingual English peers, adolescent ELLs will need much more time developing vocabulary and background knowledge. ELLs will also need integration of reading, writing, speaking, and listening across the curriculum (Genesee, Lindholm-Leary, Saunders, & Christian, 2006).

A meta-analysis for developing academic content and literacy for elementary and middle school students revealed strong evidence for teaching academic vocabulary intensively and integrating oral and written English during content area teaching (Baker et al., 2014). Instructors must be certain that ELLs have attained the basic and advanced skills of language and literacy in order for these students to participate in challenging content area coursework. In studies pertaining to academic vocabulary and science content knowledge among middle school ELLs, it was beneficial for students to learn both the general vocabulary and academic vocabulary through multiple modalities and exposures (August et al., 2014). Using visual graphic organizers and demonstrations can help these students better understand the new concepts and the new vocabulary words (August & Shanahan, 2006). In addition, using the student's native language as a resource for words that are cognates is helpful in developing English vocabulary. Instructors should therefore capitalize on the cross-language potential when teaching academic content.

Adolescent ELLs also benefit from reciprocal teaching, whereby teachers and students share responsibility for a dialogue centered on understanding the meaning of text (Rivera, Moughamian, Lesaux, & Francis, 2008).

A lesson plan for ELLs should include determining the words to teach. Teaching words that are necessary to understand the content but that can also be useful across contexts is necessary. In addition, providing multiple exposures and opportunities for experiencing the words is also beneficial. A checklist for designing an evidence-based academic vocabulary, literacy, and content area lesson is described next.

Steps for designing lessons that address academic vocabulary, literacy, and content knowledge:

1. Select the topic and a reading passage to enhance content knowledge.

2. Analyze the text to determine the vocabulary that is necessary for understanding the content and make sure the ELL has the basic literacy skills for interacting with the text.

3. Teach content-specific vocabulary as well as general vocabulary.

4. Determine cross-language correlations, and provide multiple exposures to the word.

5. Remember, multiple exposures and opportunities to use the words can be attained from explaining meanings to peers in partner pairs or small groups.

6. Provide friendly definitions and examples and nonexamples of the word meanings.

7. Use visuals and graphic organizers to further enhance understanding.

8. Use technology and video clips that can extend understanding of the content and can further engage the student and his or her understanding of the information.

Examples of how to teach academic vocabulary follow.

Word	Definition	Example	Nonexample	Connection
content	happy	Good grades	Bad grades	contento
volume	quantity of a 3D object	Volume of a cube	Length of stick	volumen
migration	move from 1 place to another	Mexico to U.S.	Stay in U.S.	migración
custom	tradition	Thanksgiving	Studying	costumbre

Instructors will need to continue to address language development as well as content knowledge. ELLs are doing twice the cognitive work—developing language and content. This is only possible when instructors have an understanding of their language proficiency skills, literacy skills, and content-area knowledge.

CLOSING THOUGHTS: DEVELOPING LANGUAGE AND LITERACY IN ENGLISH LANGUAGE LEARNERS

Reading in two languages is possible when students' strengths and knowledge base are considered. The NRP (NICHD, 2000) reported important findings regarding the development of English reading skills. The results acknowledged the importance of phonemic awareness, phonics, vocabulary, reading fluency, and reading comprehension for successful reading development. Consider the challenge of biliteracy. Learning to read in two languages can be facilitated by incorporating similar skills from one language to the next in a systematic, direct, and comprehensive instructional program that focuses on the structure of each language using instruction to facilitate learning. Implementing an RTI model will enhance the understanding of the language and literacy needs of ELLs. Differentiated instruction benefits all students, including those who are learning English as a second language.

ONLINE COMPANION MATERIALS

The following Chapter 19 resources are available at http://www.brookespublishing.com/birshcarreker/materials:

- Reflect, Connect, and Respond Questions

- Appendix 19.1: Technology Resources

- Appendix 19.2: Knowledge and Skill Assessment Answer Key

- Appendix 19.3: Resources for English Language Learners

KNOWLEDGE AND SKILL ASSESSMENT

1. If an ELL reads the word *startled* as *estart* the teacher should correct by doing what?

   a. The teacher models the correct word and asks the student to repeat the word.

   b. The teacher reviews the difference between the sounds /l/ and /t/.

   c. The teacher reviews the base word as one with an *s*-blend and reviews the suffix of each word, and then has the student re-read to note the difference between the words.

   d. The teacher reviews by using the backing procedure to read.

2. An ELL whose native language is Spanish writes the word *latter* as *larer*. What is an effective way for the teacher to respond?

   a. The teacher explains that the medial sound is /t/ not /r/.

   b. The teacher explains that the letter *t* is used to represent the /t/ sound.

   c. The teacher explains that the letter *r* is pronounced as /r/.

   d. The teacher explains that the medial Spanish *r* is written with the letter *t* in the medial position of English words between two vowels.

3. An ELL reads the word *buzz* as *bus*. What is an effective way for the teacher to respond?

   a. The teacher instructs the student on the difference between the voiced and voiceless cognates.

   b. The teacher has the student practice reading words with the letter *z*.

    c.   The teacher re-reads the word to the student.

    d.   The teacher has the student read words with the letter *s*.

4.   An ELL does not understand the word *intercommunication*. What is the preferred method for teaching the meaning of the word?

    a.   The teacher demonstrates the meaning by speaking to another person.

    b.   The teacher has the student look up the definition of the word.

    c.   The teacher has the student analyze and discover the meaning of the morphemes, provide examples and nonexamples of their use, and make a connection with the native language.

    d.   The teacher has the student write a sentence using the word in context.

5.   An ELL does not understand the phrase *run of the mill*; therefore, the student requires assistance with which component of the English language?

    a.   The phonological component

    b.   The pragmatic component

    c.   The morphological component

    d.   The syntax

REFERENCES

Anderson, R.C., & Nagy, W.I. (1992). The vocabulary conundrum. *American Educator, 16*(4), 14–18, 44–47.

Arteagoitia, I., Howard, E.R., Louguit, M., Malabonga, V., & Kenyon, D. (2005). Spanish developmental contrastive spelling test: An instrument for investigating intra-linguistic and crosslinguistic influences on Spanish-spelling development. *Bilingual Research Journal, 29*(1), 541–560.

August, D., Branum-Martin, L., Cardenas-Hagan, E., Francis, D., Powell, S., Moore, S., & Haynes, E. (2014). Helping ELLs meet the Common Core State Standards for Literacy in science: The impact of an instructional intervention focused on academic language. *Journal of Research on Educational Effectiveness, 7*(1), 54–82.

August, D., McCardle, P., & Shanahan, T. (2014). Developing literacy in English language learners: Findings from a review of the experimental research. *School Psychology Review, 43*(4), 490–498.

August, D.L., & Shanahan, T. (2006). Introduction and methodology. In D.L. August & T. Shanahan (Eds.), *Developing literacy in a second language*: *Report of the National Literacy Panel*. Mahwah, NJ: Lawrence Erlbaum Associates.

Baker, S., Lesaux, N., Jayanthi, M., Dimino, J., Proctor, C.P., Morris, J., … Newman-Gonchar, R. (2014). *Teaching academic content and literacy to English language learners in elementary and middle school* (NCEE 2014-4012). Washington, DC: U.S. Department of Education, Institute of Education Sciences, National Center for Education Evaluation and Regional Assistance (NCEE). Retrieved from the NCEE web site: https://ies.ed.gov/ncee/wwc/PracticeGuide/19

Barrutia, R., & Schwegler, A. (1994). *Fonética y fonología españolas* (2nd ed.). New York, NY: Wiley.

Bialystok, E. (2002). Acquisition of literacy in bilingual children: A framework for research. *Language Learning, 52*(1), 159–199.

Bloom, L., & Lahey, M. (1978). *Language development and language disorders.* New York, NY: Wiley.

Bowman-Perrott, L.J., Herrera, S., & Murry, K. (2010). Reading difficulties and grade retention: What's the connection for English Language Learners? *Reading and Writing Quarterly, 26*(1), 91–107.

Branum-Martin, L., Ta, S., Garnaat, S., Burta, F., & Francis, D. (2012). Meta-analysis of bilingual phonological awareness: Language, age and psycholinguistic grain size. *Journal of Educational Psychology, 104*(4), 932–944.

Camarota, S. (2012). *Immigrants in the United States: A profile of America's foreign-born population.* Washington, DC: Center for Immigration Studies.

Cárdenas-Hagan, E. (1998). *Esperanza: A multisensory Spanish language program.* Brownsville, TX: Valley Speech, Language, and Learning Center.

Cárdenas-Hagan, E. (2015). *Esperanza training manual.* Brownsville, TX: Valley Speech, Language, and Learning Center.

Cárdenas-Hagan, E. (2016). Listening comprehension: Special considerations for English learners. *Perspectives on Language and Literacy, 42,* 31–35.

Cárdenas-Hagan, E., & Carlson, C.D. (2009). *Orthography and ELLs.* Paper presented at Tejas Lee Reading Conference, San Antonio, Texas.

Chiappe, P., Siegel, L., & Wade-Woolley, L. (2002). Linguistic diversity and the development of reading skills. *Scientific Studies of Reading, 6*(4), 369–400.

Durán, L.K., Hartzheim, D., Lund, E.M., Simonsmeier, V., & Kohlmeier, T.L. (2016). Bilingual and home language interventions with young dual language learners: A research synthesis. *Language Speech and Hearing Services in Schools, 47*(4), 347–371.

Durgunoglu, A.Y., Nagy, W.E., & Hancin-Bhatt, B.J. (1993). Cross-language transfer of phonological awareness. *Journal of Education Psychology, 85,* 453–465.

Every Student Succeeds Act (ESSA) of 2015, PL 114-95, 129 Stat. 1802, 20 U.S.C. §§ 6301 *et seq.*

Fernald, A., Marchman, V.A., & Weisleder, A. (2013). SES differences in language processing skill and vocabulary are evident at 18 months. *Developmental Science, 16*(2), 234–248.

Francis, D., & Carlson, C. (2003). *The Development of a Spanish Early Reading Assessment.* Tejas Lee Spanish Reading Symposium, Houston, Texas.

Fry, R., & Gonzales, F. (2008). *One-in-five and growing fast: A profile of Hispanic public school students.* Retrieved from http://pewhispanic.org/files/reports/89.pdf

Genesee, F., Lindholm-Leary, K., Saunders, W., & Christian, D. (2006). *Educating English language learners: A synthesis of research evidence.* New York, NY: Cambridge University Press.

Gersten, R., Baker, S.K., Shanahan, T., Linan-Thompson, S., Collins, P., & Scarcella, R. (2007). *Effective literacy and English language instruction for English learners in the elementary grades: A practice guide* (NCEE 2007-4011). Washington, DC: U.S. Department of Education, Institute of Education Sciences, National Center for Education Evaluation and Regional Assistance. Retrieved from https://ies.ed.gov/ncee/wwc/PracticeGuide/6

Geva, E., & Ramirez, G. (2015). *Focus on reading.* Oxford, United Kingdom: Oxford University Press.

Giroir, S., Grimaldo, L.R., Vaughn, S., & Roberts, G. (2015). Interactive read-alouds for English learners in the elementary grades. *The Reading Teacher, 68*(8), 639–648.

Graves, M.F., August, D., & Mancilla-Martinez, J. (2013). *Teaching vocabulary to English language learners.* New York, NY: Teachers College Press.

Hancin-Bhatt, B.J., & Nagy, W.E. (1994). Lexical transfer and second language morphological development. *Applied Psycholinguistics, 15*(3), 289–310.

Hart, B., & Risley, T.R. (2003). The early catastrophe: The 30 million word gap by age 3. *American Educator, 20*(1), 4–9.

Individuals with Disabilities Education Improvement Act (IDEA) of 2004, PL 108-446, 20 U.S.C. 1400 §§ *et seq.*

Jiang, Y., Granja, M.R., & Koball, H. (2017). *Basic facts about low-income children: Children under 18 years, 2015.* New York, NY: Columbia University Mailman School of Public Health, National Center for Children in Poverty.

Kieffer, M.J., & Lesaux, N.K. (2012). Direct and indirect roles of morphological awareness in the English reading comprehension of native English, Spanish, Filipino, and Vietnamese speakers. *Language Learning, 62,* 1170–1204.

Lesaux, N.K., & Siegel, L.S. (2003) The development of reading in children who speak English as a second language. *Developmental Psychology, 39*(6), 1005–1018.

Linan-Thompson, S., Vaughn, S., Prater, K., & Cirino, P. (2006). The response to intervention of English language learners at risk for reading problems. *Journal of Learning Disabilities, 39,* 390–398.

Lindzey, G. (2003). *Why study Latin?* [Brochure]. Retrieved from http://www.promotelatin.org/latin.htm

Mancilla-Martinez, J., Gámez, P.B., Vagh, S.B., & Lesaux, N.K. (2016). Parent reports of young Spanish–English bilingual children's productive vocabulary: A development and validation study. *Language Speech and Hearing Services in Schools, 47*(1), 1–15.

Marinova-Todd, S.H., Siegel, L., & Mazabel, S. (2013). The association between morphological awareness and literacy in English language learners from different language backgrounds. *Topics in Language Disorders, 33*(1), 93–107.

McFarland, J., Hussar, B., De Brey, C., Snyder, T., Wang, X., Wilkinson-Flicker, S., ... Hinz, S. (2017). *The condition of education 2017* (NCES 2017-144). Washington, DC: U.S. Department of Education, National Center for Education Statistics. Retrieved from http://nces.ed.gov/pubsearch/pubsinfo.asp?pubid=2017144

National Institute of Child Health and Human Development (NICHD). (2000). *Report of the National Reading Panel: Reports of the subgroups. Teaching children to read: An evidence-based assessment of the scientific research literature on reading and its implications for reading instruction* (NIH Publication No. 00- 4754). Washington, DC: National Government Printing Office. Retrieved from http://www1.nichd.nih.gov/publications/pubs/nrp/documents/report.pdf

No Child Left Behind (NCLB) Act of 2001, PL 107-110, 115 Stat. 1425, 20 U.S.C. §§ 6301 *et seq.*

Pollard-Durodola, S.D., Gonzalez, J.E., Saenz, L., Soares, D., Resendez, N., Kwok, O., ... Zhu, L. (2016). The effects of content-related shared book reading on the language development of preschool dual language learners. *Early Childhood Research Quarterly, 36,* 106–121.

Prevoo, M.J., Malda, M., Mesman, J., & Ijzendoorn, M.H. (2016). Within- and cross-language relations between oral language proficiency and school outcomes in bilingual children with an immigrant background: A meta-analytical study. *Review of Educational Research, 86*(1), 237–276.

Project ELITE, Project ESTRELLA, & Project REME. (2015). *Effective practices for English learners: Brief 1, Meeting the needs of English learners through a multitiered instructional framework.* Washington, DC: U.S. Office of Special Education Programs.

Quirk, M., & Beem, S. (2012). Examining the relations between reading fluency and reading comprehension for English language learners. *Psychology in the Schools, 49*(6), 539–553.

Quiroga, T., Lemons-Britton, Z., Mostafapour, E., Abbott, R.D., & Berninger, V.W. (2000). Phonological awareness and beginning reading in Spanish-speaking ESL first grade: Research into practice. *Journal of School Psychology, 40*(1), 85–111.

Ramirez, G. (2017). Morphological awareness and second language learners. *Perspectives on Language and Literacy, 43,* 35–40.

Ramirez, G., Chen, X., Geva, E., & Luo, Y. (2011). Morphological awareness and word reading in English language learners: Evidence from Spanish speaking and Chinese speaking children. *Applied Psycholinguistics, 32,* 601–618.

Richards-Tutor, C., Baker, D.L., Gersten, R., Baker, S.K., & Smith, J.M. (2016). The effectiveness of reading interventions for English learners: A research synthesis. *Exceptional Children, 82*(2), 144–169.

Rivera, M.O., Moughamian, A.C., Lesaux, N.K., & Francis, D.J. (2008). *Language and reading interventions for English language learners and English language learners with disabilities.* Portsmouth, NH: RMC Research Corporation, Center on Instruction.

Shakkour, W. (2014). Cognitive skill transfer in English reading acquisition: Alphabetic and logographic languages compared. *Open Journal of Modern Linguistics, 4,* 544–562.

Short, D., & Fitzsimmons, S. (2007). *Double the work: Challenges and solutions to acquiring language and academic literacy for adolescent English language learners.* A report to Carnegie Corporation. Washington, DC: Alliance for Excellent Education.

Snyder, T.D., de Brey, C., & Dillow, S.A. (2018). *Digest of Education Statistics 2016* (NCES 2017-094). Washington, DC: U.S. Department of Education, Institute of Education Sciences, National Center for Education Statistics.

Vaughn, S., Cirino, P.T., Linan-Thompson, S., Mathes, P.G., Carlson, C.D., Cardenas-Hagan, E., ... Francis, D.J. (2006, Autumn). Effectiveness of a Spanish intervention and an English intervention for English language learners at risk for reading problems. *American Educational Research Journal, 43*(3), 449–487.

Vaughn, S., & Fuchs, L.S. (2003). Redefining learning disabilities as inadequate response to treatment: The promise and potential problems. *Learning Disabilities Research and Practice, 18*(3), 137–146.

Vaughn, S., Mathes, P., Linan-Thompson, S., Cirino, P., Carlson, C., Pollard-Durodola, S., ... Francis, D. (2006). Effectiveness of and English intervention for first-grade English language learners at risk for reading problems. *The Elementary School Journal, 107*(2), 153–180.

Verhoeven, L., & Perfetti, C. (2011). Morphological processing in reading acquisition: A cross-linguistic perspective. *Applied Psycholinguistics, 32,* 457–456.

Technology Resources

Elaine A. Cheesman

Effective programs/apps have the following features:

- They have a text-to-speech option when appropriate.
- They have simultaneous text highlighting and narration.

Colorín Colorado   http://www.colorincolorado.org

This web site provides research-based suggestions for teaching English vocabulary, pre-K to adult levels. Instructions are in English.

ESL Party Land   http://www.eslpartyland.com

This web site provides practice in pronunciation, conversational skills, grammar, and vocabulary. It includes lesson ideas with video, music, and Internet resources.

ESL Video   http://www.eslvideo.com

This web site provides practice in listening, speaking, grammar, and vocabulary.

Free Translation   http://www.freetranslation.com

To use this program, the user uploads several types of files for the web-based program to translate the text. The program provides an oral pronunciation to accompany text.

Google Translate   https://translate.google.com

This tool translates written text. The user can hold a smartphone above the text for an instant translation.

Grammarly   http://www.grammarly.com

This web-based writing program identifies complex writing errors in text and provides suggestions for the writer, who corrects each error manually. It automatically supports documents, e-mail, and social media posts. The free version identifies errors in contextual spelling, grammar, punctuation, and syntax. The user can export the corrected document with the same file name. The free version has many useful features; the premium upgrade detects plagiarism and provides citation suggestions. The premium upgrade provides statistics on each type of error. School site licenses are available. The program is appropriate for older writers and English language learners.

Hemingway App   http://www.hemingwayapp.com

This text editing program/app is for teachers. Teachers can enter text online to simplify written language. Color-coded highlighting identifies sentences that are difficult to read, too long, or in passive voice.

ibooks or Kindle books with Project Gutenberg   http://www.gutenberg.org

Users can download PDF files or public domain books from Project Gutenberg. Users can tap and hold a word to hear oral pronunciation and see the definition in English; users can tap the "manage" tab to download a non-English diction-ary to access definitions in other languages and tap the "search" tab to access web definitions.

Learn English Free   http://www.bravolol.com

This program/app is designed to improve vocabulary and syntax. It requires reading skills and presents words individually and within conversational phrases with matching pictures. Users can access phrases off-line.

Learn English With Lingo Arcade   http://www.alligatorapps.com

This app has the user match spoken words and sentences with pictures and/or written words with sequential and cumulative instruction. The app tracks prog-ress while it automatically branches in response to errors. The user can self-select to review or advance to another level. It includes a variety of games for review.

Mango Languages   http://www.mangolanguages.com

These courses, which can be offered free through public library or school library systems, are offered in 17 different native languages. The mobile app comple-ments the web-based program. Phrases are color-coded in English and native languages. Each course has a built-in voice-comparison tool to perfect pronun-ciation. The variable pronunciation speeds help build awareness of English speech sounds, or phonemes.

Many Things   http://www.manythings.org

This program provides narrated stories with simultaneous text highlighting, pronunciation practice and quizzes. It combines phonological awareness train-ing with vocabulary growth by contrasting minimal pairs such as 13 and 30.

Mondly   http://www.mondly.com

This web site and mobile app requires reading skills in one's native language. It matches the user with choices of several native languages. It presents conver-sational topics for oral language development. For written language, it presents words individually and within phrases with matching pictures in native language and English. It provides spoken and written verb conjugations within phrases.

PBS Kids   http://pbskids.org

This site requires reading skills. For younger users, this web site has a variety of phonological awareness (e.g., rhyme identification) and word identification games. The blending game includes blending a written onset with rimes (e.g., s + ock to form *sock*). The narrated stories have simultaneous highlighting. Users can identify adjectives/nouns ("the red piggybank") and synonyms. It includes puzzles to match letters with sounds. One error is that the letter X matches the letter name as in *x-ray*, not the most common sound /ks/ as in *box*.

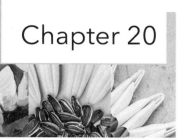

Chapter 20

Instruction for Older Students With a Word-Level Reading Disability

Barbara A. Wilson

LEARNING OBJECTIVES

1. To understand the prevalence and the challenges of word-level deficits for students beyond the elementary grades

2. To understand which key factors to consider when planning reading interventions for older students

3. To learn strategies for word-level instruction for older students, including decoding and spelling

4. To learn the importance of providing students with accommodations to access text while also teaching them to read so that they can access text independently

For students in fourth grade and beyond to be successful readers, they must be able to decode and read text fluently, understand advanced vocabulary, draw on substantial background knowledge, and comprehend diverse text structures (Biancarosa & Snow, 2006; Snow, 2002). Far too many students do not have these skills and are thus considered struggling adolescent readers. This group includes students in 4th through 12th grade who read 2 or more years below grade level (Torgesen, 2005). Many states have also defined this population as students reading at or below the 40th percentile.

The statistics on reading failure in the United States are astounding. The 2015 National Assessment of Educational Progress (NAEP) reported that 31% of 4th-grade students, 24% of 8th-grade students, and 28% of 12th-grade students scored below the basic level in overall reading skill. In addition, 33% of 4th-grade students, 42% of 8th-grade students, and 35% of 12th-grade students scored at the basic level (National Assessment Governing Board, 2015). Every day, millions of students in middle and high schools across the nation are clearly struggling to read.

When adolescents have low-level literacy skills and cannot adequately decode, it may become impossible for them to sustain participation in school. Students entering ninth grade in the lowest 25% of achievement are 20 times more likely to drop out than their higher performing peers (Carnevale, 2001). More than 500,000 students per year leave school without obtaining a high school diploma (McFarland, Stark, & Cui, 2016). Among students who lack a high school diploma, 27.5% live in poverty, which is approximately twice the percentage of high school graduates who do (U.S. Census Bureau, 2015). These facts have serious implications for individuals and society.

Although children in the primary grades who have reading difficulty usually have decoding deficits at the phoneme or word level, older students have more varied profiles. They may have **word-level deficits, comprehension deficits,** or both (Hock et al., 2009; Leach, Scarborough, & Rescorla, 2003). Although it is often assumed that adolescent readers have acquired adultlike decoding and word-recognition abilities and that their reading difficulties are due to comprehension challenges alone, research suggests that many of these students lack sufficient fluency in word recognition and can benefit from intervention targeted at word-reading strategies (Hock et al., 2009). This chapter focuses on instruction for those students beyond third grade who have word-level reading difficulty (with or without an accompanying comprehension deficit).

THE PREVALENCE OF WORD-LEVEL DEFICITS

Researchers have determined that about one third of middle school struggling readers have difficulty at the basic word level (Brasseur-Hock, Hock, Kieffer, Biancarosa, & Deshler, 2011; Scammacca, Roberts, Vaughn, & Stuebing, 2015). Other studies have shown that it is more than that (Cirino et al., 2013; Leach et al., 2003). In urban settings, where the percentages of adolescents with only basic literacy levels are especially pronounced (Hock et al., 2009; Snow & Biancarosa, 2003), most of the students have difficulty at the word level.

A study of 320 struggling high school freshmen in a large urban district found that 74% of all ninth-grade students scored at the "unsatisfactory" or "basic" levels on the state assessment test in reading. Those at the "unsatisfactory" level were at the third percentile in decoding and word recognition and the first percentile in reading comprehension. Those at the "basic" level were reading at the ninth percentile in decoding and word recognition and at the eighth percentile in reading comprehension (Hock, Deshler, Marquis, & Brasseur, 2005).

In another adolescent study in urban school settings, the domains of word level, fluency, vocabulary, and comprehension were assessed, and an analysis of the results found that 61% of the struggling adolescent readers had significant deficits in all of these reading components, including word-level skills (Hock et al., 2009). The researchers noted that the majority of all students read slowly with poor accuracy and that even students with adequate reading skills had a fluency deficit.

Students are expected to read to learn beginning in the upper elementary grades. Chall (1983) explained it well: First, students learn to read, and then students read to learn. The previously mentioned data indicates that a significant percentage of students beyond the elementary grades lack decoding and fluency skills to read grade-level text with ease and thus are unable to learn from reading. If students in 4th through 12th grade lack sufficient reading skills, then this expectation places extraordinary demands on them.

THE CHALLENGES OF HAVING A WORD-LEVEL READING DISABILITY

An adolescent struggling reader faces many academic challenges that must be addressed. Beyond Grade 3, students are expected to decode with ease, but when this is not possible, they struggle with all aspects of the school day. Although some educators may believe that it is inappropriate to provide word-level instruction to older students who cannot yet do this, Scammacca and colleagues explained, "For older students struggling at the word level, word-study intervention is an appropriate response" (2007, p. 13; see also Cirino et al., 2013).

Areas of Difficulty

Older students who do not yet have automatic single-word reading skills have difficulty at the beginning levels of reading. They are likely to have underlying phonological awareness deficits and persistent difficulty mapping the alphabetic symbols to sounds (Bruck, 1990, 1992; Spreen, 1989). As a result, they stumble over words, often even monosyllabic words, which are unfamiliar to them. The words *depth, gene, nerve,* and *source* are just a few such examples that they will encounter in their content-area courses that might cause difficulty without sufficient sound–symbol knowledge. Although it is obvious that fluent decoding alone will not result in proficient reading, it is necessary. With the ability to isolate sounds and link them to letters, students can read 70% of regular monosyllabic words (Ziegler, Stone, & Jacobs, 1997).

Without knowledge of the patterns that make up longer words, adolescent students with word-level deficits demonstrate limited orthographic awareness (Bruck, 1990). They might be able to recognize common multisyllabic words but lack understanding of syllable and affix word structure and therefore struggle with longer, unfamiliar words. They often have well-established guessing habits when reading text. They subsequently misread multisyllabic words, guessing at words using clues such as the first or last letters in the word, the length of the word, or other features.

Academic problems go well beyond decoding. If students cannot adequately map alphabetic symbols to sounds and lack orthographic awareness, then they will have a corresponding spelling deficit (Banks, Guyer, & Guyer, 1993; Bruck, 1993; Ehri, 2000). This, in turn, significantly limits their written output. Students find themselves unable to transfer their thoughts into written words, even when they know the answers.

Older students with basic decoding problems have limited experience with text despite several years of schooling. Peers who can read with ease have so much more exposure to the written word (Anderson, Wilson, & Fielding, 1988). Struggling adolescent readers tend to avoid reading so that the many benefits associated with this practice elude them. A meta-analysis looking at print exposure shows that with less exposure to print due to lack of reading, low-ability readers are unlikely to improve their reading and spelling skills to the same extent as their peers who read (Mol & Bus, 2011). The problem increases exponentially over the years. These students clearly face daily academic challenges. Without fluent decoding and limitations in reading rate, the adolescent students are unable to negotiate the demands of content areas of study. The struggling readers' lack of experience with print results in lower levels of vocabulary and significantly less background knowledge so that the deficits in word-level decoding, vocabulary, and content knowledge compound each other (Nagy & Anderson, 1984; Stanovich, 1986), resulting in significant academic challenges and, all too often, failure.

Interventions: It Is Not Too Late

Even if students are beyond the third grade, it is not too late. A meta-analysis of research by the Center on Instruction (Scammacca et al., 2007) determined that word-level interventions are appropriate for older students struggling at the word level. Learners at the initial stages of reading typically benefit from intervention targeted at word-reading strategies. This entails word-study instruction that includes phonemic awareness, phonics, word analysis, and sight word recognition as well as vocabulary, fluency, and comprehension. In fact, students beyond the elementary grades (including high school students) with significant word-level deficits should receive intensive instruction in these areas (Curtis & Longo, 1999; Deshler et al., 2001; Lovett, Barron, & Benson, 2003; Penney, 2002; Wilson & O'Connor, 1995). They may require between 50 and 90 minutes per day of reading instruction (Denton, Vaughn, Wexler, Bryan, & Reed, 2012; Shaywitz, 2003). Middle and high schools, however, typically do not address these basic skills, even in classes for struggling readers who cannot yet efficiently decode.

In order to sufficiently address the needs of this student population, literacy planning will require identifying these students and placing them into intervention classes that properly address their word-level needs (Cirino et al., 2013).

REFLECT, CONNECT, and RESPOND

Why is it important to provide instruction at the word level for some students beyond the elementary grades, even though many educators may be reluctant to do so?

ASSESSMENT TO DETERMINE NEEDS

Scammacca and colleagues noted the importance of assessing older students' reading skills and addressing their needs:

> Older students with reading difficulties benefit from interventions focused both at the word level and the text level. Identifying needs and intervening accordingly in the appropriate areas (e.g., vocabulary, word reading, comprehension strategies, and so on) is associated with improved outcomes for older students with reading difficulties. (2007, p. 12)

Students beyond third grade vary in their reading skills in more ways than younger students. For one thing, the range of overall reading levels in a given grade is much greater in the later grades. An 8th-grade class, for example, might include some students who are nonreaders as well as some who read at a high school level. This poses many challenges for instruction. It also requires schools to do more than simply identify their struggling readers through annual testing.

When designing intervention plans for older students with reading difficulties, the specific area(s) of deficit must be addressed. Simply knowing that a student is a "struggling reader" who is unsuccessful in school literacy tasks gives little information about the reader's specific areas of difficulty (Alvermann, 2001). In middle and high school settings, student performance data are central to literacy improvement efforts (Cirino et al., 2013; Irvin, Meltzer, & Dukes, 2007) because students with late-identified reading disabilities may have word-level deficits, comprehension deficits, or both (Hock et al., 2009; Leach et al., 2003).

The *Reading Next* report (Biancarosa & Snow, 2006) summarized the varying needs of adolescent struggling readers:

> Part of what makes it so difficult to meet the needs of struggling readers and writers in middle and high school is that these students experience a wide range of challenges that require an equally wide range of interventions. Some young people still have difficulty simply reading words accurately. Most older struggling readers can *read* words accurately, but they do not *comprehend* what they read for a variety of reasons. For some, the problem is that they do not yet read words with enough fluency

to facilitate comprehension. Others can read accurately and quickly enough for comprehension to take place, but they lack the strategies to help them comprehend what they read. In addition, problems faced by struggling readers are exacerbated when they are ESL [speakers of English as a second language] or have learning disabilities. (Biancarosa & Snow, 2006, p. 8)

Beyond third grade, an effective assessment plan is required in order to develop a responsive literacy plan. Although state- and districtwide English language arts and reading tests provide general reading scores and can identify struggling readers, additional assessments will allow the teacher to determine a student's mastery of sub-skills so that instruction can be properly planned and executed. Deficits in the following sub-skills indicate weaknesses at the word level that need to be addressed: phonological awareness, sound–symbol relationships, word attack (decoding), word identification, fluency, and spelling. Assessing these sub-skills will identify students who require an intervention that targets their specific needs.

A general screening will assist educators in determining students' needs. State literacy tests provide an overall reading score that can be combined with a quick universal screening of key word-level sub-skills. School districts completing this process in late spring or at the end of the school year will be prepared to schedule appropriate intervention classes for these struggling students for the following school year.

One such screening process uses three tests: the Test of Silent Reading Efficiency and Comprehension (TOSREC; Wagner, Torgesen, Rashotte, & Pearson, 2010), the Test of Silent Word Reading Fluency–Second Edition (TOSWRF-2; Mather, Hammill, Allen, & Roberts, 2014), and the spelling subtest of the Word Identification and Spelling Test (WIST; Wilson & Felton, 2004). These tests can be quickly administered in a group setting within one or two class periods. The TOSREC is a 3-minute screening assessment that helps to identify students who have difficulty with silent reading comprehension. Further screening with the TOSWRF-2 can determine if a word identification deficit is contributing to that poor reading comprehension. The TOSWRF-2 provides students with a single page of words that are presented with no spaces between them. The students are timed for 3 minutes as they put slashes between the words; see Figure 20.1 for an example. Students who

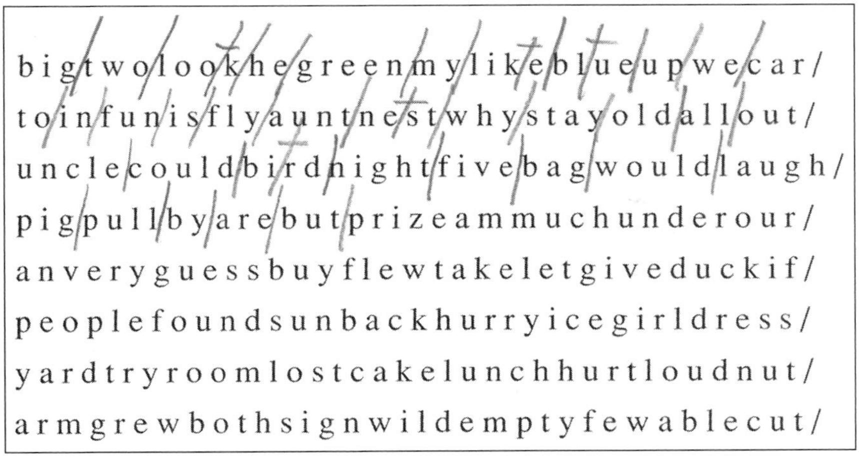

bigtwolookthegreenmylikeblueupwecar/
toinfunisflyauntnestwhystayoldallout/
unclecouldbirdnightfivebagwouldlaugh/
pigpullbyarebutprizeammuchunderour/
anveryguessbuyflewtakeletgiveduckif/
peoplefoundsunbackhurryicegirldress/
yardtryroomlostcakelunchhurtloudnut/
armgrewbothsignwildemptyfewablecut/

Figure 20.1. Sample page showing TOSWRF-2. (*Source:* From *Test of Silent Word Reading Fluency*–Second Edition, by N. Mather, D. Hammill, E.A. Allen, and R. Roberts, 2014, Austin, TX: PRO-ED, Inc. Copyright by PRO-ED, Inc. Reprinted with permission.)

can adequately decode are able to discern the division between words, whereas those who cannot decode randomly divide the letters on the page. The spelling subtest of the WIST, a nationally normed spelling assessment for older students, takes approximately 20–25 minutes in a group setting. Students with poor decoding also have poor spelling, and this subtest provides additional information on the knowledge of specific syllable patterns.

Results from this screening process help to identify students struggling with word-level deficits. To assist with instructional planning, additional WIST subtests can be administered to further determine which skills are weak or lacking. Furthermore, both a comprehension assessment and an oral reading fluency assessment that includes a prosody measure can provide valuable information for intervention planning.

Other similar screening tests can be utilized; however, it is essential to select tests that will separately examine the two different areas of reading difficulty: lack of basic decoding skills and difficulty with comprehension. Teachers need to be able to distinguish between older struggling readers who have trouble reading due to a lack of basic reading skills and those who are struggling with understanding but can sufficiently decode. (See Chapter 7 for more information about assessment; see Chapter 16 for more information about how to improve students' reading comprehension.) Following the screening, it is important to conduct a more comprehensive diagnostic evaluation for any student with a significant reading and writing deficit (see Chapter 7).

Based on assessment results, multi-tiered intervention classes (in addition to students' English language arts [ELA] classes) can be scheduled to address students' actual identified needs. This is far more effective than assigning them to a generic reading class that does not provide the differentiated instruction that they need. For adolescents who cannot yet decode efficiently, specific and skillful word-level instruction is critical (Hock et al., 2009). For students with comprehension deficits, educators must determine if they also have a word-level deficit. If that is the case, intervention will need to focus on more basic processes in addition to the comprehension (Cirino et al., 2013). Adolescents who decode fluently but have poor comprehension benefit from interventions that focus on vocabulary and comprehension instruction (Deshler et al., 2001; Moore, Bean, Birdyshaw, & Rycik, 1999; Scruggs, Mastropieri, Berkeley, & Graetz, 2010). Furthermore, students with a diagnosed reading disability, such as dyslexia, need more intensive instruction than other students (Lyon et al., 2001). See Figure 20.2 for an example of how literacy planning can address students' varied instructional needs beyond Grade 3.

INSTRUCTION FOR STUDENTS WITH WORD-LEVEL DEFICITS

Students may need word-level reading instruction at any age, a point emphasized by Boardman and colleagues:

> A student who has difficulty decoding words should receive instruction in word study whether he is in first grade, fourth grade, 12th grade or beyond. The instructional materials used may vary depending on age and grade level, but the learning objectives remain the same. (2008, p. 5)

Adolescent students with word-level deficits require instruction that targets these deficits (Cirino et al., 2013; Deshler & Hock, 2006; Hock et al., 2009; Toregesen et al., 2007). This instruction includes advanced word study that teaches the letter

Example of Literacy Planning Beyond Grade 3

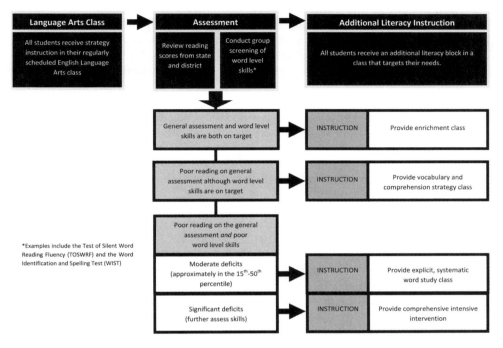

Figure 20.2. Example of literacy planning beyond Grade 3. (From Wilson, B.A. [2015]. Example of literacy planning beyond grade 3 [p.1]. Wilson Academy Resources, http://www.wilsonacademy.com; reprinted by permission. Copyright © 2015 Wilson Language Training. All rights reserved.)

patterns and structural features of predictable speech sounds. Here, students learn how to identify syllable patterns and break difficult words into manageable parts. Students also learn the recognition and meanings of prefixes, suffixes, inflectional endings, and roots. Vocabulary instruction must be interwoven into the word-study work (Boardman et al., 2008; Murray et al., 2010; Wilson & O'Connor, 1995).

Older students with decoding deficits need practice applying newfound decoding strategies. Word-level instruction provides a critical base but must include supported practice with connected text for the students to become skilled readers. Instruction must include fluency work but also must go beyond speed to include oral reading prosody with an emphasis on comprehension (Kuhn, Schwanenflugel, & Meisinger, 2010; Samuels & Farstrup, 2006; Wilson, 1996, 2018c).

For both word study and fluency instruction, students progress to more advanced work only when mastery is achieved. This principle requires the demonstration of learning by applying skills, a core element of competency-based instruction (Sturgis & Patrick, 2010).

Accuracy and Automaticity of Single-Word Reading

The difficulty of mapping alphabetic symbols to sounds can persist in older students, resulting in lingering problems with reading and spelling (Bruck, 1990, 1993; Spreen, 1989; Vaughn et al., 2008). Adolescents with decoding deficits have not fully internalized the sound system of the language, and they do not understand the structure of English words. As a result, they cannot accurately or fluently read text, and they are poor spellers. Although it may seem awkward to present basic skills to older students, this is not a good reason to let problems go unaddressed. If students who need basic skills are taught in a multisensory, systematic way, then they will make substantial progress (Campbell, Helf, & Cooke, 2008; Curtis & Longo, 1999; Penney, 2002; Wilson & O'Connor, 1995). This instruction needs to focus on developing students' understanding of the alphabetic principle; phonemic awareness (segmentation and manipulation); blending; the understanding of total word structure (syllable patterns, morphology, and rules of orthography); and automatic reading and spelling of high-frequency, irregular words.

Teach the Alphabetic Principle, Phonemic Awareness, and Blending The
ability to decode words requires phonemic awareness—the ability to hear, identify, segment, and manipulate phonemes—and mastery of the alphabetic principle, that is, the linking of sounds to letters (National Institute of Child Health and Human Development [NICHD], 2000). Phonemic awareness instruction is most effective when students are taught to manipulate phonemes by using the letters of the alphabet (NICHD, 2000). Thus, phonemic awareness training is closely linked with the direct teaching of the alphabetic principle (letter–sound/grapheme–phoneme correspondences). Accuracy with sounds is a crucial first step for students. The teacher begins instruction by teaching letter names and sounds for consonants, short vowels, and consonant digraphs.

An assessment such as the WIST can help the teacher determine a baseline of sound knowledge. Many older students know most of the consonant sounds. They often add a vowel sound to each consonant, however. For example, they may say /muh/ rather than /m/. It is more natural to say /muh/, and therefore the correct /m/ sound must be carefully taught and practiced. For this reason, be sure to teach students how to clip consonant sounds, explaining that it is important to clip sounds in order to blend them into words. It helps to explain that one should minimize the dropping of the chin when pronouncing consonant sounds. For example, say /tuh/, then /t/. When the sound is clipped, the chin does not drop.

Illustrate the importance of clipping sounds using sound or phoneme cards. For example, make the word *mat*. If the sounds are said /muh/ - /ă/ - /tuh/, then the word will not blend to make the word *mat*. The sounds /m/ - /ă/ - /t/, however, do blend to say *mat*.

Unlike younger children, older students only need key words for consonant sounds that are either unknown or are not well established. Use key words for any troublesome consonants, always linking the key word to the letter(s) and the sound—*qu, queen,* /kw/. Key words aid memory and provide a reference to help students gain access to the sound. The same key word should be consistently used to represent a sound. For example, many students say that the sound for *y* is /w/ because the name of the letter *y* starts with a /w/ sound. The key word *yellow* can help students remember that the sound for *y* is /y/, not /w/.

Typical consonants needing key words include *qu, w, x,* and *y*. Key words are also useful for the consonants *g* and *c* to emphasize the primary sound (*g, game,* /g/; *c, cat,* /k/). Students who have not mastered the sound system often say the secondary sound for these letters—/j/ for the letter *g*—when trying to decode unfamiliar words. Also, teach students the basic consonant digraphs: *sh, th, wh, ch,* and *ck*.

Using a sound card with two letters on one card, show students that digraphs are two letters that have only one sound (*sh, ship,* /sh/).

Use key words for all of the short vowels, regardless of baseline assessment results, because these sounds are critical and are easily confused. The key word helps students isolate and gain access to the sound. Also, students learn to extend the vowel sound that begins the key word. For example, the key word *apple* is used for short *a.* Say "aaaaaaaapple" and have students repeat it. Ask students to say the sound until they run out of breath or to extend the sound at the beginning of the key word until you hold up your hand. Have them repeat the letter, key word, and sound after you: "Say *a, apple,* /ă/."

Each student can develop a notebook divided into several sections to record information about the word structure of the English language. The first section of the notebook, labeled "sounds," is used for reference. Have students enter the short vowel sounds on one page, the consonants on another page, and basic digraphs on a third page. See the vowel student notebook sample in Figure 20.3. On the consonant page, the student draws key word pictures for only the consonant sounds that were unknown as indicated with pretesting. The rest of the notebook is devoted to recording syllable structure, affixes and roots, spelling rules, vocabulary, and high-frequency irregular words (Wilson, 1996, 2018c).

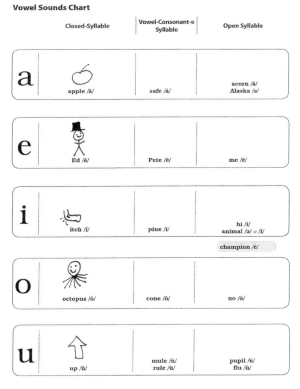

Figure 20.3. Page from a student notebook for noting key words and pictures for short vowel sounds. (From Wilson, B.A. [2018c]. In Wilson Reading System®. Oxford, MA: Wilson Language Training; reprinted by permission. Copyright © 1998, 2018 Wilson Language Training. All rights reserved.)

With most students, all consonants, short vowels, and basic digraphs can be introduced and entered into the notebook in the initial lesson. However, present other letter or sound patterns incrementally and cumulatively in a sequence that reflects frequency in the language and ease of learning. Carefully teach all sounds to mastery. At first, model the sounds and have students repeat after you until they can accurately pronounce each sound independently. As each sound is introduced, practice it in two directions: first for decoding (students look at the letter and name the sound) and second for spelling (students hear the sound and identify the letter). For spelling practice, dictate a sound, such as /m/, and have students (individually or as a group) repeat it. Then, have them name the letter (*m*) that makes that sound and write it.

Mastering sounds of the English language is critical; however, this skill is not sufficient for successful decoding or spelling. Students must also be able to blend and segment sounds. Phoneme segmentation, the ability to pull apart the sounds in a given word, is a critical skill for reading and spelling success. Poor readers often need direct teaching of this skill. Students can learn how to blend and segment three sounds, then four, five, and six sounds, using one-syllable short-vowel words. One multisensory method for phoneme blending and segmentation training utilizes a combination of phoneme cards, blank cards (for segmenting), and a finger-tapping procedure (Wilson, 1996, 2018c).

This method begins with teaching students how to segment and blend familiar three-sound words such as *map*. Put three phoneme cards (/m/, /a/, /p/) on a table surface or in a pocket chart, as shown in Figure 20.4. The card with the vowel should be represented by a different color.

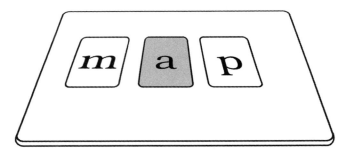

Figure 20.4. Example of phoneme cards used to segment and blend sounds within a word.

Teach students how to say each sound as they tap a finger to their thumb: As they say /m/, they tap their index finger to their thumb; as they say /ă/, they tap their middle finger to their thumb; and as they say /p/, they tap their ring finger to their thumb (see Figure 20.5). Then, have students say the sounds as they drag their thumb across their fingers, starting with their index finger for /m/. This multisensory approach has been successful in getting students to blend sounds.

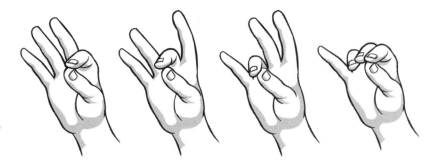

Figure 20.5. Illustration of how to tap phonemes using one's fingers. (From *Multisensory Teaching of Basic Language Skills, Third Edition* [p. 496].)

The tactile input to the fingertips appears to aid in the blending process. With a word such as *math*, the *th* digraph should be one card to represent one sound. The student also taps only three times because the digraph *th* stays together to make only one sound (and thus the word has four letters but only three phonemes). Although tapping fingers to the thumb seems to be ideal, some students prefer to tap on the table surface rather than the thumb. This still provides tactile feedback. To tap out the word *map* on the table, a student says /m/ while tapping the index finger on the table, /ă/ while tapping the middle finger, and /p/ while tapping the ring finger. The student then taps all fingers to the table while saying the word *map*.

To teach phoneme segmentation, use the same tapping method, but do not form a word. Instead, dictate a word, have the student repeat it, and then tap out each sound in a similar way as described previously for blending. After tapping it, the corresponding letters can be placed to reinforce the segmentation and the spelling–reading connection.

With older students, you should immediately show them that they can decode a word that they have never seen before. They will usually read three-sound words such as *map* without a problem, but there are many words that have three sounds that are unfamiliar. Tell the students that the tapping-out method works with these unfamiliar words as well. Examples of three-sound words that are often unknown by sight are *vat, shod, posh, thud, yen,* and *sod.* Form these words, one at a time, with cards. Be sure students say the sounds accurately with each tap, clipping the consonant sounds.

Model the blending as needed. When you make a three-sound word that the students do not know, help them decode it with tapping. Students often have an "aha" moment the first time they successfully decode an unfamiliar word—take advantage of this moment by explaining that you will be showing them ways to determine hundreds of words that they have never seen before without memorizing them. Students often feel encouraged when they are successful with some of these words that they do not know by sight. Be sure to take the time to talk about this with them and give them hope. They have tried to memorize so many words. Tell them, "See, you don't need to memorize. I'm going to show you how to figure words out."

Teach students how to identify closed syllables during this initial phase of word study. The English language uses six kinds of syllables; closed syllables are the most common. Students must learn to visually recognize when a syllable is closed, which tells them that the vowel in that syllable has a short sound. (See Chapter 9, Table 9.4 for six syllable types.) Demonstrate that these sounds can be blended into a "nonsense" syllable that is not a word by itself, such as *lish*. Explain that these syllables are part of longer words such as *publish,* and with the mastery of these short syllables, the student can then successfully learn to decode longer words.

Gradually build closed syllable, short-vowel words, and nonsense syllables with three sounds (e.g., *cap, cash, lish*), then four (e.g., *step, stash, stim*), then five (e.g., *stump, shrimp, bresk*) and six sounds (e.g., *script*). This teaching of sounds, phoneme segmentation, and blending sets the essential groundwork for successful and fluent decoding. Students should not progress to words with four sounds until they can read and spell any unfamiliar three-sound words without tapping. Tapping is a useful tool, but the goal is for students to read a word automatically without tapping. Students vary in the amount of practice needed for this automaticity.

Students must easily blend and segment the sounds in a single syllable before progressing to multisyllabic work. In addition to the methods already described, give students a lot of automaticity practice with short-vowel words and nonsense words on flashcards and on word lists. For students just learning how to decode, also provide application with these words within connected text (Partnership for Reading, 2003; Wilson, 1996, 2018c). This is just the beginning stage for decoding and encoding, but it is a crucial one.

Help students become metacognitive thinkers about word structure to develop accurate reading of words. They should be aware of what they know and understand how it helps them determine an unknown word. Use questioning techniques to facilitate this. For example, if a student reads the word *shop* instead of *chop,* ask, "What is the digraph in that word?" and "What sound does the digraph make?" to lead to the correction. When the student determines the correct word, say, "That is the word! What did you do to figure it out?" Use questioning to emphasize word structure and to correct errors, but do not overuse it. Reduce questioning as a student becomes more accurate so that you can then work on quick and automatic word recognition. When students become accurate, you can do timed drills to increase their automaticity.

Teach Syllable Structure   Students need to learn the sounds of the language, but they must also learn total word structure. Teaching the students more detail about word structure helps them accurately apply the sounds in longer words. Syllable patterns are an important part of that instruction because the type of syllable regulates the vowel sound. Also, spelling instruction that emphasizes syllable types assists older students with word-analysis skills (Bhattacharya & Ehri, 2004; Curtis & Longo, 1999; Wilson, 1996, 2018c).

It is important to give older students a feeling of accomplishment with longer words as soon as possible. Teach them how to combine closed syllables so that they succeed with multisyllabic words. The word *combat,* for example, combines two closed syllables. The word *Wisconsin* combines three closed syllables. When students master one type of syllable, teach them the next type, manipulating sound cards to teach the concept. When you introduce a new syllable type, use words combining the new and previously learned syllable types (Wilson, 1996, 2018c). For example, after students learn closed and vowel-consonant-*e* syllables, have them read and spell words such as *reptile, inflate,* and *compensate.* The word *compensate,* for example, has two closed syllables (with short vowels) and a vowel-consonant-*e* syllable. With older students, present long words containing only one or two types of syllables as soon as possible. By reading and spelling longer words, they gain confidence and a sense of success they would not achieve by only decoding short words. Students should practice reading and spelling these words in isolation as well as within sentences and passages.

Teaching basic syllable patterns should be done gradually and cumulatively. As students learn each syllable type, have them add the definition of each pattern, word examples, and corresponding rules of syllable division to their student notebooks.

Teach Morphology and Rules of Orthography   English is a morphophonemic system; thus, the spelling of English words relies on the smallest units of meaning (morphemes) in addition to the smallest units of sounds (phonemes). Between fourth grade and high school, knowing common word elements—affixes (prefixes and suffixes) and Latin and Greek base elements (*rupt, phono*)—is increasingly important to word-level reading success (Henry, 1993; Kruk & Bergman, 2013; Nagy, Diakidoy, & Anderson, 1993; Pacheco & Goodwin, 2013). These word elements make up the majority of words in text beyond Grade 4 (Egan & Pring, 2004; Nagy, Anderson, Schommer, Scott, & Stallman, 1989), and provide the key vocabulary in exemplar text (Hiebert, Goodwin, & Cervetti, 2018). As a result, they are included in the language standards of the Common Core State Standards and other college- and career-ready standards for Grades 4–8. For example, sixth-grade students are expected to "Use common, grade-appropriate Greek or Latin affixes and roots as clues to the meaning of a word (e.g., *audience, auditory, audible*)" (NGA Center for Best Practices & CCSSO, 2010, L.6.4b. Also see L.4.4b, L.5.4b, L.7.4b, L.8.4b).

Morphological awareness refers to students' ability to understand, analyze, and manipulate morphemes within words, contributing greatly to students' ability to decode, spell, and comprehend (Carlisle, 2010; Kruk & Bergman, 2013; Pacheco & Goodwin, 2013; Wolter & Dilworth, 2014). It aids in accurate and automatic word recognition as students learn to recognize a string of letters with meaning (Verhoeven & Perfetti, 2011). Research indicates that 4%–15% of students' performance on measures of word-level reading, reading comprehension, and spelling depends on the students' morphological awareness (McCutchen, Green, & Abbott, 2008; Singson, Mahony, & Mann, 2000; Wolter, Wood, & D'zatko, 2009).

Morphological awareness requires a simultaneous focus on sound, pattern, and meaning (Apel, Diehm, & Apel, 2013; Apel & Henbest, 2016; Bowers, Kirby, & Deacon, 2010). For students who do not have phonemic awareness or the alphabetic principle yet established, it is key to do that first before advancing to the more complex morphology instruction. Even with older students, mastery of the basic alphabetic principle and phonemic segmentation is critical. With these established, instruction can then interweave phonology, morphology, and orthography, which is the English spelling system that includes rules for adding affixes.

The direct teaching of morphology, then, is another effective means to help older students understand and apply word structure for decoding and spelling (Carlisle, 2010; Kruk & Bergman, 2013; National Institute for Literacy, 2007; Pacheco & Goodwin, 2013). All sounds need not be mastered prior to initiating morphology and orthography instruction. For example, even when students are only able to segment and blend three-sound words, the concept of suffixes can be introduced with nonchanging bases (*bug–bugs, box–boxes*). The first suffixes can include *-s, -es, -ed,* and *-ing.* Combined, these four suffixes comprise 65% of

Table 20.1.   Most frequently used prefixes in English

	% of all prefixed words	Total %		% of all prefixed words	Total %		% of all prefixed words	Total %
1. un-	26	26	8. over- (too much)	3	72	15. trans-	2	91
2. re-	14	40	9. mis-	3	75	16. super-	1	92
3. in-, im-, il-, ir- (not)	11	51	10. sub-	3	78	17. semi-	1	93
4. dis-	7	58	11. pre-	3	81	18. anti-	1	94
5. en-, em-	4	62	12. inter-	3	84	19. mid-	1	95
6. non-	4	66	13. fore-	3	87	20. under- (too little)	1	97
7. in-, im- (in/into)	4	69	14. de-	2	89	All others	3	100

Sources: Carroll, Davies, & Richman, 1971; White, Sowell, & Yanagihara, 1989.

words containing suffixes (White, Sowell, & Yanagihara, 1989). Explicit instruction in the most frequently used prefixes helps students decode, spell, and figure out the meaning of many longer words. There are 20 prefixes that represent 97% of prefixed words in English, and just 4 of these (*un-, re-, in-,* and *dis-*) account for 58% of prefixed words (White et al., 1989). Table 20.1 identifies these frequently used prefixes.

It is important to also introduce the Anglo-Saxon, Latin, and Greek structures to provide a more in-depth word study (see Chapters 1 and 15). The word *predict,* for example, has two morphemes: the prefix, *pre,* and the Latin root, *dict.* Build related words by adding prefixes and suffixes to root words such as *nation, national, international, multinational,* and *nationality,* directly teaching the vowel shifts that occur in words such as in the words *nation/nationality.* Graphic organizers, including word webs, word matrices, and word sums, provide wonderful visual representations of morphological word structure (Bowers, 2013; Bowers & Cooke, 2012; Bowers & Kirby, 2010).

As mentioned previously, instruction should incrementally interweave phonology, morphology, and orthography, thus systematically teaching students the rules that govern English written language. Students with a language learning disability actually can learn these rules, although they might have difficulty with the language of the rules. Words get in their way. For these students, instruction that includes demonstration and practice with manipulatives helps to clarify verbal explanations (Banks et al., 1993; Janney & Snell, 2004; Wilson, 1996, 2018c). When students add a rule that governs the written spelling of a word to their notebooks for reference, they also need to learn about this rule through the manipulation of word parts in order to facilitate the understanding of the rule by means other than memorizing the wording of it. Manipulating word parts helps them see and feel the structure. For example, the silent *e* spelling rule can be taught with sound cards and suffix cards. Present suffixes to students on individual cards. First, have the students categorize suffixes into two columns, putting those that begin with a vowel in one column and those that begin with a consonant in another column. An example is shown in Figure 20.6.

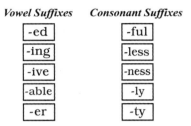

Figure 20.6. Example of suffixes categorized by whether they begin with a vowel or consonant. (From *Multisensory Teaching of Basic Language Skills, Third Edition* [p. 498].)

Next, make the word *hope* with the sound cards:

h   o   p   e

Tell the students that words ending in a silent *e* follow a rule when a vowel suffix is added. Put the *-ing* suffix card to the right of the word *hope*. Point to the column of vowel suffixes as you explain that whenever a vowel suffix is added to a word with a silent *e,* the *e* must drop from the end. Pull down the silent *e* card and move the *-ing* suffix card over to form *hoping.* Put the *e* back and make *hope* again. Point to the column of consonant suffixes as you tell the students that whenever a consonant suffix is added to a silent *e* word, the suffix is simply added and the *e* does not drop. Add the suffixes *-ful* and *-less* to demonstrate. Next, explain that this rule applies no matter when there is a silent *e.* Add suffixes to several words and again explain the addition of the vowel versus consonant suffixes. Help students to understand the dropping of the *e* because the *e* is literally dropped whenever a vowel suffix is added. Some word examples are shown in Table 20.2.

Demonstrate word structure for this and other rules of orthography using sound cards and suffix cards. This is usually necessary for students to process the information, understand it, and thus succeed in the learning and application. Teach and thoroughly practice each rule. Provide multiple opportunities to read words in isolation on flashcards and on word lists. Also, dictate the words for spelling. When students demonstrate mastery, introduce another rule, but continue to

Table 20.2. Examples of words in which silent *e* is dropped when a suffix is added

Word	Reason for silent *e*	Addition of suffixes
shape	Vowel-consonant-*e* syllable	shaped, shaping, shapeless
give	No English word ends in *v*	giving, giver, gives
settle	Consonant-*le* syllable	settling, settler, settlement
infringe	Letter *g* with a /j/ sound	infringing, infringement
nice	Two jobs: vowel-consonant-*e* and *c* with an /s/ sound	nicest, nicer, nicely

From *Multisensory Teaching of Basic Language Skills, Third Edition* (p. 498).

practice and review all rules previously taught. Students must overlearn the application of the rule as opposed to the wording of the rule. The wording is added to their notebooks for reference only.

REFLECT, CONNECT, and RESPOND
How does knowledge and an understanding of word structure improve a teacher's ability to provide instruction to older students?

Fluency

The previous sections describe the systematic and incremental teaching of total word structure. This is the key for older students who lack the word-level skills necessary to decode their grade-level text. However, students with emerging decoding skills also need sufficient reading practice to develop fluent reading of text. For older students with significant decoding challenges, fluency instruction is essential.

To promote fluency among their students, teachers should apply three strategies (Snow, Griffin, & Burns, 2005; see also Rasinski & Samuels, 2011):

1. Integrate fluency with phonemic awareness, phonics, word identification, vocabulary, and comprehension instruction.

2. Provide extensive practice with reading connected text (including repeated reading of the same material).

3. Provide extensive reading of many different things (wide reading).

See Chapter 12 for more information about building students' fluency.

Integrate Fluency Instruction   The development of fluency should start from the very beginning of reading instruction. Do not just teach phonemic awareness and phonics alone for a given period of time and then plan to begin fluency work later after decoding of single words is mastered. Rather, as soon as a new word structure is introduced, put it into context to be read accurately and with ease and comprehension (Snow et al., 2005; Wolf & Katzir-Cohen, 2001).

Some older students may be at the initial phase of reading development with very limited **word-attack skills.** At this stage, provide text that is limited to word structure that has been taught. This text should have only the letter–sound relationships, syllable patterns, and words that students have mastered for accurate decoding or recognition on sight (NICHD, 2000). **Controlled decodable text** offers this. Practice with controlled decodable text will allow students to achieve word-reading accuracy and integrate fluency instruction. The use of controlled decodable text also provides a demonstration of word structure so that students begin to "see" that there is a system to the language and that all words do not need to be memorized.

Less skilled readers improve reading rates when they read texts with a greater percentage of known high-frequency words and decodable words (Compton, Appleton, & Hosp, 2004; Hiebert & Fisher, 2007). However, few texts that are limited to taught word structure exist for older students. Seek out controlled text specifically written for older students, which should use vocabulary and themes more appropriate for their age (see Figure 20.7). If students have been introduced to the sounds of the short vowels, consonants, and basic consonant digraphs in three-sound words, then a controlled text such as "On the Job with Bill" could be used. The passage "Snack or Script?" is a sample of controlled text that can be presented when students have learned multisyllabic words combining closed syllables and vowel-consonant-*e* syllables.

On the Job with Bill	Snack or Script?
When Bill gets to his job, he has lots to do. He picks up boxes and bins, fills them, and then ships them. His boss tells him to get a pen and a pad. They have to ship ten boxes of pens to a shop at the mall. Bill tucks all the pens in the boxes and lugs them into the hall for the rig to pick up. (continued)	Dennis went to go meet Meg on campus at seven p.m. He had asked Meg to get some hummus, chips, and a cold drink at the snack shop. When Dennis got to Meg's hall, she was candid with him and told him that she had to finish her work on a script. Meg said that she had to submit the text in class on the last day of the month. That was the very next day! She still had a lot of work to do and a number of things left to publish the script... (continued)

Figure 20.7. Sample student reader passages. (From On the Job with Bill, and Snack or Script? From Wilson, B.A. [2018a]. On the Job with Bill. In Wilson Reading System® Student Reader One; and Wilson, B.A. [2018b]. Snack or script. In Wilson Reading System® Student Reader Three. Oxford, MA: Wilson Language Training; reprinted by permission. Copyright © 1998, 2018 Wilson Language Training. All rights reserved.)

Right from the beginning, appropriate controlled decodable texts present the opportunity to offer integrated instruction in all aspects of reading: accuracy, fluency, vocabulary, and comprehension. Although this type of text is limited by its nature, its purpose is to provide students with substantial practice within context, applying specific word-attack skills to develop accuracy and to break the habit of guessing. Controlled decodable passages are also used to establish fluent reading practices with the goal of reading for comprehension (Wilson, 1996, 2018c).

Provide Extensive Practice at Reading To build fluency, students need frequent practice with relatively easy, but not oversimplified, texts. The Partnership for Reading explained:

> Fluency develops as a result of many opportunities to practice reading with a high degree of success. Therefore, your students should practice orally re-reading text that is reasonably easy for them—that is, text containing mostly words that they know or can decode easily. If the text is more difficult, students will focus so much on word recognition that they will not have an opportunity to develop fluency. (2003, p. 27)

Students with emerging reading ability must read, read, read. Their fluent reading of text is affected by the proportion of words that they instantly recognize as well as by their decoding speed and accuracy (Torgesen & Hudson, 2006). As their word recognition and single-word decoding skills increase with instruction, the level of text difficulty should gradually increase as well. Students can then read **noncontrolled readable text** that is not restricted to words containing taught word structures.

Motivation to read is an important factor in getting students to practice. Students respond best when their work is challenging but at a level where they can be successful (Christensen, Horn, & Johnson, 2010). Students report that having the right materials motivates them to read (Ivey & Broaddus, 2001). If the material used with students is too difficult, then it is discouraging and frustrating. If the material is too juvenile, then it is demeaning.

Be sure that passages are read for meaning, helping the students to focus on comprehension as they successfully decode. Research indicates that fluency aids comprehension and comprehension aids fluency (Chard, Vaughn, & Tyler, 2002). Controlled decodable and noncontrolled readable text should be used to practice fluent reading with an emphasis on prosody and comprehension. Prosody is the rhythmic or tonal aspects of spoken language, and prosodic reading involves chunking groups of words into meaningful phrases according to syntax (Kuhn & Stahl, 2003). Again, comprehension is the aim of reading and must always be presented as the foremost purpose. If a student understands what he or she is reading, then he or she is likely to read it more fluently.

Providing a graphical representation of phrasing for meaning can be a way to offer fluency support. Scoop the passage into phrases to model fluent reading with prosody (Wilson, 2006). Draw scooped lines under the text to illustrate appropriate phrasing in accordance with the syntactic structure of the text. An example is shown in Figure 20.8. The text your students practice re-reading orally should be relatively short—approximately 50–200 words—ideally, with many words repeated.

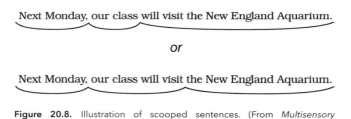

Figure 20.8. Illustration of scooped sentences. (From *Multisensory Teaching of Basic Language Skills, Third Edition* [p. 504]).

Teachers should not use repeated reading instruction without the accompaniment of specific word-level instruction if a student has word recognition and decoding deficits. Too often, this is a common practice with students beyond elementary grades. As a result, students improve their fluency on given passages but do not improve their automatic decoding of new passages. Therefore, it is important to keep in mind that fluency instruction without specific decoding instruction does not improve decoding (O'Connor, Swanson, & Geraghty, 2010; O'Connor, White, & Swanson, 2007).

Facilitate Wide Reading   Reading a wide variety of texts also helps students build fluency. Snow, Burns, and Griffin explained, "Adequate progress in learning to read beyond the initial level depends on . . . sufficient practice in reading to achieve fluency with different kinds of texts written for different purposes" (1998, p. 223).

Students need to practice reading in order to become fluent (NICHD, 2000). Unfortunately, from the early grades, poor readers are exposed to much less text than students who read well, and the gap increases dramatically as students progress into higher grades. A landmark study of fifth-grade students conducted by

Anderson, Wilson, and Fielding (1988) showed an enormous gap in independent reading practices. Students at the 98th percentile of reading read approximately 4,358,000 words per year; students at the 10th percentile read 8,000 words per year; and students at the 2nd percentile read 0 words per year. The amount or volume that a student reads makes a difference because reading builds comprehension and fluency.

Although repeated reading is useful instruction, nonrepetitive reading with a wide variety of noncontrolled readable text is also essential (Homan, Klesius, & Hite, 1993; Rashotte & Torgesen, 1985). This wide reading has the added benefit of exposing students to more vocabulary and additional background knowledge. As students demonstrate sufficient success with more challenging text, gradually increase the level of text difficulty in relation to length of passages, size of font, complexity of content, and overall level of difficulty.

Increasing students' independent ability to fluently read a passage and comprehend it at the same time is the primary aim of instruction with noncontrolled readable text. In order to provide students with more challenging text, sufficient supports must be in place. Without scaffolds and instructional supports to assist students, outcomes may decline. However, with supports in place, students may be able to perform as well as they did with less difficult texts (Morgan, Wilcox, & Eldredge, 2000; O'Connor et al., 2010).

When you initially select noncontrolled readable text for students to work with, use their areas of interest and background knowledge to guide your selection because the more students know about a topic, the more likely they will be able to successfully determine the words. Students can read several things on that same topic with the teacher providing scaffolding.

Also use several nonfiction, informational passages, again staying on the same topic. By reading aloud to students a text on an unfamiliar subject that is written on their grade level, you can build their vocabularies, schema, and comprehension about that topic. You can then introduce additional passages on the same topic, gradually increasing the difficulty of the text. Because you have provided the schema, or background information, you will have the opportunity to teach students how to use context clues in combination with their emerging decoding strategies to determine unfamiliar words. (See Figures 20.9 and 20.10 for sample passages that address the same topic at different levels of text difficulty.) As the students progress in word identification skill, they can eventually read, with your assistance, the same passage that you originally read to them.

Most of the reading that students will do in their lives will be silent, not oral, especially from middle school on. Therefore, as students increase their word recognition skills, it is important to add scaffolded silent reading to your instruction. Independent silent reading, with student scaffolding and accountability, differs from many of the sustained silent reading practices with little teacher support (Armbruster & Wilkinson, 1991; Reutzel, Fawson, & Smith, 2008). Carefully selected and scaffolded silent reading, including follow-up comprehension checks and discussion, is an important component of instruction for struggling adolescent readers.

All reading opportunities (both oral and silent) initially must be with direct teacher instruction. Interactively work with students as they orally read in order to help them integrate their decoding skills. Model both fluent reading and thinking. Also provide short, appropriate passages to read silently to help students

A Hidden World in New Guinea

During an *expedition* in December of 2005 to the Foja Mountains located on the western side of New Guinea Island, a team of American, Indonesian and Australian scientists uncovered dozens of *exotic* plants, new *species* of frogs, birds, and butterflies.

The team was dropped by helicopter to the *isolated* mountainous tropical forest that is about the size of the state of Rhode Island. It is said to be one of the largest *pristine* forests in Asia and remains free of hunting, logging, and human *impact* because of its *remote* location and *restricted access*. No one has ever built *dwellings* there.

Many new *species* were discovered in their *natural habitat* during the month-long *expedition*. At least 20 new *species* of frog, several butterfly *species* and 5 new palm plants were found...

Figure 20.9. A Hidden World in New Guinea (enriched version). (From Wilson, B.A. [2006]. A hidden world in New Guinea. *Wilson Fluency®/Basic, Instructor Manual* [p. 41]. Oxford, MA: Wilson Language Training; reprinted by permission. Copyright © 2006 Wilson Language Training. All rights reserved.)

A Hidden World in New Guinea

In 2005, people visited New Guinea to find many hidden things. There were a lot of plants and insects that no one had ever been able to see before this visit to this land.

People have not traveled to this spot because it is very remote with big mountains that are difficult to cross. People do not inhabit the land there. Plus, the government is not fond of visitors. People have not hunted, fished, or put dwellings there. There has been no logging. This land has not had people there for all these years.

Figure 20.10. A Hidden World in New Guinea (decodable version). (From Wilson, B.A. [2006]. A hidden world in New Guinea. *Wilson Fluency®/Basic, Basic Reader* [p. 30]. Oxford, MA: Wilson Language Training; reprinted by permission. Copyright © 2006 Wilson Language Training. All rights reserved.)

begin to develop reading independence. Both the text complexity and the length of these passages should be gradually increased so that students build their reading stamina. In all cases, comprehension needs to remain the goal and should be assessed.

Assess Fluency   Using curriculum-based measurement to assess oral reading fluency on a regular basis can help identify students' instructional levels and their progress (Hosp, Hosp, & Howell, 2007; see also Chapters 7, 9, and 12). Oral reading proficiency rates at the 50th percentile for students in 4th and 5th grade are 120–140 words correct per minute (WCPM) and 150 WCPM for students in 6th through 12th grade (Hasbrouck & Tindal, 2006). For Grade 6 on, this corresponds to the rate of typical speech production of adults in the United States (Schmidt & Flege, 1995). Silent reading norms were determined on data from the 1950s and need to be updated. However, those norms indicate a silent reading rate much faster than an oral rate, with a 50th percentile range from 185 WPM in Grade 6 to 250 WPM in Grade 12 (Taylor, Frankenpohl, & Pettee, 1960).

Students must practice to achieve these goals. The trajectory of growth in fluency may take longer with older students and therefore takes considerable practice to achieve (O'Connor et al., 2010; O'Connor et al., 2007). Fluency growth rates for middle school students are at a much lower rate than for elementary students, but progress can be made (Solis, Miciak, Vaughn, & Fletcher, 2014; Vaughn et al., 2011).

Increasing evidence indicates that any assessment of fluency should also include a prosody measure. Otherwise, fluency instruction might simply address correct words per minute, which is inadequate and incomplete (Kuhn et al., 2010; Samuels & Farstrup, 2006). The National Assessment of Educational Progress (NAEP) uses a rubric to rate prosody that can help guide instruction (National Center for Education Statistics [NCES], 2002).

See Chapters 7 and 12 for more information about oral reading fluency instruction and assessment.

Vocabulary, Background Knowledge, and Comprehension

Reading develops general language skills, vocabulary, background knowledge, and familiarity with complex syntax structures (Cunningham & Stanovich, 1997). Good readers may read up to 10 times as many words as poor readers (Nagy & Anderson, 1984). Students who do not learn to read fluently in elementary school are at a major disadvantage in terms of growing their background knowledge and vocabularies. Vocabulary depends more on exposure to written text than oral language because it is developed largely through print (Nagy & Anderson, 1984; Stanovich, 1986). Students at the bottom percentiles of reading ability cannot read independently, and if they do not read, they will have limited exposure to new vocabulary terms. Over time, they exhibit what has become widely known as the Matthew Effect (Stanovich, 1986); that is, students who are behind grow even further behind.

Older students who are just entering a multisensory structured language (MSL) program have a lot of catching up to do. True, they need to learn how to decode and read text fluently in a multisensory, sequential manner. This will not happen overnight, however. In the meantime, these students need as much exposure to enriched text as possible in order to develop their background knowledge, vocabulary, and comprehension.

Provide Access to Curriculum and Other Enriched Text   An essential element of teaching the older struggling reader is ensuring that while intervention is happening to remediate the reading disability, a good plan is in place to expose the student to rich content and access to the standard curriculum. Students who are not yet able to sufficiently read grade-level text must have the printed word read to them, either by an individual or through technological means. Reading to students, unfortunately, often ends in the primary grades. However, students who listen to more sophisticated text than they are able to read independently are exposed to more advanced vocabulary, substantially more background knowledge, more complex syntax structure, and higher level thinking. Older students still working on their decoding skills should listen to enriched text that is at a higher level than they can independently decode. Therefore, choices for them should include both narrative and expository selections.

Provide Access by Reading to Students   One option is to read grade-level text to students. This is the necessary choice for students with poor auditory processing skills and/or students who have not been extensively read to in the past. In addition to decoding, these students need assistance with comprehension. When reading enriched text to students, do not have them follow along while listening. They can simply listen and visualize or create a mental image of the text. Because they are listening to text at a much higher level than they can independently decode, students will likely lose their place if they try to follow along, hindering their understanding. Having them try to stay on track and attempt to decipher the words will distract them from the meaning. As skills increase, students benefit from following along, but not initially.

Help students to establish a coherent mental model through periodic discussion, modeling of thinking, and retelling of the story using mental imagery as a guide for words (Beck, Kucan, & McKeown, 2002; Wilson, 1996, 2018c). Help them with challenging vocabulary, providing student-friendly explanations using everyday language. Draw simple picture representations of the concepts to aid students' understanding of the content. Literally pull apart the text with them to create understanding by using comprehension strategies such as retelling and making graphic organizers (see Chapters 15 and 16).

Provide Exposure to Print Through Technology   **Digital** or **electronic text** can be extremely useful in assisting students who struggle with reading (Higgins, Boone, & Lovitt, 1996; Raskind, Goldberg, Higgins, & Herman, 1999). Studies have found that adding **speech synthesis** to the print material presented on computers is an effective practice for reading instruction (NICHD, 2000). This digital text can be read aloud by **screen-reading software** (also called **text-to-speech software**).

Also, if the text is digital, it can be enlarged, which is very helpful to students who are just learning to read. Studies have indicated that students with dyslexia benefit from features that include font size and spacing of lines (Kraft, 2015) as well as shorter lines of text on reduced-size screens such as the iPod touch (Schneps, as cited in Johnson, 2013).

For students with language-based disabilities and an active **individualized education program (IEP),** one of the best free sources for digital access to educational texts is https://www.bookshare.org. Bookshare provides access to more than half a million book titles, as well as access to the National Instructional Materials

Access Center (NIMAC). Another free source for digital access is http://www
.gutenberg.org. Learning Ally (https://www.learningally.org) offers audio and digital access to text. Although there is a cost associated with their product, some students benefit from the human voice and other features of this product. Audible,
iBooks, Kindle, and other vendors also offer audio and/or digital versions of many
books for a fee.

For web-based text, a computer can read the words aloud to the student. This
is done differently based on the type of computer being used. Apple products
currently have a text-to-speech feature built into the operating system. Chromebook computers offer text-to-speech as an added extension. Some older models of
PC computers may have text-to-speech built into their operating systems. Newer
versions have followed the Chromebook model, making text-to-speech applications available through the Microsoft Web Store. Users should try several options
to figure out which one fits the student's learning style the best.

Kurzweil 3000™ (http://www.kurzweiledu.com) is another software program
that reads printed text aloud, highlighting the sentence and words being read in
color. For writing assistance, the software provides templates, word prediction,
spellcheck and graphic organizers. Kurzweil also has a tablet version called Firefly.
Both versions offer many metacognitive features to support the older reader.

Screen-reading software and e-books are appropriate for students who have
poor decoding but adequate listening comprehension, giving them access to curricular materials in a form that they can use. This has exciting potential for all students, allowing them to participate more fully in their academic classes. Caution
must be used with students who have poor decoding and poor comprehension,
however. These tools might be helpful only if these students are closely monitored
and given much assistance with comprehension.

Students with decoding challenges also have difficulty with spelling and cannot easily keep up with notetaking in the classroom. Although there are several
assistive technology products designed to support notetaking, it is best to think
about tools that will generalize to most, if not all, notetaking settings. Thus, choosing a web-based tool frees the learner from being dependent on one electronic
device.

Regardless of the methods chosen to access educational materials digitally,
the key is to find the person at the student's school who will teach him or her how
to effectively use these tools and also advocate for the student so that access to the
curriculum is always available.

Technology can provide struggling readers with application and practice
opportunities but cannot replace a skilled teacher (Fisher & Ivey, 2006). Teachers
provide interactive dialogue and essential instruction to develop deep understanding of text. Furthermore, it is critical that these tools not supplant classes that
provide direct, systematic instruction in word-level skills and fluency, which will
ultimately lead to the student's reading independence.

OTHER CONSIDERATIONS

It is hard to imagine the daily challenges faced by older students who are unable
to read grade-level text. They require a tremendous amount of support throughout the day to gain access to the content in their classes and succeed in school.
Content-area teachers need professional development to assist them with these
challenges.

Provide Successful Classroom Practices

As discussed in this chapter, students in fourth grade and beyond with gaps in their independent reading skills, as indicated by testing, should have intervention classes to close those gaps. In addition, these students should participate in ELA and content-area classes with differentiated instruction that provides the supports necessary to succeed. If their reading levels are below that of the textbooks and other printed materials presented in classes, then students cannot independently gain access to that information. These students require instruction that integrates reading with subject-area content.

All students can benefit from reading comprehension instruction that integrates the specific content area being studied, although content-area teachers have resisted an integrated approach over the years (Kosanovich, Reed, & Miller, 2010; O'Brien, Dillon, Wellinski, Springs, & Stith, 1997; Ratekin, Simpson, Alvermann, & Dishner, 1985). Although Anderson, Hiebert, Scott, and Wilkinson (1985) noted long ago that reading should be part of content-area instruction, that integration does not occur widely in today's practice (ACT, 2007; Biancarosa & Snow, 2006; Kosanovich et al., 2010; Lovette, 2013; see also Chapter 18).

Address the Needs of English Language Learners

National and state assessment scores reveal a significant discrepancy in reading proficiency levels between English language learners (ELLs) and native English speakers, which only widens as students progress through school (NCES, 2011).

Research on struggling ELLs suggests that the most effective interventions correspond to the skills that are the basis of their difficulties, utilizing developmentally appropriate instruction that builds on students' current abilities in those skills (Gerber et al., 2004; Leafstedt, Richards, & Gerber, 2004). For ELLs with reading difficulties, this instruction should include explicit and scaffolded teaching in targeted skill areas (Pollard-Durodola, Mathes, Vaughn, Cardenas-Hagan, & Linan-Thompson, 2006). This research also indicates that word-level instruction should be available for ELLs with decoding deficits.

All ELLs need intensive and intentional vocabulary instruction—even more so than other, native-speaking struggling readers. Their literacy instruction should provide cultural schema and offer substantial background information (Short & Fitzsimmons, 2007). However, ELLs with decoding deficits present increased instructional needs.

In addition, Francis, Rivera, Lesaux, Kieffer, and Rivera (2006) recommended that interventions for ELLs follow these research-based practices:

- Provide explicit phonological awareness and phonics to build decoding skills. (Delaying intervention until students gain proficiency in English is discouraged.)

- Increase instruction and opportunities to develop vocabulary, including academic vocabulary.

- Teach strategies to comprehend and monitor understanding because many ELLs passively read text.

- Provide exposure to print and fluency work with repeated oral readings, emphasizing vocabulary.

- Engage students in academic talk and structured opportunities.

- Provide independent reading with structure and a careful selection of text to match reading ability (90% accuracy), with follow-up discussion.

Furthermore, classroom demonstrations of concepts can be particularly effective (Janney & Snell, 2004). These demonstrations are characterized by a teacher's verbal explanation of concepts enhanced by visual, physical, and kinesthetic involvement. Thus, the multisensory instruction described in this chapter offers multiple examples of the kinds of demonstrations that can benefit ELLs.

Spanish is by far the most prevalent language of the ELL population in the United States (Ruiz Soto, Hooker, & Batalova, 2015). Spanish-speaking ELLs can benefit from direct instruction on the similarities and differences between the sound and spelling systems of the two languages; educators should clearly teach key words to assist with any differences. For example, a key word for the consonant *h* is important (*h, hat,* /h/) because it is silent in Spanish. Also, there are thousands of cognates (words with shared etymological roots) between English and Spanish, including many academic vocabulary words (Lubliner & Hiebert, 2011). Direct instruction of these cognates is highly useful.

The lack of English vocabulary and background knowledge presents additional challenges to comprehension (August, Carlo, Dressler, & Snow, 2005; Bernhardt, 2005). One way to overcome this is for teachers to interactively dialogue with students in their native language, relating the material to their experiences and discussing background information and vocabulary. Although research is inconclusive, several studies suggest that students who receive instruction in both their native language and in English outperform students in English-only programs on English reading proficiency measures (August & Shanahan, 2006; Genesee, Lindholm-Leary, Saunders, & Christian, 2006). For further information, see Chapter 19.

REFLECT, CONNECT, and RESPOND
Discuss the important components of instruction for ELLs with a word-level deficit.

Develop Students' Belief in Their Potential

Students with significant word-level deficits cannot function at the literacy levels expected of them on a daily basis. This problem is often accompanied by heightened stress, behavior and social problems, a lack of motivation, and low self-esteem (Alexander-Passe, 2008; Daniel et al., 2006). The teacher must help establish clear goals, provide relevant and timely feedback, and find a balance between the right level of challenge and students' abilities to meet that challenge. Students must not become either overwhelmed by expectations beyond their reach or bored by a slow introduction of concepts (VanDeWeghe, 2009).

Older students who are struggling with reading have likely met with failure throughout the years. Yet, students in middle school still have a high interest in learning to read, regardless of their failure and varied reasons for it (McCray, 2001). It is hard to imagine the feelings these students have when facing undecodable words on a page. Most do not believe they can improve, so they do not want to show their interest. Expect this. Students protect their self-esteem by resisting instruction. It has failed them in the past; why should this be different? For this reason, teachers must not feel thwarted in the beginning. Instead, they should respond sympathetically and help students understand that they are beginning a detailed and sophisticated study of the English language and will learn the structure of the English language in depth. Teachers can explain that abundant research now indicates that many people share the difficulty of mastering the sound system and that systematic, sequential instruction has been proven to make mastery of it possible.

Explain to students that English is based on a sound system in which 44 sounds are put together to make thousands and thousands of words. Most people think of English as a jumbled mix of words, formed without rhyme or reason. A study conducted by Hanna, Hanna, Hodges, and Rudorf (1966), however, determined that the spellings of a majority of words in English follow a system. Explain that English is logical if one carefully and systematically studies phonology (sound–symbol correspondence as related to syllable patterns); morphology (word elements—prefixes, suffixes, and Latin and Greek base elements), and orthography (spelling rules). Tell students that they will learn more about English than most people know and that this will help them tremendously with both reading and spelling.

Older students with a history of academic failure need help to motivate them and program them for success. Today's adolescents may be motivated to master reading and writing basics for different reasons than students in the past. Some students may want to read text on the Internet as well as various interactive communications. Access to the written word in technology environments can increase students' motivation to become independent readers and writers (Kamil, Intrator, & Kim, 2000).

Several studies have demonstrated that students with learning disabilities who possess certain personal attitudes and behaviors have more successful life outcomes. The attributes of self-awareness, perseverance, proactivity, emotional stability, goal setting, and the use of support systems are powerful predictors of success (Goldberg, Higgins, Raskind, & Herman, 2003; Raskind et al., 1999; Reiff, Gerber, & Ginsberg, 1997; Wehmeyer, 1996; Werner & Smith, 1992). Help students become aware of their strengths while working with them to overcome their difficulties.

Students with phonological weaknesses potentially have strengths in areas other than phonological coding (Fink, 1998; Geschwind, 1982; Shaywitz, 2003; West, 2009). Some studies show that individuals who have chosen fields that benefit from visual-spatial skills (e.g., math, engineering) also have a higher than average incidence of reading problems (Colangelo, Assouline, Kerr, Huesman, & Johnson, 1993; Sowell, 1997; Steffert, 1998; Winner, Casey, DaSilva, & Hayes, 1991). This has not yet been fully verified, and further research is needed to determine if indeed there is a link between dyslexia and talents in nonverbal areas. This is a current area of interest in the field of research, and hopefully more information will be forthcoming because it would be helpful for older students to more clearly understand their strengths.

The writing sample and drawing shown in Figure 20.11 demonstrate the strengths of a sixth-grade student diagnosed with dyslexia. Although he has difficulty with the basics of written language, his creativity shines through with his choice of words, such as "I scream and the echo fades into the dark void in my heart." The same student quickly copied the illustration by freehand within minutes.

The goal of instruction should include an increased understanding of students' strengths so that they can have a clearer direction for their future. Combined with the skills that will develop as a result of sufficient multisensory structured

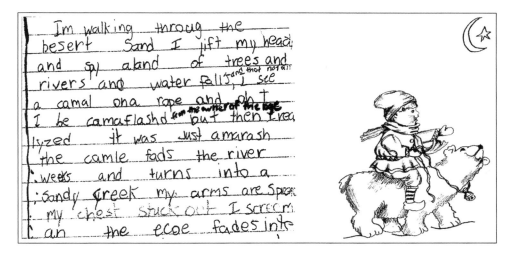

Im walking throug the
besert Sand I lift my head
and spy aland of trees and
rivers and water falls, I see
a camal ona rope and oh I
I be camaflashd but then I rea
lyzed it was just amarash
the camle fads the river
weeks and turns into a
sandy greek my arms are Sprea
my chest stuck out I scream
an the ecoe fades int

Figure 20.11.   Sample writing and illustration from sixth-grade student with dyslexia. (From *Multisensory Teaching of Basic Language Skills, Third Edition* [p. 512].)

language instruction, students can begin to believe in themselves. Given appropriate instruction and time, teachers can help them set goals and develop support systems for success.

REFLECT, CONNECT, and RESPOND
What key factors should be taken into consideration when planning an intervention class in middle school?

Prepare Teachers in Word-Level Instruction

One of the most important conclusions from research is that learning is hard work for children with learning problems. A corollary to this finding is that instruction is hard work for teachers and requires an enormous amount of training and support.

There are many factors involved in properly addressing the literacy needs of all students beyond the elementary grades. Because the challenges of students who cannot yet decode are great, instruction from a highly trained teacher is critical. Semrud-Clikeman explained, "Children who have difficulty learning to read will likely not benefit from 'more of the same' but require an alternative method of teaching to assist their learning" (2005, p. 567).

Teachers who work with struggling readers beyond the elementary grades are generally not familiar with word-level instruction. Most teachers are uncomfortable presenting older students with phonics—they may resist or avoid this instruction. Their discomfort comes partly from the expectation that older students will not want to work on basic skills, but mostly it comes from their lack of preparation and inexperience in teaching basic skills. Unfortunately, all too often, teachers lack core information about phonology, orthography, and morphology and do not know how to teach word structure in depth (American Federation of Teachers, 1999; Lovette, 2013; McCutchen et al., 2002). This makes basic skills instruction challenging for a teacher working with elementary school students, but it makes it even more difficult for a teacher working with older students.

Adolescents at the initial stages of reading who require intensive interventions in alphabetics must have a teacher who has been trained specifically in those methods (Curtis, 2004). Because older students will hesitate to work on basic skills, precise, experienced teaching is necessary. To begin with, teachers should be skilled and proficient with multisensory structured language teaching methods. It is also important for the teacher to present the systematic language instruction with confidence and with no hint of apology. In order to do this, the teacher must believe strongly that this teaching is appropriate and necessary.

Given the demands, teachers cannot be expected to implement a program for struggling readers without substantial targeted professional development and ongoing support. The International Dyslexia Association's (2018) *Knowledge and Practice Standards for Teachers of Reading* offers guidance on content knowledge and application skills that teachers require to be effective. Among the knowledge and skills already mentioned, those standards also note that teachers should be well prepared in understanding how the "relationships among the major components of literacy development change with reading development" and be able to "identify the most salient instructional needs of students who are at different points of reading and writing development" (IDA, 2018, p. 6).

CLOSING THOUGHTS: TEACHING OLDER STUDENTS WHO STRUGGLE WITH WORD READING

The effect of inadequate reading skills on the lives of individuals and on society is great. These students are much more likely to drop out of school, have trouble finding employment, and experience ongoing challenges in society (National Association of State Boards of Education [NASBE], 2006; RAND Reading Study Group, 2002). Many of these students have severe difficulties that need a more intensive level of instruction from someone other than the content-area classroom teacher (Deshler et al., 2001). To make this happen, school policies and structures need to be in place to support an action plan. In particular, effective interventions need to be selected, and then proper scheduling and staffing is needed to allow for the literacy interventions to be delivered as designed. Leadership support at the building and district level are necessary to assure success. These leaders must make literacy a priority and provide professional development for teachers to succeed with students who bring varied literacy skills into the classroom (Irvin et al., 2007).

The cost of low literacy in terms of human suffering has not been fully measured. However, it is all too clear that middle and high schools need to respond. Failure must not be the continued path. Students must be provided with the instruction that they require in order to develop proficient reading and writing skills for success in school and beyond. Given appropriate multisensory structured language instruction and sufficient time, teachers can help students set goals and develop skills for their success.

REFLECT, CONNECT, and RESPOND
Discuss the effects on the individual level and the society level for students with unaddressed literacy issues.

ONLINE COMPANION MATERIALS

The following Chapter 20 resources are available at http://www.brookespublishing.com/birshcarreker/materials:

- Reflect, Connect, and Respond Questions

- Appendix 20.1: Technology Resources for Older Students and High-Functioning Adults

- Appendix 20.2: Knowledge and Skill Assessment Answer Key

- Appendix 20.3: Supplemental Information

KNOWLEDGE AND SKILL ASSESSMENT

1. Older students without automatic single-word reading skills likely have which of the following?

    a. Phonological awareness deficits

    b. Difficulty mapping letters to sounds

    c. Difficulty with spelling

    d. All of the above

2. Which is the best instructional approach for struggling adolescent readers with word-level deficits that inhibit their reading?

    a. Focus mostly on building vocabulary and background knowledge

    b. Focus mostly on comprehension strategies

    c. Focus mostly on word-study instruction, including phonemic awareness, phonics, word analysis, and sight-word recognition

    d. Address word-study instruction in combination with vocabulary, fluency with connected text, and comprehension of text

3. Which of the following is true about the delivery of instruction to struggling adolescent readers?

    a. They should be placed in intervention groups to correspond with their grade-level reading.

    b. They should be placed in intervention groups based on their specific area(s) of deficit.

    c. They do not need to be placed in specific intervention groups but should receive extra support in their general education classrooms.

    d. They often outgrow their word-level challenges by the time they enter high school, so they likely need motivational support.

4. Word-study instruction is defined to include all the following *except:*

     a. Repeated reading of connected text

     b. Sight word instruction

     c. Segmentation, manipulation, and blending of phonemes

     d. Study of syllable patterns, morphology, and rules of orthography

5. Older readers with word-level difficulties need teachers who:

     a. Have received training in how to teach word structure in depth using multisensory structured language teaching methods

     b. Can provide targeted instruction in an intervention setting and reading support in subject-area classes

     c. Can develop students' confidence and motivation by communicating a plan of study on the structure of the English language, setting clear goals, and helping students meet the challenges set

     d. All of the above

REFERENCES

ACT. (2007). *Aligning postsecondary expectations and high school practice: The gap defined.* Iowa City, IA: Author.

Alexander-Passe, N. (2008). Sources and manifestations of stress amongst school-aged dyslexics, compared with sibling controls. *Dyslexia, 14*(4), 291–313.

Alvermann, D.E. (2001). *Effective literacy instruction for adolescents.* Chicago, IL: National Reading Conference.

American Federation of Teachers. (1999). *Teaching reading is rocket science: What expert teachers of reading should know and be able to do.* Washington, DC: Author.

Anderson, R.C., Hiebert, E.H., Scott, J.A., & Wilkinson, I.A.G. (1985). *Becoming a nation of readers: The report of the Commission on Reading.* Washington, DC: National Academy of Education, Commission on Education and Public Policy.

Anderson, R.C., Wilson, P.T., & Fielding, L.G. (1988). Growth in reading and how children spend their time outside of school. *Reading Research Quarterly, 23,* 285–303, 611–626.

Apel, K., Diehm, E., & Apel, L. (2013). Using multiple measures of morphological awareness to assess its relation to reading. *Topics in Language Disorders, 33*(1), 42–56.

Apel, K., & Henbest, V.S. (2016). Affix meaning knowledge in first through third grade students. *Language, Speech, and Hearing Services in Schools, 47*(2), 148–156.

Armbruster, B.B., & Wilkinson, I.A.G. (1991). Silent reading, oral reading, and learning from text. *The Reading Teacher, 45,* 154–155.

August, D., Carlo, M., Dressler, C., & Snow, C. (2005). The critical role of vocabulary development for English language learners. *Learning Disabilities: Research and Practice, 20*(1), 50–57.

August, D., & Shanahan, T. (Eds.). (2006). *Developing literacy in second-language learners: Report of the National Literacy Panel on Language-Minority Children and Youth.* Mahwah, NJ: Lawrence Erlbaum Associates.

Banks, S.R., Guyer, B.P., & Guyer, K.E. (1993). Spelling improvement for college students who are dyslexic. *Annals of Dyslexia, 43,* 186–193.

Beck, I.L., Kucan, L., & McKeown, M.G. (2002). *Bringing words to life: Robust vocabulary instruction.* New York, NY: Guilford.

Bernhardt, E. (2005). Progress and procrastination in second language reading. *Annual Review of Applied Linguistics, 25,* 133–150.

Bhattacharya, A., & Ehri, L.C. (2004). Graphosyllabic analysis helps adolescent struggling readers read and spell words. *Journal of Learning Disabilities, 37*(4), 331–348.

Biancarosa, C., & Snow, C.E. (2006). *Reading next: A vision for action and research in middle and high school literacy. A report to Carnegie Corporation of New York.* Washington, DC: Alliance for Excellent Education.

Boardman, A.G., Roberts, G., Vaughn, S., Wexler, J., Murray, C.S., & Kosanovich, M. (2008). *Effective instruction for adolescent struggling readers: A practice brief.* Portsmouth, NH: RMC Research Corporation, Center on Instruction. Retrieved from http://www.centeroninstruction.org/files/Practice%20Brief-Struggling%20Readers.pdf

Bowers, P.N. (2013). *Teaching how the written word works.* Kingston, ON: Word Works Literacy Centre.

Bowers, P.N., & Cooke, G. (2012, Fall). Morphology and the Common Core: Building students' understanding of the written word. *Perspectives on Language and Literacy,* 31–35.

Bowers, P.N., & Kirby, J.R. (2010). Effects of morphological instruction on vocabulary acquisition. *Reading and Writing: An Interdisciplinary Journal, 23,* 515–537.

Bowers, P.N., Kirby, J.R., & Deacon, S.H. (2010). The effects of morphological instruction on literacy skills: A systematic review of the literature. *Review of Educational Research, 80,* 144–179.

Brasseur-Hock, I., Hock, M., Kieffer, M., Biancarosa, G., & Deshler, D. (2011). Adolescent struggling readers in urban schools: Results of a latent class analysis. *Learning and Individual Differences, 21,* 438–452. doi:10.1016/j.lindif.2011.01.008

Bruck, M. (1990). Word recognition skill of adults with childhood diagnoses of dyslexia. *Developmental Psychology, 26,* 439–454.

Bruck, M. (1992). Persistence of dyslexics' phonological awareness deficits. *Developmental Psychology, 28,* 874–886.

Bruck, M. (1993). Component spelling skills of college students with childhood diagnoses of dyslexia. *Developmental Psychology, 16,* 171–184.

Campbell, M.S., Helf, S., & Cooke, N.L. (2008). Effects of adding multisensory components to a supplemental reading program on the decoding skills of treatment resisters. *Education and Treatment of Children, 31*(3), 267–295.

Carlisle, J.F. (2010, Oct./Nov./Dec.). Review of research: Effects of instruction in morphological awareness on literacy achievement: An integrative review. *Reading Research Quarterly, 45*(4), 464–487.

Carnevale, A.P. (2001). *Help wanted: College required.* Washington, DC: Educational Testing Service, Office for Public Leadership.

Carroll, J.B., Davies, P., & Richman, B. (1971). *The American heritage word frequency book.* Boston, MA: Houghton Mifflin.

Chall, J.S. (1983). *Stages of reading development.* New York, NY: McGraw-Hill.

Chard, D.J., Vaughn, S., & Tyler, B.J. (2002). A synthesis of research on effective interventions for building reading fluency with elementary students with learning disabilities. *Journal of Learning Disabilities, 35,* 386–406.

Christensen, C.M., Horn, M.B., & Johnson, C.W. (2010). *Rethinking student motivation: Why understanding the "job" is crucial for improving education.* Retrieved from https://www.christenseninstitute.org/wp-content/uploads/2013/04/Rethinking-student-motivation.pdf

Cirino, P.T., Romain, M.A., Barth, A.E., Tolar, T.D., Fletcher, J.M., & Vaughn, S. (2013). Reading skill components and impairments in middle school struggling readers. *Reading and Writing, 26*(7), 1059–1086.

Colangelo, N., Assouline, S.G., Kerr, B., Huesman, R., & Johnson, D. (1993). Mechanical inventiveness: A three phase study. In G. Bock & K. Ackrill (Eds.), *The origins and development of high ability* (pp. 160–174). New York, NY: Wiley.

Compton, D.L., Appleton, A.C., & Hosp, M.K. (2004). Exploring the relationship between text-leveling systems and reading accuracy and fluency in second-grade students who are average and poor decoders. *Learning Disabilities Research & Practice, 19*(3), 176–184.

Cunningham, A.E., & Stanovich, K.E. (1997). Early reading acquisition and its relation to reading experience and ability 10 years later. *Developmental Psychology, 33,* 934–935.

Curtis, M.E. (2004). Adolescents who struggle with word identification: Research and practice. In T.L. Jesson & J.A. Dole (Eds.), *Adolescent literacy research and practice* (pp. 119–134). New York, NY: Guilford.

Curtis, M.E., & Longo, A.M. (1999). *When adolescents can't read: Methods and materials that work.* Cambridge, MA: Brookline Books.

Daniel, S.S., Walsh, A.K., Goldston, D.B., Arnold, E.M., Reboussin, B.A., & Wood, F.B. (2006). Suicidality, school dropout and reading problems amongst adolescents. *Journal of Learning Disabilities, 39*(6), 507–514.

Denton, C.A., Vaughn, S., Wexler, J., Bryan, D., & Reed, D. (2012). *Effective instruction for middle school students with reading difficulties: The reading teacher's sourcebook.* Baltimore, MD: Paul H. Brookes Publishing Co.

Deshler, D.D., & Hock, M.F. (2006). *Shaping literacy achievement.* New York, NY: Guilford.

Deshler, D.D., Schumaker, J.B., Lenz, B.K., Bulgren, J.A., Hock, M.F., Knight, J., & Ehren, B. J. (2001). Ensuring content-area learning by secondary students with learning disabilities. *Learning Disabilities Research and Practice, 16*(2), 96–108.

Egan, J., & Pring, L. (2004). The processing of inflectional morphology: A comparison of children with and without dyslexia. *Reading and Writing, 17*(6), 567–591.

Ehri, L.C. (2000). Learning to read and learning to spell: Two sides of a coin. *Topics in Language Disorders, 20*(3), 19–36.

Fink, R. (1998). Literacy development in successful men and woman with dyslexia. *Annals of Dyslexia, 48,* 311–346.

Fisher, D., & Ivey, G. (2006). Evaluating the interventions for struggling adolescent readers. *Journal of Adolescent and Adult Literacy, 50,* 180–189.

Francis, D.J., Rivera, M., Lesaux, N., Kieffer, M., & Rivera, H. (2006). *Practical guidelines for the education of English language learners: Research-based recommendations for instruction and academic interventions.* Retrieved from http://www.centeroninstruction.org/resources.cfm? category=ell&subcategory=research&grade_start =0&grade_end=12

Genesee, F., Lindholm-Leary, K., Saunders, W., & Christian, D. (Eds.). (2006). *Educating English language learners: A synthesis of research evidence.* New York, NY: Cambridge University Press.

Gerber, M., Jimenez, T., Leafstedt, J.M., Villaruz, J., Richards, C., & English, J. (2004). English reading effects of small-group intensive intervention in Spanish for K–1 English learners. *Learning Disabilities Research & Practice, 19*(4), 239–251.

Geschwind, N. (1982). Why Orton was right. *Annals of Dyslexia, 32,* 13–20.

Goldberg, R.J., Higgins, E.L., Raskind, M.H., & Herman, K.L. (2003). Predictors of success in individuals with learning disabilities: A quantitative analysis of a 20-year longitudinal study. *Learning Disabilities Research & Practice, 18*(4), 222–236.

Hanna, P.R., Hanna, J.S., Hodges, R.E., & Rudorf, E.H., Jr. (1966). *Phoneme-grapheme correspondences as cues to spelling improvement* (USOE Pub No. 32008). Washington, DC: U.S. Government Printing Office.

Hasbrouck, J.E., & Tindal, G.A. (2006). Oral reading fluency norms: A valuable assessment tool for reading teachers. *The Reading Teacher, 59*(7), 636–644.

Henry, M K. (1993). Morphological structure: Latin and Greek roots and affixes as upper grade code strategies. *Reading and Writing: An Interdisciplinary Journal, 5*(2), 227–241.

Hiebert, E.H., & Fisher, C.W. (2007). Critical Word Factor in texts for beginning readers. *The Journal of Educational Research, 101,* 3–11.

Hiebert, E.H., Goodwin, A.P., & Cervetti, G.N. (2018). Core vocabulary: Its morphological content and presence in exemplar texts. *Reading Research Quarterly, 53*(1). Advance online publication. Retrieved from http://textproject.org/library/research-articles/vocabulary-research-articles/core-vocabulary-its-morphological-content-and-presence-in-exemplar-texts-2/

Higgins, K., Boone, R., & Lovitt, T. (1996). Hypertext support for remedial students and students with learning disabilities. *Journal of Learning Disabilities, 29*(4), 402–412.

Hock, M.F., Brasseur, I.F., Deshler, D.D., Catts, H.W., Marquis, J.G., Mark, C.A., & Stribling, J. (2009). What is the reading component skill profile of adolescent struggling readers in urban schools? *Learning Disability Quarterly, 32*(1), 21–38.

Hock, M.F., Deshler, D.D., Marquis, J.G., & Brasseur, I.F. (2005). *Reading component skills of adolescents attending urban schools.* Lawrence: University of Kansas, Center for Research on Learning.

Homan, S.P., Klesius, J.P., & Hite, C. (1993). Effects of repeated readings and nonrepetitive strategies on students' fluency and comprehension. *Journal of Educational Research, 87,* 94–99.

Hosp, M.K., Hosp, J.L., & Howell, K.W. (2007). *The ABC's of CBM: A practical guide to curriculum-based measurement.* New York, NY: Guilford.

International Dyslexia Association, The. (2018, March). *Knowledge and practice standards for teachers of reading.* Retrieved from https://dyslexiaida.org/knowledge-and-practices/

Irvin, J.L., Meltzer, J., & Dukes, M. (2007). *Taking action on adolescent literacy: An implementation guide for school leaders.* Alexandria, VA: Association for Supervision and Curriculum Development.

Ivey, G., & Broaddus, K. (2001). Just plain reading: A survey of what makes students want to read in middle school classrooms. *Reading Research Quarterly, 36,* 350–377.

Janney, R., & Snell, M.E. (2004). *Teachers' guides to inclusive practices: Modifying schoolwork* (2nd ed.). Baltimore, MD: Paul H. Brookes Publishing Co.

Johnson, C. (2013, July 3). Personal discovery on dyslexia may aid many: Scientist explores how small screens can make difference. *The Boston Globe.* Retrieved from https://www.bostonglobe.com

Kamil, M.L., Intrator, S.M., & Kim, H.S. (2000). The effects of other technologies on literacy and literacy learning. In M.L. Kamil, P.B. Mosenthal, P.D. Pearson, & R. Barr (Eds.), *Handbook of reading research* (Vol. 3, pp. 771–788). Mahwah, NJ: Lawrence Erlbaum Associates.

Kosanovich, M.L., Reed, D.K., & Miller, D.H. (2010). *Bringing literacy strategies into content instruction: Professional learning for secondary-level teachers.* Portsmouth, NH: RMC Research Corporation, Center on Instruction.

Kraft, A. (2015, December 14). Books vs. e-books: The science behind the best way to read. *CBS News.* Retrieved from http://www.cbsnews.com/news/kindle-nook-e-reader-books-the-best-way-to-read/

Kruk, R.S., & Bergman, K. (2013). The reciprocal relations between morphological processes and reading. *Journal of Experimental Child Psychology, 114*(1), 10–34.

Kuhn, M.R., Schwanenflugel, P.J., & Meisinger, E.B. (2010, April/May/June). Review of research: Aligning theory and assessment of reading fluency: Automaticity, prosody, and definitions of fluency. *Reading Research Quarterly, 45*(2), 230–251.

Kuhn, M.R., & Stahl, S.A. (2003). Fluency: A review of developmental and remedial practices. *Journal of Educational Psychology, 95*(1), 3–21.

Leach, J., Scarborough, H., & Rescorla, L. (2003). Late-emerging reading disabilities. *Journal of Educational Psychology, 95,* 211–224.

Leafstedt, J.M., Richards, C.R., & Gerber, M.M. (2004). Effectiveness of explicit phonological awareness instruction for at-risk English learners. *Learning Disabilities Research and Practice, 19,* 252–261.

Lovett, M.W., Barron, R.W., & Benson, N.J. (2003). Effective remediation of word identification and decoding difficulties in school-age children with reading disabilities. In H.L. Swanson, K.R. Harris, & S. Graham (Eds.), *Handbook of learning disabilities* (pp. 273–292). New York, NY: Guilford.

Lovette, G.E. (2013). Reading preparation of secondary ELA teachers: A U.S. Survey of state licensure requirements. *Journal of Adolescent & Adult Literacy, 57*(3), 193–203.

Lubliner, S., & Hiebert, E.H. (2011). An analysis of English-Spanish cognates as a source of general academic language. *Bilingual Research Journal, 34*(1), 76–93.

Lyon, G.R., Fletcher, J.M., Shaywitz, S.E., Shaywitz, B.A., Torgesen, J.K., Wood, F.B., … Olson, R. (2001). Rethinking learning disabilities. In C.E. Finn, Jr., A.J. Rotherham, & C.R. Hokanson, Jr. (Eds.), *Rethinking special education for a new century* (pp. 259–287). Washington, DC: Thomas B. Fordham Foundation and Progressive Policy Institute.

Mather, N., Hammill, D.D., Allen, E.A., & Roberts, R. (2014). *Test of Silent Word Reading Fluency–Second Edition* (TOSWRF-2). Austin, TX: PRO-ED.

McCray, A.D. (2001, November). Middle school students with learning disabilities. *Reading Teacher, 55*(3), 298–310.

McCutchen, D., Green, L., & Abbott, R.D. (2008). Children's morphological knowledge: Links to literacy. *Reading Psychology, 29*(4), 289–314.

McCutchen, D., Harry, D.R., Cunningham, A.E., Cox, S., Sidman, S., & Covill, A.E. (2002). Reading teachers' knowledge of children's literature and English phonology. *Annals of Dyslexia, 52,* 207–228.

McFarland, J., Stark, P., & Cui, J. (2016). *Trends in high school dropout and completion rates in the United States: 2013* (NCES 2016-117). Washington, DC: U.S. Department of Education, National Center for Education Statistics. Retrieved from http://nces.ed.gov/pubsearch

Mol, S.E., & Bus, A.G. (2011). To read or not to read: A meta-analysis of print exposure from infancy to early adulthood. *Psychological Bulletin, 137*(2), 267–296.

Morgan, A., Wilcox, B.R., & Eldredge, J.L. (2000). Effect of difficulty levels on second-grade delayed readers using dyad reading. *The Journal of Educational Research, 94*, 113–119.

Moore, D.W., Bean, T.W., Birdyshaw, D., & Rycik, J.A. (1999). *Adolescent literacy: A position statement for the Commission on Adolescent Literacy of the International Reading Association.* Newark, DE: International Reading Association.

Murray, C.S., Wexler, J., Vaughn, S., Roberts, G., Tackett, K. K., Boardman, A.G., . . . Kosanovich, M. (2010). *Effective instruction for adolescent struggling readers: Professional development module facilitator's guide* (2nd ed.). Portsmouth, NH: RMC Research Corporation, Center on Instruction. Retrieved from http://www.centeroninstruction.org/files/EIASR%20FG%20 2nd%20Ed.pdf

Nagy, W.E., & Anderson, R.C. (1984). How many words are there in printed school English? *Reading Research Quarterly, 19*, 304–330.

Nagy, W.E., Anderson, R.C., Schommer, M., Scott, J.A., & Stallman, A.C. (1989). Morphological families in the internal lexicon. *Reading Research Quarterly, 24*, 262–282.

Nagy, W.E., Diakidoy, I.N., & Anderson, R.C. (1993). The acquisition of morphology: Learning the contribution of suffixes to the meanings of derivatives. *Journal of Reading Behavior, 25*, 155–170.

National Assessment Governing Board. (2015). *National Assessment of Educational Progress: The Nation's Report Card, 2015 Reading Assessment.* Retrieved from https://www .nationsreportcard.gov/reading_math_2015/#reading?grade=8 and http://www.nations reportcard.gov/reading_math_g12_2015/#reading

National Association of State Boards of Education (NASBE). (2006). *Reading at risk: The state response to the crisis in adolescent literacy.* Arlington, VA: Author.

National Center for Education Statistics (NCES). (2002). *NAEP–Oral Reading Fluency Scale.* Washington, DC: U.S. Department of Education, Institute of Education Sciences. Retrieved from https://nces.ed.gov/nationsreportcard/studies/ors/scale.aspx

National Center for Education Statistics (NCES). (2011). *English language learners in public schools.* Washington, DC: U.S. Department of Education. Retrieved from https://nces .ed.gov/programs/coe/pdf/coe_cgf.pdf

National Governors Association (NGA) Center for Best Practices & Council of Chief State School Officers (CCSSO). (2010). *Common core state standards for English language arts & literacy in history/social studies, science, and technical subjects.* Washington, DC: Author. Retrieved from http://www.corestandards.org/ELA-Literacy/

National Institute of Child Health and Human Development (NICHD). (2000). *Report of the National Reading Panel: Reports of the subgroups. Teaching children to read: An evidence-based assessment of the scientific research literature on reading and its implications for reading instruction* (NIH Pub No. 00-4769). Washington, DC: Government Printing Office.

National Institute for Literacy. (2007). *Adapted from what content-area teachers should know about adolescent literacy.* Retrieved from http://www.nifl.gov/nifl/publications/adolescent_ literacy07.pdf

O'Brien, D.G., Dillon, D.R., Wellinski, S.A., Springs, R., & Stith, D. (1997). *Engaging "at-risk" high school students.* Athens, GA: National Reading Research Center.

O'Connor, R.E., Swanson, H.L., & Geraghty, C. (2010). Improvement in reading rate under independent and difficult text levels: Influences on word and comprehension skills. *Journal of Educational Psychology, 102*, 1–19.

O'Connor, R.E., White, A., & Swanson, H.L. (2007). Repeated reading versus continuous reading: Influences on reading fluency and comprehension. *Exceptional Children, 74*(1), 31–46.

Pacheco, M.B., & Goodwin, A.P. (2013). Putting two and two together: Middle school students' morphological problem-solving strategies for unknown words. *Journal of Adolescents & Adult Literacy, 56*(7), 541–553.

Partnership for Reading. (2003, June). *Put reading first: The research building blocks for teaching children to read: Kindergarten through grade 3* (2nd ed.). Washington, DC: Author.

Penney, C. (2002). Teaching decoding skills to poor readers in high school. *Journal of Literacy Research, 34*, 99–118.

Pollard-Durodola, S.D., Mathes, P.G., Vaughn, S., Cardenas-Hagan, E., & Linan-Thompson, S. (2006). The role of oracy in developing comprehension in Spanish-speaking English language learners. *Topics in Language Disorders, 26*(4), 365–384.

RAND Reading Study Group. (2002). *Reading for understanding: Toward a research and development program in reading comprehension.* Santa Monica, CA: RAND Corporation.

Rashotte, C.A., & Torgesen, J.K. (1985). Repeated reading and reading fluency in learning disabled children. *Reading Research Quarterly, 20,* 180–188.

Rasinski, T.V., & Samuels, S.J. (2011). Reading fluency: What it is and what it is not. In S.J. Samuels & A.E. Farstrup (Eds.), *What research has to say about reading instruction* (4th ed., pp. 94–114). Newark: DE: International Reading Association.

Raskind, M.H., Goldberg, R.J., Higgins, E.L., & Herman, K.L. (1999). Patterns of change and predictors of success in individuals with learning disabilities: Results from a twenty-year longitudinal study. *Learning Disabilities Research and Practice, 14*(1), 35–49.

Ratekin, N., Simpson, M., Alvermann, D., & Dishner, E. (1985). Why teachers resist content reading instruction. *Journal of Reading, 28,* 432–437.

Reiff, H.B., Gerber, P.J., & Ginsberg, R. (1997). *Exceeding expectations: Successful adults with learning disabilities.* Austin, TX: PRO-ED.

Reutzel, D.R., Fawson, P.C., & Smith, J.A. (2008). Reconsidering silent sustained reading: An exploratory study of scaffolded silent reading. *Journal of Educational Research, 102*(1), 37–50.

Ruiz Soto, A.G., Hooker, S., & Batalova, J. (2015). *Top languages spoken by English language learners nationally and by state.* Washington, DC: Migration Policy Institute.

Samuels, S.J., & Farstrup, A.E. (Eds.). (2006). *What research has to say about fluency instruction.* Newark, DE: International Reading Association.

Scammacca, N., Roberts, G., Vaughn, S., Edmonds, M., Wexler, J., Reutebuch, C.K., & Torgesen, J. (2007). *Intervention for adolescent struggling readers: A meta-analysis with implications for practice.* Portsmouth, NH: RMC Research Corporation, Center on Instruction.

Scammacca, N., Roberts, G., Vaughn, S., & Stuebing, K. (2015). A meta-analysis of interventions for struggling readers in grades 4–12: 1980–2011. *Journal of Learning Disabilities, 48*(4), 369–390.

Schmidt, A., & Flege, J. (1995). Effects of speaking rate changes on native and non-native production. *Phonetica, 52,* 41–54.

Scruggs, T.E., Mastropieri, M.A., Berkeley, S., & Graetz, J. (2010). Do special education interventions improve learning of secondary content? A meta-analysis. *Remedial and Special Education, 31*(6), 437–449.

Semrud-Clikeman, M. (2005). Neuropsychological aspects for evaluating learning disabilities. *Journal of Learning Disabilities, 38,* 563–568.

Shaywitz, S. (2003). *Overcoming dyslexia: A new and complete science-based program for reading problems at any level.* New York, NY: Alfred A. Knopf.

Short, D., & Fitzsimmons, S. (2007). *Double the work: Challenges and solutions to acquiring language and academic literacy for adolescent English language learners—A report to Carnegie Corporation of New York.* Washington, DC: Alliance for Excellent Education.

Singson, M., Mahony, D., & Mann, V. (2000). The relation between reading ability and morphological skills: Evidence from derivational suffixes. *Reading and Writing: An Interdisciplinary Journal, 12,* 219–252. doi:10.1023/A:1008196330239

Snow, C.E. (2002). *Reading for understanding: Toward an R & D program in reading comprehension.* Santa Monica, CA: Science and Technology Policy Institute.

Snow, C., & Biancarosa, G. (2003). *Adolescent literacy and the achievement gap: What do we know and where do we go from here?* New York, NY: Carnegie Corporation.

Snow, C.E., Burns, M.S., & Griffin, P. (Eds.). (1998). *Preventing reading difficulties in young children.* Washington, DC: National Academies Press.

Snow, C.E., Griffin, P., & Burns, M.S. (Eds.). (2005). *Knowledge to support the teaching of reading.* San Francisco, CA: Jossey-Bass.

Solis, M., Miciak, J., Vaughn, S., & Fletcher, J. (2014). Why intensive interventions matter: Longitudinal studies of adolescents with reading disabilities and poor reading comprehension. *Learning Disability Quarterly* [Advance online publication]. doi:10.1177/0731948714528806

Sowell, T. (1997). *Late-talking children.* New York, NY: Basic Books.

Spreen, O. (1989). Learning disability, neurology, and long-term outcome: Some implications for the individual and for society. *Journal of Clinical and Experimental Neuropsychology, 11*(3), 389–408.

Stanovich, K.E. (1986). Matthew effects in reading: Some consequences of individual differences in the acquisition of literacy. *Reading Research Quarterly, 21,* 369–407.

Steffert, B. (1998). Sign minds and design minds. In S. Dingli (Ed.), *Creative thinking: Towards broader horizons.* Proceedings of the third international conference on creative thinking. Msida: Malta University Press.

Sturgis, C., & Patrick, S. (2010). *When success is the only option: Designing competency-based pathways for next generation learning.* Vienna, VA: International Association for K–12 Online Learning (iNACOL).

Taylor, S.E., Frackenpohl, H., & Pettee, J.L. (1960). Grade level norms for the components of the fundamental reading skill. *EDL Research and Information Bulletin, 3,* 22.

Torgesen, J.K. (2005). *Essential features of effective reading instruction for struggling readers in grades 4–12* [PowerPoint]. Presentation at meetings of the Utah Branch of the International Dyslexia Association, Salt Lake City. Retrieved from http://www.fcrr.org/science/pdf/torgesen/Utah_remediation.pdf

Torgesen, J.K., & Hudson, R.R. (2006). Reading fluency: Critical issues for struggling readers. In S.J. Samuels & A.E. Parstrup (Eds.), *What research has to say about fluency instruction* (pp. 130–158). Newark, DE: International Reading Association.

Torgesen, J.K., Houston, D.D., Rissman, L.M., Decker, S.M., Roberts, G., Vaughn, S., . . . Lessaux, N. (2007). *Academic literacy instruction for adolescents: A guidance document from the Center on Instruction.* Portsmouth, NH: RMC Research Corporation, Center on Instruction.

U.S. Census Bureau. (2015). *2011–2015 American community survey 5-year estimates.* Retrieved from https://factfinder.census.gov/faces/tableservices/jsf/pages/productview.xhtml?pid=ACS_15_5YR_S1501&src=pt

VanDeWeghe, R. (2009). *Engaged learning.* Thousand Oaks, CA: Corwin Press.

Vaughn, S., Fletcher, J.M., Francis, D.J., Denton, C.A., Wanzek, J., Wexler, J., . . . Romain, M.A. (2008). Response to intervention with older students with reading difficulties, *Learning and Individual Differences, 18*(3), 338–345.

Vaughn, S., Wexler, J., Roberts, G., Barth, A., Cirino, P., Romain, M., & Denton, C.A. (2011). Effects of individualized and standardized interventions on middle school students with reading disabilities. *Exceptional Children, 77*(4), 291–407.

Verhoeven, L., & Perfetti, C. (2011). Morphological processing in reading acquisition: A cross-linguistic perspective. *Applied Psycholinguistics, 32*(3), 457–466.

Wagner, R.K., Torgesen, J.K., Rashotte, C.A., & Pearson, N.A. (2010). *Test of Silent Reading Efficiency and Comprehension (TOSREC): Examiner's Manual.* Austin, TX: PRO-ED, Inc.

Wehmeyer, M.L. (1996). Self-determination as an educational outcome: Why is it important to children, youth, and adults with disabilities? In D.J. Sands & M.L. Wehmeyer (Eds.), *Self-determination across the lifespan: Independence and choice for people with disabilities* (pp. 17–36). Baltimore, MD: Paul H. Brookes Publishing Co.

Werner, E.E., & Smith, R.S. (1992). *Overcoming the odds: High risk children from birth to adulthood.* Ithaca, NY: Cornell University Press.

West, T.G. (2009). *In the mind's eye: Creative visual thinkers, gifted dyslexics, and the rise of visual strategies* (2nd ed.). Buffalo, NY: Prometheus Books.

White, T.G., Sowell, J., & Yanagihara, A. (1989). Teaching elementary students to use word-part clues. *The Reading Teacher, 42*(4), 302–308.

Wilson, B.A. (1996). *Wilson Reading System instructor manual* (3rd ed.). Oxford, MA: Wilson Language Training.

Wilson, B.A. (2006). *Wilson Fluency/Basic.* Oxford, MA: Wilson Language Training.

Wilson, B.A. (2015). *Example of literacy planning beyond grade 3.* Oxford, MA: Wilson Language Training. Retrieved from http://www.wilsonacademy.com

Wilson, B.A. (2018a). On the job with Bill. In *Wilson Reading System student reader one.* Oxford, MA: Wilson Language Training.

Wilson, B.A. (2018b). Snack or script? In *Wilson Reading System student reader three.* Oxford, MA: Wilson Language Training.

Wilson, B.A. (2018c). *Wilson Reading System instructor manual* (4th ed.). Oxford, MA: Wilson Language Training.

Wilson, B.A., & Felton, R. (2004). *Word Identification and Spelling Test (WIST).* Austin, TX: PRO-ED.

Wilson, B.A., & O'Connor, J. (1995). Effectiveness of the Wilson Reading System used in public school training. In C. McIntyre & J. Pickering (Eds.), *Clinical studies of multisensory structured language education for students with dyslexia and related disorders* (pp. 247–254). Salem, OR: International Multisensory Structured Language Education Council.

Winner, E., Casey, M., DaSilva, D., & Hayes, R. (1991). Spacial abilities and reading deficits in visual arts students. *Empirical Studies of the Arts, 9*(1), 51–63.

Wolf, M., & Katzir-Cohen, T. (2001). Reading fluency and its intervention. *Scientific Studies of Reading (Special Issue on Fluency), 5,* 211–238.

Wolter, J.A., & Dilworth, V. (2014). The effects of morphological awareness approach to improve language and literacy. *Journal of Learning Disabilities, 47,* 76–85.

Wolter, J.A., Wood, A., & D'zatko, K. (2009). The influence of morphological awareness on first-grade children's literacy development. *Language, Speech, and Hearing Services in Schools, 40*(3), 1–13.

Ziegler, J.C., Stone, G.O., & Jacobs, A.M. (1997). What's the pronunciation for *-ough* and the spelling for /u/? A database for computing feedforward and feedback inconsistency in English. *Behavior Research Methods, Instruments, and Computers, 29*(4), 600–618.

Chapter 21

Working With High-Functioning Adults With Dyslexia and Other Academic Challenges

Susan H. Blumenthal

LEARNING OBJECTIVES

1. To understand the long-standing learning difficulties and the emotional repercussions experienced by high-functioning students with dyslexia and other academic challenges

2. To learn how to tailor one's teaching to these students' specific needs

3. To understand the necessity of differentiating adults' goals for remediation from those of children and to apply this understanding as an instructor

4. To learn how to encourage adults to become active learners and to progress in their work or advanced study in their professions

The population of high-functioning adults with dyslexia is a specific but quite diverse group of individuals. They study and work in a variety of fields and are college students, graduate students, physicians, lawyers, and members of the clergy. Some adults, especially those in graduate school, are required to do tremendous amounts of reading each week. Other graduate students conduct experiments in science research, which may require less reading than is necessary in liberal arts programs. In science settings, however, graduate students need to perform sequential, multistep experiments with relative independence over a period of several days. Frequent shifting from abstract conceptualization to sequenced detail and back again requires a high degree of organization, which can be troublesome for some adults with dyslexia.

Not all high-functioning individuals with dyslexia are in a school environment. Some adults with dyslexia have already completed school and are working in a business setting. Whether an individual runs his or her own business or is in a corporate setting, he or she usually has to do background reading in trade or professional journals to keep abreast of developments in the field. In addition,

---

A note from Dr. Judith R. Birsh: Although this chapter has not been updated in the same way as the others, it continues to have relevance and value in this fourth edition. The learning objectives help guide the reader through the necessary steps in working with this unique population of high-functioning adults and students who have dyslexia and other academic challenges beyond high school.

individuals in professional positions often have to write memos and reports on a regular basis as part of their job.

Virtually all high-functioning adults with dyslexia are ambitious and highly motivated, but they also experience chronic feelings of inadequacy, stress, and low self-esteem regarding their ability to learn. Almost all of them had a difficult beginning in the early grades of elementary school and continued to function quite unevenly during their school years.

EMOTIONAL REPERCUSSIONS

Despite being above average or quite superior in general ability, nearly all of the high-functioning adults with dyslexia who seek help with reading and writing skills experience anxiety about some aspects of their work and learning. They often do not know why they have so much difficulty with written language. Through the years, they have tried to both compensate for and hide the problem. They may have never read a book all of the way through but will rarely miss class so that they can pick up the necessary information from discussion. They may have to write multiple drafts of a term paper but often will ask and be allowed to give an oral presentation or work in tandem with another student. So many of these students have been told to "try harder" throughout their school careers. Nearly every adult with dyslexia who goes for a psychoeducational consultation or evaluation thinks that he or she is "lazy," that everyone else is smarter, or that there is something wrong with his or her brain. It does not matter whether these individuals graduated from a state school or an Ivy League school, nor does it matter whether they were inducted into Phi Beta Kappa. They almost always are plagued by varying degrees of self-doubt.

There are important differences between children and adults who have learning difficulties that can affect intervention. First, their basic attitudes are generally different. When children are referred for language intervention, they often are resistant at first. They have been identified as not doing well in school, and both the children and the parents may be upset with the children's school performance and/or with the school staff. In contrast, adults usually are highly motivated to improve their language skills. Many are self-referred or are referred by other professionals, such as psychotherapists or college teachers. As a consequence, adults with learning difficulties often have definite goals. In addition, they often are relieved when they realize that they can get help.

A sense of awareness is the second difference between children and adults with learning difficulties. Children's awareness of their learning needs and difficulties usually is unformulated. In some way, the children sense that there is something wrong. They say, "Reading is not hard for me—I just don't like it." Adults are much more aware of how learning difficulties, especially reading difficulties, have affected their lives. They may feel self-conscious in a social group—not because they lack social skills but because they do not make the same kind of contributions as others. They may not make the same mental associations because they lack the underlying foundation of knowledge, which is often derived from reading. For example, a 35-year-old physician with a persistent reading problem who came for help had this comment: "I feel I am shallow, compared with all my friends. They read all of the time."

Coping is another difference between children and adults with learning disabilities. Children are part of an established support system; they are evaluated, tested, promoted to or held back from the next grade, and are often the focus of parent–teacher conferences. The responsibility of learning or not learning is shared.

Adults with learning disabilities invariably seem to have a secret life. They do not have the same support system as children. Adults have to work in an increasingly independent manner, and they worry about being "found out." Many adults with learning disabilities have learned to hide their problems and compensate as much as possible. Often, they focus on avoidance in order to escape potential humiliation.

Finally, the beginning of the referral process is also different for adults and children. Children are usually referred or evaluated because they are failing or not doing well in school. Adults are referred for a variety of reasons. Some adults experience a change in their work requirements or in their educational setting, and they find that they cannot meet the expected level of the new requirements. For example, a member of the Coast Guard with severe dyslexia was promoted to petty officer. Instead of working on machines, at which he was an expert, he now had to do considerable paperwork and report writing. His performance ratings, which were consistently high, fell below average. In another instance, an ambitious 31-year-old account executive who had a history of dyslexia was quite successful on her job. She had excellent verbal skills and was effective at meetings. Her new boss, however, insisted that there be more memos and outlines of marketing goals and fewer face-to-face meetings. The account executive knew that if she wanted to be promoted, then she would have to get her ideas down in writing.

Some adults who return to school for a higher degree refer themselves for a psychoeducational evaluation. For example, a successful 47-year-old businesswoman with a bachelor of arts degree decided to apply for a master of business administration program. She referred herself for evaluation because she suspected that she had a previously undiagnosed learning problem. When her son was diagnosed with dyslexia, she recognized similar patterns in her own academic life.

More adults are being referred by mental health workers, personnel in the workplace, and college and university faculty to explore whether there is an undetected learning problem. As awareness increases about the different forms that learning problems can take, psychotherapists, job supervisors, and professors have begun to notice areas of discrepancy in individuals who otherwise are functioning well. For example, an administrator at a university was referred for a psychoeducational evaluation after his boss wrote, "The communication area is of great concern and an obstacle to Mr. K's career development. He exceeds expectations in personal skills and in commitment to all aspects of his job. I recommend that he get help for problems in writing and other communications skills."

REFLECT, CONNECT, and RESPOND
What impact might a reading disability have on an adult's day-to-day life, in terms of everyday tasks, professional responsibilities, and emotional repercussions? Why do you suppose adults are typically more aware of their disability than children and sometimes more receptive to the idea of seeking help?

EVALUATION AND ASSESSMENT

Gathering information about the individual's early developmental, educational, and medical histories and, if appropriate, employment history is the first component of a comprehensive assessment for an adult. The individual's own perception of the problem is particularly helpful. The latter information can be obtained from a writing sample called Educational Memories (Blumenthal, 1981a), which is described later in this section.

The purpose of the assessment is to try to understand and evaluate the client's presenting problems in order to develop a treatment plan. The assessor tries to determine why the person is having difficulty functioning in an academic or a work setting and explores the client's capabilities and learning patterns to see what interferes with learning. Current information is as important as the individual's history. If the individual is in school, then it is important to read several recent term papers as well as look over class notes from lectures. Individuals with jobs can bring in reports, memos, or letters that are representative of work demands.

There is no specific test battery for diagnosing learning disabilities. Psychologists who specialize in working with individuals who have dyslexia or other types of learning disabilities use many of the same tests in their evaluation as are used in traditional psychological evaluations, but they view the results in a particular way. That is, during assessment of learning disabilities, qualitative information is always an important supplement to the quantitative results. The evaluator wants to know exactly what the client said and how he or she responded to each task. A trained diagnostician always administers tests in a standardized manner according to the test manual but views each test as a vehicle for deriving other important, perhaps subtle, currents of information. By listening carefully and recording precisely what the client says, an evaluator can pick up clues about receptive and expressive language problems, confusion in using prepositions, word substitutions, and so forth. Although this ancillary information may not directly affect the overall test results, it is important because it helps show vulnerabilities in the client's learning and performance and often illuminates why his or her performance in school or on the job has been uneven.

A typical test battery to identify learning disabilities in adults includes the Wechsler Adult Intelligence Scale–III (Wechsler, 1991); a silent reading test such as the Nelson-Denny Reading Test (Brown, Bennett, & Hanna, 1981) or the Gates-MacGinitie Reading Tests–Third Edition (MacGinitie & MacGinitie, 1989); the Wide Range Achievement Test–Third Edition (Wilkinson, 1993), which has Word Recognition, Spelling, and Math Computation subtests; a test of oral reading such as the Gray Oral Reading Test–Third Edition (GORT–3; Wiederholt & Bryant, 1992) or the Diagnostic Assessments of Reading with Trial Teaching Strategies (DARTTS; Roswell & Chall, 1992); a design copying test such as the Bender Visual Motor Gestalt Test (Bender, 1938); and several writing samples (usually one written during the session and two written at home between testing sessions), including Educational Memories (Blumenthal, 1981a). Other tests may be included, depending on the client's presenting problems, such as The House-Tree-Person Drawing (Buck, 1978), selected cards from the Thematic Apperception Test (TAT; Murray & Bellak, 1973), and a sentence completion test such as the Rotter Incomplete Sentences Blank–Second Edition (Rotter, Lah, & Rafferty, 1992). Sometimes a client has had a prior psychological examination but has not undergone reading tests or a writing evaluation. Although it is not necessary to redo what has been done already, a reading and writing assessment should be done before the specialist begins to work with the client.

After the testing is completed, the evaluator interprets the findings and explains them to the client. It is important for the evaluator as well as the remedial specialist (if the specialist is different from the evaluator) to present the results in as constructive a manner as possible. When the evaluator uses trial teaching techniques and judiciously chosen teaching materials, the client can begin to sense how he or she can make progress. After test findings were explained to one young physician and he had begun working on his problems, he wrote the following:

My diagnosis as dyslexic, i.e., reading more slowly in order to understand, was both difficult and refreshing. At first I had attached a stigma to it, yet it was also refreshing, because it validated my life experience. I now feel in control. Adequate time to read translates into adequate time to process and understand.

EDUCATIONAL MEMORIES

The Educational Memories writing sample measure provides information that cannot be obtained through typical diagnostic tests. Between the initial telephone call and the time of the first testing appointment, clients receive a writing assignment that focuses on their school memories. Clients are asked to relate their own version of their educational experience, including both positive and negative memories. They write a first draft only, by hand, on 8.5" × 11" paper. They should avoid talking to family members or using a dictionary or any other reference source. Educational Memories allows evaluators to get to know more about a client and at the same time obtain a writing sample for close examination. Most individuals write seven to nine handwritten pages.

Educational Memories serves as a valuable part of the diagnostic examination for a number of reasons. First, it is possible to find out what insights the client has about his or her own difficulties. Second, the writing sample reveals information about the individual's tendency to blame him- or herself or others for any difficulties faced. Third, the sample gives a sense of the emotional impact of years of struggling with school and/or work. Finally, the writing sample offers an initial view of the person's ability to organize information. This sample also allows an examination of handwriting, grammar, syntax, vocabulary, and spelling. The Educational Memories sample also is a useful part of the diagnostic process because it helps diagnosticians differentiate between individuals who have learning difficulties and those who do not. Individuals with learning difficulties rarely report positive memories about school. Their negative memories always center around difficulties with mastery. In contrast, individuals with no learning difficulties have many more positive memories of school, and their negative memories relate not to mastery but instead to specific social problems (e.g., I was never popular. I didn't get invited to parties) or to the harshness of particular teachers.

Following are excerpts from the Educational Memories samples of four individuals that illustrate how painful the introduction to school can be, particularly in the beginning years when children are especially vulnerable.

Bobbie

Bobbie, a 45-year-old woman with learning and memory problems, admitted during her first session that she has never read a book all of the way through.

She is now in a graduate program with approximately 1,000 pages per week of assigned reading, such as Freud, D.W. Winnicott, and Melanie Klein. Bobbie wrote,

I always have difficulty remembering what I read, and also I have trouble with facts and names. The memory of my education goes back to my very first day at school. I sat there and they debated whether or not I was retarded, because I did not know my name. I had been called Bobbie all my life, and had no idea my given name was Roberta.

Lana

Lana, a 30-year-old woman studying for her bachelor of science degree in physical therapy, wrote the following:

From the time I was around 8 years old, I have had this underlying feeling of inadequacy and inferiority, which is very tied into my feelings about school. The two are almost synonymous. My driving force to get my B.S. is to rid myself of this burden.

Derek

Derek, a 27-year-old law student, recalled the following in his write-up:

I attended private school from nursery through third grade, and it was there where I encountered the most academic difficulty. The school told my parents that I was "unteachable." This attitude is reflected in a progress report from the third grade in which it was stated they no longer measured my advancement on a scale with other students: "His grades reflect individual progress rather than third-grade expectations." These are particularly painful years to remember as my self-esteem was significantly diminished.

Mark

Mark, a 22-year-old dental student, wrote the following:

My earliest academic memories are filled with anxiety—feeling the inability to master all of the spelling words for the Monday morning quiz. As I grew older, reading quickly and accurately became more important. I always had to work longer and concentrate more intently than my peers. Finally, my compensatory mechanisms of using extra time were inadequate because I was confronted with timed exams, and no matter how much I prepared I was faced with my nemesis, only a limited amount of time to read. This forced me to skim over material rather than master it, and I therefore could not answer questions on topics I was familiar with.

REFLECT, CONNECT, and RESPOND
What information can a teacher who works with adult learners gather from the Educational Memories writing sample? Based on the excerpts, what principles are important to keep in mind when working with adult learners who have experienced learning difficulties since childhood?

THE MOST COMMON NEEDS OF HIGH-FUNCTIONING STUDENTS WITH DYSLEXIA AND OTHER ACADEMIC CHALLENGES

Experimental research on adult literacy has lagged behind the abundance of experimental research on childhood literacy. As McCardle and Chhabra (2004) pointed out, the extent of the need for adult literacy intervention, especially among adults who are black, Hispanic, and non–native speakers of English, is known, but there is little that informs educators on what kind of programs or instruction are effective. The need for this kind of research and the training of specialists on scientifically based methods in adult literacy are priorities.

Individuals with learning difficulties or dyslexia usually need help in one or more of the following areas: silent reading comprehension skills, vocabulary development, expressive language (writing) skills, spelling, study skills, and managing or allocating time in a constructive manner. Each person may have a greater or lesser degree of difficulty with any one of these areas and may not have difficulty with all of them. It is particularly important to remember that each person presents a unique combination of strengths as well as weaknesses. The remediation plan has to be tailored to that person's specific needs. Often, the client manifests competence in unexpected areas as well as surprising gaps in background knowledge. Information gathered from the individual's history, diagnostic study, and examination of current work as well as trial teaching helps to pinpoint areas that need attention.

There are several important goals in treatment. The first goal is to change the individual's perception of him- or herself from someone who cannot learn to one who can learn by helping the person become an active learner. Many readers who have learning and reading problems are too passive in relation to the material they read. As a result, their retention, understanding, and even appreciation are affected. Being an active learner means thinking about and evaluating the material being read. Active learning involves bringing prior information to the discussion of the subject at hand. The active reader tries to discern the author's point of view. Encouraging making the transition from a passive to a more active approach to reading requires guidance from the remedial specialist. The remedial specialist needs to know when to pose evocative questions, how to elicit information, and when to prepare the client to develop insights about the material.

For example, Evelyn, an ambitious college graduate, was running a successful business and wanted to go to graduate school for her master of business administration degree. The evaluation showed that she had a slow reading rate and had difficulty retaining what she read. Evelyn thought that she often missed main ideas, which undermined her confidence in general. An intelligent woman, she was quite interested in world affairs. She was encouraged to read the editorial columns in the daily newspaper to improve her reading comprehension and retention of information. Instead of skimming articles and retaining a minimal amount, as she had done formerly, Evelyn was asked to approach the reading material differently, using a four-step approach.

1. First, she should read the headline and subhead and before reading further, ask herself, "What do I think this article is about?" By posing this question, she immediately became more active and focused on the article's topic.

2. Next, she should read the article and then ask herself, "What did the author say?"

3. Then, she should ask, "What did I learn that was new?"

4. Finally, she should ask, "What is my opinion about this subject? Do I agree or disagree?"

After using this approach with one newspaper article, Evelyn wrote a one-page essay about the article, which she brought to the next session. The entire assignment took her about 1 hour at home. This active approach stimulated her ability to concentrate, fostered her retention, and improved her writing skills. After approximately 2 months of remediation, Evelyn commented, "At first it seemed like I was taking baby steps, but the way I read is really changing. When we went out to dinner with friends, it was amazing, I found I had facts and opinions and held my own in the discussion." Evelyn also worked with a variety of other standard-ized reading comprehension materials, such as Six-Way Paragraphs (Advanced) by Pauk (1983), and in doing so improved her concentration, reading comprehen-sion, and writing skills. At the end of the year, she took the Graduate Management Admissions Test with extended time and was accepted into business school, where she did well.

Progress can be made when the therapeutic alliance is optimal and the demands of the remedial work are challenging but not overwhelming. The cli-ent often will report a sense of excitement about his or her own potential being realized. For example, one graduate student declared, "I looked at this assign-ment and said, 'I know you, you sucker! I can do it.'" Another client said, "I know that what is coming next will be hard, but now I think there is nothing I can't handle."

Helping the individual develop an awareness of his or her own thinking process is the second goal of remediation. Positive changes occur as individuals become aware of their own thinking, and thinking, reading, and writing become more efficient. It is possible to stimulate and activate cognitive processes such as reasoning, organizing, generalizing, and planning so that they are enhanced across a broad range of content areas. One way to encourage this kind of awareness of how one thinks is through the use of process notes (Blumenthal, 1981b).

Clients can be taught to be more aware of how they think, what interrupts their reasoning, and what helps them to continue their work. When clients face obstacles in doing their work, the remedial specialist can encourage them to write process notes; that is, to evaluate in writing their reactions to the assignment. This often helps clients to develop organizing principles, which facilitates their work.

For example, Ted, a doctoral student with dyslexia, referred himself for evalu-ation after he failed his written comprehensive exams. The members of the exam-ining committee had harsh comments and remarked on how "poorly written" and how "disorganized" Ted's written effort was. They raised questions about Ted's suitability in a doctoral program, perhaps forgetting that he had completed all of the coursework up to that point with excellent grades. None of the committee mem-bers thought about the discrepancy between Ted's record and his performance on the comprehensives, yet unevenness in performance is the hallmark of almost all learning disabilities.

Reading Ted's comprehensive exam was one of the first steps the remedial specialist took in helping Ted. Although the exam was more than 35 handwritten pages long, it was necessary to read it carefully to understand how Ted performed under pressure, evaluate exactly where he needed help, and develop a treatment plan. Although Ted experienced both anger and mild depression in reaction to his failure, his drive to improve his writing was prodigious. He responded well to the varied writing assignments that the remedial specialist gave him, most of which he completed in the library between sessions. During sessions, all completed work was read aloud, sentence by sentence, and discussed in relation to clarity, organization, and effectiveness. Although the remedial specialist made no marks on Ted's paper, every unclear sentence was discussed. In essence, the remedial specialist modeled an active approach for Ted by questioning unclear areas rather than by writing correct answers. After the 20th session, the specialist encouraged Ted to write process notes. Ted wrote the following passage after the 21st session of work:

I began writing this time before I began typing—I began to frame this essay in my mind ahead of time. I asked a main question, and then made myself ask, "What does another person reading this have to know in order to understand both the question and the answer?" I asked myself, "Does the piece follow a logical and easily understood order?" and "Does each paragraph contain a logical order too? Do all the paragraphs fit together?" Although there were a good many spelling lapses, the general ordering of the ideas seem okay to me—and this is encouraging to me. I would have to say a guarded yes to my questions.

The working relationship between the remedial specialist and the client is never a static one. It draws its strength from the balance between necessary support and the increasing autonomy of the student as he or she becomes more able to compensate for his or her difficulties. In this case, Ted developed an awareness of the elements of effective and communicative writing. The revelation that his writing always needs to be understood by others continued to transform Ted's efforts, and Ted eventually integrated this principle into most of his writing. By the end of the year, he retook the comprehensive exams and passed with high commendations.

Finally, reducing anxiety related to learning is the third goal of treatment. A client can decrease anxiety while working on the area of his or her greatest vulnerability if a positive therapeutic alliance has been established, materials appropriate to the client's intellectual level are used, and each defined goal or task is broken down into manageable parts. Achieving all three goals of treatment—helping the individual to change his or her self-perception, develop an awareness of his or her thought processes, and reduce anxiety—can help the individual to achieve a degree of mastery. The following three case examples illustrate these points.

REFLECT, CONNECT, and RESPOND
What are the three main goals of treatment when working with adult learners, and why are these goals important? What additional goals would you add to the list?

Janet

The emotional repercussions of learning disabilities can interfere with a sense of positive self-worth and cause a person to feel intense shame. Janet, a friendly 30-year-old who works for a large corporation, graduated from a small liberal arts college with a degree in marketing.

Early History   Janet had difficulty learning to read in the early grades. During reading instruction, she was placed in a corrective reading group that met 5 times per week for 1 hour each time. Janet recalls that reading was always difficult for her. In high school, her parents helped her with assignments. They helped her review before tests and made editorial and spelling changes on her papers. She graduated from high school with a *C* average. Janet's anxiety heightened in college, and she often stayed up all night before an exam. She made it a point to find a study group. Her friends read her papers and made corrections before she handed them in. She did well enough so that no professor ever identified her as someone who needed to be referred for psychoeducational evaluation. After passing all of her courses, she graduated in 4 years.

Work History   After college, Janet worked in sales. Her organizational ability was praised, but she decided to change jobs because she wanted a position that included some travel. She took a job with the large corporation for whom she currently works. Her new job required interpersonal and organizational skills and also involved some travel. After 1 year, she had her first job review. She was rated outstanding in interpersonal skills and in working as a member of a team. In fact, she was rated well above average in every category except writing and communication skills. The job review noted, "Written work is dramatically inadequate for her level of responsibility." Janet was told that the quality of her written work would keep her from being promoted. Janet's boss told her that she thought that Janet had some kind of learning disability and strongly urged her to get help if she wanted to advance on the job.

Testing and Remediation   Janet was extremely anxious when she first consulted the psychoeducational diagnostician and wept helplessly when she talked about her learning problems. Confronting her problems with learning was so traumatic that a month passed after the first interview before she called to begin work. Her parents were supportive both emotionally and financially. Janet asked her parents not to tell anyone else in her family that she was getting help for her learning problems. She told her boss but did not tell any of her close friends. She felt stigmatized and very ashamed.

An intelligence test showed that Janet had average ability, but the unevenness of her subtest scores showed that she had higher potential ability. For example, her general knowledge clearly had been inhibited by lack of background reading. She also experienced considerable anxiety when asked to answer questions and do specific tasks; this anxiety had a definite negative impact on the intelligence test results.

On the Word Recognition subtest of the Wide Range Achievement Test–Third Edition (Wilkinson, 1993), Janet scored at the sixth percentile, which is equivalent to approximately an eighth-grade skill level. Her oral and silent reading were approximately at the 10th-grade level. When answering questions about the silent reading passages, Janet read the passages and had to look back at them to find every answer.

She was asked to write several short summaries. Although it was evident that she could express herself verbally, she was uncertain about how to put what she wanted to say in writing. Her fear about making spelling errors made her choose simple vocabulary that made her writing seem less mature.

The evaluation was stressful. The findings were interpreted and explained to her in as positive a manner as possible, but Janet felt despair about making progress. It seemed likely that Janet had experienced severe reading problems when she was a child. There was no indication in her history or in the current evaluation, however, that suggested that she would be unable to make progress during remediation, and the evaluator conveyed this positive outlook to her.

The Work   The first goal of treatment was to change Janet's perception of herself from someone who could not learn to someone who could learn by having Janet work on appropriate materials within the context of a supportive relationship. It was also necessary to reduce Janet's anxiety and despair related to learning.

Because of Janet's intense anxiety in relation to reading, writing, and words in general, it was particularly important for the remedial specialist to be supportive and nonpressuring and at the same time choose materials that were mature in format and content and appropriate to Janet's reading level. Janet and the remedial specialist met once per week, before Janet was due at work. Remediation focused on oral reading, vocabulary development, silent reading comprehension, and expressive language skills, including letter and memo writing, spelling, and word analysis. Janet reviewed expressive writing and vocabulary activities during the week at home.

Janet's first writing assignments were to write about members of her family. These assignments required no advance reading. Writing impressions about family and friends usually tends to be less stressful than a more formal assignment. The remedial specialist made no corrections on these first few writing assignments. After a few weeks, the specialist asked Janet to summarize an article of her choice from a newspaper. Janet was able to find articles she could read in *USA Today*. Because she rarely had looked at a newspaper, she and the specialist looked at one together to see how to locate news articles, the weather section, and human-interest stories. The specialist asked her to choose a newspaper article that appealed to her, read the article at home, and then summarize it in writing. Janet underlined any words in the article that she did not know or words that she thought she would have trouble defining. She read the summary aloud each week at her remedial session. Again, the specialist made no corrections at the time of the reading. Instead, the specialist chose one aspect of the writing—usually grammar, spelling, or general usage—for teaching during the next session. In this way, Janet felt less threatened because she was not corrected during her presentation and because skills were taught separately from the presentation. She began incorporating the grammar and usage lessons into her writing. After approximately 8 months, Janet started reading *The New York Times* instead of *USA Today*. This change boosted her self-esteem because her family and friends also read *The New York Times*. She generally found at least one article of interest to write about.

The newspaper reading was important to remediation because Janet avoided reading in general and never read the newspaper at all. After she had been attending remediation sessions for a while, Janet started to read the newspaper once per week and, as a consequence, had more to contribute when she socialized with her co-workers. Each week she added new words to her vocabulary by underlining new words at home. During remediation sessions, she and the specialist discussed and defined each word with the aid of a dictionary. By herself, Janet felt intimidated by the dictionary, but she did use it during sessions. She wrote each new word on a 3″ × 5″ index card with the definition on the reverse side. She also added a sentence using the word to help her to retain the word. The specialist also encouraged Janet to keep and bring to her sessions a list of any unknown words that she might hear at work. In this way, all of the new words studied were ones that Janet herself had selected rather than words from a list in a vocabulary book.

During each session Janet read a short selection silently and answered accompanying comprehension questions. She and the remedial specialist discussed any incorrect responses. The questions that posed the most problems for Janet were questions that required inferential thinking, a skill that is essential for advanced reading comprehension. Inferential thinking involves making accurate judgments and drawing conclusions about what is read. It was necessary for Janet to approach the text in a more interactive manner than she was accustomed to. She also tended to make literal interpretations that limited her understanding of subtleties. The remedial specialist helped her make more accurate inferences in the following way. Through guided discussion, Janet was encouraged to identify relationships between events in a passage as she and the specialist returned to the text for additional analysis of the content. The specialist helped Janet recognize that she often could use some prior knowledge to figure out an answer. Increased self-monitoring of her own thought processes was also encouraged. In this way, Janet began to derive more meaning from what she read.

Misspelled words were identified in Janet's weekly writing assignments and in the memos or reports that she wrote for her job so that she could improve her spelling skills. When the words were common and likely to be used frequently, she copied them in a small, alphabetized notebook that she could carry in her pocketbook. The remedial specialist reviewed the words with Janet during the weekly sessions and added to the list each week so that Janet became familiar with the words. When she needed to use a word in her writing, she referred to her personal dictionary. As time went on, she memorized many of the words, and they were dropped from the list. New words were added as Janet began to expand her vocabulary. In this way, her spelling skills improved steadily and so did her confidence in including a more varied vocabulary in her writing.

Although Janet was reading at the high school level, she was not confident about applying word analysis skills or syllabication skills to figure out new multisyllabic words. Because review of basic word analysis skills was a painful reminder of early school failures, word analysis was taught in conjunction with the words from newspaper articles that Janet mispronounced. For example, when she was not able to pronounce *mirth,* an opportunity arose for the remedial specialist to introduce the pronunciation of the special letter combinations *ir, ur,* and *er* and select different words for teaching and practice at the following session. Teaching was thus tied to use and did not take on the qualities of drills. All of the necessary word analysis skills were eventually reviewed.

Although Janet was motivated and conscientiously completed her writing and vocabulary review at home, she continued to hide her efforts from her friends and close family members. After approximately 8 months of remediation, Janet received a promotion and a pay bonus. Her boss no longer criticized her writing and communication skills. Janet was more confident and handled pressure and stress on her job with greater equanimity. She still tended to procrastinate when she had to write memos and letters, but she brought them to the remedial sessions more readily to work on them with her remedial specialist. Janet still found reading to be a struggle, but she was more willing to try to get information from books and began to read some self-help books related to career advancement.

After 1 1/2 years of remedial sessions, Janet had less anxiety and had increased confidence about reading and writing. As a result, she was able to learn and retain information more easily. She became more willing to write memos and letters at work and did not automatically think that whatever she wrote was of poor quality. Her vocabulary expanded, and she realized that she was aware of words in a way that she had not been before. She made an effort to retain what she knew by reviewing and trying to use the words in conversation.

Roy

Many individuals with learning disabilities or symptoms of mild dyslexia who have struggled for years in school tend to become discouraged and take an increasingly passive approach to academic work. This was the case with Roy, an articulate 24-year-old college graduate who was distressed about his future. He wanted to decide on a career but did not think he could do anything well.

Early History   Roy's earliest memory of school was of feeling frightened. In the first and second grade, he did not make sufficient progress in reading and was assigned to remedial reading classes. In addition, he went to tutors periodically throughout elementary school. He never read for pleasure and read only what was assigned. Roy described elementary school as frustrating. Roy chose to attend an alternative high school that offered smaller classes and more individual attention to each student. He became a student government leader but never excelled in his studies. In college, he graduated with a *B*-minus average and felt he had not learned as much as he would have liked. Roy stated that he never put his full effort into schoolwork. He told himself that if he did not do well, then he could also comfort himself with the fact that he had not tried very hard.

Testing and Remediation   After college, Roy was evaluated by a neuropsychologist who administered a comprehensive testing battery. Roy had done mediocre academic work throughout college, and the testing showed Roy to have uneven abilities. He had above-average ability in verbal and math areas, but he read very slowly and had a relatively limited vocabulary. He had extensive word retrieval problems and also had difficulty interpreting visual or pictorial material. The neuropsychologist discouraged Roy from attempting graduate school. No silent reading test was administered at the evaluation. Instead of choosing a career, Roy, with the encouragement of his family, decided to seek remediation for his learning difficulties.

Roy was interested in learning more about his problem and wanted to improve his reading skills, but he was ambivalent about working on anything academic. The remedial specialist needed a baseline measure because there was no current information about how well Roy could read textbook-like material. The Nelson-Denny Reading Test (Brown et al., 1981) was administered. The specialist made a mark on Roy's answer sheet when the standard time had passed but then allowed Roy to complete the test to find out his accuracy if he had sufficient time to finish the test. The results (relative to the results of typical college seniors) are shown in Table 21.1.

Table 21.1.   Roy's results on the Nelson-Denny Reading Test (Brown, Bennett, & Hanna, 1981), relative to the results of typical college seniors

Area tested	Standard time percentile	Extended time percentile
Vocabulary	12	82
Reading comprehension	31	85

From *Multisensory Teaching of Basic Language Skills, Third Edition* (p. 598).

The results indicated that although Roy had a slow rate of reading, he definitely could understand difficult material when he had sufficient time. At this point, Roy was quite discouraged and did not see himself as capable of doing well in school because he had never done so.

Many students who read slowly and struggle constantly to keep up with their work also never learn how to study effectively or sustain effort in order to master material for a difficult course of study. Roy had shown very uneven ability on the intelligence test, but he had average ability, and the pattern of scores suggested that he had higher potential ability. The silent reading test helped confirm his good basic ability. When devising a plan of treatment, the remedial specialist took into account Roy's statement that he had never put in full effort. The specialist interpreted and explained the results of the reading test to Roy in as positive a manner as possible; that is, she told him that the results showed that he had good basic ability and that although he had a slow rate of reading, he definitely could improve. She also told him that he expressed his ideas well in writing.

It is possible to help an individual change from being a passive reader to being an active one if appropriate materials are chosen and if assignments are presented both supportively and incrementally. It was important that Roy not be overwhelmed. The plan was to help him gradually perceive himself as a learner, as someone who could sustain effort even with difficult material. The plan also incorporated Roy's enjoyment of expressing his ideas in writing.

Roy came to weekly 1-hour remedial sessions and spent approximately 2 hours per week working at home. Each week he was assigned a short story by a writer such as Raymond Carver, Ernest Hemingway, George Orwell, Eudora Welty, or Italo Calvino. Roy was always able to complete each assignment because the stories were short. He felt positive about being able to do the assignments and, at the same time, learned about many new authors. After reading the week's story at home, he wrote a one- or two-page summary that included a discussion about the story's main theme. After a few weeks, he was also assigned to read an editorial essay in *The New York Times* by a regular editorial writer. Roy read and summarized these point-of-view articles at home. He was encouraged to agree or disagree with the columnist at the end of his summary. Roy was slowly but systematically beginning to acquire information both from literature and from current events. Roy liked to write, and the act of writing required him to become more interactive with the text. He began to discuss the new information with his family and his friends and engage more actively in discussion about politics.

Each week, Roy brought in a list of new words from the reading selection. Roy had an excellent speaking vocabulary but had a much more limited reading vocabulary because of his limited reading experience. He, therefore, had many new words to discuss each week. He and the remedial specialist chose 10 words per week to write on 3" x 5" cards and wrote the definitions on the reverse sides along with sentences from the article or book that included the new words. Roy and the remedial specialist discussed the meanings in the sessions, and Roy reviewed the words at home. Roy's vocabulary gradually improved. Other topical articles were introduced, for example, essays by Elisabeth Kübler-Ross and Betty Friedan, to broaden both his interests and his knowledge base. Finally, the remedial specialist asked Roy to get a book by a professional photographer. Every other week he wrote an essay about a photograph of his choice. He had to discern the story the photographer appeared to convey. The book contained no explanatory text, so Roy's entire essay had to be rooted in what he saw in the photograph. He got practice in interpreting visual and pictorial material, which had been identified as a problem area in his neuropsychological testing. His observations became more acute, and with practice, he began producing integrated essays that incorporated most of the visual details as well as the underlying drama in the photographs.

Roy's anxiety about learning and reading gradually lessened. All of Roy's written assignments were read aloud and discussed at the remedial sessions. He received general positive feedback as well as specific suggestions for improving his essays. At the end of 3 months, Roy began to think of himself as both well informed and well read. He saw that he had learned a great deal and had developed his own opinions about world events. He felt so energized by all of the information that he was absorbing and learning that he declared, "This has been the most exciting 3 months of my life!"

At this point, Roy began to have hope for his future. He decided that he might like to go to medical school. First, he had to prove to himself that he could put forth the effort in a sustained way. He and his remedial specialist found an undergraduate science course that he could take on a noncredit basis. He attended each week, did the reading and assignments, took the exams, and saw that he could master the material.

Next, as part of this new long-range plan, Roy had to apply for a program in which he could take all of his premed requirements because he had not been a science major in college. He took these background science courses over a 2-year period so that he and his remedial specialist could concentrate on effective study skills. It was necessary for him not only to become an active learner but also to begin to work in an increasingly independent manner. The remedial specialist encouraged him to sit near the front of the lecture room, prepare for class before going to the lecture, take complete notes, and review the notes after the lecture, underlining important points in red pencil. He learned to apply these study skills as the first term progressed. Before the midterm exams, the specialist encouraged Roy to go to his professors during office hours to ask questions about anything that was not clear. He first wrote out a list of the questions and left space for the answers. Roy was surprised to find that he was the only student who visited during office hours, so each professor spent the entire hour with him. In addition, Roy and the remedial specialist looked over the questions together to see whether his questions were based on insufficient information, misreading the text, or topics that were not covered in lectures. He could then focus on any vulnerable area when he studied.

During his first term, Roy definitely became a more active learner. He was introduced to the Survey, Question, Read, Recite, Review (SQ3R) method of study (Robinson, 1946), which helped him to be less overwhelmed by the science texts. These texts were difficult, but it was particularly helpful for Roy to find out that most of the information in each paragraph is represented in the first sentence of the paragraph and that the remaining sentences in the paragraph support the first sentence with details.

Roy remained motivated throughout the 2 years, even though the premed courses were difficult and demanding. At the end of the 2 years, he had earned seven *A*s and one *B*. He took the Medical College Admissions Test (MCAT) with extended time because he had a diagnosis of dyslexia. His score on the MCAT was above average, and Roy was accepted to medical school. Although Roy's reading rate had improved, it still was slower than that of the average student. As a consequence, he requested and was granted extended time on examinations in medical school. Roy continued to do well in medical school.

Evan

A student's reading comprehension, expressive writing, and mathematical skills can be above average, and the student still may not do well in college. Puzzled parents and teachers often call these students "underachievers." Positive changes can occur when these students are helped to become more attentive to their own thinking processes, however. These cognitive processes are usually related to organizational, attentional, and strategy issues. Executive function, a concept from clinical **neuropsychology,** has been useful in understanding and working with these students. Often included under the rubric executive function are activities such as planning, prioritizing, sequencing, organizing, being able to shift focus, and following a project through to completion (Denckla, 1996). These students may not have actual deficits, but they seem unaware of what they need to do in order to be successful. First, they tend to be passive learners and are overly dependent on their teachers or professors to provide them with information. They do not seem conscious of the fact that it is up to them to initiate ideas, create outlines, and organize their time so that all of the work can get done. They have trouble prioritizing the steps of a task, and they are not flexible in shifting their focus when the task demands it. These issues become increasingly important as the students advance through school. Evan is an example of a student with a mild learning disability combined with problems in executive functioning.

Early History Evan, a well-spoken 20-year-old, reported that he always had difficulty concentrating in school and was easily distracted. He did not enjoy reading and tended to read only what was assigned for a class. In elementary school, he had been diagnosed as having mild dyslexia, but he did not receive any specialized help, probably because his grades were consistently above average. He did not excel in high school, but he graduated with a *B*-minus average and high SAT scores (Verbal, 680; Math, 710). When Evan was accepted at a competitive liberal arts college, he did not anticipate any difficulty with coursework. Not particularly self-reflective, Evan did not give much thought as to how to plan his time or how to study effectively when he began college. To his dismay, he did not do well in his academic subjects. The required reading was much more complex and dense than in high school, and the amount of new information to be absorbed and integrated was considerably higher. He found that he could not sustain his concentration long enough to study and retain material at a satisfactory level. He was not used to organizing his time, and often he did not leave sufficient time to complete long assignments, much less do a first draft and revisions. He had trouble working independently, something that is increasingly necessary as a student advances through college. Notetaking was not easy for him. If his attention wavered in class, then he often could not get back on track again for that class period.

Sensing he might be in academic trouble, he began to put extra time into studying in the library and in doing his schoolwork, but much to his disappointment, the results were not commensurate with his effort. He began to experience anxiety about his ability to do well in college, and his confidence plummeted. By the end of his sophomore year, Evan had achieved a *C*-plus average. He decided to take an official leave of absence and be evaluated for learning disabilities.

Testing and Remediation   The results of the neuropsychological evaluation showed Evan to be a cooperative and motivated student who was above average in general intelligence. He expressed a wish to do well in school, and he did not understand why his efforts did not result in better grades. He scored higher than the 85th percentile on a reading comprehension test and seemed to have good overall ability in reading. He could solve mental arithmetic problems quickly and accurately, was higher than average in abstract thinking, and had an excellent vocabulary. He was found to have mild organizational weaknesses, however. When a lot of unfamiliar information was presented, Evan seemed rattled and had difficulty deciding where to begin the task. Also, it was noted that, when encountering any degree of challenge in a task, Evan tended to give up easily rather than plan an approach and then generate strategies to solve the problem. Finally, although Evan did well on reading the relatively short reading comprehension passages, he was slow to apply phonic principles to multisyllabic, unfamiliar words that he had to read. This suggested that there was a lack of automaticity in his reading ability that might account, in part, for some of his problems with assignments. In college, reading material is usually much more difficult than in high school and requires reading original sources as well as the ability to sustain attention over time.

According to the evaluation, Evan was both puzzled and demoralized by his college performance. He pictured himself as a good student, but, at this point, his confidence was quite low. He had put in effort, but the results did not bear him out. He had tried studying by himself and with a small group of fellow students. Neither method led to success. A recurring comment by professors was that his papers were superficial and did not go deep enough.

After the results of the evaluation were interpreted to Evan, it was recommended that he begin work with a remedial specialist. Evan first found a part-time job, and then he began remediation. He had a wry, self-deprecating sense of humor, and from the start, it was clear that he was eager to collaborate in finding ways to be a more effective student. The remedial specialist's first goal was to help Evan see himself as someone who could learn and succeed in an academic setting. As part of the remediation plan, Evan was asked to summarize and comment on one chapter per week from *Into Thin Air* by Jon Krakauer (1997), a true adventure account of climbing Mt. Everest. He also was given a newspaper essay on a stimulating topic, which he was asked to summarize and critique. In the past, he had tended to procrastinate, and now he was urged to complete his assignments during the week, not at the last minute, so that he could improve and revise his writing if he wanted to. Evan and the remedial specialist particularly discussed the consequences of the themes included in both the essay and in the book. By starting his work in advance and looking for the ramifications and consequences in the essays, Evan began to spend more time on his own interpretations. As the weeks went on, he became more committed to the work.

During the session, Evan and the remedial specialist worked on improving inferential reading skills, expanding vocabulary, and focusing on writing as a way to communicate ideas. Evan began to care more about the words he chose to express himself and to re-read to decide if he had communicated effectively.

After 15 sessions, Evan had to decide whether to reenroll at his college or transfer to a nearby university. Instead of making an impulsive decision, Evan was persuaded to write two essays: one to support reenrollment at his college and the other about whether to transfer to the nearby university. He wrote two detailed essays for and against reenrollment. Evan and the remedial specialist talked about the pros and cons, and he discussed the options with his family. In the end, he decided to enroll as a nonmatriculated student at a nearby university, with the understanding that if he did well he would apply as a matriculated student.

Evan registered for three courses, which he chose himself. All of the courses required a term paper, plus a good deal of reading. To Evan's surprise, he found the lectures, the reading, and the assignments much more stimulating and compelling than he had ever experienced before. Together, he and the remedial specialist worked on planning a study schedule that he agreed he could adhere to. They discussed the topics for the assigned papers, and he chose his topic early in the term. He was encouraged to keep up with the required reading, to participate in class discussions, and to begin the research for his assigned papers early in the semester. The therapeutic alliance was positive, and he liked talking over the ideas from his courses. He was receptive to suggestions regarding how to study effectively. He began to function increasingly as an organized student. Procrastination ceased to be a major problem, and he started to set priorities among the demands of his schedule. After two semesters as a nonmatriculated student, Evan had maintained a GPA of 3.5 and was able to matriculate as a regular student.

Evan was feeling much more confident in general, and he began to look to the future and consider law as a career. In preparation, he decided on political science as a major area of study. By this time, Evan's approach toward mastering his coursework was much more organized. He set aside blocks of time for writing papers. On occasion, he would procrastinate, but that became much less of a problem. He found his courses interesting, and his attitude toward schoolwork continued to be positive. His written assignments and term papers were no longer criticized for being superficial. Instead, his professors tended to write "Good point" and "You write well." After 2 years, Evan graduated with a GPA of 3.5. Instead of going immediately to graduate school, Evan decided to work for 2 years as a paralegal. He found legal work interesting and was given increased responsibility and an opportunity to do legal research. At the end of 2 years, he began law school. Law school demands a student's full attention because of the sheer quantity of reading material and the special requirements of detailed written briefs and notes. Evan experienced the academic work as challenging but manageable. He was conscious of allocating his time so that he could complete his work in a timely manner. He was particularly satisfied with the praise he received for his analytic reasoning ability and for the clarity of his writing.

REFLECT, CONNECT, and RESPOND
Review the three main goals of treatment you identified earlier. How were these goals reflected in the experiences of Janet, Roy, and Evan? Of the three, which learner's story yielded the most information or insights for you as a teacher? Explain.

CLOSING THOUGHTS: WORKING
WITH HIGH-FUNCTIONING ADULTS WITH DYSLEXIA

Although the three individuals described in these case studies (Janet, Roy, and Evan) are quite different, they made a lot of progress and developed a greater sense of self-confidence. Although learning differences in high-functioning adults with dyslexia and other academic challenges vary greatly, all individuals have the potential to make progress. Each client should have a thorough and competent evaluation (which is interpreted to the client in the most positive manner possible), from which an effective treatment plan can be developed. When a treatment plan is successfully implemented, the client can take an active role in his or her own learning. Often, when clients understand their strengths and weaknesses, they can advocate for the necessary accommodations in school or on the job. When these accommodations are made, clients can show the extent of their knowledge better. They perform better, receive recognition for their improved performance, can sustain hope about the future, and often achieve their goals.

REFLECT, CONNECT, and RESPOND
Regardless of whether you work (or plan to work) with adults, how might you use what you have learned in this chapter to become a better teacher?

ONLINE COMPANION MATERIALS

The following Chapter 21 resources are available at http://www.brookespublishing .com/birshcarreker/materials:

- Reflect, Connect, and Respond Questions

- Appendix 21.1: Knowledge and Skill Assessment Answer Key

KNOWLEDGE AND SKILL ASSESSMENT

1. Who initiates the referral process for adults with learning difficulties or disabilities?

    a. Employers

    b. College or university faculty

    c. Mental health workers

    d. The adults themselves

    e. Any of the above

2. In which area do adults with learning difficulties or dyslexia typically *not* need help?

    a. Silent reading comprehension

    b. Spelling

    c. Rapid automatic naming tasks

    d.   Time management

    e.   Writing skills

3.   Which of the following types of assessments might be used with an adult who seeks help for learning difficulties?

    a.   Standard intelligence tests, such as the Wechsler Adult Intelligence Scale

    b.   Tests of oral reading ability

    c.   Writing samples

    d.   Psychological assessments such as the Thematic Apperception Test

    e.   All of the above

4.   When administering assessments to adults, how important is it to pay attention to qualitative information?

    a.   It is unimportant; a skilled evaluator can identify problems based on quantitative data alone.

    b.   It is important; the evaluator can use qualitative information to identify issues that might not be apparent from quantitative data alone.

    c.   It is extremely important; qualitative information usually is more significant than quantitative data.

    d.   Researchers disagree on whether paying attention to qualitative information is important.

    e.   The evaluator should always ignore qualitative information; to do otherwise compromises the assessment's validity.

REFERENCES

Bender, L. (1938). *Bender Visual Motor Gestalt Test.* San Antonio, TX: The Psychological Corporation.

Blumenthal, S. (1981a). *Educational Memories.* Unpublished manuscript.

Blumenthal, S. (1981b). *Process Notes.* Unpublished manuscript.

Brown, J.I., Bennett, J.M., & Hanna, G.S. (1981). *The Nelson-Denny Reading Test.* Chicago, IL: Riverside.

Buck, J.N. (1978). *The House-Tree-Person Technique* (Rev. manual). Los Angeles, CA: Western Psychological Services.

Denckla, M.B. (1996). A theory and model of executive function: A neuropsychological perspective. In G.R. Lyon & N.A. Krasnegor (Eds.), *Attention, memory, and executive function* (pp. 263–278). Baltimore, MD: Paul H. Brookes Publishing Co.

Krakauer, J. (1997). *Into thin air.* New York, NY: Villard Books.

MacGinitie, W.H., & MacGinitie, R.H. (1989). *Gates-MacGinitie Reading Tests–Third Edition.* Chicago, IL: Riverside.

McCardle, P., & Chhabra, V. (Eds.). (2004). *The voice of evidence in reading research.* Baltimore, MD: Paul H. Brookes Publishing Co.

Murray, H.A., & Bellak, L. (1973). *Thematic Apperception Test (TAT).* San Antonio, TX: The Psychological Corporation.

Pauk, W. (1983). *Six-way paragraphs (advanced).* Providence, RI: Jamestown Publishers.

Robinson, F.P. (1946). *Effective study.* New York, NY: HarperCollins.

Roswell, F.G., & Chall, J.S. (1992). *Diagnostic Assessments of Reading with Trial Teaching Strategies (DARTTS).* Chicago, IL: Riverside.

Rotter, J.B., Lah, M.I., & Rafferty, J.E. (1992). *Rotter Incomplete Sentences Blank–Second Edition.* San Antonio, TX: The Psychological Corporation.

Wechsler, D. (1991). *Wechsler Adult Intelligence Scale–III.* San Antonio, TX: Harcourt Assessment.

Wiederholt, J.L., & Bryant, B.R. (1992). *Gray Oral Reading Test–Third Edition (GORT–3).* Austin, TX: PRO-ED.

Wilkinson, G.S. (1993). *Wide Range Achievement Test–Third Edition: Manual.* Wilmington, DE: Jastak Associates.

Glossary

Robin Anderson Singer

3PV 3RQ Evidence-based strategy for reading comprehension with adaptations for English language learners (ELLs): determining purpose, preparing a connection, predicting, working with vocabulary, reading, and answering questions.

academic vocabulary Language of the classroom; an essential part of the oral and written discourse necessary for academic success that should be used liberally throughout the school day.

accent Stress or emphasis on one syllable in a word or on one or more words in a phrase or sentence. The accented part is spoken louder, longer, and/or in a higher tone. The speaker's mouth opens wider while saying an accented syllable. *See also* suprasegmental.

accommodations Accommodations change *how* a student learns material. Changes within the general education classroom to enable students to keep up with the education program, such as intensive instruction; reduced assignments; adapted test procedures; and the use of computers, calculators, and audio recorders. The term *accommodations* is not used in the Individuals with Disabilities Education Improvement Act (IDEA) of 2004 (PL 108-446). That law, however, generally refers to supplemental services that are, for the most part, what Section 504 of the Rehabilitation Act Amendments of 1998 (PL 105-220) and the Americans with Disabilities Act (ADA) of 1990 (PL 101-336) call reasonable accommodations.

active learning Learning in which the learner mentally searches for connections between new and already known information. Also students are more involved in the process of learning.

ADD *See* attention deficit disorder.

adding A manipulation task that requires inclusion of another syllable or phoneme to a given word.

ADHD *See* attention-deficit/hyperactivity disorder.

affix A letter or a group of letters attached to the beginning or ending of a base word or root that creates a derivative with a meaning or grammatical form that is different than the base word or root. *See also* prefix; suffix.

affricate A consonant speech sound that is articulated with the tongue touching the roof of the mouth (e.g., /ch/ in *chair*, /j/ in *judge*) (Henry, 2003; Moats, 2010).

agnosia *See* finger agnosia.

air writing *See* sky writing.

alliteration　The repetition of the initial sound in two or more words such as "laughing llamas."

allophones　Slight variations in production of vowels or consonants that are predictable variants of a phoneme (e.g., /p/ in *pot* and *spot*, /ă/ in *fast* and *tank*).

alphabet　A series of letters or signs arranged in a fixed sequence, each of which represents a spoken sound of that language. Knowing the 26 letters of the English alphabet is essential to the language skills—phonics, reading, writing, and spelling.

alphabet knowledge　A student's ability to identify and name the letters of the alphabet.

alphabetic language　A language, such as English, in which letters are used systematically to represent speech sounds, or phonemes.

alphabetic principle　The concept that letters and letter patterns represent the sounds of spoken language.

alveolar　Pertaining to sounds produced with the tongue placed against the alveolar ridge behind the upper front teeth (e.g., /n/, /s/).

alveolar ridge　The gum ridge behind the upper front teeth.

amanuensis　A person, such as a teacher, who writes while another person, such as a student, dictates words, sentences, or stories.

analytic　Pertaining to instruction or a process that separates the whole into its constituent parts to reveal the relationships of the parts. Analytic phonics separates the whole word into its constituent parts so that students can deduce the phonic relationships of the separate orthographic patterns. *See also* synthetic.

anaphora　Using a pronoun or a definite article to refer to something already mentioned (e.g., The turtle moved slowly. *It* crept along the road).

Anglo-Saxon　The language of the Germanic peoples (Angles, Saxons, and Jutes) who settled in Britain in the 5th and 6th centuries A.D. Anglo-Saxon was the dominant language in Britain until the Norman Conquest in 1066 and is a major contributor to the English language.

antonyms　Words of opposite meaning.

appositive　A noun or noun phrase that is placed after a noun to explain it more fully; it usually contains modifiers (e.g., Susan B. Anthony, an influential suffragist, appears on the silver dollar).

argumentative writing　Writing whose purpose is to convince the reader to accept a certain viewpoint through evidence, such as the use of facts and statistics, reasons, and quotes from experts. This writing appeals to logic and lacks an emotional appeal.

articulation　The vocal production of speech in which the mouth, tongue, lips, teeth, and other parts of the vocal tract are used in specific ways.

aspiration The push of air that accompanies the production of some stop consonants (e.g., /t/ in *top*) (Moats, 2010).

assessment Collection of information to make decisions about learning and instruction.

assistive technology Any item, piece of equipment, or product that is used to increase, maintain, or improve the functional capabilities of individuals with disabilities.

attention deficit disorder (ADD) Disorder characterized by difficulty with attending to and completing tasks.

attention-deficit/hyperactivity disorder (ADHD) Disorder characterized by difficulty with attending to and completing tasks, impulsivity, and/or hyperactivity that frequently co-occurs with but is not a learning disability. *See also* learning disability.

auditory discovery Listening and responding to guided questions to discover new information, such as when students echo words dictated by the teacher to discover a new common sound.

automaticity Ability to respond or react without attention or conscious effort. Automaticity in word recognition permits full energy to be focused on comprehension.

background knowledge The prior knowledge a student brings to a reading task. For example, if a student is reading a passage about the American Revolution, then his or her prior knowledge about the war will bolster comprehension.

base element The morphological base of a word that holds the core to its meaning (e.g., *struct* is the base element in *construction*). Also called *root word*.

base word A word to which affixes are added (e.g., *whole* in *unwholesome*). A base word can stand alone. *See also* free morpheme.

bilabial Pertaining to consonant sounds produced with the two lips contacting each other.

biliteracy The ability to speak, read, and write in two languages.

blend Two or more adjacent consonants (a consonant blend) or two or more adjacent vowels (a vowel blend) whose sounds flow smoothly together. *See also* blending.

blending Fusing individual sounds, syllables, or words to produce meaningful units or to sound out (e.g., saying /m/ /ă/ /p/ as "map," saying "tooth" and "brush" as "toothbrush").

blocked *See* continuant.

bound morpheme A morpheme that must be attached to other morphemes (e.g., *-ed* in *spotted*, *-s* in *boys*, *pre-* in *preview*). *See also* free morpheme.

breve   The curved diacritical mark (˘) above a vowel in a sound picture or phonic/dictionary symbol notation that indicates a short vowel sound (e.g., ĭt, căt, blĕnd, dĭvide').

Broca's area   Region of the brain responsible for speech.

CBMs   *See* curriculum-based measures.

CCSS   *See* Common Core State Standards.

chaining   An activity in which a phoneme in a word changes in a string of words (e.g., "Say *hat* and change the /h/ to /k/ to get *cat*, change the /k/ to /p/ to get *pat*, change the /p/ to /r/ to get *rat*").

checkpoint   *See* marker.

choral reading   Reading in which the instructor and the student(s) read the passage aloud together. *See also* echo reading; shared reading.

circumflex   A diacritical mark (ˆ) placed over certain vowels when coding or when writing a sound picture to indicate an unexpected pronunciation. The circumflex is used in Alphabetic Phonics (Cox, 1992) coding to indicate when a vowel-*r* combination is accented (e.g., âr, êr, îr, ôr, ûr). The circumflex is also used over the circled *a* to indicate the /aw/ pronunciation before /l/ in a monosyllabic word (e.g., b â ll).

close reading   A deep examination of a text.

closed syllable   A syllable ending with one or more consonants after one vowel (e.g., *mat, hand*). The vowel is usually short. *See also* open syllable.

cloze technique   Any of several ways of measuring a student's ability to restore omitted portions of an oral or written message from its remaining context. Also called *fill-in-the blank technique.*

clue   *See* context clue; *see also* marker.

coarticulation   The phenomenon of word pronunciation in which adjacent sounds often are spoken in such a way that one phoneme seems to overlap, is changed by, and/or modifies another.

cognates   *See* voiced-voiceless cognates. Also words in different languages that are derived from the same morphome or morphemes (e.g., *geography* in English, *geografía* in Spanish).

cognitive flexibility   Ability to shift attention among competing stimuli and consider alternatives.

cognitive strategies   Self-regulating mechanisms, including planning, testing, checking, revising, and evaluating, during an attempt to learn or to problem-solve. Using cognitive strategies is a higher order cognitive skill that influences and directs the use of lower order skills.

collaborative learning   Learning by working together in small groups to understand new information or to create a common product.

combination   *See* letter cluster.

combining form   Greek combining forms are meaning-carrying units that compound to form words (e.g., *autograph, microscope*).

Common Core State Standards (CCSS)   These standards define educational goals for what students should know and be able to do in language arts and mathematics by the end of each grade level.

compare-and-contrast composition   Writing that explores the similarities and differences between related or unrelated objects, concepts, or categories. For example, writing that describes how dogs and foxes are the same and different.

compound word   A word composed of two or more smaller words (e.g., *doghouse*). A compound word may or may not be hyphenated depending on its part of speech and conventions of usage (e.g., in modern usage, *football* is not hyphenated).

comprehension   Making sense of what we read. Comprehension depends on good word recognition, fluency, vocabulary, worldly knowledge, and language ability.

comprehension monitoring   The active awareness of whether one is understanding or remembering text being processed.

concepts of print   The ability of a child to know and recognize the ways in which print "works" for the purposes of reading, particularly with regard to books.

conjunction   A part of speech that serves to connect words, phrases, clauses, or sentences (e.g., *and, but, as, because*). Also called *connectives*.

consolidated alphabetic   Phase when a reader can instantly recognize entire words (rather than sequences of letters).

consonant   One of a class of speech sounds in which sound moving through the vocal tract is constricted or obstructed by the lips, tongue, or teeth during articulation.

consonant blend   *See* blend.

consonant digraph   *See* digraph.

consonant prefix   A prefix that ends with a consonant. The spelling of a consonant prefix may change for euphony (e.g., *ad-* becomes *at-* in *attraction*, *in-* becomes *ir-* in *irresponsible*). *See also* euphony.

consonant suffix   A suffix beginning with a consonant (e.g., *-ful, -ness*).

consonant-*le* syllable   A syllable in final position of a word that ends in a consonant, an *l*, and final silent *e* (e.g., *middle, rifle*). *See also* final stable syllable.

consonant-vowel-consonant (CVC)   Pertaining to a word or syllable composed of letters with a consonant-vowel-consonant pattern. Short words or syllables with this pattern are a common starting point for reading phonetically regular words.

content   In Multisensory Structured Literacy instruction, the elements of Structured Literacy to be taught: phonology, phonics, morphology, handwriting, composition, syntax, text reading fluency, vocabulary, and semantics-comprehension. *See also* context; process.

context   In Multisensory Structured Literacy instruction, the learning environment or setting for teacher instruction and student learning. *See also* content; process.

context clue   Information from the immediate setting in which a word occurs, such as surrounding words, phrases, sentences, illustrations, syntax, or typography, that might be used to help determine the meaning and/or pronunciation of the word. Also called *contextual clue, visual hint.*

context processor   In the Four-Part Processing Model for Word Recognition, this is the neural processing system involved in the use of language experiences and context to confirm word recognition and meaning. *See also* Four-Part Processing Model for Word Recognition; meaning processor; orthographic processor; phonological processor.

continuant   Pertaining to speech sounds that are sustained in their production (e.g., /f/, /m/, /s/)

continuous text   Linked words such as the wording found in sentences, phrases, and paragraphs. Also known as *connected text.*

controlled decodable text   Text that is written with 95%–100% of the words already taught, either through word structure or by memory as a high-frequency word; used to apply phonics in reading of text. Also called *controlled text.*

convergence of evidence   Evidence from the identical replication of a study in a similar population by other researchers. Convergence of evidence is important in drawing conclusions from research because the outcomes from a single study are not sufficient to generalize across all populations.

cooperative learning   Instructional approach in which students work together rather than compete to solve a problem or to complete a task.

co-normed   When a test is created, it is administered to the same students along with one or more other tests so that results can be compared without using different population samples.

corrective feedback   Teacher responses during and following performance of a skill that is sensitive to the student's level and that guides him or her closer to mastery.

criterion-referenced scores   Test scores that examine whether the student has met a goal, such as reading a certain number of words per minute with a text.

criterion-referenced test   Test in which performance is assessed in terms of the kind of behavior expected of a person with a given score. A criterion-referenced test permits descriptions of a child's domain of knowledge represented in the test and allows an item-by-item description of knowledge attained and knowledge yet to be acquired. *See also* informal assessment or test.

critical thinking   An attitude of deep, focused thought, along with knowledge of strategies of logical reasoning.

cross-modal integration   Combination of information received as visual, auditory, kinesthetic, and tactile input.

Cuisenaire rods   Published educational material of wooden rods of different sizes used to make mathematical concepts and learning concrete and able to be manipulated.

cumulative   Describes instruction that is presented in a sequence that begins with the simplest skills and concepts and progresses systematically to the more difficult.

curriculum-based measures (CBMs) Assessments that measure how well a student performs for the standards of a particular curriculum.

curriculum-referenced assessment Test in which items are taken from the curriculum used in the child's classroom so that he or she is not tested on material that has not been taught. A curriculum-referenced test provides a good match between assessment and instruction and may be standardized or informal. *See also* informal assessment or test; standardized assessment or test.

cursive handwriting Handwriting with the slanted strokes of successive characters joined and the angles rounded.

CVC *See* consonant-vowel-consonant.

DAP *See* developmentally appropriate practice.

decodable text Text that is written at the independent reading level of a student; for the text to be decodable the student should be able to read 95%–100% of the words independently, with no more than 1 error per 20 words.

decode To break the phonic code (to recognize a word); to determine the pronunciation of a word by noting the position of the vowels and consonants.

deductive Pertaining to the blending of individual sounds (phonemes) into a whole syllable (or word). *See* synthetic.

deep *See* opaque.

deictic term A word whose use and meaning change based on context (e.g., *I, you, tomorrow, here, there*).

deletion *See* elision; *see also* sound deletion.

derivation The process of building a new word from another word by adding affixes. For example, *deconstructing* is a derivative of *deconstruct*, which in turn is derived from *construct*. *See also* etymology.

derivational morpheme Morpheme added to a base word that creates a new word that is a different part of speech from that of the base word (e.g., *-ness* changes adjective *careless* into noun *carelessness*).

derivational suffix Suffix added to a base word or root and changes the part of speech or the function of the base word or root (e.g., *-ful*).

derivative A word made from a base word by adding one or more affixes.

descriptive writing Writing that describes a person, place, object, or event, often using sensory or figurative language; for example, a description of someone's pet.

developmentally appropriate practice (DAP) An approach to teaching grounded in the research on how young children develop and learn and in what is known about effective early education. Its framework is designed to promote young children's optimal learning and development through interaction with both adults and the environment. It has three elements: knowing about child development and learning, knowing the individual child, and knowing the cultural context of the child.

diachronic   Describes etymology pertaining to the influence that roots of words (e.g., Latin, Greek, Old English) have on the meanings and spellings of words currently in the language.

diacritical marking   A distinguishing mark used in dictionaries and phonics programs to indicate the pronunciation of a letter or combination of letters. *See also* breve; circumflex; macron.

diagnostic   Pertaining to instruction in which the teacher is constantly taking notice of how students are handling the lesson concepts. Diagnostic instruction is sometimes used in conjunction with prescriptive instruction. *See also* diagnostic and prescriptive instruction.

diagnostic and prescriptive instruction   Instruction in which students are engaged in components of the lesson while the teacher observes how students are handling the discrete components (diagnostic instruction) so that the teacher may plan instruction. The prescriptive part of the lesson may involve changes to permit additional practice, review, and/or multisensory activities.

dialogic reading   A reading activity that involves an adult reading a book to an individual or a small group of children with the level of interaction more extensive and interactive.

differentiated instruction   An approach to instruction in which the teacher adapts content and teaching practices in response to individual student readiness, interests, ability, and learning profile.

digital text   *See* electronic text.

digraph   Two adjacent consonants (a consonant digraph) or two adjacent vowels (a vowel digraph) in the same syllable representing a single speech sound (e.g., *sh* in *wish*, *ee* in *feet*). *See also* diphthong; quadrigraph; trigraph.

diphthong   Two adjacent vowels in the same syllable whose sounds blend together with a slide or shift during the production of the syllable (e.g., *oy* in *toy*, *ow* in *cow*). *See also* digraph.

directionality   The direction used in a language for reading and writing. English is governed by left-to-right directionality.

discovery learning   *See* Socratic method.

discovery words   Group of related words used during guided discovery teaching to help students perceive a principle, pattern, or feature of the language. *See also* guided discovery teaching.

discrepancy model   A means of identifying a learning disability by using a combination of cognitive and achievement tests. A student is diagnosed with a learning disability and therefore eligible for special education services when he or she exhibits a severe discrepancy between intellectual ability and academic achievement.

discrimination   The process of noting differences between stimuli. Auditory discrimination involves listening for the position of a particular sound in a word.

dorsal pathway   Region of the brain that codes for the location in space of letters and words and programs eye movements and attention directed toward letters and words.

dysarthria Neurological oral-motor dysfunction including weaknesses of the musculature necessary for making the coordinated movements of speech production.

dyscalculia Specific learning disability in learning and understanding mathematical concepts.

dysgraphia Extremely poor handwriting or the inability to perform the motor movements required for handwriting. The condition is associated with neurological dysfunction.

dyslexia According to Lyon, Shaywitz, and Shaywitz, "Dyslexia is a specific learning disability that is neurobiological in origin. It is characterized by difficulties with accurate and/or fluent word recognition and by poor spelling and decoding abilities. These difficulties typically result from a deficit in the phonological component of language that is often unexpected in relation to other cognitive abilities and the provision of effective classroom instruction. Secondary consequences may include problems in reading comprehension and reduced reading experience that can impede growth of vocabulary and background knowledge" (2003, p. 2).

dyspraxia Sensorimotor disruption in which the motor signals to the muscles, such as those necessary for speech production, are not consistently or efficiently received.

echo reading Reading in which the instructor reads a paragraph aloud and has the student(s) read it aloud after the instructor has finished reading. *See also* choral reading; shared reading.

ecological validity A test's resemblance to the contexts of everyday life. *See also* face validity; validity.

effect size The degree to which a form of instruction is found through research to be more effective than another form.

electronic text Text material that has been converted to a digital format on a computer. Also called *e-text.*

elision A language task in which a part is taken away. Also called *deletion.*

Elkonin boxes An instructional technique to build phonemic awareness in which the teacher draws a series of squares, repeats a word, and then asks the student to place a token in the appropriate number of boxes to indicate how many phonemes in the target word. For example, for the target word *wish,* the student would select three tokens and place each of them in three different boxes.

ELL *See* English language learner.

ellipsis The omission of one or more words in a statement that must be supplied by the reader so the construction makes sense (e.g., "Do you like tortillas? I do").

embedded clause A clause enclosed within a sentence (e.g., The hummingbird, whose wings beat very rapidly, has brilliant plumage). *See also* relative clause.

embedded phonics Phonological awareness and phonics taught implicitly through reading real words in text.

emergent literacy The cognitive maturation characterized by well-developed oral language ability, exposure to written language, and metalinguistic awareness.

encode   To spell a word.

English language learner (ELL)   A student who is learning English, who comes from a language background other than English, and whose English proficiency is not fully developed.

epilinguistic   Pertaining to implicit sensitivity to word structure.

eponym   A word for a place, an object, or an action that is named after an individual (e.g., *sandwich, Fahrenheit, diesel*).

ERP   *See* event-related potential.

ethnographic observation   A type of qualitative research in which researchers observe, listen, and ask questions to collect descriptive data in order to understand the content, context, and dynamics of an environment. *See also* qualitative research.

etymology   The study of the origins and historical development of words.

euphony   Beautiful or pleasing sound (from Greek). A desire for euphony may explain why, in the development of the English language, the last letter of certain prefixes drop or change to match the first letter of the base words or stems (e.g., *emit*, not *exmit*; *irregular*, not *inregular*). Knowing this phenomenon is an aid to spelling.

event-related potential (ERP)   The measured brain response that is the direct result of a specific sensory, cognitive, or motor event.

evidence   Information in the text to support a claim, typically as answers to text-dependent questions.

evidence-based research   *See* scientifically based research.

exaggerated pronunciation   Overpronunciation of a word as an aid to spelling. Students with dyslexia are encouraged to develop and practice exaggerated pronunciation at first as needed to strengthen auditory memory. Thus, vowel sounds in unaccented syllables are not reduced to the indistinguishable schwa sound but are pronounced phonetically (e.g., the closed syllable in *vital* is exaggerated as /tal/ to emphasize the *a*). Also called *spelling-based pronunciation, spelling pronunciation,* or *spelling voice.*

executive function   The mental processes that allow individuals to regulate their thinking and behaviors.

executive function difficulties   Difficulties with certain cognitive skills such as poor planning, disorganization of time and materials, difficulty narrowing a topic in writing, and procrastination.

experimental research   Experimental educational research raises a question based on a theory, which determines the experimental design for directly investigating the question using scientific methods of collecting data using rigorously applied methods of instruction, with detailed descriptions of the participants and measures used. In this kind of experimental research, the data are interpreted to yield results of the impact of the manipulation and control of the conditions of observation. Studies thus designed can be analyzed for knowledge gained and can be replicated.

explicit instruction Teaching a specific skill step by step, also known as direct instruction.

expository writing Writing that explains or informs, including persuasive or descriptive writing and compare-and-contrast compositions.

expressive language This type of language refers to the words a child speaks and then later writes.

face validity The appearance of an assessment's measuring an aspect or of having meaning (e.g., if a test looks as if it must be measuring reading comprehension, one might assume that is what it is doing). However, it is possible for a test to appear valid without being reliable or valid. *See also* ecological validity; validity.

fast mapping Picking up from context an initial impression of the meaning of a word.

figurative language *See* nonliteral language.

fill-in-the-blank technique *See* cloze technique.

final Pertaining to or occurring at the exact end; pertaining to the very last letter or sound in a word or syllable. Z is the final letter of the alphabet.

final stable syllable A syllable with nonphonetic spelling and relatively stable pronunciation that occurs frequently in final position in English words (e.g., *-tle, -sion, -cial*).

fine motor skills The strategic control of small sets of voluntary muscles such as in writing, grasping small objects, controlling eye movements, or producing speech.

finger agnosia A kinesthetic feedback disorder in which the fingers do not report their location to the brain.

flap The reduction of /t/ and /d/, such as in the American English pronunciations of *ladder* and *latter,* formed by the tongue flapping on the alveolar ridge.

fluency Reading words at an adequate rate, with a high level of accuracy, appropriate expression, and understanding.

fMRI *See* functional magnetic resonance imaging.

formal test *See* standardized assessment or test.

formative assessment Assessment administered on a regular basis to guide daily or weekly instruction, in effect helping to "form" or "inform" instruction.

formative data collection Procedure to gather information about a child's progress in acquiring particular skills or knowledge to be applied to short-term instructional goals; usually collected using criterion- and curriculum-referenced tests. *See also* criterion-referenced test; curriculum-referenced assessment; summative data collection.

Four-Part Processing Model for Word Recognition Model in which four unique, complex, yet interrelated systems contribute to word recognition: the phonological, orthographic, meaning, and context processors.

fragment   A phrase or subordinate clause that is not a sentence (e.g., The girl who was standing).

free morpheme   A morpheme that can stand alone as a whole word (e.g., *box, plant, tame*). Also called *unbound morpheme*. *See also* bound morpheme.

frequency   The number of times an event occurs in a given category (e.g., frequency in English of multiple spellings of the long /ū/ sound as in *cube, human,* and *statue*) that guides the order of introduction for reading and spelling.

fricative   A consonant produced by a partial obstruction of the airflow, which creates friction and slight hissing noise (e.g., /s/, /f/).

full alphabetic   Phase when a reader has full knowledge of sound–symbol relationships and can use that information to decode unknown words.

functional magnetic resonance imaging (fMRI)   Detects fluctuations in the blood flow to specific areas of the brain to measure neural activity.

functional neuroimaging   Pictures of brain activity of awake individuals performing specific tasks that allow researchers to investigate which brain areas are used during certain tasks. *See also* neuroimaging.

gerund   An English word ending in *-ing* when used as a noun (e.g., She loves dancing and singing).

glide   A vowel-like consonant (i.e., /w/ and /y/) produced with little or no obstruction of the air stream in the mouth. Also called *semivowel*.

grapheme(s)   A written letter or letter cluster representing a single speech sound (e.g., *i, igh*). *See also* digraph; quadrigraph; trigraph.

graphic organizers   Visual displays of information to help a student bolster comprehension and compose written material or study for tests (e.g., outlines, semantic maps, story grammars/diagrams).

graphomotor   Pertaining to the skillful coordination of the muscle groups involved in handwriting.

graphophonemic   Pertaining to letter–sound patterns.

guide letter   The letter in a word that guides the reader in alphabetizing a word or finding it in the dictionary (e.g., when determining if *plow* appears on a dictionary page with the guide words *please* and *prison*, the second letter is the guide letter).

guided discovery teaching (learning)   Manner of presenting new material or concepts so that they can be deduced or discovered by the students. Only material that relates logically to their previous learning or that evolves through reason or sequence will lend itself to the students' discovery. Students will remember more readily that which they have been allowed to discover. Successful discovery teaching requires careful preparation. *See also* Socratic method.

guided oral reading   An instructional strategy in which an adult or peer reads a passage out loud to model fluent reading and then asks the student to re-read the same passage while providing feedback. Also called *repeated reading*.

heterogeneous practice   A spelling or reading practice session with more than one focus that is used only after the student has mastered each of the concepts contained in the practice.

high-frequency word   A word that is encountered numerous times in text and is important to know.

Hispanic   Relating to individuals descended from Spanish or Latin American people or their culture.

homogeneous practice   A spelling or reading practice in which every word contains the same pattern or rule that is the single focus of the practice.

homographs   Words that have the same spelling but sound different and have different meanings (e.g., *tear* meaning "to rip"; *tear* meaning "a drop of liquid from the eye").

homonyms   Words that sound the same and often have the same spelling but have different meanings (e.g., *lie* meaning "to not tell the truth"; *lie* meaning "to be in a resting position").

homophones   Words that sound alike but have different spellings and meanings (e.g., *bare* and *bear*; *fourth* and *forth*).

hybrid writers   Writers who use both keyboard and hands for producing written language.

I Do   First phase of the I Do, We Do, You Do instructional sequence, in which a teacher models an activity or skill for students before having them practice it with the teacher ("We do") and then do it without the teacher's help ("You do"). *See also* We Do; You Do.

IDEA   *See* Individuals with Disabilities Education Improvement Act of 2004 (PL 108-446).

IEP   *See* individualized education program.

impulsivity   Inability to inhibit behaviors.

incidental learning   Learning that takes place without any intent to learn. Informal learning.

individualized education program (IEP)   A document that sets out the child's placement in special education as well as the specific goals, short-term objectives, and benchmarks for measuring progress each year. Creating and implementing the IEP must include the opportunity for meaningful participation by the parents.

Individuals with Disabilities Education Improvement Act (IDEA) of 2004 (PL 108-446), reauthorized in 2015 (PL 114-95) Every Student Succeeds Act   Special education legislation, originally passed in 1975 (PL 94-142) and amended in 1990 (PL 101-476) and 1997 (PL 105-17), that serves as a mechanism to help fund special education. This legislation mandates that states receiving federal monies must provide special education and other services to qualified children (from birth through age 21) with disabilities or risk the loss of these dollars. IDEA 2004 protects a child's right to a free appropriate public education (FAPE) in the least restrictive environment (LRE).

Indo-European   A family of languages consisting of most of the languages of Europe, as well as those of Iran, the Indian subcontinent, and other parts of Asia. Most English words are ultimately of Indo-European origin.

inductive   Pertaining to how the whole can be broken down into its component parts. *See* analytic.

inflectional morpheme   A morpheme added to the end of a word that shows tense, number, or person of a verb; plural or possessive of a noun; or comparative or superlative form of an adjective (e.g., *-ed* in *floated*, *-s* in *tales*, *-er* in *thinner*).

inflections or inflectional endings   Endings that are added to base words (e.g., *-s, -ed, -er, -est, -ing*) and change their number, tense, voice, mood, or comparison.

informal assessment or test   A test that is structured but not standardized; it typically follows the format of a standardized test, but presentation can be modified to probe the students' responses in ways that are not permissible with standardized tests. *See also* standardized assessment or test.

inhibitory control   The ability to not act on specific emotions or ideas.

initial   The first or beginning sound or letter in a word or syllable. *A* is the initial letter of the alphabet.

instant word recognition   The ease and automaticity with which a skilled reader is able to read individual words.

interrater reliability   The agreement in scores between different individuals giving the same test. *See also* reliability.

intersensory   Involving neurological organization for the automatic linkage of auditory, visual, and kinesthetic–motor impressions.

intonation   The pattern or melody of pitch changes revealed in connected speech.

invented spelling   Spelling that is not the same as conventional orthography and that may be encouraged from preschool to first grade to help students develop phonemic awareness and apply their knowledge of sounds, symbols, and letter patterns. Using invented spelling is temporary until regular orthography is learned. Also called transitional spelling.

irregular word   A word that has an unexpected spelling either because its orthographic representation does not match its pronunciation (e.g., *colonel, Wednesday*) or because it contains an infrequent orthographic representation of a sound (e.g., *soap*).

juncture   The transition or mode of transition from one sound to another in speech; a pause that contributes to meaning of words (e.g., to make a *name* distinguishable from an *aim*) or rising intonation, as in a question.

key word   A word emphasizing a particular letter–sound association that serves as the key to unlock the student's memory for that association (e.g., *apple* for /ă/, *itch* for /ĭ/).

kinesthetic   Pertaining to the sensory experience stimulated by bodily movements and tensions; often pertaining to the student's feeling of letter shapes while moving parts of the body through space.

kinesthetic feedback   Sensory feedback from the tactile sense when movement is involved, for example, finger and hand movement in letter formation.

language content   Knowing the vast array of objects, events, and relationships and the way they are represented in language.

language-based learning disability (LBLD)   A language-based learning disability is defined as a disorder in one or more of the basic processes involved in understanding or producing spoken or written language.

latency of response   A delay in responding.

laterality   The tendency to use either the left or the right side of the body; handedness.

lax vowel   *See* short vowel.

LBLD   *See* language-based learning disability.

learning disability   According to the Interagency Committee, "a generic term that refers to a heterogeneous group of disorders manifested by significant difficulties in the acquisition and use of listening, speaking, reading, writing, reasoning, and mathematics abilities, or of social skills. These disorders are intrinsic to the individual and presumed to be due to central nervous system dysfunction. Even though a learning disability may occur with other handicapping conditions (e.g., sensory impairment, intellectual disability, social and emotional disability), with socioenvironmental influences (e.g., cultural factors), and especially with attention deficit disorder, all of which may cause learning problems, a learning disability is not the direct result of those conditions or influences" (1985, as cited in Kavanagh & Truss, 1988, pp. 550–551).

letter cluster   Group of two or more letters that regularly appear adjacent in a single syllable (e.g., *oo, ng, th, sh, oi, igh*). In spelling instruction, a pattern of letters in a single syllable that occurs frequently together. The pronunciation of at least one of the component parts may be unexpected, or the letters may stand in an unexpected sequence (e.g., *ar, er, ir, or, qu, wh*). A cluster may be a blend (two or more letters that represent more than one sound) or a digraph (two letters that represent one sound). Also called *combination. See also* blend; digraph; diphthong; quadrigraph; trigraph.

letter combinations   *See* letter cluster.

letter–sound correspondences   *See* phonics.

lexical   Relating to words or the vocabulary of a language or the meaning of the base word in inflected and derived forms.

lexical cohesion   The planning and organizing of the content of a message before it is communicated.

lexicon   A body of word knowledge in linguistic memory, either spoken or written.

linguistic   Denoting language processing and language structure.

linguistic hierarchy   The progression of syllable and phoneme awareness development along the segmental levels of 1) word boundaries within sentences, 2) syllables in words, 3) onset–rime units, and 4) phonemes in words.

linguistics   Study of the production, properties, structure, meaning, and/or use of language.

linkages   The associations developed in language training between students' visual, auditory, kinesthetic, and tactile perceptions by seeing the letter, naming it, saying its sound, and writing it in the air and on paper. Connections between cursive letters. Students may need extra practice with the more difficult linkages such as the bridge stroke after the letters *b, o, v,* and *w.*

liquid   A class of consonant sounds that contains /l/ and /r/ of American English.

literacy   The ability to read and write.

literacy socialization   As a result of being read to, the development of the sense that marks on a page relate to the words being said, that there is a correct way to manipulate books, and that there is a positive connection between reading and nurturing experiences (Snow & Dickinson, 1991).

long vowel   A vowel sound that is produced by a slightly higher tongue position than the short vowels. The long sounds represented by the written vowels (i.e., *a, e, i, o, u*) are usually the same as their names. When coding or writing a sound picture, any long vowel is marked by a macron. Also called *tense vowel.*

long-term memory   Permanent storage of information by means of primarily semantic links, associations, and general organizational plans; includes experiential, semantic, procedural, and automatic habit memories.

macron   The flat diacritical mark (¯) above a vowel in a sound picture or phonic/dictionary notation that indicates a long sound (e.g., /fāvor/).

manner   In phonology, the articulation and perceptual character of speech sounds.

manuscript handwriting   *See* printing.

marker   A distinguishing feature of a word that signals the need to apply a spelling rule or a coding for reading. The student may literally place a mark at each crucial point as a reminder. Also called *checkpoint, clue.*

mastery   Proficiency in specific sub-skills of a new task. Based on the bottom–up notion of gaining automatic recall of basic information or learning to automaticity. Also called *overlearning.*

Matthew effect   A term coined by Stanovich (1986) to describe a phenomenon observed in findings of cumulative advantage for children who read well and have good vocabularies and cumulative disadvantage for those who have inadequate vocabularies and read less and thus have lower rates of achievement. The term is named after a passage from the New Testament: "For unto everyone that hath shall be given, and he shall have abundance: but from him that hath not shall be taken away even that which he hath" (Matthew 25:29).

meaning processor   In the Four-Part Processing Model for Word Recognition, this is the neural processing system involved in providing access to the semantic network and varied meanings. *See also* context processor; Four-Part Processing Model for Word Recognition; orthographic processor; phonological processor.

medial   The letters or sounds that occur in the interior of a word or syllable or somewhere between the first and last letters. All of the letters in the sequential alphabet are medial except *a* and *z.* Medial is not a synonym for middle. *See also* middle.

meta-analysis   A statistical technique that allows comparisons of results across many studies.

metacognition   The deliberate rearrangement, regrouping, or transfer of information; the conscious choice of the strategies used to accomplish a task and processes to provide feedback on learning and performance.

metacognitive   Pertaining to executive functions that govern how people think about thinking.

metacognitive strategies   Strategies that students may use to think about what they are reading and the factors that influence their thinking.

metalinguistic   Pertaining to an awareness of language as an entity that can be contemplated; crucial to early reading ability, to understanding discourse patterns in the classroom, and to analyzing the language being used to teach the language that must be learned.

metalinguistics   One kind of metacognition: analyzing, thinking, and talking about language independent of the meanings of words.

metaphor   A word or phrase that is used to compare one thing to something else (e.g., America is a melting pot, all the world's a stage). *See also* simile.

middle   Equidistant from two extremes (e.g., first and last). Middle and medial are not synonymous. The middle letters of the alphabet are *m* and *n*. *See also* medial.

miscue   Used by reading specialists to refer to inaccurate reading responses to written text during oral reading.

mnemonics, mnemonic strategies   Formal schemes designed to improve memory, including using key words, chunking, rhyming, and visualizing. Arbitrary learning is more difficult for the student with dyslexia than learning that is related and logical, so devices such as mnemonic strategies for grouping needed facts are essential.

modality   A specific sensory pathway. Multisensory instruction simultaneously engages the student's visual, auditory, and kinesthetic/tactile senses.

model   A standard or example provided by the teacher for imitation or comparison (e.g., a model of syllable division procedure before a reading practice); a structure or design to show how something is formed (e.g., teacher skywrites a cursive letter).

modifications   Modifications change *what* a student is taught or expected to learn. *See also* accommodations.

monosyllabic   Pertaining to a one-syllable word containing one vowel sound.

morpheme   The smallest meaningful linguistic unit. A morpheme may be a base word or root (e.g., *child; graph*), a suffix (e.g., *-hood* in *childhood*), or a prefix (e.g., *un-* in *untie*). *See also* derivational morpheme; inflectional morpheme.

morphological   In linguistic terms, pertaining to the meaningful units of speech; for example, a suffix is a morphological ending.

morphological awareness   Ability to recognize the meaningful units of speech.

morphology   The internal structure of the meaningful units within words and the relationships among words in a language. The study of word formation patterns.

morphophonemic relationships   The conditions in which morphemes change their phonemic forms or pronunciations when they are combined to form words (e.g., let*s* /s/, leg*s* /z/, lense*s* /ĕz/; in + legal = illegal).

morphophonemics   The interaction between morphological and phonological processes (Venezky, 1999).

MPO   *See* Multiple Paragraph Outline.

MSL   *See* Multisensory Structured Literacy.

multi-modal   Involving multiple sensory pathways. Multisensory instruction simultaneously engages the student's visual, auditory, and kinesthetic/tactile senses.

multi-motor   Pertaining to feeling the unique sequence of movements during speech production as each letter name (or phoneme) is pronounced (kinesthetic–motor) and feeling the unique sequence of movements as each letter is formed (kinesthetic–motor).

multiple meanings   Different meanings for the same word; characteristic of English language. Students with learning disabilities often have difficulty with multiple meanings of words.

Multiple Paragraph Outline (MPO)   Outline format used for developing compositions of three or more paragraphs as students are preparing to write more advanced compositions and argumentative essays.

multiple spellings   The various ways in which a sound may be spelled (e.g., long /ā/ may be spelled *a, ay, ei, eigh, ey,* or *ai*).

multisensory   Referring to any learning activity that includes using two or more sensory modalities simultaneously for taking in or expressing information.

multisensory integration   The mental process of combining information through multiple senses.

multisensory strategies   Explicit instructional procedures using visual, auditory, tactile–kinesthetic sensory systems to learn the phonological, morphemic, semantic, and syntactic layers of language along with the articulatory–motor components of language.

Multisensory Structured Literacy (MSL)   Instructional approach that incorporates systematic, cumulative, explicit, and sequential approaches taught by teachers trained to instruct language structure at the levels of sounds, syllables, meaningful parts of words, sentence structure, and paragraph and discourse organization.

multisyllabic   Pertaining to a word of more than one syllable (e.g., *fantastic*). Also called *polysyllabic*.

narrative   Composition containing a sequence of events, usually in chronological order.

narrative writing   Writing that describes an experience or event from a personal perspective, often in story form.

nasal A sound produced in which air is blocked in the oral cavity but escapes through the nose. The consonants in *mom* and *no* are nasal sounds.

naturalistic assessment Assessment involving activities that are commonly participated in at school, which are used for evaluative purposes and would yield more ecological validity.

NCLB *See* No Child Left Behind Act of 2001 (PL 107-110).

neural correlates of typical reading and reading disability Brain activity that corresponds with, and is necessary to produce, typical reading or reading disability.

neuroimaging Diagnostic and research method of viewing brain structures and activity through the use of advanced medical technology, such as magnetic resonance imaging, in which the patient's body is placed in a magnetic field and resulting images are processed by computer to produce an image of contrasting adjacent tissues. *See also* functional neuroimaging; structural neuroimaging.

neuropsychology The study of areas of the brain and their connecting networks involved in learning and behavior.

No Child Left Behind (NCLB) Act of 2001 (PL 107-110) Federal legislation that established standards and the creation of measurable outcomes for learning.

noncontrolled readable text Text that is narrative or informational that is not restricted to words with taught word structures, but which students can read with at least 80%–90% accuracy and preferably higher than 85%.

nonliteral language Language that avoids using the exact meanings of words and uses exaggeration, metaphors, and embellishments. Also called *figurative language*.

nonsense word A word having no meaning by itself, the spelling of which is usually phonetic (e.g., *vop*). Reading and spelling nonsense words are phonic reinforcement for students who have already memorized a large number of words. Nonsense words can be used for teaching older students to apply phonetic decoding. Also called *nonsense syllable, nonword, pseudoword*.

norm-referenced assessment or test Assessment of performance in relation to that of the norm group (cohort) used in the standardization of the test. Norm-referenced tests produce scores that permit comparisons between a student and other children of the same age or grade level. All norm-referenced tests are standardized. *See also* standardized assessment or test.

norms Comparison to a stable reference base such as age or grade level.

OGA *See* Orton-Gillingham Approach.

onset The initial written or spoken single consonant or consonant cluster before the first vowel in a syllable (e.g., /s/ in *sit*, /str/ in *strip*). Some syllables do not have an onset (e.g., *on, ask*). *See also* rime.

opaque Describes a more complex system of phoneme–grapheme and phoneme–grapheme correspondences. There are multiple pronunciations (phonemes) associated with a single grapheme (e.g., *oo* is pronounced differently in *moon*, *book*, and *blood*); likewise, there are multiple spellings (graphemes) that represent a single phoneme (e.g., *ai, ay, a_e,* and *a* are all common spellings, or graphemes, that represent /ā/).

open syllable   A syllable ending in one vowel; the vowel is long (e.g., the first syllables in *labor* and *i/tem*). *See also* closed syllable.

oral and written language learning disability (OWL LD)   Unusual difficulty with listening comprehension and reading comprehension and oral and written expression at the syntax level. *See also* specific language impairment (SLI).

oral language   A spoken system of words with rules for their use that includes listening and speaking.

orthographic memory   Memory for letter patterns and word spellings.

orthographic processing   Mental processing of letter patterns and word spellings.

orthographic processor   In the Four-Part Processing Model for Word Recognition, this is the neural processing system involved in recognition of letter and letter patterns (graphemes). *See also* context processor; Four-Part Processing Model for Word Recognition; meaning processor; phonological processor.

orthography   The writing system of a language. Correct or standardized spelling according to established usage.

Orton-Gillingham Approach (OGA)   Multisensory method of teaching language-related academic skills that focuses on the structure and use of sounds, syllables, words, sentences, and written discourse. Instruction is explicit, systematic, cumulative, direct, and sequential.

outcomes   In assessment, the measured results of an educational program.

overlearning   *See* mastery.

OWL LD   *See* oral and written language learning disability.

palatal   Pertaining to sounds produced by the tongue touching the hard palate.

PALS   *See* Peer-Assisted Learning Strategies.

paralinguistic   *See* suprasegmental.

partial alphabetic   Phase or stage in which children know some sound–symbol relationships but not enough to process an entire word phonetically.

partially blocked   *See* stop.

pause   A break, stop, or rest in spoken language; one of the suprasegmental aspects of language. *See also* juncture; suprasegmental.

peer review   Scrutiny and evaluation of the results of a research study by a group of independent researchers with expertise and credentials in that field of study before the research findings are publicly reported.

Peer-Assisted Learning Strategies (PALS)   Research-supported cooperative learning strategy in which a higher performing student is paired with a lower performing student from the same class and they work together frequently as reading partners in highly structured sessions. *See also* cooperative learning.

perseverate   To get "stuck" on one idea or activity and have difficulty making the transition from one activity to another.

persuasive writing   Writing whose purpose is to sway the reader's way of thinking through an emotional appeal that uses persuasive techniques (e.g., inclusive language, repetition, rhetorical questions).

phoneme   The smallest unit of speech that makes one word distinguishable from another in a phonetic language such as English (e.g., /f/ makes *fat* distinguishable from *vat*; /j/ makes *jump* distinguishable from *chump*).

phoneme awareness   *See* phonemic awareness.

phoneme deletion   *See* sound deletion.

phonemic awareness   Awareness of the smallest units of sound in the speech stream and the ability to isolate or manipulate the individual sounds in words. Phonemic awareness is one aspect of the larger category of phonological awareness. Also called *phoneme awareness*. *See also* phonological awareness.

phonetic   Pertaining to speech sounds and their relation to graphic or written symbols.

phonetic stage   Stage in spelling development in which every sound is represented, but the complete knowledge of conventional orthography is not (e.g., *kik* for *kick*; *brij* for *bridge*). *See also* prephonetic stage; semiphonetic stage.

phonetics   The system of speech sounds in any specific language.

phonics   Paired association between letters and sounds; an approach to teaching of reading and spelling that emphasizes sound–symbol relationships, especially in early instruction.

phonological   Pertaining to sounds and sound patterns in a language.

phonological awareness   The sensitivity to the sound structure in spoken language. Phonological awareness progresses from rhyming; to syllable counting; to detecting first, last, and middle sounds; to phonemic awareness, which includes segmenting, adding, deleting, and substituting sounds in words. *See also* phonemic awareness.

phonological memory   Ability to immediately process and recall sound-based information (i.e., something you have heard) in short-term memory for temporary storage.

phonological naming   Ability to efficiently retrieve words stored in long-term memory using phonological information.

phonological processing   Ability to perceive, understand, and use the sound structures of words in both oral and written language.

phonological processor   In the Four-Part Processing Model for Word Recognition, this is the neural processing system involved in identification of sounds (phonemes). *See also* context processor; Four-Part Processing Model for Word Recognition; meaning processor; orthographic processor.

phonological representation   The quality or distinctness of how well words are stored in long-term memory and the ability to access word representations in a conscious manner.

phonological retrieval   *See* phonological naming.

phonological rules   Implicit rules governing speech sound production and the sequence in which sounds can be produced in a language.

phonological sensitivity   Awareness of the syllables and phonemes of language.

phonological working memory   Part of one's working memory for verbal information, involving short-term storage of phonological input and rehearsal of this information.

phonology   The science of speech sounds, including the study of the development of speech sounds in one language or the comparison of speech sound development across different languages.

PL 107-110   *See* No Child Left Behind (NCLB) Act of 2001.

PL 108-446   *See* Individuals with Disabilities Education Improvement Act (IDEA) of 2004.

place of articulation   The place in the oral cavity where the stream of air is obstructed or changed during the production of a sound.

place value   The position of a digit in a numeral or series (e.g., the ones place, the tens place, the hundreds place).

polyglot   A person who knows and uses several languages. Also, a language influenced by several languages; English is a polyglot of Anglo-Saxon, Latin (Romance), and Greek.

polysyllabic   *See* multisyllabic.

pragmatic language   Language as it is used in interactional contexts.

pragmatics   The set of rules that dictates behavior for communicative intentions in a particular context and the rules of conversation or discourse.

pre-alphabetic   The first phase of word recognition when a child begins to recognize words in connection with images they are associated with (e.g., McDonald's) or visual features of letters (e.g., a dog has a tail and the *g* in a printed word looks like a tail).

prefix   An affix attached to the beginning of a word that changes the meaning of that word (e.g., *tri-* in *tricycle*). *See also* consonant prefix; vowel prefix.

preliteracy   Early experiences with skills associated with learning to read, such as singing the alphabet, identifying letters, playing with rhyming words, and understanding the difference between a word and an image in a book.

prephonetic stage   A stage of early spelling that demonstrates a lack of understanding of the concept of a word, the alphabetic principle, or the conventions of print, such as spaces between words and the left-to-right progression of writing.

prescriptive   When used in the context of instruction, entailing the changes made to a lesson to tailor it for more practice, review, and/or multisensory activities.

print awareness   Children's appreciation and understanding of the purposes and functions of written language.

printing   Unconnected letters formed using arcs and straight lines. Also called *manuscript handwriting, manuscript print, print handwriting*.

print-rich environment   An environment filled with many varieties of printed materials used for multiple purposes, including nonacademic purposes.

procedural memory   Memory that stores and retrieves how to perform a task.

process   In Multisensory Structured Literacy instruction, the instructional process (Orton-Gillingham Approach). *See also* content; context; Orton-Gillingham Approach (OGA).

pro/con writing   *See* argumentative writing.

progress monitoring assessment   Assessment used with students identified as not meeting learning expectations who participate in specialized instruction to help them develop needed skills. Progress monitoring tasks are administered after short intervals of instruction. Their purpose is to measure students' learning and determine the impact of the instruction.

proprioception   An individual's subconscious perception of movement and spatial orientation coming from stimuli within the body.

prosody   Features of spoken language, such as intonation and stress, that fluent readers use for appropriate phrasing of text into meaningful units.

pseudoword   *See* nonsense word.

psycholinguistic strategies   Strategies related to learning relevant knowledge about language.

psychometric assessment   Relating to the objective measurement of knowledge and skills.

psychometricians   Professionals who create tests that are intended to assess the construct of executive function.

quadrigraph   Four adjacent letters in a syllable that represent one speech sound (e.g., *eigh*). *See also* digraph; trigraph.

qualitative research   Research that involves observing individuals and settings and relies on observation and description of events in the immediate context.

quantitative research   Research using experimental or quasi-experimental design methods to gather data. *See also* quasi-experimental research.

quasi-experimental research   Research that determines cause and effect without strict randomized controlled trials and is valid but less reliable than randomized controlled trials.

RAN   *See* rapid automatic naming.

randomized controlled trial   An intervention study in which subjects are randomly assigned to experimental and control groups; all variables are held constant except the one variable that is hypothesized to cause a change.

rapid automatic naming (RAN)   *See* rapid serial naming.

rapid serial naming   A speed naming task, most often administered to prereaders, in which the individual is asked to quickly name a series of printed letters, numbers, or blocks of color repeated in random order. Also called *rapid automatized naming, rapid automatic naming.*

raw score   An unaltered measurement from an assessment (e.g., 16 items correct); assessment result data that has not been transformed in any way.

r-controlled   Pertaining to the phenomenon in English in which the letter *r* affects the way a preceding vowel is pronounced. For example, the *a* in *bar* is influenced by the *r* and sounds different from the *a* in *bad.*

r-controlled syllable   A syllable containing the combination of a vowel followed by *r.* The sound of the vowel often is not short but instead may represent an unexpected sound (e.g., *dollar, star, her*). This kind of syllable is also called a *vowel-r syllable,* a term which focuses on the orthographic pattern (whereas the term *r-controlled syllable* focuses on the sound pattern).

reader's theatre   Fluency-building activity in which students read literature presented in a dramatic form without sets, costumes, or the need to memorize lines.

reading disability   *See* dyslexia.

reading fluency   *See* fluency.

receptive language   This type of language includes the words a child hears and then later reads.

recognition   The act of identifying a stimulus as the same as something previously experienced (e.g., auditory recognition is involved in listening for a particular sound).

regrouping   New mathematical term for carrying (in addition) and borrowing (in subtraction); necessary in the base-10 positional notation system.

regular word   A word that is spelled the way it sounds. Also called *phonetically regular word.*

relative clause   A dependent clause introduced by a relative pronoun such as *who, that, which, or whom* (e.g., We bought ice cream from the man who was standing on the corner). A relative clause is not a complete sentence on its own. *See also* embedded clause.

reliability   In assessment, the consistencies of the following: 1) the test results across individuals administering it; 2) the results between various forms of the test; 3) the test items to each other; and 4) the results on retesting (usually for a short period, to avoid changes in what is being measured). *See also* interrater reliability.

repeated reading   *See* guided oral reading.

response to intervention (RTI)   An integrated model of assessment and intervention with a multilevel prevention system to identify students at risk as well as monitor their progress, supply evidence-based interventions, and allow for appropriate adjustments based on student responsiveness. An alternative way to identify students with learning disabilities. Also called *response to instruction.*

review Look over again; bring back to awareness. Used repeatedly in a multisensory lesson to increase automatic reaction to symbols for reading and spelling and to make a brief reference to the day's new material.

rime The vowel and the consonant(s) after the vowel in a written or spoken syllable (e.g., *at* in *cat, itch* in *switch*). *See also* onset.

root A morpheme to which affixes can be added (e.g., *hat, group, green, fast*). Some roots, usually of Latin origin, are morphemes that generally cannot stand alone as words in English (e.g., *cred, dict, struct, vis*). *See also* base word; bound morpheme; free morpheme.

RTI *See* response to intervention.

rule word A word that carries information indicating when a letter should be dropped, doubled, or changed (e.g., *shiny, rabbit, bountiful*).

run-on sentence Two adjacent main clauses without a conjunction or punctuation to join them together (e.g., It began raining they parked the car).

scaffolding An educational strategy in which the teacher models and guides students' learning and then gradually decreases supports to increase students' independence in the learning process.

scatter The range and uneven alignment of test scores.

schema A student's prior knowledge and experience relevant to a new topic insofar as it contributes to a frame of reference, factual or attitudinal, for the new information, thus creating links or structures through which the new information can be assimilated. Also called *schemata*.

schwa An unaccented vowel (ə) whose pronunciation approximates the short /ŭ/ sound, such as the sound that corresponds to the first and last *a* in *America* or the second *a* in *sandal*.

scientifically based research A process that gathers evidence to answer questions and bring new knowledge to a field so that effective practices can be determined and implemented. Also called *evidence-based research*.

screeners Broad-based assessments designed to identify students who have developed expected skills to an established benchmark and those who have not.

screen-reading software *See* text-to-speech software.

segmental Pertaining to a feature of language that can be divided or organized into a class (e.g., place of articulation, voicing).

segmentation Separating a word into smaller units, such as syllables, onsets, and rimes, or individual phonemes. Also called *unblending*.

segmenting *See* segmentation.

selective attention The ability to attend to certain stimuli while ignoring other stimuli; in working memory, putting ideas on hold while working on other ideas.

self-regulation The inhibitory control needed to determine when an emotional response can be initiated or should be inhibited.

semantic map A graphic organizer that focuses on the relationship of words.

semantic organizer Visual representations of information in expository or narrative text (e.g., webs, charts, diagrams) to help readers focus on specific concepts and their relationship to other concepts. *See also* graphic organizer.

semantics The meaning of words and the relationships among words as they are used to represent knowledge of the world.

semiphonetic stage Stage in spelling development that demonstrates the use of incomplete but reasonable phonetic representations of words (e.g., *nf* for *enough*; *left* for *elephant*).

sentence expansion Addition of details explaining who, what, where, when, and/or how to a sentence kernel (e.g., *Yesterday when I was at the store, I saw the woman with the brown dog* is an expansion of *I saw the woman*).

sentence kernel A simple sentence without modifiers.

sequencing In multisensory structured language education, the orderly presentation of linguistic concepts based on frequency and ease of learning in a continuous series of connected lessons or retrieving names of things such as letters of the alphabet or the act of ordering information.

sequential *See* sequencing.

shallow *See* transparent.

shared reading Reading in which the instructor reads a paragraph aloud and then the student reads a paragraph aloud, with the instructor assisting with words as needed. *See also* choral reading; echo reading.

short vowel A vowel that usually occurs in a closed syllable and is marked with a breve. Also called *lax vowel*.

short-term memory Memory that lasts only briefly, has rapid input and output, is limited in capacity, and depends directly on stimulation for its form. Short-term memory enables the reader to keep parts of the reading material in mind until enough material has been processed for it to make sense. Also called *working memory*.

sight word A word that is immediately recognized as a whole and does not require decoding to identify. A sight word may or may not be phonetically regular, such as *can, would,* and *the*.

simile An explicit comparison of two unlike things using the word *like* or *as* (e.g., Her tousled hair was like an explosion in a spaghetti factory). *See also* metaphor.

Simple View of Reading Model that defines reading comprehension as a product of lower level skills such as word recognition and higher level thinking processes such as listening comprehension.

simultaneous multisensory strategies Strategies that incorporate the simultaneous use of visual, auditory, kinesthetic (speech and handwriting), and tactile sensory modalities to link listening, speaking, reading, and writing.

Simultaneous Oral Spelling (S.O.S.) A structured sequence of procedures to teach the student how to think about the process of spelling. The student listens to the word while looking at the speaker's mouth, segments the word, spells it aloud, writes it while naming each letter, codes it, and reads it aloud for proof-reading (Cox, 1992).

Single Paragraph Outline (SPO)   Outline format used for developing a single paragraph, intended to help students discern the basic structure of a paragraph: topic sentence, supporting details, and concluding sentence.

situational   Used in reading and spelling instruction to describe a feature in a word that provides clues about how to spell or read a word. The situation refers to the position of letters or sounds, placement of accent, and the influence of sur-rounding sounds or letters.

sky writing   Technique of "writing" a letter or word in the air using the arm and writing hand. Use of upper arm muscles during sky writing helps the student retain kinesthetic memory of the shape of letters. Also called *air writing*.

SLI   *See* specific language impairment.

social cognition   Cognition that involves how one perceives, processes, and recalls social information and applies knowledge in social contexts.

Socratic method   A teaching method that leads learners to discover information through carefully guided questioning based on information they already pos-sess. Also called *discovery learning, Socratic questioning. See also* guided discovery teaching.

Socratic questioning   *See* Socratic method.

S.O.S.   *See* Simultaneous Oral Spelling.

sound deletion   Early literacy task in which the student is presented with a word and is asked to say all of the sounds in the word except one (e.g., "Say *bat* without /b/"). Ability to delete sounds is an important component of phonemic aware-ness. Also called *phoneme deletion*.

sound dictation   Procedure in which the teacher dictates individual pho-nemes, words, or sentences and the student repeats and responds by writing them down. Sound dictation may involve oral and/or written review with a sound or spelling deck to develop automaticity in translating sounds to spellings.

sound–symbol associations; sound–symbol correspondences   *See* phonics.

special education   A federally defined type of education for a qualified child with a disability that is specially designed instruction, at no cost to the parents, to meet the unique needs of the child with a disability, including—(A) instruction conducted in the classroom, in the home, in hospitals and institutions, and in other settings; and (B) instruction in physical education (PL 108-446, 20 U.S.C. § 1401 [29][a–b]).

specific language impairment (SLI)   A spoken language disorder not accompa-nied by any other disorder, disability, or medical condition.

specific learning disability   A disorder in one or more of the basic processes involved in understanding or producing spoken or written language.

speech synthesis   Software in which synthetic speech is added to the printed material presented on computers or other electronic devices. *See also* text-to-speech software.

SPO   *See* Single Paragraph Outline.

standard scores   Test scores that address a student's change in performance relative to the mean rate of change for other students of his or her age or grade.

standardized assessment or test   A test that is standardized using a carefully selected sample of individuals representative of the larger group of individuals for whom the test was created; such a test must be administered and scored following procedures prescribed in the manual accompanying the test. *See also* informal assessment or test.

statistical significance   A result that is likely to have occurred due to something other than random chance.

Stern blocks   Wooden blocks of different sizes that are manipulated to aid in the understanding of mathematical concepts.

stop   In terms of speech sounds, a consonant that is produced with a complete obstruction of air (e.g., /p/, /t/, /k/).

story map   A graphic organizer that highlights different categories of content in narrative text (e.g., characters, setting, events, problem, solution). *See also* graphic organizer.

story structure   Term used in discussing reading comprehension strategies; students use the structure of the text (story) to aid in the recall of content to answer questions about the text (story).

strategy   An individual's approach to a task, including how the person thinks and acts when planning, executing, and evaluating performance on a task and its subsequent outcomes.

stress   *See* accent.

structural analysis   The perception and examination of syllables and morphemes. Structural analysis enables the reader to decode long, unfamiliar words.

structural neuroimaging   Technique used to obtain images of the brain.

Structured Literacy   A research-based approach to instruction that involves the simultaneous use of multisensory teaching strategies.

study skills   Those competencies associated with acquiring, recording, organizing, synthesizing, remembering, and using information and ideas learned in school or other instructional arenas.

sublexical   Pertaining to component parts of a word.

sub-skill   A skill that is part of a more complex skill or group of skills. Sub-skills of reading include phonological awareness and knowledge of letter–sound correspondences.

substitution   The activity of both deleting a syllable or phoneme from a word and adding a new one to a say a different word.

subvocalize   To move the lips with vocalization that is not audible.

suffix   A morpheme attached to the end of a base word that creates a word with a different form, use (e.g., *-s* in *cats, -ing* in *lettering*), or meaning (e.g., *helpful, helpless*). Inflectional suffixes indicate tense, number, person, voice, mood, or comparatives. Derivational suffixes change the part of speech or function of the base word. *See also* consonant suffix; vowel suffix.

summative assessment   An assessment that summarizes what has been learned. An example might be a mid-term or final exam.

summative data collection   Procedure to gather information about the accumulation and integration of knowledge to be applied to long-term comprehensive teaching goals; typically collected using norm-referenced measures but sometimes collected with curriculum- and criterion-referenced tests. *See also* criterion-referenced test; curriculum-referenced assessment; formative data collection; norm-referenced assessment or test.

suprasegmental   Pertaining to the singular musical or prosodic qualities of spoken language, including intonation, expression, accent, pitch, juncture, and rhythm, which are significant in our ability to communicate and comprehend emotions and attitudes. Also called *paralinguistic*.

syllable(s)   A spoken or written unit that has a vowel or vowel sound and may include consonants or consonant sounds that precede or follow the vowel. Syllables are units of sound made by one opening of the mouth or one impulse of the voice.

syllable division   The process of breaking multisyllabic words into separate syllables using a reliable pattern to aid pronunciation.

syllable division patterns   Patterns for dividing words into syllables. There are four major syllable division patterns in English: VCCV, VCV, VCCCV, and VV.

syllable types   Orthographic classifications of syllables. There are six syllable types in English: closed, open, vowel-consonant-*e*, vowel pair (vowel team), vowel-*r* (*r*-controlled), and consonant-*le*. *See also specific syllable types*.

synchronic   Describes etymology pertaining to the current spelling of a word in a language at a given time in history.

synonyms   Words having the same or a similar meaning.

syntactic awareness   Conscious ability to manipulate or judge word order within the context of a sentence based on the application of grammatical rules.

syntactic processing   The mental ability to manipulate or judge word order within the context of a sentence based on the application of grammatical rules.

syntax   The system by which words may be ordered in phrases, clauses, and sentences; sentence structure; grammar.

synthetic   Pertaining to instruction or a process that begins with the parts and builds to the whole. Synthetic phonics starts with individual letter sounds that are blended together to form a word. *See also* analytic.

systematic   *See* sequential.

tactile   Relating to the sense of touch.

target word   A word that is being looked for in a dictionary or other reference source. A word that is the focus of reading, spelling, vocabulary, handwriting, or other instruction.

tense vowel   *See* long vowel.

text-dependent questions   Questions that require the reader to look for evidence in a text to analyze, evaluate, and synthesize.

text-to-speech software   Software that can convert computer-based text into spoken words.

thesis statement   A short statement, usually appearing in an essay's opening paragraph in which the writer expresses the main idea, purpose, and intent of a piece of writing.

think-aloud   Strategies to enhance learning by talking about content aloud.

three-cueing systems   The use of a hierarchy of cues—first semantic, then syntactic, and finally graphophonemic—to identify an unfamiliar word.

toxic stress   What happens when children experience severe, prolonged adversity without adult support; significant adversity early in life can alter a child's capacity to learn.

Transition Outline   Outline format that is effective to use with younger students who are beginning to write compositions of two or three paragraphs.

transition words   Words that aid in changing a thought within a sentence or paragraph (e.g., *first, next, then, finally*).

transitions   Words that signal, or indicate, a relationship between ideas and help to begin sentences, link thoughts within sentences, or help unify sentences and paragraphs.

transparent   Describes orthography with a one-to-one relationship between graphemes and phonemes, so both word identification and spelling of words are very consistent.

trigraph   Three adjacent letters in a syllable that represent one speech sound (e.g., *tch, dge*). *See also* digraph; quadrigraph.

Triple Word Form Theory (TWFT)   Learning to read and write words is a process of increasing awareness and coordination (integration) of three different types of word forms and their parts: phonemes, graphemes, and morphemes (Richards et al., 2006).

typography   The physical appearance of written letters such as whether they are upper- or lowercase or formed in cursive or manuscript.

unblend, unblending   *See* segmentation.

unbound morpheme   *See* free morpheme.

universal design for learning   An educational approach that concentrates on designing instructional practices, teaching materials, and educational environments that meet the needs and maximize the learning of all students, including those with disabilities.

universal screening   Broad-based assessments administered to all students to identify students who may be at risk for reading difficulties.

unvoiced   *See* voiceless.

VAKT (visual, auditory, kinesthetic, tactile)   *See* Multisensory Structured Literacy (MSL).

validity   In assessment, the meaning that can be assigned to a test result. *See also* ecological validity; face validity.

VCE   *See* vowel-consonant-*e* syllable.

velar   Pertaining to sounds produced when the tongue and roof of the mouth contact near the soft palate.

velum   The soft palate.

ventral visual pathway   Region of the brain that recognizes the identity of letters and words.

verbal reasoning   The ability to use words to consider events and information, to think about circumstances, and to solve problems by using language.

verbalization   The saying aloud of a pattern or rule for reading or spelling or strokes of a letter shape after that pattern or rule or letter shape has been discovered or learned.

virgules   Two slash marks / / with printed phonemes represented in between.

visual, auditory, kinesthetic–motor, and tactile (VAKT)   *See* Multisensory Structured Literacy (MSL).

visual word form area (VWFA)   Left occipito-temporal area of the brain that plays an essential role in the rapid recognition (visual analysis) of letters and letter sequences (graphemes) and then distributes this visual information to numerous other cortical regions—spread over the left hemisphere—that encode word meaning, articulation (i.e., pronunciation), and sound patterns (Dehaene, 2009).

vocabulary   A large store of words that a person recognizes and/or uses in his or her oral and written language for communication and comprehension.

voice recognition software   Computer software recognizes the user's voice and provides an alternative to handwriting or keyboarding while drafting text.

voiced   Pertaining to a consonant articulated with vocal vibration (e.g., /z/, /m/, /n/).

voiced-voiceless cognates   Phonemes produced in the same place of the mouth and in the same manner but that vary in the voicing characteristic (e.g., /k/, /g/; /j/, /ch/).

voiceless   Pertaining to a consonant articulated with no vocal vibration (e.g., /s/, /t/). Also called *unvoiced*.

vowel   A class of open speech sounds produced by the easy passage of air through a relatively open vocal tract. English vowels include *a, e, i, o, u,* and sometimes *y.*

vowel blend   *See* blend.

vowel digraph   *See* digraph.

vowel pair syllable   A syllable containing two adjacent vowels that have a long, short (e.g., *meet, head*), or diphthong sound (*loud, coin*). Also called *vowel team syllable*.

vowel prefix   A prefix that ends with a vowel. The spelling of a vowel prefix does not change when it is added to a base word or a root.

vowel suffix   A suffix beginning with a vowel, such as *-ing* and *-ed*.

vowel team syllable   *See* vowel pair syllable.

vowel-consonant-*e* syllable (VCE)   A one-syllable word or a final syllable of a longer word in which a final silent *e* signals that the vowel before the consonant is long (e.g., *cake, rope, cube, five, athlete*).

vowel-*r* syllable   See *r*-controlled syllable.

VWFA   *See* visual word form area.

Watch Our Writing (W.O.W.)   A checklist designed to help students write accurately and legibly: Place feet flat on the floor, sit up straight, slant the paper at a 45-degree angle, rest arms on the desk, and hold the pencil lightly while pointing its upper end toward the shoulder of writing arm (Phelps & Stempel, 1985).

We Do   Second phase of the I Do, We Do, You Do instructional sequence, in which a teacher does an activity or skill with students for practice, after having first modeled it for students ("I do") and before having them do it without the teacher's help ("You do"). *See also* I Do; You Do.

Wernicke's area   Region of the brain responsible for comprehension.

whole language   A perspective on teaching literacy based on beliefs about teaching and learning that include the following: Reading can be learned as naturally as speaking; reading is focused on constructing meaning from text using children's books rather than basal or controlled readers; reading is best learned in the context of the group; phonics is taught indirectly during integration of reading, writing, listening, and speaking; teaching is child centered and emphasizes motivation and interest; and instruction is offered on the basis of need.

word bank   A list of vocabulary words that can be used as answer choices on a vocabulary test.

word blindness   Term used in the late 19th and early 20th centuries for dyslexia. Word blindness now refers to acquired alexia, "the loss or diminution of ability of reading ability resulting from of brain trauma, a tumor, or a stroke" (Shaywitz, 2003, p. 140).

word consciousness   An interest in and awareness of words.

word prediction software   Software that uses spelling knowledge, grammar rules, and context clues to predict what word a student wants to type as he or she enters the first few letters into the computer.

word recognition   Ability to read written words accurately and effortlessly.

word-attack skills   Strategies to employ to accurately read words.

word-finding problem   Circumstance in which a speaker knows the word he or she needs to say but cannot recall it at the moment. Also called *word-retrieval problems*.

word-retrieval problems   *See* word-finding problems.

working memory   The process of holding onto (i.e., short-term memory) and manipulating information.

W.O.W.   *See* Watch Our Writing.

written language disorder   Disability that involves impairment in reading decoding, sight word recognition, reading comprehension, written spelling, and/or written expression. Written language disorders, as with spoken language disorders, can involve any of the five language domains (phonology, morphology, syntax, semantics, and pragmatics).

You Do   Third phase of the I Do, We Do, You Do instructional sequence, in which students perform an activity or skill independently or with a peer after having first seen the skill modeled by the teacher ("I do") and then practiced with the teacher ("We do"). *See also* I Do; We Do.

REFERENCES

Americans with Disabilities Act (ADA) of 1990, PL 101-336, 42 U.S.C. §§ 12101 *et seq.*

Cox, A.R. (1992). *Foundations for literacy: Structures and techniques for multisensory teaching of basic written English language skills.* Cambridge, MA: Educators Publishing Service.

Dehaene, S.D. (2009). *Reading in the brain: The science and evolution of a human invention.* New York, NY: Viking Adult.

Education for All Handicapped Children Act of 1975, PL 94-142, 20 U.S.C. §§ 1400 *et seq.*

Henry, M.K. (2003). *Unlocking literacy: Effective decoding and spelling instruction* (2nd ed.). Baltimore, MD: Paul H. Brookes Publishing Co.

Individuals with Disabilities Education Act Amendments (IDEA) of 1997, PL 105-17, 20 U.S.C. §§ 1400 *et seq.*

Individuals with Disabilities Education Act (IDEA) of 1990, PL 101-476, 20 U.S.C. §§ 1400 *et seq.*

Individuals with Disabilities Education Improvement Act (IDEA) of 2004, PL 108-446, 20 U.S.C. §§ 1400 *et seq.*

Kavanagh, J.F., & Truss, T.J. (Eds.). (1988). *Learning disabilities: Proceedings of the National Conference.* Timonium, MD: York Press.

Lyon, G.R., Shaywitz, S.E., & Shaywitz, B.A. (2003). A definition of dyslexia. *Annals of Dyslexia, 53,* 1–14.

Moats, L.C. (2010). *Speech to print: Language essentials for teachers* (2nd ed.). Baltimore, MD: Paul H. Brookes Publishing Co.

Phelps, J., & Stempel, L. (1985). *CHES's Handwriting Improvement Program* (CHIP). Dallas, TX: Children's Handwriting Evaluation Scale.

Rehabilitation Act Amendments of 1998, PL 105-220, 29 U.S.C. §§ 701 *et seq.*

Richards, T.L., Aylward, E.H., Field, K.M., Grimme, A.C., Raskind, W., Richards, A.L., ... Berninger, V.W. (2006). Converging evidence for Triple Word Form Theory in children with dyslexia. *Developmental Neuropsychology, 30*(1), 547–589.

Shaywitz, S. (2003). *Overcoming dyslexia: A new and complete science-based program for reading problems at any level.* New York, NY: Alfred A. Knopf.

Snow, C., & Dickinson, D. (1991). Skills that aren't basic in a new conception of literacy. In A. Purves & E. Jennings (Eds.), *Literate systems and individual lives: Perspectives on literacy and schooling* (pp. 175–213). Albany, NY: SUNY Press.

Stanovich, K.E. (1986). Matthew effects in reading: Some consequences of individual differences in the acquisition of literacy. *Reading Research Quarterly, 21,* 360–407.

Venezky, R.L. (1999). *The American way of spelling.* New York, NY: Guilford.

Index

Page numbers followed by *t* indicate tables; those followed by *f* indicate figures.